MANUAL OF
NURSING
THERAPEUTICS

Applying Nursing Diagnoses
to Medical Disorders

MANUAL OF
NURSING THERAPEUTICS

Applying Nursing Diagnoses to Medical Disorders

Pamela L. Swearingen, R.N.
Special Project Editor

Second edition

The C. V. Mosby Company

St. Louis • Baltimore • Philadelphia • Toronto   1990

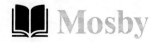

Executive Editor: Don Ladig
Developmental Editor: Robin Carter
Production Editor: Cindy Miller

Second edition

Printed in the United States of America

The C.V. Mosby Company
11830 Westline Industrial Drive, St. Louis, MO 63146

Library of Congress Cataloging-in-Publication Data

Manual of nursing therapeutics: applying nursing diagnoses to medical
    disorders / special project editor, Pamela L. Swearingen.— 2nd ed.
        p.   cm.
    Includes bibliographical references.
    ISBN 0-8016-5847-0
    1. Byrsubg—Handbooks, manuals, etc.   2. Diagnosis—Handbooks.
manuals, etc.   I. Swearingen, Pamela L.
    [DNLM: 1. Nursing—handbooks.   2. Nursing Assessment—handbooks.
WY 39 M2946]
RT48.M36   1990
    610.73—dc20
    DNLM/DLC
    for Library of Congress   89-13333
                                                                      CIP

C/C/D   9   8   7   6   5   4   3

Contributors

Lolita M. Adrien, R.N., M.S., C.E.T.N.
Clinical Nurse Specialist
Stanford University Hospital
Stanford, California

Linda S. Baas, R.N., M.S.N., C.C.R.N.
Cardiac Clinical Nurse Specialist
Consultation Department
University Hospital, University of
 Cincinnati Medical Center
Cincinnati, Ohio

Patricia Brown, R.N., C., Ph.D.
Associate Professor, School of Nursing
Adelphi University
Garden City, New Jersey

Bertie Chuong, R.N., M.S., C.C.R.N.
Head Nurse, Medical Intensive Care Unit
Yale-New Haven Hospital
New Haven, Connecticut

Mary E. Cooley, R.N., M.S.N., O.C.N.
Oncology Clinical Nurse Specialist
Hospital of the University of Pennsylvania
Philadelphia, Pennsylvania

Barbara J. Deveau, R.N., B.A., M.A.
Director of Nursing
Massachusetts Eye and Ear Infirmary
Boston, Massachusetts

Michelle M. Ferguson, R.N., M.S.N., O.C.N.
Clinical Nurse Specialist
Hospital of the University of Pennsylvania
Philadelphia, Pennsylvania

Ursula Easterday Heitz, R.N., M.S.N., C.C.R.N.
Clinical Nurse Specialist
Community Hospital North
Indianapolis, Indiana

Mima M. Horne, R.N., M.S.
Lecturer
University of North Carolina, Wilmington
School of Nursing
Wilmington, North Carolina

Cheri Howard, R.N., M.S.N.
Unit Director
Indiana University Hospitals
Indianapolis, Indiana

Patricia E.R. Jansen, R.N., M.S.N.
Geriatric Nurse Specialist/Staff
 Development Specialist
El Camino Hospital
Mountain View, California

Janet Hicks Keen, R.N., M.S., C.C.R.N., C.E.N.
Trauma Clinical Nurse Specialist
Georgia Baptist Medical Center
Atlanta, Georgia

Donna Kershner, R.N., M.S.
Nursing Instructor
Cabrillo College
Santa Cruz, California

Carol E. Lang, R.D., M.S.
Director of Dietetics
New England Deaconess Hospital
Boston, Massachusetts

CONTRIBUTORS

Debra Haire-Joshu, R.N., Ph.D.
Diabetes Research and Training Center
Washington University School of Medicine
St. Louis, Missouri

Janet H. Keen, R.N., M.S., C.E.N., C.C.R.N.
Georgia Baptist Medical Center
Atlanta, Georgia

Mary McCarthy, R.N., N.P.
Owen Clinic
University of California, San Diego Medical Center
San Diego, California

Edwina A. McConnell, R.N., Ph.D.
Independent Nurse Consultant
Madison, Wisconsin

Kenneth Miller, R.N., Ph.D.
University of California, San Francisco
San Francisco, California

Nancy E. Mooney, R.N., M.A., O.C.N.
Columbia-Presbyterian Medical Center
New York, New York

Joyce Powers, R.N., M.S.N.
Cardiology Consultants, P.A.
Albuquerque, New Mexico

Susan A. Reed, R.N.C.S., M.S.N.
Veterans' Administration Medical Center
Baltimore, Maryland

Roberta Ronayne, R.N., BScN(ed), MSc(A)
University of Ottawa
Ottawa, Ontario

Mary Jo Sagaties, R.N., F.N.P.-C., Ph.D.
New England Medical Center Hospitals
Boston, Massachusetts

Brenda K. Shelton, R.N., B.S., C.C.R.N., O.C.N.
The Johns Hopkins Oncology Center
Baltimore, Maryland

Linda Shepherd, R.N., M.N., O.C.N.
Northeast Georgia Medical Center, Inc.
Gainesville, Georgia

Ann Coghlan Stowe, R.N., M.S.N.
West Chester University, Department of Nursing
West Chester, Pennsylvania

Debbie Thompson, R.N., Ed.D.
University of North Carolina, Chapel Hill
Chapel Hill, North Carolina

Sara Jane Tobiason, R.N., M.A.
Arizona State University
Tempe, Arizona

Gayle R. Whitman, R.N., M.S.N.
The Cleveland Clinic Foundation
Cleveland, Ohio

Preface

Using a convenient pocket-sized format, the second edition of **Manual of Nursing Therapeutics:** *Applying Nursing Diagnoses to Medical Disorders,* offers nurses quick, easy access to clinical information formerly found only in medical-surgical textbooks or large manuals. It is the first pocket-sized reference to feature the application of nursing diagnoses and interventions to over 175 specific medical disorders. Written by clinical experts, it was designed to help both staff and student nurses plan and evaluate care of the adult medical-surgical patient. Focusing on NANDA-approved nursing diagnoses that are specific to each disorder, the manual also provides a quick review of pathophysiology, physical assessment, diagnostic testing, medical and surgical management, and patient-family teaching and discharge planning data. The outcome criteria are specific, positive statements that facilitate evaluation of care. The order of presentation of the information in each disorder provides a hierarchy of information that enables the nurse to make nursing diagnoses and plan interventions specific to each patient. If the patient has care needs that are not addressed under the specific medical disorder, we invite the reader to find the appropriate nursing diagnosis in the appendicized section, "Nursing Diagnoses Used in this Manual," where all the diagnoses are listed along with their "related to" and "secondary to" data. Additional, more generic information can be found in the appendix, where nursing diagnoses and interventions for preoperative and postoperative patients, patients on prolonged bed rest, and patients with cancer and other life-disrupting illnesses are discussed.

Finally, a word about the medical-surgical disorders that we selected for discussion: those chosen are either commonly seen as primary admission diagnoses or those seen frequently as secondary diagnoses in hospitalized patients. To control the number of pages and ensure a portable, pocket-sized reference, we did not include specific discussions of pediatric, critical care, mental health, or other specialized areas. Medical disorders added to this edition include abdominal trauma and acquired immune deficiency syndrome (AIDS).

Manual of Nursing Therapeutics was designed to help students and staff nurses apply nursing diagnoses in the "real world" of the acute care hospital. Reviewers indicate that it achieves this objective. The ultimate judgment rests with those nurses who read and use the manual on a daily basis. We welcome comments on how we might enhance its usefulness in subsequent editions.

Pamela L. Swearingen

Acknowledgments

The contributors and I want to thank the many individuals whose input was of value in the development of this manuscript. In particular, we wish to acknowledge the first edition contributions of Deborah G. Althoff, R.N., B.S.N., C.N.O.R.; Janet Lederer, R.N., M.N.; Sheryl Michelson, R.N., M.S.; Julie Randolph Miller, R.N., B.S.N.; Lorraine Walters, R.N., B.A.; and Rosemary Watt, R.N., M.S. The contributions of Susan Clausen Stone and Ursula Easterday Heitz from *Manual of Critical Care: Applying Nursing Diagnoses to Adult Critical Illness* helped us tremendously in the preparation of the respiratory chapter and the section "Caring for Patients with Cancer and Other Life-Disrupting Illnesses."

P.L.S.

Contents

Chapter 3   Renal-Urinary Disorders
Mima M. Horne
and Patricia E.R. Jansen

Chapter 8 Musculoskeletal Disorders
Dennis Ross

Chapter 9 Reproductive Disorders
Diane Wind Wardell
and Patti R. Jansen

Chapter 12   Providing Care for Patients with Special
                  Needs
                  Carol E. Lang
                  and Nancy A. Stotts

Appendices   Janet Hicks Keen,
                  Linda S. Baas,
                  Dennis Ross,
                  Mary E. Cooley,
                  Michelle M. Ferguson,
                  and Julie Klausen Moe

1
CHAPTER

Respiratory disorders

Section One   ACUTE RESPIRATORY DISORDERS

Acute respiratory disorders are short-term diseases or acute complications of chronic conditions. They can occur once and respond to treatment or recur to further complicate an underlying disease process.

Atelectasis

Atelectasis is a spontaneous collapse of all or part of the lung. It is most commonly seen following major abdominal or thoracic surgery as a result of hypoventilation of dependent portions of the lungs or inadequate clearing of secretions. Atelectasis can be either an acute or chronic condition, and it occurs most frequently in individuals with chronic

1

obstructive pulmonary disease (COPD). In the postoperative period it can be precipitated by the effects of anesthesia, sedation, and decreased mobility. Other precipitating factors include mucus plugs, foreign objects in the airways, pleural effusion, bronchogenic carcinoma, history of smoking, and obesity. Atelectasis can lead to pulmonary infection.

ASSESSMENT

The clinical picture is determined by the site of collapse, rate of development, and size of the affected area.

Signs and symptoms: Pleuritic chest pain, tachypnea, shortness of breath (SOB), fever, dyspnea.

Physical assessment: Decreased chest wall movement, dullness to percussion, decreased or absent breath sounds, crackles after deep inspiration or cough.

DIAGNOSTIC TESTS

1. *Chest x-ray:* Reveals higher density in affected lung, elevation of the hemidiaphragm on affected side, and compensatory hyperinflation of adjacent lobes on the opposite side.
2. *Arterial blood gas (ABG) values:* May reveal acute respiratory acidosis, with pH <7.35 and $Paco_2$ >45 mm Hg. Pao_2 may be <80 mm Hg, which is consistent with hypoxemia.

MEDICAL MANAGEMENT

Medical management is aimed at preventing this condition in all patients. If atelectasis occurs and is left untreated, the affected lung area may become fibrotic and functionless.
1. **Deep breathing and coughing exercises:** To expand alveoli deep in the lungs and mobilize/clear secretions.
2. **Chest physiotherapy:** To mobilize secretions.
3. **Hyperinflation therapy:** For example, incentive spirometry and intermittent positive pressure breathing to expand partially collapsed lung areas.
4. **Analgesics:** To reduce pain, thereby facilitating production of an effective cough.
5. **Bronchoscopy:** Procedure in which patient is intubated and a fiberoptic scope is passed into the bronchi to visualize the area and remove mucus plugs, retained secretions, or foreign objects.
6. **Oxygen therapy:** To maintain Pao_2 >80 mm Hg or within patient's normal baseline range.

NURSING DIAGNOSES AND INTERVENTIONS

For patients with atelectasis

Impaired gas exchange related to decreased perfusion of oxygen or increased retention of CO_2 secondary to ventilation/perfusion mismatch occurring as a result of alveolar collapse

Desired outcome: Patient has adequate gas exchange as evidenced by normal breath sounds, absence of adventitious breath sounds, pH 7.35-7.45, Pao_2 ≥80 mm Hg, $Paco_2$ <45 mm Hg (or ABG results consistent with patient's baseline parameters), and orientation to person, place, and time.

1. Auscultate breath sounds at least q2h. Report any decrease in breath sounds or an increase in adventitious breath sounds.
2. Monitor patient for signs and symptoms of hypoxia: restlessness, agitation, and changes in LOC. Report significant changes to MD.
3. Position patient for comfort and to promote optimal gas exchange (usually semi-Fowler's position).

4. Monitor serial ABG values. Be alert to decreasing Pao_2 or increasing $Paco_2$, both of which can signal respiratory failure.

For patients at risk for atelectasis

Potential for ineffective breathing pattern related to hypoventilation secondary to inactivity or omission of deep breathing

Desired outcome: Patient demonstrates deep breathing and effective coughing at desired intervals and exhibits eupnea (RR 12-20 breaths/min with normal depth and pattern).

1. Auscultate breath sounds at least q2h. Report any decrease in breath sounds or presence of/increase in adventitious breath sounds to MD.
2. Request respiratory therapy consultation to instruct patient in the use of incentive spirometry or other hyperinflation device. Ensure that patient inhales slowly and deeply and holds the breath at least 5 seconds at the end of inspiration. Encourage deep breathing, followed by coughing, at least q2h. Monitor patient's progress and document in nurses' notes.
3. Administer analgesics as prescribed to reduce pain, which may facilitate patient's ease with coughing and deep breathing exercises.
4. Encourage activity as prescribed to help mobilize secretions and promote effective airway clearance.

PATIENT-FAMILY TEACHING AND DISCHARGE PLANNING

Provide patient and significant others with verbal and written instructions for the following:
1. Use of hyperinflation device if patient is to continue this therapy at home. As appropriate, request that respiratory therapy staff conduct a predischarge check of patient's technique and document an assessment in the progress notes.
2. Importance of maintaining activity level as prescribed to promote optimal lung expansion.
3. Medications, including name, purpose, dosage, schedule, precautions, and potential side effects.
4. Precipitating factors in the development of atelectasis.
5. Importance of notifying MD if signs and symptoms recur.
6. Importance of medical follow-up. Review date and time of next appointment.

Pneumonia

Pneumonia is an acute bacterial or viral infection that causes inflammation of the lung parenchyma (alveolar spaces and interstitial tissue). As a result of the inflammation the involved lung tissue becomes edematous and the air spaces fill with exudate (consolidation). Bacterial pneumonias involve all or part of a lobe, whereas viral pneumonias appear diffusely throughout the lungs.

Pneumonias generally are classified into two groups: community-acquired and hospital-associated (nosocomial). A third type that occurs is pneumonia in the immunocompromised individual.

Community-acquired: Individuals with this type of pneumonia generally do not require hospitalization unless an underlying medical condition, such as COPD, cardiac disease, diabetes mellitus, or an immunocompromised state, contributes to the illness.

Hospital-associated (nosocomial): These pneumonias usually occur following aspiration of oropharyngeal flora in an individual whose resistance is altered or whose coughing mechanisms are impaired (e.g., a patient who has undergone thoracoabdominal surgery). Bacteria invade the lower respiratory tract *via* three routes: aspiration of oropharyngeal organisms (most common route), inhalation of aerosols that contain bacteria, or hematogenous spread to the lung from another site of infection (rare). Gram-negative pneumonias have a high mortality rate, even with appropriate antibiotic therapy. *Aspiration pneumonia* is a nonbacterial cause of hospital-associated pneumonia that occurs when gastric contents are aspirated. If the alveolar-capillary membrane is affected, adult respiratory distress syndrome (ARDS) may be seen.

Pneumonia in the immunocompromised individual: Immunosuppression and neutropenia are predisposing factors in the development of nosocomial pneumonias from both common and unusual pathogens. Severely immunocompromised patients are affected not only by bacteria but also by fungi *(Candida, Aspergillus)*, viruses (Cytomegalovirus), and protozoa *(Pneumocystis carinii)*. Most commonly, *Pneumocystis carinii* is seen in patients with AIDS or in those who are immunosuppressed therapeutically following organ transplants.

ASSESSMENT

Findings are influenced by the patient's age, extent of the disease process, underlying medical condition, and pathogen involved. Generally, any factor that alters the integrity of the lower airways, thereby inhibiting ciliary activity, increases the likelihood of developing pneumonia (see Table 1-1).

General signs and symptoms: Cough (productive and nonproductive); increased sputum (rust-colored, purulent, bloody, or mucoid) production; fever; pleuritic chest pain (more common in community-acquired bacterial pneumonias); dyspnea; chills; headache; myalgia. Elderly individuals may be confused or disoriented and run low-grade fevers but may present with few other signs and symptoms.

General physical assessment findings: Presence of nasal flaring and expiratory grunt; use of accessory muscles of respiration (scalene, sternocleidomastoid, external intercostals); decreased chest expansion caused by pleuritic pain; dullness on percussion over affected (consolidated) areas; tachypnea (RR >20 breaths/min), tachycardia (HR >100 bpm), increased vocal fremitus, decreased breath sounds, high-pitched and inspiratory crackles (increased by or heard only after coughing), low-pitched inspiratory crackles caused by airway secretions, and circumoral cyanosis (a late finding). **Note:** Findings may be normal, even with an abnormal chest x-ray.

DIAGNOSTIC TESTS

1. *Chest x-ray:* Confirms the presence of pneumonia (i.e., vague haziness to consolidation in the affected lung fields).
2. *Sputum for gram stain and culture and sensitivity tests:* Sputum is obtained from the lower respiratory tract before initiation of antibiotic therapy. It can be obtained *via* expectoration, suctioning, transtracheal aspiration, bronchoscopy, or open-lung biopsy.
3. *WBC:* Will be increased (>11,000 μl) in the presence of bacterial pneumonias. Normal or low WBC count may be seen with viral or mycoplasma pneumonias.
4. *Blood culture and sensitivity:* To determine presence of bacteremia and aid in the identification of the causative organism.
5. *ABG values:* May vary, depending on the presence of underlying pulmonary or other debilitating disease. Hypoxemia (Pao_2 <80 mm Hg) and hypocarbia ($Paco_2$ <35 mm Hg), with a resultant respiratory alkalosis (pH >7.45), will be seen in the absence of an underlying pulmonary disease.
6. *Serologic studies:* Acute and chronic titers are drawn to diagnose viral pneumonia. A relative rise in antibody titers is suggestive of a viral infection.
7. *Acid-fast stains and cultures:* To rule out tuberculosis.

MEDICAL MANAGEMENT

1. **Oxygen therapy:** Administered when ABGs demonstrate presence of hypoxemia. Special care must be taken not to abolish the drive to breathe if patient has a chronic lung disorder and is known to retain CO_2. (Normally, the drive to breathe occurs with increased $Paco_2$ levels; in patients with CO_2 retention the drive to breathe occurs with

T A B L E 1 - 1　Assessment guidelines by pneumonia type

Type/ pathogen	Risk groups	Onset	Defining characteristics	Complications/ comments
Community acquired				
Pneumococcal *(Pneumococcus pneumoniae, Streptococcus pneumoniae)*	Aged people with debilitating diseases, (e.g., diabetes mellitus, CHF)	Abrupt	Single shaking chill, fever, pleuritic chest pain, severe cough, SOB, rust-colored sputum	Herpes labialis, abdominal distention, meningitis, empyema, pericarditis, impaired liver function, septicemia. Mortality rate increases if more than one lobe is involved
Mycoplasma *(Mycoplasma pneumoniae)*	School-aged children to young adult (5-30 yr). Intrafamilial spread is common	Gradual	Cough, sore throat, fever, lower lobe involvement, ear involvement (usually in children)	Rare. Persistent cough and sinusitis are possible
Legionnaires' *(Legionella pneumophila)*	Middle-aged, elderly (males at increased risk) populations; cigarette smokers; individuals with malignancy, immunosuppression, chronic renal failure	Abrupt	Malaise, headache within 24 hrs, fever with normal HR, shaking chills, nonproductive cough progressing to purulent sputum, GI symptoms	Respiratory failure, hypotension, shock, acute renal failure
Viral influenza A	Elderly people with chronic diseases (e.g., COPD, diabetes mellitus, CHF); pregnancy	One week after onset of influenza symptoms	Severe dyspnea, cyanosis, scant sputum with gross blood	Rapid course leading frequently to acute respiratory failure; secondary bacterial pneumonia

From Easterday U and Howard C. In Swearingen PL et al: Manual of critical care, St Louis, 1988, The CV Mosby Co.

Continued.

TABLE 1-1 Assessment guidelines by pneumonia type—cont'd

Type/ pathogen	Risk groups	Onset	Defining characteristics	Complications/ comments
Nosocomial				
Klebsiella *(Klebsiella pneumoniae)**	Males >40 yrs, alcoholics; patients with diabetes mellitus or COPD	Abrupt	Chills, fever, productive cough (copious gray-green, brick-red). Severe pleuritic chest pain, delirium, tenacious dark-brown or red-current jelly sputum. Cyanosis and dyspnea, jaundice, vomiting, and diarrhea	Lung abscess and empyema, necrotizing pneumonitis with cavitation, acute respiratory failure. High mortality rate
Pseudomonas	Patients receiving sedatives, endotracheal intubation, IPPB, numerous courses of antibiotic therapy	Gradual	Fever, shaking, chills, hyperventilation, confusion, delirium, bradycardia, green foul-smelling sputum	Primary *Pseudomonas* is rare. Bacteremic *Pseudomonas* can result in circulatory collapse and has a high mortality rate
Proteus	Patients receiving antibiotics or who have undergone urinary tract instrumentation	Abrupt	High fever, chills, pleuritic chest pain	Rare. Localizes to areas that already are damaged. Presents as a mixed infection. Has 4 pathogenic species with differing antibiotic susceptibilities

*Enterobacter and *Serratia* are enteric organisms that cause pneumonia with the same clinical pattern as *Klebsiella*.

T A B L E 1 - 1 Assessment guidelines by pneumonia type—cont'd

Type/ pathogen	Risk groups	Onset	Defining characteristics	Complications/ comments
Staphylo-coccus aureus	Patients with debilitating diseases (e.g., diabetes mellitus, renal failure, liver disease, malnutrition, influenza, measles, COPD)	Abrupt with community acquired; insidious with hospital associated	Cough, early peripheral vascular collapse, chills, high fever, progressive dyspnea, cyanosis, pleuritic pain, bloody sputum	Pulmonary abscesses or empyema. Response to antibiotics is slow
Aspiration of gastric contents	Patients with impaired gag/cough reflexes; general anesthesia; presence of NG/ET tube	Gradual: latent period between aspiration and onset of symptoms	Fever, wheezes, crackles (rales), rhonchi, dyspnea, cyanosis	Physiologic response depends on pH of material aspirated: ≥ 2.5, little necrosis occurs; <2.5, atelectasis, pulmonary edema, hemorrhage, and necrosis can occur.
Immunocompromised patient				
Pneumocystis (Pneumocystis carinii)	Patients with AIDS or organ transplants	Insidious	Severe dyspnea and tachypnea. Nonproductive cough, progressive hypoxemia, few auscultatory signs, minimal or absent fever. Cyanosis is a late sign	Open lung biopsy is most reliable method of diagnosis. High mortality rate
Aspergillosis (Aspergillus)	Patients with AIDS, transplants, or COPD; those receiving cytotoxic agents or steroids	Abrupt with immunosuppression; insidious with COPD	Hemoptysis; fungal ball within lung cyst or cavity	Biopsy necessary for definitive diagnosis. Hematogenous spread common in immunocompromised patient

decreased Pao_2 levels. Therefore giving high concentrations of oxygen to an individual with COPD will decrease the drive to breathe.) Initially, oxygen is delivered in low concentrations, and ABG levels are watched closely. If Pao_2 does not rise to acceptable levels ($\geq$60 mm Hg), Fio_2 is increased in small increments, with concomitant checks of ABG levels.

2. **Antibiotic agents:** Prescribed empirically, based on presenting signs and symptoms, clinical findings, and chest x-ray results until sputum or blood culture results are available. Erythromycin is the most commonly used antibiotic in community-acquired pneumonia. Many of the organisms responsible for nosocomial pneumonias are resistant to multiple antibiotics. Proper identification of the organism and determination of sensitivity to specific antibiotics are critical for appropriate therapy.

3. **Hydration:** IV fluids may be necessary to replace fluids lost from insensible sources (e.g., tachypnea, diaphoresis, fevers).

4. **Percussion and postural drainage:** Indicated if deep breathing and coughing are ineffective in mobilizing secretions.

5. **Hyperinflation therapy:** Prescribed for patients with inadequate inspiratory effort.

6. **Antitussives:** Given in the absence of sputum production if coughing is continuous and exhausting to the patient.

7. **Antipyretics and analgesics:** Prescribed to reduce fever and provide relief from pleuritic pain or pain from coughing.

8. **Body substance isolation:** A relatively new concept in infection control, this procedure advocates treating *all* patients in an identical manner. Gloves are worn when contact with body substances, nonintact skin, or mucous membranes is anticipated, regardless of the patient's diagnosis. A mask may be required if the suspected or diagnosed disease is transmitted by an airborne route. Mask and eye protection are necessary if splashing of body substances into the eyes or mucous membranes is likely to occur (e.g., with suctioning). A gown is required only if soiling of clothing is anticipated.

NURSING DIAGNOSES AND INTERVENTIONS

Impaired gas exchange related to decreased diffusion of oxygen secondary to inflammatory process in the lungs

Desired outcome: Patient has adequate gas exchange as evidenced by Pao_2 $\geq$60 mm Hg, $Paco_2$ 35-45 mm Hg, pH 7.35-7.45, and RR 12-20 breaths/min with normal depth and pattern (or values consistent with patient's baseline).

1. Observe for signs and symptoms of respiratory distress (e.g., restlessness, anxiety, SOB, tachypnea, use of accessory muscles of respiration). Remember that cyanosis of the lips and nailbeds is a late indicator of hypoxia.

2. Monitor and document VS q2-4h. Be alert to a rising temperature and other changes in VS that may be indicative of infection (e.g., increased HR, increased RR, changing BP).

3. Auscultate breath sounds at least q2h. Monitor for decreased or adventitious sounds (e.g., crackles or wheezes).

4. Monitor ABG results. A decreasing Pao_2 often is indicative of the need for oxygen therapy.

5. Position patient for comfort (usually semi-Fowler's position) to optimize lung expansion and decrease work of breathing (WOB).

6. Deliver oxygen as prescribed; monitor Fio_2 to ensure that oxygen is within prescribed concentrations.

7. Provide periods of rest between care activities to decrease oxygen demand.

Ineffective airway clearance related to presence of viscous pulmonary secretions or pain and fatigue secondary to lung consolidation

Desired outcome: Patient's airway is free of adventitious breath sounds.

1. Auscultate breath sounds q2-4h and report changes in the patient's ability to clear pulmonary secretions.

2. Follow up with respiratory therapy department to ensure that patient gets prescribed chest physiotherapy. Document patient's response to treatment.
3. Teach patient to splint chest with pillow or crossed arms when coughing to reduce pain.
4. Assess need for hyperinflation therapy (i.e., patient's inability to take deep or sustained breaths). Report complications of hyperinflation therapy to MD, including hyperventilation, gastric distention, headache, signs and symptoms of pneumothorax (see p. 19), and hypotension.
5. Inspect sputum for quantity, color, and consistency; document findings. As the patient's condition worsens, the sputum can change in color from clear→white→yellow→green.
6. Assist patient with position changes q2h to help mobilize secretions. If the patient is ambulatory, encourage ambulation to patient's tolerance.
7. Ensure that patient performs deep breathing and coughing exercises at least q2h. Assist patient into position of comfort, usually semi-Fowler's position, to facilitate effectiveness and ease of these exercises.
8. Suction as prescribed and indicated.

Potential fluid volume deficit related to increased need secondary to infection or loss secondary to tachypnea, fever, or diaphoresis

Desired outcome: Patient is normovolemic as evidenced by urine output $\geq$30 ml/hr with specific gravity 1.010-1.030, stable weight, HR and BP within patient's normal limits, CVP >2 mm Hg (5 cm H_2O), moist mucous membranes, and normal skin turgor.

1. Monitor I&O. Consider insensible losses if patient is diaphoretic and tachypneic. Be alert to urinary output <30 ml/hr.
2. Weigh patient daily, at the same time of day and on the same scale. Report weight decreases of 1-1.5 kg/day.
3. Encourage fluid intake (at least 2-3 L/day in the unrestricted patient) to ensure adequate hydration.
4. Maintain IV fluid therapy as prescribed.
5. Promote oral hygiene, including lip and tongue care to moisten dried tissues and mucous membranes.

Alteration in nutrition Less than body requirements related to decreased intake secondary to anorexia

Desired outcome: Patient has adequate nutrition as evidenced by stable weight, balanced or positive nitrogen state per nitrogen studies, and serum albumin 3.5-5.5 g/dl.

1. Provide small, frequent feedings of nutritious foods that are easy to consume. Monitor and record amount of nutrients consumed.
2. Request dietitian consultation so that patient can verbalize food likes and dislikes.
3. Request that MD prescribe dietary supplements if patient is unable to consume adequate diet.
4. Discuss with patient and significant others the importance of good nutrition in the treatment of pneumonia.
5. For other interventions, see section "Providing Nutritional Support," p. 611.

For patients at risk for pneumonia

Potential for infection (nosocomial pneumonia) related to high risk secondary to recent thoracoabdominal surgery, aspiration, exposure to contaminated respiratory equipment, respiratory instrumentation, colonization of oropharynx with aerobic gram-negative bacilli, or immunosuppression

Desired outcome: Patient is free of infection as evidenced by body temperature $\leq$37.56° C (99.6° F), WBC count $\leq$11,000 μl, and sputum clear to whitish in color.

1. Perform good handwashing after contact with respiratory secretions (even though gloves were worn) and before and after contact with patient who has a tracheostomy or is intubated.

2. Identify presurgical candidate who is at increased risk for nosocomial pneumonia: individuals who are >70 years old or obese; who have COPD or history of smoking, abnormal pulmonary function tests (especially decreased forced expiratory flow rate), tracheostomy, or will be intubated for a prolonged period of time; or who will have upper abdominal or thoracic operations.

   □ Before surgery provide patient with verbal and written instructions and demonstrations of exercises to perform after surgery to prevent respiratory tract infection. Make sure that patient verbalizes knowledge of the exercises and their rationale and *returns* the demonstrations appropriately. Encourage smokers to discontinue smoking, especially during preoperative and postoperative periods.

   □ Be aware that most patients can expand their lungs effectively after surgery but won't do so unless they are encouraged. At frequent intervals, enforce the following regimens that expand the lungs: deep-breathing exercises, coughing, turning in bed, and walking. In addition, use of hyperinflation devices promotes periodic, voluntary lung expansion greater than tidal volume.

   □ For patient who cannot remove secretions effectively by coughing, perform procedures that stimulate coughing, such as chest physiotherapy, which may include percussion and postural drainage.

   □ In the high-risk patient who is too weak to deep-breathe independently, confer with MD regarding use of intermittent positive pressure breathing (IPPB). However, the role of IPPB in preventing pneumonia following surgery has not been determined.

   □ If pain interferes with lung expansion, control it by administering medications ½ hour before deep-breathing exercises and providing support of wound areas with hands or pillows placed firmly across site of incision.

3. Identify patients who are at high risk for aspiration: individuals with a depressed LOC, dysphagia, or who have an NG tube in place.

   □ For patient with depressed LOC, confer with MD regarding need for a method of feeding in which risk of aspiration is minimal, for example, enteral feedings or IV hyperalimentation.

   □ For patient with NG tube in place, elevate HOB at least 30 degrees during feedings and turn patient onto side rather than back. Provide small, frequent feedings rather than large ones.

4. Recognize the following ways in which nebulizer reservoirs can contaminate patient: introduction of nonsterile fluids or air, manipulation of nebulizer cup, or backflow of condensate from delivery tubing into reservoir or into patient when tubing is manipulated.

   □ Use only sterile fluids and dispense them aseptically.

   □ Replace (rather than replenish) solutions and equipment at frequent intervals. For example, empty reservoir completely and refill with sterile solution q8-24h, according to agency protocol.

   □ Change breathing circuits q48h; if used for multiple patients, replace breathing circuit with sterilized or disinfected breathing circuit between patients.

   □ Fill fluid reservoirs immediately before use (not far in advance).

   □ Discard any fluid that has condensed in tubing; do not allow it to drain back into reservoir or into patient.

5. Recognize risk factors for patients with tracheostomy: presence of underlying lung disease or other serious illness, increased colonization of oropharynx or trachea by aerobic gram-negative bacteria, greater access of bacteria to lower respiratory tract, and cross-contamination due to manipulation of tracheostomy tube.

   □ Employ "no-touch" technique or use of sterile gloves on both hands until tracheostomy wound has healed or formed granulation tissue around the tube.

   □ Suction on an "as needed" rather than routine basis because frequent suctioning increases risk of trauma and cross-contamination.

   □ Use sterile catheter for each suctioning procedure and sterile solutions if secretions are tenacious and catheter flushing is necessary.

   □ Always wear gloves on both hands to suction.

PATIENT-FAMILY TEACHING AND DISCHARGE PLANNING

Provide patient and significant others with verbal and written information for the following:

1. Techniques that promote gas exchange and minimize stasis of secretions (e.g., deep breathing, coughing, use of incentive spirometry, increasing activity level as much as possible for patient's medical condition, and percussion and postural drainage, as necessary).
2. Medications, including drug name, purpose, dosage, frequency, precautions, and potential side effects, particularly of antibiotics.
3. Signs and symptoms of pneumonia and the importance of reporting them promptly to health professional should they recur. Teach patient's significant others that changes in sensorium may be the only indicator of pneumonia if patient is elderly.
4. Importance of preventing fatigue by pacing activities and allowing for frequent rest periods.
5. Importance of avoiding exposure to individuals known to have flu and colds. Recommend that patient get annual flu and pneumococcal vaccines.
6. Minimizing factors that can cause reinfection, including close living conditions, poor nutrition, and poorly ventilated living quarters or work environment.

Pleural effusion

A pleural effusion is an accumulation of fluid (blood, pus, chyle, serous fluid) in the pleural space. It is caused by a number of inflammatory, circulatory, or neoplastic diseases. Transudate effusion results from changes in hydrodynamic forces in the circulation and usually is caused by congestive heart failure or cirrhosis. Exudate effusion results from irritation of the pleural membranes secondary to inflammatory, infective, or malignant processes.

ASSESSMENT

Clinical indicators of pleural effusion are related to the underlying disease. Dyspnea is present when there is a large effusion. With a small effusion the patient may be asymptomatic.

Signs and symptoms: Pleuritic chest pain, diaphoresis, cough, fever.

Physical assessment: Decreased breath sounds, dullness to percussion, decreased tactile fremitus, tracheal deviation away from affected side.

DIAGNOSTIC TESTS

1. *Chest x-ray:* Will show evidence of effusion if there is >300 ml of fluid in the pleural space. The costophrenic angle will be obliterated and opacification of the hemithorax, as evidenced by shadiness on the x-ray, increases as the effusion increases. With a large effusion the x-ray may show mediastinal shift toward the normal lung.
2. *Thoracentesis:* Removal of fluid from the pleural space for examination to provide the definitive diagnosis and determine type of effusion.
3. *Pleural biopsy:* Determines cause of effusion. Tissue is removed *via* biopsy needle and sent to the pathologist for examination.

MEDICAL MANAGEMENT AND SURGICAL INTERVENTIONS

1. Therapeutic thoracentesis: Removal of fluid, thereby allowing the lung to reexpand. The rate of recurrence and time span for return of symptoms is recorded.
2. Chest tube insertion: To provide continuous drainage of larger effusions through a 26-30 F catheter that is connected to a closed chest-drainage system.
3. Sclerosing pleurodesis: Instillation of sclerosing agent (tetracycline, bleomycin, or ni-

trogen mustard) *via* the chest tube to produce pleural fibrosis and symphysis (a line of fusion below the pleura and chest wall).

NURSING DIAGNOSES AND INTERVENTIONS

Ineffective breathing pattern related to decreased lung expansion secondary to fluid accumulation in the pleural space

Desired outcome: Patient becomes eupneic.

1. Auscultate breath sounds q2-3h, monitoring for decreasing breath sounds or the presence of a pleural friction rub.
2. Ensure patency of chest drainage system (see guidelines, p. 20, in "Pneumothorax/ Hemothorax").
3. Position patient for maximum chest expansion, generally semi-Fowler's position.
4. If hyperinflation therapy is prescribed, request a respiratory therapy consultation, as appropriate, to instruct patient in its use. Reinforce teaching, and document patient's progress.
5. For patients with gross pleural effusion, provide the following instructions for apical expansion breathing exercises:
   □ Sit upright.
   □ Position fingers just below the clavicles.
   □ Inhale and attempt to push upper chest wall against the pressure of the fingers.
   □ Hold breath for a few seconds and then exhale passively. When performed at frequent intervals, this exercise will help expand the involved lung tissues, minimize flattening of the upper chest, and mobilize secretions.

See "Pneumonia" for **Alteration in nutrition:** Less than body requirements, p. 9. See "Pneumothorax/Hemothorax" for **Pain** related to impaired pleural integrity, inflammation, or presence of chest tube, p. 21.

PATIENT-FAMILY TEACHING AND DISCHARGE PLANNING

Provide patient and significant others with verbal and written instructions for the following:

1. Importance of smoking cessation. As indicated, arrange for a consultation with a cardiac or pulmonary rehabilitation team member to give patient resources related to smoking cessation programs.
2. Signs of respiratory distress, such as restlessness, agitation, changes in behavior, and complaints of SOB or dyspnea, and the importance of notifying MD if these signs occur.
3. Use of equipment at home (e.g., hyperinflation device, nebulizer, oxygen).
4. Medications, including drug name, dosage, purpose, schedule, precautions, and potential side effects.

Pulmonary embolus

The most common pulmonary perfusion abnormality, a pulmonary embolus (PE) is caused by the passage of a foreign substance (blood clot, fat, air, or amniotic fluid) into the pulmonary artery or its branches, with subsequent obstruction of blood supply to lung tissue. The most common occurrence is a dislodged blood clot from the systemic circulation, typically the deep veins of the legs or pelvis. Thrombus formation is the result of one or more of the following factors: blood stasis, alterations in clotting factors, and injury to vessel walls. A fat embolus is the most common nonthrombotic cause of pulmonary perfusion disorders. It is the result of the release of free fatty acids, causing a toxic vasculitis, followed by thrombosis and obstruction of small pulmonary arteries by fat.

Total obstruction leading to pulmonary infarction is rare because the pulmonary circulation has multiple sources of blood supply. Early diagnosis and appropriate treatment reduce mortality to under 10%. Although most pulmonary emboli resolve completely and leave no residual deficits, some patients may be left with chronic pulmonary hypertension.

ASSESSMENT

Signs and symptoms often are nonspecific and variable, depending on the extent of the obstruction and whether or not the patient has infarction as a result of the obstruction.

Pulmonary embolus: Sudden onset of dyspnea and sharp chest pain, restlessness, anxiety, nonproductive cough, palpitations, nausea, and syncope. With a large embolism, oppressive substernal chest discomfort will be present.

Pulmonary infarction: Fever, pleuritic chest pain, and hemoptysis.

Physical assessment: Tachypnea, tachycardia, hypotension, crackles (rales), decreased chest wall excursion secondary to splinting, S_3 and S_4 gallop rhythms, transient friction rub, jugular venous distention, diaphoresis, edema, and cyanosis. Temperature may be elevated if infarction has occurred.

History and risk factors

1. *Prolonged immobilization:* Especially significant when it coexists with surgical or nonsurgical trauma, carcinoma, or cardiopulmonary disease. Risk increases as length of immobilization increases.
2. *Cardiac disorders:* Atrial fibrillation, congestive heart failure, myocardial infarction, rheumatic heart disease.
3. *Surgical intervention:* Risk increases in postoperative period, especially for patients with pelvic, thoracic, and abdominal surgery, and for those with extensive burns or musculoskeletal injuries of the hip or knee.
4. *Pregnancy:* Especially during the postpartum period.
5. *Chronic pulmonary disease.*
6. *Trauma:* Especially fractures of the lower extremities and burns. The degree of risk is related to the severity, site, and extent of trauma.
7. *Carcinoma:* Particularly neoplasms involving the breast, lung, pancreas, and genitourinary and alimentary tracts.
8. *Obesity:* A 20% increase in ideal body weight is associated with an increased incidence of PE.
9. *Varicose veins or prior thromboembolic disease.*
10. *Age:* Risk of thromboembolism is greatest between 55-65 years of age.

Specific findings for fat embolus: Typically, patient is asymptomatic for a period lasting 12-24 hours following embolization; this period ends with sudden cardiopulmonary and neurologic deterioration: restlessness, confusion, delirium, coma, and dyspnea.

Physical assessment for fat embolus: Tachypnea, tachycardia, and hypertension; fever; petechiae, especially of the upper torso and axillae; inspiratory crowing; and expiratory wheezes.

History and risk factors for fat embolus

1. *Multiple long bone fractures:* Especially fractures of the femur and pelvis.
2. *Trauma to adipose tissue or liver.*
3. *Burns.*
4. *Osteomyelitis.* Bone infection
5. *Sickle cell crisis.*

DIAGNOSTIC TESTS

General findings for pulmonary emboli

1. *ABG values:* Hypoxemia (Pao_2 <80 mm Hg), hypocarbia ($Paco_2$ <35 mm Hg), and respiratory alkalosis (pH >7.45) usually are present. A normal Pao_2 does not rule out the presence of pulmonary emboli.

2. *Chest x-ray:* Initially, the chest x-ray is normal or an elevated hemidiaphragm may be present. After 24 hours the x-ray may reveal small infiltrates secondary to atelectasis that results from the decrease in surfactant. If pulmonary infarction is present, infiltrates and pleural effusions may be seen within 12-36 hours.
3. *EKG:* If PE is extensive, signs of acute pulmonary hypertension may be present: right-shift QRS axes, tall and peaked P waves, ST-segment changes, and T-wave inversion in leads V_1-V_4.
4. *Pulmonary ventilation-perfusion scan:* Used to detect presence of abnormalities of ventilation or perfusion in the pulmonary system. The patient inhales radioactive-tagged gases and radioactive particles are injected peripherally. If there is a mismatch of ventilation and perfusion (e.g., normal ventilation with decreased perfusion), vascular obstruction is likely.
5. *Pulmonary angiography:* The definitive study for pulmonary emboli. It is an invasive procedure that involve right heart catheterization and injection of dye into the pulmonary artery (PA) to visualize pulmonary vessels. An abrupt vessel "cut off" may be seen at the site of embolization. Usually, filling defects are seen. More specific findings are abnormal blood vessel diameters (i.e., obstruction of right pulmonary artery would cause dilatation of left pulmonary artery) and shapes (i.e., the affected blood vessel may taper to a sharp point and disappear).

Findings specific for fat emboli
1. *ABG values:* Hypoxemia (Pao_2 <80 mm Hg) and hypercarbia ($Paco_2$ >45 mm Hg) will be present with a respiratory acidosis (pH <7.35).
2. *Chest x-ray:* A pattern similar to adult respiratory distress syndrome is seen: diffuse, extensive bilateral interstitial and alveolar infiltrates.
3. *CBC:* May reveal decreased hemoglobin and hematocrit secondary to hemorrhage into the lung, in addition to thrombocytopenia.

MEDICAL MANAGEMENT

The three goals of therapy are as follows: 1) prophylaxis for individuals at risk for development of pulmonary emboli; 2) treatment during the acute embolic event; and 3) prevention of future embolic events in the individual who has experienced a pulmonary embolus.

General management of pulmonary emboli
1. Oxygen therapy: Delivered at appropriate concentration to maintain a Pao_2 of >60 mm Hg.
2. IV heparin therapy: Treatment of choice; it is started immediately in patients without bleeding or clotting disorders and in whom PE is strongly suspected.
   □ *Initial dose:* IV bolus of 5,000-10,000 units.
   □ *Maintenance dose:* 2 to 4 hours after initial dose, either a continuous infusion of 1,000 units/hr or 5,000-7,500 units IV q4h.
   □ *Goals of therapy:* To inhibit thrombus growth, promote resolution of the formed thrombus, and prevent further embolus formation. These goals are achieved by keeping partial thromboplastin time (PTT) at 1.5-2.5 times the normal. This test should be done just prior to each bolus and q4-6h thereafter.
   □ *Protamine sulfate:* Heparin antidote, which should be readily available during heparin therapy. Fatal hemorrhage occurs in 1%-2% of patients undergoing heparin therapy. Risk of bleeding is greatest in women who are >60 years of age.
3. Oral anticoagulants (warfarin sodium): Started 48-72 hours after initiation of heparin therapy. The two are given simultaneously for 6-7 days to allow time for warfarin to inhibit vitamin K-dependent clotting factors before heparin is discontinued.
   □ *Prothrombin time (PT):* Monitored daily, with the goal of 1.25-1.50 times normal. Once the patient has stabilized and the heparin is discontinued, weekly monitoring of PT is acceptable. After hospital discharge the PT should be monitored q2weeks for as long as the patient continues to take oral anticoagulants.

□ *Maintenance:* Usually 10 mg/day continued for 3-6 months, based on the continued presence of risk factors. Certain tumors (e.g., Trousseau syndrome) necessitate lifetime therapy.

□ *Vitamin K:* Reverses the effects of warfarin in 24-36 hours. Fresh frozen plasma may be required in cases of serious bleeding.

□ **Caution:** Warfarin crosses the placental barrier and can cause spontaneous abortion and birth defects.

4. Thrombolytic therapy (i.e., streptokinase and urokinase): May be given in the first 24-72 hours after PE to speed the process of clot lysis *via* conversion of plasminogen to plasma. After the first 24-72 hours of thrombolytic therapy, heparin therapy is initiated. Thrombolytic therapy may be preferred for initial treatment of PE in patients with hemodynamic compromise, >30% occlusion of pulmonary vasculature, and in whom therapy has been initiated no later than 3 days after onset of PE.

□ *Streptokinase:* Loading dose of 250,000 IU in normal saline or D_5W given IV over a 30-minute period. Maintenance dose is 100,000 IU/hr given IV for 24-72 hours.

□ *Urokinase:* Loading dose of 4,400 IU/kg of body weight in 5 ml of solution given IV over a 10 minute period. Maintenance dose is 4,400 IU/kg/hr for 12 hours.

□ *Thrombin time:* Monitors therapy for both drugs. The test is repeated q4h during therapy to ensure adequate response, which should be between 2-5 times normal. PTT can be used instead of thrombin time and should be 2-5 times control. Once thrombolytic therapy is stopped, thrombin time or PTT should be checked frequently until values fall below 2 times normal. When the values are below 2 times normal, heparin is started and continued as described under "heparin therapy."

□ *Contraindications:* Active internal bleeding, cerebrovascular accident, or intracranial bleeding within 2 months of PE. Other contraindications include trauma or surgery within 15 days of PE, diastolic hypertension >100 mm Hg, recent cardiopulmonary resuscitation, pregnancy, and <10 days postpartum.

Note: Up to 33% of patients receiving thrombolytic therapy have hemorrhagic complications. Discontinuing the drug and administering fresh frozen plasma are the appropriate treatments.

---

5. Surgical interventions: Used only in select cases owing to the success rate of anticoagulant therapy.

□ *Vena caval interruption/ligation:* Multiple methods that share the common purpose of interrupting passage of venous thrombi through the inferior vena cava.

□ *Pulmonary embolectomy:* To remove clots from the pulmonary circulation. Generally, the use of thrombolytic agents eliminates the need for this procedure.

Management of fat emboli

1. Oxygen: Concentration of oxygen is based on clinical picture, ABG results, and patient's prior respiratory status. Intubation and mechanical ventilation may be required.

2. Steroids: Cortisone 100 mg or methylprednisolone 30 mg/kg is used to decrease local injury to pulmonary tissue and pulmonary edema.

3. Diuretics: Approximately 30% of patients with fat emboli develop pulmonary edema, necessitating use of diuretics.

NURSING DIAGNOSES AND INTERVENTIONS

Impaired gas exchange related to decreased diffusion of oxygen secondary to ventilation-perfusion mismatch occurring with pulmonary embolus

Desired outcome: Patient exhibits adequate gas exchange and ventilatory function as evidenced by RR 12-20 breaths/min with normal pattern and depth (eupnea), Pao_2 ≥60 mm Hg, $Paco_2$ 35-45 mm Hg, and pH 7.35-7.45 (or values consistent with acceptable baseline parameters).

1. Monitor serial ABG values, assessing for the desired response to treatment: increased Pao_2 and correction of respiratory alkalosis. Report lack of response to treatment or worsening ABG values.
2. Monitor patient for signs and symptoms of increasing respiratory distress: respiratory rate increased from baseline, increasing dyspnea, anxiety, and cyanosis.
3. Ensure delivery of prescribed concentrations of oxygen.
4. Position patient for comfort and optimal gas exchange. Ensure that the area of the lung affected by the emboli is not dependent when patient is in the lateral decubitus position. Elevate HOB 30 degrees to ensure a better ventilation-perfusion match, thereby improving Pao_2.
5. Avoid positioning patient with knees bent (i.e., gatching the bed) because this impedes venous return from the legs and can increase the risk of pulmonary emboli.
6. Decrease metabolic demands for oxygen by limiting or pacing patient's activities and procedures.
7. Ensure that patient performs deep-breathing and coughing exercises 3-5 times q2h.

Potential for injury related to increased risk of bleeding or hemorrhage secondary to anticoagulation therapy

Desired outcome: Patient is free of frank or occult bleeding.

1. Monitor VS for indicators of profuse bleeding or hemorrhage resulting from anticoagulant therapy: hypotension, tachycardia, and tachypnea.
2. Monitor serial PTT (desired range is 1.5-2.5 times normal) or PT (desired range is 1.25-1.50 times normal) as appropriate. Report values outside the desired therapeutic ranges.
3. Ensure easy access to antidotes for prescribed treatment.
   - □ *Protamine sulfate:* 1 mg counteracts 100 units of heparin. Usually, the initial dose is 50 mg.
   - □ *Vitamin K:* 20 mg given subcutaneously to counteract the effects of oral anticoagulants.
   - □ *E-aminocaproic acid (e.g., Amicar):* Reverses the fibrinolytic condition related to thrombolytic therapy. Note: Use of this drug as an antidote has not been documented in humans. It might, however, be used in emergency situations.
4. At least once a shift, inspect the following sites for evidence of bleeding: any entry site of an invasive procedure, oral mucous membranes, wounds, and nares.
5. At least once a shift, inspect the skin and mucous membranes for petechiae.
6. At least once a shift, check stool, urine, sputum, and vomitus for occult blood, using agency-approved method for testing.
7. Apply pressure to ail venipuncture or arterial puncture sites until bleeding stops completely.
8. To prevent hematoma formation, avoid giving an IM injection unless it is unavoidable.
9. To avoid negative interactions with anticoagulants or thrombolytic therapy, establish compatibility of all drugs before administering them.
   - □ *Heparin:* Digitalis, tetracyclines, nicotine, and antihistamines decrease the effect of heparin therapy. Consult with pharmacist regarding compatibility before infusing other IV drugs through heparin IV line.
   - □ *Warfarin sodium:* Numerous drugs result in a decrease or increase in response to treatment with warfarin. Consult with pharmacist to obtain specific information about patient's medication profile.
   - □ *Thrombolytic therapy:* No specific drug interactions are noted. However, consult with pharmacist before infusing any other medication through the same IV line.
10. Because aspirin and nonsteroidal antiinflammatory drugs (e.g., ibuprofen) are platelet aggregation inhibitors and can prolong episodes of bleeding, avoid use of *any* drug that contains these medications.
11. Discuss with patient and significant others the importance of reporting promptly the presence of bleeding from any source.
12. Teach patient the necessity of using sponge toothettes and mouthwash for oral care

to minimize the risk of gum bleeding. Instruct patient to shave with an electric rather than straight razor.

13. If patient is restless and combative, provide a safe environment: pad the side rails, restrain patient as necessary to prevent falls, and use extreme care when moving patient to avoid bumping of extremities into side rails.

Knowledge deficit: Oral anticoagulant therapy, potential side effects, and foods and medications to avoid during therapy

Desired outcome: Patient verbalizes knowledge of his or her prescribed anticoagulant drug, the potential side effects, and foods and medications to avoid while on oral anticoagulant therapy.

1. Determine patient's knowledge of oral anticoagulant therapy. As appropriate, discuss the drug name, purpose, dosage, and schedule.
2. Inform patient of the potential side effects of anticoagulant therapy: easy bruising, prolonged bleeding from cuts, spontaneous nose bleeds, black and tarry stools, and blood in urine and sputum.
3. Discuss with patient the importance of laboratory testing and follow-up visits with MD.
4. Explain the importance of informing all health-care providers (e.g., dentists and other physicians) that patient is on anticoagulant therapy. Suggest that patient wear a Medic-Alert tag or other method of informing health-care providers about the anticoagulant therapy.
5. Teach patient about foods high in vitamin K (e.g., fish, bananas, dark green vegetables, tomatoes, and cauliflower), which can interfere with anticoagulation.
6. Caution patient that a soft-bristled, rather than hard-bristled, toothbrush and an electric, rather than straight, razor should be used during anticoagulant therapy.
7. Instruct patient to consult with physician before taking OTC or prescribed drugs that were used prior to initiation of anticoagulants. Aspirin, cimetidine, and trimethaphan are among many drugs that enhance the response to warfarin. Drugs that decrease the response include antacids, diuretics, oral contraceptives, and barbiturates, among others.

Also, if appropriate, see the appendix for nursing diagnoses and interventions for the care of patients on prolonged bed rest, p. 651, and the care of preoperative and postoperative patients, p. 637.

PATIENT-FAMILY TEACHING AND DISCHARGE PLANNING

Provide patient and significant others verbal and written instructions for the following:
1. Risk factors related to the development of thrombi and embolization, and preventive measures to reduce the risk.
2. Signs and symptoms of *thrombophlebitis:* swelling of the calf, tenderness or warmth in the involved area, possible presence of pain in affected calf when ankle is flexed, slight fever, distention of veins in affected leg; signs and symptoms of *pulmonary embolism:* sudden onset of dyspnea and anxiety, nonproductive cough, palpitations, nausea, syncope.
3. Rationale and application procedure for antiembolism hose. Explain that patient should put them on in the morning before getting out of bed.
4. Importance of preventing impairment of venous return from the lower extremities by avoiding prolonged sitting, crossing legs, and constrictive clothing.
   Note: Rehabilitation and family teaching concepts for fat emboli are nonspecific.

Pneumothorax/Hemothorax

Pneumothorax is an accumulation of air in the pleural space. Risk factors include blunt or penetrating chest injury, COPD, previous pneumothorax, and positive pressure ventilation. There are three types:

Spontaneous: Also referred to as closed pneumothorax because the chest wall remains intact with no leak to the atmosphere. It results from the rupture of a bleb or bulla on the visceral pleural surface, usually near the apex. Generally, the cause of the rupture is unknown, although it may result from a weakness related to a respiratory infection or from an underlying pulmonary disease (e.g., COPD, tuberculosis, malignant neoplasm). The affected individual is usually young (20-40 years), previously healthy, and male. Generally, onset of symptoms occurs at rest, rather than with vigorous exercise or coughing. Potential for recurrence is great, with the second pneumothorax occurring an average of 2-3 years after the first.

Traumatic: Can be open or closed. An open pneumothorax occurs when air enters the pleural space from the atmosphere through an opening in the chest wall, such as with a gunshot wound, stab wound, or invasive medical procedure (e.g., lung biopsy, thoracentesis, or placement of a central line into a subclavian vein). A sucking sound may be heard during inspiration over the area of penetration. A closed pneumothorax occurs when the visceral pleura is penetrated, but the chest wall remains intact with no atmospheric leak. This usually occurs with blunt trauma that results in a fracture and dislocation of the ribs. It also may occur from the use of positive end expiratory pressure (PEEP) or after cardiopulmonary resuscitation (CPR).

Tension: Occurs with open pneumothorax when pleural tissue acts as a one-way valve. Air enters the pleural space through the pleural tear when the individual inhales and continues to accumulate but cannot escape during expiration because the pleural flap closes. As the pressure in the thorax and mediastinum increases, it produces a shift in the affected lung and mediastinum toward the unaffected side, which further impairs ventilatory efforts. The increase in pressure also compresses the vena cava, which impedes venous return, leading to a decrease in cardiac output and, ultimately, to circulatory collapse if it is not diagnosed and treated quickly. Tension pneumothorax is a life-threatening medical emergency.

Hemothorax is an accumulation of blood in the pleural space. Hemothorax generally results from blunt trauma to the chest wall, but it can occur following thoracic surgery as a result of anticoagulant therapy, after the insertion of a central venous catheter, or following various thoracoabdominal organ biopsies. Mediastinal shift, ventilatory compromise, and lung collapse can occur, depending on the amount of blood accumulated.

ASSESSMENT

Clinical presentation will vary, depending on the type and size of the pneumothorax/hemothorax (see Table 1-2).

DIAGNOSTIC TESTS

1. *Chest x-ray:* Will reveal the presence of air or blood in the pleural space on the affected side, size of the pneumothorax/hemothorax, and any shift in the mediastinum.
2. *ABG values:* Hypoxemia (Pa_{O_2} <80 mm Hg) may be accompanied by respiratory acidosis (pH <7.35) and hypercarbia (Pa_{CO_2} >45 mm Hg). Arterial oxygen saturation may be decreased initially but usually returns to normal within 24 hours.
3. *CBC:* May reveal a decreased hemoglobin proportionate to the amount of blood lost in a hemothorax.

MEDICAL MANAGEMENT AND SURGICAL INTERVENTIONS

Management is determined by the signs and symptoms. A small pneumothorax may heal itself *via* reabsorption of the free air, making medical management unnecessary. A hemothorax nearly always requires intervention.

1. Oxygen therapy: Administered when ABG values demonstrate the presence of hypoxemia, which usually occurs when the pneumothorax/hemothorax is large.
2. Thoracentesis: For hemothorax to remove blood from the pleural space. In cases of

T A B L E 1 - 2   Assessment of the patient with pneumothorax or hemothorax

	Spontaneous or Traumatic Pneumothorax		Tension pneumothorax	Hemothorax
	Closed	**Open**		
Signs and symptoms	SOB, cough, chest tightness, chest pain	SOB, sharp chest pain	Dyspnea, chest pain	Dyspnea, chest pain
Physical assessment	Tachypnea, decreased thoracic movement, cyanosis, subcutaneous emphysema, hyperresonance over affected area, diminished breath sounds, paradoxical movement of chest wall (may signal flail chest)	Agitation, restlessness, tachypnea, cyanosis, presence of chest wound, hyperresonance over affected area, sucking sound on inspiration, diminished breath sounds	Anxiety, tachycardia, cyanosis, jugular vein distension, tracheal deviation toward the unaffected side, absent breath sounds on affected side, distant heart sounds, hypotension	Tachypnea, pallor, cyanosis, dullness over affected side, tachycardia, hypotension

tension pneumothorax it is performed immediately to remove air from the pleural space. A large-bore needle is inserted in the second intercostal space, midclavicular line, which correlates to the superior portion of the anterior axillary lobe. A sudden rushing out of air confirms the diagnosis of tension pneumothorax. To decrease risk of further pleural laceration as the chest reexpands, a stylet introducer needle with a plastic sheath may be used. The needle is removed after penetration and the plastic catheter sheath is left in place to allow decompression of the chest cavity. Following air aspiration, chest tubes are inserted.

3. **Chest tube placement:** A chest tube (thoracic catheter) may be inserted in any patient who is symptomatic. During insertion the patient should be in an upright position so that the lung falls away from the chest wall. The position of the thoracic catheter will depend on whether the physician wants to drain air, fluid, or both. The thoracic catheter must be connected to an underwater-seal drainage system. Usually, simple underwater-seal drainage is all that is necessary for 6-24 hours. Suction may be used, depending on size of the pneumothorax/hemothorax, patient's condition, and amount of drainage. If drainage is minimal and no suction is required, a one-way flutter valve may be used instead of an underwater-seal drainage system. After chest tube insertion and removal of air or fluid from the pleural space, the lung begins to reexpand. A chest tube may produce inflammation of the pleura, causing pleuritic pain, slight temperature elevation, and pleural friction rub.

4. **Thoracotomy:** Often indicated if patient has had two or more spontaneous pneumothoraces on one side, owing to the risk of continuous recurrence, or if resolution of the pneumothorax does not occur within 7 days. With a hemothorax it is performed to locate the source and control bleeding if blood loss exceeds 200 ml/hr over 2 hours. Thoracotomy may involve mechanical abrasion of the pleural surfaces with a

dry sterile sponge or chemical abrasion *via* an agent such as tetracycline solution or talc, both of which result in pleural adhesions to prevent recurrence. A partial pleurectomy may be performed instead of mechanical or chemical abrasion.

5. **IV therapy:** If there is significant loss of fluids or blood.
6. **Analgesia:** Provides relief of pain from the pneumothorax/hemothorax or its treatment.

NURSING DIAGNOSES AND INTERVENTIONS

Impaired gas exchange related to decreased diffusion of oxygen secondary to ventilation-perfusion mismatch

Desired outcome: Patient exhibits adequate gas exchange and ventilatory function as evidenced by Pao_2 ≥ 80 mm Hg and $Paco_2$ 35-45 mm Hg (or values within acceptable baseline parameters, which are dependent on underlying pathophysiology), RR ≤ 20 breaths/min with normal depth and pattern (eupnea), and orientation to person, place, and time.

1. Monitor serial ABG results to detect decreasing Pao_2 and increasing $Paco_2$, a situation that can signal impending respiratory failure. Report significant findings to MD.
2. Observe for indicators of hypoxia, including increased restlessness, anxiety, and changes in mental status. Cyanosis is a late sign.
3. Assess patient's VS and breath sounds q2h (patient will require checks q15min after thoracotomy until stable) for signs of respiratory distress: increased RR, diminished or absent movement of chest wall on affected side, paradoxical movement of the chest wall, increased work of breathing, use of accessory muscles of respiration, complaints of increased dyspnea, and cyanosis. Evaluate HR and BP for indications of shock state (i.e., tachycardia and hypotension).
4. Position patient to allow for full expansion of the unaffected lung. Semi-Fowler's position usually provides comfort and allows adequate expansion of chest wall.
5. Change patient's position q2h to promote drainage and lung reexpansion and facilitate alveolar perfusion.
6. Encourage patient to take deep breaths, providing necessary analgesia to decrease discomfort during deep-breathing exercises. Deep breathing will promote full lung expansion and may decrease the risk of atelectasis. Coughing will facilitate mobilization of tracheobronchial secretions, if present.
7. Deliver oxygen and monitor oxygen delivery as indicated.

Potential for ineffective breathing pattern related to malfunction of chest drainage system

Desired outcome: Patient remains eupneic.

1. Monitor patient at frequent intervals (q2-4h, as appropriate) to assess breathing pattern while chest-drainage system is in place. Auscultate breath sounds, reporting a decrease, and be alert to and report signs of respiratory distress, including restlessness, anxiety, and changes in mental status.
2. Assess and maintain the closed chest-drainage system.
   □ Tape all connections and secure chest tube to thorax with tape.
   □ Avoid all kinks in the tubing, and ensure that the bed and equipment are not compressing any component of the system.
   □ Maintain fluid in underwater-seal chamber and suction chamber at appropriate levels.
3. Be aware that the suction apparatus does not regulate the amount of suction applied to the closed chest-drainage system. The amount of suction is determined by the water level in the suction control chamber. Minimal bubbling is acceptable.
   □ **Note:** Suction aids in the reexpansion of the lung, but removing suction for short periods of time, such as for transporting, will not be detrimental or disrupt the closed chest-drainage system.

4. Follow institution's policy regarding chest tube stripping. Be aware that this mechanism for maintaining chest tube patency is controversial and has been associated with creating high negative pressures in the pleural space, which can damage fragile lung tissue. Chest tube stripping may be indicated when bloody drainage or clots are visible in the tubing. Squeezing alternately hand-over-hand along the drainage tube may generate sufficient pressure to move fluid along the tube.

5. Be aware that fluctuations in the long tube of the underwater-seal chamber are indicative of a patent chest tube. Fluctuations stop when either the lung has reexpanded or there is a kink or obstruction in the chest tube.

  ☐ Bubbling in the underwater-seal chamber occurs on expiration and is a sign that air is leaving the pleural space.

  ☐ Continuous bubbling on expiration in the underwater-seal chamber may be a signal that air is leaking into the drainage system. Locate and seal the system's air leak, if possible.

6. Keep necessary emergency supplies at the bedside: petrolatum gauze pad, to apply over insertion site if the chest tube becomes dislodged, and sterile water, in which to submerge the chest tube if it becomes disconnected from the underwater-seal system. *Never* clamp a chest tube without a specific directive from the MD because clamping may lead to tension pneumothorax since the air can no longer escape.

Pain related to impaired pleural integrity, inflammation, or presence of a chest tube

Desired outcome: Patient's subjective evaluation of pain improves, as documented by a pain scale.

1. At frequent intervals, assess patient's degree of discomfort using patient's verbal and nonverbal cues. Devise a pain scale with patient, rating pain from 0 (no pain) to 10. Medicate with analgesics as prescribed, evaluating and documenting the effectiveness of the medication, again using the pain scale.

2. Premedicate patient 30 minutes before initiating coughing, exercising, or repositioning.

3. Teach patient to splint affected side when coughing, moving, or repositioning.

4. Schedule activities to provide for 90-minute periods of undisturbed rest, which may increase patient's pain threshold.

5. Stabilize chest tube to reduce pull or drag on latex connector tubing. Tape chest tube securely to thorax, eliminating any obstructions on the latex tubing.

Also see appropriate psychosocial nursing diagnoses and interventions in "Caring for Patients with Cancer and Other Life-Disrupting Illnesses," p. 690-700.

PATIENT-FAMILY TEACHING AND DISCHARGE PLANNING

Give patient and significant others verbal and written instructions for the following:
1. Purpose for chest tube placement and maintenance.
2. Potential for recurrence of spontaneous pneumothorax. Average time between occurrences is 2-3 years. Explain the importance of seeking medical care immediately if the symptoms recur (see Table 1-2, p. 19).
3. Medications, including drug name, purpose, dosage, schedule, precautions, and potential side effects.

Section Two ACUTE RESPIRATORY FAILURE

Acute respiratory failure (ARF) develops when the lungs are unable to exchange oxygen and carbon dioxide adequately. Clinically, respiratory failure exists when Pao_2 is <50 mm Hg with the patient at rest and breathing room air. $Paco_2$ ≥50 mm Hg or pH <7.35 is significant for respiratory acidosis, which is the common precursor to ARF.

TABLE 1-3   Disease processes leading to the development of respiratory failure

Impaired alveolar ventilation
A.   COPD (emphysema, bronchitis, asthma, cystic fibrosis)
B.   Restrictive pulmonary disease (interstitial fibrosis, pleural effusion, pneumothorax, kyphoscoliosis, obesity, diaphragmatic paralysis)
C.   Neuromuscular defects (Guillain-Barré syndrome, myasthenia gravis, multiple sclerosis, muscular dystrophy)
D.   Depression of respiratory control centers (drug-induced cerebral infarction, inappropriate use of high-dose oxygen therapy)

Diffusion disturbances
A.   Pulmonary/interstitial fibrosis
B.   Pulmonary edema
C.   Adult respiratory distress syndrome
D.   Anatomic loss of functioning lung tissue (tumor pneumonectomy)

Ventilation or perfusion disturbances
A.   Pulmonary emboli
B.   Atelectasis
C.   Pneumonia
D.   Emphysema
E.   Chronic bronchitis
F.   Bronchiolitis
G.   Adult respiratory distress syndrome

Right-to-left shunting
A.   Atelectasis
B.   Pneumonia
C.   Pulmonary edema
D.   Pulmonary emboli
E.   Oxygen toxicity

From Easterday U and Howard C: In Swearingen PL et al: Manual of critical care: applying nursing diagnoses to adult critical illness, St Louis, 1988, The CV Mosby Co.

While a variety of disease processes can lead to the development of respiratory failure (see Table 1-3), four basic mechanisms are involved:

Alveolar hypoventilation: Occurs secondary to reduction in alveolar minute ventilation. Because differential indicators (cyanosis and somnolence) occur late in the process, the condition may go unnoticed until hypoxia is severe.

Ventilation-perfusion mismatch: Considered the most common cause of hypoxia. Normal alveolar ventilation occurs at a rate of 4 L/min, with normal pulmonary vascular blood flow occurring at a rate of 5 L/min. Normal ventilation/perfusion ratio is 0.8. Any disease process that interferes with either side of the equation upsets the physiologic balance and can lead to respiratory failure as a result of reduction in arterial oxygen levels.

Diffusion disturbances: Processes that physically impair gas exchange across the alveolar-capillary membrane. Diffusion is impaired owing to the increase in anatomic distance the gas must travel from alveoli to capillary and capillary to alveoli.

Right-to-left shunt: Occurs when the above processes go untreated. Large amounts of blood pass from the right side of the heart to the left and out into the general circulation without adequate ventilation; therefore blood is poorly oxygenated. This mechanism occurs when alveoli are atelectatic or fluid-filled, as these conditions interfere with gas exchange. Unlike the first three responses, hypoxia secondary to right-to-left shunting does not improve with the administration of oxygen because the additional FIO_2 is unable to cross the alveolar-capillary membrane.

ASSESSMENT

Clinical indicators of acute respiratory failure vary according to the underlying disease process and severity of the failure. ARF is one of the most common causes of impaired LOC. Often, it is misdiagnosed as CHF, pneumonia, or CVA. Sometimes the onset of ARF is so insidious that it is missed because the staff does not want to disturb the patient who appears to be sleeping.

Early indicators: Restlessness, anxiety, headache, fatigue, cool and dry skin, increased BP, tachycardia, and cardiac dysrhythmias.

Intermediate indicators: Confusion, lethargy, tachypnea, hypotension caused by vasodilatation, cardiac dysrhythmias.

Late indicators: Cyanosis, diaphoresis, coma, respiratory arrest.

DIAGNOSTIC TESTS

1. *ABG analysis:* Assesses adequacy of oxygenation and effectiveness of ventilation and is the most important diagnostic tool. Typical results are Pao_2 $\leq$60 mm Hg, $Paco_2$ $\geq$45 mm Hg, and pH <7.35, which are consistent with severe respiratory acidosis.
2. *Chest x-ray:* Ascertains presence of underlying pathophysiology or disease process that may be contributing to the failure.

MEDICAL MANAGEMENT

Treatment is aimed at correcting the acid-base disturbance, while at the same time treating the underlying pathophysiology in an effort to prevent or correct ARF. While the general rule is to bring the Pao_2 to >60 mm Hg and the $Paco_2$ to <45 mm Hg, patients with COPD may be clinically stable with a $Paco_2$ >45 mm Hg, so determination of pH is critical with these individuals. For example, the patient with a chronically high $Paco_2$ whose pH drops is headed for danger.

1. Oxygen therapy: As determined by ABG values. Oxygen therapy at an Fio_2 of 0.50 or less and chest physiotherapy, in conjunction with pharmacotherapy (e.g., bronchodilators, steroids, antibiotics), often improve ABGs sufficiently to get the patient out of danger. Persistent respiratory acidosis following medical intervention may be an indicator of the need for intubation and mechanical ventilation.
2. IV aminophylline: To treat bronchospasms. Therapeutic range is 10-20 μg/ml. Daily serum levels are drawn to evaluate the patient.
3. Bronchodilator therapy: Delivered *via* nebulizer or IPPB machine q2-4h to minimize CO_2 retention.
4. Chest physiotherapy: To assist in mobilization of secretions.
5. Coughing/deep breathing exercises: To mobilize secretions and promote full lung expansion. If the cough is ineffective, suctioning may be necessary to stimulate cough reflex and clear secretions.
6. IV fluids: To maintain fluid balance and prevent dehydration.
7. Antibiotics: If infection is present.
8. Intubation and mechanical ventilation: To prevent further airway collapse and tissue injury. The patient may require intubation and mechanical ventilation to provide adequate respiratory function and stabilize ABGs if ARF progresses. Mechanical support is used until the underlying cause of the failure can be corrected and the patient can resume ventilatory efforts independently.

NURSING DIAGNOSES AND INTERVENTIONS

Ineffective airway clearance related to impaired coughing ability secondary to fatigue or decreased LOC

Desired outcome: Patient's airways are clear.

1. Auscultate breath sounds at least q2h. Report any increase in adventitious breath sounds or sudden absence of breath sounds in the presence of increasing respiratory distress.
2. Teach patient the following coughing technique:
   □ Sit upright with the upper body flexed slightly forward.
   □ Take two deep breaths and exhale passively.
   □ Then take a deep breath, hold it, and cough forcefully. **Caution:** To avoid small airways collapse, patients with COPD should cough twice sharply from the midinspiratory point rather than after a deep breath.
3. Administer chest physiotherapy as prescribed to assist with mobilization of secretions.
4. If the patient is unable to clear secretions with coughing, obtain a physician's order for nasotracheal or pharyngeal suction. Suction may stimulate the cough reflex and enhance airway clearance.

See "Pneumonia" for **Potential fluid volume deficit,** p. 9. See "Nursing Diagnoses Used in This Manual," p. 717, for discussions of **impaired gas exchange** and the pathologic process that can cause impaired gas exchange, as they may be precursors to ARF. Also see COPD section, p. 24-32, as appropriate. For psychosocial nursing diagnoses and interventions, see "Caring for Patients with Cancer and Other Life-Disrupting Illnesses," p. 690-700.

PATIENT-FAMILY TEACHING AND DISCHARGE PLANNING

ARF is an acute condition that is symptomatically treated during the patient's hospitalization. Discharge planning and teaching should be directed at educating the patient and significant others about the underlying pathophysiology and treatment specific for that process. See sections in this chapter that relate specifically to the underlying pathophysiology contributing to the development of ARF.

Section Three CHRONIC OBSTRUCTIVE PULMONARY DISEASE (COPD)

COPD is the second leading cause of disability in the United States. It is a chronic respiratory condition that obstructs the flow of air to or from the bronchioles. Causative factors include smoking, allergens, and environmental and occupational pollutants. This section will discuss the following types of COPD: asthma, chronic bronchitis, and emphysema.

Asthma

Asthma is a disorder in which there is obstruction of airflow in the bronchioles and smaller bronchi secondary to bronchospasm, mucosal edema, and excessive mucus production. It can occur in any age group, and its symptoms are intermittent and usually alleviated with treatment. Extrinsic asthma is precipitated by environmental allergens (pollens, dust, feathers, animal dander, foods, etc.). Intrinsic asthma is believed to be caused by an infection in the upper or lower respiratory tract and occurs more frequently in individuals over age 35.

ASSESSMENT

Signs and symptoms: Coughing, chest tightness, increased sputum production, dyspnea.

Physical assessment: Agitation, prolonged expiratory phase, use of accessory muscles of respiration, tachypnea, chest retractions, nasal flaring, expiratory wheezing. **Note:** If symptoms are untreated, the condition can progress to status asthmaticus (SA), a severe and unrelenting asthma attack. If SA is not reversed, death can ensue.

DIAGNOSTIC TESTS

1. *ABG values:* Reveal status of oxygenation and acid-base balance. Generally, acute respiratory acidosis is present during an acute asthma attack ($Paco_2$ >45 mm Hg and pH <7.35).
2. *Chest x-ray:* The x-ray usually shows lung hyperinflation due to air trapping and a flat diaphragm related to increased intrathoracic volume.
3. *Sputum:* Gross exam may show viscosity or actual mucus plugs. Culture and sensitivity may show microorganisms if infection was the precipitating event.
4. *CBC:* Differential may show increased eosinophiles (in patients not on corticosteroids), which is indicative of allergic response.
5. *Serum theophylline level:* Important baseline indicator for patients who are on this therapy. Acceptable therapeutic range is 10-20 µg/ml. The therapeutic level is close to the toxic level and the patient must be monitored for toxic side effects (e.g., nausea, CNS stimulation, dysrhythmias). Serial levels are drawn at frequent intervals.
6. *Pulmonary function testing:* To evaluate the degree of obstruction. Forced expiratory volume (FEV) is decreased during acute episodes because of severely narrowed airways that prevent forceful exhalation of inspired volume (see Table 1-4).
7. *EKG:* Presence of sinus tachycardia is an important baseline indicator because the use of some bronchodilators (e.g., metaproterenol) may produce cardiac stimulant effects and dysrhythmias.

MEDICAL MANAGEMENT

Primarily, management is directed toward decreasing bronchospasm and increasing pulmonary ventilation.

Acute phase
1. Oxygen therapy: Generally, these patients experience mild to moderate hypoxia. Low-flow (1-3 L/min) oxygen is delivered *via* nasal cannula.
2. Pharmacotherapy: Initiated to relieve bronchospasm and continued until wheezing subsides and pulmonary function tests return to baseline.
   □ *Bronchodilators:* Dilate smooth muscles of the airways (see Table 1-5).
   □ *Corticosteroids:* To decrease the inflammatory response. Dosage varies according to severity of the episode and whether patient is currently taking steroids. **Note:** Acute adrenal insufficiency can develop in patients who take steroids routinely at home if these drugs are not given to the patient during hospitalization.
   □ *Antibiotics:* Given if infectious pulmonary process is present as evidenced by fever, purulent sputum, or leukocytosis.
3. Fluid replacement: To maintain adequate hydration. Generally, crystalloid fluids (i.e., D_5W or D_5NS) are used.
4. Chest physiotherapy: Generally contraindicated in acute phases owing to hyperreactive state of airways. The patient may benefit from the cautious use of percussion and postural drainage to help mobilize secretions.

Chronic phase
1. Aminophylline: Dosage is determined by blood levels of theophylline.
2. Nebulizer/aerosolized bronchodilators: For short-term, acute exacerbations of symptoms.
3. Steroids: May be prescribed, depending on severity of symptoms. Generally, physicians try to wean patients completely off steroids but some patients may require low-dose steroids indefinitely.

NURSING DIAGNOSES AND INTERVENTIONS

Impaired gas exchange related to decreased alveolar ventilation secondary to narrowed airways

TABLE 1-4 Pulmonary function tests used in individuals with asthma

Test	Description	Normal values	Parameters in asthma
Forced vital capacity (FVC)	Total amount of gas exhaled as forcefully and as rapidly as possible after maximal inspiration	≥80% of predicted normal	Normal or slightly decreased due to air trapping
Forced expiratory volume in one second (FEV$_1$)	Volume of gas exhaled over first second of FVC. (FEV$_2$ and FEV$_3$ also may be measured at two and three seconds, respectively)	≥75% of predicted normal	Decreased due to airway obstruction. It may return to normal after administration of aerosolized bronchodilator
Forced midexpiratory flow (FEF). Formerly this was called maximal midexpiratory flow (MMF)	Average rate of flow during middle half of FEV. It is an accurate estimate of airway resistance	≥80% of predicted normal	Decreased due to small airways obstruction. It may return to normal after administration of aerosolized bronchodilator

From Easterday U and Howard C. In Swearingen PL et al: Manual of critical care: applying nursing diagnoses to adult critical illness, St Louis, 1988, The CV Mosby Co.

Desired outcome: Patient has adequate gas exchange as evidenced by Pao$_2$ ≥60 mm Hg, Paco$_2$ 35-45 mm Hg, pH 7.35-7.45, and RR 12-20 breaths/min (or values consistent with patient's baseline).

1. Observe for signs and symptoms of hypoxia (e.g., restlessness, agitation, changes in LOC). Remember that cyanosis of the lips and nailbeds is a late indicator of hypoxia.
2. Position patient for comfort and to promote optimal gas exchange. Usually this is accomplished using high-Fowler's position, with the patient leaning forward and elbows propped on the over-the-bed table to promote maximal chest excursion. Record patient's response to positioning.
3. Auscultate breath sounds q2-4h. Monitor for decreased or adventitious sounds (e.g., crackles or wheezes).
4. Monitor ABG results. Be alert to decreasing Pao$_2$ and increasing Paco$_2$, which can signal respiratory failure.
5. Deliver oxygen as prescribed; monitor Fio$_2$ to ensure oxygen is within prescribed concentrations.

See "Chronic Bronchitis" for **Ineffective airway clearance** related to excessive mucus production and ineffective cough, p. 29. See "Emphysema" for **Ineffective breathing pattern** related to dyspnea, p. 31. For nursing diagnoses and interventions related to fear and anxiety see "Caring for Patients with Cancer and Other Life-Disrupting Illnesses," pp. 690-700.

TABLE 1-5 Bronchodilators used in the treatment of acute asthma

Medication	Usual dosage	Action	Side effects
Epinephrine	0.2-0.5 ml of a 1:1000 solution given SC q15-30min	Immediate adrenergic effects; activates adrenergic sympathomimetic receptors; acts on alpha, beta-one, and beta-two receptors; relieves bronchospasm	Cardiac stimulation, palpitations, anxiety
Terbutaline	0.2-0.3 ml given SC q30min × 3 doses	Selective beta-adrenergic; relaxes bronchial smooth muscle	Fewer than with epinephrine and usually transient; increased HR (>20 bpm), nervousness, tremor, palpitations, nausea, vomiting, headache
Methylxanthine	*Loading dose:* 6 mg/kg given IV bolus. *Maintenance dose:* 0.1-0.5 µg/kg/hr given *via* continuous IV infusion	Short-acting nonadrenergic; directly relaxes smooth muscle of bronchial airways and pulmonary vasculature	Nausea, vomiting, GI bleeding, gastric distress, HR >20 bpm, decreased BP, restlessness. **Note:** Because toxic levels are close to therapeutic levels, serum levels should be monitored to ensure correct dosage adjustment. Dysrhythmias may result from toxic levels of theophylline
Isoproterenol/isoetharine	Inhalants usually avoided during acute SA as gas flow may be too minimal to provide adequate distribution of medication		

From Easterday U and Howard C. In Swearingen PL et al: Manual of critical care: applying nursing diagnoses to adult critical illness, St Louis, 1988, The CV Mosby Co.

PATIENT-FAMILY TEACHING AND DISCHARGE PLANNING

Give patient and significant others verbal and written instructions for the following:

1. Irritants that can precipitate an attack, and the importance of removing these irritants from patient's environment.
2. Signs and symptoms of pulmonary infection (e.g., increased cough, increasing sputum production, change in color of sputum from clear-white to yellow-green, fever) or bronchial irritation (e.g., dry, hacking cough).
3. Medications, including name, route, purpose, dosage, precautions, and potential side effects. In addition, teach patient the proper use of metered-dose inhalers, documenting accurate return of demonstration before hospital discharge. Remind patient that OTC inhalers contain medications that can interfere with the prescribed therapy. Instruct patient to contact MD before taking any OTC medications.
4. Importance of avoiding contact with infectious individuals, especially those with respiratory infections. Encourage patient to get yearly flu and pneumococcoal vaccines.
5. Importance of follow-up care. Confirm date and time of next appointment.

Chronic bronchitis

Chronic bronchitis is the most common respiratory disease in the United States. It occurs in individuals who have smoked cigarettes for a long period of time or lived in areas of severe air pollution. The extent of the disease is somewhat dependent on the length of time the lungs have been exposed to these pollutants.

Lung changes that occur with this disease include airway inflammation, loss of ciliary action, hypertrophy of mucosal glands, hyperinflation of the alveoli, and edema of bronchial mucosa, all of which result in increased mucus production. When this occurs, mucus plugs develop in the stretched alveoli, causing obstruction of the bronchioles. As the disease progresses there is further destruction of the lungs, causing inadequate ventilation. Recurrent upper respiratory infections (URIs) are common in this population. As the disease progresses acute exacerbations of the disease increase in severity and duration. Respiratory failure and cardiac problems can develop.

ASSESSMENT

Chronic indicators: Morning cough, clear and copious secretions, anorexia, cyanosis, dependent edema.

Acute indicators (exacerbation): Fever, dyspnea, thick and tenacious sputum.

Physical assessment: Use of accessory muscles of respiration, prolonged expiratory phase, digital clubbing, decreased thoracic expansion, dullness over areas of consolidation, adventitious breath sounds (especially coarse rhonchi and wheezing).

DIAGNOSTIC TESTS

1. *Chest x-ray:* Will reveal normal A-P diameter, nearly normal diaphragm position, and increased peripheral lung markings.
2. *ABG values:* Will reveal hypoxemia (Pao_2 <60 mm Hg) and hypercapnia ($Paco_2$ >50-60 mm Hg) in most patients. Baseline pH may be 7.35-7.38, but during acute exacerbation, as the $Paco_2$ increases, it may fall below 7.35.
3. *Sputum culture:* May reveal presence of infective organisms.
4. *CBC:* Will reveal chronically elevated hemoglobin in the presence of chronic hypoxemia and elevated WBC count in the presence of acute bacterial infection.
5. *Pulmonary function tests:* Will show reduced capacity, increased residual volume due to trapping of air, and increased expiratory reserve volume. For descriptions and normal values of these tests, see Table 1-4, p. 26.

MEDICAL MANAGEMENT

1. **Oxygen therapy:** To treat hypoxemia. It is used cautiously and at a low flow rate (1-2 L/min) in patients with chronic CO_2 retention for whom hypoxemia, rather than hypercapnia, stimulates the respiratory drive.
2. **Pharmacotherapy**
   - □ *Bronchodilators:* To open the airways by relaxing smooth muscles. The resultant increased airflow may help loosen mucus.
   - □ *Steroids (i.e., prednisone):* To decrease inflammation, thereby increasing airflow.
   - □ *Antibiotics:* Based on sensitivity studies from sputum cultures.
3. **Chest physiotherapy:** To help loosen and mobilize pulmonary secretions.
4. **IV or oral fluids:** To promote adequate hydration.
5. **Diuretics or sodium restriction:** To reduce fluid overload in the presence of cardiac complications, such as congestive heart failure (CHF).

NURSING DIAGNOSES AND INTERVENTIONS

Ineffective airway clearance related to excessive mucus production and ineffective coughing

Desired outcome: Patient demonstrates effective cough and is free of adventitious breath sounds.

1. Auscultate breath sounds q2-4h and after coughing. Be alert to and report changes in adventitious breath sounds.
2. Teach patient the "double cough" technique:
   - □ Sit upright with upper body flexed forward slightly.
   - □ Take 2-3 breaths and exhale passively.
   - □ Inhale again, but only to the midinspiratory point.
   - □ Exhale by coughing quickly 2-3 times.
   This technique prevents small airway collapse, which can occur with forceful coughing.
3. Administer chest physiotherapy as prescribed to mobilize secretions.

Alteration in nutrition: Less than body requirements related to decreased intake secondary to fatigue and anorexia

Desired outcome: Patient has adequate nutrition as evidenced by stable weight, positive nitrogen state on nitrogen studies, and serum albumin 3.5-5.5 μg/dl.

1. Monitor patient's food intake. If indicated, obtain dietary consultation for calorie counts.
2. Provide diet in small, frequent meals that are nutritious and easy to consume.
3. Request a dietitian consultation so that the patient can verbalize food likes and dislikes.
4. Unless otherwise indicated, provide calories from more unsaturated fat sources than from carbohydrate sources. During the process of carbohydrate metabolism, the body uses oxygen and produces CO_2, which is then excreted by the lungs. The patient with COPD takes in less oxygen and retains CO_2. A high-fat diet minimizes this problem because fat generates the least amount of CO_2 for a given amount of oxygen used, while carbohydrates generate the most. See Table 1-6 for foods high in fat.
5. Discuss with the patient and significant others the importance of good nutrition in the treatment of chronic bronchitis.

Also see "Asthma" for **Impaired gas exchange** related to chronic tissue hypoxia, p. 25. See "Emphysema" for **Ineffective breathing pattern** related to dyspnea, p. 31, and **Activity intolerance** related to fatigue, p. 32. See "Heart Failure" for **Fluid volume excess:** Edema related to retention secondary to decreased cardiac output, p. 56.

TABLE 1-6 Recommended calorie sources for patients with COPD

Foods high in fat	Foods to avoid
whole milk	cakes
cream	cookies
evaporated milk	jams
cream soups	pastries
custards	sugar-concentrated snacks
cheese	
salad and cooking oils	
margarine	
mayonnaise	
nuts	
meat	
poultry	
fish	

PATIENT-FAMILY TEACHING AND DISCHARGE PLANNING

Provide patient and significant others with verbal and written instructions for the following:
1. Use of home oxygen, including instructions for when to use it, importance of not increasing prescribed flow rate, precautions, and community resources for oxygen replacement when necessary. Request respiratory therapy consultation to assist with teaching related to oxygen therapy, if indicated.
2. Medications, including name, route, purpose, dosage, schedule, precautions, and potential side effects.
3. Signs and symptoms of CHF that necessitate medical attention: increased dyspnea; fatigue; increased coughing; changes in the amount, color, or consistency of sputum; swelling of the ankles and legs; fever; and sudden weight gain. Patients with COPD often have right-sided heart failure secondary to cardiac effects of the disease. For more information, see "Heart Failure," p. 54.
4. Avoiding individuals who are known to be infectious, especially those with URIs.
5. Review of sodium-restricted diet (see Table 11-3, p. 550) and other dietary considerations, as indicated.
6. Importance of pacing activity level to conserve energy.
7. Importance of yearly flu and pneumococcal vaccines.
8. Follow-up appointment with MD; confirm date and time of next appointment.
9. Introduction to local chapter of American Lung Association activities and pulmonary rehabilitation programs.

Emphysema

Pulmonary emphysema is a degenerative process characterized by enlargement of the air spaces distal to the terminal bronchioles accompanied by destruction of the alveolar walls. Because of the destruction of the alveoli, air becomes trapped and distal airways become hyperinflated and may rupture or collapse. Emphysema is a progressive disease and affected individuals can become totally disabled because they use all available energy for breathing. In later stages of the disease pulmonary hypertension develops, leading to cor pulmonale, a condition that produces cardiac as well as respiratory problems.

ASSESSMENT

Chronic indicators: Nonproductive cough (unless patient also has bronchitis), dyspnea on exertion.

Acute indicators (exacerbation): Increased dyspnea, productive cough, fever, peripheral edema, fatigue.

Physical assessment: Emaciation, increased A-P chest diameter, pursed-lip breathing, hypertrophy of accessory muscles of respiration, decreased fremitus over affected lung fields, decreased thoracic excursion, hyperresonance over affected lung fields, decreased breath sounds, and prolonged expiratory phase. Digital clubbing occurs late in the disease.

DIAGNOSTIC TESTS

1. *Chest x-ray:* Will show hyperinflation of the lungs, an increased A-P diameter, lowered and flattened diaphragm, and a small cardiac silhouette.
2. *ABG values:* May reveal a slight decrease in Pao_2. As the disease progresses, the Pao_2 will continue to decrease and $Paco_2$ may increase because of hypoventilation and CO_2 retention. Early in the disease process, however, the $Paco_2$ may be normal if the patient has good ventilation-perfusion matching. The pH will be low-normal once CO_2 retention begins.
3. *CBC:* May reveal a chronically elevated RBC count (polycythemia) later in the disease process as a compensatory response to chronic hypoxemia.
4. *Pulmonary function tests:* Will show an increased total lung capacity, increased residual volume, and decreased forced expiratory reserve volume. The vital capacity will be normal or slightly decreased. For descriptions and normal values of these tests, see Table 1-4, p. 26.
5. *EKG:* May reveal atrial and ventricular dysrhythmias. Most patients will have an atrial dysrhythmia as a result of atrial dilatation and right ventricular hypertrophy caused by pulmonary hypertension.
6. *Sputum culture:* May be ordered to determine presence of pulmonary infection.

MEDICAL MANAGEMENT

See "Chronic Bronchitis," p. 29.

NURSING DIAGNOSES AND INTERVENTIONS

Ineffective breathing pattern related to dyspnea secondary to chronic airflow limitations

Desired outcome: Patient verbalizes a reduction in dyspnea.

1. Assess patient's respiratory status q2-4h, being alert to indicators of respiratory distress (i.e., agitation, restlessness, decreased LOC, and use of accessory muscles of respiration). Auscultate breath sounds; report a decrease in breath sounds or an increase in adventitious breath sounds.
2. Instruct patient in the use of pursed-lip breathing, which provides internal stability to the airways and may prevent airway collapse during expiration:
   □ Sit upright with hands on thighs or lean forward with elbows propped on the over-the-bed table.
   □ Inhale slowly through the nose with the mouth closed.
   □ Form lips in an "O" shape as though whistling.
   □ Exhale slowly through pursed lips. Exhalation should take twice as long as inhalation.
   Record patient's response to breathing technique.
3. Administer bronchodilator therapy as prescribed. Monitor patient for side effects, including tachycardia and dysrhythmias.

4. Monitor patient's response to prescribed oxygen therapy. Be aware that high concentrations of oxygen can depress the respiratory drive in individuals with chronic CO_2 retention.
5. Monitor serial ABG values. Patients with chronic CO_2 retention will have chronically compensated respiratory acidosis with a low-normal pH (7.35-7.38) and a $Paco_2$ >45 mm Hg.

Activity intolerance related to decreased energy levels secondary to inefficient work of breathing

Desired outcome: Patient reports decreasing dyspnea at his or her optimal level of activity.

1. Maintain prescribed activity levels and explain rationale to patient.
2. Monitor patient's respiratory response to activity. Activity intolerance would be indicated by excessively increased respiratory rate (e.g., >10 breaths/min above baseline) and depth, dyspnea, and use of accessory muscles of respiration. If activity intolerance is noted, instruct patient to stop the activity and rest.
3. Organize care so that periods of activity are interspersed with periods (at least 90 minutes) of undisturbed rest.
4. Assist patient with active ROM exercises to build stamina and prevent complications of decreased mobility.

See "Asthma" for **Impaired gas exchange**, p. 25. See "Chronic Bronchitis" for **Ineffective airway clearance** related to excessive mucus production and ineffective coughing, p. 29, and **Alteration in nutrition:** Less than body requirements, p. 29. Also see psychosocial nursing diagnoses and interventions in "Caring for Patients with Cancer and Other Life-Disrupting Illnesses," p. 690.

PATIENT-FAMILY TEACHING AND DISCHARGE PLANNING

See "Chronic Bronchitis," p. 30.

Section Four   RESTRICTIVE PULMONARY DISORDERS

Restrictive lung disease is a category of pulmonary pathologies that impair lung function by restricting alveolar inflation. Restrictive disorders are characterized by decreased vital capacity, reduced resting volumes, and normal airway resistance. Lung compliance (distensibility) decreases and elastic recoil (deflating force) increases, resulting in an increase in the work of breathing. Physiologic consequences are similar for all restrictive processes and can be mildly, moderately, or severely debilitating for the patient. See Table 1-7 for some of the pathologies identified as etiologies for restrictive lung disease. This section discusses pulmonary fibrosis.

Pulmonary fibrosis

The physiologic mechanisms in the development of pulmonary fibrosis are not clearly defined. It is theorized that pulmonary fibrosis occurs as a reaction to the inhalation of noxious materials or exposure to radiation. The fibrotic process is a continuous one and does not abate, even when the causative agent is no longer present. Fibrotic tissue forms as a natural process of tissue repair following infection, inflammation, or destruction of tissue. The fibrosis primarily affects the alveoli and causes an increase in the bronchial diameter in relation to lung volume. Work of breathing is increased because of decreased lung compliance, and affected individuals adopt a rapid, shallow breathing pattern since it requires less energy. Cardiac complications can occur as a result of pulmonary hypertension.

T A B L E 1 - 7   Etiologic factors in the development of pulmonary fibrosis

Extrapulmonary (involves respiratory muscles, pleura, and chest wall)	Intrapulmonary (involves lung parenchyma)
Bony deformities	Alveolar fibrosis (secondary to:)
scoliosis	infection
ankylosing spondylitis	chronic aspiration
Neuromuscular disorders	inhalation of toxins
Guillain-Barré syndrome	chemotherapy
amyotrophic lateral sclerosis	radiation therapy
(ALS)	alveolar cell cancer
myasthenia gravis	Goodpasture's syndrome
muscular dystrophy	idiopathic
Pleural effusion	Pneumoconioses
Pleural thickening	asbestosis
Pneumothorax	silicosis
Ascites	black lung
Obesity	Atelectasis
Pregnancy	Pulmonary edema
	Lung resection

ASSESSMENT

The etiology of pulmonary fibrosis is very difficult to uncover. Meticulous history of lifestyle, occupation, habits, and background can provide valuable information.

Signs and symptoms: Dyspnea, cough.

Physical assessment: Tachypnea, shallow respirations, cyanosis, digital clubbing, use of accessory muscles of respiration, and crackles.

Risk factors: See Table 1-7.

DIAGNOSTIC TESTS

1. *Chest x-ray:* Reveals the extent of the fibrosis as evidenced by diffuse, mottled shadowing of the lung fields (honeycombing).
2. *Pulmonary function tests:* Will demonstrate concentric reduction in lung volumes; normal airway resistance.
3. *ABG analysis:* Pao_2 may be normal at rest but may decrease with exercise. $Paco_2$ may be within normal limits secondary to tachypnea but may increase in late stages of the disease.
4. *Lung biopsy:* To determine etiology and pathologic mechanism of the process.

MEDICAL MANAGEMENT

1. Oxygen therapy: To correct the hypoxemia, which will relieve the dyspnea. Generally, low-flow (2-4 L/min) oxygen therapy is indicated.
2. Corticosteroids: To decrease inflammation. Prednisone usually is given at 1 mg/kg daily.

NURSING DIAGNOSES AND INTERVENTIONS

Ineffective breathing pattern related to dyspnea secondary to decreased lung expansion

Desired outcomes: Patient's breathing pattern improves, as evidenced by Pao_2 >60 mm Hg. Patient verbalizes a subjective relief of dyspnea.

1. Assess respiratory status q2-4h. Auscultate breath sounds and report increasing crackles or other adventitious sounds.
2. Monitor serial ABGs for decreasing Pao_2 and be alert to early signs of hypoxemia in the patient (restlessness, anxiety, dyspnea), especially with activity.
3. Assist patient in identifying ways to conserve energy during daily activities (e.g., planning frequent rest periods before and after activities as needed, stopping the activity and resting if dyspnea increases, and waiting for 1 hour after eating before engaging in activities because digestion draws blood and hence oxygen away from the muscles). As indicated, arrange for a consultation with OT or PT for evaluation.
4. Deliver oxygen as prescribed. Remember that the Pao_2 may be normal at rest but may decrease with exercise. The patient may require supplemental oxygen with activity.

See "Chronic Bronchitis" for **Alteration in nutrition:** Less than body requirements related to decreased intake secondary to fatigue and anorexia, p. 29. See "Glomerulonephritis" for **Knowledge deficit:** Negative side effects of corticosteroids, p. 104. Also see psychosocial nursing diagnoses in "Caring for Patients with Cancer and Other Life-Disrupting Illnesses," p. 690.

PATIENT-FAMILY TEACHING AND DISCHARGE PLANNING

Provide patient and significant others with verbal and written instructions for the following:

1. Importance of pacing activities to tolerance and avoiding strenuous exercises that would increase cardiac and respiratory symptoms.
2. Medications, including drug name, dosage, purpose, schedule, precautions, and potential side effects. It is likely that the patient will take corticosteroids while at home. Provide instructions accordingly to ensure that the patient takes the correct amount, particularly during the period in which the medication will be tapered.
3. Use of oxygen and the necessary precautions if it is to be used at home.
4. Avoiding exposure to individuals known to have pulmonary infections. Recommend annual flu and pneumococcal vaccines.
5. Date and time of follow-up visit.

Section Five   BRONCHOGENIC CARCINOMA

In 1986 lung cancer became the number one cause of cancer deaths in American women. For nearly 40 years it has been the leading cancer killer in men. Of individuals diagnosed with lung cancer, 87% die in less than 5 years. The length of survival depends on the tumor histology and stage of the disease at the time treatment begins. Statistically, 80%-90% of lung cancer occurs among people who smoke tobacco. Environmental and occupational exposure to chemicals, toxins, and pollutants also may contribute to the development of this disease.

Lung cancer can be categorized as small cell or non-small cell cancer. *Small cell lung cancer* (SCLC) is composed of classic or "oat" cell, intermediate cell, and mixed cell. SCLC comprises 25%-30% of all lung cancers and has the following characteristics: 1) it arises from basal lining of bronchial mucusa; 2) it has rapid cell growth (highly proliferative); 3) it has propensity for widespread dissemination; and 4) it is highly sensitive to cytotoxic drugs and radiation therapy. Approximately 60% of patients with SCLC present with extensive disease and 40% with limited disease. The period of time between onset of symptoms and diagnosis is approximately 3-4 months, with a change in the character of a chronic cough being the typical presenting symptom. Tumors generally form in larger, central bronchi, causing obstruction, wheezing, coughing, and dyspnea. Hemoptysis occurs as cancers erode blood vessels and capillaries in the airways. The tumors can compress nerves, causing radiating chest pain.

Non-small cell lung cancer (NSCLC) is composed of epidermoid (squamous cell), adenocarcinoma, and large cell cancer. NSCLC comprises approximately 70%-75% of all lung cancers and possesses the following characteristics: 1) it arises from large bronchi (squamous) or periphery of lung (adenocarcinoma); 2) it is slower growing (less proliferative); 3) squamous cell generally is less disseminated; 4) adenocarcinoma and large cell often have distant metastases; 5) response to therapy is limited, except for surgical excision (only form of treatment currently considered curative); and 6) it is generally not curable once metastasized outside the thoracic cavity.

Most patients have advanced disease at the time of diagnosis and receive multimodality therapy with minimal or partial response. Ultimately patients succumb to both local and distant disease with multiple complications. Tumors generally grow in the small peripheral bronchi and alveoli and may press against nerves in the pleural tissues. Typical presenting symptoms include shortness of breath and sharp chest pain on inspiration.

ASSESSMENT

Patients often are asymptomatic in early stages of the disease process. When symptoms do occur they are likely to be vague and easily confused with other pulmonary conditions.

Early indicators: Cough, dyspnea, change in character of sputum, hemoptysis, fatigue, dull chest pain, frequent respiratory infections.

Advanced disease: Weakness, anorexia, dysphagia, hoarseness, weight loss.

Physical assessment: Presence of adventitious breath sounds and pleural friction rub. In advanced disease, the patient may exhibit use of accessory muscles of respiration, nasal flaring, cyanosis, and severe muscle wasting.

DIAGNOSTIC TESTS

1. *Sputum for cytology:* Generally, a first morning specimen is obtained for three consecutive days. Sputum contains cells that shed from the tumor, which aids in identifying tumor type.
2. *Chest x-ray:* To define tumor outline. X-ray may reveal presence of solitary nodules and possibly pleural effusion, atelectasis, and lymph node enlargement.
3. *Bronchoscopy:* To visualize central tumor directly and take tissue samples for biopsy, along with bronchial washings.
4. *Fine-needle aspiration:* Needle biopsy to obtain tissue samples from peripheral tumor for histologic exam.
5. *Lung tomogram:* To locate tumor and determine depth and extent.
6. *Other tests:* Once the cancer has metastasized from the primary site to nearby lymph nodes or distant organs, tests may include fluoroscopy, rib x-ray, abdominal and chest CT scan, bone studies, radionuclide studies, and bone marrow aspiration.

MEDICAL MANAGEMENT

The most effective intervention is prevention. Treatment is planned according to histology, location, and extent of the disease.
1. Surgery: To excise a tumor confined to lung tissue and remove involved lymph nodes.
2. Radiation therapy: Use can be curative, adjuvant to chemotherapy/surgery, or palliative. It is used if the tumor has grown to adjacent tissues or if cancer has produced clearly defined secondary tumors elsewhere in the body. Usual dose is 2,500-6,000

rads delivered over a 5-6 week period. This therapy generally shrinks tumors more often than eradicating them. Side effects include anorexia, esophagitis, dysphasia, radiation pneumonitis, and skin changes.

3. **Chemotherapy:** Used when the primary tumor extends beyond the lungs into surrounding tissues or metastasizes outside the lungs. It is also given to patients with SCLC whose disease has not yet spread beyond the lung. Agents generally are used in combination for treatment. Drugs commonly used include cyclophosphamide, doxorubicin, methotrexate, procarbazine, mitomycin C, vinblastine, cisplatin, and bleomycin.
4. **Antiemetics:** To control nausea and vomiting associated with chemotherapy. Generally, phenothiazines, metoclopramide, and steroids are used.
5. **Analgesics:** To control pain.
6. **Sedatives:** Benzodiazepines are given for their amnesic effects, helping patients forget unpleasantness of the chemotherapy and thus promoting therapy continuation.

NURSING DIAGNOSES AND INTERVENTIONS

Pain related to compression of nerves by the tumor

Desired outcome: Patient's subjective evaluation of pain improves, as documented by a pain scale.

1. Assess and document the following: location, description, onset, duration, and factors that precipitate and alleviate patient's pain. Devise a pain scale with the patient, rating pain from 0 (no pain) to 10.
2. Encourage patient to ask for pain medication before pain becomes severe. If patient has more than one analgesic, confer with patient regarding which would be more beneficial for pain control. Document the amount of pain relief obtained using the pain scale.
3. Position patient for comfort.
4. Encourage patient to use relaxation techniques (e.g., deep breathing, imagery, and biofeedback) and diversional activities (e.g., television, books, radio, and crafts). For a description of an effective relaxation technique, see p. 49, **Health-seeking behaviors:** Relaxation technique effective for stress reduction.
5. For other effective pain interventions, see the appendix, p. 638, **Pain.**

See "Pulmonary Fibrosis" for **Ineffective breathing pattern** related to dyspnea secondary to decreased lung expansion, p. 34. Also see "Caring for Preoperative and Postoperative Patients," p. 637, and "Caring for Patients with Cancer and Other Life-Disrupting Illnesses," p. 659.

PATIENT-FAMILY TEACHING AND DISCHARGE PLANNING

Provide patient and significant others with verbal and written instructions for the following:

1. Signs and symptoms of respiratory complications that may necessitate medical attention: increased dyspnea, cyanosis, agitation.
2. If surgery was performed, the indicators of wound infection: redness at wound site, local warmth, purulent drainage, pain, fever.
3. Medications, including name, purpose, dosage, schedule, precautions, and potential side effects.
4. Use of all equipment that will be used at home.
5. Need for follow-up care with MD; confirm date and time of next appointment.
6. Local American Cancer Society and American Lung Society programs. Provide available literature.

SELECTED REFERENCES

Armstrong D: Lung cancer: the diagnostic work-up, Am J Nurs 86(11):1429-1430, 1986.

Cerrato PL: The special nutritional needs of a COPD patient, RN 50:75-76, 1987.

Comis RL and Martin G: Small cell carcinoma of the lung: an overview, Semin Oncol Nurs 3(3):174-182, 1987.

Conner P et al: Two stages of care for pleural effusion, RN 52:30-34, 1989.

Easterday U and Howard C: Respiratory dysfunctions. In Swearingen PL et al: Manual of critical care: applying nursing diagnoses to adult critical illness, St Louis, 1988, The CV Mosby Co.

Eubanks DH and Bone RC: Comprehensive respiratory care, St Louis, 1985, The CV Mosby Co.

Fishman AP: Pulmonary diseases and disorders, ed 2, New York, 1988, McGraw-Hill Book Company.

Foote M et al: Dyspnea: a distressing sensation in lung cancer, Oncol Nurs For 13(5):25-30, 1986.

Gerdes L: Recognizing the multisystem effects of embolism, Nursing 87(12):34-41, 1987.

Hahn K: Slow teaching the COPD patient, Nursing 87(4):34-42, 1987.

Harwood K: Non-small cell lung cancer: issues in diagnosis, staging, and treatment, Semin Oncol Nurs 3(3):183-193, 1987.

Hopp L and Williams M: Ineffective breathing pattern related to decreased lung expansion, Nurs Clin North Am 22(1):193-205, 1987.

Horne M, Heitz U, and Swearingen PL: Practical guide to fluids and electrolytes: a case study approach, St Louis, 1990, The CV Mosby Co.

Lareau S and Larson J: Ineffective breathing pattern related to airflow limitation, Nurs Clin North Am 22(1):1428-1429, 1987.

McNaull F: Lung cancer: what are the odds? Am J Nurs 87(11):1428-1429, 1987.

McNaull F: Radiation therapy for lung cancer: nursing considerations, Semin Oncol Nurs 3(3):194-201, 1987.

Moseley JR: Nursing management of toxicities associated with chemotherapy for lung cancer, Semin Oncol Nurs 3(3):202-210, 1987.

Oncology: Programmed modules for nurses, vol 3, types of cancer, part A, New York, 1988, LP Communications, Inc.

Roberts S: Pulmonary tissue perfusion altered: emboli, Heart Lung 16(2):128-137, 1987.

2

CHAPTER

Cardiovascular disorders

Arterial embolism
Venous thrombosis/thrombophlebitis
Varicose veins
SELECTED REFERENCES

Section One DEGENERATIVE CARDIOVASCULAR DISORDERS

Pulmonary hypertension

As blood passes through the pulmonary vasculature, it exchanges carbon dioxide and particulate matter for oxygen. Normally the pulmonary vascular bed offers little resistance to blood flow, but when resistance occurs, pulmonary hypertension results. Pulmonary hypertension can be primary (rare), causing severe fibrosis of the pulmonary vasculature, or secondary (most common), owing to some other condition. Possible causes include increased pulmonary blood flow from a ventricular or atrial shunt, left ventricular failure, chronic hypoxia related to COPD, pulmonary embolus, pulmonary stenosis, or any physiologic occurrence that increases pulmonary vascular resistance or constriction of the vessels in the pulmonary tree.

ASSESSMENT

Acute indicators: Exertional dyspnea, syncope, and precordial chest pain, all of which result from low cardiac output or hypoxia. Cough and palpitations also can occur.

Chronic indicators: Signs of right or left ventricular failure.

☐ *Right ventricular failure:* Peripheral edema, increased venous pressure and pulsations, liver engorgement, distended neck veins.
☐ *Left ventricular failure:* Dyspnea; SOB, particularly on exertion; decreased BP; oliguria; orthopnea; anorexia.

Physical assessment: Cyanosis from decreased cardiac output and subsequent systemic vasoconstriction, systolic murmur caused by tricuspid regurgitation or pulmonary stenosis, diastolic murmur due to pulmonary valvular incompetence, and accentuated S_2 heart sound.

DIAGNOSTIC TESTS

1. *Chest x-ray:* Will show enlargement of the pulmonary artery and right atrium and ventricle.
2. *Echocardiography:* Often valuable for showing increased right ventricular dimension, thickened right ventricular wall, and possible tricuspid or pulmonary valve dysfunction.
3. *Radionuclide imaging:* For example, equilibrium-gated blood pool imaging and thallium imaging to assess function of the right ventricle.
4. *Cardiac catheterization with angiography:* Necessary to confirm pulmonary hypertension. Pulmonary vascular resistance will be very high, and pulmonary artery and right ventricular pressures can approach or equal systemic arterial pressures. (See "Cardiac Catheterization," p. 81, for further detail.)
5. *Pulmonary perfusion scintigraphy* (perfusion scan): A noninvasive way to assess pulmonary blood flow. This study involves IV injection of serum albumin tagged with trace amounts of a radioisotope, most often technetium. The particles pass through the circulation and lodge in the pulmonary vascular bed. Subsequent scanning reveals concentrations of particles in areas of adequate pulmonary blood flow.
6. *EKG:* Will show evidence of right atrial enlargement and right ventricular enlarge-

ment (evidenced by right axis deviation and tall, peaked P waves) secondary to the increased pressure needed to force blood through the hypertensive pulmonary vascular bed.

7. *Pulmonary function test:* Results usually are normal, although some individuals will have increased residual volume, reduced maximum voluntary ventilation, and decreased vital capacity.

8. *ABG analysis:* May show low $Paco_2$ and high pH, which occur with hyperventilation, or increased $Paco_2$ with decreased gas exchange.

9. *CBC:* Usually normal, although polycythemia can occur in the presence of hypoxemia due to compensation.

10. *Liver function tests:* May be abnormal if venous congestion is significant. Examples include increased SGOT, SGPT, and bilirubin.

11. *Open lung biopsy:* May be done to establish the type of disorder causing the hypertension.

MEDICAL MANAGEMENT AND SURGICAL INTERVENTIONS

1. **Oxygen:** Usually 2-5 L/min by nasal cannula. If hypoxia is severe, oxygen is administered by mask. **Caution:** Use care when administering oxygen to patients with a history of COPD.

2. **Diet:** Low in sodium (see Table 11-3, p 550) if signs of heart failure are present.

3. **Pharmacotherapy**
   - *Diuretics:* If indicators of right- or left-sided heart failure are present.
   - *Anticoagulants (warfarin sodium):* Although prophylactic use is controversial, it may be administered if pulmonary emboli are present.
   - *Vasodilators and calcium antagonists:* To decrease cardiac workload by vasodilatation.
   - *Bronchodilators (aminophylline):* Have been shown to reduce pulmonary artery and right ventricular pressures in some cases.
   - *Beta adrenergic agents such as terbutaline:* To decrease pulmonary vascular resistence.

4. **Treatment of causative factor if possible:** For example, by surgically closing arteriovenous shunts or replacing defective valves.

5. **Heart-lung transplantation:** For advanced pulmonary vascular disease.

NURSING DIAGNOSES AND INTERVENTIONS

Impaired gas exchange related to reduced oxygen transport secondary to pulmonary capillary constriction and restricted blood flow

Desired outcome: Patient has improved gas exchange as evidenced by RR 12-20 breaths/min with normal depth and pattern (eupnea), lung fields clear to auscultation, and Pao_2 ≥80 mm Hg.

1. Every 4 hours, assess respiratory rate, pattern, and depth; chest excursion; and use of accessory muscles of respiration.

2. Auscultate lung fields q4-8h to assess lung sounds. Note the presence of adventitious sounds, which can occur with fluid extravasation.

3. Monitor ABG results for evidence of hyperventilation: low $Paco_2$ and high pH; and for hypoventilation: decreased Pao_2, increased $Paco_2$, and decreased pH.

4. Observe for and document presence of cyanosis or skin color change, which can occur with decreased gas exchange.

5. Teach patient to take slow, deep breaths to enhance gas exchange.

6. Assist patient into Fowler's position, if possible, to decrease work of breathing and maximize chest excursion.

7. Administer prescribed low-flow oxygen as indicated.

Activity intolerance related to fatigue and weakness secondary to right and left ventricular failure

Desired outcome: Patient exhibits cardiac tolerance to increasing activity levels as evidenced by RR <24 breaths/min, HR <120 bpm, and BP within 20 mm Hg of normal range.

1. Observe for and document any changes in VS. Monitor systemic BP at least q4h. Report drops >10-20 mm Hg, which can signal decompensation of the cardiac muscle. Also be alert to other signs of left ventricular failure, including dyspnea, SOB, and crackles (rales).
2. Measure and document I&O, as well as weight, reporting any steady gains or losses. Be alert to other signs of right ventricular failure including peripheral edema, both pedal and sacral; ascites; distended neck veins; and increased CVP (>12 cm H_2O).
3. Administer diuretics, vasodilators, and calcium channel blockers as prescribed.
4. Provide periods of undisturbed rest; limit visitors as appropriate.
5. Keep frequently used items within patient's reach so that exertion can be avoided as much as possible.
6. Assist patient with maintenance of prescribed activity level and progress as tolerated. If activity intolerance is observed, stop activity and have patient rest.
7. Assist patient with ROM exercises at frequent intervals. To help prevent complications caused by immobility, plan progressive ambulation and exercise based on patient's tolerance and prescribed activity restrictions. For examples, see the appendix for the following: **Potential activity intolerance** related to deconditioning secondary to prolonged bed rest, p. 651, and **Potential for disuse syndrome,** p. 653.

Knowledge deficit: Disease process and treatment

Desired outcome: Patient and significant others verbalize knowledge of the disease, its treatment, and measures that promote wellness.

1. Assess the patient's level of knowledge of the disease process and its treatment.
2. Discuss the purposes of the medications: to ease the workload of the heart (vasodilators); "relax" the heart (calcium antagonists); and prevent fluid accumulation (diuretics).
3. Support the patient in dealing with the concept of having a chronic disease.
4. If the etiology of pulmonary hypertension is known, reinforce explanations of the disease process, treatment, and the need for changing lifestyle, if appropriate.
5. Explain the value of relaxation techniques, including tapes, soothing music, meditation, and biofeedback. See **Health-seeking behaviors:** Relaxation technique effective for stress reduction, p. 49.
6. If the patient smokes, explain that smoking increases the workload of the heart by causing vasoconstriction. Provide materials that explain the benefits of quitting smoking, such as the pamphlets prepared by the American Heart Association.
7. Confer with MD regarding the type of exercise program that will benefit the patient; provide patient teaching as indicated.
8. If appropriate, involve the dietitian to assist patient with planning meals that are low in sodium (see Table 11-3, p. 550).

See "Heart Failure" for the following: **Fluid volume excess:** Edema, p. 56, **Knowledge deficit:** Precautions and negative side effects of diuretic therapy, p. 56, and **Knowledge deficit:** Precautions and negative side effects of vasodilators, p. 57. Also see "Caring for Patients with Cancer and Other Life-Disrupting Illnesses," p. 690.

PATIENT-FAMILY TEACHING AND DISCHARGE PLANNING

Provide patient and significant others with verbal and written information for the following:
1. Indicators that necessitate medical attention: decreased exercise tolerance, increasing SOB or dyspnea, swelling of ankles and legs, steady weight gain.
2. Medications, including drug name, purpose, dosage, schedule, precautions, and potential side effects.

3. For additional information see **Knowledge deficit:** Disease process and treatment, p. 42.

Cardiomyopathy

Cardiomyopathy is a disorder of the heart muscle, usually of unknown origin. It is classified according to abnormalities in structure and function. The disorder involves the heart muscle and usually results in heart failure (see p. 54).

Dilated (or congestive) cardiomyopathy: Characterized by dilatation of all four of the heart chambers, especially the ventricles. Contractile dysfunction usually is the first sign, followed by congestive heart failure. There is progressive deterioration of cardiac muscle function caused by toxic (e.g., alcohol), metabolic (e.g., thyrotoxicosis), or infectious (bacterial, viral) agents. Pathophysiologic changes include loss of functioning myofibrils, decreased contractile strength, and dilatation followed by sympathetic nervous system (SNS) stimulation, increased myocardial oxygen consumption, increased pulmonary pressures, increased venous pressures, and failure.

Hypertrophic cardiomyopathy: Characterized by an abnormally hypertrophied left ventricle that is not accompanied by a concomitant increase in cavity size. Therefore filling is restricted, and there is the potential for outflow obstruction. This causes increased left atrial and left ventricular pressures, resulting in increased workload and increased pulmonary pressures causing dyspnea. Cardiac function can remain normal for varying periods of time before decompensation occurs. Symptoms include increased diastolic BP, decreased cardiac output, pulmonary hypertension, and right ventricular failure. Although it is theorized that hypertrophic cardiomyopathy has a strong hereditary link, the etiology is unknown. Possible causes include increased circulating catecholamine levels, subendocardial ischemia, or abnormal conduction patterns that lead to abnormal ventricular contraction.

Restrictive cardiomyopathy: Least common in Western countries, it is characterized by restrictive ventricular filling caused by fibrosis, infiltration, hypertrophy, and cardiac stiffness.

ASSESSMENT

Signs and symptoms: Dyspnea usually is the symptom that brings the patient to the physician. Decreased exercise tolerance, fatigue, weakness, syncope, peripheral edema, palpitations, right or left ventricular failure, and peripheral or pulmonary emboli also can occur. Chest pain may occur owing to ischemia of the hypertrophied muscle.

Physical assessment: Presence of S_3 or S_4 heart sounds and valve murmurs, systolic murmur, prominent apical pulse, increased venous pressure and pulsations, crackles (rales), decreased BP, and increased HR and RR related to decreased cardiac output. In addition, hepatomegaly and mild to severe cardiomegaly may be present.

DIAGNOSTIC TESTS

1. *Chest x-ray:* To detect cardiac enlargement, particularly of the ventricle and left atrium. Pulmonary hypertension also may be seen.
2. *EKG results:* Determined by the extent and location of myocardial involvement. EKG changes indicative of cardiomyopathy include left ventricular hypertrophy, conduction defects, nonspecific ST segment changes, and Q waves that resemble those found with infarction.
3. *Echocardiography:* Will identify thickened ventricular walls, septal thickening, and chamber dilatation or restriction, depending on the type of cardiomyopathy. Poor contractility also may be seen if myocardial muscle deterioration has progressed.
4. *Cardiac catheterization:* Does not confirm cardiomyopathy, but it can be valuable for ruling out other disorders such as ischemic heart disease. Findings may include decreased cardiac output, decreased ventricular movement, increased filling pres-

sures, and valvular regurgitation. For detail, see "Cardiac Catheterization," p. 81.

5. *Endomyocardial biopsy:* Sometimes necessary to identify the type of pathologic agent; it can be done during the cardiac catheterization procedure.

6. *Radionuclide studies:* May demonstrate contractile dysfunction.

MEDICAL MANAGEMENT AND SURGICAL INTERVENTIONS

Medical management is aimed toward support, maintenance of normal function for as long as possible, and delaying disease progression.

1. Controlling symptoms of heart failure: See "Heart Failure," p. 54.
2. Limiting or restricting activity: To decrease oxygen demand. Activity is increased gradually.
3. Prohibiting alcohol intake: Alcohol can worsen myopathy.
4. Pharmacotherapy
   □ *Antiarrhythmic agents:* To control dysrhythmias.
   □ *Beta blockers:* To decrease outflow obstruction during exercise.
   □ *Calcium antagonists:* To produce arterial vasodilatation, decrease cardiac workload, and improve symptoms and exercise capacity.
   □ *Anticoagulants (warfarin sodium):* To prevent embolus formation.
   □ *Diuretics:* To decrease pulmonary congestion.
   □ *Vasodilators:* To decrease cardiac workload.
   □ *Inotropic agents:* To increase contractile strength.
5. Surgical replacement of valves: See "Cardiac Surgery," p. 84.
6. Cardiac transplant.

NURSING DIAGNOSES AND INTERVENTIONS

Activity intolerance related to weakness and fatigue secondary to decrease in cardiac muscle contractility

Desired outcome: Patient exhibits cardiac tolerance to increasing activity levels as evidenced by RR <24 breaths/min, BP within 20 mm Hg of normal range, HR within 20 bpm of resting HR, and absence of chest pain.

1. Monitor BP and VS q4h, and report changes such as irregular HR, HR >110 bpm, or decreasing BP.
2. Observe for and report signs of acute decreased cardiac output, including oliguria, decreasing BP, decreased mentation, and dizziness.
3. Assess integrity of peripheral perfusion by monitoring peripheral pulses and urine output. Report changes such as decreased amplitude of pulses and decreased urinary output.
4. In the presence of acute decreased cardiac output, ensure that the patient's needs are met so that activity can be avoided, for example, by keeping water at the bedside and urinal or commode nearby, maintaining a quiet environment, and limiting visitors as appropriate.
5. Plan nursing care to allow for 90-minute periods of undisturbed rest.
6. Administer medications as prescribed.
7. To help prevent complications caused by immobility, assist patient with passive and some active or assistive ROM and other exercises, depending on patient's tolerance and prescribed limitations. For discussion of a progressive in-bed exercise program, see the appendix for the following: **Potential activity intolerance,** p. 651, and **Potential for disuse syndrome,** p. 653.
8. Monitor patient's physiologic response to activity. Report chest pain, increased SOB, increased HR >20 bpm over resting HR, and RR >24 breaths/min.

Decreased cardiac output related to impaired contractility secondary to cardiac muscle changes

Desired outcome: Patient has adequate cardiac output as evidenced by systolic BP >90 mm Hg, HR <100 bpm, urinary output ≥30 ml/hr, RR ≤20 breaths/min, normal breath sounds, edema ≤1+ on a 0-4+ scale, and orientation to person, place, and time.

1. Assess for and document evidence of decreased cardiac output, such as edema, jugular venous distention, adventitious breath sounds, SOB, decreased urinary output, changes in LOC, cool extremities, hypotension, tachycardia, and tachypnea.
2. Keep accurate I&O records.
3. Help minimize patient's cardiac workload by assisting with ADLs and ensuring 90-minute periods of undisturbed rest.
4. Administer medications as prescribed, such as beta blockers, calcium channel blockers, and antiarrhythmics.
5. Assist patient into position of comfort, usually semi-Fowler's.

Potential alteration in tissue perfusion: Cardiopulmonary and peripheral, related to impaired circulation secondary to embolus formation

Desired outcome: Patient's tissue perfusion is adequate as evidenced by peripheral pulses >2+ on a 0-4+ scale, warm extremities, and absence of chest pain.

1. Observe for and report indicators of pulmonary emboli (e.g., sudden onset of chest pain, dyspnea, SOB, and hemoptysis). For more information, see "Pulmonary Embolus," p. 12.
2. Observe for and report indicators of peripheral emboli (e.g., decreased peripheral pulses and calf pain or tenderness).
3. In the *absence* of decreased peripheral pulses and calf pain or tenderness, assess for a positive Homan's sign by flexing the knee 30 degrees and dorsiflexing the foot. Pain elicited in the calf signifies a positive Homan's sign, which occurs in the presence of deep vein thrombosis. Report significant findings to MD.
Note: For patients who are asymptomatic of embolization, see interventions for prevention of this disorder in the appendix: **Alteration in tissue perfusion:** Peripheral, related to compromised circulation secondary to prolonged immobility, p. 655.

See "Pulmonary Embolus" in Chapter 1 (Respiratory Disorders) for **Potential for injury** related to increased risk of bleeding secondary to anticoagulant therapy, p. 16. See "Pulmonary Hypertension" for **Activity intolerance,** p. 41. See "Coronary Artery Disease" for **Knowledge deficit:** Precautions and negative side effects of beta blockers, p. 50. See "Heart Failure" for **Knowledge deficit:** Precautions and negative side effects of diuretic therapy, p. 56, **Fluid volume excess:** Edema, p. 56, and **Knowledge deficit:** Precautions and negative side effects of vasodilators, p. 57. See psychosocial nursing diagnoses and interventions for the care of patients on prolonged bed rest, p. 651, and for the care of patients with cancer and other life-disrupting illnesses, p. 690-700.

PATIENT-FAMILY TEACHING AND DISCHARGE PLANNING

Provide patient and significant others with verbal and written information for the following:
1. Medications, including drug name, purpose, dosage, schedule, precautions, and potential side effects.
2. Signs and symptoms that necessitate immediate medical attention: dyspnea, decreased exercise tolerance, alterations in pulse rate/rhythm, loss of consciousness (caused by dysrhythmia or decreased cardiac output), and steady weight gain (caused by heart failure).
3. Reinforcement that cardiomyopathy is a chronic disease requiring lifetime treatment.
4. Importance of abstaining from alcohol, which increases cardiac muscle deterioration.
5. Need for physical support from family and outside agencies as disease progresses.
6. Availability of community and medical support such as American Heart Association.

Coronary artery disease

The coronary arteries are the vessels that supply the myocardial muscle with oxygen and nutrients necessary for optimal function. Atherosclerotic lesions within these arteries are a major cause of obstruction and subsequent ischemia, which ultimately can lead to

TABLE 2-1 Classification of angina

Stable: Pattern of frequency, duration, and severity stable over several months.
Unstable: Pattern of frequency, duration, or severity changed or increased; associated with decreased exercise or exertion.
Preinfarction (also called crescendo): Unstable, with progression to myocardial infarction (MI) possible (term sometimes used interchangeably with "unstable").
Prinzmetal's (also called variant): Often occurs at rest, unrelated to exercise, or during sleep; usually caused by coronary artery spasm.
Intractable: Continuous or frequent; unrelieved by therapy.

myocardial infarction. Other mechanisms include spasm, platelet aggregation, and thrombus formation. The most common symptom of coronary artery disease (CAD) is angina (see Table 2-1, below), a result of decreasing blood flow and decreased oxygen supply through narrowed or obstructed arteries (ischemia). This often occurs during exercise, but it may occur at rest or during a condition of decreased perfusion, such as an episode of hypotension. Often, CAD is diagnosed only after the patient presents with angina or myocardial infarction.

ASSESSMENT

Chronic indicators: Stable or progressively worsening angina that occurs when myocardial demand for oxygen is more than the supply, such as during exercise. The pain usually is described as pressure or a crushing or burning substernal pain that radiates down one or both arms. It also can be felt in the neck, cheeks, and teeth. Usually, it is relieved with discontinuation of exercise or administration of nitroglycerine.

Acute indicators: CAD is considered unstable (acute) when angina becomes more frequent and is unrelieved by nitroglycerine and rest, when it occurs during sleep or rest, or when it occurs with progressively lower levels of exercise.

Risk factors: Family history, increasing age, male gender, smoking, diet high in sodium and cholesterol, hypertension, obesity, abnormal glucose tolerance, "type A" behavior, sedentary and stressful lifestyle.

DIAGNOSTIC TESTS

1. *EKG:* Usually normal unless MI has occurred or the individual is experiencing angina at the time of the test. If performed during angina, characteristic changes include ST segment depression in leads over the area of ischemia.
2. *Chest x-ray:* Usually normal unless heart failure is present.
3. *Treadmill exercise test:* To determine the amount of exercise that causes angina, as well as the degree of ischemia and EKG changes produced. Significant findings can include 1 mm or more ST segment depression or elevation and ventricular ectopic beats.
4. *Radionuclide studies*
   □ Infarct imaging: Use of an imaging agent, usually technetium pyrophosphate, that concentrates in the infarcted zone.
   □ Myocardial perfusion imaging: Use of an imaging agent, usually thallium, that concentrates in "normal" tissue.
   □ Radionuclide ventriculography: Enables visualization of the ventricular muscle during the cardiac cycle.
5. *Ambulatory monitoring:* A 24-hour EKG monitoring that can show activity-induced ST segment changes or ischemia-induced dysrhythmias.
6. *Coronary arteriography via cardiac catheterization:* Provides the ultimate diagnosis of CAD. Arterial lesions (plaque) are located and the amount of occlusion is determined. At this time, feasibility for coronary artery bypass grafting (CABG) or angio-

plasty is determined. For details, see "Cardiac Surgery," p. 84 and "Medical Management," below.

7. *Serum enzymes:* To rule out myocardial infarction (see p. 51).

MEDICAL MANAGEMENT AND SURGICAL INTERVENTIONS

1. **Management of risk factors:** Eliminating tobacco, reducing BP, reducing serum lipid levels, controlling weight and stress, and initiating an exercise program.
2. **Oxygen by nasal cannula:** During angina attacks.
3. **Pharmacotherapy**
   □ *Sublingual nitroglycerine:* During angina to increase microcirculation, perfusion to the myocardium, and venodilatation.
   □ *Beta blockers:* To decrease oxygen demand of the myocardium.
   □ *Calcium antagonists such as enalapril:* To reduce oxygen demands.
   □ *Long-acting nitrates or topical nitroglycerine:* For anginal prophylaxis.
   □ *Calcium channel blockers such as nifedipine, diltiazem:* To decrease coronary artery vasospasm and decrease oxygen demand.
4. **Diet:** Low in cholesterol (see Table 2-2), sodium (see Table 11-3, p. 550), calories, and triglycerides, as appropriate.
5. **Percutaneous transluminal coronary angioplasty:** A procedure that improves coronary blood flow by using a balloon inflation catheter to compress plaque material into the vessel wall. Performed in the cardiac catheterization laboratory with a local anesthetic and mild sedation, it is becoming a common alternative to bypass surgery for individuals with discrete lesions.

NURSING DIAGNOSES AND INTERVENTIONS

Pain related to angina secondary to decreased oxygen supply to the myocardium

Desired outcome: Patient's subjective evaluation of angina improves, as documented by a pain scale.

1. Assess the location, character, and severity of the pain. Record the severity on a subjective 0 (no pain) to 10 scale. Also record the number of nitroglycerine tablets needed to relieve each episode, the factor or event that precipitated the pain, and alleviating factors. Document angina relief obtained, using the pain scale.
2. Keep sublingual nitroglycerine within reach of patient, and explain that it is to be administered as soon as angina begins, repeating q5min × 3 if necessary.
3. Stay with patient and provide reassurance during periods of angina. If indicated, request that visitors leave the room.
4. Monitor HR and BP during episodes of chest pain. Be alert to and report irregularities in HR and changes in systolic BP >20 mm Hg from baseline.
5. Monitor for presence of headache and hypotension after administration of nitroglycerine. Keep patient recumbent during angina, as well as during nitroglycerine administration.
6. Administer oxygen as prescribed to increase the oxygen supply to the myocardium.
7. Emphasize to patient the importance of immediately reporting to staff any manifestations of angina.
8. Avoid activities and factors that are known to cause stress for the patient and may precipitate angina.
9. Discuss the value of relaxation techniques, including tapes, soothing music, biofeedback, meditation, or yoga. See **Health-seeking behaviors:** Relaxation technique effective for stress reduction, p. 49.

Activity intolerance related to weakness and fatigue secondary to tissue ischemia (myocardial infarction)

Desired outcome: Patient exhibits cardiac tolerance to increasing levels of activity as evidenced by RR <24 breaths/min, HR ≤120 bpm (or within 20 bpm of resting HR), systolic BP within 20 mm Hg of patient's resting systolic BP, and absence of chest pain.

TABLE 2-2 Guidelines for a low-cholesterol diet

Foods to avoid	Foods allowed
Egg yolks (no more than 3 per week)	Egg whites; cholesterol-free egg substitutes
Foods made with many egg yolks (e.g., sponge cakes)	Lean, well-trimmed meats; minimize servings of beef, lamb, and pork
Fatty cuts of meat; fat on meats	Fish (except shellfish), chicken and turkey (without the skin)
Skin on chicken and turkey	Dried peas and beans as meat substitutes
Luncheon meats or cold cuts	Nonfat (skim) or lowfat (2%) milk
Sausage, frankfurters	Partially skim-milk cheeses
Shellfish (e.g., lobster, shrimp, crab)	Ice milk and sherbet
Whole milk, cream, whole milk cheese	Polyunsaturated oils for cooking and food preparation: corn, safflower, cottonseed, sesame, and sunflower
Ice cream	Margarines that list one of the above oils as their first ingredient
Commercially prepared foods with hydrogenated shortening. This is saturated fat.	Foods prepared "from scratch" with the above suggested oils
Coconut and palm oils and products made with them (e.g., cream substitutes)	Meats (in acceptable quantity) and vegetables prepared by broiling, steaming, or baking (never frying).
Butter, lard, hydrogenated shortening	Spices, herbs, lemon juice, wine, flavored wine vinegars
Meats and vegetables prepared by frying	
Seasonings containing large amounts of sugar and saturated fats	
Sauces and gravies	
Salad dressings containing cream, cheeses, or mayonnaise	

1. Observe for and report the following: increasing frequency of angina, angina that occurs at rest, angina that is unrelieved by nitroglycerine, or decreased exercise tolerance without angina.
2. Assess patient's response to activity. Be alert to chest pain, increase in HR (>20 bpm), change in systolic BP (20 mm Hg over or under resting BP), excessive fatigue, and SOB.
3. Assist patient with recognizing and limiting activities that increase oxygen demands, such as exercise and anxiety.
4. Maintain oxygen as prescribed for angina episodes.
5. Have patient perform ROM exercises, depending on tolerance and prescribed activity limitations. Because cardiac intolerance to activity can be further aggravated by prolonged bed rest, consult with MD regarding in-bed exercises and activities that can

be performed by the patient as the condition improves. Examples are found in **Potential for activity intolerance** related to deconditioning secondary to prolonged bed rest, p. 651, and **Potential for disuse syndrome,** p. 653, in the appendix.

Alterations in nutrition: More than body requirements related to excessive intake of calories, sodium, or fats

Desired outcome: Patient demonstrates knowledge of the dietary regimen by planning a 3-day menu that includes and excludes appropriate foods.

1. If patient is over ideal body weight explain that a low-calorie diet is necessary.
2. Teach patient how to decrease dietary intake of saturated (animal) fats and increase intake of polyunsaturated (vegetable oil) fats.
3. Teach patient to limit dietary intake of cholesterol to <300 mg/day. See Table 2-2, p. 48.
4. Teach patient to limit dietary intake of refined/processed sugar.
5. Teach patient to limit dietary intake of sodium chloride to <4 g/day (mild restriction). See Table 11-3, p. 550.
6. Encourage intake of fresh fruits, natural carbohydrates, fish, poultry, legumes, fresh vegetables, and grains for a healthy, balanced diet.

Health-seeking behaviors: Relaxation technique effective for stress reduction

Desired outcome: Patient reports subjective relief of stress following relaxation technique.

1. Discuss with patient the importance of relaxation for decreasing nervous system tone (sympathetic), energy requirements, and oxygen consumption.
2. There are many techniques that use breathing, concentration, or imagery to promote relaxation and decrease energy requirements. The following is an example of a technique that can be used easily by anyone. Give patient the following guidelines, speaking slowly and softly.
   □ Find a comfortable position. Close your eyes.
   □ Relax all your muscles. First, concentrate on your toes. Relax your toes. Now move to your feet. Relax the muscles of your feet. Continue with each muscle group, moving up your body, until finally you reach your facial muscles. Concentrate on your facial muscles and relax them.
   □ Now breath through your nose. Concentrate on feeling the air move in and out. As you exhale, say the word "one" silently to yourself. Again, continue feeling the air move in and out of your lungs. Continue for approximately 20 minutes.
   □ Try to clear your mind of worries; be passive. Let relaxation occur. If distractions appear, gently push them away. Continue breathing through your nose, repeating "one" silently.
   □ When approximately 20 minutes have passed, slowly begin to allow yourself to become aware of your surroundings. Keep your eyes closed for a few moments.
   □ Open your eyes.
3. Encourage patient to practice this technique 2-3 times a day or whenever feeling stressed or tense. Acknowledge that this technique may feel strange at first but that it becomes easier and more effective with each practice.
4. Mention that the use of baroque music, played softly, helps many individuals achieve an even greater state of relaxation.

Knowledge deficit: Precautions and negative side effects of nitrates

Desired outcome: Patient verbalizes understanding of the precautions and side effects of the prescribed medication.

1. Instruct patient to report to MD or staff the presence of a headache associated with nitroglycerine, in which case the MD may alter the dosage.
2. Teach patient to assume a recumbent position if a headache occurs. Explain that the vasodilatation effect of the drug causes a decrease in BP, which can result in orthostatic hypotension and transient headache.

Knowledge deficit: Precautions and negative side effects of beta blockers

Desired outcome: Patient verbalizes understanding of the precautions and side effects of beta blockers.

1. Instruct patient to be alert to depression, fatigue, dizziness, erythematous rash, respiratory distress, and sexual dysfunction, which can occur as side effects of beta blockers. Explain the importance of notifying MD promptly should they occur.
2. Explain that weight gain and peripheral and sacral edema can occur as side effects of beta blockers. Teach patient how to assess for edema and the importance of reporting signs and symptoms promptly should they occur.
3. Explain that BP and pulse rate are assessed before administration of beta blockers because the drug can cause hypotension and excessive slowing of the heart.
4. Caution patient about skipping or abruptly stopping beta blockers, which can result in rebound angina or even MI.

PATIENT-FAMILY TEACHING AND DISCHARGE PLANNING

Provide patient and significant others with verbal and written information for the following:

1. Medications, including drug name, dosage, purpose, schedule, precautions, and potential side effects. Discuss the potential for headache and dizziness after nitroglycerine administration. Caution patient about using nitroglycerine more frequently than prescribed and notifying MD if three tablets do not relieve angina.
2. Importance of reducing intake of caffeine, which causes vasoconstriction and increases the heart rate.
3. Dietary changes: low salt (see Table 11-3, p. 550), low saturated fat, and low cholesterol (see Table 2-2, p. 48); the need for weight loss if appropriate.
4. Prescribed exercise program and importance of maintaining a regular exercise schedule. Remind patient of the need to measure pulse, stop if pain occurs, and stay within prescribed exercise limits. See Table 2-3 for a progressive at-home walking program.
5. Indicators that necessitate medical attention: progression to unstable angina, loss of consciousness, decreased exercise tolerance, unrelieved pain, angina that is unrelieved by nitroglycerine, increasing frequency of angina, and need to increase the number of nitroglycerine tablets to relieve angina.
6. Elimination of smoking; refer patient to a "stop smoking" program, as appropriate.
7. Importance of involvement and support of significant others in patient's lifestyle changes.
8. Importance of getting BP checked at regular intervals (at least once a month if the patient is hypertensive).
9. Avoiding strenuous activity for at least an hour after meals to avoid excessive oxygen demands.

TABLE 2-3 Guidelines for a progressive at-home walking program

Week	Distance	Time
1	100-200 feet	2 times a day
2	200-400 feet	2 times a day
3	¼ mile	8-10 minutes
4	½ mile	15 minutes
5	1 mile	30 minutes
6	1¾ mile	30 minutes
7	2 miles	40 minutes

From Gawliniski A. In Swearingen PL et al: Manual of critical care: applying nursing diagnoses to adult critical illness, St Louis, 1988, The CV Mosby Co.

10. Importance of reporting to health care provider any change in the pattern or frequency of angina.

Myocardial infarction

Ischemic heart disease accounts for approximately one third of all deaths in the United States, and of patients with ischemic heart disease, half die because of MI. Most MIs are caused by critical narrowing of the coronary arteries due to atherosclerosis (see "Coronary Artery Disease," p. 45). Occlusion also can be caused by thrombus formation or coronary artery spasm. When ischemia is prolonged and unrelieved, irreversible damage (infarction) occurs. MI can occur in various areas of the heart, depending on the location of the coronary artery occlusion and distribution of blood supply.

ASSESSMENT

Signs and symptoms: Chest pain, substernal pressure and burning, pain that radiates to the jaw and arm. Weakness, diaphoresis, nausea, vomiting, and acute anxiety also can occur. The HR can be abnormally slow (bradycardia) or rapid (tachycardia).

Physical assessment: Possible minor hypotension, increasing RR, and crackles (rales) if ventricular failure occurs. Temperature elevations to 39.4° C (104° F) can occur secondary to the inflammatory process. Intensity of S_1 and S_2 heart sounds may be decreased and pulmonary congestion will occur if papillary muscle rupture has occurred. S_3 and S_4 sounds may be present if heart failure has occurred.

History of: Sudden onset of intense chest pain that is unrelieved by nitroglycerine, positive family history, cigarette smoking, hypercholesterolemia, obesity, stressful or sedentary lifestyle.

DIAGNOSTIC TESTS

1. *Serum enzymes:* Will reveal myocardial muscle damage. The following enzyme levels will increase: creatinine phosphokinase (CPK), the MB isoenzyme, SGOT, and lactic dehydrogenase (LDH).
2. *Serial EKGs:* For comparison to the baseline. Lead changes, including ST segment elevation, T wave inversion, and formation of Q waves, identify the area of infarct.
3. *Chest x-ray:* Usually reveals cardiomegaly and signs of left ventricular failure.
4. *Radionuclide studies (using technetium pyrophosphate):* May help localize area of infarct. The imaging agent concentrates in the infarcted zone, enabling visualization by scan.
5. *Echocardiography:* Detects abnormalities of left ventricular wall motion, which usually correspond to the EKG site of infarction.
6. *Hemodynamic monitoring in the CCU:* Measures cardiac output and pulmonary artery pressures, which usually are reflective of infarction.
7. *Coronary angiography:* Determines areas of stenosis or occlusion and suitability for coronary artery bypass grafting or percutaneous transluminal coronary angioplasty (PTCA). See discussion in "Cardiac Catheterization," p. 82.
8. *ABG analysis:* May reveal hypoxemia (decreased Pao_2) and hyperventilation (decreased $Paco_2$).
9. *Multiple-gated acquisition (MUGA) scan:* Evaluates left ventricular function and detects aneurysms and wall motion abnormalities.
10. *CBC:* May reveal leukocytosis secondary to the inflammatory process.
11. *Erythrocyte sedimentation rate (ESR) and WBC count:* Increase in the presence of an inflammatory process.

MEDICAL MANAGEMENT AND SURGICAL INTERVENTIONS

1. Relief of acute pain: Usually with IV morphine sulfate in small increments (2 mg) until relief is obtained or nitroglycerine by IV drip.
2. Oxygen: Usually 2-4 L/min by nasal cannula or mask for 2-3 days to increase the

patient's oxygen supply. Hypoxia is common and adds stress to the compromised myocardium.

3. Limiting infarct size by decreasing cardiac workload: Beta blockade, controlled exercise program, risk-factor management, bed rest with commode privileges.
4. Treatment and prevention of dysrhythmias: Antiarrhythmic agents (e.g., lidocaine) for ventricular premature beats; atropine for bradycardias.
5. Management of fluid imbalance: Oral or IV fluids for dehydration; diuretics for fluid overload.
6. Treatment of ventricular failure: See "Heart Failure," p. 54.
7. Medical reperfusion
   □ *Thrombolytic therapy with streptokinase or tissue plasminogen activator (TPA):* To lyse (break down) the fibrin clot. Usually, it is done in the cardiac catheterization laboratory, ICU, or emergency room.
   □ *PTCA:* To compress plaque in the coronary artery. See discussion under "Cardiac Catheterization," p. 82.
8. Surgical reperfusion: Coronary artery bypass graft (see "Cardiac Surgery," p. 84).
9. Transfer to CCU: For close monitoring, if needed.

NURSING DIAGNOSES AND INTERVENTIONS

Pain related to ischemia and infarction of myocardial tissue

Desired outcome: Patient's subjective evaluation of pain improves as documented by a pain scale.

1. Assess location, character, and intensity of pain, using a pain scale of 0 (no pain) to 10.
2. Administer prescribed pain medications (usually morphine sulfate) and document quality of relief obtained, using the pain scale, and the time interval from administration to expressed relief.
3. Provide reassurance during episodes of pain; stay with patient if possible.
4. Observe for and report side effects of pain medications, such as hypotension, slowed RR, and difficulty with urination.
5. Administer oxygen as prescribed, usually 2-4 L/min per nasal cannula.

Fluid volume excess: Edema (pulmonary or peripheral) related to retention of fluids secondary to decreased cardiac output

Desired outcome: Patient becomes normovolemic as evidenced by balanced I&O, stable weights, urinary output ≥30 ml/hr, RR 12-20 breaths/min with normal depth and pattern (eupnea), edema ≤1+ on a 0-4+ scale, and absence of crackles.

1. Record I&O, and report imbalances.
2. Observe for and report any indicators of fluid accumulation in the lungs, such as dyspnea, crackles (rales), and SOB.
3. Be alert to and report decreasing urine output (particularly <30 ml/hr) and increasing specific gravity (>1.030).
4. Assess for peripheral (sacral, pedal) edema.
5. Maintain IV infusion as prescribed. Usually, fluids are monitored closely to prevent failure and circulatory overload.
6. If fluids are limited, help control thirst by offering ice chips or popsicles, if they are allowed; record the amount of intake. Teach patient and significant others the importance of fluid limitation.

Activity intolerance related to fatigue and weakness secondary to decreased strength of cardiac contraction and decreased cardiac output

Desired outcome: Patient exhibits cardiac tolerance to activity as evidenced by systolic BP within 20 mm Hg of resting BP, RR <24 breaths/min, and HR <120 bpm (or <20 bpm over resting HR).

1. Observe for and report any symptoms of decreased cardiac output or cardiac failure, such as decreasing BP, cold extremities, oliguria, decreased peripheral pulses, and increased HR.
2. Monitor I&O, and be alert to urinary output <30 ml/hr. Auscultate lung fields q2h for presence of crackles (rales), which can occur with fluid retention and cardiac failure.
3. Palpate peripheral pulses at frequent intervals. Be alert to irregularities and decreased amplitude, which can signal cardiac failure.
4. Administer oxygen and medications as prescribed.
5. During acute periods of decreased cardiac output and as prescribed, support patient in maintaining bed rest by keeping personal articles within reach, providing a calm and quiet atmosphere, and limiting visitors to ensure periods of undisturbed rest.
6. Assist patient to commode if bathroom privileges are allowed.
7. Assist patient with passive or assistive ROM exercises, as determined by tolerance and activity limitations. Consult with MD regarding the type and amount of in-bed exercises the patient can perform as the condition improves. Examples of in-bed exercises can be found in the nursing diagnosis **Potential activity intolerance** related to deconditioning secondary to prolonged bed rest, p. 651, and **Potential for disuse syndrome,** p. 653.
8. As appropriate, teach patient self-measurement of pulse rate for gauging exercise tolerance.

Potential impaired gas exchange related to tissue hypoxia secondary to fluid accumulation in the lungs

Desired outcome: Patient has adequate gas exchange as evidenced by Pao_2 ≥80 mm Hg, $Paco_2$ 35-45 mm Hg, oxygen saturation ≥95%, BP within patient's baseline range, HR <100 bpm, and RR 12-20 breaths/min with normal pattern and depth (eupnea).

1. Auscultate lung fields q2h for presence of crackles (rales), which occur with fluid accumulation.
2. Assess ABG levels, and be alert to evidence of hypoxemia (decreased Pao_2), decreased oxygen saturation, or hyperventilation (decreased $Paco_2$).
3. Monitor for sudden changes in respiratory pattern (increased dyspnea or decreased RR), which can occur with an extension of the infarction and should be reported immediately.
4. Administer oxygen as prescribed. Deliver oxygen with humidity to help prevent its drying effects on oral and nasal mucosa.
5. Monitor BP. In the absence of marked hypotension, place patient in semi-Fowler's position to ease dyspnea.
6. Administer prescribed analgesics (usually morphine sulfate) or antianxiety agents (usually diazepam) to relax patient, decrease cardiac workload, and ease respiratory effort.

Sleep pattern disturbance related to awakening for VS assessment or medication administration

Desired outcome: Patient relates the attainment of adequate rest.

1. Plan care activities so that they do not interfere with patient's rest.
2. Provide periods of at least 90 minutes for undisturbed sleep.
3. Administer mild sedatives, if prescribed, to facilitate sleep.
4. Involve significant others in the care plan; coordinate visiting times.
5. If necessary, limit visitors so that patient can attain rest/sleep.
6. Question patient about interventions used at home that promote sleep.

See the appendix for nursing diagnoses and interventions in "Caring for Preoperative and Postoperative Patients," p. 637. See psychosocial nursing diagnoses and interventions in the section "Caring for Patients with Cancer and Other Life-Disrupting Illnesses, p. 690.

PATIENT-FAMILY TEACHING AND DISCHARGE PLANNING

Provide patient and significant others with verbal and written information for the following:

1. Process of myocardial infarction and extent of the patient's injury.
2. Indicators that necessitate immediate medical attention: unrelieved pain, decreased activity tolerance, sudden onset of SOB, weight gain.
3. Medications, including drug name, purpose, dosage, schedule, precautions, and potential side effects.
4. Exercise program specific to patient's condition. Guidelines for walking are provided in Table 2-3, p. 50. Caution patient to start slowly, walk 3-5 times/week, warm up and cool down with stretching exercises, notify MD of any change in exercise tolerance, not to overexert, and stop when tired.
5. Importance of avoiding overexertion and getting rest when tired.
6. Resumption of sexual activity as directed, usually after 2-4 weeks, but will vary with each patient.
7. Diet regimen as prescribed. See Table 2-2, p. 48, for a description of a low-cholesterol diet.
8. Cessation of smoking; refer patient to programs that specialize in this process.
9. Phone number or address for local American Heart Association branch, local heart rehabilitation programs, family physician, and primary nurse.
10. Referral to stress management programs, if appropriate. See **Health-seeking behaviors:** Relaxation technique effective for stress reduction, p. 49.

Heart failure

Heart (cardiac) failure is the state in which the heart is unable to pump blood at a rate sufficient to meet metabolic requirements of the tissues. Heart failure can occur as a result of myocardial or cardiac muscle damage such as after large infarcts, or when an adequate cardiac muscle is stressed or forced to work harder over a period of time. When the heart is unable to pump sufficient blood to meet metabolic demands, it relies on three main compensatory mechanisms:

□ *Increasing cardiac fluid* to increase fiber length and subsequent force of contraction (Frank-Starling law). The fluid that fills the ventricles before systole is termed "preload," and it is a critical factor in patients with cardiac failure. It is important to have enough volume to stretch the fibers, but not so much of a stretch that decreased contractility and decreased cardiac output occur.

□ *Increasing catecholamine discharge* (epinephrine and norepinephrine) to increase contractility. This causes systemic vasoconstriction, which in turn increases workload of the heart by increasing resistance. This is called "afterload."

□ *Myocardial hypertrophy* to increase the mass of working contractile tissue. The hypertrophy will be either right sided, left sided, or both, depending on the cause of failure. Conditions that can result in primary right-sided heart failure include right ventricular MI, COPD, left-to-right shunts, and pulmonary valve stenosis. Primary left-sided heart failure is caused by such conditions as left ventricular MI, aortic valve stenosis, mitral regurgitation, and hypertension. Over time, left-sided failure can result in the involvement of both sides of the heart.

ASSESSMENT

Signs and symptoms: Orthopnea, fatigue, weakness, nocturia, cardiac cachexia (malnutrition/wasting), and confusion, which can occur late in the disease. In addition, decreased right ventricular output can cause increased CVP, distended neck veins, and peripheral edema; decreased left ventricular output can cause dyspnea and SOB, as well as other indicators of pulmonary edema.

Physical assessment: Decreased BP, dysrhythmias, tachycardia, tachypnea, increased venous pulsations and pressure, crackles (rales), pitting edema, ascites, galloping heart sounds, and pulsus alternans (alternating strong and weak heart beats). Hepatomegaly may occur in the presence of right-sided or left-sided heart failure.

History of: Noncompliance with medication or diet regimen, sleeping on extra pillows to enhance respirations, decreased exercise tolerance, increasing SOB, CAD, and risk factors for CAD (see p. 46).

DIAGNOSTIC TESTS

1. *Chest x-ray:* Will show the presence of cardiomegaly and engorged pulmonary vasculature.
2. *Serum electrolytes:* May reveal hyponatremia (dilutional); hyperkalemia if glomerular filtration is decreased; or hypokalemia, which can result from some diuretics. See "Fluid and Electrolyte Disturbances," p. 546-563, for more information.
3. *Serum enzymes:* May reveal an elevated SGOT level with hepatic congestion and decreased liver function.
4. *Serum bilirubin:* May reveal hyperbilirubinemia in the presence of liver dysfunction.
5. *CBC:* May reveal decreased hemoglobin and hematocrit levels in the presence of anemia.

MEDICAL MANAGEMENT AND SURGICAL INTERVENTIONS

1. Treatment of underlying cause: Surgical repair of abnormalities such as valvular lesions or treatment of conditions such as hypertension or endocarditis.
2. Treatment of precipitating factors such as infection or dysrhythmias.
3. Physical and emotional rest.
4. Low-sodium diet: In less severe disease states, this may mean elimination of table salt only. See Table 11-3, p. 550.
5. Weight control: If appropriate.
6. Pharmacotherapy
   □ *Diuretics:* To control fluid accumulation and reduce blood volume.
   □ *Vasodilators:* To decrease cardiac workload by decreasing sympathetic nervous system vasoconstriction. Although there is some controversy about when to initiate vasodilator therapy, it is believed that it is appropriate when patients develop symptoms with light activity or when they are being treated with digitalis. This provides a combination of increased contractility (digitalis) and decreased afterload (vasodilator). The administration of IV vasodilators such as sodium nitroprusside and nitroglycerine necessitates the patient's transfer to the CCU.
   □ *Inotropic drugs:* Administered during acute exacerbation to increase the strength of contractions (usually digitalis). Administration of inotropic drugs necessitates the patient's transfer to the CCU for close monitoring of vasoactive effects.

NURSING DIAGNOSES AND INTERVENTIONS

Activity intolerance related to weakness and fatigue secondary to decreased strength of cardiac contraction

Desired outcome: Patient exhibits cardiac tolerance to increasing levels of activity as evidenced by RR <24 breaths/min with normal depth and pattern (eupnea), HR <120 bpm (or within 20 bpm of resting HR), systolic BP within 20 mm Hg of resting systolic BP, and absence of chest pain.

1. Monitor VS q2h or as necessary, and report decreasing BP, increasing HR, or increasing RR, which can occur with worsening failure related to sympathetic nervous system discharge and fluid retention.
2. Administer vasodilators and other cardiac drugs as prescribed.
3. If symptoms worsen, discuss the need for activity limitations with patient. Assist patient with ADL to prevent SOB, and plan nursing care and limit visitors to allow for periods of undisturbed rest.

4. Monitor HR, BP, and RR during periods of patient activity. Note signs of activity intolerance such as HR >120 bpm, RR ≥24 breaths/min, and systolic BP >20 mm Hg from normal range.
5. Discuss ways to decrease activities at home, such as not climbing stairs.
6. If appropriate, refer patient to an occupational therapist (OT) to learn how to conserve energy so that ADLs can be performed with a minimum of exertion.
7. Assist patient with passive or assistive ROM exercises, depending on tolerance and prescribed activity limitations. Because cardiac intolerance to activity can be further aggravated by prolonged bed rest, consult with MD regarding the type and amount of in-bed exercises that can be initiated as the patient's condition improves. For details, see **Potential activity intolerance** related to deconditioning secondary to prolonged bed rest, p. 651, and **Potential for disuse syndrome,** p. 653.

Fluid volume excess: Edema related to retention of fluid secondary to decreased cardiac output

Desired outcome: Patient is normovolemic as evidenced by urinary output ≥30 ml/hr, balanced I&O, stable weight (or weight loss attributable to fluid loss), edema ≤1+ on a 0-4+ scale, HR <100 bpm, and absence of crackles.

1. Auscultate lung fields at least qshift; report presence of crackles (rales), which occur with fluid volume excess.
2. Monitor and document I&O at least qshift. Report imbalances, including urinary output <30 ml/hr, which can occur with decreased renal blood flow.
3. Monitor weight daily, and report unusual gains. Be alert to the presence of pitting edema. To assess for pitting edema, apply firm pressure to the edematous area with a finger. If the indentation remains after the finger has been removed, pitting edema is present.
4. Auscultate heart sounds; be alert to S_3 gallop, an early sign of heart failure.
5. Administer diuretics as prescribed. Observe for indicators of decreased effective circulating volume such as hypotension, decreased CVP (<5 cm H_2O), and tachycardia.
6. If appropriate, teach patient the importance of decreasing intake of sodium (or table salt). See Table 11-3, p. 550.
7. If fluids are limited, help relieve patient's thirst by offering ice chips or popsicles. Record the amount of intake on the I&O record.

Knowledge deficit: Precautions and negative side effects of diuretic therapy

Desired outcome: Patient verbalizes knowledge of the precautions and negative side effects of diuretic therapy.

1. Depending on type of diuretic used, teach patient to report signs and symptoms of the following:
   □ *Hypokalemia:* Anorexia, irregular pulse, nausea, apathy, muscle cramps.
   □ *Hyperkalemia:* Muscle weakness, hyporeflexia, and irregular heart rate, which can occur with potassium-sparing diuretics.
   □ *Hyponatremia:* Fatigue, weakness, and edema (owing to fluid extravasation).
2. For patients on long-term diuretic therapy, explain the importance of follow-up monitoring of blood levels of sodium and potassium.
3. As appropriate, instruct patient to use care when rising from a sitting or recumbent position to prevent injury from orthostatic hypotension.

Knowledge deficit: Precautions and negative side effects of digitalis therapy

Desired outcome: Patient verbalizes understanding of the precautions and negative side effects associated with digitalis therapy.

1. Teach patient the technique and importance of assessing pulse rate before taking digitalis. Explain that he or she should obtain pulse rate parameters from MD, but that digitalis is usually withheld when it is <60 bpm if the usual heart rate before digitalis administration is greater.

2. Explain that serum potassium levels are monitored routinely because low potassium levels can potentiate digitalis toxicity.
3. Explain that the apical heart rate and peripheral pulses are assessed for irregularity, which is a sign of digitalis toxicity.
4. Teach patient to be alert to other indicators of digitalis toxicity, including nausea, vomiting, anorexia, diarrhea, blurred vision, and mental confusion. Explain the importance of reporting signs and symptoms promptly to MD or staff should they occur.

Knowledge deficit: Precautions and negative side effects of vasodilators

Desired outcome: Patient verbalizes knowledge of the precautions and negative side effects associated with vasodilators.

1. Explain that a headache can occur after administration of a vasodilator and that lying down will help alleviate the pain.
2. Teach the importance of assessment for weight gain and signs of peripheral or sacral edema, any of which can occur as side effects of vasodilator therapy.
3. Instruct patient to alert MD to negative side effects of this therapy.

See "Coronary Artery Disease" for **Alteration in nutrition:** More than body requirements related to excessive intake of salt, calories, and fats, p. 49, and **Knowledge deficit:** Precautions and negative side effects of beta blockers, p. 50. See "Myocardial Infarction" for **Sleep pattern disturbance,** p. 53, and **Impaired gas exchange,** p. 53. See Caring for Patients on Prolonged Bed Rest, p. 651, and Caring for Patients with Cancer and Other Life-Disrupting Illnesses, p. 690.

PATIENT-FAMILY TEACHING AND DISCHARGE PLANNING

Provide patient and significant others with verbal and written information for the following:
1. Medications, including drug name, purpose, dosage, schedule, precautions, and potential side effects. Stress the importance of taking medications regularly and not stopping them without MD consultation. Teach patient and significant others how to measure pulse rate for digitalis therapy.
2. Diet: Advise patient that sodium restriction may be lessened as cardiac function improves. Assist patient with diet planning or refer to a nutrition specialist if major dietary changes are necessary. Low-sodium guidelines are found in Table 11-3, p. 550.
3. Signs and symptoms that necessitate medical attention: irregular pulse, bradycardia, unusual SOB, increased orthopnea, decreased exercise tolerance, and unusual or steady weight gain.
4. Importance of quitting smoking, which causes vasoconstriction and increases cardiac workload. As appropriate, refer patient to programs that specialize in smoking cessation.
5. Importance of limiting exertional activities at home (e.g., minimize bending and lifting and avoid stair climbing).
6. Emergency telephone numbers to call if needed.
7. Importance of follow-up care; confirm date and time of next medical appointment.

Section Two   INFLAMMATORY HEART DISORDERS

The disorders described in this section are inflammations or infections involving mainly the heart muscle and linings: pericardium, myocardium, and endocardium. The inflammation can be acute or chronic, and prognosis usually depends on extent of the involvement, structures involved, and secondary disorders that occur.

Pericarditis

Pericarditis is an inflammation of the stiff, fibrous sac (pericardium) that surrounds, supports, and protects the heart. The pericardium is composed of a fibrous outer layer and a serous inner layer. The inflammatory condition produces friction between the layers during cardiac movement. Acute pericarditis causes exudate production and formation of chronic fibrinous adhesions. Pericarditis also may involve formation of pericardial effusions. Pericarditis occurs in a vast number of medical disorders. The most common causes are viral or bacterial infections, uremia, acute myocardial infarction, neoplastic disease, and trauma.

ASSESSMENT

Chronic indicators: Elevated CVP and signs secondary to systemic venous congestion including edema, ascites, and hepatic congestion. If fibrous constriction is severe, symptoms of left-sided heart failure may appear, such as dyspnea, cough, and orthopnea.

Acute indicators: Chest pain localized to the retrosternal and left precordial regions, or pain that mimics acute abdominal pain or ischemic pain. Unlike ischemic pain, however, it is often increased with deep inspirations, movement, or lying down and eased by sitting up and leaning forward. Other indicators include dyspnea, if the increased pericardial fluid is severe enough to cause constriction of the bronchi, and fever.

Physical assessment: Characteristic pericardial friction rub (a scratching, grating, high-pitched sound) heard on auscultation.

DIAGNOSTIC TESTS

1. *Serial EKGs:* Typically show widespread ST elevation in most leads, unlike localized ischemic ST segment elevation.
2. *CBC and other hematologic studies:* Often show presence of increased WBCs (leukocytosis) and increased ESR in the presence of inflammation.
3. *Cardiac enzymes:* Probably will be normal, although the MB fraction of CPK may increase with epicardial inflammation.
4. *Echocardiogram:* Reveals increase in pericardial fluid, which occurs with infection or irritation.

MEDICAL MANAGEMENT AND SURGICAL INTERVENTIONS

1. Treatment of underlying disorder:
2. Bed rest: Until pain and fever are relieved.
3. Pharmacotherapy
   □ *Nonsteroidal antiinflammatory agents:* See Table 8-1, p. 432.
   □ *Corticosteroids:* For example, prednisone 60-80 mg qd in divided doses for 5-7 days and tapered thereafter, if symptoms are unrelieved by nonsteroidal anti-inflammatory agents.
   □ *Antibiotics:* Given only in the presence of purulent pericarditis.
4. Emergency pericardiocentesis: If cardiac tamponade (accumulation of fluid that restricts ventricular filling and reduces cardiac output) develops. This procedure involves needle aspiration of the fluid in the pericardial sac to relieve pressure and allow for normal cardiac muscle contraction. Usually it is done under local anesthetic in the ICU, operating room, or cardiac catheterization lab.
5. Partial or total pericardectomy: To allow normal cardiac movement and function if pericarditis is recurrent and has produced scar tissue and constriction. This procedure involves the removal of part (pericardial "window") or all of the pericardium to prevent constriction by scar tissue, exudate, or bleeding.

NURSING DIAGNOSES AND INTERVENTIONS

Activity intolerance related to weakness and dyspnea secondary to inflammation of the cardiac muscle and restriction of contraction

Desired outcome: Patient's cardiac tolerance to increasing levels of activity improves as evidenced by systolic BP within 20 mm Hg of resting systolic BP, RR <24 breaths/min, HR ≤20 bpm above resting HR, and absence of dyspnea and pain.

1. Ensure that patient maintains bed rest during febrile period and understands the rationale for doing so.
2. Anticipate patient's needs by placing personal articles within easy reach.
3. Advise patient about the importance of frequent periods of rest during convalescence.
4. Monitor VS for changes that are indicative of cardiac or pulmonary decompensation, such as decreasing BP and increasing heart and respiratory rates.
5. Assist patient with turning at least q2h, and provide passive ROM exercises at frequent intervals to help prevent complications of immobility. As the patient's condition improves, consult with MD regarding in-bed exercises that require more cardiac tolerance. Examples are found with the nursing diagnosis **Potential activity intolerance** related to deconditioning secondary to prolonged bed rest, p. 651, and **Potential for disuse syndrome,** p. 653, in the appendix.

Potential alteration in tissue perfusion: Peripheral, cardiopulmonary, cerebral, and renal related to impaired circulation secondary to dysfunctional cardiac muscle

Desired outcome: Patient has adequate tissue perfusion as evidenced by distal pulses >2+ on a 0-4+ scale; HR <100 bpm; BP >90/60 mm Hg; RR ≤20 breaths/min with normal depth and pattern (eupnea); normal heart sounds (see appendix, p. 710); orientation to person, place, and time; and urinary output ≥30 ml/hr.

1. Observe for and report increasing restlessness or anxiety and changes in mentation, which can occur with decreased cerebral perfusion.
2. Palpate peripheral pulses at least q2-4h to assess peripheral perfusion.
3. Be alert to signs of cardiac tamponade, including narrowed pulse pressure, rapid pulse, hypotension, dyspnea, distended neck veins, and distant or decreased heart sounds. Report positive findings to MD and prepare for emergency pericardiocentesis.
4. Assess for pulsus paradoxus (decrease in pulse volume and systolic BP >10 mm Hg during inhalation as compared to exhalation), which is produced by pericardial restriction and subsequent decreased ventricular filling. The assessment is performed as follows:
   □ Apply BP cuff to the patient's arm; palpate the brachial pulse.
   □ Place the stethoscope over the pulse point and inflate the cuff to above the level of the patient's normal systolic BP.
   □ Slowly deflate the cuff. Ask patient to exhale.
   □ Listen for the first sound that occurs after the patient exhales. Note the manometer reading and tell patient to breathe normally.
   □ Continue to deflate the BP cuff slowly until sounds are heard during inhalation and exhalation. Note the reading.
   □ Calculate the difference in mm Hg between the two readings. This is the measurement of pulsus paradoxus.
5. Monitor urinary output to determine renal perfusion. Be alert to output <30 ml/hr for 2 consecutive hours.
6. Instruct patient to perform foot and leg exercises q4h to enhance venous circulation.
7. If patient exhibits signs of decreased cerebral perfusion, reorient and institute safety precautions as necessary.

Pain related to friction rub secondary to inflammatory process

Desired outcome: Patient's subjective evaluation of pain improves, as documented by a pain scale.

1. Assess and document character, intensity, and duration of pain. Establish a pain scale with the patient, rating the pain on a scale of 0 (no pain) to 10. Administer pain medications as prescribed, and document their effectiveness, again using the pain scale. Advise patient to notify staff as soon as pain occurs so that the medication can be administered early.
2. Use the following interventions to enhance the effectiveness of the medication: Support the patient in a side-lying position with pillows, or place the patient in Fowler's position; provide emotional support; and control environmental stimuli by limiting visitors, dimming the lights, and providing a quiet environment.
3. Administer oxygen as prescribed, typically 2-3 L/min by nasal cannula.

Ineffective breathing pattern related to guarding secondary to pericardial pain

Desired outcome: Patient's RR is 12-20 breaths/min with normal depth and pattern (eupnea).

1. Assess breath sounds and respirations at least q4h. Report the presence of crackles or areas of diminished breath sounds, which may occur due to atelectasis caused by decreased depth of respirations (guarding).
2. Assess the breathing effort for adequate depth at least q2h, and teach the patient to breathe deeply. Teach the use of an incentive spirometer.
3. Place the patient in semi-Fowler's or high-Fowler's position to ease pressure on the heart, which will help decrease the effort of breathing.

See "Caring for Patients on Prolonged Bed Rest," p. 651.

PATIENT-FAMILY TEACHING AND DISCHARGE PLANNING

Provide patient and significant others with verbal and written information for the following:
1. Importance of frequent rest periods during convalescence.
2. Importance of prompt treatment if symptoms of pericarditis recur.
3. Procedure for measuring temperature, which can be an indicator of recurring inflammation.
4. Importance of avoiding individuals with URI and promptly seeking medical attention if flu or cold symptoms occur.
5. Medications, including drug name, purpose, dosage, schedule, precautions, and potential side effects.
In addition,
6. Explain that feelings of wellness do not necessarily mean that the inflammation has completely resolved.

Myocarditis

Myocarditis is an inflammation of the myocardium (middle layer of the heart walls, composed of cardiac muscle), often caused by a virus, bacteria, or protozoa. Clinical consequences range from focal inflammation with spontaneous recovery to more severe processes, such as acute congestive cardiomyopathy and chronic dilated cardiomyopathy. The condition can be acute or chronic.

ASSESSMENT

Chronic indicators: Signs of congestive heart failure may appear, including distended neck veins, pulmonary congestion, dyspnea, and tachycardia.

Acute indicators: Fatigue, dyspnea, palpitations, continuous precordial discomfort, fever.

Physical assessment: Cardiomegaly with diffuse point of maximal impulse (PMI), soft heart sounds, heart murmur of tricuspid or mitral regurgitation, S_3 and S_4 heart sounds.

History of: URI or GI complaints.

DIAGNOSTIC TESTS

1. *EKG:* Changes are usually transient and involve the ST segment and T wave or intraventricular conduction defects.
2. *Chest x-ray:* Heart varies in size from normal to enlarged, depending on extent of involvement and subsequent muscle damage.
3. *Radionuclide scans:* May identify areas of the myocardium that are necrotic or akinetic.
4. *Cardiac enzymes:* To assess for elevated CPK or CPK isoenzyme.
5. *Cultures and sensitivities by blood studies or muscle biopsy:* To identify causative organism.

MEDICAL MANAGEMENT AND SURGICAL INTERVENTIONS

1. Oxygenation and bed rest: Hypoxia and exercise contribute to muscle damage. Usually, oxygen is administered by nasal cannula at 2-3 L/min.
2. Pharmacotherapy
   □ *Antibiotics:* Type is determined by the causative organism.
   □ *Diuretics and digitalization:* To treat congestive heart failure. Close observance for digitalis toxicity is important because these patients are particularly sensitive to digitalis.
   □ *Antiarrhythmic agents:* For prompt treatment of dysrhythmias. Drugs with negative inotropic action (such as propranolol), which further decrease the strength of contraction, should be avoided because of the weakness of the already compromised myocardial muscle.
   □ *Steroids:* Controversial with this disorder, and are used mostly for patients with acute viral myocarditis.

NURSING DIAGNOSES AND INTERVENTIONS

Activity intolerance related to weakness and fatigue secondary to dysfunction of myocardial muscle

Desired outcome: Patient's cardiac tolerance to activity improves, as evidenced by HR <120 bpm, systolic BP within 20 mm Hg of baseline systolic BP, and RR <24 breaths/min with normal pattern and depth (eupnea).

1. Observe for and immediately report signs of congestive heart failure, including dyspnea, distended neck veins, and crackles (rales).
2. Be alert to a steady weight gain, which can occur with heart failure. Monitor I&O and report imbalances. For more detail, see **Decreased cardiac output,** p. 44, in "Cardiomyopathy."
3. Administer and maintain oxygen as prescribed.
4. Ensure that the patient maintains bed rest during the febrile period; teach the importance of frequent periods of rest during convalescence.
5. Anticipate patient's needs by placing personal items within reach.
6. Assist patient with turning q2h, and provide assistance with ROM exercises at frequent intervals to help prevent complications of immobility. As the patient's condition improves, consult with MD regarding progressive in-bed exercises that require increasing cardiac tolerance. These are discussed with the nursing diagnosis **Potential activity intolerance** related to deconditioning, p. 651, and **Potential for disuse syndrome,** p. 653, in the appendix.

See "Heart Failure" for **Knowledge deficit:** Precautions and negative side effects of digitalis therapy, p. 56. See "Pericarditis" for **Pain** related to friction rub, p. 59. See "Infective Endocarditis" for **Knowledge deficit:** Disease process and therapeutic regimen, p. 63. See "Osteomyelitis" in Chapter 8 (Musculoskeletal Disorders) for **Knowledge deficit:** Adverse side effects from prolonged use of potent antibiotics, p. 447. See "Caring for Patients on Prolonged Bed Rest," p. 651.

PATIENT-FAMILY TEACHING AND DISCHARGE PLANNING

Provide patient and significant others with verbal and written information for the following:

1. Indicators of recurring inflammation or heart failure. The signs of heart failure, which must be reported *stat,* include steady weight gain, decreased exercise tolerance, fatigue, dyspnea, and SOB.
2. Medications to be taken at home, including drug name, purpose, dosage, schedule, precautions, and potential side effects.
3. Importance of helping to fight infection with a well-balanced diet that includes vegetables, fruits, and protein. Advise patients with congestive heart failure not to add salt to their food.
4. Importance of immunization and vaccination as preventive measures.
5. Technique for measuring body temperature and importance of regular measurement to detect elevations, which can signal recurring infection. Suggest that the patient measure body temperature at least once a week if asymptomatic, and more frequently if symptoms of colds and flu, fatigue, or weakness occur.
6. Notifying MD if URI or viral infections occur, because they can precipitate myocarditis.
7. Importance of regular follow-up; confirm date and time of next medical appointment.

Infective endocarditis

Inflammation of the inner lining of the atria, ventricles, and covering of the heart valves is called infective endocarditis. This infection involves the left side of the heart more frequently than the right side and is characterized by vegetations (fibrous network of platelets, blood cells, and pathogenic organisms), which are found most frequently on the mitral and aortic valves. Vegetations on the valves can prevent adequate closure and adherence of the valve flaps, resulting in regurgitation or stenosis. When the vegetations affect the chamber lining, muscle fibers eventually undergo degenerative changes, and the patient becomes at risk for emboli because parts of the vegetations can break off. In addition, there is a tendency for fibrin and platelets to deposit on the vegetations, and these may embolize as well. Endocarditis usually is classified as acute or subacute. Manifestations of infective endocarditis are the result of infection (systemic and local), the effects of emboli or valvular dysfunction, or antigen-antibody complexes causing injury to the microvasculature.

ASSESSMENT

Chronic indicators: Murmurs (sign of valvular involvement); and dyspnea, distended neck veins, peripheral edema, pulmonary congestion, splenomegaly, and activity intolerance (signs of congestive heart failure).

Acute indicators: Temperature elevation, malaise, anorexia, weight loss, tachycardia, pallor, diaphoresis, and joint pain.

Physical assessment: Presence of a murmur. If heart failure has developed as a result of valvular dysfunction, the following may be present: crackles, SOB, edema, neck vein distention, and hepatomegaly. **Note:** If embolization has occurred, signs may include evidence of decreased renal, cerebral, and peripheral perfusion.

History of: URI, flu, or other infectious process.

DIAGNOSTIC TESTS

1. *Blood cultures:* To identify causative organism.
2. *ESR:* Usually elevated owing to inflammatory process.
3. *WBC count:* May be normal in subacute forms and can range from 15,000-20,000 μl in acute disease.
4. *Two-dimensional echocardiography:* May be used to detect intracardiac complications such as valvular disorders or wall motion abnormalities. This test uses sound waves (or echoes), which allow visualization of the cardiac wall and valvular movement.
5. *Echo with Doppler:* May be performed to evaluate valvular involvement. Adding the Doppler to the echocardiogram provides more or different information than would be found using the echo alone.

MEDICAL MANAGEMENT AND SURGICAL INTERVENTIONS

1. Specific antibiotic therapy: Will depend on the causative organism and its susceptibility or sensitivity to drugs. In the subacute form of the disorder, it is satisfactory to wait until the organism is identified, but with acute endocarditis, broad-spectrum antibiotic therapy is instituted immediately after blood cultures are drawn and then adjusted if necessary after organism identification. Intermittent IV antibiotics are given q4-6h. The duration of therapy usually is 4-6 weeks.
2. Bed rest.
3. Well-balanced diet: To maintain resistance to infection.
4. Surgical repair or valve replacement: Performed when congestive heart failure does not respond to medical management; when an infection does not respond to antimicrobial therapy within 1 week; when repeated episodes of embolization occur, especially when vascular occlusions are found in the eyes, brain, coronary arteries, and kidneys; when repeated infections occur (e.g., relapse after 3 months); and when fungal endocarditis is found. (See discussion of mitral valve replacement in "Mitral Stenosis," p. 65.)
5. Treatment of heart failure, if present. See page 54.

NURSING DIAGNOSES AND INTERVENTIONS

Potential for infection (secondary) related to decreased immune response secondary to prolonged antibiotic therapy and vulnerability secondary to invasive procedures

Desired outcome: Patient is free of secondary infection as evidenced by normothermia, normal skin temperature and color at IV sites, HR ≤100 bpm, and urine that is straw-colored, clear, and with normal odor.

1. Use aseptic technique when working with IV lines, urinary catheters, and wounds.
2. Monitor patient's temperature and WBC count for increases from baseline assessment. Both already may be increased as a result of the primary infection, but unexplained increases may occur after resolution of the acute phase as a result of a secondary infection.
3. For patients with indwelling urinary catheters, monitor urine for signs of infection, including cloudiness and foul odor. Cleanse the urethral meatus and surrounding area daily, using soap and water.
4. Rotate IV sites and change tubing and dressings q48-72hr, or per agency protocol.

Knowledge deficit: Disease process, therapeutic regimen, and assessment for infection

Desired outcome: Patient verbalizes understanding of the disease process and measures that are taken to prevent bacteremia.

1. Assess patient's level of knowledge about the disease and therapy.
2. As indicated, explain the disease process and the need for prolonged antibiotic therapy.

3. Because of the increased risk for bacteremia, discuss the need for antibiotic prophylaxis before dental procedures and all major and minor surgical procedures and early treatment of common infections (e.g., urinary tract infections, upper respiratory infection, and wound infection [see Table 5-3, p. 298]).
4. Teach patient the early indicators of infection (e.g., low-grade fever and malaise), and the importance of reporting indicators to MD promptly. Teach patient how to measure body temperature and the importance of monitoring temperature weekly if asymptomatic and more frequently if weakness, fatigue, or symptoms of a cold or flu occur.

See "Pulmonary Embolus" in Chapter 1 for **Potential for injury** related to increased risk of bleeding or hemorrhage secondary to anticoagulant therapy, p. 16. See "Cardiomyopathy" for **Potential alteration in tissue perfusion** (embolus formation), p. 45. See "Myocardial Infarction" for **Impaired gas exchange**, p. 53. See "Pericarditis" for **Activity intolerance**, p. 59. See "Mitral Stenosis" for **Decreased cardiac output**, p. 65. See "Osteomyelitis" in Chapter 8 for **Knowledge deficit:** Adverse side effects from prolonged use of potent antibiotics, p. 447. See "Caring for Preoperative and Postoperative Patients," p. 637, and "Caring for Patients on Prolonged Bed Rest," p. 651.

PATIENT-FAMILY TEACHING AND DISCHARGE PLANNING

Provide patient and significant others with verbal and written information for the following:
1. Need for prolonged antibiotic therapy, including prophylaxis before dental and surgical procedures.
2. Other medications to be taken at home, including drug name, purpose, dosage, schedule, precautions, and potential side effects. **Note:** The patient may be required to self-administer IV antibiotics at home to decrease the length of hospital stay; teach the technique if indicated.
3. Importance of medical follow-up to check valve function; confirm date and time of next medical appointment.
4. Signs and symptoms of URI (see Chapter 1) and other infections that can precipitate recurrence of endocardial infection, and indicators of recurrence of endocarditis and the importance of getting prompt medical attention if they occur.
5. Importance of reporting signs of increasing cardiac failure *stat*. These include steady weight gain, decreased exercise tolerance, fatigue, and dyspnea.
6. Importance of regular temperature measurement (e.g., weekly if asymptomatic and more frequently if weakness, fatigue, or symptoms of a cold or flu occur).

Section Three   VALVULAR HEART DISORDERS

Mitral stenosis

The most common cause of mitral valve stenosis is rheumatic heart disease, although it also can be caused by a virus or malignancy. In the diseased mitral valve the orifice becomes narrowed either by calcification or thickening of the valve leaflets. Because the mitral valve is located between the left atrium and ventricle, stenosis results in decreased ventricular filling and increased left atrial and pulmonary pressures. As the severity of the stenosis increases, maintenance of cardiac output becomes more difficult. In addition, high pulmonary pressures cause fluid extravasation into the alveoli, which results in pulmonary edema.

Patients with valvular disorders are predisposed to endocarditis (see "Infective Endocarditis," p. 62). Bacteria in the bloodstream have a tendency to lodge in the malfunctioning valves because of calcium deposits or turbulent blood flow, so special care should be taken whenever a systemic infection is present or the patient is undergoing major or minor surgical procedures, such as dental work.

ASSESSMENT

Chronic indicators: Decreased exercise tolerance secondary to decreased cardiac output; increased pulmonary artery pressures.

Acute indicators: Dyspnea usually is the first symptom of worsening stenosis. Orthopnea, hemoptysis, thromboembolism, and chest pain with subsequent right ventricular failure may occur with elevated pulmonary pressure. In some patients, chest pain occurs secondary to decreased oxygen perfusion.

Physical assessment: Decreased arterial pulse volume, as determined by palpation or Doppler ultrasonic probe; increased venous pulsations; low-pitched diastolic murmur; elevated CVP; and hepatomegaly. Left ventricular impulse (the point of maximal impulse [PMI]) may be displaced by an enlarged right ventricle. Normally, it is best heard over the mitral area, fifth intercostal space, midclavicular line.

DIAGNOSTIC TESTS

1. *Chest x-ray:* May reveal an enlarged left atrium and right ventricle.
2. *Echocardiography:* Can readily diagnose mitral stenosis by poor valve leaflet separation and thickened leaflets; also may demonstrate pulmonary hypertension.
3. *EKG:* Although not useful for a definitive diagnosis, it will demonstrate characteristic changes associated with left atrial and right ventricular enlargement such as tall P waves and right axis deviation.
4. *Cardiac catheterization:* To determine extent of the stenosis (see "Cardiac Catheterization," p. 81).

MEDICAL MANAGEMENT AND SURGICAL INTERVENTIONS

1. Restriction of physically strenuous activities.
2. Antibiotic prophylaxis for endocarditis: Before and after invasive procedures, including dental work (see "Infective Endocarditis," p. 62).
3. Pharmacotherapy
   □ *Oral diuretics:* To reduce pulmonary artery pressures and relieve dyspnea.
   □ *Positive inotropic drugs such as digitalis glycosides:* To increase the strength of contraction for patients with ventricular failure.
   □ *Oral anticoagulants (warfarin sodium):* May be prescribed to prevent thromboemboli.
4. Mitral commissurotomy: To relieve stenosis by incising the valve and removing calcifications. This procedure involves a heart-lung bypass. Usually the chest is entered through the left fifth intercostal space. The left atrial appendage is incised and a dilator is inserted and guided through the mitral orifice.
5. Percutaneous mitral valve balloon valvuloplasty: An alternative to surgery for some patients, this procedure is done in the cardiac catheterization laboratory, using local anesthetic. A balloon dilating catheter is inserted into the valve and inflated across the area of stenosis.
6. Mitral valve replacement: For patients who continue to be symptomatic after a commissurotomy. Using a midline sternotomy incision, a prosthetic mitral valve is inserted while the patient is on a heart-lung bypass machine. Usually the patient remains in the ICU for 48 hours after the procedure.

NURSING DIAGNOSES AND INTERVENTIONS

Potential for decreased cardiac output related to decreased strength of contractions secondary to ventricular dysfunction

Desired outcome: Patient has adequate cardiac output as evidenced by urine output ≥ 30 ml/hr, systolic BP within 20 mm Hg of baseline systolic BP, HR 60-100 bpm with regular rhythm, pedal pulses $>2+$ on a 0-4+ scale, extremities warm and of normal color, and orientation to person, place, and time.

1. Monitor BP and HR q4h unless patient is unstable. Report changes such as irregular heart rhythm, HR <60 bpm or >100 bpm, or systolic BP >20 mm Hg over or under baseline.
2. Monitor urine output, noting amount that is <30 ml/hr for 2 consecutive hours.
3. Assess pedal pulses and color and temperature of the extremities along with other assessment parameters. Be alert to pulses ≤2+ and to extremities that are cool, pale, and mottled.
4. Administer inotropic drugs as prescribed to increase cardiac contractility.

Activity intolerance related to fatigue and weakness secondary to decreased left ventricular filling

Desired outcome: Patient exhibits cardiac tolerance to increasing levels of activity as evidenced by HR ≤20 bpm over resting HR, systolic BP within 20 mm Hg of baseline systolic BP, and RR ≤24 breaths/min with normal depth and pattern (eupnea).

1. Monitor VS with patient activity, and report significant (20 mm Hg or greater) decrease or increase in BP. Assess for orthostatic changes in BP that occur when the patient moves from supine to standing position.
2. Assess peripheral pulses, capillary refill, and temperature and color of the extremities as indicators of cardiac output.
3. Provide rest periods at frequent intervals, especially between care activities.
4. Confer with MD regarding in-bed exercises that can be incorporated as the patient's condition improves. Examples are found in **Potential activity intolerance** related to deconditioning secondary to prolonged bed rest, p. 651, and **Potential for disuse syndrome,** p. 653. Increase ambulation progressively and to the patient's tolerance; be alert to indicators of activity intolerance including SOB, dyspnea, and fatigue.

Potential fluid volume excess: Edema related to retention of fluid secondary to right-sided heart failure

Desired outcome: Patient is normovolemic as evidenced by balanced I&O, stable weight, urine output ≥30 ml/hr, edema ≤1+ on a 0-4+ scale, flattened neck veins, and lungs clear on auscultation.

1. Observe for and report the following indicators of right-sided heart failure: increasing CVP (≥12 cm H_2O), peripheral edema, dyspnea, hepatic enlargement on palpation, and jugular vein distention.
2. Monitor I&O and administer fluids only as prescribed to ensure that patient maintains adequate volume without overload. Weigh patient daily and report significant I&O imbalance.
3. If fluids are limited, offer ice chips and popsicles to help patient control thirst. Record the amount of intake.
4. As prescribed, administer inotropic drugs such as digitalis to increase the strength of cardiac contraction.
5. Administer diuretics as prescribed to decrease volume load.

Potential for infection (with concomitant endocarditis) related to increased susceptibility secondary to valvular disorder

Desired outcome: Patient is free of infection as evidenced by normothermia, WBC count ≤11,000 µl, and HR ≤ 100 bpm.

1. Maintain aseptic technique for all invasive procedures.
2. Monitor temperature q4h and report significant increases to MD.
3. Be alert to rising HR, which can signal the presence of an infection.
4. Administer prescribed antibiotics on time.
5. Maintain hydration, as prescribed, through oral and prescribed IV fluids, making sure that patient has adequate volume without overload.

Knowledge deficit: Potential for development of endocarditis

Desired outcome: Patient verbalizes knowledge of the potential for endocarditis, indicators of the disorder, and measures that prevent it.

1. Assess patient's knowledge of the disease process and potential for endocarditis. As indicated, explain how endocarditis affects the heart and its valves and why individuals with valvular disorders are predisposed toward developing this disorder.
2. Discuss the importance of antibiotic prophylaxis before and after any major or minor surgical procedures.
3. Teach patient the following indicators of endocarditis: temperature increases, malaise, anorexia, tachycardia, and pallor. Explain the importance of reporting the symptoms early.
4. Teach patient the indicators of frequently encountered infections (e.g., URI, UTI, and wounds [(see Table 5-3, p. 298]), and stress the importance of reporting them to MD promptly should they occur.

See "Pulmonary Embolus" in Chapter 1 for **Potential for injury** related to increased risk of bleeding secondary to anticoagulant therapy, p. 16. See "Heart Failure" for **Knowledge deficit:** Precautions and negative side effects of diuretic therapy, p. 56, and **Knowledge deficit:** Precautions and negative side effects of digitalis therapy, p. 56. As appropriate, see nursing diagnoses and interventions in "Cardiac Catheterization," p. 82, and "Cardiac Surgery," p. 84. Also see "Caring for Preoperative and Postoperative Patients," p. 637.

PATIENT-FAMILY TEACHING AND DISCHARGE PLANNING

Provide patient and significant others with verbal and written information for the following:
1. Medications, including drug name, purpose, dosage, schedule, precautions, and potential side effects
2. Gradually increasing exercise, avoiding heavy lifting (>5 pounds), incorporating rest periods.
3. Name and phone number of a resource person (e.g., MD, primary nurse) should questions arise after hospital discharge.
4. Referral to cardiac rehabilitation program if appropriate.
5. Resumption of sexual activity as directed by MD.
6. Indicators that necessitate immediate medical attention: decreased exercise tolerance, signs of infection, SOB, bleeding.
7. Importance of consulting MD before using OTC medications, especially aspirin products for individuals taking oral anticoagulants. Aspirin can affect coagulation times.
8. Importance of follow-up care; confirm date and time of next medical appointment.

Mitral regurgitation

Abnormalities of the mitral valve can cause mitral regurgitation (MR). MR can be caused by a number of conditions, including MI, CAD, papillary muscle dysfunction, cardiomyopathy, or inflammatory heart disorders. The significant effects of MR occur during ventricular systole. Normally, the mitral valve is closed during ventricular systole, but with MR the valve allows approximately half of the ventricular volume back into the left atrium rather than forcing it forward into the aorta. The heart may be able to compensate for a period of time, but eventually cardiac output decreases and heart failure occurs. Additionally, the increase in pulmonary vascular volume causes pulmonary hypertension (see p. 40).

ASSESSMENT

Chronic indicators: A majority of patients with MR remain asymptomatic, although weakness and low exercise tolerance secondary to low cardiac output may be present. Anxiety and patient complaints of intermittent palpitations and chest discomfort also can occur.

Acute indicators: Fatigue, exhaustion, dyspnea, palpitations, and signs of pulmonary edema (see p. 76) and heart failure (see p. 54).

Physical assessment: Holosystolic murmur heard at the apex, radiating toward the axilla; possible presence of S_3 heart sounds; characteristic ejection click.

DIAGNOSTIC TESTS

1. *EKG:* Will show left atrial enlargement, possibly with atrial fibrillation.
2. *Chest x-ray:* Will demonstrate cardiomegaly with left ventricular and left atrial enlargement.
3. *Echocardiography:* Provides a definitive diagnosis and reveals severity of the disorder.
4. *Radionuclide imaging:* Often useful in follow-up; progressive increases in end-systolic or end-diastolic volumes can indicate a worsening condition.
5. *Angiography and ventriculogram:* Will show decreased contraction and dilatation.

MEDICAL MANAGEMENT AND SURGICAL INTERVENTIONS

1. Endocarditis prophylaxis with antibiotics: Initiated before major or minor surgical procedures, dental procedures, or any activity that may result in bacteremia.
2. Pharmacotherapy
   □ *Beta blockade:* To decrease cardiac workload and prevent chest pain and irregularities in rhythm.
   □ *Digitalis:* To increase strength of contraction.
   □ *Vasodilators:* To decrease afterload and increase cardiac output.
   □ *Diuretics:* To control fluid accumulation and prevent pulmonary edema.
   □ *Anticoagulants (heparin or warfarin):* To prevent embolization.
3. Diet: Low in sodium (see Table 11-3, p. 550).
4. Mitral valve replacement: If necessary (see "Mitral Stenosis," p. 65).
5. Medical treatment for heart failure: As appropriate. See p. 55.

NURSING DIAGNOSES AND INTERVENTIONS

Activity intolerance related to fatigue and weakness secondary to decreased cardiac output with valvular regurgitation

Desired outcome: Patient exhibits cardiac tolerance to increased activity levels as evidenced by HR ≤20 bpm over resting HR, systolic BP within 20 mm Hg of baseline systolic BP, and RR ≤24 breaths/min with normal depth and pattern (eupnea).

1. Assess patient's VS during activities, being alert to HR ≥20 bpm over resting HR, systolic BP >20 mm Hg over or under resting systolic BP, and RR >24 breaths/min with normal depth and pattern (eupnea).
2. Provide frequent rest periods, especially between care activities.
3. As necessary, assist patient with ADL to avoid shortness of breath.
4. Discuss ways to decrease energy output at home.
5. Progressively increase ambulation to patient's tolerance. Be alert to dyspnea, fatigue, and SOB with activity. Modify or restrict activities, as indicated. Also see the appendix for the following: **Potential activity intolerance,** p. 651, and **Potential for disuse syndrome,** p. 653.

See "Pulmonary Embolus" for **Potential for injury** related to increased risk of bleeding or hemorrhage secondary to anticoagulant therapy, p. 16. See "Coronary Artery Disease" for **Knowledge deficit:** Precautions and negative side effects of beta blockers, p. 50. See "Heart Failure" for **Fluid volume excess:** Edema, p. 56, **Knowledge deficit:** Precautions and negative side effects of diuretic therapy, p. 56, **Knowledge deficit:** Precautions and negative side effects of digitalis therapy, and **Knowledge deficit:** Precautions and negative side effects of vasodilators, p. 57. See "Mitral Stenosis" for **Knowl-**

edge deficit: Potential for development of endocarditis, p. 66, and **Potential for infection** (with concomitant endocarditis), p. 66. As appropriate, see nursing diagnoses and interventions in "Cardiac Catheterization," p. 82, "Cardiac Surgery," p. 84, and "Caring for Preoperative and Postoperative Patients," p. 637.

PATIENT-FAMILY TEACHING AND DISCHARGE PLANNING

See "Heart Failure," p. 57, and "Cardiac Surgery," p. 85, depending on patient's clinical course.

Aortic stenosis

Aortic stenosis is a condition that obstructs outflow from the left ventricle. It is either congenital or acquired and it results from adhesions and fusion of the valve cusps. Usually, normal left ventricular output can be maintained by compensatory left ventricular hypertrophy, but eventually progressive stenosis causes signs of low cardiac output, such as cool extremities, fluid accumulation, decreased urinary output, and cardiac failure.

ASSESSMENT

Signs and symptoms: Often, patients are asymptomatic until approximately age 60 when angina, orthostatic hypotention, syncope with exertion, orthopnea, signs of pulmonary edema, and cardiac failure are seen. Signs of left ventricular failure also may be present, including dyspnea and SOB.

Physical assessment: Decreased systolic BP, decreased pulse pressure (the difference between the systolic and diastolic pressures), increased left ventricular impulse ([PMI] palpable at fifth intercostal space, midclavicular line as a "lift" of the chest wall during ventricular systole), and systolic ejection murmur (best heard at the apex of the heart, second intercostal space).

DIAGNOSTIC TESTS

1. *EKG:* Will show presence of left ventricular hypertrophy as evidenced by left axis deviation and increased amplitude of QRS complexes.
2. *Chest x-ray:* May reveal aortic valve calcification.
3. *Cardiac catheterization with angiography:* Demonstrates degree of thickness of the stenotic valve and the pressure gradient across the valve.
4. *Echocardiography:* Allows visualization of the narrowed valve opening. Two-dimensional echocardiography can be helpful in determining severity of the stenosis.

MEDICAL MANAGEMENT AND SURGICAL INTERVENTIONS

1. Antibiotics: As a prophylaxis against endocarditis.
2. Treatment of congestive heart failure: If present. See "Medical Management and Surgical Interventions" in "Heart Failure," p. 55.
3. Aortic valve replacement: Appropriate for patients with left ventricular dysfunction and symptoms of decreased cardiac output and functional disability. Aortic valve replacement is performed using heart-lung bypass, and the patient is in ICU for 2-3 days postoperatively. **Note:** Artificial mechanical valves, as well as those obtained from animals may be used. Patients with artificial valves are maintained on lifetime anticoagulant therapy.
4. Percutaneous aortic valve valvuloplasty: An alternative to surgery for some patients. The procedure uses a balloon dilating catheter, which is advanced to the stenotic valve and then inflated to dilate the valve. The procedure is performed under local anesthetic in the cardiac catheterization laboratory.

NURSING DIAGNOSES AND INTERVENTIONS

See "Pulmonary Embolus" for **Potential for injury** related to increased risk of bleeding or hemorrhage secondary to anticoagulant therapy, p. 16. See "Coronary Artery Disease" for **Knowledge deficit:** Precautions and negative side effects of beta blockers, p. 50. See "Heart Failure" for **Fluid volume excess:** Edema, p. 56, **Knowledge deficit:** Precautions and negative side effects of diuretic therapy, p. 56, **Knowledge deficit:** Precautions and negative side effects of digitalis therapy, and **Knowledge deficit:** Precautions and negative side effects of vasodilators, p. 57. See "Mitral Stenosis" for **Decreased cardiac output,** p. 65, **Activity intolerance,** p. 66, **Knowledge deficit:** Potential for development of endocarditis, p. 66, and **Potential for infection** (with concomitant endocarditis), p. 66. As appropriate, see nursing diagnoses and interventions in "Cardiac Catheterization," p. 82, "Cardiac Surgery," p. 84, and "Caring for Preoperative and Postoperative Patients," p. 637.

PATIENT-FAMILY TEACHING AND DISCHARGE PLANNING

See "Heart Failure," p. 57, and "Cardiac Surgery," p. 85, depending on patient's clinical course.

Aortic regurgitation

Many disorders can cause aortic valve regurgitation, but the most common is rheumatic fever. The cusps of the valve become fibrotic and retract, preventing valve closure during diastole. Incompetence of this valve allows backward flow, which results in a large ventricular volume. If the condition develops slowly the patient remains asymptomatic longer because the left ventricle hypertrophies to accommodate a larger volume.

ASSESSMENT

Signs and symptoms: With slowly developing regurgitation, the patient can remain asymptomatic for years. When the heart begins to fail, signs associated with left ventricular failure develop, including dyspnea, orthopnea, decreasing BP, changes in mentation, peripheral vasoconstriction, and pulmonary edema.

Physical assessment: Widened aortic pulse pressure (the difference between systolic and diastolic pressures), low diastolic BP, high systolic BP until heart failure develops, low-pitched diastolic murmur located in the second intercostal space to the right of the sternum, tachycardia, crackles (rales), and increased pulmonary arterial pressures.

DIAGNOSTIC TESTS

1. *EKG:* Will demonstrate left axis deviation and left ventricular conduction defects with chronic aortic regurgitation. With acute regurgitation, nonspecific ST-segment changes or left ventricular hypertrophy will be seen.
2. *Chest x-ray:* Results depend on the severity and duration of the disorder, but it eventually demonstrates cardiac enlargement and left ventricular dilatation.
3. *Cardiac catheterization with angiography:* Useful in determining severity of the regurgitation.
4. *Echocardiography:* May identify the cause of regurgitation by revealing damaged cusps or vegetations caused by endocarditis.

MEDICAL MANAGEMENT AND SURGICAL INTERVENTIONS

1. Pharmacotherapy
   ☐ *Positive inotropic agents, such as digitalis:* To maintain ventricular function by increasing the strength of ventricular contractions.
   ☐ *Vasodilators:* To decrease afterload.

2. Treatment of heart failure: See "Heart Failure," p. 55.
3. Surgical interventions: Heart failure is not uncommon in patients with aortic regurgitation, even with aggressive medical treatment. Therefore aortic valve replacement is usually recommended. Indications for this surgery include chronic aortic regurgitation that has become symptomatic and ventricular dysfunction during exercise.

NURSING DIAGNOSES AND INTERVENTIONS

See "Pulmonary Embolus" for **Potential for injury** related to increased risk of bleeding or hemorrhage secondary to anticoagulant therapy, p. 16. See "Coronary Artery Disease" for **Knowledge deficit:** Precautions and negative side effects of beta blockers, p. 50. See "Heart Failure" for **Fluid volume excess:** Edema, p. 56, **Knowledge deficit:** Precautions and negative side effects of diuretic therapy, p. 56, **Knowledge deficit:** Precautions and negative side effects of digitalis therapy, and **Knowledge deficit:** Precautions and negative side effects of vasodilators, p. 57. See "Mitral Stenosis" for **Knowledge deficit:** Potential for development of endocarditis, p. 66, and **Potential for infection** (with concomitant endocarditis), p. 66. As appropriate, see nursing diagnoses and interventions in "Cardiac Catheterization," p. 82, "Cardiac Surgery," p. 84, and "Caring for Preoperative and Postoperative Patients," p. 637.

PATIENT-FAMILY TEACHING AND DISCHARGE PLANNING

See "Heart Failure," p. 57, and "Cardiac Surgery," p. 85, depending on patient's clinical course.

Section Four   CARDIOVASCULAR CONDITIONS SECONDARY TO OTHER DISEASE PROCESSES

Cardiac and noncardiac shock (circulatory failure)

A shock state exists when tissue perfusion decreases to the point of cellular metabolic dysfunction. Shock is classified according to the causative event.

Hematogenic (hemorrhagic or hypovolemic) shock: Occurs when blood volume is insufficient to meet metabolic needs of the tissues, for example, with severe hemorrhage.

Cardiogenic shock: Occurs when cardiac failure results in decreased tissue perfusion, such as in MI.

Neurogenic shock: Result of a neurologic event (e.g., head injury) that causes massive vasodilatation and decreased perfusion pressures.

Anaphylactic shock: A severe systemic response to an allergen (foreign protein), resulting in massive vasodilatation, decreased perfusion, decreased venous return, and subsequent decreased cardiac output.

Septic shock: Occurs when bacterial toxins cause an overwhelming systemic infection. Regardless of the cause, shock results in cellular hypoxia secondary to decreased perfusion and ultimately to cellular, tissue, and organ dysfunction. A prolonged shock state can result in death, so early recognition and intervention are essential.

ASSESSMENT

Early signs and symptoms: Cool, pale, and clammy skin; decreased pulse strength; dry and pale mucous membranes; restlessness; hyperventilation; anxiety; nausea; thirst; weakness.

Physical assessment: Rapid HR; decreased systolic BP and increased diastolic BP secondary to catecholamine (sympathetic nervous system) response.

T A B L E 2 - 4   Shock: systemic clinical signs

	Cardiogenic	Septic	Hypovolemic	Neurogenic	Anaphylactic
Cardio-vascular	↓ BP, ↑ HR, ↓ pulses	*Early:* ↑ BP ↑ pulses *Late:* ↓ BP ↓ pulses	↓ BP, ↑ HR Flat neck veins	Vasodilation, ↑ BP (early)	↓ BP, ↑ HR, ↓ pulses
Respiratory	Dyspnea, rales	*Early:* ↑ RR *Late:* ↓ RR- Crackles	Lungs clear	Lungs clear	Dyspnea to air hunger; wheezes and complete obstruction
Neurologic	Confusion, lethargy, drowsiness	↓ LOC	↓ LOC	Normal or ↓ LOC	↓ LOC
Renal	↓ Urinary output	↓ Urinary output	↓ Urinary output	Normal or ↓ urinary output	↓ Urinary output
Cutaneous	Cool skin	*Early:* warm *Late:* cool	Cool skin	Warm, secondary to vasodilation	Urticaria, angioedema

Late signs and symptoms: Decreased urinary output, hypothermia, drowsiness, diaphoresis, confusion, and lethargy, all of which can progress to a comatose state.

Physical assessment: Irregular HR; continually decreasing BP, usually with systolic pressure palpable at 60 mm Hg or less; rapid and possibly irregular RR.

DIAGNOSTIC TESTS

Diagnosis usually is based on the presenting symptoms and clinical signs.
1. *ABG values:* Will reveal metabolic acidosis caused by anaerobic metabolism.
2. *Serial measurement of urinary output:* Less than 30 ml/hr is indicative of decreased perfusion and decreased renal function.
3. *BUN & creatinine:* Increase with decreased renal perfusion.
4. *Blood glucose:* Hyperglycemia may be present owing to epinephrine-induced glycogenolysis.

For septic shock
5. *Serial creatinine and BUN levels:* To assess for potential renal complications and dysfunction.
6. *Serum electrolyte levels:* Identify renal complications and dysfunctions as evidenced by hyperkalemia and hypernatremia.
7. *Blood culture:* To identify the causative organism.
8. *WBC and ESR:* Elevated in the presence of infection.

For hematogenic shock
9. *CBC:* Hematocrit and hemoglobin will be decreased because of decreased blood volume.

For anaphylactic shock

10. *WBC count:* Will reveal increased eosinophils, a type of granulocyte that appears in the presence of allergic reaction.

MEDICAL MANAGEMENT

Interventions are determined by clinical presentation and severity of the shock state. Patients are transferred to ICU to assess severity of the shock state and closely monitor status.

For cardiogenic shock

1. **Vascular support:** Intraaortic balloon counterpulsation is used to augment perfusion pressures.
2. **Optimize blood volume:** Either with volume expanders such as dextran or with diuretics if fluid overload is the problem.
3. **Pharmacotherapy**
   □ *Sympathomimetics:* For example, dopamine infusion at low doses (2-5 μg/kg/min) to increase renal perfusion and decrease systemic vasoconstriction. Moderate doses (5-8 μg/kg/min) help strengthen cardiac contraction.
   □ *Vasopressors:* To stimulate vasoconstriction. Usually they are used in conjunction with vasodilators to achieve the desired effect without the negative effects of one drug alone. Levophed, for example, may be used in combination with regitine, which counteracts the severe end-organ and peripheral damage caused by the severe vasoconstriction associated with Levophed.
   □ *Vasodilators:* To increase peripheral perfusion and reduce afterload vasoconstriction caused by the vasopressors (see above).
   □ *Osmotic diuretics:* To increase renal blood flow.
4. **Oxygen support:** As needed, to increase oxygen availability to the tissues.
5. **Correction of acidosis and electrolyte imbalances.**

For anaphylactic shock

1. **Pharmacotherapy**
   □ *Epinephrine (0.5 ml, 1:1000 in 10 ml saline):* To promote vasoconstriction and decrease the allergic response by counteracting vasodilatation caused by histamine release.
   □ *Bronchodilators:* To relieve bronchospasm.
   □ *Antihistamines:* To prevent relapse and relieve urticaria.
   □ *Hydrocortisone:* For its antiinflammatory effects.
   □ *Vasopressors:* May be necessary for reversing shock state.
2. **Oxygen and airway support:** As needed.

For hemorrhagic shock

1. **Control of hemorrhage.** If possible, depending on the location and cause.
2. **Fresh whole blood:** To increase oxygen delivery at the tissue level when >2 L of blood have been lost.
3. **Albumin or dextran:** Sometimes used to increase vascular volume.
4. **Ringer's solution:** Often used as an isotonic solution to replace electrolytes and ions lost with bleeding in hemorrhagic shock.

For septic shock

1. **Antibiotic therapy:** Specific to causative organism.
2. **Fluid administration:** To maintain adequate vascular volume.
3. **Vasopressors:** May be required to reverse vasodilatation and maintain perfusion.
4. **Positive inotropic drugs:** To augment cardiac contractility.

NURSING DIAGNOSES AND INTERVENTIONS

Alteration in tissue perfusion: Peripheral, cardiopulmonary, cerebral, and renal, related to impaired circulation secondary to decreased circulating blood volume

Desired outcome: Patient has adequate perfusion as evidenced by palpable peripheral pulses (>2+ on a 0-4+ scale); brisk capillary refill (<3 seconds); BP within patient's normal range; CVP ≥4 cm H_2O; HR regular and ≤100 bpm; orientation to person, place, and time; and urine output ≥30 ml/hr.

1. Assess and document peripheral pulses. Report significant findings, such as coolness and pallor of the extremities, decreased amplitude of pulses, and delayed capillary refill.
2. Monitor BP at frequent intervals; be alert to readings >20 mm Hg below patient's normal or to other indicators of hypotension, such as dizziness, altered mentation, or decreased urinary output.
3. If hypotension is present, place patient in a supine position to promote venous return. Remember that BP must be at least 80/60 mm Hg for adequate coronary and renal artery perfusion.
4. Monitor CVP (if line is inserted) to determine adequacy of venous return and blood volume; 4-10 cm H_2O usually is considered an adequate range. Values near zero can indicate hypovolemia, especially when associated with decreased urinary output, vasoconstriction, and increased HR.
5. Observe for indicators of decreased cerebral perfusion, such as restlessness, confusion, and decreased LOC. If positive indicators are present, protect patient from injury by raising side rails and placing bed in its lowest position. Reorient patient as indicated.
6. Monitor for indicators of decreased coronary artery perfusion, such as chest pain and an irregular HR.
7. Monitor urinary output hourly. Notify MD if it is <30 ml/hr in the presence of adequate intake. Check weight daily for evidence of gain.
8. Monitor lab results for elevated BUN and creatinine levels; report increases.
9. Monitor serum electrolyte values for evidence of imbalances, particularly sodium and potassium. Be alert to signs of hyperkalemia, such as increased serum levels, muscle weakness, hyporeflexia, and irregular HR. Also monitor for signs of hypernatremia, such as increased serum levels, fluid retention, and edema. For more information, see "Fluid and Electrolyte Disturbances," p. 546.
10. Administer fluids as prescribed to increase vascular volume. The type and amount of fluid will depend on the type of shock and the patient's clinical situation.
    □ *Cardiogenic shock:* Fluids probably will be limited to prevent overload, yet dehydration must be avoided to ensure support of vascular space and cardiac muscle.
    □ *Hypovolemic shock:* The amount lost is replaced. As much as 1,000 ml/hr of Ringer's solution may be administered if volume loss is severe. Most often, this includes blood replacement.
    □ *Septic shock:* Ringer's solution, plasma, and blood are administered.

Impaired gas exchange related to decreased diffusion of oxygen secondary to decreased respiratory muscle function occurring with altered metabolism

Desired outcome: Patient has adequate gas exchange as evidenced by RR ≤20 breaths/min with normal depth and pattern (eupnea), oxygen saturation ≥95%, Pao_2 ≥80 mm Hg, $Paco_2$ ≤45 mm Hg, and pH ≥7.35.

1. Monitor respirations q30min; note and report presence of tachypnea or dyspnea.
2. Teach patient to breathe slowly and deeply to promote oxygenation.
3. Ensure that the patient has a patent airway; suction secretions as needed to assist with gas exchange.
4. Administer oxygen as prescribed.
5. Monitor ABG results. Be alert to and report presence of hypoxemia (decreased oxygen saturation, decreased Pao_2), hypercapnia (increased $Paco_2$), and acidosis (decreased pH, increased $Paco_2$). Report significant findings to MD.

See psychosocial nursing diagnoses and interventions in "Caring for Patients with Cancer and Other Life-Disrupting Illnesses," p. 690.

PATIENT-FAMILY TEACHING AND DISCHARGE PLANNING

For interventions, see discussion with patient's primary diagnosis.

Cardiac arrest

Note: *This section is intended as an overview only. In the event of a cardiac arrest, the reader should refer to cardiac arrest procedures established by the institution.*

Cardiac arrest occurs when the heart stops beating, or when the contraction is ineffective (such as in ventricular tachycardia or ventricular fibrillation) in maintaining cardiac output. Many conditions can precipitate cardiac arrest, including myocardial infarction, heart failure, shock state, severe electrolyte disturbances, drowning, electrocution, drug overdose, and hypoxia. Often, the events that precipitate cardiac arrest occur in a "vicious cycle." For example, a cardiac rhythm disturbance leads to decreased cardiac output, which leads to decreased tissue perfusion, which results in hypoxia, which leads to more rhythm disturbances, and the cycle goes on. Management of the pre-arrest stage is directed toward breaking this cycle and correcting the condition to prevent cardiac arrest. To help prevent an arrest from occurring, accurate and prompt nursing assessment is crucial. However, an arrest can occur without prior warning. This is an emergency situation, which requires *immediate* medical intervention.

ASSESSMENT

Signs and symptoms: Loss of consciousness—inability to arouse the patient by shaking and shouting.

Physical assessment: Absence of carotid pulse; loss of audible or palpable BP; and usually, absence of respirations.

MEDICAL MANAGEMENT

1. **Management of pre-arrest phase:** Includes treatment for shock, oxygen therapy or airway support, transfer to ICU, antiarrhythmic drugs, and pain relief.
2. **Basic life support:** Cardiopulmonary rescusitation (CPR) to maintain ventilation and circulation until normal cardiac rhythm is restored.
3. **Ventilation:** To prevent hypoxia and subsequent anaerobic metabolism. The method depends on the patient's clinical presentation. Mouth-to-mask breathing, oxygen mask with 100% oxygen if the patient is breathing, oral or nasal airways, endotracheal intubation, and manual ventilation may be used. **Note:** Mouth-to-mask breathing is the preferred method of providing adjunct ventilation (rather than mouth-to-mouth). It is the nurse's responsibility to ensure availability of a mask prior to an emergency and know how to use it properly.
4. **Closed chest compressions:** An adjunct to circulation. If done properly, cardiac compression can provide 25%-30% of the normal cardiac output.
5. **IV access line:** In arrest situations, it is often difficult to establish a peripheral IV line because of vascular collapse or constriction. In addition, with decreased peripheral perfusion, absorption of drugs can be variable. The MD may instead insert a central venous catheter into the femoral, jugular, or subclavian vein.
6. **Treatment of cardiac rhythm abnormalities:** Lidocaine to suppress ventricular ectopic beats; atropine for bradycardias; defibrillation or epinephrine to combat ventricular fibrillation.
7. **Stimulation of effective cardiac contractions**
   - □ *Inotropic drugs:* To increase strength of cardiac contractions.
   - □ *Maintenance of acid-base and electrolyte balance:* Disorders such as acidosis, hyperkalemia, hypocalcemia, and hypomagnesemia are identified and corrected. For treatment information, see "Fluid and Electrolyte Disturbances," p. 546, and "Acid-Base Disorders," p. 563.

8. Restoration of effective ventilation and circulation and stable cardiac rhythm before transfer to ICU.

NURSING DIAGNOSES AND INTERVENTIONS

Decreased cardiac output related to ineffective ventricular contractions secondary to cardiac arrest

Desired outcome: Patient has adequate cardiac output as evidenced by systolic BP >90 mm Hg, HR 60-100 bpm with normal rhythm, peripheral pulses >2+ on a 0-4+ scale, equal radial/apical pulse, RR 12-20 breaths/min with normal depth and pattern (eupnea).

1. Ensure adequate oxygenation by hyperextending the neck of stuporous patients and providing oxygen support as prescribed.
2. Maintain or establish an IV line. Typically, 5% dextrose in water (D_5W) is run at a rapid rate unless otherwise prescribed.
3. Assess and document BP at frequent intervals (q5-15min) and report changes in pressure to MD immediately.
4. Assess and document HR; report irregularities or apical/radial deficit (e.g., apical rate 80 bpm/radial rate 50 bpm).
5. Administer antiarrythmic agents such as quinidine and procainamide and inotropic drugs such as dopamine hydrochloride as prescribed.
6. Maintain closed chest compressions until cardiac rhythm is restored.
7. Observe ventilatory status and be alert to indicators of hypoxia or inadequate ventilation, such as changes in breathing rhythm, adventitious breath sounds, or breath sounds that are not equal in both lungs. Be alert to ABG results that signal hypoxemia, hypercapnia, or acidosis, such as low pH (<7.35), low Pao_2 (<80 mm Hg), decreased oxygen saturation (<90%-95%), and high $Paco_2$ (>45 mm Hg). Report significant findings.
8. Monitor peripheral perfusion (femoral pulses). Be alert to and report decreasing amplitude of pulse pressures.

See psychosocial nursing diagnoses and interventions in "Caring for Patients with Cancer and Other Life-Disrupting Illnesses," p. 690.

PATIENT-FAMILY TEACHING AND DISCHARGE PLANNING

See discussion under patient's primary diagnosis.

Pulmonary edema

Acute pulmonary edema is an emergency situation in which hydrostatic pressure in the pulmonary vessels is greater than the vascular colloid osmotic pressure that holds fluid in the vessels. As a result, fluid floods the alveoli. When the alveoli contain fluid, their ability to participate in gas exchange is reduced and hypoxia will occur. The most common cause or precipitating factor in acute pulmonary edema is acute left ventricular failure, or an acute exacerbation of congestive heart failure. Other causes include hypertension, volume overload, or such nervous system disorders as head trauma and grand mal seizures, which result in sympathetic nervous system hyperactivity and produce shifts in blood volume to the pulmonary system to increase pulmonary capillary pressure. Pulmonary edema can develop suddenly, or it can develop slowly over a period of hours or days. Prompt determination of cause and treatment are critical.

ASSESSMENT

Signs and symptoms: Anxiety, restlessness, frothy and blood-tinged sputum, orthopnea, extreme dyspnea. The patient exhibits "air hunger" and may thrash about and describe a sensation of drowning.

Physical assessment: Crackles (rales), tachycardia, tachypnea, engorged neck veins, S_3 heart sound, and murmurs (with valve dysfunction, such as mitral regurgitation).

History of: Recent myocardial infarction or "heart problems" in the past; hypertension; fluid overload, often from IV fluids.

DIAGNOSTIC TESTS

1. *ABG values:* Will reveal hypoxemia.
2. *Chest x-ray:* Will delineate interstitial fluid and may reveal an increased heart size or pericardial tamponade (fluid accumulation in the pericardial space, resulting in compression of the heart muscle and interference with normal cardiac function).
3. *EKG:* May reveal evidence of old or new MI.

MEDICAL MANAGEMENT

1. Transfer to ICU.
2. Oxygen: High flow either by non-rebreathing mask or endotracheal intubation and mechanical ventilation.
3. High-Fowler's position: To decrease venous return.
4. Morphine sulfate: In small increments (2-4 mg IV slowly) to decrease anxiety, work of breathing, and sympathetic vasoconstriction. **Note:** Morphine is avoided when pulmonary edema is associated with bronchial asthma, COPD, or CO_2 retention.
5. Diuretics: To reduce fluid volume and decrease venous return to the heart. Usually they are injected over a 2-minute period.
6. Rotating tourniquets: Occasionally used to decrease venous return. Wide, soft rubber tubing or BP cuffs are applied in a rotating system to three of the four extremities and inflated to approximately 10 mm Hg below diastolic pressure. This allows arterial flow but impedes venous return from the extremity. Every 15 minutes the tourniquets are rotated so that each extremity is relieved of a tourniquet one out of every four rotations.
7. Other pharmacotherapy
   □ *Vasodilators, such as nitroprusside:* May be used to reduce systemic and venous pressures. Nitroglycerine (0.3-0.6 mg sublingual or transdermal) also may be given for venodilatation and to decrease preload.
   □ *Digitalis:* To decrease ventricular rate and strengthen contractions for patients who are not already using the drug.
   □ *Theophylline:* To reduce bronchodilatation if bronchospasm further complicates the pulmonary edema.
8. Identification and treatment of precipitating factors.

NURSING DIAGNOSES AND INTERVENTIONS

Fear related to life-threatening situation

Desired outcomes: Patient and significant others communicate fears and concerns. Patient relates the attainment of increasing physical and psychologic comfort.

1. Provide the opportunity for patient and significant others to express feelings and fears. Be reassuring and supportive.
2. Help make the patient as comfortable as possible with prompt pain relief and positioning, typically high Fowler's.
3. Keep the environment as calm and quiet as possible.
4. Explain all treatment modalities, especially those that may be uncomfortable (e.g., oxygen face mask and rotating tourniquets).
5. Remain with patient if at all possible, providing emotional support both for the patient and significant others.

Alteration in tissue perfusion: Cardiopulmonary, peripheral, and cerebral, related to impaired circulation secondary to decreased cardiac output

Desired outcome: Patient has adequate tissue perfusion as evidenced by BP within 20 mm Hg of patient's baseline, HR ≤100 bpm with regular rhythm, RR ≤20 breaths/min with normal depth and pattern (eupnea), brisk capillary refill (<3 seconds), urine output ≥30 ml/hr, and orientation to person, place, and time.

1. Monitor BP q15min, or more frequently if unstable. Be alert to decreases >20 mm Hg over patient's baseline or associated changes, such as dizziness and altered mentation.
2. Check pulse rate q15-30min. Monitor for irregularities, increased HR, or skipped beats, which can signal decompensation and decreased function.
3. Monitor for indicators of peripheral vasoconstriction (from sympathetic nervous system compensation), such as cool extremities, pallor, and diaphoresis. Evaluate capillary refill. Optimally, pink color should return within 1-3 seconds after applying pressure to the nail beds.
4. Monitor for indicators of decreased cerebral perfusion, such as restlessness, anxiety, confusion, lethargy, stupor, and coma. Institute safety precautions accordingly.
5. Administer inotropic drugs such as digitalis as prescribed.
6. Administer vasodilators as prescribed, and monitor the effects closely. Be alert to problems such as hypotension and irregular heart beats.
7. Implement measures for decreasing venous return and increasing peripheral perfusion, such as placing patient in high-Fowler's position.

Impaired gas exchange related to decreased diffusion of oxygen secondary to fluid accumulation in the alveoli

Desired outcome: Patient has adequate gas exchange as evidenced by RR ≤20 breaths/ min with normal depth and pattern (eupnea), normal breath sounds (see p. 713) and skin color, HR ≤100 bpm, Pao_2 ≥80 mm Hg, and $Paco_2$ ≤45 mm Hg.

1. Auscultate lung fields for breath sounds; be alert to the presence of crackles (rales), which signal alveolar fluid congestion.
2. Assist patient into high-Fowler's position to decrease work of breathing and enhance gas exchange.
3. Teach patient to take slow, deep breaths to increase oxygenation.
4. Administer oxygen as prescribed. If ABGs are drawn, monitor the results for the presence of hypoxemia (decreased Pao_2) and hypercapnia (increased $Paco_2$).
5. Be alert to signs of increasing respiratory distress: increased RR, gasping for air, cyanosis, or rapid HR.
6. Administer diuretics as prescribed. Monitor potassium levels because of the potential for hypokalemia in patients taking certain diuretics. See "Hypokalemia," p. 555.
7. As indicated, have emergency equipment (e.g., airway and manual rescusitator) available and functional.

Fluid volume excess: Edema related to retention secondary to decreased cardiac output

Desired outcome: Patient is normovolemic as evidenced by balanced I&O, stable weight, normal breath sounds, urine output ≥30 ml/hr, and edema ≤1+ on a 0-4+ scale.

1. Closely monitor I&O, including insensible losses from diaphoresis and respirations.
2. Record weight daily, and report steady gains.
3. Assess for edema (interstitial fluids), especially in dependent areas, such as the ankles and sacrum.
4. Assess the respiratory system for indicators of fluid extravasation, such as crackles (rales) or pink-tinged, frothy sputum.
5. Monitor IV rate of flow to prevent volume overload. Use a commercial infusion controller, if possible.
6. Unless contraindicated, provide ice chips or popsicles to help patient control thirst. Record the amount on the I&O record.
7. Administer diuretics as prescribed, and record patient's response.

See "Coronary Artery Disease" for **Knowledge deficit:** Precautions and negative side effects of nitrates, p. 49. See "Heart Failure" for **Knowledge deficit:** Precautions and negative side effects of vasodilators, p. 57, **Knowledge deficit:** Precautions and negative side effects of digitalis therapy, p. 56, and **Knowledge deficit:** Precautions and negative side effects of diuretic therapy, p. 56. See psychosocial nursing diagnoses and interventions in "Caring for Patients with Cancer and Other Life-Disrupting Illnesses," p. 690.

PATIENT-FAMILY TEACHING AND DISCHARGE PLANNING

See the patient's primary diagnosis.

Section Five   SPECIAL CARDIAC PROCEDURES

Pacemakers

A mechanical pacemaker delivers an electrical impulse to the heart to stimulate contraction when the heart's natural pacemakers fail to maintain normal rhythm. Patients for whom pacemakers are indicated have a history of syncopal episodes, dizziness, intolerance to exercise, blacking out, or an episode of cardiac arrest. When patients suffer from temporary or transient rhythm disturbances, such as severe bradycardia or a conduction block, a temporary pacemaker can be inserted. Temporary pacemakers are seen most often in ICUs and on an emergency basis. The lead wire is inserted through a peripheral vein into the right side of the heart where it lodges in the tissue to deliver the electrical impulse.

Some patients who have had temporary pacemakers inserted are observed for the possibility of permanent pacing. Permanent pacemakers are indicated for patients with a complete or incomplete conduction block that recurs or is not transient. Stokes-Adams syncope (an intermittent heart block), symptomatic bradycardia, and uncontrollable tachydysrhythmias also are indications for permanent pacing. The pacemaker is implanted subcutaneously under local anesthesia, and it is completely internal.

UNIVERSAL CODING

The increasing complexity of pacemakers has led to the development of a five-letter code for universal language by the International Commission on Heart Disease. However, the first three letters remain the basis for classification.
1. First letter: Chamber that is paced.
   □ V: Ventricle.
   □ A: Atrium.
   □ D: Dual/both.
2. Second letter: Chamber that is sensed.
   □ V: Ventricle.
   □ A: Atrium.
   □ D: Dual/both.
   □ O: None.
3. Third letter: Mode of response.
   □ T: Triggered by ventricular activity.
   □ I: Inhibited by ventricular activity.
   □ D: Dual/both — atrial triggered, ventricular inhibited.
   □ O: Neither (works continuously).
   □ R: Reverse. Pacing occurs when tachycardia is sensed.
4. Fourth letter: Programmable functions.
   □ P: Programmable.
   □ M: Multiprogrammable.
   □ O: None.

5. Fifth letter: Special antitachycardia functions.
   □ B: Burst ventricular pacing to break ventricular tachycardia.
   □ N: Silent during normal rates.
   □ S: Scans and delivers progressive stimuli.
   □ E: Externally activated.

PACEMAKER TYPES

1. **Asynchronous or fixed rate:** Discharges an impulse to the ventricle at a prescribed rate, without a sensing mechanism. Asynchronous or fixed-rate pacemakers can be VOO, AOO, or DOO.
2. **Ventricular demand:** Senses intrinsic cardiac function and discharges only when the ventricle fails to do so (at the prescribed rate). This type of pacemaker is coded VVI or VVT.
3. **Synchronous:** Senses the activity in the atrium and stimulates the ventricle. This type of pacemaker is coded VAT.
4. **Sequential:** Senses the activity in the atrium and ventricle and stimulates both sequentially if no intrinsic activity occurs. This type of pacemaker is coded DVI, VDD, or DDD.

   Temporary pacemakers often are inserted in the ICU where the patient can be monitored continuously. Permanent pacemakers are implanted in the operating room, after which the patient is transferred to the telemetry unit for 24-48 hours of close monitoring. After implantation, physical activity, especially arm movement, is restricted for approximately 48 hours to allow the lead and pacemaker to affix and imbed in the ventricular wall. A sling or other immobilizer may be used to restrict movement of the affected arm and shoulder.

NURSING DIAGNOSES AND INTERVENTIONS

Knowledge deficit: Pacemaker insertion procedure and pacemaker function

Desired outcome: Patient verbalizes knowledge of the insertion procedure and function of the pacemaker.

1. Assess patient's knowledge of the insertion procedure and function of the pacemaker. As appropriate, describe the procedure and explain that the pacemaker stimulates the patient's own heart to beat when the heart becomes lazy or slows down.
2. Begin a teaching program specific to the patient's rhythm disorder and type of pacemaker inserted, including normal function of the heart, patient's disorder of rhythm that requires a pacemaker, and how the patient's pacemaker works.
3. Reinforce explanation by MD of the length of time of the procedure, use of local anesthetic, and postprocedure care.

Potential alteration in tissue perfusion: Peripheral and cardiopulmonary, related to impaired circulation secondary to pacemaker malfunction

Desired outcome: Patient has adequate perfusion as evidenced by BP within 20 mm Hg of patient's baseline BP, peripheral pulses >2+ on a 0-4+ scale, apical/radial pulse regular, equal, and at rate ≥ than that established for pacemaker.

1. Monitor perfusion by assessing BP at frequent intervals.
2. Assess rate and regularity of apical and radial pulses. At minimum, it should be the rate established for the pacemaker.
3. Assess for apical/radial deficit, which if present indicates that the heart is mechanically contracting but there is no peripheral perfusion (e.g. if the apical pulse rate is 80 bpm with auscultation but the palpable radial pulse is 42 bpm).
4. Be alert to pulse irregularity, which can signal pacemaker malfunction or decreasing patient response.
5. Ensure that patient maintains strict bed rest for 48 hours postoperatively to prevent pacemaker dislodgement.

6. Maintain patient's arm in a sling or other immobilizer to prevent pacemaker dislodgement caused by arm movement.
7. Alert MD to significant findings.

Pain related to pacemaker insertion

Desired outcome: Patient's subjective evaluation of pain improves, as documented by a pain scale.

1. Assess for pain, using a pain scale of 0 (no pain) to 10, and medicate as prescribed. Evaluate relief obtained, using the pain scale.
2. Assist patient with positioning for comfort, using pillows for support as needed.
3. Adjust the sling or shoulder support to avoid incisional pressure and other pressure areas.

PATIENT-FAMILY TEACHING AND DISCHARGE PLANNING

Provide patient and significant others with verbal and written information for the following:
1. Activity restrictions as directed by MD, such as heavy lifting, and instructions about the amount and type of exercise allowed. Resumption of sexual activity probably will not be affected, but will depend on patient's underlying condition.
2. Technique for measuring radial pulse.
3. Signs and symptoms that necessitate medical attention, such as decreasing pulse rate, irregular pulse, dizziness, passing out, and signs of infection.
4. Necessity of follow-up care, usually at pacemaker clinic; confirm date of next appointment. Telephonic monitoring of pacemakers is used frequently as a method of assessing patients between visits. If this method is to be used, inform patient about this type of monitoring.
5. Medications, including drug name, purpose, dosage, schedule, precautions, and potential side effects.
6. Importance of using caution around strong magnetic fields, which can alter the function of the pacemaker (this is not a problem for newer pacemakers). **Note:** Strong magnetic fields such as microwave ovens can convert some pacemakers to a "fixed-rate" mode. Once the patient moves away from the magnetic field, the pacemaker will return to the normal programmed function.
7. Expected life of the pacemaker battery, which is approximate and can vary from 5-10 years, depending on the type of battery. It is important to know the manufacturer of the specific pacemaker because some start to show signs of battery failure 2 years before absolute failure.

Cardiac catheterization

Cardiac catheterization is an invasive diagnostic procedure used to assess the extent of coronary artery disease or valvular heart disease. It involves the insertion of a radiopaque catheter through a peripheral vessel into the heart. *With left heart catheterization,* the catheter is advanced retrogradely, usually through the femoral artery, into the left ventricle and the coronary arteries. Subsequently, pressure measurements are made and the amount of cardiac output is determined to diagnose valvular stenosis and resistance to blood flow. Then dye is injected so that the heart structures, including ventricular chambers, coronary arteries, great vessels, and valves, can be visualized with fluoroscopy. *Right heart catheterization* involves advancement of a catheter from a peripheral vein into the right side of the heart to the pulmonary artery. This catheter measures pulmonary vascular pressures.

Associated procedures may include *electrophysiologic studies (EPS)* to assess conduction system abnormalities and ectopic (irregular) beats. If indicated, *transvenous intracardiac pacing wires* also may be inserted to assess conduction defects and determine the exact location of the disorder. Another procedure performed in the cardiac catheterization laboratory is the *intracoronary injection of streptokinase,* a therapeutic measure used to dissolve a clot or thrombus that is occluding a coronary artery. This procedure restores circulation to the myocardial muscle distal to the occlusion.

Patients are sedated before cardiac catheterization and given a local anesthetic so that they can be awake to alert the MD to any chest pain and cooperate with position changes. Usually, cardiac catheterization is an elective, scheduled procedure, but it also might be performed in emergency situations.

Percutaneous transluminal coronary angioplasty (PTCA): A treatment similar to cardiac catheterization that offers an alternative to cardiac surgery for some patients with coronary artery occlusions and disease. After basic procedures (e.g., coronary artery visualization) are performed, a balloon catheter is inserted until it is positioned at the point of stenosis. The balloon is then inflated in increments of pressure to compress the plaque and allow distal perfusion.

Laser angioplasty: A newer treatment for some patients with coronary artery occlusions. It is similar to cardiac catheterization and involves application of a laser beam to the occlusion or lesion in the coronary artery to ablate the lesion and allow reperfusion.

NURSING DIAGNOSES AND INTERVENTIONS

Knowledge deficit: Catheterization procedure and postcatheterization regimen

Desired outcome: Patient verbalizes knowledge of the catheterization procedure and postcatheterization regimen.

1. Assess patient's knowledge of the catheterization procedure. As appropriate, reinforce MD's explanation of the procedure, and answer any questions or concerns the patient and significant others have. If possible, arrange for an orientation visit to the catheterization laboratory before the procedure.
2. Before the cardiac catheterization, have the patient practice techniques (e.g., Valsalva maneuver, coughing, and deep breathing) that will be used during the catheterization.
3. Explain that after the procedure bed rest will be required, and that VS, circulation, and the insertion site will be checked at frequent intervals to ensure integrity. In addition, explain that sandbags may be used over the insertion site, and that flexing of the insertion site (arm or groin) is contraindicated to prevent bleeding.
4. Stress the importance of reporting signs and symptoms of hemorrhage, hematoma formation, or embolization promptly.

Potential alteration in tissue perfusion: Peripheral, cardiopulmonary, and cerebral, related to impaired circulation secondary to the catheterization procedure

Desired outcome: Patient has adequate perfusion as evidenced by HR regular and within 20 bpm of baseline HR, apical/radial pulse equality, BP within 20 mm Hg of baseline BP, peripheral pulses >2+ on a 0-4+ scale, warmth and normal color in the extremities, and urine output ≥30 ml/hr.

1. Monitor BP q15min until stable on three successive checks, q2h for the next 12 hours, and q4h thereafter. If the systolic pressure drops 20 mm Hg below previous recordings, lower the head of the bed and notify MD. **Note:** If the insertion site was the antecubital space, measure BP in the unaffected arm.
2. Be alert to and report indicators of decreased perfusion, including cool extremities, cyanosis, decreased LOC, and SOB.
3. Monitor patient's HR, and notify MD if dysrhythmias occur. If the patient is not on a cardiac monitor, auscultate apical and radial pulses with every BP check, and report irregularities or apical/radial discrepancies.

Potential fluid volume deficit related to risk of hemorrhage or hematoma formation secondary to arterial puncture

Desired outcomes: Patient is normovolemic as evidenced by HR ≤100 bpm, BP ≥90/60 mm Hg (or within 20 mm Hg of baseline range), and orientation to person, place, and time. The patient's dressing is dry and there is absence of swelling at the puncture site.

1. Be alert to indicators of shock or hemorrhage, such as a decrease in BP, increase in pulse rate, and decreasing LOC.
2. Inspect dressing on the groin or antecubital space for presence of frank bleeding or hematoma formation (fluctuating swelling).
3. Monitor peripheral perfusion and be alert to decreased amplitude or absence of distal pulses, delayed capillary refill, coolness of the extremities, and pallor, which can signal embolization or hemorrhagic shock.
4. To minimize the risk of bleeding, caution patient about flexing the elbow or hip for 6-8 hours, or as prescribed.
5. If bleeding occurs, maintain pressure at the insertion site as prescribed. Typically, this is done with a pressure dressing or a 2½-5 pound sandbag.

Potential alteration in tissue perfusion: Peripheral, related to impaired circulation secondary to embolization

Desired outcome: Patient has adequate perfusion in the involved extremity as evidenced by peripheral pulses in involved extremity >2+ on a 0-4+ scale; normal color, sensation, and temperature in the involved extremity; and brisk capillary refill (<3 seconds).

1. Assess peripheral perfusion by palpating peripheral pulses q15min for 30 minutes, then q30min for 1 hour, then qh for 2 hours, or per protocol.
2. Monitor for and report any indicators of embolization in the involved limb, such as faintness or absence of pulse, coolness of extremity, mottling, decreased capillary refill, cyanosis, and complaints of numbness, tingling, and pain at the insertion site. Instruct patient to report any of these indicators promptly.
3. If there is *no* evidence of an embolus or thrombus formation, instruct patient to move fingers or toes and rotate wrist or ankle to promote circulation.
4. Ensure that patient maintains bed rest for 4-6 hours, or as prescribed.

Potential alteration in tissue perfusion: Renal, related to impaired circulation secondary to decreased cardiac output or reaction to contrast dye

Desired outcome: Patient has adequate renal perfusion as evidenced by urinary output ≥30 ml/hr, good skin turgor, and moist mucous membranes.

1. Because contrast dye for cardiac catheterization may cause osmotic diuresis, monitor for indicators of dehydration, such as poor skin turgor, dry mucous membranes, and high urine specific gravity.
2. Monitor I&O. Notify MD if urinary output is <30 ml/hr in the presence of an adequate intake.
3. If urinary output is insufficient despite adequate intake, restrict fluids. Be alert to and report indicators of fluid overload, such as crackles (rales) on auscultation of lung fields, distended neck veins, and SOB. Notify MD of significant findings.
4. If patient does not exhibit signs of cardiac or renal failure, encourage daily intake of 2-3 L of fluids, or as prescribed, to flush the contrast dye out of the system.

See "Coronary Artery Disease" for **Pain** related to angina, p. 47, **Knowledge deficit:** Precautions and negative side effects of nitrates, p. 49, and **Knowledge deficit:** Precautions and negative side effects of beta blockers, p. 50.

PATIENT-FAMILY TEACHING AND DISCHARGE PLANNING

Provide patient and significant others with verbal and written information for the following:

1. Use of nitroglycerine, including purpose, dosage, schedule, precautions, and potential side effects, such as headache and dizziness. Caution patient to avoid using nitroglycerine more frequently than prescribed and to notify MD if three tablets do not relieve pain.

2. Use of calcium antagonists, beta blockers, antiarrhythmic agents, and antihypertensive agents, including the drug name, purpose, dosage, schedule, precautions, and potential side effects. Advise patient about the importance of taking the medications regularly and not discontinuing them without MD approval.

3. Signs and symptoms necessitating immediate medical attention, including chest pain unrelieved by nitroglycerine, decreased exercise tolerance, increasing SOB, and loss of consciousness.

4. Activity and dietary limitations as prescribed.

5. Importance of follow-up with MD; confirm date and time of next appointment.

Cardiac surgery

Cardiac surgery is performed to correct a variety of heart disorders. For example, *coronary artery bypass grafting* (CABG) is a technique used to treat blocked coronary arteries; a portion of the saphenous vein or internal mammary artery is used to shunt blood around the blocked portions of arteries to maintain flow to the heart muscle. *Valve replacement*, another type of cardiac surgery, is performed for patients with valvular stenosis or valvular incompetence of the mitral, tricuspid, pulmonary, or aortic valve. Cardiac surgery is also performed to correct heart defects that are either acquired or congenital, such as ventricular aneurysm, ventricular or atrial septal defects, transposition of great vessels, and tetralogy of Fallot.

Unless an emergency occurs, patients usually are admitted to the hospital the day before surgery. Most institutions that perform cardiac surgery have special units called transitional care, special care, or "step-down" units where preoperative cardiac patients are admitted. After surgery, most patients are in an ICU for 24-72 hours and then transferred to a medical-surgical unit. However, this is highly variable and depends on the patient's postoperative course and need for close cardiac monitoring.

NURSING DIAGNOSES AND INTERVENTIONS

Knowledge deficit: Diagnosis, surgical procedure, preoperative routine, and postoperative course

Desired outcome: Patient verbalizes knowledge of the diagnosis, surgical procedure, and the preoperative and postoperative regimen.

1. Assess patient's level of knowledge pertaining to the diagnosis and surgical procedure, and provide information where necessary. Encourage questions, and allow time for verbalization of concerns and fears.

2. If appropriate for the patient, provide orientation to the ICU and equipment that will be used postoperatively.

3. Provide instructions for deep breathing and coughing in the preoperative teaching.

4. Reassure patient that postoperative discomfort will be relieved with medication.

5. Advise patient that in the immediate postoperative period, speaking will be impossible because of the presence of an endotracheal tube, which will assist with breathing. Also explain that a chest tube will be present. Teach patient how he or she will move, deep breathe, and cough with a chest tube in place. (Refer to Chapter 1 for care considerations for patients with chest tubes.)

Activity intolerance related to weakness secondary to cardiac surgery

Desired outcome: Patient exhibits cardiac tolerance to increasing levels of activity following cardiac surgery as evidenced by HR ≤120 bpm, systolic BP within 20 mm Hg of baseline systolic BP, and RR ≤24 breaths/min.

1. Monitor VS at frequent intervals and be alert to indicators of cardiac failure, including hypotension, tachycardia, crackles (rales), tachypnea, and decreased peripheral pulses. Notify MD of significant findings.

2. To help minimize myocardial oxygen consumption, ensure that the patient has frequent rest periods.

3. Assess perfusion to the brain by checking patient's orientation to time and place.

4. As prescribed, administer medications that decrease myocardial oxygen consumption, such as beta blockers or calcium antagonists.
5. Assist patient with ROM and other exercises, depending on tolerance and prescribed activity limitations. Consult with MD regarding patient's readiness to participate in exercises that require increased cardiac tolerance. For a discussion of in-bed exercises that may be used, see **Potential for activity intolerance** related to deconditioning secondary to prolonged bed rest, p. 651, and **Potential disuse syndrome,** p. 655.

See "Pulmonary Embolus" in Chapter 1 for **Potential for injury** related to increased risk of bleeding or hemorrhage secondary to anticoagulant therapy, p. 16. See "Coronary Artery Disease" for **Alteration in nutrition:** More than body requirements related to excessive intake of salt, calories, and fat, p. 49, and **Health-seeking behaviors:** Relaxation technique effective for stress reduction, p. 49. See "Atherosclerotic Arterial Occlusive Disease" for **Potential impairment of tissue perfusion:** Renal, p. 89. See "Caring for Preoperative and Postoperative Patients," p. 637, and **Potential alteration in tissue perfusion:** Peripheral, p. 655.

PATIENT-FAMILY TEACHING AND DISCHARGE PLANNING

Provide patient and significant others with verbal and written information for the following:
1. Medications, including drug name, dosage, schedule, purpose, precautions, and potential side effects.
2. Untoward symptoms requiring medical attention for patients taking warfarin, such as bleeding from the nose, hemoptysis, hematuria, melena, and excessive bruising. In addition, stress the following: Take warfarin at the same time every day; notify MD if *any* signs of bleeding occur; keep appointments for PT checks; avoid OTC medications unless approved by MD; carry a Medic-Alert bracelet or card; avoid constrictive or restrictive clothing; and use soft-bristled toothbrushes and electric razors.
3. Maintenance of low-sodium (see Table 11-3, p. 550), low-fat, low-cholesterol (see Table 2-2, p.48) diet.
4. Importance of pacing activities at home and allowing frequent rest periods.
5. Technique for assessing radial pulse, temperature, and weight, if these indicators require monitoring at home, and reporting significant changes to MD.
6. Introduction to local American Heart Association activities.
7. Telephone number of nurse available to discuss concerns and questions or clarify instructions that are unclear.
8. Importance of follow-up visits with MD; confirm date and time of next appointment.
9. Signs and symptoms that necessitate immediate medical attention: chest pain, dyspnea, SOB, weight gain, and decrease in exercise tolerance.
10. Activity restrictions (e.g., lifting ≥5-20 pounds, pushing, and pulling for at least 6 weeks); prescribed exercise program; and resumption of sexual activity, work, and driving a car, as directed.
11. Care of the incision site; importance of assessing for signs of infection, such as drainage, fever, persistent redness, and local warmth and tenderness.

Section Six DISORDERS OF THE PERIPHERAL VASCULAR SYSTEM

Atherosclerotic arterial occlusive disease

Arteriosclerosis is a normal aging process of changes occurring in the arteries, including thickening of the walls, loss of elasticity, increase in calcium deposits, and usually, an increase in external diameter and a decrease in internal diameter. In contrast, *atherosclerosis* refers to a pathologic process of focal changes in the arteries, usually involving the accumulation of lipids, carbohydrates, calcium, blood components, and fibrous tissue. Although the two processes differ, they usually occur simultaneously.

The process of atherosclerotic disease results in narrowing of the arterial lumen, which limits blood flow. Thrombosis or aneurysm can occur, depending on the reaction of the tissue that is supplied by the atherosclerotic vessels. Arterial occlusion and insufficiency are usually found in the lower extremities in patients over age 50. *Thromboangiitis obliterans* (Buerger's disease) is an arterial occlusive disease that differs from atherosclerosis in that there is recurrent arterial inflammation. The cause is unknown, but the risk factors appear to be the same as those for atherosclerosis. It usually occurs in individuals 20-35 years of age and begins in the small arteries. *Raynaud's disease* is another type of impairment that tends to affect younger individuals and women. It is characterized by vasospasm of small arteries and arterioles in the extremities, particularly associated with an oversensitivity to the sympathetic nervous system effects of cold. The cause of Raynaud's disease is unknown.

ASSESSMENT

Signs and symptoms: Severe, cramping pain (called intermittent claudication) that follows exercise and is usually relieved by rest, although some patients continue to experience pain at rest. It is indicative of ischemia secondary to decreased blood flow. The patient also can have delayed healing, collapsed veins, decreased sensory or motor function, leg ulcers, or gangrene.

Physical assessment: Decreased pulse amplitude, decreased hair distribution, and bluish discoloration of the extremities and areas of decreased circulation. The skin may appear shiny and the nails thickened. Audible bruits may be assessed with a stethoscope over partially occluded vessels. Capillary filling will be >3 seconds (with normal circulation, capillary filling occurs in 1-3 seconds) and amplitude of peripheral pulses will be decreased. Peripheral pulses often are assessed on a 0-4+ scale, using the following parameters:

☐ 0: Pulse is not palpable.
☐ 1+: Pulse is weak, thready, or intermittent or difficult to palpate.
☐ 2+: Pulse is obliterated easily with slight digital pressure.
☐ 3+: Pulse is easily palpable; considered "normal."
☐ 4+: Pulse is strong, bounding; considered "hyperdynamic."

Risk factors: Hypertension, cigarette smoking, diabetes mellitus, family history of atherosclerotic disease, and hyperlipoproteinemia. Use of beta blocker drugs can exacerbate patient's symptoms because of their peripheral vasoconstricting effect.

DIAGNOSTIC TESTS

1. *Angiography of peripheral vasculature:* Will locate obstruction and reveal extent of vascular lesions. This invasive study usually is done only if surgery is planned.
2. *Doppler flow studies:* Uses a transducer that emits sound waves through a probe to determine the amount of blood flow in arteries in which palpable pulses are difficult to obtain.
3. *Digital subtraction angiography:* Uses computerized tomography to visualize arteries radiologically and determine presence and extent of occlusion.
4. *Exercise testing:* To determine the amount of exercise that precipitates ischemia and claudication.
5. *Oscillometry:* Uses a BP cuff connected to a manometer to locate occlusive sites, as evidenced by decreased pressure readings.

MEDICAL MANAGEMENT AND SURGICAL INTERVENTION

1. Regular lower extremity exercise program: To increase circulation. This can include a walking program or Buerger-Allen exercises. Activity may be contraindicated for

some patients with severe disease, who may instead require bed rest to decrease oxygen demands to the tissues.

2. **Cessation of cigarette smoking:** To prevent increased vasoconstriction and severity of the circulation deficit.

3. **Control of hyperlipidemia and cholesterol levels:** To help prevent progression of atherosclerosis. This is accomplished through low-fat, low-cholesterol diets (see Table 2-2, p. 48) or the controversial antilipemic drugs, which may be used if diet control is ineffective. Examples of these drugs include clofibrate and cholestyramine.

4. **Control of hypertension:** Administration of agents such as thiazide diuretics.

5. **Provision of warmth:** To promote arterial flow. **Caution:** Care must be taken not to apply extreme heat because the patient's sensitivity to temperature is often decreased and burns can result.

6. **Pharmacotherapy**
   □ *Mild analgesics:* For relief of pain.
   □ *Antiplatelet agents such as aspirin and dipyridamole:* May be used to help prevent platelet adherence and thromboembolism. The use of anticoagulants such as warfarin to prevent thrombus formation is controversial.
   □ *Thrombolytics:* For example, streptokinase, to lyse the clot.
   □ *Pentoxyphylline:* To increase flexibility of erythrocytes, which enhances their movement through the microcirculation, prevent aggregation of RBCs and platelets, and decrease viscosity. This has the potential to increase circulation at the capillary level.
   □ *Calcium channel blockers:* For example, diltiazem, to reduce vasospasm.

7. **Surgical management:** For patients who are severely limited by the occlusion and for whom the occlusion is fairly localized.
   □ *Endarterectomy:* Removal of the atheromatous obstruction *via* an arterial incision.
   □ *Bypass vascular grafting:* Removal or bypass of the obstructed segment by suturing a graft proximally and distally to the obstruction.
   The most common procedures are aortofemoral, aortoiliac, and femoropopliteal bypasses. Graft material may be the patient's saphenous vein or prosthetic materials such as Gortex or dacron.
   □ *Percutaneous transluminal angioplasty (PTA):* May be used to treat focal arterial obstruction. A balloon-tipped catheter is inserted through the vein or artery to the area of the occlusion. The balloon is gradually inflated to ablate the obstruction.
   □ *Laser angioplasty:* Technique similar to PTA. A fiberoptic catheter is inserted and threaded to the area of occlusion. Energy from a laser is applied and the occlusion is obliterated.
   □ *Sympathectomy:* Relief of arterial vasoconstriction to help improve circulation. Nerves that stimulate vasoconstriction (sympathetic) are incised and ligated to decrease constriction and relax the vessels.
   □ *Amputation:* See discussion, p. 465, in Chapter 8.

NURSING DIAGNOSES AND INTERVENTIONS

Impaired skin and tissue integrity related to tissue ischemia secondary to decreased arterial circulation

Desired outcome: Patient's skin and tissue in the extremities remain intact.

1. Assess leg(s) for ulcerations that can occur with decreased arterial circulation.
2. Teach patient to elevate HOB to increase circulation to the lower extremities. Explain that this can be accomplished at home by raising the HOB on 6-inch blocks.
3. Teach patient that walking and ROM exercises to the hip, knee, and ankle promote collateral circulation.
4. Discuss an exercise program with MD, and describe the routine to the patient. Often, this includes walking to the patient's tolerance (without pain).
5. If prescribed, teach the patient Buerger-Allen exercises:
   □ Teach patient to lie flat in bed with the legs elevated above the level of the heart for 2-3 minutes.

☐ Have the patient sit on the edge of the bed for 2-3 minutes with the legs relaxed and dependent.

☐ In the same position, instruct patient to flex, extend, invert, and evert the feet, holding each position for 30 seconds each.

☐ Finally, have the patient lie flat with the legs at heart level and covered with a warm blanket for approximately 5 minutes.

Note: Bed rest without exercise may be prescribed to decrease oxygen demand in acute, severe cases.

6. Teach patient to assess peripheral pulses, warmth, color, hair distribution, and capillary filling. To check for capillary filling, teach the patient to press on a nail bed until blanching occurs and release the pressure. Explain that with normal capillary filling, color (pink) returns in 1-3 seconds.

7. As appropriate, teach patient that smoking results in both a decrease in blood flow to the extremities and a decrease in extremity temperature, particularly to the fingers and toes.

8. Discuss the importance of keeping warm by wearing socks when walking or in bed. Caution patient about using heating pads, which increase metabolism and may promote ischemia if circulation is limited.

Chronic pain related to tissue ischemia secondary to atherosclerotic obstructions

Desired outcomes: Patient's subjective evaluation of pain improves as documented by a pain scale.

1. Assess for the presence of pain, using a pain scale from 0 (no pain) to 10. Administer pain medications as prescribed, documenting effectiveness using the pain scale.

2. Teach patient to rest and stop exercising before claudication (severe, cramping pain) occurs.

3. Because the pain may be chronic and continuous, explore alternate methods of pain relief, such as visualization, guided imagery, biofeedback, meditation, and relaxation exercises or tapes. An example of a relaxation exercise is the following: **Health-seeking behaviors:** Relaxation technique effective for stress reduction, p. 49.

4. Institute measures to increase circulation to ischemic extremities, such as Buerger-Allen exercises and walking.

Knowledge deficit: Potential for infection and impaired skin and tissue integrity due to decreased arterial circulation

Desired outcome: Patient verbalizes knowledge of the potential for infection and impaired skin and tissue integrity, as well as measures to prevent these problems.

1. Teach patient how to assess for signs of infection or problems with skin integrity and to report significant findings to MD.

2. Caution patient about the increased potential for easily traumatizing the skin, for example, from bumping the lower extremities.

3. Stress the importance of wearing shoes or slippers that fit properly.

4. Instruct patient to cut toenails straight across to prevent ingrown toenails.

5. Advise patient to cover corns or callouses with pads to prevent further injury.

6. Encourage patient to keep the feet clean and dry, using mild soap and warm water for cleansing, and applying a mild lotion to prevent dryness.

7. Advise patient not to scratch or rub the skin on the feet as this can result in abrasions that easily can become infected.

8. Suggest that patient keep the feet warm with loose-fitting socks and warm soaks. Caution the patient to check the temperature of warm soaks and bath water carefully to protect the skin from burns.

Potential alteration in tissue perfusion: Peripheral, related to impaired circulation secondary to graft occlusion

Desired outcome: Patient has adequate peripheral perfusion as evidenced by peripheral pulses ≥2+ on a 0-4+ scale, BP within 20 mm Hg of baseline BP, and absence of the five "Ps" in the involved extremities.

1. Assess peripheral pulses and the involved extremity for the five "Ps": pain, pallor, pulselessness, paresthesia, and paralysis. Report significant findings.
2. Monitor BP, another indicator of peripheral perfusion pressure. Report to MD any significant increase or decrease (>15-20 mm Hg, or as directed).
3. If necessary, use the Doppler ultrasonic probe to check pulses, holding the probe to the skin at a 45-degree angle to the blood vessel. In the presence of blood flow, wavelike "whooshing" sounds will be heard. Record the presence or absence of pulsations, as well as the rate, character, frequency, and intensity of the sounds.
4. To prevent pressure on the tissue, keep sheets and blankets off the legs and feet with an overbed cradle.
5. For the first 48-72 hours after surgery (or as directed), prevent acute joint flexion in the presence of a graft, which can occlude blood flow.

Potential alteration in tissue perfusion: Renal, related to impaired circulation secondary to decreased blood supply during surgery and potential embolization

Desired outcome: Patient has adequate renal perfusion as evidenced by urinary output ≥30 ml/hr.*:* **Note:** During many vascular surgical procedures, the aorta is clamped temporarily to facilitate endarterectomy and grafting. Although all body systems are affected to a degree, the renal system is especially sensitive to the lack of blood flow.

1. Monitor I&O. Report urinary output <30 ml/hr.
2. Monitor results of renal function tests. Be alert to increases in serum creatinine and BUN, which occur with decreasing renal function.
3. Monitor for signs of fluid retention (e.g., distended neck veins, crackles [rales], and peripheral edema).
4. In the absence of acute cardiac or renal failure, encourage adequate fluid intake (2-3 L/day) to help maintain adequate renal blood flow and promote fluid balance.

See "Caring for Preoperative and Postoperative Patients," p. 637.

PATIENT-FAMILY TEACHING AND DISCHARGE PLANNING

Provide patient and significant others with verbal and written information for the following:
1. "Stop Smoking" programs, if appropriate.
2. Importance of avoiding factors and activities that cause vasoconstriction (e.g., tight clothing and crossing the legs at the knee).
3. Exercise program as prescribed by MD; importance of rest periods if claudication occurs.
4. Skin and foot care.
5. Measures that optimize arterial blood flow, such as keeping warm and raising HOB on blocks to promote circulation to the lower extremities.
6. Medications, including drug name, purpose, dosage, schedule, precautions, and potential side effects.

Aneurysms: abdominal, thoracic, and femoral

An aneurysm is a localized, outpouching sac that is formed at a weak point in an arterial wall. The most common cause of aneurysm is atherosclerosis, although vessel wall trauma, congenital defect, and infection are other causes. Loss of vessel wall elasticity and atherosclerotic deposits cause the vessel to weaken, resulting in gradual dilatation. Unless this condition is recognized and surgically treated, rupture and exsanguination can occur. Although aneurysms can develop in any vessel, peripheral vessel aneurysms are most commonly found in the abdominal aorta, thoracic aorta, and femoral arteries.

Dissecting aneurysms occur in aortic vessels that have atherosclerotic lesions and develop intimal tears, allowing bleeding into the layers of the vessel, which causes weakening and hematoma formation.

Until the aneurysm reaches sufficient size to press on adjacent organs, the individual may be asymptomatic. Complications include rupture and bleeding, exsanguination, and embolization. Most individuals with aneurysms are hypertensive.

ASSESSMENT

Chronic indicators

☐ *Abdominal aneurysm:* Patient describes sensation of "heart beat" in the abdomen. Chronic abdominal pain in the middle or lower abdomen also may be present.

☐ *Thoracic aneurysm:* Patient may be asymptomatic for years. Pressure from the aneurysm on adjacent structures can result in dull pain in the upper back, dyspnea, cough, dysphagia, and hoarseness.

☐ *Femoral aneurysm:* Signs of decreased distal arterial blood flow. See the indicators discussed with "Atherosclerotic Arterial Occlusive Disease," p. 86.

Acute indicators (rupture or dissection): Sudden onset of severe pain, often described as tearing or ripping; pallor; diaphoresis; and sudden loss of consciousness.

☐ *Pain with aneurysm at ascending aorta:* Nonradiating, central chest pain.
☐ *Pain with aneurysm at distal aorta:* Radiation to back, abdomen, and legs.

Physical assessment: Decreased BP and peripheral pulses, tachycardia, cyanosis, and cool and clammy skin. Patient may have pulsating abdominal mass or systolic bruit over the abdomen (abdominal aneurysm) or a diastolic murmur (thoracic aneurysm).

DIAGNOSTIC TESTS

1. *Chest x-ray:* May reveal the outline of an aneurysm, especially if there is calcification.
2. *Aortography:* Uses contrast dye to locate the lesion and identify its size as well as the condition of the proximal and distal vessels.
3. *Sonogram:* May assist in diagnosis when x-ray and physical exam are inconclusive. The sound waves may help determine the size, shape, and location of the aneurysm.
4. *Digital subtraction angiography:* To confirm diagnosis *via* computerized tomography, which visualizes the arteries radiographically.
5. *EKG:* May help differentiate the pain of thoracic aneurysm from that of MI.
6. *CT scan:* To determine the site of the intimal tear.

MEDICAL MANAGEMENT AND SURGICAL INTERVENTIONS

1. Decrease BP: Using antihypertensive agents such as atenolol or hydralazine.
2. Decrease aortic pulsatile flow: Using medications that decrease myocardial contractility, such as propranolol.
3. Analgesics: For pain relief.
4. Surgical interventions: Indicated if the aneurysm is larger than 4 cm in diameter, peripheral embolization has occurred, there is rupture (a surgical emergency), or a stable aneurysm suddenly becomes tender or causes severe pain. The procedure involves resection of the aneurysm and restoration of vascular flow with an autogenous graft, such as the patient's saphenous vein or a synthetic graft.

NURSING DIAGNOSES AND INTERVENTIONS

Knowledge deficit: Potential for aneurysm rupture (if surgery is not immediately planned)

Desired outcome: Patient and significant others verbalize knowledge of the potential for aneurysm rupture, the symptoms of rupture, and the importance of seeking immediate medical attention should symptoms occur.

1. Assess patient's knowledge of the potential for rupture, and intervene accordingly. Teach patient and significant others the symptoms of rupture.
2. Emphasize the importance of seeking immediate medical attention should any signs and symptoms of rupture occur. Provide numbers of emergency services in the area.
3. Encourage questions, and answer them clearly.

Potential fluid volume deficit related to loss secondary to postsurgical bleeding/hemorrhage

Desired outcome: Patient is normovolemic as evidenced by systolic BP >90 mm Hg (or within 20 mm Hg of patient's baseline), HR ≤100 bpm, peripheral pulses >2+ on a 0-4+ scale, balanced I&O, and urine output ≥30 ml/hr.

1. After the patient has been transferred from the ICU, monitor BP and peripheral pulses q30min during the first hour; then q2h or as necessary.
2. Check the operative site for the presence of frank bleeding.
3. Assess apical and peripheral pulses, and report the presence of tachycardias or a decreased amplitude of peripheral pulses, which can occur with bleeding.
4. Monitor abdomen for increasing girth.
5. Be alert to patient complaints of low back pain, which, in addition to signs of hypovolemic shock, may signal retroperitoneal hemorrhage.
6. Monitor urine output hourly and report volume <30 ml/hr.
7. Instruct patient to alert staff promptly to untoward signs and symptoms such as dizziness, lightheadedness, or palpitations (tachycardia), which may occur with hemorrhage due to sympathetic nervous system compensation.

Potential alteration in tissue perfusion: Peripheral, related to impaired circulation secondary to postoperative embolization

Desired outcome: Patient has adequate peripheral circulation as evidenced by peripheral pulses >2+ on a 1-4+ scale, brisk capillary refill (<3 seconds), and normal extremity sensation, motor function, color, and temperature.

1. Assess peripheral pulses at least qh, and report decreases in amplitude or absence of a pulse.
2. Report to MD any changes in color, capillary refill, temperature, sensation, and motor function of the extremities.
3. Maintain patient on bed rest until otherwise directed.
4. Keep patient flat to maintain graft patency and ensure healing with decreased risk of embolization.
5. Instruct patient to report untoward signs and symptoms, such as impaired sensation, promptly to staff.

See "Caring for Preoperative and Postoperative Patients," p. 637.

PATIENT-FAMILY TEACHING AND DISCHARGE PLANNING

Provide patient and significant others with verbal and written information for the following:
1. Importance of regular medical follow-up to ensure graft patency and prompt identification of the development of a new aneurysm.
2. Prevention of recurrence of aneurysm by avoiding factors that accelerate atherosclerosis, such as cigarette smoking, obesity, and hypertension.
3. Necessity of a regularly scheduled exercise program that alternates exercise with rest.

4. Indicators of wound infection and thrombus or embolus formation, and the need to report them promptly to MD should they occur.
5. Medications, including drug name, purpose, dosage, schedule, precautions, and potential side effects.
6. Telephone number of nurse available to discuss concerns and questions or clarify instructions that are unclear.
7. Importance of follow-up visits with MD; confirm date and time of next appointment.

Arterial embolism

An embolus is a fragment of a thrombus, globule of fat, clump of tissue, fragment of an atherosclerotic lesion, bacteria, or a bubble of air that moves in the circulation, lodges in a vessel, and ultimately obstructs flow.

Emboli can be venous (see "Venous Thrombosis/Thrombophlebitis," p. 93) or arterial. An arterial embolism most commonly arises from thrombi that develop in the chambers of the heart secondary to valvular heart disease, atrial fibrillation (a dysrhythmia with ineffective atrial contraction), MI, congestive or chronic cardiac failure, or vascular injury or disease. Emboli also can arise from atherosclerotic plaque lesions in any vessel. The clinical course following embolism depends on the size of the embolus, the vessel(s) affected, the degree of obstruction, and whether distal tissue is involved. Also see "Pulmonary Embolus," p. 12.

ASSESSMENT

Signs and symptoms: Sudden onset of severe pain and a gradual decrease in sensory and motor functioning; presence of tingling, numbness, blanching, coolness, and cyanosis.

Physical assessment: Possible presence of a darkened or mottled extremity; diminished or absent pulse(s). Necrosis or gangrene can occur if there is total occlusion and absence of collateral flow.

History of: Vascular injury or surgery, infection such as cellulitis, valvular heart disease, cardiac dysrhythmias.

DIAGNOSTIC TESTS

1. *Ultrasonic Doppler flow studies:* Will reveal decreased or absent arterial blood flow distal to the embolus.
2. *Angiography:* Provides visualization of the embolus in the arterial tree and collateral circulation.

MEDICAL MANAGEMENT

1. Bed rest: To prevent further embolization.
2. Anticoagulation with oral anticoagulant or heparin *via* continuous IV drip: To prevent further embolization.
3. Thrombolytic drugs such as streptokinase: To speed up the process of clot lysis.
4. Analgesics: To relieve pain caused by distal vasospasm and ischemia.
5. Embolectomy: Surgical removal of the embolus.

NURSING DIAGNOSES AND INTERVENTIONS

Potential alteration in tissue perfusion: Peripheral, related to impaired circulation secondary to embolization (preoperative period)

Desired outcome: Patient's peripheral perfusion is adequate as evidenced by peripheral pulses >2+ on a 0-4+ scale and normal extremity color, temperature, sensation, and motor function.

1. Maintain patient on bed rest to prevent further embolization.
2. Monitor peripheral circulation. Keep extremities warm (room temperature). Advise patient to avoid chilling by wearing socks or slippers.
3. Protect extremities from trauma. Provide an overbed cradle to keep sheets and blankets off tissue that has decreased circulation.
4. If prescribed, keep the lower extremities slightly dependent (but not >45 degrees) to promote circulation.
5. Teach patient signs and symptoms of embolization, which necessitate immediate medical attention.

See "Pulmonary Embolism" in Chapter 1 for the following: **Potential for injury** related to increased risk of bleeding or hemorrhage secondary to anticoagulant therapy, p. 16. See "Caring for Preoperative and Postoperative Patients," p. 637.

PATIENT-FAMILY TEACHING AND DISCHARGE PLANNING

Provide patient and significant others with verbal and written information for the following:
1. Prescribed exercise plan to prevent stasis of the blood.
2. Signs and symptoms that necessitate immediate medical attention: extremity pain, coolness, pallor, and cyanosis.
3. Indicators of wound infection, if surgery was performed.
4. Oral anticoagulant therapy: need for regular medical checkups and immediate reporting of epistaxis, ecchymosis, hemoptysis, melena, or hematuria; administration at the same time every day; not changing regular dietary habits (e.g., becoming a vegetarian without first consulting MD or nurse [many green, leafy vegetables are high in vitamin K, which reverses the effect of warfarin; vegetarian diets may necessitate an increase in warfarin dosage to achieve therapeutic anticoagulation]); importance of consulting with MD before taking any OTC medications, especially aspirin products, which affect platelet aggregation and potentiate the anticoagulant effect of warfarin.
5. Other medications, including drug name, purpose, dosage, schedule, precautions, and potential side effects.

Venous thrombosis/thrombophlebitis

Although venous thrombosis and thrombophlebitis are different disorders, clinically they are referred to as a single entity, and the terms are used interchangeably to refer to the development of a venous thrombus or thrombi, with associated inflammation. Disturbances in the venous system can have a variety of causes and precipitating factors, including stasis of blood, hemoconcentration, venous trauma, inflammation, or altered coagulation. Venous stasis can occur with heart failure, shock states, immobility from prolonged bed rest, structural disorders of the veins, or as a side effect of anesthesia. Vessel trauma can result from chemical irritation caused by IV solutions or direct trauma. Altered coagulation states usually are related to liver disease or withdrawal from anticoagulants. Venous thrombosis and thrombophlebitis most often occur in the lower extremities, and the most serious complication is embolization.

ASSESSMENT

Signs and symptoms: Pain, edema, tenderness, erythema, local warmth, and prominence of superficial veins. Sometimes the first sign is a pulmonary embolus (see "Pulmonary Embolus," p. 12).

Physical assessment: A knot or bump occasionally can be felt on palpation. **Caution:** Because of the risk of embolization, never test for a positive Homans's sign in the presence of clinical indicators of venous thrombosis or thrombophlebitis.

Risk factors: Prolonged bed rest and immobility, leg trauma, recent surgery, use of oral contraceptives, obesity, varicose veins.

DIAGNOSTIC TESTS

1. *Contrast phlebography (venography):* A contrast dye is injected into the venous system that is to be studied, allowing visualization of the veins by showing filling or absence of filling.
2. *Doppler ultrasound:* Identifies changes in blood flow secondary to presence of a thrombus.
3. *I-fibrinogen injection test:* Useful screening device for early detection of thrombosis because the isotope identifies clots that are forming.
4. *Impedence plethysmography (IPG):* Estimates blood flow using measures of resistance and normal changes that occur during pulsatile blood flow.

MEDICAL MANAGEMENT AND SURGICAL INTERVENTIONS

1. Prevention: Involves identifying patients at risk, increasing fluid intake to at least 2-3 L/day, promoting leg exercises to prevent stasis, and prescribing elastic stockings and early ambulation.
2. Therapeutic anticoagulation: Prevents development of a pulmonary embolus. Heparin is used during the acute phase, and long-term warfarin therapy is used after the acute phase.
3. Thrombolytic therapy: Instituted in some medical centers to lyse and digest the clot. Streptokinase or urokinase may be used.
4. Bed rest: During the acute phase, with support hose and leg elevation to decrease venous stasis.
5. Analgesics for pain: Usually acetaminophen.
6. Exercise regimen: Walking or leg exercises after the acute phase.
7. Warm moist packs: To reduce discomfort and pain.
8. Thrombectomy: Necessary when the danger of pulmonary embolism is extreme, the patient cannot tolerate anticoagulation, or extremity damage from the absence of venous drainage is imminent.

NURSING DIAGNOSES AND INTERVENTIONS

Potential alteration in tissue perfusion: Pulmonary and peripheral, related to impaired circulation secondary to embolization from thrombus formation

Desired outcome: Patient has adequate pulmonary and peripheral perfusion as evidenced by normal extremity color, temperature, and sensation; RR 12-20 breaths/min with normal depth and pattern (eupnea); HR ≤100 bpm; BP within 20 mm Hg of baseline BP; and normal breath sounds.

1. Be alert to and promptly report early indicators of peripheral thrombus formation: pain, edema, erythema, and impaired sensation. If indicators appear, maintain patient on bed rest and notify MD promptly.
2. Monitor for and immediately report signs of pulmonary embolus: sudden onset of chest pain, dyspnea, tachypnea, tachycardia, hypotension, hemoptysis, shallow respirations, crackles, decreased breath sounds, and diaphoresis. Should they occur, prompt medical attention is crucial.
3. Administer anticoagulants as prescribed. Double-check drip rates and dosages with a colleague.
4. Minimize the risk of pulmonary embolism by keeping patient on bed rest, providing ROM exercises, and applying support hose as prescribed.

Pain related to inflammatory process secondary to thrombus formation

Desired outcomes: Patient's subjective evaluation of pain improves, as documented by a pain scale.

1. Monitor patient for the presence of pain. Document the degree of pain, using a pain scale from 0 (no pain) to 10. Administer analgesics as prescribed and document relief obtained using the pain scale.
2. Ensure that the patient maintains bed rest during the acute phase to minimize painful engorgement and the potential for embolization.
3. If prescribed, apply warm, moist packs. Be sure that the packs are warm (but not extremely so) and not allowed to cool. If appropriate, use a Kock-Mason dressing (warm towel covered by plastic wrap and a K-pad to provide continuous moist heat).
4. To enhance venous drainage and reduce engorgement, keep the legs elevated above heart level (but not >45 degrees).

Alteration in tissue perfusion: Peripheral, related to impaired circulation secondary to venous engorgement or edema

Desired outcome: Patient has adequate peripheral perfusion as evidenced by absence of discomfort and normal extremity temperature, color, sensation, and motor function.

1. Assess for signs of inadequate peripheral perfusion, such as pain and changes in skin temperature, color, motor, or sensory function.
2. Elevate patient's legs above heart level (not >45 degrees) to promote venous drainage.
3. As prescribed for patients without evidence of thrombus formation, apply antiembolic hose, which compress superficial veins to increase blood flow to the deeper veins. Remove the stockings for approximately 15 minutes q8h. Inspect the skin for evidence of irritation.
4. Encourage patient to perform ankle circling and active or assisted ROM exercises on the lower extremities to prevent venous stasis. Perform passive ROM if patient is unable to do this. **Caution:** If there are any signs of acute thrombus formation such as calf hardness or tenderness, the exercises are contraindicated because of the risk of embolization. Notify MD.
5. Encourage deep breathing, which creates increased negative pressure in the lungs and thorax to assist in the emptying of large veins.
6. Arterial circulation usually will not be impaired unless there is arterial disease or severe edema compressing arterial flow. Assess pulses regularly, however, to confirm the presence of good arterial flow.

See "Pulmonary Embolus" in Chapter 1 for **Potential for injury** related to increased risk of bleeding or hemorrhage secondary to anticoagulant therapy, p. 16. See "Varicose Veins" for **Altered skin and tissue integrity** related to impaired tissue nutrition secondary to venous engorgement, p. 97.

PATIENT-FAMILY TEACHING AND DISCHARGE PLANNING

Provide patient and significant others with verbal and written information for the following:

1. Exercise program as prescribed by MD. Usually, walking is the best exercise.
2. Avoiding restrictive clothing (e.g., tight socks, stockings, and pants).
3. Avoiding prolonged periods of standing still.
4. If possible, elevating legs above heart level when sitting.
5. Weight reduction program, if appropriate. Provide consultation with a nutritional therapist, if indicated.
6. Keeping extremities and feet clean and dry; being alert to early signs of venous stasis ulcers, such as redness and skin breakdown.
7. Importance of avoiding trauma to the extremities.
8. Wearing antiembolic hose, if prescribed. The hose must fit properly and should be snug over the feet and progressively less snug as they reach the knee or thigh. Stress the importance of avoiding wrinkles in the hose.
9. Signs and symptoms that require medical attention: persistent redness, swelling, tenderness, weak or absent pulses, and ulcerations on the extremity.

In addition:

10. If the patient is discharged from the hospital on warfarin therapy, provide information about the following:
    □ As directed, see MD for scheduled PT checks.
    □ Take warfarin at same time each day; do not skip days unless directed to by MD.
    □ Wear a Medic-Alert bracelet.
    □ Avoid alcohol consumption and changes in diet (e.g., changing to a vegetarian diet), both of which can alter the body's response to warfarin.
    □ Inform other physicians and dentists that warfarin is being taken when making appointments with them.
    □ Be alert to indicators that necessitate immediate medical attention: hematuria, melena, epistaxis, ecchymosis, hemoptysis, dizziness, and weakness.
    □ Avoid taking OTC medications (e.g., aspirin, which potentiates the anticoagulant effect of warfarin) without consulting MD or nurse.

Varicose veins

Varicose veins are enlarged, tortuous, and dilated, and they occur as a result of incompetent valves or increased venous pressure. As the vessels dilate, they lose their elasticity and become less functional. This can result in venous stasis and subsequent thrombus formation. Varicose veins are most often found in the lower extremities.

ASSESSMENT

Signs and symptoms: If only the superficial veins are involved, the patient can be asymptomatic except for the appearance of dilated veins. Increases in venous pressure can cause swelling, pain, leg fatigue, and muscle aches and cramps. As the condition progresses, discomfort increases and ulcerations can develop.

Physical assessment: Increased firmness of calf muscles, redness, and swelling; tenderness elicited at the affected site; leg ulcer(s).

Risk factors: Pregnancy, prolonged periods of standing, familial history, obesity, lack of exercise.

DIAGNOSTIC TESTS

1. *Brodie-Trendelenburg test:* Demonstrates the presence of backward flow through incompetent venous valves. While the patient is supine, the leg is elevated to empty the venous system. A tourniquet is then applied to occlude the superficial veins and the patient is asked to stand. If the communicating valves are incompetent, blood will flow superficially and engorge the superficial veins. This test determines the appropriate treatment.
2. *Doppler flow studies:* Detects backward blood flow through incompetent valves.
3. *Phlebography:* Allows visualization of veins *via* injection of contrast medium to reveal dilatations, incompetent valves, and thrombi.

MEDICAL MANAGEMENT AND SURGICAL INTERVENTIONS

1. Prevention through health teaching.
2. Support hose or antiembolic hose: To compress the superficial veins, decrease engorgement, and shunt venous flow to the deeper, stronger veins.
3. Weight reduction program: If obesity is a contributing factor.
4. Walking or leg-exercise program: To prevent venous stasis.
5. Vein ligation and stripping: When pain from the varicose veins is severe or the risk of thrombus formation increases. Usually this involves ligation of the saphenous vein at the groin, where the saphenous and femoral veins meet. Another small incision is made at the ankle, and a wire is passed into the vein, "stripping" it as it passes. For tortuous veins, multiple incisions may be required.

6. **Injection sclerotherapy:** Injection of a sclerosing agent into the vein to obliterate and cause permanent fibrosis.

NURSING DIAGNOSES AND INTERVENTIONS

Pain related to preoperative venous engorgement or surgical procedure

Desired outcome: Patient's subjective evaluation of pain improves, as documented by a pain scale.

1. Monitor patient for the presence of pain using a pain scale from 0 (no pain) to 10. Administer analgesics as prescribed and document their effectiveness, using the pain scale.
2. To prevent increased venous pressure and promote venous drainage, encourage patient to keep the legs elevated above the level of the heart.
3. Maintain elastic wraps and antiembolic hose for support and venous drainage.
4. To promote circulation and prevent venous stasis, initiate postoperative leg exercises and ambulation as soon after surgery as possible (as directed by MD). To minimize discomfort, advise patient not to sit with the legs dependent or to stand still for prolonged periods.
5. Suggest to patient that for long periods of sitting when the legs cannot be elevated above heart level, elevation of the feet 5-10 inches off the floor (for example, by resting the feet on several books) may help decrease venous stasis.

Altered skin and tissue integrity related to impaired tissue nutrition secondary to venous engorgement

Desired outcome: Patient's skin and tissue remain intact.

1. Apply elastic stockings when the veins are most likely to be empty, for example, after patient has been recumbent or legs have been elevated for 20 minutes. This will help minimize distention.
2. Remove the stockings at prescribed intervals to minimize swelling proximal to the hose. Assess the skin during the period the hose are removed and be alert to signs of stasis dermatitis: skin that is thin, shiny, and bluish in color, and for ulcerations. Be sure that the patient's skin is cleansed and dried thoroughly before reapplying the stockings.
3. Ensure that the tops of the stockings do not roll as this would cause a tourniquet effect and compromise circulation further. Also be sure that there are no creases or wrinkles in the hose, which would cause pressure areas.
4. Protect the extremities from trauma. If indicated, use a bed cradle to keep bedding off the compromised tissues.
5. Teach patient not to cross legs, which worsens venous stasis.

See "Venous Thrombosis/Thrombophlebitis" for **Alteration in tissue perfusion:** Peripheral related to impaired circulation secondary to venous engorgement or edema, p. 95. See "Caring for Preoperative and Postoperative Patients," p. 637.

PATIENT-FAMILY TEACHING AND DISCHARGE PLANNING

Provide patient and significant others with verbal and written information for the following:
1. Medications, including drug name, purpose, dosage, schedule, precautions, and potential side effects.
2. Importance of preventive measures, including the following: Wear support hose, elevate legs when possible, avoid prolonged periods of sitting and standing still, initiate a walking or exercise program, change positions at frequent intervals, and start a weight reduction program, if appropriate.
3. Necessity of frequent rest periods for at least the first 6 weeks after surgery.
4. Importance of regular medical follow-up.

5. Avoiding constricting clothing or "knee-high" stockings, which can obstruct venous flow.

SELECTED REFERENCES

Brooks-Brunn J: Thrombolytic intervention and its effect on mortality in acute myocardial infarction: review of clinical trials, Heart Lung 17(6):756-760, 1988.

Burke CM and Morris AJ: Perfusion scans and pulmonary angiography, Heart Lung 15(4):357-360, 1986.

Casey PE: Pathophysiology of dilated cardiomyopathy: nursing implications, J Cardiovasc Nurs 2(1):1-12, 1987.

Cicciu JV: Aortic and mitral valvuloplasty: nursing grand rounds, J Cardiovasc Nurs 1(3):70-78, 1987.

Courtney-Jenkins A: The patient with hypertrophic cardiomyopathy, J Cardiovasc Nurs 2(1):33-47, 1987.

Dixon MB and Nunelee J: Arterial reconstruction for atherosclerotic occlusive disease, J Cardiovasc Nurs 1(2):36-49, 1987.

Doyle JE: Treatment modalities in peripheral vascular disease, NCNA 21(2):241-254, 1986.

Finkelmeier BA and Salinger MH: Dual-chamber cardiac pacing: an overview, Crit Care Nurse 6(5):12-31, 1986.

Gawlinski A: Cardiovascular dysfunctions. In Swearingen PL et al: Manual of critical care: applying nursing diagnoses to adult critical illness, St Louis, 1988, The CV Mosby Co.

Guyton AC: Textbook of medical physiology, ed 7, Philadelphia, 1986, WB Saunders Co.

Herman J: Nursing assessment and nursing diagnosis in patients with peripheral vascular disease, NCNA 21(2):219-232, 1986.

Hubner C: Exercise therapy and smoking cessation for intermittent claudication, J Cardiovasc Nurs 1(2):50-58, 1987.

Lababidi Z et al: Percutaneous balloon aortic valvuloplasty: results in 23 patients, Am Journal Cardiol 53:194-197, 1984.

Lewis N: Monitoring the patient with acute myocardial infarction, NCNA 22(1):15-32, 1984.

Marrie TJ: Infective endocarditis: a serious and changing disease, Crit Care Nurse, 7(2):31-46, 1987.

Massey JA: Diagnostic testing for peripheral vascular disease, NCNA 1(2):207-218, 1986.

McHugh MJ: The patient with alcoholic cardiomyopathy, J Cardiovasc Nurs 2(1):13-23, 1987.

Metcalfe K: Understanding cardiac pacing: a guide for nurses, Norwalk, CT/San Mateo, CA, 1986, Appleton & Lange.

Misinski M: Pathophysiology of acute myocardial infarction: a rationale for thombolytic therapy, Heart Lung 17(6):743-740, 1988.

Moynihan M: Assessing the needs of postmyocardial infarction patients, NCNA 19(3):441-448, 1984.

Niederman MS and Matthay RA: Cardiovascular function in secondary pulmonary hypertension, Heart Lung 15(4):341-351, 1986.

Peil ML and Rubin LJ: Therapy of secondary pulmonary hypertension, Heart Lung 15(45):450-455, 1986.

Porth CM: Pathophysiology: concepts of altered health states, ed 2, Philadelphia, 1986, JB Lippincott Co.

Rodriguez SW and Reed RL: Thrombolytic therapy for MI, AJN 87(5):631-640, 1987.

Scrima DA: Infective endocarditis: nursing considerations, Crit Care Nurse 7(2):47-57, 1987.

Shinn JA: Heart and lung transplantation of end-stage pulmonary vascular hypertension, NCNA 19(3):547-558, 1984.

Tueller BL: Cardiovascular dysfunctions. In Swearingen PL et al: Manual of critical care: applying nursing diagnoses to adult critical illness, St Louis, 1988, The CV Mosby Co.

Turner J: Nursing intervention in patients with peripheral vascular disease, NCNA 21(2):233-240, 1986.

Whitman GR: Prosthetic cardiac valves, Prog Cardiovasc Nurs 2(4):116-124, 1987.

3
CHAPTER

Renal-urinary disorders

Section One   RENAL DISORDERS

Glomerulonephritis

Glomerulonephritis (GN) is the name of a group of diseases that damage the renal glomeruli. When the glomerulus is injured, protein and RBCs are allowed to enter the renal tubule and be excreted in the urine. GN can be acute or chronic. Most individuals with acute GN improve dramatically within weeks and recover completely within 1-2 years, but renal damage continues to progress for those with chronic GN. Chronic GN is the most common cause of chronic renal failure. Most forms of GN are the result of immunologic processes (e.g., poststreptococcal infection, systemic lupus erythematosus).

See "Acute Renal Failure," p. 116, and "Chronic Renal Failure," p. 121, as appropriate.

ASSESSMENT

Indicators can range from subtle to blatant, depending on the patient's level of renal function.

Acute indicators: Hematuria, proteinuria, oliguria, dull bilateral flank pain, headache, low-grade fever.

Chronic indicators: Fatigue, lethargy, anorexia, nausea, nocturia, headache, weakness.

Physical assessment: Presence of edema (peripheral, periorbital, sacral), crackles (rales), elevated BP, pallor.

History of: Recent URI or other infection; systemic lupus erythematosus or other autoimmune disease; bloody urine.

DIAGNOSTIC TESTS

1. *Urinalysis and 24-hour urinary protein excretion:* Hematuria with red cell casts and proteinuria are the cardinal findings.
2. *BUN and serum creatinine:* If elevated, may indicate decreased renal function.
3. *Plasma complement, antinuclear antibody titer, antistreptolysin 0 titer, throat and blood cultures, hepatitis B antigen, and immunoelectrophoresis of the serum and urine:* Optional tests to determine cause of GN.
4. *Renal biopsy:* Indicated when tissue diagnosis is needed to direct therapy or provide prognostic data. Usually a percutaneous (closed) renal biopsy is performed. Postbiopsy care includes keeping the patient supine with a rolled towel under the biopsy site for 12 hours and frequent monitoring of VS (q15min initially). **Note:** Two possible complications are bleeding and infection. Severe pain, hypotension, persistent gross hematuria, or fever should be reported to the MD immediately.

MEDICAL MANAGEMENT

1. Bed rest: For patients with acute GN. Limited activity may be necessary for weeks to months.
2. Decrease level of antigen availability: When possible (e.g., treat infections with antibiotics).
3. Pharmacotherapy
   □ *Corticosteroids and cytotoxic agents:* To suppress the immune system and reduce antibody formation.
   □ *Anticoagulants:* To reduce nonimmunologic mediators of glomerular damage.
   □ *Antibiotics:* If causative factor is bacterial.
   □ *Diuretics:* To remove excess fluid (see Table 3-1).
   □ *Antihypertensives:* To control BP.
4. Plasmapheresis: To remove immune complexes or antiglomerular basement antibodies. It is used only in patients with severe or rapidly progressing GN.

TABLE 3-1 Diuretics

Generic name	Common brand names	Usual dosage/24 hr (mg)
acetazolamide	Diamox	250-375(qod)
amiloride HCl*	Midamor	5-10
chlorothiazide sodium	Diuril	250-1,000
chlorthalidone	Hygroton	25-100
ethacrynic acid	Edecrin	25-200
furosemide	Lasix	20-160
hydrochlorothiazide	Esidrix	25-100
metolazone	Zaroxolyn, Diulo	2.5-10
spironolactone*	Aldactone	25-200
triamterene*	Dyrenium	50-300

*Although most diuretics can cause hypokalemia, these diuretics might cause hyperkalemia. For this reason they are often used in combination with thiazide diuretics.

5. Diet: Restriction of sodium (see Table 11-3, p. 550) and fluids if edema or hypertension is present. A high-carbohydrate diet is encouraged to maintain nutrition and prevent tissue catabolism. If renal function is markedly decreased, protein and phosphorus may be limited to prevent retention of excess nitrogenous wastes and hyperphosphatemia.
6. Peritoneal dialysis or hemodialysis: To maintain homeostasis or prevent uremic complications if renal function is markedly decreased (see "Renal Dialysis," p. 126).

NURSING DIAGNOSES AND INTERVENTIONS

Activity intolerance related to weakness secondary to prolonged bed rest and disease process

Desired outcomes: Patient maintains bed rest until BP and protein excretion are normal or near normal. Patient demonstrates ability to assume normal activity levels after enforced bed rest.

1. During the period of enforced bed rest, assist patient with ADL as necessary. For patients with acute GN, bed rest usually lasts 10 days–2 weeks.
2. Provide bed exercises within the prescribed activity limitations. Establish a progressive activity regimen that will allow patient to return to normal activities without complications. For more information, see the appendix for **Potential for disuse syndrome** related to inactivity secondary to prolonged bed rest, p. 653, and **Potential activity intolerance,** p. 651.
3. Before patient resumes activities, ensure that BP is within patient's normal range and urine protein excretion is near normal. Normal ranges for protein excretion are 2-8 mg/dl (random) and 40-150 mg/24 hr. Notify MD if elevations occur after patient resumes activities.

Fluid volume excess: Edema and hypertension related to retention secondary to decreased renal function

Desired outcomes: Patient is normovolemic as evidenced by urine output of at least 30-60 ml/hr (or patient's norm), stable weights, and edema $\leq 1+$ on a 0-4+ scale. BP and HR are within patient's normal range, CVP is 5-12 cm H_2O, and RR is 12-20 breaths/min with normal depth and pattern (eupnea). Patient states that thirst is controlled, can list foods that are high in sodium, and plans a 3-day menu that excludes foods high in sodium.

1. Monitor I&O closely. Notify MD of sudden changes in output.
2. Monitor weight daily. Report unusual or steady gains or losses (e.g., 0.5-1 kg/day).
3. Observe for indicators of fluid overload: edema, hypertension, crackles (rales), tachycardia, lethargy, distended neck veins, SOB, and increased CVP. **Note:** Not all patients with edema are fluid-overloaded. Edema also can occur because of decreased serum albumin secondary to urinary losses.
4. Offer ice chips or popsicles to minimize thirst in the fluid-restricted patient; be sure to record the amount on the intake record. Frequent mouth care also may help minimize thirst.
5. Provide patient with data regarding foods high in sodium (see Table 11-3, p. 550), which should be avoided. In addition, many OTC preparations are also high in sodium (e.g., mouthwashes and antacids). Advise patient and significant others to read all labels carefully.

Knowledge deficit: Signs and symptoms of fluid and electrolyte imbalance (caused by decreased renal function or diuretic therapy)

Desired outcome: Patient verbalizes knowledge of the signs and symptoms of fluid and electrolyte imbalance and the importance of reporting them promptly to MD or staff should they occur.

1. Alert patient and significant others to the following signs and symptoms of fluid and electrolyte imbalance:
   □ *Hypokalemia:* Muscle weakness, lethargy, dysrhythmias, nausea, and vomiting.
   □ *Hyperkalemia:* Abdominal cramping, diarrhea, irritability, and muscle weakness (if severe).
   □ *Hypocalcemia:* Neuromuscular irritability, such as twitching.
   □ *Hyperphosphatemia:* Excessive itching.
   □ *Uremia:* Confusion, lethargy, restlessness, and itching.
2. Instruct patient to report the above signs and symptoms to MD or staff promptly should they occur.

Knowledge deficit: Negative side effects of corticosteroids and cytotoxic agents

Desired outcome: Patient verbalizes knowledge of the negative side effects of corticosteroids and cytotoxic agents and the importance of reporting them promptly to staff or MD should they occur.

1. Corticosteroids and cytotoxic agents are potent medications with potentially serious side effects. For the patient on corticosteroids, alert him or her to the potential for the following: infection, increasing BP, mental changes, and hyperglycemia and GI bleeding.
2. For the patient on cytotoxic agents, alert him or her to the potential for the following: infection, cystitis with hematuria, and abnormal hair loss. See "Caring for the Patient with Cancer and Other Life-Disrupting Illnesses," p. 659, for more information.
3. Stress the importance of notifying MD or staff promptly should any of the above occur.

Potential for infection related to increased susceptibility secondary to corticosteroid therapy, immobility, invasive techniques, and impaired skin integrity

Desired outcome: Patient is free of infection as evidenced by normothermia and absence of adventitious breath sounds. Respiratory secretions are of normal color, consistency, and quantity.

1. Because the respiratory system is a common site for infection in the immunocompromised patient, be alert to indications of infection, such as increased body temperature, adventitious breath sounds, and increased, thickened, or colored airway secretions. If secretions are noted, encourage coughing or provide suctioning at frequent intervals. **Note:** Uremic and elderly individuals tend to run subnormal temperatures, so even slight fevers can be significant. Remember that steroids may mask the signs and symptoms of infection.

2. Use meticulous, sterile technique when performing invasive procedures or manipulating urinary catheters, IV lines, or venous catheters.
3. Provide oral hygiene and skin care at frequent intervals. Edema, bed rest, and uremia all increase the potential for skin breakdown, which further increases the risk of infection.

See "Pulmonary Embolus" in Chapter 1 for **Potential for injury** related to increased risk of bleeding secondary to anticoagulation therapy, p. 16. See the appendix for nursing diagnoses and interventions for the care of patients on prolonged bed rest, p. 651.

PATIENT-FAMILY TEACHING AND DISCHARGE PLANNING

Provide patient and significant others with verbal and written information for the following:
1. Medications, including drug name, purpose, dosage, schedule, precautions, and potential side effects.
2. Diet, including fact sheet listing foods that should be avoided or limited. Inform patient that diet and fluid restrictions may be altered as renal function changes.
3. Indicators that require medical attention: irregular pulse, fever, unusual SOB or edema, sudden change in urine output, or unusual weakness.
4. Technique for measuring temperature and pulse and recording I&O.
5. Necessity for continued medical evaluation; confirm date and time of next MD appointment, if known.
6. Importance of adjusting and gradually increasing activities to avoid fatigue.
7. Necessity of avoiding infections and seeking treatment promptly should they occur.

Teach the signs and symptoms of URI, otitis media, UTI, and impetigo (see **Potential for infection,** p. 125, in "Care of the Renal Transplant Patient").

In addition:
8. Coordinate family and social service support for the patient who must continue bed rest or restrict activity at home. Consider such factors as meals, loss of income, housework, child care, and transportation.

Nephrotic syndrome

Nephrotic syndrome (NS) is a complex of symptoms that can occur with any disease that causes glomerular damage and consequent increased glomerular permeability to protein. The hallmarks of NS are increased urinary excretion of protein, decreased serum albumin, increased serum lipids, and edema. The two main causes of NS are glomerulonephritis and diabetic nephropathy, and its course and prognosis depend on the status of the disease that caused it. In adults, NS usually progresses to chronic renal failure.

See "Glomerulonephritis," p. 102, and "Chronic Renal Failure," p. 121, as appropriate.

ASSESSMENT

Signs and symptoms: Anorexia, nausea, diarrhea, lethargy, fatigue. Patient also may have ascites, pleural effusion, decreased urinary output, and weight gain.

Physical assessment: Pallor; edema (periorbital, abdominal, sacral, dependent); and either hypertension or hypotension, depending on the primary renal disease and effective circulating volume.

History of: Glomerulonephritis, diabetes mellitus, lupus erythematosus, or infectious disease.

DIAGNOSTIC TESTS

1. *24-hour protein excretion:* To diagnose the syndrome. NS is defined as the urinary excretion of >3.5 g/day of protein. Protein loss can be >10 g/day.
2. *Urinalysis.* Will show sediment-containing casts, oval fat bodies, and RBCs.

Note: All urine samples should be sent to the lab immediately after they are obtained or refrigerated if this is not possible. Urine left at room temperature has greater potential for bacterial growth, turbidity, and alkalinity, any of which can distort the results. Specimens for urine culture should *not* be refrigerated.

3. *Serum tests:* Will show low albumin, elevated cholesterol and triglycerides, and low total calcium. BUN and creatinine may be elevated. Additional lab tests might be performed, depending on the suspected cause of NS.
4. *Renal biopsy:* Often necessary to determine the cause, direct the therapy, and indicate the prognosis of NS.

MEDICAL MANAGEMENT

1. Bed rest: During periods of severe edema.
2. Diet: Low in sodium (see Table 11-3, p. 550), rich in high biologic value protein (1.5 g/kg body weight/day), with adequate caloric intake. Liberal protein intake is required to provide necessary amino acids for albumin synthesis.
3. Pharmacotherapy may include the following:
   □ *Diuretics:* Used cautiously to reduce edema (see Table 3-1, p. 103).
   □ *Antibiotics:* To treat infection.
   □ *Corticosteroids, anticoagulants, or cytotoxic agents:* To treat glomerulonephritis. See "Glomerulonephritis," p. 102. Anticoagulants also may be used in patients with thromboembolic complications.
   □ *Antihypertensive agents:* To treat hypertension.

NURSING DIAGNOSES AND INTERVENTIONS

Potential alterations in fluid volume: *Deficit* related to decreased vascular volume secondary to pharmacotherapy; *excess* related to fluid retention secondary to decreased serum albumin and renal retention of sodium and water

Desired outcomes: Patient is normovolemic as evidenced by balanced I&O, urine output of at least 30-60 ml/hr (or patient's normal range), stable weight, normal breath sounds, edema ≤1+ on a 0-4+ scale, CVP 5-12 cm H_2O, and BP and HR within patient's normal range. Patient verbalizes knowledge of foods high in sodium and the rationale for avoiding them.

1. Monitor I&O closely; document every shift.
2. Monitor patient's weight daily. Report unusual or steady gains or losses.
3. Observe for and document changes in hydration and VS after administration of diuretics, antihypertensives, or osmotic agents.
4. Limit sodium intake as prescribed. Instruct patient about foods that are high in sodium (see Table 11-3, p. 550).
5. Measure abdominal girth every shift in patients with ascites.
6. Auscultate lung fields every shift for evidence of pleural effusion (i.e., bronchial or decreased breath sounds), and be alert to signs of respiratory distress, such as increased RR and SOB. Notify MD of significant changes.
7. Observe for indicators of decreased effective circulating volume (e.g., hypotension or hypotension with position changes, tachycardia, and decreased CVP), which can occur as a result of sodium restriction and the administration of diuretics or certain antihypertensives.

Alteration in nutrition: Less than body requirements related to decreased intake secondary to anorexia and increased need secondary to urinary losses of protein

Desired outcomes: Patient has adequate nutrition as evidenced by stable weights, normal or near normal values of serum albumin (3.5-5.5 g/dl), and a positive nitrogen state. Patient maintains a diet high in protein and relates knowledge of foods high in protein.

1. Provide prescribed high-protein diet in small, frequent feedings.
2. Teach patient about foods high in protein (e.g., meat, poultry, fish, lentils, and eggs).
3. Develop diet plan with dietitian, patient, and significant others, adjusting it to patient preference.
4. Encourage significant others to bring in patient's favorite high-protein foods as allowed.
5. Record calorie intake and weigh patient daily.

Potential for infection related to vulnerability secondary to treatment with immunosuppressive agents, prolonged immobility, invasive procedures, and disease process

Desired outcomes: Patient is free of infection as evidenced by normothermia, normal breath sounds, and respiratory secretions of normal consistency, color, and odor. Patient verbalizes knowledge of the indicators of infection and the importance of seeking medical attention promptly should they occur.

Note: NS causes an increased susceptibility to infection, which is believed to occur because of the loss of serum-immune globulins in the urine. The risk of infection is further increased if the patient is being treated with immunosuppressive agents.

---

1. Minimize the risk of exposing patient to individuals with infections by providing a private room, if possible. Alert significant others to this concern.
2. For other interventions, see the same nursing diagnosis in "Glomerulonephritis," p. 104.

See "Pulmonary Embolus" in Chapter 1 for **Potential for injury** related to increased risk of bleeding secondary to anticoagulant therapy, p. 16. See Glomerulonephritis for **Activity intolerance,** p. 103, **Knowledge deficit:** Signs and symptoms of fluid and electrolyte imbalance, p. 104, and **Knowledge deficit:** Negative side effects of corticosteroids and cytotoxic agents, p. 104. See the appendix for nursing diagnoses and interventions for the care of patients on prolonged bed rest, p. 651.

PATIENT-FAMILY TEACHING AND DISCHARGE PLANNING

Provide patient and significant others with verbal and written information for the following:

1. Medications, including drug name, purpose, dosage, schedule, precautions, and potential side effects.
2. Diet: Advise patient and significant others that diet and fluid restrictions may be altered as renal function changes. Provide lists of advocated and restricted foods.
3. Signs and symptoms that require medical attention: irregular pulse, fever, unusual SOB or edema, sudden change in urinary output, unusual weakness, and increase in weight of >1 kg/week.
4. Need for continued medical evaluation; confirm time and date for the next MD appointment, if known.
5. Importance of avoiding infections and seeking treatment promptly should signs and symptoms appear. Teach the indicators of URI, otitis media, impetigo, and UTI. For details, see **Potential for infection,** p. 125, in "Care of the Renal Transplant Patient."
6. Importance of skin care, especially over edematous areas.

In addition:

7. Coordinate family and social service support for the patient who must continue bed rest or limited activity at home. Consider such factors as meals, loss of income, housework, child care, and transportation.

Acute pyelonephritis

Acute pyelonephritis is an infection of the renal parenchyma and pelvis, which usually occurs secondary to an ascending UTI. UTIs typically result from anatomic or functional obstruction to urine flow (e.g., from prostatic hypertrophy or renal calculi, or instrumentation, such as catheterization or cystoscopy). Hematogenous infection also can occur in acute pyelonephritis when bacteria reach the kidney *via* the bloodstream.

The incidence of acute pyelonephritis increases with advancing age. In the absence of anatomic obstruction or instrumentation, acute pyelonephritis is almost exclusively a disease of females. The infecting organism may be a type of fecal flora, such as *Escherichia* or *Klebsiella,* or normal flora from the periurethral skin (e.g., *Staphylococcus saprophyticus)*. Recurrent infections are common; chronic renal failure is a rare complication.

ASSESSMENT

Signs and symptoms: Fever, chills, flank pain, nausea, vomiting, malaise, frequency and urgency of urination, dysuria, cloudy and foul-smelling urine. **Note:** These indicators can be nonspecific, especially in the elderly.

Physical assessment: Tender, enlarged kidneys; abdominal rigidity; and costovertebral tenderness.

History of: UTI or obstruction; recent urologic procedure.

DIAGNOSTIC TESTS

Unless an anatomic or preexisting renal disease is present, renal function should remain normal.
1. *Urine culture:* Should be positive for the causative organism. **Note:** Asymptomatic bacteriuria is common in the elderly.
2. *Urinalysis:* Will reveal presence of WBCs, WBC casts, RBCs, and bacteria.

Note: All urine samples should be sent to the lab immediately after they are obtained or refrigerated if this is not possible. Urine left at room temperature has greater potential for bacterial growth, turbidity, and alkalinity, any of which can distort the test results. Urine cultures should *not* be refrigerated.

3. *Blood culture:* Positive for the causative organism in hematogenous infection. It is obtained from patients who appear septic or are hypotensive.
4. *IVP or retrograde pyelogram:* May be performed if there are recurrent episodes or if obstruction is suspected.

MEDICAL MANAGEMENT AND SURGICAL INTERVENTIONS

1. Bed rest.
2. Pharmacotherapy
   □ *Antibiotics:* For the infection; initially parenteral, then oral.
   □ *ASA or acetaminophen:* To control the fever and treat the discomfort.
3. Surgical intervention: May be necessary if an obstruction is present.

NURSING DIAGNOSES AND INTERVENTIONS

Pain related to dysuria secondary to infection

Desired outcome: Patient relates relief from discomfort and pain when voiding.

1. Monitor patient for the presence of dysuria. As appropriate, administer the prescribed analgesics, and document their effectiveness.
2. If it is not contraindicated, increase the patient's fluid intake to help relieve dysuria.

3. Notify MD of unrelieved or increasing flank pain.
4. As appropriate, assist patient with repositioning if it is effective in relieving discomfort.
5. Use nonpharmacologic interventions when possible (e.g., relaxation techniques, guided imagery, and distraction).

Potential for infection (or its recurrence) related to increased susceptibility secondary to disease process

Desired outcomes: Patient is free of infection as evidenced by normothermia, urine that is clear and of normal odor, HR ≤100 bpm, BP ≥90/60 mm Hg, and absence of flank or labial pain, dysuria, urgency, and frequency. Patient verbalizes knowledge of the signs and symptoms of infection and the importance of reporting them promptly should they occur.

1. Monitor patient's temperature at least q4h. Report temperature >37.78° C (100° F) to MD. Monitor for the presence of flank or labial pain, foul-smelling or cloudy urine, and frequency and urgency of urination. Teach these indicators to the patient and stress the importance of reporting them promptly to MD or staff should they occur.
2. Monitor BP and pulse at least q4h. The presence of hypotension and tachycardia can be indicative of sepsis and bacteremic shock.
3. Administer prescribed antibiotics as scheduled. Draw prescribed antibiotic serum levels at correct times to ensure reliable results. **Note:** Most antibiotics are measured at peak (30-60 minutes after infusion) and trough (30-60 minutes before the next dose) levels.
4. Use urinary catheters only when mandatory. Use meticulous, sterile technique when inserting and irrigating. Provide perineal care at least every shift. For indwelling catheters, maintain unobstructed flow, and always keep the urinary collection container below the level of the patient's bladder to prevent reflux of urine. Tape the catheter to the thigh or abdomen to decrease meatal irritation. **Note:** Intermittent catheterization carries less of a risk of UTI than indwelling catheterization.
5. Offer cranberry, plum, or prune juices, which leave an acid ash in the urine and inhibit bacteriuria.
6. Teach female patients the importance of wiping the perianal area from front to back and voiding before and immediately after sexual intercourse to minimize the risk of introducing bacteria into the urinary tract.
7. Treat fever with prescribed antipyretics and tepid baths as needed.

Alteration in nutrition: Less than body requirements related to decreased intake secondary to nausea and anorexia

Desired outcome: Patient maintains an adequate diet as evidenced by normal food intake and stable weight.

1. Provide nauseated or anorexic patient with frequent, small meals and carbonated beverages.
2. Treat nausea and vomiting with prescribed medications.
3. Record accurate calorie intake, and weigh patient daily.
4. Alert MD to inadequate nutritional intake.

Fluid volume deficit related to decreased intake secondary to anorexia or abnormal loss secondary to vomiting and diaphoresis

Desired outcomes: Patient is normovolemic as evidenced by balanced I&O, stable weight, urinary output ≥30-60 ml/hr, and BP and HR within patient's normal range. Patient verbalizes knowledge of the importance of a fluid intake of at least 2-3 L/day.

1. Maintain adequate fluid intake to avoid fluid volume deficit. An intake of at least 2-3 L/day is usually indicated; however, the appropriate amount depends on the patient's output, which includes NG, fecal, urinary, sensible, and insensible losses. Obtain parameters for the desired amount of fluid intake/restriction from MD. Teach nonrestricted patients the importance of maintaining a fluid intake of at least 2-3 L/day.

2. Monitor I&O and daily weight as indicators of hydration status.
3. Report indicators of volume deficit: poor skin turgor, thirst, dry mucous membranes, tachycardia, or orthostatic hypotension.

PATIENT-FAMILY TEACHING AND DISCHARGE PLANNING

Provide patient and significant others with verbal and written information for the following:

1. Medications, including drug name, purpose, dosage, schedule, precautions, and potential side effects.
2. Importance of taking medications for prescribed length of time, even if feeling "well."
3. Necessity of reporting the following indicators of UTI to MD: urgency, frequency, dysuria, flank pain, cloudy or foul-smelling urine, and fever.
4. Importance of perineal hygiene for female patients and the necessity of wiping from front to back, wearing undergarments with cotton crotch, and voiding before and after intercourse.
5. Importance of emptying the bladder at least q3-4h and once during the night to help prevent UTI caused by residual urine.
6. Necessity of maintaining a fluid intake of at least 2-3 L/day and drinking fruit juices (cranberry, plum, prune) that leave an acid ash in the urine.
7. Importance of continued medical follow-up because of the high incidence of recurrence.

Renal calculi

The kidneys excrete several substances that singly or in combination are highly insoluble. Normally, these substances are excreted with minimal crystal formation, but diet, medications, metabolic abnormalities, systemic disease, or infection can increase the tendency for crystals to form and stones to develop. Altered urine pH and concentration also can be important factors in stone formation.

Stones can lodge and cause obstruction or be passed in the urine. Giant staghorn calculi occasionally develop and fill the entire renal pelvis. The most common types of stones are made of calcium, struvite, uric acid, and cystine. Renal calculi are often recurrent and a common medical problem. Complications include infection and hydronephrosis.

ASSESSMENT

Signs and symptoms: The primary symptom is pain, with the location and severity depending on the area in which the stone has lodged. Vague back pain occurs when the stone lodges in the calyces or pelvis. Renal colic (severe flank pain radiating to the groin) is typical when the stone has lodged at the junction of the pelvis and ureter. Other indicators are hematuria, nausea, vomiting, syncope, and fever.

Physical assessment: Diaphoresis, pallor, and obvious distress.

History of: Previous stone formation, UTI, or urinary tract obstruction; diet high in calcium, purine, or oxalate; gout or administration of uricosuric agents; or treatment of neoplastic disease (due to increased production of uric acid).

DIAGNOSTIC TESTS

See "Ureteral Calculi," p. 132.

MEDICAL MANAGEMENT AND SURGICAL INTERVENTIONS

1. See "Ureteral Calculi," p. 132, for a discussion of medical management, including extracorporeal shock wave lithotripsy.

2. Surgical interventions: Indications for surgery include complete obstruction; persistent infection; severe, uncontrollable pain; renal pelvic calculus that is too large to pass spontaneously.

☐ *Pyelolithotomy* (incision into the renal pelvis).

☐ *Nephrolithotomy* (incision into the renal parenchyma).

☐ *Nephrectomy* (removal of the kidney if it is severely damaged).

NURSING DIAGNOSES AND INTERVENTIONS FOR THE SURGICAL PATIENT

Potential fluid volume deficit related to abnormal loss secondary to postoperative bleeding

Desired outcome: Patient is normovolemic as evidenced by balanced I&O, stable weight, good skin turgor, and BP and HR within patient's normal range.

1. Monitor I&O, daily weight, VS, and skin turgor as indicators of volume status. **Note:** Skin turgor is not a reliable indicator of volume deficit in the elderly owing to decreased elasticity of the skin.
2. Observe for signs of hemorrhage. Urine usually is dark red or pink for approximately 48 hours postoperatively in the patient who has had a pyelolithotomy or nephrolithotomy. Urine should not be bright red or contain clots. **Note:** The postnephrectomy patient should have clear urine. Alert MD to inappropriate hematuria.
3. Monitor BP and pulse for signs of hidden bleeding (e.g., hypotension and rapid pulse rate).
4. Check dressings and sheets under the dressing q4h for evidence of bleeding from the incision.

Potential impaired skin integrity related to irritation secondary to wound drainage

Desired outcome: Patient's skin remains clear and intact.

1. After a pyelolithotomy, there can be drainage of urine from the incision for several days to 2 weeks. Apply an ostomy pouch with a skin barrier to collect drainage and protect the skin.
2. Closely monitor skin integrity, especially in elderly patients who are at increased risk for skin breakdown.
3. Ensure that the drainage tube remains in its proper position; notify MD immediately if it dislodges, as it can be difficult to reinsert after 30 minutes.

See the appendix for nursing diagnoses and interventions for the care of preoperative and postoperative patients, p. 637.

PATIENT-FAMILY TEACHING AND DISCHARGE PLANNING

Provide patient and significant others with verbal and written information for the following:
1. Medications, including drug name, purpose, dosage, schedule, precautions, and potential side effects.
2. When appropriate, a diet that prevents recurrence of stones. Provide lists of foods that should be limited or avoided, including those that are high in calcium (e.g., dairy products), purine (e.g., meats, fish, poultry), and oxalate (e.g., beets, figs, nuts, spinach, black tea, chocolate). Encourage a daily fluid intake of at least 3 L/day in nonrestricted patients. A high fluid intake is especially important in preventing recurrent stones in patients with cystinuria.
3. Need for continued use of medications and medical follow-up because of the high rate of recurrence.
4. Requirements for maintaining alterations in urinary pH to prohibit stone precipitation and the necessity of urine pH testing.

5. Importance of seeking prompt medical treatment for signs and symptoms of UTI (e.g., fever, flank or labial pain, cloudy or foul-smelling urine) or obstruction (e.g., anuria, oliguria, and pain that is dull and aching or sharp and sudden).
6. Care of drains or catheters if patient is discharged with them.
7. Care of the surgical incision and indicators of wound infection, which necessitate medical attention: persistent erythema, swelling, pain, local warmth, and purulent drainage.
8. Postoperative activity precautions: avoiding heavy lifting (>5 lb) for the first 6 weeks, being alert to fatigue, getting maximum amounts of rest, and gradually increasing activities to tolerance.

Hydronephrosis

Hydronephrosis is the dilatation of the renal pelvis and calyces secondary to the obstruction of urinary flow. It results from any condition or abnormality that causes urinary tract obstruction. If the obstruction is not corrected, the affected kidney eventually atrophies and fails. Obstruction in the urethra or bladder will affect both kidneys, while obstruction in a single ureter or kidney will affect only the involved kidney.

Dramatic postobstructive diuresis can occur after the release of the obstruction. Inappropriate loss of sodium and water can in turn lead to volume depletion.

ASSESSMENT

Indicators are determined by the level, severity, and duration of obstruction.

Kidney/ureteral obstruction: Flank pain and abdominal tenderness, renal colic, gross hematuria.

Bladder neck/urethral obstruction: Frequency, hesitancy, dribbling, incontinence, nocturia, signs and symptoms of renal insufficiency, suprapubic pain, anuria.

Physical assessment: Enlarged kidney(s), distended bladder (if bladder neck obstruction is present), crackles (rales), and possibly hypertension and edema if patient is fluid overloaded.

History of: UTI or obstruction.

DIAGNOSTIC TESTS

1. *BUN and serum creatinine:* To determine level of renal function.
2. *Urinalysis:* To determine the presence of stone formation or infection.
3. *Renal ultrasound:* Noninvasive technique that uses high-frequency sound waves to assess renal size, contour, and structural changes. Because it does not rely on dye uptake, it can be used to evaluate poorly functioning kidneys.
4. *Abdominal x-ray, IVP, and retrograde pyelogram:* To identify cause of obstruction.

MEDICAL MANAGEMENT AND SURGICAL INTERVENTIONS

Management of hydronephrosis depends on the cause and duration of the urinary tract obstruction. Major causes of obstruction in the pelvis and ureter are calculi (see "Renal Calculi," p. 110) and neoplasms. Major causes of obstruction in the bladder and urethra are neoplasm (see "Cancer of the Bladder," p. 138), neurogenic bladder (see "Neurogenic Bladder," p. 147), and prostatic hypertrophy (see "Prostatic Hypertrophy," p. 509). Also see "Urinary Tract Obstruction," p. 135, for a general discussion of urinary tract obstruction. See "Chronic Renal Failure," p. 121, and "Acute Renal Failure," p. 116, as appropriate.

Management of hydronephrosis might include the insertion of a nephrostomy tube into the renal pelvis to drain urine and relieve pressure. It is inserted percutaneously under local anesthesia or in an open surgical procedure. The tube may be permanent or temporary.

NURSING DIAGNOSES AND INTERVENTIONS

Potential for infection related to vulnerability secondary to insertion/presence of nephrostomy tube

Desired outcome: Patient is free of infection as evidenced by normothermia, BP and HR within patient's normal range, urine that is clear and normal in odor and color, and absence of dysuria.

1. Maintain sterile technique when providing dressing changes and nephrostomy tube care.
2. Observe for and report indicators of infection, such as fever, pain, purulent drainage, and tachycardia. Document changes in color, odor, or clarity of urine. Infection is common with hydronephrosis.
3. Do not change, clamp, or irrigate the nephrostomy tube unless specifically prescribed by MD. **Caution:** Because of the tiny renal pelvis, never insert more than 5 ml at one time into the tube unless a larger amount has been specifically prescribed by the MD.
4. Keep the urine collection container and tubing in a dependent position. Avoid kinks in the tubing.

Potential for impaired tissue integrity related to insertion/presence of nephrostomy tube

Desired outcome: Patient is free of nephrostomy tube complications as evidenced by urine that is clear and of normal color after the first 24-48 hours, absence of pain, and a urine output of 30-60 ml/hr.

1. Report gross hematuria (urine that is bright red, possibly with clots). Transient hematuria can be expected for 24-48 hours after tube insertion.
2. Notify MD of leakage around the catheter, which can occur with blockage, as well as a sudden decrease in urine output, which can signal a dislodged catheter.
3. Report a sudden onset of or increase in pain, which can indicate perforation of a body organ by the catheter.
4. Keep the tube securely taped to the patient's flank with elastic tape. If the tube becomes accidentally dislodged, cover the site with a sterile dressing; notify MD immediately.

Note: Before removing the nephrostomy tube, the MD may request that it be clamped for several hours at a time to evaluate patient tolerance. While the tube is clamped, monitor the patient for the following indications of ureteral obstruction: flank pain, diminished urinary output, and fever.

Fluid volume deficit related to abnormal loss secondary to postobstructive diuresis

Desired outcome: Patient is normovolemic as evidenced by stable weight, good skin turgor, BP $\geq$90/60 mm Hg, HR $\leq$100 bpm, and CVP $\geq$5 cm H_2O (or VS within patient's normal range).

1. Monitor I&O hourly. Initially, output should exceed intake.
2. Monitor weight daily. Alert MD to steady weight loss.
3. Observe for and report indicators of volume depletion, including postural hypotension, tachycardia, poor skin turgor, elevated hematocrit, and decreased CVP. Monitor VS q30min for the first few hours after release of obstruction.
4. As prescribed, encourage fluids in nonrestricted patients who are hypovolemic.

See "Glomerulonephritis" for **Knowledge deficit:** Signs and symptoms of fluid and electrolyte imbalance, p. 104.

PATIENT-FAMILY TEACHING AND DISCHARGE PLANNING

Provide patient and significant others with verbal and written information for the following:

1. Medications, including drug name, purpose, dosage, schedule, precautions, and potential side effects.
2. Care of the nephrostomy catheter, if discharged with one; procedure to follow should the catheter become dislodged.
3. Frequency of and procedure for dressing changes. Patient or significant others should demonstrate safe dressing change technique before hospital discharge.
4. Need for continued medical follow-up; confirm date and time of next MD appointment, if known.
5. Signs and symptoms that necessitate medical attention: fever, cloudy or foul-smelling urine, flank or labial pain, increased catheter drainage, and drainage around the catheter site.

Renal artery stenosis

Stenosis of the renal artery or one of its main branches usually is the result of congenital fibromuscular hyperplasia or arteriosclerotic changes. A reduction in the lumen of the renal artery causes a decrease in blood flow to the affected kidney, which in turn stimulates the renin-angiotensin system, causing systemic hypertension. The elevation in blood pressure usually is proportional to the degree of ischemia in the affected kidney. If the hypertension is left untreated, the nonischemic kidney will develop arteriolar hyperplasia. When both kidneys are involved, renal failure can occur.

ASSESSMENT

Signs and symptoms: Headache, nose bleeds, tinnitus.

Physical assessment: Auscultation of a bruit in the midepigastric area. BP can be severely elevated.

DIAGNOSTIC TESTS

1. *IVP:* Visualizes kidneys *via* excretion of iodine-containing contrast medium; will demonstrate an ischemic kidney.
2. *Renal arteriography:* Injection of contrast medium into the renal arteries to visualize renal vasculature. The arteriogram can be false positive in the older adult. Complications include allergic reaction to the contrast medium, contrast medium-induced acute renal failure, hemorrhage, embolus, and infection.
3. *Radioisotope renogram:* Will demonstrate a delayed transit time of the radioisotope through the affected kidney.
4. *Renal vein renin levels:* Will show a difference between the two kidneys in unilateral disease. The renin level from the ischemic kidney should be 1.5 times that of the nonischemic kidney.
5. *Plasma renin level:* Will be increased owing to stimulation of the renin-angiotensin system.
6. *Captopril test:* A significant increase in plasma renin levels after a dose of captopril suggests renovascular hypertension. Captopril inhibits the enzyme that converts angiotensin I to angiotensin II. Individuals with hypertension caused by increased renin levels will respond to captopril by producing more renin.
7. *BUN and serum creatinine:* To determine the level of renal function.

MEDICAL MANAGEMENT AND SURGICAL INTERVENTIONS

Renovascular hypertension can be treated medically (see "Hypertension," p. 40), invasively *via* percutaneous transluminal angioplasty, or surgically. Patients with diffuse arteriosclerotic vascular disease or bilateral renal artery lesions may be considered poor surgical risks. Type and duration of the disease are additional factors that can contribute to the decision to treat patients medically.

Invasive procedure

Percutaneous transluminal angioplasty: Performed if the patient is a suitable candidate and the necessary equipment and personnel are available. Angioplasty involves the insertion of a balloon-tipped catheter to dilate the narrowed vessel. It can be performed under local anesthesia and requires minimal hospitalization.

Surgical interventions
1. Arterial endarterectomy with follow-up anticoagulant therapy.
2. Resection or bypass of the lesion (aortorenal bypass graft): Performed for those patients who are unsuitable candidates for endarterectomy or angioplasty, or when angioplasty has been unsuccessful or is unavailable.

NURSING DIAGNOSES AND INTERVENTIONS

Knowledge deficit: Rationale for frequent assessments after angioplasty, endarterectomy, or resection and the technique for measuring BP

Desired outcome: Patient verbalizes knowledge of the potential complications of angioplasty and the importance of frequent VS checks, and demonstrates BP measurement technique prior to hospital discharge.

1. Monitor BP frequently during the first 48 hours after aortorenal bypass graft. Explain to patient and significant others that hypertension during this period is temporary but may require treatment.
2. Explain the rationale for measuring VS q15min immediately after angioplasty. Monitor the integrity of the pulses distal to the angioplasty site.
3. Alert patient and significant others to the potential for bleeding and hematoma formation at the angioplasty site, as well as symptoms of hidden bleeding, including hypotension and tachycardia. Explain that if a hematoma is noted, it will be circled with ink and the time will be noted to detect further bleeding.
4. Explain the rationale for measuring BP under the same conditions each day: sitting, standing, lying down. Teach the technique for measuring BP to the patient and significant others prior to hospital discharge.

See the appendix for nursing diagnoses and interventions for the care of preoperative and postoperative patients, p. 637.

PATIENT-FAMILY TEACHING AND DISCHARGE PLANNING

Provide patient and significant others with verbal and written information for the following:
1. Medications, including drug name, purpose, dosage, schedule, precautions, and potential side effects.
2. Diet: low in sodium (see Table 11-3, p. 550). Include lists of foods high in potassium if patient is taking diuretics that cause hypokalemia (see Table 11-4, p. 555). Provide sample menus, and have the patient demonstrate understanding of the diet by planning meals for 3 days.
3. Technique for measuring BP. Patient or significant others should demonstrate proficiency before discharge.
4. Care of incision or angioplasty site. Teach patient the indicators of wound infection (e.g., erythema, purulent discharge, local warmth, fever) and the importance of reporting them promptly to the MD.
5. Need for continued medical follow-up to evaluate effectiveness of the treatment.

Section Two   RENAL FAILURE

Acute renal failure

Acute renal failure (ARF) is a sudden loss of renal function, which may or may not be accompanied by oliguria. The kidney loses its ability to maintain biochemical homeostasis, causing retention of metabolic wastes and dramatic alterations in fluid and electrolyte and acid-base balance. Although the renal damage usually is reversible, ARF has a high mortality rate.

The most common cause of ARF is acute tubular necrosis (ATN), which usually is caused by ischemia or nephrotoxins (antibiotics, heavy metals, or radiographic contrast media.) ATN also can occur after transfusion reactions, septic abortions, or crushing injuries. The clinical course of ATN can be divided into the following three phases: oliguric (lasting approximately 7-21 days); diuretic (7-14 days); and recovery (3-12 months). Causes of ARF other than ATN include acute poststreptococcal glomerulonephritis, malignant hypertension, and hepatorenal syndrome. The mortality rate of ARF varies greatly with etiology, the patient's age, and other medical problems. The overall mortality rate for ATN is 40%-60%.

A decrease in renal function secondary to decreased renal perfusion, but without kidney damage, is called *prerenal failure*. A reduction in urine output because of obstruction of urine flow is called *postrenal failure*. Prolonged prerenal or postrenal problems can lead to kidney damage and ARF, so early detection and correction of these problems are critical.

ASSESSMENT

Electrolyte disturbance: Muscle weakness, dysrhythmias, pruritus.

Fluid volume excess: Oliguria, pitting edema, hypertension, pulmonary edema.

Metabolic acidosis: Kussmaul respirations (hyperventilation), lethargy, headache.

Uremia (retention of metabolic wastes): Altered mental state, anorexia, nausea, diarrhea, pale and sallow skin, purpura, decreased resistance to infection, anemia, fatigue.

Note: Uremia adversely affects all body systems.

Physical assessment: Pallor; edema (peripheral, periorbital, sacral); crackles (rales); and elevated BP in patient who has fluid overload.

History of: Exposure to nephrotoxic substances, recent blood transfusion, prolonged hypotensive episodes or decreased renal perfusion, abortion, or a recent URI.

DIAGNOSTIC TESTS

1. *BUN and serum creatinine:* Assess the progression and management of ARF. Although both BUN and creatinine will increase as renal function decreases, creatinine is a better indicator of renal function because it is not affected by diet, hydration, or tissue catabolism.
2. *Creatinine clearance:* Measures the kidney's ability to clear the blood of creatinine and approximates the glomerular filtration rate. It will decrease as renal function decreases. Creatinine clearance is normally decreased in the elderly. **Note:** Failure to collect all urine during the period of study can invalidate the test.
3. *Urinalysis:* Can provide information about the cause and location of renal disease as reflected by abnormal urinary sediment (casts and cellular debris).
4. *Urinary osmolality and urinary sodium:* To rule out renal perfusion problems (prerenal). In ATN the kidney loses the ability to adjust urine concentration and conserve sodium.

Note: All urine samples should be sent to the lab immediately after collection or refrigerated if this is not possible. Urine left at room temperature has greater potential for bacterial growth, turbidity, and alkalinity, any of which can distort the reading.

5. _Renal ultrasound:_ Provides information about renal anatomy and pelvic structures, evaluates renal masses, and detects obstruction and hydronephrosis.
6. _Renal scan:_ Provides information about the perfusion and function of the kidneys.

MEDICAL MANAGEMENT

The goal is to remove the precipitating cause, maintain homeostatic balance, and prevent complications until the kidneys are able to resume function. Initially, prerenal or postrenal causes are ruled out or treated. A trial of fluid and diuretics may be used to rule out prerenal problems.
1. **Restrict fluids:** Replace losses plus 400 ml/24 hr. **Note:** Insensible fluid losses are only partially replaced to offset the water formed during the metabolism of protein, carbohydrates, and fats.
2. **Pharmacotherapy**

Note: Medications that are handled primarily by the kidney (see Table 3-2) will require modification of dosage or frequency to prevent medication toxicity. Renal failure also may decrease hepatic metabolism and protein binding of certain medications, resulting in increased medication effect.

☐ _Diuretics:_ In nonoliguric ARF for fluid removal (see Table 3-1, p. 103).

T A B L E 3 - 2 **Drug usage in renal failure**

Drugs that are handled primarily by the kidney have an increased effect in patients with renal failure. Usually they require modification of dosage or frequency. Some of these medications are:

Antibiotics	**Sedatives**	**Antiarrhythmics**
carbenicillin*	phenobarbital	digoxin
cefazolin*		procainamide*
gentamicin*		
kanamycin*	**Hypoglycemic agents**	
tobramycin*	insulin	
vancomycin		

Drugs that usually do not require dosage modification include:

Antibiotics	**Antihypertensive agents**	**Sedatives**
chloramphenicol*	hydralazine	diazepam
clindamycin	clonidine HCl	chlordiazepoxide HCl
dicloxacillin	prazosin HCl	
erythromycin	minoxidil	
nafcillin sodium	methyldopa*	
Diuretics	**Hypoglycemic agent**	**Antiinflammatory**
furosemide	tolbutamide	indomethacin
metolazone		
Narcotics	**Antiarrhythmics**	
codeine	propranolol	
morphine	quinidine gluconate*	

*Dialyzable drugs, which might require extra dosage after dialysis

☐ *Furosemide (Lasix) or mannitol:* May be given early in ARF to prevent the development of oliguria.

☐ *Antihypertensives:* To control BP.

☐ *Aluminum hydroxide antacids or calcium carbonate antacids:* To control hyperphosphatemia.

☐ *Cation exchange resins* (Kayexalate): To control hyperkalemia (see "Fluid and Electrolyte Disturbances," p. 558, for additional treatment).

☐ *Calcium or vitamin D supplements:* For hypocalcemic patients.

☐ *Sodium bicarbonate:* To treat acidosis. It is used cautiously in hypocalcemic or fluid-overloaded patients.

☐ *Vitamins B and C:* To replace losses if patient is on dialysis.

3. **Packed cells:** For active bleeding or if anemia is poorly tolerated.

4. **Diet:** High carbohydrate, low protein (high biologic value), low potassium (see Table 11-4, p. 555), and low sodium (see Table 11-3, p. 550). Sodium is limited to prevent thirst and fluid retention. Potassium is limited because of the kidney's inability to excrete excess potassium. Protein is limited to minimize retention of nitrogenous wastes. **Note:** Because of the loss of potassium during the diuretic phase, potassium might need to be increased during this time.

5. **TPN:** May be necessary for patients unable to maintain adequate oral/enteral intake.

6. **Peritoneal dialysis or hemodialysis:** Administered if the above therapy is inadequate for maintaining homeostatis or preventing complications (see "Renal Dialysis," p. 126).

NURSING DIAGNOSES AND INTERVENTIONS

Fluid volume excess: Edema related to fluid retention secondary to renal dysfunction: Oliguric phase

Desired outcome: Patient adheres to prescribed fluid restrictions and is normovolemic as evidenced by stable weight (patient should lose 0.5 kg/day if not eating), normal breath sounds, edema ≤1+ on a 0-4+ scale, CVP ≤12 cm H_2O, and BP and HR within patient's normal range.

1. Closely monitor and document I&O.
2. Monitor weight daily. A steady weight gain suggests excessive fluid volume.
3. Observe for indicators of fluid volume excess, including edema, hypertension, crackles (rales), tachycardia, distended neck veins, SOB, and increased CVP.
4. Carefully adhere to prescribed fluid restriction. Provide oral hygiene at frequent intervals, and offer fluids in the form of ice chips or popsicles to minimize thirst. Hard candies also may be given to decrease thirst. Spread allotted fluids evenly over a 24-hour period, and record the amount given. Instruct patient and significant others about the need for fluid restriction.

Note: Patients nourished *via* total parenteral nutrition (TPN) are at increased risk for fluid overload because of the necessary fluid volume.

Fluid volume deficit related to abnormal loss secondary to excessive urinary output: Diuretic phase

Desired outcome: Patient is normovolemic as evidenced by stable weight, balanced I&O, good skin turgor, CVP ≥5 cm H_2O, and BP and HR within patient's normal range.

1. Closely monitor and document I&O.
2. Monitor weight daily. A weight loss ≥0.5 kg/day may reflect excessive volume loss.
3. Observe for indicators of volume depletion, including poor skin turgor, hypotension, tachycardia, and decreased CVP.
4. As prescribed, encourage fluids in the dehydrated patient.
5. Report significant findings to MD.

Alteration in nutrition: Less than body requirements related to nausea, vomiting, anorexia, and dietary restrictions

Desired outcome: Patient has stable weight and demonstrates normal intake of food within restrictions, as indicated.

1. The presence of nausea, vomiting, and anorexia may signal increased uremia. Alert MD to symptoms and monitor BUN levels. BUN levels >80-100 mg/dl usually require dialytic therapy.
2. Provide frequent, small meals.
3. Administer prescribed antiemetics as necessary.
4. Coordinate meal planning and dietary teaching with patient, significant others, and renal dietitian.

Activity intolerance related to fatigue and weakness secondary to uremia and anemia

Desired outcome: Patient verbalizes decreases in weakness and fatigue and exhibits signs of improving endurance as evidenced by HR ≤20 bpm over resting HR, systolic BP ≤20 mm Hg over or under resting systolic BP, and RR ≤20 breaths/min with normal depth and pattern (eupnea).

1. Hematocrit will decrease and stabilize at around 20%-25%. Usually, patients are not transfused unless their hematocrit drops below 20%-25% or their anemia is poorly tolerated. Notify MD of increased weakness, fatigue, dyspnea, chest pain, or a further decrease in hematocrit. **Note:** Muscle weakness can be an indicator of dangerous hyperkalemia and should be reported immediately.
2. Assist with ADL as necessary; encourage independence to patient's tolerance.
3. Establish a progressive activity regimen within patient's activity limitations that will help patient to return to normal activities without complications. For more information, see **Potential for disuse syndrome** related to inactivity secondary to prolonged bed rest, p. 653.

Potential sensory/perceptual alterations related to mentation and motor disturbances secondary to uremia, electrolyte imbalance, and metabolic acidosis

Desired outcomes: Patient verbalizes orientation to person, place, and time, is asymptomatic of dysrhythmias and muscle weakness, and has a RR of 12-20 breaths/min with normal depth and pattern (eupnea). Patient verbalizes the signs and symptoms of electrolyte imbalance and metabolic acidosis and the importance of reporting them promptly should they occur.

1. Assess for and alert patient to indicators of the following:
   □ *Hypokalemia* (may occur during the diuretic phase): Muscle weakness, lethargy, dysrhythmias, and nausea and vomiting (secondary to ileus). See "Fluid and Electrolyte Disturbances," p. 556, for treatment.
   □ *Hyperkalemia:* Muscle cramps, dysrhythmias, muscle weakness, peaked T waves on EKG. **Note:** A normal serum potassium level is necessary for normal cardiac function. Hyperkalemia is a common and potentially fatal complication of ARF during the oliguric phase. See "Fluid and Electrolyte Disturbances," p. 558, for treatment.
   □ *Hypocalcemia:* Neuromuscular irritability and paresthesias.
   □ *Hyperphosphatemia:* Excessive itching.
   □ *Uremia:* Confusion, lethargy; restlessness.
   □ *Metabolic acidosis:* Rapid, deep respirations; confusion.
2. Avoid giving patient foods high in potassium (see Table 11-4, p. 555).
3. Minimize tissue catabolism by controlling fevers, maintaining adequate nutritional intake (especially calories), and preventing infections. If caloric intake is inadequate, body protein will be used for energy. A high carbohydrate diet helps to minimize tissue catabolism and production of nitrogenous wastes.
4. Prepare patient for the possibility of altered taste and smell.
5. Patients with renal failure tend to have increased magnesium levels because of decreased urinary excretion of dietary magnesium, and thus magnesium-containing medications should be avoided. For example, patients using magnesium-containing antacids, such as Maalox, are typically switched to aluminum hydroxide preparations, such as AlternaGel or Amphojel.

6. Administer aluminum hydroxide antacids as prescribed. Experiment with different brands or try capsules for patients who refuse certain liquid antacids.
7. Assure patient and significant others that irritability, restlessness, and altered thinking are temporary. Facilitate orientation through calendars, radios, familiar objects, and frequent reorientation.
8. Ensure safety measures (e.g., padded side rails, airway, tongue blade) for patients who are confused or severely hypocalcemic. For patients who exhibit signs of hyperkalemia, have emergency supplies (e.g., manual resuscitator bag, crash cart, and emergency drug tray) available.

Potential for infection related to increased susceptibility secondary to uremia

Desired outcome: Patient is free of infection as evidenced by normothermia, WBCs $\leq 11,000$ μl, urine that is clear and of normal odor, normal breath sounds, and absence of adventitious breath sounds and erythema, swelling, and drainage at the catheter sites.

Note: One of the primary causes of death in ARF is sepsis.

---

1. Monitor temperature and secretions for indicators of infection. Even minor increases in temperature can be significant because uremia masks the febrile response and inhibits the body's ability to fight infection.
2. Use meticulous, aseptic technique when changing dressings or manipulating venous catheters, IV lines, or indwelling catheters.
3. Avoid the use of indwelling urinary catheters since they are a common source of infection. When it is indicated, use intermittent catheterization instead.
4. Provide oral hygiene and skin care at frequent intervals. Use emollients and gentle soap to avoid drying and cracking of skin, which can lead to breakdown and infection. Take care to rinse off all soap when bathing, since soap residue may further irritate skin.

Constipation related to restrictions of fresh fruit and fluids, prolonged bed rest, and negative side effects of drugs (e.g., phosphate binders)

Desired outcomes: Patient relates that bowel movements are within normal pattern. Patient relates the foods and activities that promote bowel movements.

1. Monitor and record the quality and number of bowel movements.
2. Provide prescribed stool softeners and bulk-building supplements (e.g., Metamucil) as necessary.
3. Suggest alternate dietary sources of fiber, such as unsalted popcorn or unprocessed bran.
4. Encourage exercise and activity as appropriate.
5. Provide Fleet, oil retention, or tap water enemas as prescribed, *only* if the above measures fail. Avoid use of large-volume water enemas because excess fluid can be absorbed from the GI tract.

PATIENT-FAMILY TEACHING AND DISCHARGE PLANNING

Provide patient and significant others with verbal and written information for the following:
1. Medications, including drug name, purpose, dosage, schedule, precautions, and potential side effects.
2. Diet: Include fact sheet that lists foods to restrict.
3. Care and observation of the dialysis access if the patient is being discharged with one (see "Renal Dialysis," p. 126).
4. Importance of continued medical follow-up of renal function.
5. Instructions regarding the signs and symptoms of potential complications. These should include indicators of infection (see **Potential for infection,** above), electrolyte imbalance (see **Potential sensory/perceptual alterations,** p. 119), fluid volume excess (see p. 118), and bleeding (especially from the GI tract for patients who are uremic).

In addition:

6. If the patient requires dialysis after discharge, coordinate discharge planning with dialysis unit staff. Arrange visit to dialysis unit if possible.

Chronic renal failure

Chronic renal failure (CRF) is a progressive, irreversible loss of kidney function, which can develop over days to years. Eventually it may progress to end-stage renal disease (ESRD). The patient with ESRD requires dialysis or a kidney transplant to sustain life. Prior to ESRD, the patient can lead a relatively normal life with CRF, managed by diet and medications. This period can last from days to years, depending on the cause of renal failure and the patient's level of renal function at the time of diagnosis.

There are many causes of CRF. Some of the most common include glomerulonephritis, diabetes mellitus, hypertension, and polycystic kidney disease. In some patients the etiology of CRF is unknown.

ASSESSMENT

Fluid volume abnormalities: Crackles (rales), hypertension, edema, oliguria, or anuria.

Electrolyte disturbances: Muscle weakness, dysrhythmias, pruritus, tetany.

Uremia—retention of metabolic wastes: Weakness, malaise, anorexia, dry and discolored skin, peripheral neuropathy, irritability, clouded thinking, ammonia odor to breath.

Note: Uremia adversely affects all body systems.

Metabolic acidosis: Rapid respirations, lethargy, headache.

Potential acute complications

☐ *Congestive heart failure:* Crackles, dyspnea, orthopnea.
☐ *Pericarditis:* Chest pain, SOB.
☐ *Cardiac tamponade:* Hypotension, distant heart sounds, pulsus paradoxus (exaggerated inspiratory drop in systolic BP).

Physical assessment: Pallor, dry and discolored skin, edema (peripheral, periorbital, sacral). With fluid overload, crackles and elevated BP may be present.

History of: Glomerulonephritis, diabetes mellitus, polycystic kidney disease, hypertension, systemic lupus erythematosus, chronic pyelonephritis, and analgesic abuse, especially the combination of phenacetin and aspirin.

DIAGNOSTIC TESTS

1. *BUN and serum creatinine:* Both will be elevated. **Note:** Nonrenal problems, such as dehydration or GI bleeding, also can cause the BUN to increase, but there will not be a corresponding increase in creatinine.
2. *Creatinine clearance:* Measures the kidney's ability to clear the blood of creatinine and approximates the glomerular filtration rate. Creatinine clearance will decrease as renal function decreases. Dialysis is usually begun when the creatinine clearance is less than 10 ml/min. Creatinine clearance normally is decreased in the elderly. **Note:** Failure to collect all urine specimens during the period of study will invalidate the test.
3. *X-ray of the kidneys, ureters, and bladder (KUB):* Documents the presence of two kidneys, changes in size or shape, and some forms of obstruction.
4. *IVP, renal ultrasound, renal biopsy, renal scan (using radionuclides), and CT scan:* Additional tests for determining the cause of renal insufficiency. Once the patient has reached ESRD, these tests are not performed.
5. *Serum chemistries, chest and hand x-rays, and nerve conduction velocity test:* To assess for development and progression of uremia and its complications.

MEDICAL MANAGEMENT AND SURGICAL INTERVENTIONS

Prior to ESRD, medical management is aimed at slowing the progression of CRF and avoiding complications. Once the patient reaches ESRD, management is aimed at alleviating uremic symptoms and providing dialysis or renal transplantation.

1. **Diet:** Carbohydrates are increased in protein-restricted patients to ensure adequate caloric intake and prevent catabolism. Depending on existing renal function, sodium is limited to prevent thirst and fluid retention (see Table 11-3, p. 550), potassium is limited because of the kidney's inability to excrete excess potassium (see Table 11-4, p. 555), and protein is limited to minimize retention of nitrogenous wastes. Protein restriction may slow the progression of CRF in some patients. Protein intake should be that of high biologic value only.
2. **Fluid restriction:** For patients at risk for developing fluid volume excess. Fluid weight gain should be limited to 3%-4% of an individual's "dry" weight (i.e., weight with stable fluid balance).
3. **Pharmacotherapy**
   - □ *Aluminum hydroxide or calcium carbonate antacids:* To control hyperphosphatemia.
   - □ *Antihypertensives:* To control BP.
   - □ *Multivitamins and folic acid:* For patients with dietary restrictions or who are on dialysis (water-soluble vitamins are lost during dialysis).
   - □ *Anabolic steroids, parenteral iron, or ferrous sulfate:* To treat anemia.
   - □ *Recombinant human erythropoietin (Epogen):* A newly developed medication used to treat anemia of CRF.
   - □ *Diphenhydramine:* To treat pruritus.
   - □ *Sodium bicarbonate:* To treat acidosis.
   - □ *Vitamin D preparations and calcium supplements:* To treat hypocalcemia and prevent bone disease.
   - □ *Deferoxamine:* To treat iron or aluminum toxicity.

Note: Medications that are excreted primarily by the kidney require modification of dosage or frequency. Dialyzable medications may need to be increased or held and given postdialysis (see Table 3-2, p. 117).

---

4. **Packed cells:** To treat severe or symptomatic anemia.
5. **Maintenance of homeostasis and prevention of complications** by avoiding the following: Volume depletion, hypotension, use of radiopaque contrast medium, and nephrotoxic substances. Pregnancy is contraindicated.
6. **Renal transplant or dialysis:** If the above therapies are inadequate.

NURSING DIAGNOSES AND INTERVENTIONS

Activity intolerance related to weakness and fatigue secondary to anemia and uremia

Desired outcome: Patient verbalizes decreases in weakness and fatigue and exhibits improving endurance as evidenced by HR ≤20 bpm over resting HR, systolic BP ≤20 mm Hg over or under resting systolic pressure, and RR ≤20 breaths/min with normal depth and pattern (eupnea).

1. Anemia is usually proportional to the degree of azotemia. Hematocrit can be as low as 20% or less, but usually stabilizes at around 20%-25%. Typically, these patients are not transfused unless hematocrit drops below 20% or anemia is poorly tolerated. Notify MD of increased weakness, fatigue, dyspnea, chest pain, or further decreases in hematocrit. **Note:** Anemia is better tolerated in the uremic than in the nonuremic patient.
   - □ Provide and encourage optimal nutrition.
   - □ Administer anabolic steroids (e.g., nandrolone, if prescribed). Prepare female patients for side effects, including increasing facial hair, deepening voice, and menstrual irregularities.

☐ Coordinate lab studies to minimize blood drawing.
☐ Observe for and report evidence of occult blood and blood loss.
☐ Report symptomatic anemia: weakness, SOB, chest pain.
☐ Do not administer ferrous sulfate at the same time as antacids. The two medications should be given at least 1 hour apart to maximize absorption of the ferrous sulfate.
☐ Administer parenteral iron if prescribed. Anaphylaxis is a possible complication.

2. Assist patient with identifying activities that cause increased fatigue and adjusting those activities accordingly.
3. Assist the patient with ADL while encouraging maximum independence to the patient's tolerance.
4. Establish with the patient realistic, progressive exercises and activity goals that are designed to increase endurance. Ensure that they are within the patient's prescribed limitations. Examples are found in **Potential for disuse syndrome, p.** 653, and **Potential for activity intolerance,** p. 651, in the appendix.

Impaired skin integrity related to pruritus and dry skin secondary to uremia and edema

Desired outcome: Patient's skin remains intact and free of erythema and abrasions.

1. Pruritus is common in uremic patients, causing frequent and intense scratching. Pruritus often decreases with a reduction in BUN and improved phosphorus control. Encourage the use of phosphate binders and the reduction of dietary phosphorus if elevated phosphorus level is a problem. Give phosphate binders with meals for maximum effects. If necessary, administer antihistamines as prescribed. Keep patient's fingernails short.
2. Because uremia retards wound healing, instruct the patient to monitor scratches for evidence of infection and seek early medical attention should signs and symptoms of infection appear.
3. Uremic skin is often dry and scaly because of reduction in oil gland activity. Encourage the use of skin emollients. Patients should avoid hard soaps and excessive bathing. Advise patient to bathe every other day and use bath oils as needed if dry skin is a problem.
4. Clotting abnormalities and capillary fragility place the uremic patient at increased risk for bruising. Advise patient and significant others that this can occur.
5. Provide scheduled skin care and position changes for individuals with edema.

Knowledge deficit: Need for frequent BP checks and adherence to antihypertensive therapy and the potential for change in insulin requirements for diabetics

Desired outcome: Patient verbalizes knowledge of the importance of frequent BP checks and adherence to antihypertensive therapy. Diabetic patient verbalizes knowledge of the potential for change in insulin requirements.

Note: Patients with CRF may experience hypertension because of fluid overload, excess renin secretion, or arteriosclerotic disease.

1. Teach patient the importance of getting BP checked at frequent intervals and adhering to the prescribed antihypertensive therapy.
2. Teach diabetic patients that insulin requirements often decrease as renal function decreases. Instruct diabetic patients to be alert to indicators of hypoglycemia, including confusion, diaphoresis, and hypotension.

Potential sensory/perceptual alterations related to mentation and motor disturbances secondary to electrolyte and acid-base imbalance

Desired outcomes: Patient verbalizes orientation to person, place, and time and is asymptomatic of dysrhythmias and muscle weakness. Patient relates the importance of avoiding foods and products that are high in potassium.

1. Hyperkalemia is a common complication of ESRD. Avoid salt substitutes (KCl) and "light" salts (contain KCl) and potassium-containing medications, such as potassium

penicillin G. (For a list of foods that are high in potassium, see Table 11-4, p. 555.) Teach patient and significant others to read all OTC labels.

2. If the patient requires multiple blood transfusions, observe for indicators of hyperkalemia, because old banked blood may contain as much as 30 mEq/L of potassium. Use fresh packed cells when possible.

3. For other interventions, see the same nursing diagnosis in "Acute Renal Failure," p. 119.

See "Acute Renal Failure" for **Fluid volume excess** (oliguric phase), p. 118, **Alteration in nutrition**, p. 118, **Potential for infection**, p. 120, and **Constipation**, p. 120. See the appendix, p. 690, for psychosocial nursing diagnoses and interventions for the care of patients with life-disrupting illnesses.

PATIENT-FAMILY TEACHING AND DISCHARGE PLANNING

Provide patient and significant others with verbal and written information for the following:

1. Medications, including drug name, purpose, dosage, schedule, precautions, and potential side effects.

2. Diet, including fact sheet listing foods that are to be restricted or limited. Inform patient that diet and fluid restrictions may be altered as renal function decreases. Provide sample menus and have the patient demonstrate understanding by preparing 3-day menus that incorporate dietary restrictions.

3. Care and observation of dialysis access if the patient has one (see "Renal Dialysis," p. 130).

4. Signs and symptoms that necessitate medical attention: irregular pulse, fever, unusual SOB or edema, sudden change in urine output, and unusual muscle weakness.

5. Need for continued medical follow-up; confirm date and time of next MD appointment.

6. Importance of avoiding infections and seeking treatment promptly should one develop. Instruct the patient in the indicators of frequently encountered infections, including URI, UTI, impetigo, and otitis media. For details, see **Potential for infection**, p. 125, in "Care of the Renal Transplant Patient."

In addition:

7. For the patient with or approaching ESRD, provide data concerning the various treatment options and support groups. The local chapter of the National Kidney Foundation can be helpful in identifying support groups and organizations in the area. Patient and significant others should meet with the renal dietitian and social worker before discharge.

8. Coordinate discharge planning and teaching with the dialysis unit or facility. If possible, have patient visit dialysis unit before discharge.

9. For the individual with ESRD, the importance of coordinating all medical care through the nephrologist and the importance of alerting all medical and dental personnel to ESRD status, owing to the increased risk of infection and the need to adjust medication dosages. In addition, dentists may want to premedicate ESRD patients with antibiotics prior to dental work and avoid scheduling dental work on the day of dialysis owing to the heparinization that is used with dialytic therapy.

Section Three CARE OF THE RENAL TRANSPLANT PATIENT

Annually, approximately 9,000 patients with ESRD receive renal transplants. Although patients receive transplants at major medical centers and are cared for postoperatively in specialized units, they may be admitted to any hospital for treatment of a rejection episode, medication complication, or unrelated illness. The majority of the transplanted kidneys come from cadavers, although living family members might also donate. Unless the graft is donated from an identical twin, transplant success depends on the suppression of graft rejection. This is accomplished by carefully matching donors to recipients through tissue typing before transplantation and immunosuppression after transplantation. Rejection is the major complication of renal transplant.

IMMUNOSUPPRESSION

1. Necessary for the life of the graft.
2. Puts patient at increased risk for infection and development of malignancy in the long term.
3. Usual immunosuppressive medications
   □ *Azathioprine* (Imuran): Side effects include decreased WBC and platelet counts.
   □ *Prednisone:* Side effects include muscle wasting, aseptic necrosis of bone, cataracts, bleeding, sodium retention, altered carbohydrate metabolism, mood and behavior changes, and Cushingoid changes.
   □ *Cyclosporine* (Sandimmune): Side effects include nephrotoxicity, hepatotoxicity, hirsutism, tremors, gum hyperplasia, hypertension, infection, malignancy. Route is either PO or IV. If IV, administer slowly over period of 2-4 hours and monitor for anaphylaxis. If route is PO, use a glass container; mix with orange juice or chocolate milk to make it more palatable. Do not allow solution to stand.
   □ *Antilymphocyte sera* (ATGAM): Given IV. Side effects include increased risk of infection and malignancy. In addition, immediate side effects include chills, fever, rash, and joint pain.
   □ *Monoclonal antibody* (Orthoclone OKT3): Given IV. Side effects include increased risk of infection and malignancy. In addition, immediate side effects include fever, chills, headache, nausea, and bronchospasm. Patients receiving initial doses require close monitoring owing to the high incidence of side effects.

REJECTION

1. Acute: 1 week-4 months after surgery; potentially reversible; treated with increased immunosuppression.
2. Chronic: Months to years after transplant; irreversible; managed conservatively with diet and antihypertensives until dialysis is required.
3. Indicators of rejection: Oliguria, tenderness over kidney (located in iliac fossa), sudden weight gain, fever, malaise, hypertension, and increased BUN and serum creatinine.

NURSING DIAGNOSES AND INTERVENTIONS

Potential for infection related to vulnerability secondary to invasive procedures, exposure to infected individuals, and immunosuppression

Desired outcomes: Patient is free of infection as evidenced by normothermia, HR ≤100 bpm (or within patient's normal range), and absence of erythema or purulent drainage at wounds or catheter exit sites. Patient relates the indicators of infection and the importance of reporting them promptly to MD or staff.

1. Observe for indicators of infection, such as fever and unexplained tachycardia. Instruct the patient to be alert to signs and symptoms of commonly encountered infections and the importance of reporting them promptly. These include *urinary tract infection:* cloudy and malodorous urine; urinary burning, frequency, and urgency; *upper respiratory tract infection:* malodorous, purulent, colored, and copious sputum; productive cough; *otitis media:* malaise, earache; *impetigo:* inflamed or draining areas on the skin.
2. Teach patient to avoid exposure to individuals known to have infections.
3. Use aseptic technique with all invasive procedures and dressing changes.

Knowledge deficit: Signs and symptoms of rejection, negative side effects of immunosuppressive agents, and importance of protecting the fistula

Desired outcome: Patient verbalizes knowledge of the signs and symptoms of rejection, the side effects of immunosuppressive therapy, and the importance of protecting the hemodialysis vascular access.

1. Explain the importance of renal function monitoring: I&O, daily weight, and BUN and serum creatinine values. As renal function decreases, BUN and creatinine values will increase.
2. Alert patient to the signs and symptoms of rejection (see p. 125) and the importance of reporting them promptly should they occur.
3. Explain that significant decreases in WBC and platelet counts can be a side effect of immunosuppressive agents, and therefore serial monitoring is essential.
4. Explain that GI bleeding is a potential side effect of immunosuppressive agents. Alert patient to the signs and symptoms of GI bleeding (e.g., tarry stools, "coffee-ground" emesis, increasing fatigue and weakness) and the importance of reporting them promptly should they occur.
5. If the patient has a patent fistula or graft (hemodialysis vascular access), explain that it must be handled with care, since the patient will need it if a return to dialysis is indicated. Explain that taking blood pressures, drawing blood, and starting IVs are contraindicated in the fistula arm; and therefore, patient should warn others about these contraindications.

Section Four   RENAL DIALYSIS

Note: This section does not include care of the patient during dialysis, but rather it provides essential background data, including nursing therapeutics for the care of patients who undergo dialysis.

Peritoneal dialysis and hemodialysis are lifesaving procedures used to treat severely decreased or absent renal function. Dialysis can be either temporary, until the kidneys are able to resume adequate function, or permanent. Dialysis is defined as the selective movement of water and solutes from one fluid compartment to another across a semipermeable membrane. The two fluid compartments are the patient's blood and the dialysate (electrolyte and glucose solution). With hemodialysis, the semipermeable membrane is an artificial one; while with peritoneal dialysis, the peritoneum serves as a natural dialysis membrane.

Indications for dialysis: Acute renal failure or acute episodes of renal insufficiency that cannot be managed by diet, medications, and fluid restriction; ESRD; drug overdose; hyperkalemia; fluid overload; or metabolic acidosis.

Functions of dialysis: Correction of electrolyte abnormalities; removal of excess fluid and metabolic wastes; correction of acid-base abnormalities. **Note:** Dialysis does not compensate completely for the lack of functioning kidneys. Medications and dietary and fluid restrictions are often necessary to supplement dialysis.

Peritoneal dialysis: Slower, does not require heparinization; can be performed by trained floor nurses; requires a minimum of equipment.

Hemodialysis: Faster, requires heparinization, specially trained staff, expensive and complex equipment; patient must have adequate vasculature for access.

Care of the peritoneal dialysis patient

Peritoneal dialysis uses the peritoneum as the dialysis membrane. Dialysate is instilled into the peritoneal cavity *via* a special catheter, and movement of solutes and fluid occurs between the patient's capillary blood and the dialysate. At set intervals the peritoneal cavity is drained and new dialysate is instilled.

COMPONENTS OF PERITONEAL DIALYSIS

1. **Catheter:** Silastic tube that is either implanted as a surgical procedure for chronic patients or inserted at the bedside for acute dialysis.
2. **Dialysate:** Sterile electrolyte solution similar in composition to normal plasma. The electrolyte composition of the dialysate can be adjusted according to individual need. The most commonly adjusted electrolyte is potassium. Glucose is added to the dialysate in varying concentrations to remove excess body fluid *via* osmosis. **Note:** Some glucose crosses the peritoneal membrane and enters the patient's blood. Diabetic patients may require additional insulin. Observe for and report indicators of hyperglycemia (e.g., complaints of thirst or changes in sensorium).

TYPES OF PERITONEAL DIALYSIS

1. **Intermittent peritoneal dialysis (IPD):** The patient is dialyzed for periods of 8-10 hours, 4-5 times per week. A predetermined amount of dialysate (usually 2 L) is instilled for a set length of time (usually 20-30 min). It is then allowed to drain by gravity, and the process is repeated. IPD can be performed manually with individual bottles and bags, or mechanically using a proportioning machine or cycler. The patient is restricted to a chair or bed. Peritoneal dialysis also can be performed as an acute, temporary procedure. Continuous hourly exchanges are performed for 48-72 hours. This type of dialysis usually requires a critical care setting. The patient is restricted to bed.
2. **Continuous ambulatory peritoneal dialysis (CAPD):** The patient attaches a specialized bag of dialysate to the peritoneal catheter; allows the dialysate to drain in; clamps the catheter, leaving the bag attached; and goes about his or her daily routine. After 4 hours (8 hours at night) the clamp is opened and the dialysate is allowed to drain out. Using aseptic technique, the patient attaches a new bag of dialysate and the process is repeated. Dialysis exchanges are done continuously, 7 days a week. CAPD is used primarily for ESRD.
3. **Continuous cycling peritoneal dialysis (CCPD):** This is a combination of IPD and CAPD. A cycler performs three dialysate exchanges at night. In the morning a fourth exchange is instilled and left in the peritoneal cavity for the entire day. At the end of the day, the fourth exchange is allowed to drain out and the process is repeated. The patient is ambulatory by day and restricted to bed at night.

NURSING DIAGNOSES AND INTERVENTIONS

Potential for infection related to vulnerability secondary to direct access of the catheter to the peritoneum

Desired outcomes: Patient is free of infection as evidenced by normothermia and absence of the following: abdominal pain, cloudy outflow, nausea, malaise, and erythema, drainage, and tenderness at the exit site. Patient relates the signs and symptoms of infection and demonstrates sterile technique for bag, tubing, and dressing changes.

1. The most common complication of peritoneal dialysis is peritonitis. Observe for and report indications of peritonitis, including fever, abdominal pain, cloudy outflow, nausea, and malaise. **Caution:** It is essential that sterile technique be used when connecting and disconnecting the catheter from the dialysis system.
2. The dialysate must remain sterile because it is instilled directly into the body. Maintain sterile technique when adding medications to the dialysate.
3. Follow agency policy for dressing the catheter exit site.
4. Observe for and report redness, drainage, or tenderness at exit site. Culture any exudate and report the results to the MD.
5. Report to MD if dialysate leaks around the catheter exit site. This can indicate an obstruction or the need for another purse-string suture around the catheter site. Continued leakage at the site can lead to peritonitis.
6. Instruct the patient in the above interventions and observations if peritoneal dialysis will be used after discharge.

Potential alterations in fluid volume: *Excess* related to fluid retention or inadequate exchange secondary to catheter problems or peritonitis; *deficit* related to abnormal loss secondary to hypertonicity of the dialysate

Desired outcomes: Patient is normovolemic as evidenced by balanced I&O, stable weight, good skin turgor, CVP 5-12 cm H_2O, RR 12-20 breaths/min with normal depth and pattern (eupnea), and BP and HR within patient's normal range. The volume of dialysate outflow is $\geq$ inflow.

1. Fluid retention can occur because of catheter complications that prevent adequate outflow, or a severely scarred peritoneum that prevents adequate exchange. Observe for and report indicators of fluid overload, such as hypertension, tachycardia, distended neck veins, or increased CVP. Also be alert to incomplete dialysate returns. Accurate measurement and recording of outflow is critical.
2. Outflow problems can occur because of the following:
   ☐ *Full colon:* Use stool softeners, high-fiber diet, or enemas if necessary.
   ☐ *Catheter occlusion by fibrin* (usually occurs soon after insertion): Obtain order to irrigate with heparinized saline.
   ☐ *Catheter obstruction by omentum:* Turn patient from side to side, elevate HOB, or apply firm pressure to the abdomen.

Note: Notify MD for unresolved outflow problems.

---

3. Monitor I&O and weight daily. A steady weight gain is indicative of fluid retention.
4. Respiratory distress can occur because of compression of the diaphragm by the dialysate. If this occurs, elevate the HOB, drain the dialysate, and notify MD.
5. Bloody outflow may appear with initial exchanges. Report gross bloody outflow.
6. Coordinate lab studies to limit blood drawing, since patients with renal failure are anemic due to alteration in erythropoietin, causing decreased RBC production and longevity.
7. Volume depletion can occur with excessive use of hypertonic dialysate. Observe for and report indicators of volume depletion, including poor skin turgor, hypotension, tachycardia, and decreased CVP.

Alteration in nutrition: Less than body requirements related to increased need secondary to protein loss in the dialysate

Desired outcome: Patient has adequate nutrition as evidenced by stable weight, serum albumin 3.5-5.5 g/dl, and protein intake of 1.2-1.5 g/kg body weight/day.

1. Protein crosses the peritoneum and a significant amount is lost in the dialysate. An increased intake of protein is necessary to prevent excessive tissue catabolism. Protein loss increases with peritonitis. Ensure adequate dietary intake of protein: 1.2-1.5 g/kg body weight daily.
2. Peritoneal dialysis patients typically have fewer dietary restrictions than those on hemodialysis. Ensure that a dietary evaluation and teaching program is performed when the patient changes from one type of dialysis to the other.
3. Provide a list of restricted and encouraged foods with menus that illustrate their integration into the daily diet. Ensure patient's understanding by having him or her plan a 3-day menu that incorporates the appropriate foods and restrictions.

Potential for sensory/perceptual alterations related to mentation and motor changes secondary to uremia and serum electrolyte imbalance

Desired outcome: Patient verbalizes orientation to person, place, and time and is free of dysrhythmias.

1. Instruct patient and staff to observe for and report indications of the following:
   ☐ *Increased uremia:* Confusion, lethargy, and restlessness. Monitor BUN and serum creatinine values. Increases in value can signal the need for increased dialysis. BUN should be <80-100 mg/dl. Serum creatinine values will vary, depending on the individual's muscle mass.

□ *Hyperkalemia:* Muscle cramps and muscle weakness. Monitor serum potassium values. Normal range is 3.5-5.0 mEq/L.

□ *Hypokalemia* (secondary to dialysis): Abdominal pain, lethargy, and dysrhythmias. Monitor serum potassium values. Normal range is 3.5-5.0 mEq/L. **Note:** Alert MD to the development of an irregular pulse, since it can be indicative of dangerous hypokalemia. This is especially important for patients on digitalis, as hypokalemia potentiates digitalis toxicity.

2. Promptly report abnormal lab values to the MD. The dialysate or length of dialysis time may require adjustment to compensate for the abnormal lab values.

3. For other interventions, see the same nursing diagnosis in "Acute Renal Failure," p. 119.

Care of the hemodialysis patient

During hemodialysis, blood is removed *via* a special vascular access, heparinized, pumped through an artificial kidney (dialyzer), and then returned to the patient's circulation. Hemodialysis is either a temporary, acute procedure performed as needed, or it is performed chronically 2-4 times a week for 2-5 hours each treatment.

COMPONENTS OF HEMODIALYSIS

1. **Artificial kidney** (dialyzer): Composed of a blood compartment and dialysate compartment, separated by a semipermeable membrane that allows the diffusion of solutes and the filtration of water. Protein and bacteria do not cross the artificial membrane.

2. **Dialysate:** An electrolyte solution similar in composition to normal plasma. Each of the constituents may be varied according to patient need. The most commonly altered component is potassium. Glucose may be added to prevent sudden drops in serum osmolality and serum glucose during dialysis.

3. **Vascular access:** Necessary to provide a blood flow rate of 200-500 ml/min for an effective dialysis.

NURSING DIAGNOSES AND INTERVENTIONS

Potential alterations in fluid volume: *Excess* related to fluid retention secondary to renal failure; *deficit* related to excessive fluid removal or increased risk of bleeding secondary to dialysis

Desired outcomes: Patient is normovolemic as evidenced by balanced I&O, stable weight, RR 12-20 breaths/min with normal depth and pattern (eupnea), CVP 5-12 cm H_2O, HR and BP within patient's normal range, and absence of abnormal breath sounds and abnormal bleeding. Patient relates the signs and symptoms of fluid volume excess and deficit.

1. Monitor I&O and daily weight as indicators of fluid status. A steady weight gain is indicative of retained fluid. The patient's weight is an important guideline for determining the quantity of fluid that needs to be removed during dialysis. Weigh patient at the same time each day, using the same scale, and wearing the same amount of clothing (or with same items on the bed if using a bed scale).

2. Instruct patient and staff to observe for and report indications of fluid volume excess: edema, hypertension, crackles (rales), tachycardia, distended neck veins, SOB, and increased CVP.

3. After dialysis observe for and report indicators of fluid volume deficit, including hypotension, decreased CVP, and tachycardia. Describe the signs and symptoms to the patient and explain the importance of reporting them promptly should they occur. **Note:** Because of autonomic neuropathy, the uremic patient may not develop a compensatory tachycardia when hypovolemic.

Note: Antihypertensive medications usually are held before and during dialysis to help prevent hypotension during dialysis. Clarify medication prescriptions with the MD.

4. Observe for bleeding (gums, needle sites, incisions) postdialysis, which can occur because of use of heparin during dialysis. Alert patient to the potential for bleeding from these areas.
5. To prevent hematoma formation, do not give IM injection for at least 1 hour postdialysis.
6. GI bleeding is common in patients with renal failure, especially after heparinization. Test all stools for the presence of blood. Report significant findings.

Potential for altered tissue perfusion and infection related to susceptibility secondary to the creation of the vascular access for hemodialysis

Desired outcomes: Patient has adequate tissue perfusion as evidenced by normal skin temperature and color and brisk capillary refill (<3 seconds) distal to the vascular access. Patient is free of infection as evidenced by normothermia and absence of erythema, local warmth, exudate, swelling, and tenderness at the exit site. Patient's access is patent as evidenced by presence of bright red blood within shunt tubing or presence of thrill with palpation and bruit with auscultation of fistula.

1. After the surgical creation of the vascular access, assess for patency, auscultate for bruit, and palpate for thrill. Report severe or unrelieved pain, and observe for and report numbness, tingling, and swelling of the extremity distal to the access, any of which can signal impaired tissue perfusion. Expect postoperative swelling along the fistula; elevate the extremity.
2. Notify MD if the extremity distal to vascular access becomes cool, has decreased capillary refill, or is discolored, as these problems can occur with vascular insufficiency.
3. Follow the three principles of nursing care common to all types of vascular access: prevent bleeding, prevent clotting, and prevent infection. Explain the monitoring and care procedures to the patient. Remember that the vascular access is the patient's lifeline. Monitor it closely and handle it with care. Vascular accesses include the following:

Shunt: An external, temporary connection between an artery and a vein
☐ *Prevent bleeding:* Keep shunt securely wrapped with gauze, exposing a portion of the loop to allow evaluation of patency. Tape shunt connection. Do not puncture tubing. Never cut dressings off. Keep bulldog or other smooth rubber-shod clamps at the bedside in case the shunt becomes disconnected. If shunt is pulled out, apply firm pressure at site and call MD *stat.* If necessary, apply tourniquet above the site.
☐ *Prevent clotting:* Do not kink tubing. Do not take BP, start IVs, or draw lab work from shunt arm. Document patency at least once a shift. Blood within shunt tubing should be warm and bright red. Palpate for thrill and auscultate for bruit above venous cannula exit site. Observe for and immediately report indications of clotting: dark or separated blood within the shunt, shunt cool to the touch, absence of thrill and bruit.
☐ *Prevent infection:* Use aseptic technique with dressing changes. Observe for and report indications of infection: presence of erythema, swelling, local warmth, exudate, and tenderness at the exit site. Culture any drainage.

Subclavian or femoral lines: External, temporary catheters inserted into a large vein
☐ *Prevent bleeding:* Anchor catheter securely since it might not be sutured in. Tape all connections. Keep clamps at bedside in case line becomes disconnected. If the line is removed or accidentally pulled out, apply firm pressure to site for at least 10 min.

Caution: An air embolus can occur if a subclavian line accidentally becomes disconnected. If this occurs, immediately clamp the line. Then turn the patient into a left side-lying position to help prevent the air from blocking the pulmonary artery, and lower the HOB into Trendelenburg's position to increase intrathoracic pressure. This will decrease the flow of inspiratory air into the vein. Notify MD *stat!*

☐ *Prevent clotting:* Keep line patent by priming with heparin or by constant infusion with a heparinized solution. Follow protocol or obtain specific order from MD. Attach a label to all lines that are primed with heparin to alert other personnel.

☐ *Prevent infection:* Perform aseptic dressing changes according to agency protocol. Observe for and report indications of infection, including presence of erythema, local warmth, exudate, swelling, and tenderness at exit site. Report and culture any drainage.

Fistula: Internal, permanent connection between an artery and a vein, or the insertion of an internal graft that is joined to an artery and vein. Grafts can be straight or U-shaped. They are located in the arm or thigh.

☐ *Prevent bleeding:* Inspect needle puncture sites postdialysis for bleeding. Should it occur, apply just enough pressure over the site to stop it. Release the pressure and check for bleeding q5-10min.

☐ *Prevent clotting:* Do not take BP, start IV, or draw blood in the fistula arm. Avoid tight clothing, jewelry, name bands, or restraint on fistula extremity. Palpate for thrill and auscultate for bruit at least every shift and after hypotensive episodes. Notify MD *stat* if bruit or thrill is absent.

☐ *Prevent infection:* Observe for and report indications of infection: presence of erythema, local warmth, swelling, exudate, and unusual tenderness at the fistula site. Culture and report any drainage.

See "Care of the Peritoneal Dialysis Patient" for **Potential sensory/perceptual alterations, p. 128.**

Section Five   DISORDERS OF THE URINARY TRACT

Ureteral calculi

Ureteral calculi (stones) are a common urologic condition. Although the cause of stones is unknown in 50% of reported cases, it is believed that they originate in the kidney and are passed through the kidney to the ureter. About 90% of all stones pass from the ureter into the bladder and out of the urinary system spontaneously.

See "Renal Calculi," p. 110, for related information.

ASSESSMENT

Signs and symptoms: Pain that is sharp, sudden, and intense, or dull and aching. Pain can be intermittent as the stone moves along the ureter and subside when it enters the bladder. Nausea, vomiting, diarrhea, abdominal pain, and paralytic ileus can occur. Patient may experience frequency, void in small amounts, and have hematuria.

Physical assessment: Pallor, diaphoresis, tachycardia, and tachypnea may be noted; chills and fever may be present in the acute stage. There can be absence of bowel sounds secondary to ileus, and the abdomen may be distended and tympanic. The patient will be restless and unable to find a position of comfort.

History of: Sedentary lifestyle; residence in geographic area in which water supply is high in stone-forming minerals; vitamin A deficiency; vitamin D excess; hereditary cystinuria; treatment with acetazolamide, which is given for glaucoma; inflammatory bowel disease; recurrent UTI; prolonged periods of immobilization; gout; decreased fluid intake; and familial history of calculi or renal disease such as renal tubular acidosis.

DIAGNOSTIC TESTS

1. *Serum tests:* To assess calcium levels >5.3 mEq/L, phosphorus levels >2.6 mEq/L, and uric acid levels >7.5 mg/dl, which have been implicated in the formation of stones.

2. *BUN and creatinine tests:* To evaluate renal-urinary function. Abnormalities are reflected by high BUN and serum creatinine and low urine creatinine. **Note:** Be aware that BUN results are affected by fluid volume excess and deficit. Volume excess will reduce BUN levels, while volume deficit will increase levels. For the older adult, serum creatinine level may not be a reliable measure of renal function because of reduced muscle mass and a decreased glomerular filtration rate. These tests must be evaluated based on an adjustment for the patient's age, hydration status, and in comparison to other renal-urinary tests.

3. *Urinalysis:* To provide baseline data on the functioning of the urinary system, detect metabolic disease, and assess for the presence of UTI. A cloudy or hazy appearance, foul odor, pH >8.0, and the presence of WBCs and WBC casts indicate the presence of UTI.

4. *Urine culture:* To determine the type of bacteria present in the genitourinary tract. To avoid contamination, a midstream specimen should be collected.

5. *24-hour urine collection:* To test for high levels of uric acid, cystine, oxalate, calcium, phosphorus, or creatinine.

Note: All urine samples should be sent to lab immediately after they are obtained, or refrigerated if this is not possible (specimens for culture are *not* refrigerated). Urine left at room temperature has greater potential for bacterial growth, turbidity, and alkaline pH, any of which can distort the reading.

6. *KUB x-ray:* To outline gross structural changes in the kidneys and urinary system. Typically, calcification is seen. Serial radiography monitors progressive movement of the stone.

7. *IVP/excretory urogram:* Used to visualize the kidneys, kidney pelvis, ureters, and bladder, this test also outlines radiopaque stones within the ureters.

8. *CT scan with or without injection of contrast medium:* To distinguish cysts, tumors, calculi, and other masses; and determine presence of ureteral dilatation and bladder distention.

MEDICAL MANAGEMENT AND SURGICAL INTERVENTIONS

1. Pharmacotherapy during the acute stage
   - □ *Narcotic and antispasmodic agents:* To relieve pain and ureteral spasms.
   - □ *Antiemetics:* For nausea and vomiting.
   - □ *Antibiotics:* For infection.

2. Prophylactic pharmacotherapy
   - □ *For uric acid stones:* Allopurinol or sodium bicarbonate is given to reduce uric acid production or alkalinize the urine, keeping the pH at ≥6.5.
   - □ *For calcium stones:* Sodium cellulose phosphate, when used with a calcium-restricted diet, reduces risk of stone formation. Orthophosphates (potassium acid phosphate and disodium and dipotassium phosphates) are given to decrease urinary excretion of citrate and pyrophosphate, and thus inhibit stone formation. Thiazides also reduce excretion of citrate and reduce urinary calcium.
   - □ *For cystine stones:* Sodium bicarbonate or sodium-potassium citrate solution is given to increase urinary pH (≥7.5). Penicillamine can be given to lower cystine levels in the urine. Alpha-mercaptopropionylglycine produces similar action to penicillamine but produces fewer side effects.

3. IV therapy: For patients who are dehydrated.

4. Increase fluid intake: To help flush stone from ureter to the bladder and out through the system.

5. Diet: Specific to patient's stone type. (See **Health-seeking behaviors:** Diet regimen and its relationship to stone formation, p. 134, for detail.)
6. Endoscopic removal of calculi *via* cystoscope: A basketing catheter is placed beyond the stone and rotated in a downward movement to capture and remove the stone.
7. Ureteral catheters (stents): Positioned above the stone to promote ureteral dilatation, allowing the calculus to pass. These catheters also can be used for intermittent or continuous irrigation with an acidic solution to combat alkalinity. They may be placed temporarily after removal of the stone to allow for healing and promote patency of the ureter in the presence of edema.
8. Ureterolithotomy: Removal of calculi that are unable to pass through the ureter. The ureter is surgically incised and the stone is manually removed.
9. Percutaneous ultrasonic lithotripsy (PUL): Used when the stone is easily accessible, such as in the renal pelvis, calyx, or upper ureter. A small tube is placed through a nephrostomy tract against the stone. An ultrasonic probe is passed through this tube, allowing ultrasound waves to shatter the stone. Fragments are removed by suction or irrigation.
10. Extracorporeal shock wave lithotripsy (ESWL): The patient is anesthetized (epidural or general) and placed in a water bath. The affected area is positioned under an electric shock generator, which shatters the calculi. Usually, 500-1,500 shock waves over a period of 30-60 seconds are adequate to break the calculi into fine particles. The fragments pass naturally in the patient's urine within a few days.

NURSING DIAGNOSES AND INTERVENTIONS

Pain related to presence of calculus or the surgical procedure to remove it

Desired outcome: Patient's subjective evaluation of pain improves, as documented by a pain scale.

1. Assess and document quality, location, intensity, and duration of the pain. Devise a pain scale with the patient that ranges from 0 (no pain) to 10. Notify MD of sudden onset of pain.
2. Notify MD of a sudden cessation of pain, which can signal the passage of the stone. (Strain all urine for solid matter and send it to the laboratory for analysis.)
3. Medicate patient with prescribed analgesics, narcotics, and antispasmodics; evaluate and document the response, based on the pain scale.
4. Provide warm blankets, heating pad to affected area, or warm baths to increase regional circulation and relax tense muscles.
5. Provide back rubs. These are especially helpful for postoperative patients who were in the lithotomy position during surgery.

Alteration in pattern of urinary elimination: Dysuria, urgency, or frequency in the presence of a ureteral calculus

Desired outcomes: Patient relates the return of normal voiding pattern within 2 days. Patient demonstrates the ability to self-record I&O and self-strain urine for stones.

1. Determine and document patient's normal voiding pattern.
2. Monitor the quality and color of the urine. Optimally it is straw colored, clear, and has a characteristic urine odor. Dark urine is often indicative of dehydration, and blood-tinged urine can result from the rupture of ureteral capillaries as the calculus passes through the ureter.
3. In patients for whom fluids are not restricted, encourage a fluid intake of at least 2 L/day to help flush the calculus through the ureter into the bladder and out through the system.
4. Record accurate I&O; teach patient how to self-record I&O.
5. Strain all urine for evidence of solid matter; teach patient the procedure.
6. Send any solid matter to the laboratory for analysis.

Potential alteration in pattern of urinary elimination: Obstruction or positional problems of the ureteral catheter

Desired outcome: Patient has output from the ureteral catheter and denies the presence of spasms or flank pain, which could denote obstruction or dislodgement.

1. Occasionally, patients return from surgery with a ureteral catheter. If patient has more than one, label one "right" and the other "left"; keep all drainage records separate.
2. Monitor output from ureteral catheter. Amount will vary with each patient and depend on catheter dimension. If drainage is scanty or absent, milk the catheter and tubing gently to try to dislodge the obstruction. If this fails, notify MD.
3. **Caution:** Never irrigate this catheter without specific MD instructions to do so. If irrigation is prescribed, use gentle pressure and aseptic technique. Always aspirate with sterile syringe prior to instillation to prevent ureteral damage from overdistention. Use another sterile syringe to insert amounts no greater than 3 ml per instillation.
4. Typically, patient will require bed rest if ureteral catheter is indwelling. Explain to patient that semi-Fowler's and side-lying positions are acceptable. Fowler's position should be avoided, however, because sutures are seldom used and gravity can cause catheter to move into the bladder.
5. Ureteral catheters are often attached to the urethral catheter after placement in the ureters. Carefully monitor the urethral catheter for movement, and ensure that it is securely attached to the patient.

Note: After the ureteral catheters have been removed (usually simultaneously with the urethral catheter), monitor for indicators of ureteral obstruction, including flank pain, nausea, and vomiting.

Potential impairment of skin integrity related to irritation secondary to wound drainage

Desired outcome: Patient's skin surrounding the wound site remains intact.

1. Monitor incisional dressings frequently during the first 24 hours and change or reinforce as needed. Excoriation can result from prolonged contact of urine with the skin.
2. Note and document odor, consistency, and color of drainage. Immediately after surgery, drainage may be red.
3. To facilitate frequent dressing changes, use Montgomery straps rather than tape to secure dressing.
4. If drainage is copious after drain removal, apply wound drainage or ostomy pouch with a skin barrier over the incision. Use a pouch with an antireflux valve to prevent contamination from reflux.

Health-seeking behavior: Dietary regimen and its relationship to stone formation

Desired outcome: Patient verbalizes knowledge of foods to limit to prevent stone formation and demonstrates this knowledge by planning a 3-day menu that excludes or limits these foods from the diet.

1. Assess patient's knowledge of diet and its relationship to stone formation.
2. As appropriate, provide the following information:
   □ *For uric acid stones:* Limit intake of foods high in purines, such as lean meat, legumes, whole grains. Limit protein intake to 90 g/day.
   □ *For calcium stones:* Limit intake of foods high in calcium, such as milk, cheese, green leafy vegetables, yogurt. Limit sodium intake (see Table 11-3, p. 550). Explain to patient that a low-sodium diet helps reduce intestinal absorption of calcium. Limit intake of refined carbohydrates and animal proteins, which cause hypercalciuria. Encourage patient to eat foods high in natural fiber content (e.g., bran, prunes, apples). Foods high in natural fiber content provide phytic acid, which binds dietary calcium.

☐ *For oxalate stones:* Limit intake of foods high in oxalate, such as chocolate, caffeine-containing drinks, beets, spinach. Large doses of pyridoxine may help with certain types of oxalate stones. Explain that vitamin C supplements should be avoided because as much as half is converted to oxalic acid.

See the appendix for nursing diagnoses and interventions for the care for preoperative and postoperative patients, p. 637.

PATIENT-FAMILY TEACHING AND DISCHARGE PLANNING

Provide patient and significant others with verbal and written information for the following:

1. Medications, including drug name, purpose, dosage, schedule, precautions, and potential side effects.
2. Indicators of UTI or recurrent calculi, which necessitate medical attention: chills, fever, hematuria, flank pain, cloudy and foul-smelling urine, frequency, and urgency.
3. Care of incision, including cleansing and dressing. Teach patient signs and symptoms of local infection, including redness, swelling, local warmth, tenderness, and purulent drainage.
4. Care of drains or catheters if patient is discharged with them.
5. Importance of daily fluid intake of at least 2 L/day in nonrestricted patients.
6. Dietary changes as specified by MD.
7. Activity restrictions as directed for patient who has had surgery: avoid lifting heavy objects (>5 lb) for the first 6 weeks, be alert to fatigue, get maximum rest, increase activities gradually to tolerance.
8. Use of nitrazine paper to assess pH of urine. Desired pH will be determined by type of stone formation to which the patient is prone. Instructions for use are on nitrazine container.
9. Importance of walking or other exercise to decrease risk of stone formation.

Urinary tract obstruction

Urinary tract obstruction usually is the result of blockage from pelvic tumors, calculi, and urethral strictures. Additional causes include neoplasms, benign prostatic hypertrophy, ureteral or urethral trauma, inflammation of the urinary tract, and pelvic or colonic surgery in which ureteral damage has occurred. The obstruction acts like a dam, causing urine to collect and pool. Muscles in the area contract to push urine around the obstruction, and dilatation of the structures behind the obstruction begins to occur. Hydrostatic pressure increases, and filtration and concentration processes within the urinary system are compromised. Obstructions can occur anywhere along the urinary tract, but the most common sites are the ureteropelvic and ureterovesical junctions, bladder neck, and urethral meatus. Obstructions in the upper urinary tract can lead to bilateral involvement of the ureters and kidneys as well as of the bladder, resulting in hydronephrosis, renal insufficiency, and kidney destruction.

ASSESSMENT

Signs and symptoms: Anuria, pain that is sharp and intense or dull and aching, nausea, vomiting, local abdominal tenderness, hesitancy, straining to start a stream, dribbling, oliguria, and nocturia.

Physical assessment: Bladder distention, mass in flank area, and "kettle drum" sound over bladder with percussion.

History of: Recent fever (possibly caused by the obstruction); hypertensive episodes (caused by increased hormone production from the body's attempt to increase renal blood flow).

DIAGNOSTIC TESTS

1. *Serum potassium and sodium:* To determine renal function. Normal range for potassium is 3.5-5.0 mEq/L; normal range for sodium is 137-147 mEq/L.
2. *BUN and creatinine:* To evaluate renal-urinary status. Normally, their values will be elevated with decreased renal-urinary function. **Note:** These values must be considered based on the patient's age and hydration status. For the older adult, serum creatinine level may not be a reliable indicator, owing to decreased muscle mass and a decreased glomerular filtration rate. Hydration status can affect BUN: fluid volume excess can result in reduced values, while volume deficit can cause higher values.
3. *Urinalysis:* To provide baseline data on the functioning of the urinary system, detect metabolic disease, and assess for the presence of UTI. A cloudy, hazy appearance; foul odor; pH >8.0; and presence of WBCs and WBC casts are signals of a UTI.
4. *Urine culture:* To determine type of bacteria present in the genitourinary tract. To minimize contamination, a sample should be obtained from a midstream collection.
5. *Hemoglobin and hematocrit:* To assess for systemic bleeding and anemia, which may be related to decreased renal secretion or erythropoietin.
6. *KUB radiography:* This x-ray identifies the size, shape, and position of the kidneys, ureters, and bladder and abnormalities such as tumors, calculi, or malformations.
7. *IVP:* To evaluate the cause of urinary dysfunction by visualizing the kidneys, kidney pelvis, ureters, and bladder.
8. *Cystoscopy:* To determine degree of bladder outlet obstruction and facilitate visualization of any tumors or masses.
9. *Cystogram:* Radiopaque dye is instilled *via* cystoscope or catheter. This allows visualization of the bladder and evaluation of the vesiculoureteral reflex.

MEDICAL MANAGEMENT AND SURGICAL INTERVENTIONS

1. Catheterization: To establish drainage of urine.
2. Pharmacotherapy
   □ *Narcotics:* For pain relief.
   □ *Antispasmodics:* For relief of spasms.
   □ *Antibiotics:* For bacterial infection.
   □ *Corticosteroids:* For reduction of local swelling.
3. IV therapy: For acutely ill, dehydrated patients.
4. Surgically establish drainage: *Via* catheters or drains (ureteral, urethral, or suprapubic) above point of obstruction.
5. Surgical removal of obstruction or dilatation of strictures.

NURSING DIAGNOSES AND INTERVENTIONS

Potential fluid volume deficit related to excessive urinary loss or hematuria secondary to postobstructive diuresis or rapid bladder decompression after catheterization procedure

Desired outcomes: Patient is normovolemic as evidenced by HR ≤90 bpm (or within patient's normal range), BP ≥90/60 mm Hg (or within patient's normal range), RR ≤20 breaths/min, and orientation to person, place, and time (within patient's normal range). Within 2 days following bladder decompression, output approximates input, patient's urinary output is normal for patient (or 30-60 ml/hr), and weight becomes stable.

1. Closely monitor initial bladder decompression. Clamp or partially clamp drainage tubing to slow the decompression process if urine flow exceeds 800-1,000 ml within the first 5 minutes after catheterization. **Caution:** Rapid decompression can lead to vascular bleeding within the bladder, causing postobstructive hematuria.
2. Monitor I&O qh for 4 hours and then q2h for four hours following bladder decompression. Notify MD if output exceeds 200 ml/hr or 2 L over an 8-hour period. This can signal postobstructive diuresis, which can lead to major electrolyte imbalance. If this occurs, anticipate initiation of IV infusion.

3. Monitor VS for signs of shock: decreasing BP, changes in LOC or mentation, tachycardia, tachypnea, thready pulse.
4. Anticipate the need for urine specimens for analysis of electrolytes and osmolality and blood specimens for analysis of electrolytes.
5. Observe for and report indicators of the following:
   □ *Hypokalemia:* Abdominal cramps, lethargy, dysrhythmias.
   □ *Hyperkalemia:* Diarrhea, colic, irritability, nausea, muscle cramps, weakness, irregular apical or radial pulses.
   □ *Hypocalcemia:* Muscle weakness and cramps, complaints of tingling in fingers, positive Trousseau and Chvostek signs.
   □ *Hyperphosphatemia:* Excessive itching.
   Note: See section "Fluid and Electrolyte Disturbances," p. 546, for further information and treatment.
6. Monitor mentation, noting signs of disorientation, which can occur with electrolyte imbalance.
7. Weigh patient daily using the same scale and at the same time of day (e.g., before breakfast). Weight fluctuations of 2-4 lb (0.9-1.8 kg) normally occur in a diuresing patient.

Pain related to bladder spasms

Desired outcome: Patient's subjective evaluation of pain improves, as documented by a pain scale.

1. Assess for and document patient complaints of pain in the suprapubic or urethral area. Devise a pain scale with the patient, rating the pain from 0 (no pain) to 10. Reassure patient that spasms are normal with obstruction.
2. Medicate with antispasmodics or analgesics as prescribed. Document the pain relief obtained, using the pain scale.
3. Teach patient the procedure for slow, diaphragmatic breathing.
4. If the patient is losing urine around the catheter and has a distended bladder (with or without bladder spasms), check the catheter and drainage tubing for evidence of obstruction. Inspect for kinks and obstructions in drainage tubing, compress and roll catheter gently between fingers to assess for gritty matter within catheter, milk drainage tubing to release obstructions, or instruct patient to turn from side to side. Obtain prescription for catheter irrigation if these measures fail to relieve the obstruction.
5. In nonrestricted patients, encourage intake of at least 2-3 L/day of fluids to help reduce frequency of spasms.
6. Instruct patient in the use of nonpharmacologic methods of pain relief, such as guided imagery, relaxation techniques, and distraction. See relaxation technique described on p. 49, **Health-seeking behaviors:** Relaxation technique effective for stress reduction.

See "Hydronephrosis" for **Potential for impaired tissue integrity** related to insertion/presence of nephrostomy tube, p. 113. See "Ureteral Calculi" for **Potential impaired skin integrity** (from wound drainage), p. 134. See the appendix for nursing diagnoses and interventions for the care of preoperative and postoperative patients, p. 637.

PATIENT-FAMILY TEACHING AND DISCHARGE PLANNING

Provide patient and significant others with verbal and written information for the following:
1. Medications, including drug name, dosage, purpose, schedule, precautions, and potential side effects.
2. Indicators that signal recurrent obstruction and require prompt medical attention: pain, fever, decreased urinary output.
3. Necessity of limiting activities during postoperative period.
4. Care of drains or catheters if patient is discharged with them; care of the surgical incision.

5. Indicators of wound infection: persistent redness, local warmth and tenderness, drainage, swelling; and *UTI:* dysuria, flank or suprapubic pain, cloudy or foul-smelling urine, chills, and fever.

Cancer of the bladder

Cancer of the bladder is the most common form of urinary system cancer, and it occurs most often in persons 50-70 years of age. Causes are not clearly understood, but individuals with a history of industrial exposure to such chemicals as β-naphthylamine or benzidine or occupational exposure to dyes, rubber, leather and leather products, and paint are at a higher risk to develop this disease. Additional environmental factors affecting the development of bladder cancer are cigarette smoking, diets high in fat and protein, and deficiency in vitamin A. Other factors, including coffee drinking, chronic bladder infection, vesical calculus disease, phenacetin and cyclophosphamide use, and pelvic radiation therapy, are under investigation.

Bladder cancer often begins in the bladder lumen, but the bladder neck wall and ureteral orifices also can be involved. Cellular proliferation can occur throughout the transitional epithelium, which lines the kidneys, ureters, and mucosa of the bladder. Metastasis most commonly occurs in the bones, liver, and lungs and spreads throughout the lymph nodes.

ASSESSMENT

Signs and symptoms: Painless hematuria, dysuria, burning with urination, increased frequency, and nocturia. Depending on tumor size, the patient may experience suprapubic pain. If the tumor causes urinary obstruction, see "Urinary Tract Obstruction," p. 135, for further data.

Physical assessment: Usually normal. A tumor can be palpated only after the disease has become deeply invasive.

DIAGNOSTIC TESTS

1. *Urinalysis, urine culture:* To check for pus, RBCs, WBCs, WBC casts, and a pH >8.0, which occur with infection.
2. *Urine cytology:* To assess for cells that have been sloughed off from tumors/neoplasms. The urine sample is taken from a voided specimen.
3. *CBC:* To check for presence of infection (WBC >11,000 μl) and anemia (RBCs, hct, and hgb less than normal).
4. *IVP:* Can reveal filling defects within the urinary tract and presence of tumor obstruction.
5. *Ultrasonography/MRI:* These tests are used to diagnose the cancer. Ultrasonography helps determine degree of tumor invasion in the bladder wall and MRI can facilitate recognition of early bladder cancer and assist in staging of the bladder neoplasm.
6. *Biopsy in conjunction with cystoscopy:* A cystoscope is inserted through the urethra and into the bladder to visualize the structures. If abnormalities are seen, a section of the tissue is removed for biopsy. Because the procedure is very uncomfortable under a local anesthetic, general anesthesia is usually used.
7. *Cystogram (cystography):* To outline tumors that are present in the bladder. A radiopaque medium is introduced into the bladder *via* a urethral catheter. X-rays are taken both before and after urination.

MEDICAL MANAGEMENT AND SURGICAL INTERVENTIONS

1. Grading and staging the disease: To formulate a prognosis and guide treatment. The degree of grading and staging is determined by the extent of metastasis and tissue involvement: the greater the metastasis, the higher the grade and stage.
2. Transurethral resection of the bladder and tumor (TURBT): Removal of the tumor with electrocautery *via* cystoscope and rectoscope. Water is used during this procedure,

as it causes the tumor cells released by the procedure to swell and lyse. TURBT is used to treat superficial bladder tumors.

3. Chemotherapy: With superficial bladder tumors, the patient may receive a bladder instillation of thiotepa *via* catheter 24-48 hours postoperatively. Mitomycin or doxorubicin also is used. These drugs reduce the recurrence rate of tumor growth. For invasive tumors, cisplatin and methotrexate are the most commonly used single agents for treatment and palliation of symptoms. Doxorubicin, vinblastine, 5-fluorouracil, and cyclophosphamide also are used.

4. Palliative radiation therapy: Used primarily in the late stages for pain relief, but it also can be used early in treatment.

5. Radon seeds: May be implanted around the base of the tumor in an attempt to eradicate the bladder tumor and prevent regrowth. Typically, this is done after a transurethral resection (TUR) and fulguration of the bladder tumor. Severe cystitis is likely to occur from the irradiation.

6. Supervoltage radiation therapy: Often used in conjunction with surgery or chemotherapy to shrink very large tumors or for pain relief if the cancer has metastasized widely.

7. Pharmacotherapy
   □ *Analgesics* and *narcotics:* For pain relief.
   □ *Antibiotics:* For therapy-induced infections.

8. Segmental resection: Performed if the dome of the bladder is involved. The top half of the bladder is removed *via* an abdominal incision.

9. Cystectomy: Removal of the entire bladder. Radical cystectomy involves removal of the entire bladder, portions or all of the urethra, and the distal ends of both ureters. In addition, seminal vesicles and the prostate gland are removed in males.

10. Urinary diversion: See p. 151 for discussion.

NURSING DIAGNOSES AND INTERVENTIONS

Potential alterations in fluid volume: *Excess* related to fluid retention secondary to irrigation; *deficit* related to loss secondary to postsurgical hemorrhage (after TURBT or segmental resection)

Desired outcome: Patient is normovolemic as evidenced by BP $\geq$90/60 mm Hg (or within patient's normal range), HR $\leq$100 bpm (or within patient's normal range), and orientation to person, place, and time (within patient's normal range).

1. Monitor and record VS and I&O; record color and consistency of catheter drainage at least q8h. Drainage may be dark red after surgery, but it should lighten to pink or blood-tinged within 24 hours. **Note:** Patients with a TURBT may have clots passing through the drainage tubing. Continuous bladder irrigation (CBI) is often used to flush bloody drainage from the bladder to prevent clot formation, which can occlude the urethral catheter. For more information about patient care following a transurethral resection, see "Benign Prostatic Hypertrophy," p. 509.

2. Be alert to hypotension and rapid pulse rate, and watch for bright red, thick drainage or drainage that does not lighten after irrigation, any of which can signal arterial bleeding within the operative area and necessitate immediate surgical intervention.

3. Monitor TURBT patient's postoperative mental status, being alert to changes in mentation, such as confusion, which can denote a change in electrolyte balance and necessitate medical intervention. Water intoxification and hyponatremia can occur because of the high volumes of irrigation fluid that are used with a TUR. See "Fluid and Electrolyte Disturbances," p. 546, for more information.

Potential for infection related to vulnerability secondary to presence of suprapubic catheter and opening of a closed drainage system

Desired outcome: Patient is free of infection as evidenced by WBC $\geq$11,000 μl, normothermia, and orientation to person, place, and time (within patient's normal range).

1. Using aseptic technique, cleanse the area surrounding the suprapubic catheter with an antimicrobial solution, such as povidone-iodine. Apply sterile 4×4 gauze pad(s) over

the catheter exit site and tape securely. Change the dressing as soon as it becomes wet, and use a pectin wafer skin barrier to protect the insertion site if indicated. **Note:** If a trocar system is used, clean around the plastic cover and keep the area dry. Tape the plastic edges securely to the skin to prevent accidental removal.

2. Wash hands *before* and *after* manipulating the catheter, and use aseptic technique when opening the closed drainage system, changing dressings, and irrigating the catheter.
3. Irrigate catheter *only* if there is an obstruction and by MD prescription.
4. Protect the catheter by keeping it securely taped to the patient's lateral abdomen.
5. If the catheter is accidentally pulled out of the insertion site, immediately cover the site with a sterile 4×4 gauze pad and notify MD.
6. To keep urine dilute to help prevent UTI, encourage a fluid intake of at least 2-3 L/day in nonrestricted patients.
7. Keep the drainage collection container below the level of the patient's bladder to prevent infection from reflux of urine.

Potential for altered patterns of urinary elimination: Obstruction of suprapubic catheter or anuria/dysuria secondary to removal of catheter

Desired outcome: Patient's urinary output is appropriate for the amount of intake within 3 days following surgery.

1. Keep drainage from suprapubic catheter separate from that of other catheters and drains.
2. Prevent external obstruction of the catheter, assessing frequently for patency. Irrigate *only* if internally obstructed and with MD order.
3. Before removal of suprapubic catheter, MD may request a 3-4–hour clamping routine to assess patient's ability to void normally. After patient has voided, unclamp the catheter and measure the residual urine that flows into the drainage collection container. Once the residual urine is <100 ml after each of two successive voidings, notify MD. Usually the catheter can be removed at that time.
4. After removal of the catheter, evaluate patient's ability to void by recording the time and amount during the first 24 hours. Patients with segmental resections will void frequently and in small amounts at first because the bladder capacity is approximately 60 ml. Explain to the patient the bladder will expand to 200-400 ml within a few months.
5. If patient cannot void 8-12 hours after catheter removal and experiences abdominal pain or has a distended bladder, notify MD for intervention.
6. If patient experiences burning with urination, encourage an increased intake of fluids and apply heat over the bladder area with a warm blanket, heating pad, or sitz bath, any of which will increase circulation to the area and relax the muscles.

See "Urinary Tract Obstruction" for **Pain** related to bladder spasms, p. 137. See the appendix for nursing diagnoses and interventions for the care of preoperative and postoperative patients, p. 637; and patients with cancer and other life-disrupting illnesses, p. 659.

PATIENT-FAMILY TEACHING AND DISCHARGE PLANNING

See discussion with "Urinary Tract Obstruction," p. 137.

Section Six URINARY DISORDERS SECONDARY TO OTHER DISEASE PROCESSES

Urinary incontinence

Urinary incontinence occurs when an individual experiences involuntary loss of urine. The ability to urinate requires complex interactions between nerve pathways, the detrusor muscle, the internal sphincter, and the external sphincter. Since incontinence occurs when bladder pressure exceeds urethral resistance, structural or musculature weakness or damage places an individual at increased risk. A spinal cord lesion above S-2 through S-4 may result in loss of sensation or awareness of bladder filling because of interruption of the nerve pathways. Thus, the bladder acts in response to bladder pressure. Urinary incontinence can be short term, caused by an acute illness, or it can be chronic. General causes can be classified as follows: interference with neural control (e.g., cerebrovascular accident [CVA], spinal cord injury); interference with bladder function (e.g., inflammatory states, loss of contractility); interference with urethral sphincter mechanism (e.g., "stress" incontinence in women, post TURP incontinence in males); and environmental interferences (e.g., radiation therapy, medications such as diuretics or anticholinergics).

ASSESSMENT

Signs and symptoms: Polyuria; dysuria; low back or flank pain; loss of urine with increased intraabdominal pressure, such as during laughing, sneezing, coughing, lifting; involuntary urination occurring soon after the urge to void is sensed; involuntary passage of urine occurring at predictable intervals; inability to reach the commode on time when environmental barriers exist or disorientation occurs; nocturia.

History of: Neurologic dysfunctions, such as Parkinson's disease, CVA, brain injury, normal pressure hydrocephalus, spinal cord injury (SCI) or lesions, multiple sclerosis (MS); acute or chronic diminishing of cerebral functioning; abdominal or bladder surgery; use of such medications as loop diuretics, anticholinergics, and adrenergic agents; radiation therapy for bladder cancer; meningitis; impaired mobility; diabetes mellitus (due to autonomic neuropathy and decreased detrusor contractility); multiparity; and low back syndrome.

DIAGNOSTIC TESTS

1. *Urinalysis:* To provide baseline data on the functioning of the urinary system, detect metabolic disease, and assess for the presence of UTI. A cloudy or hazy appearance, foul odor, pH >8.0, and presence of WBCs and WBC casts are indicative of UTI.
2. *Urine culture:* To determine the type of bacteria present in the genitourinary tract. To minimize the risk of contamination, a specimen should be obtained from a midstream collection.
3. *Urodynamic studies:* To evaluate cause and extent of the incontinence
   □ *Uroflowmetry:* Provides information about bladder strength and the opening ability of the urethral sphincter. The force of the urine stream is tested, using a specially designed commode.
   □ *Cystometry:* Measures the pressure-volume relationship of the bladder. The bladder is filled at a rate of 50 ml/min to the maximum capacity of the bladder, and the bladder's ability to accommodate pressure changes is evaluated. In a normal individual, the bladder will fill smoothly without contractions and empty when the individual desires. The ability of the patient to detect bladder fullness also is noted.
   □ *Urethral pressure profile:* Most helpful in detecting stress incontinence, this test identifies the amount of closing pressure the urethra can produce, *via* a dual-tip, microtip, pressure-sensitive catheter, which enables simultaneous measurement of the intraurethral and intravesical pressures.
   □ *Sphincter electromyography:* Evaluates the function of the striated urinary sphincter. Results of this test are compared to the results from cystometry to identify abnormalities in coordination between the bladder and sphincter function.
4. *BUN and creatinine:* Serum values increase as renal-urinary function declines. **Note:** These values can be affected by hydration status and age. Fluid volume deficit can falsely increase the values, while volume excess can decrease the values. Creatinine values may be misleading in the older adult because of the loss of muscle mass and decreased glomerular filtration rate.

MEDICAL MANAGEMENT AND SURGICAL INTERVENTIONS

1. Habit/bladder scheduling program: Focuses on emptying the bladder at set intervals. This can be supervised by the staff and taught to the patient.
2. Catheter drainage of urine: Either intermittent or continuous.
3. Pubococcygeal (Kegel) exercise program: To increase strength of perineal muscles.
4. Fluid intake: At least 2-3 L/day in nonrestricted patients.
5. External (condom) catheter: For male patients, if appropriate.
6. Surgical procedures to restore bladder-urethral structure: There are many surgical procedures that may be employed to reestablish normal vesicourethral structure. Examples of the most common include the following:
   □ *Urethral suspension (Marshall-Marchetti-Krantz; Stamey) procedure:* For stress incontinence. The bladder is elevated in the abdominal cavity *via* suprapubic transverse incision to lengthen the urethra, thereby creating resistance in the urethral lumen. The *Pereya* procedure uses both vaginal and suprapubic approaches.
   □ *Pubovaginal sling urethropexy:* After harvesting a small strip of rectus fascia through a small suprapubic incision, a transvaginal approach is used. The area lateral to the urethra is joined to the junction of the pelvic floor and the overlying symphysis pubis.
   □ *Artificial urinary sphincter.*
7. Medications used for urge incontinence: Anticholinergics or antispasmodics, such as imipramine or oxybutynin, may be prescribed to inhibit uncontrolled bladder contractions and enhance functional bladder capacity. **Note:** Anticholinergics must be used cautiously in the older adult because they can increase the occurrence of acute confusion.

NURSING DIAGNOSES AND INTERVENTIONS

Note: Patients may have overlapping conditions. For example, they may experience functional incontinence, which is made more severe by UTI, superimposed on urge incontinence.

Stress incontinence: Loss of urine <50 ml secondary to decreased pelvic muscle tone due to menopause, childbirth, obesity, or surgical procedure interfering with normal vesicourethral structure

Desired outcome: Patient remains dry between voidings.

Habit/bladder scheduling program
1. Assess and document the patient's voiding pattern: time, amount voided, amount of fluid intake, timing of fluid intake followed by voiding, and related information, such as the degree of wetness experienced (e.g., number of incontinence pads used in a day, degree of underwear dampness) and the exertion factor causing the wetness (e.g., laughing, sneezing, bending, lifting). Teach patient to keep a voiding record that incorporates this information.
2. Determine the amount of time between voidings to estimate how long the patient can hold urine. Establish a voiding schedule that does not exceed this time period.
3. Estimate and document urinary output when patient is incontinent in clothes or bed linens. For example, a wet spot of approximately 2 inches in diameter is equal to approximately 5 ml urine.
4. Teach patient techniques that strengthen the sphincter and structural supports of the bladder, such as the Kegel exercises (see **Knowledge deficit:** Pubococcygeal (Kegel) exercise program, p. 144).
5. Assist patient with scheduling times for emptying the bladder, such as q1-2h when awake and q4h at night. If successful, attempt to lengthen the time intervals between voiding. Provide patient and significant others with a written copy of the schedule.

6. Teach patient to drink measured amounts of fluids about q2h and then attempt to void 30 minutes later. In nonrestricted patients, encourage a fluid intake of at least 2-3 L/day. Be aware that patients with urinary incontinence often will reduce their fluid intake to avoid incontinence at the risk of dehydration and UTI.
7. Educate patient regarding dietary irritants (e.g., caffeine, alcoholic beverages) that may increase stress incontinence.

In addition:
8. Administer diuretics in the morning or early afternoon to reduce the risk of night-time incontinence.
9. If the patient has an intravenous infusion, consult with MD regarding advisability of reducing the infusion rate at nighttime.
10. For bedridden patients, keep call light within patient's reach and answer call quickly.
11. If patient is acutely confused, attempt to reorient by keeping clock and calendar in room and reminding patient of the time and date. Toilet patient as described above.
12. If the patient has permanent or severe cognitive impairment, reorient to baseline and toilet the patient as described above.

Urge incontinence: Involuntary passage of urine secondary to bladder irritation or reduced bladder capacity following radiation treatment for bladder cancer, UTI, increased urine concentration, use of caffeine or alcohol, or enlarged prostate

Desired outcome: Patient reports a decrease in or absence of incontinent episodes.

1. Assess and document patient's usual pattern of voiding, including frequency and timing of incontinent episodes.
2. Adhere to the toileting program (see interventions with **Stress incontinence,** above).
3. Teach patient to increase fluid intake to ≥2 L/day but to avoid caffeinated drinks or alcohol, which are natural diuretics and bladder irritants.
4. Explain the types of fluids patient should drink that are not irritating to the bladder, such as water, fruit juices, herbal drinks, and decaffeinated sodas, teas, and coffees.
5. Encourage the intake of cranberry juice, prunes, and plums, which leave an acid ash in the urine to minimize the occurrence of UTI.
6. Teach patient to keep a voiding record for at-home use, documenting accurate information regarding frequency and timing of incontinent episodes.
7. Encourage patient to decrease fluid intake a few hours prior to bedtime and to void before sleep.
8. Keep a urinal or bedpan at the bedside and instruct patient in its use.
9. If the patient is ambulatory but has a cognitive impairment, label the bathroom door with signs that denote "toilet" to the patient, such as a picture of a commode. Adhere closely to the toileting program, reminding patient to void at the scheduled intervals.

Functional incontinence related to impaired mobility secondary to bed rest or impaired motor, sensory, or cognitive capacity

Desired outcome: Patient does not experience episodes of incontinence.

1. Assess and document patient's usual pattern of voiding.
2. Determine environmental obstacles that would prevent patient from toileting appropriately and intervene accordingly. For example, remove obstacles between the bed and bathroom, leave a light on in the bathroom, and attach the call light apparatus to the bed sheet.
3. Monitor patient for the increased need to void after taking such medications as diuretics, which increase urine production or the sensation of urgency.
4. Offer bedpan, urinal, or assistance to the bathroom at least q2h.
5. Determine need for bedside commode.
6. Answer call light promptly.

Potential for impaired skin integrity related to irritation of the perineum secondary to incontinence of urine

Desired outcome: Patient's perineal skin remains intact.

1. Assess the patient for wetness of the perineal area at frequent intervals. Inform the patient that prolonged exposure to urine can cause maceration and to alert staff as soon as wetness occurs.
2. Keep bed linen dry. As necessary, use and change absorbent materials, such as protective underwear or underpads.
3. Keep the perineum clean with mild soap and water; dry it well.
4. Expose the perineum to air whenever possible by using a sheet draped over a bed cradle; ensure the patient's privacy.
5. Use sealants and moisture-barrier ointments to protect the patient's skin.
6. Sprinkle cornstarch into patient's skin folds, but do not allow it to accumulate and cake into moisture-holding lumps.
7. Make sure that plastic pads or sheet protectors do not contact the patient's skin directly because maceration can result from the increased perspiration they cause. Cover these pads with pillow cases or place them under the sheets.
8. Educate patient in the use of containment devices, such as briefs with pads, adult absorptive briefs, and external catheters.

Body image disturbance related to odor, discomfort, and embarrassment secondary to incontinence

Desired outcomes: Patient verbalizes feelings and frustrations without self-deprecating statements. Patient verbalizes knowledge of actions that will either control incontinence or control odor and discomfort.

1. Encourage patient to discuss feelings and frustrations.
2. Offer reassurance and encouragement, and provide information regarding treatment, especially about those activities that are within the patient's own control.
3. Be realistic with the patient; if incontinence cannot be controlled, reassure patient that odor and discomfort *can* be.
4. Explore with patient the methods for relief of discomfort and odor control: maintenance of good hygiene, frequent changes of undergarments, use and frequent changes of incontinence pads.
5. Although fluid intake of at least 2-3 L/day in essential for minimizing the risk of UTI, suggest that the patient limit fluids when away from the home environment and increase them on return. A decrease also should be incorporated into the evening hours to prevent nighttime incontinence.
6. Refer patient to support groups, such as HIP (Help for Incontinent People): Box 544, Union, South Carolina 29379, 803-579-7900; and The Simon Foundation: Box 835, Wilmette, Illinois, 60091, 800-23-SIMON.

Knowledge deficit: Pubococcygeal (Kegel) exercise program to strengthen perineal muscles (effective for individuals with mild-moderate stress incontinence or for those with functional incontinence who are able to participate)

Desired outcome: Patient verbalizes and demonstrates knowledge of the pubococcygeal (Kegel) exercise program.

1. Explain that Kegel exercises will strengthen the pelvic area muscles, which will help regain bladder control.
2. Assist patient with identifying the correct muscle group:
   □ To strengthen the proximal muscle, instruct patient to attempt to shut off urinary flow after beginning urination, hold for a few seconds, and then start the stream again. Explain to patient that if this can be done, the correct muscle is being exercised.
   □ To strengthen the distal muscle, teach patient to contract the muscle around the anus as though to stop a bowel movement.

Note: Common errors when attempting to identify the correct muscle group include contraction of the buttocks, quadriceps, and abdominal muscles.

---

3. Teach patient to repeat these exercises from front to back 10-20 times, 4 times a day.

Knowledge deficit: Use of external (condom) catheter

Desired outcomes: Patient or significant other successfully returns demonstration of condom catheter application and verbalizes knowledge of the rationale for its use.

1. Instruct male patients or significant other in the procedure for application of a condom catheter.
2. Teach the importance of keeping pubic hair trimmed or moved away from the penis to avoid contact with the adhesive used with the catheter.
3. Instruct patient to cleanse and dry the penis thoroughly before and after every condom application. With uncircumcised patients, the foreskin should be retracted to cleanse the area under the prepuce, and then returned to its original position.
4. For ambulatory patients, demonstrate connecting the condom catheter to a leg drainage bag; for patients on bed rest, demonstrate connecting the catheter to a bedside urinary collection container, such as that used with an indwelling catheter.
5. Advise patient to remove and replace the catheter as directed. Most manufacturers recommend that external catheters be changed and replaced daily.
6. If appropriate for the patient, suggest that the condom catheter be used only during the night.

See "Neurogenic Bladder" for **Reflex incontinence,** p. 149. For surgical patients, see the appendix for nursing diagnoses and interventions for the care of preoperative and postoperative patients, p. 637.

PATIENT-FAMILY TEACHING AND DISCHARGE PLANNING

Provide patient and significant others with verbal and written information for the following:
1. Medications, including drug name, dosage, purpose, schedule, precautions, and potential side effects.
2. Indicators of UTI, which necessitate medical attention: fever, chills, cloudy or foul-smelling urine, frequency, urgency, burning with urination, hematuria, increasing or recurring incontinence.
3. Care of catheters and drains if the patient is discharged with them.
4. Importance of maintaining fluid intake of at least 2 L/day.
5. Maintenance of schedule for bladder training program.
6. Use of perineal muscles to improve bladder tone.
7. Care of perineal skin.
8. Support groups (see **Body image disturbance,** p. 144).

For surgical patients:
9. Care of the incision, including cleansing and dressing; and indicators of infection: purulent drainage, persistent redness, swelling, warmth along incision line.
10. Activity restrictions: no heavy lifting (>5 lb) and resting when fatigued. Explain that prolonged periods of sitting can cause relaxation of the musculature of the bladder and sphincter, leading to incontinence. Encourage mild activity, such as walking, to improve muscle tone.

Urinary retention

When urine is produced and accumulates in the bladder but is not released, the condition is called urinary retention. In the acute care setting, urinary retention most commonly is seen as a postoperative complication following surgical procedures using general or spinal anesthesia. Another major cause is obstruction (e.g., from benign prostatic hypertrophy, tumor, calculi, urethral stricture, fibrosis, meatal stenosis, or fecal impaction). Other causes include decreased sensory stimulation to the bladder, anxiety, or muscular tension. Medications such as opiates, sedatives, antihistamines, antispasmodics, major tranquilizers and antidepressants, and antidyskinetics also can interfere with the normal micturition reflex.

ASSESSMENT

Signs and symptoms: Sudden inability to void, intense suprapubic pain, restlessness, diaphoresis, voiding small amounts (20-50 ml) at frequent intervals.

Physical assessment: "Kettle drum" sound with bladder percussion, bladder distention, bladder displacement to one side of the abdomen.

DIAGNOSTIC TESTS

1. *Urinalysis:* Provides baseline data regarding urinary system function, detects metabolic disease, and evaluates for the presence of UTI. A cloudy or hazy appearance, foul odor, pH >8.0, and the presence of WBCs and WBC casts are all signals of UTI.
2. *Urine culture:* To determine the type of bacteria present in the genitourinary tract. To minimize contamination, a midstream specimen should be collected.
3. *BUN and creatinine:* To evaluate renal-urinary function. Generally, serum values increase in the presence of dysfunction. **Note:** BUN values are affected by the patient's hydration status: fluid volume excess can result in decreased values, while volume deficit can result in increased values. Creatinine may not be a reliable indicator of renal function in the older adult owing to decreased muscle mass and decreased glomerular filtration rate.
4. *Urinary function tests:* To evaluate cause of the urinary retention.
   □ *Cystoscopy:* A lighted, tubular scope is inserted into the bladder to allow visualization of tumors or masses.
   □ *Cystogram:* Radiopaque dye is instilled into the bladder *via* cystoscope or catheter to enable visualization of the bladder and evaluation of the vesiculoureteral reflex.
   □ *Cystometrogram:* Water or saline is instilled into the bladder *via* a catheter to create pressure against the bladder wall to evaluate bladder tone.
5. *KUB radiography:* Used diagnostically, this x-ray identifies the size, shape, and position of the kidneys, ureters, and bladder and abnormalities such as tumors, calculi, or malformations.
6. *IVP:* Visualizes the kidney, kidney pelvis, ureters, and bladder to evaluate for the cause of urinary dysfunction.

MEDICAL MANAGEMENT

1. Catheterization: For drainage of urine.
2. Pharmacotherapy
   □ *Cholinergics:* To stimulate bladder contractions.
   □ *Analgesia:* For pain relief.
   □ *Antibiotics:* If infection is present.
3. IV therapy: For hydration of the acutely ill patient.
4. Surgery: Performed if obstruction is the cause of the retention. (See "Urinary Tract Obstruction," p. 135.)

NURSING DIAGNOSES AND INTERVENTIONS

Urinary retention: Incomplete emptying of or inability to empty the bladder secondary to weak detrusor muscle, blockage, inhibition of reflex arc, or anxiety

Desired outcome: Patient reports a normal voiding pattern within 2 days; or, if appropriate, the patient demonstrates self-catheterization.

1. Assess the bladder for distention by inspection, percussion, and palpation; measure and document I&O.
2. If appropriate, try noninvasive measures for release of urine: position patient in a normal position for voiding; have patient listen to the sound of running water or place hands in a basin of warm water. If these measures are ineffective, try pouring

warm water over the perineum. Unless contraindicated, the *Credé* maneuver (pressure applied from the umbilicus to the pubis) may be used to stimulate a weak micturitional reflex.

3. Maintain privacy for patient who is trying to use the commode, bedpan, or urinal. Remember that cold bedpans can cause muscle tension, so use a plastic bedpan or warm a metal bedpan before giving it to the patient. Encourage relaxation technique, such as deep breathing or visualization, to relax the body.

4. Provide an adequate amount of time for the patient's urge to void to occur. Do not rush the patient.

5. Notify MD if patient is unable to void, has bladder distention, or has suprapubic or urethral pain.

6. If catheterization is prescribed, maintain aseptic technique and ensure that the bladder is decompressed slowly to prevent acute fluid and electrolyte imbalance, shock, or hematuria. Allow no more than 800-1,000 ml of urine to drain during the first 5 minutes by clamping or partially clamping the catheter and unclamping after 15-30 minutes. For more information, see nursing diagnosis **Potential fluid volume deficit** related to excessive urinary loss or hematuria secondary to postobstructive diuresis or rapid bladder decompression in "Urinary Tract Obstruction," p. 136.

7. Catheterization may be difficult beyond the prostatic gland in men with benign prostatic hypertrophy (BPH) or in those over age 65, a large percentage of whom have undiagnosed BPH. For these patients, use a coudé (bent tip) catheter instead of a straight catheter. The tip on this catheter is stiff and does not bend against an obstacle. Lubricate the catheter tip generously with a minimum of 5 ml of lubricating jelly before insertion.

8. Teach patient the technique for intermittent self-catheterization, if appropriate. Catheterization should be accomplished on a set q4h schedule to prevent bladder distention, which can injure the bladder mucosa and increase the risk of infection. Teach the patient clean technique for use at home.

See "Urinary Tract Obstruction" for **Pain** related to bladder spasms, p. 137.

PATIENT-FAMILY TEACHING AND DISCHARGE PLANNING

Provide patient and significant others with verbal and written information for the following:

1. Medications, including drug name, purpose, dosage, schedule, precautions, and potential side effects.

2. Indicators of UTI and recurrent retention, which necessitate medical attention: suprapubic or urethral pain, fever, recurring or increasing difficulty with voiding.

3. Self-catheterization technique, if appropriate.

Neurogenic bladder

Neurogenic bladder, also known as neuromuscular bladder dysfunction, neurologic bladder dysfunction, or neuropathic bladder disorder, is a complex phenomenon that can be caused by a myriad of diseases or injuries. It occurs when the transmission of signals from the bladder to the cerebral cortex is interrupted or delayed. Lesions, injury, or diseases affecting the relay of the signal above the level of the spinal cord will cause bladder spasticity. The sacral reflex remains intact, but the loss of the brain's ability to respond to signals sent from the bladder results in a spastic or a mixed spastic/flaccid bladder. Conditions leading to this type of response are dementias, vascular accidents, multiple sclerosis (MS), tumors, and Parkinson's disease. SCI above the level of S-3-S-4 results in a spastic/mixed spastic bladder. Flaccid neuropathic bladder is caused most commonly by an SCI at level S-3-S-4 or below, but it also can be caused by such conditions as diabetes mellitus, pernicious anemia, and posterior spinal lesions. Poliovirus, herpes zoster, and iatrogenic factors, such as radiation and surgery, also can affect innervation and lead to neuropathic bladder dysfunction.

ASSESSMENT

Upper motor neuron disturbance (spastic bladder): Urinary frequency, residual urine, urinary retention, recurrent UTIs, spontaneous loss of urine, urge incontinence, and lack of urinary control.

Lower motor neuron disturbance (flaccid bladder): Urinary retention, recurrent UTIs, inability to perceive the need to void.

History of: SCI, spinal tumor, MS, diabetes mellitus, CVA, Parkinson's disease, Alzheimer's disease, herpes zoster.

DIAGNOSTIC TESTS

1. *Urinalysis:* To provide baseline date on the functioning of the urinary system, detect metabolic disease, and assess for the presence of UTI. A cloudy or hazy appearance, foul odor, pH >8.0, and presence of WBCs and WBC casts are indicative of UTI.
2. *Urine culture:* To determine the type of bacteria present in the genitourinary tract. To minimize the risk of contamination, a specimen should be obtained from a midstream collection.
3. *Urodynamic studies:* To evaluate cause and extent of the incontinence.
   □ *Uroflowmetry:* Provides information about bladder strength and the opening ability of the urethral sphincter. The force of the urine stream is tested, using a specially designed commode.
   □ *Cystometry:* Measures the pressure-volume relationship of the bladder. The bladder is filled at a rate of 50 ml/min to its maximum capacity and the bladder's ability to accommodate pressure changes is evaluated. In a normal individual, the bladder will fill smoothly without contractions and empty when the individual desires. The ability of the patient to detect bladder fullness also is noted.
   □ *Urethral pressure profile:* Most helpful in detecting stress incontinence, this test identifies the amount of closing pressure the urethra can produce. For a description of this test, see "Urinary Incontinence," p. 141.
   □ *Sphincter electromyography:* Evaluates the function of the striated urinary sphincter. Results of this test are compared to the results from cystometry to identify abnormalities in coordination between the bladder and sphincter function.
4. *BUN and creatinine:* Serum values increase as renal-urinary function declines. **Note:** These values can be affected by hydration status and age. Fluid volume deficit can falsely increase the values, while volume excess can decrease the values. Creatinine values may be misleading in the older adult because of the loss of muscle mass and decreased glomerular filtration rate.
5. *IVP:* Enables visualization of the kidneys, kidney pelvis, ureters, and bladder to determine cause of the dysfunction.
6. *Catheterization for residual urine:* The patient is catheterized 15-20 minutes after voiding to assess for residual urine >100 ml.
7. *Cystoscopy:* To determine loss of muscle fibers and elastic tissue.

MEDICAL MANAGEMENT AND SURGICAL INTERVENTIONS

1. Pharmacotherapy
   □ *Parasympatholytics or anticholinergics (e.g., propantheline bromide and oxybutynin chloride):* To treat hyperreflexive neurologic conditions.
   □ *Parasympathomimetics (e.g., bethanechol chloride):* To treat hypotonic bladders by increasing bladder tone.
   □ *Antibiotics:* For infection, if indicated.
2. Catheterization: Either intermittent or continuous.
3. Increase fluid intake: To prevent infection, minimize calcium concentration in urine, and prevent formation of urinary calculi.
4. Increase patient mobility: To augment renal blood flow and minimize urinary stasis.
5. Low-calcium diet: To prevent calculus formation.

6. Neuroprosthetics (bladder pacemaker): Electrodes are implanted on the ventral (motor) nerve roots of the sacral nerves that will produce detrusor contraction when stimulated. These electrodes are then connected to a subcutaneous receiver that can be controlled from outside the body. The bladder can be controlled selectively by the external transmitter.
7. Continent vesicostomy: Surgical closure of urethral neck of the bladder to form an internal reservoir for urine and create an opening or valve in the bladder wall so that the patient can insert a catheter intermittently to remove urine.
8. Artificial urinary sphincter implantation: Surgical placement of a hydraulically activated sphincter mechanism around the bladder neck or urethra. To empty the bladder, patient activates the device by squeezing the bulbs, which are implanted under the labia or scrotum.

NURSING DIAGNOSES AND INTERVENTIONS

Reflex incontinence: Involuntary passage of urine occurring with neurologic impairment following injury or disease that affects the transmission of signals from the reflex arc to the cerebral cortex

Desired outcomes: Patient or significant other participates in habit/bladder scheduling program. Patient experiences a decrease or absence in incontinent episodes.

Habit/bladder scheduling program
1. Assess patient's voiding pattern: time, amount voided, amount of fluid intake, timing of fluid intake followed by voiding, and other related factors.
2. Determine the amount of time between voidings to estimate the time period patient can hold urine. Establish a voiding schedule that does not exceed this time period.
3. Regulate fluids to achieve adequate hydration and a desirable voiding pattern. For example, teach patient to drink measured amounts of fluids (e.g., 8 ounces every 2 hours) and attempt to avoid 30 minutes later.
4. Assist patient with scheduling times for emptying the bladder, such as q1-2h when awake and q4h at night. If successful, attempt to lengthen the time intervals between voidings. Provide patient and significant others with a written copy of the schedule.
5. Monitor for bladder retention by assessing I&O, inspecting the suprapubic area, and percussing and palpating the bladder. Be alert to the presence of swelling proximal to the symphysis pubis, a "kettle drum" sound with percussion, and dribbling of urine.
6. As appropriate, teach the patient techniques that stimulate the voiding reflex. Examples include tapping the suprapubic area with the fingers, pulling the pubic hair, or digitally stretching the anal sphincter. The latter is effective because the rectal nerves follow a path that is basically the same as that of the urethral nerves; however, it is contraindicated in patients with an SCI at or above T-6 because it can cause autonomic dysreflexia. The Valsalva maneuver also can be used to stimulate voiding: the patient bears down as though having a bowel movement to increase intrathoracic and intraabdominal pressure.
7. If an artificial inflatable sphincter is used, instruct the patient to deflate the valve q4h, which allows the bladder to empty. Remind the patient to wear a Medic-Alert tag or bracelet to alert emergency personnel to the presence and use of the device.
8. If a condom catheter is used, see **Knowledge deficit:** Use of external (condom) catheter in "Urinary Incontinence," p. 145, for appropriate nursing interventions.
9. For males with extensive sphincter damage, a Cunningham (penile) clamp might be prescribed. Before and after use, instruct patient (or significant other) to cleanse the penis with soap and water, dry it thoroughly, and sprinkle powder along the shaft. Explain that the clamp is placed horizontally behind the glans after voiding, and removed q4h. Stress the importance of inspecting the skin for redness along the area in which the clamp presses. If breakdown occurs (i.e., redness does not disappear after massage), the clamp must be discontinued. If swelling appears along the

glans, advise patient to set the clamp at a looser setting. **Caution:** Minimize the potential for injury by alternating the clamp with a condom catheter.

10. If intermittent catheterization is prescribed, teach the procedure to the patient or significant other. Emphasize the necessity of following a routine, for example, q4h to minimize the potential for UTI caused by stasis and bladder distention.

11. If the *Credé* maneuver is prescribed, patients with arm and hand strength should be taught the procedure as an alternative to self-catheterization: Place the ulnar surface of the hand horizontally along the umbilicus; while bearing down with the abdominal muscles, press the hand downward and toward the bladder in a kneading motion until urination is initiated; continue q30 seconds until urination ceases.

12. Autonomic dysreflexia is a life-threatening condition that can occur in patients with neurogenic bladder, especially in those with spinal cord injuries at or above level T-6. Be alert to the following indicators of this condition: headache, bradycardia, excessively high BP, blurred vision, flushing above the level of injury, and nausea. If signs of autonomic dysreflexia occur, assess for bladder distention and have the patient empty the bladder or rectum in the accustomed manner, or check for patency of the indwelling catheter. **Caution:** Do not irrigate the catheter as this would increase bladder pressure and intensify the condition. Give appropriate medications as prescribed, such as phenoxybenzamine hydrochloride, a long-acting vasodilator that increases blood flow to the skin, mucosa, and abdominal viscera and lowers both supine and standing BP. Notify MD if symptoms do not disappear after the bladder or rectum is emptied, if the bladder or rectum is full and cannot be emptied, or if the medication does not relieve symptoms. For further information see nursing diagnosis **Potential for dysreflexia** in "Spinal Cord Injury," p. 200.

13. Encourage a fluid intake of at least 2-3 L/day, which dilutes the urine and increases output, thereby minimizing the risk of developing an infection and calculi.

14. To help prevent urinary stasis, which can lead to UTI, and to increase cardiac output, which nourishes the kidneys, encourage as much mobility as the patient can tolerate.

In addition

15. If diuretics are prescribed, administer them in the morning or early afternoon to reduce the risk of nighttime incontinence.

16. If the patient has an intravenous infusion, consult with MD regarding advisability of reducing infusion rate at night to minimize the risk of nighttime incontinence.

17. If the patient has a permanent cognitive impairment, use visual clues, such as a sign on the bathroom door that says "toilet" or a picture of a toilet.

Total incontinence: Continuous and unpredictable loss of urine occurring with lower motor neuron disturbance secondary to SCI below S-3–S-4 or neurologic dysfunction caused by disease

Desired outcome: Patient or significant other follows bladder training program; incontinent episodes decrease to less than 3 per week.

Habit/bladder scheduling program

1. Assess and document patient's voiding pattern: time, amount voided, amount of fluid intake, timing of fluid intake followed by voiding, and other related factors.

2. Determine the amount of time between voidings to estimate how long the patient can hold urine. Establish a voiding schedule that does not exceed this time period.

3. Assist patient with scheduling times for emptying the bladder, such as q1-2h when awake and q4h at night. If successful, attempt to lengthen the time intervals between voiding. Provide patient and significant other with a written copy of the schedule.

4. If the patient takes fluids orally, provide the necessary amounts for optimal hydration (2-3 L/day) during the day and decrease the amount given during the evening and nighttime hours.

5. Provide information about incontinence aids, such as incontinence pads and easy-to-remove clothing.

6. Demonstrate use of external (condom) catheters for nighttime use (see p. 145).

In addition

7. Administer diuretics in the morning or early afternoon to reduce the risk of nighttime incontinence.

8. If the patient has an intravenous infusion, consult with MD regarding advisability of reducing the infusion rate at nighttime.

Knowledge deficit: Function and care of long-term indwelling catheters after continent vesicostomy

Desired outcomes: Patient verbalizes rationale for the use of a suprapubic catheter and vesicostomy tube, including the approximate amount of time they will be indwelling. Patient or significant other demonstrates such procedures as tube irrigation and dressing changes.

1. Preoperatively, explain that the patient will return from surgery with a suprapubic catheter and vesicostomy tube in place.

2. Explain that the patient will be discharged with the catheter and readmitted for catheter removal in approximately 6 weeks. After removal of the indwelling catheter, intermittent catheterization will be performed hourly, progress to 2-4 hours, and ultimately to 4-6 hours. Continuous drainage will be used overnight.

3. Encourage patient's participation in care, including tube irrigation and dressing changes. Explain that backflow is normal and ensures patency of the tube. Demonstrate the procedure for irrigation once it has been prescribed. Typically, sterile normal saline (30-50 ml) is used for irrigation. Instruct the patient to wash hands before handling the catheters to help prevent contamination, and to cleanse around catheter site daily with an antimicrobial solution, such as povidone-iodine.

As appropriate, see "Urinary Incontinence" for **Potential for impaired skin integrity,** p. 143, and **Body image disturbance,** p. 144.

PATIENT-FAMILY TEACHING AND DISCHARGE PLANNING

Provide patient and significant others with verbal and written information for the following:

1. For patients with artificial sphincters, the indicators of UTI and erosion: pain, fever, swelling, urinary retention, or incontinence.

2. For other interventions, see discussion in "Urinary Incontinence," p. 145.

Section Seven   URINARY DIVERSIONS

Surgical interventions

When the bladder must be bypassed or is removed, a urinary diversion is created. Urinary diversions most commonly are created for individuals with bladder cancer (see p. 138). However, malignancies of the prostate, urethra, vagina, uterus, or cervix (see Chapter 9) may require the creation of a urinary diversion if anterior, posterior, or total pelvic exenteration must be done. Individuals with severe, nonmalignant urinary problems, such as radiation damage to the bladder, vesicovaginal fistula, urethrovaginal fistula, neurogenic bladder, radiation or interstitial cystitis, or urinary incontinence that cannot be managed conservatively, also are candidates for urinary diversion. A radical cystectomy may or may not accompany the placement of a urinary diversion. While most urinary diversions are permanent, some act as a temporary bypass of urine, and undiversion (reversal) can be performed if there is a change in the patient's condition.

The urinary stream may be diverted at multiple points: the renal pelvis (pyelostomy or nephrostomy); the ureter (ureterostomy); the bladder (vesicostomy); or *via* an intestinal "conduit." Cutaneous ureterostomy was the diversion most commonly performed in the past, while vesicostomies are more commonly performed in children as a temporary diversion. Continent urinary diversions are the most recently developed procedure, but the most common form of urinary diversion in the adult is the intestinal conduit.

Intestinal (ileal) conduit: Any segment of bowel may be used to create a passageway for urine, but the ileal conduit is the usual procedure. A 15-20 cm section of the ileum is resected from the intestine to form a passageway for the urine. The proximal end is closed and the distal end is brought out through the abdomen, forming a stoma. The ureters are resected from the bladder and anastomosed to the ileal segment. The intestine is reanastomosed, and therefore bowel function is unaffected.

Cutaneous ureterostomy: The ureters are resected from the bladder and brought out through the surface of the abdomen either separately, or with one attached to the other inside the body, resulting in only one abdominal stoma. Typically, the stoma is flush with the abdomen rather than protruding. Stenosis and ascending UTIs are a common problem with this diversion.

Continent urinary diversion: There are several different continent procedures, but the two that are most commonly performed are the Koch continent urostomy and the Indiana (ileocecal) reservoir. All continent urinary diversions are constructed with the following three components: a reservoir, a continence mechanism, and an antireflux mechanism. For example, with the Koch urostomy the reservoir is formed from a 78 cm segment of the ileum chosen within 15 cm of the ileocecal valve. The center portion of the ileum is arranged in a U position and stabilized by sutures to form the reservoir. The continence and antireflux mechanisms are established by intussuscepting a portion of bowel at each end of the reservoir to form "one-way" passages: the distal valve (nipple) in the reservoir and the proximal valve (stoma) at skin level. The ureters are attached to the proximal end of the ileum, which has been sutured closed.

NURSING DIAGNOSES AND INTERVENTIONS

Anxiety related to anticipated loss of body part/function and threat to self-concept secondary to urinary diversion surgery

Desired outcome: Patient communicates fears and concerns, relates the attainment of increased psychologic and physical comfort, and exhibits effective coping mechanisms.

1. Assess patient's perceptions of his or her impending surgery and resulting body function changes. Provide opportunities for patient to express fears and concerns. ("You seem very concerned about next week's surgery.") Listen actively to the patient. Recognize that anger, denial, withdrawal, and demanding behaviors may be coping responses.
2. Acknowledge patient's fears and concerns.
3. Provide brief, basic information regarding physiology of the procedure and the equipment that will be used after surgery, including tubes and drains.
4. Show patient pouches that will be used after surgery. Assure patient that the pouch usually cannot be seen through clothing and that it is odor resistant.
5. Discuss ADL with patient. Inform patient that showers, baths, and swimming can continue and that diet is not affected after the early postoperative period.
6. As appropriate, ask patient what information has been relayed by the surgeon about the sexual implications of the surgery. This will help establish an open relationship between the patient and primary nurse and inform the nurse if the patient has understood the information given by the surgeon. Males undergoing radical cystectomy with urinary diversion will be impotent. The pelvic plexus that innervates the corpora cavernosa will be damaged permanently. Autonomic nerve damage results in loss of erection and ejaculation; however, because sensation and orgasm are mediated by the pudendal nerve (sensorimotor), they are not affected.
7. Arrange for a visit by the ET nurse during the preoperative period. Collaborate with the surgeon, ET nurse, and patient to identify and mark the most appropriate site for the stoma. This information may help alleviate anxiety because it will show the patient the actual spot for placement and thus reinforce that the impact on lifestyle and body image will be minimal.

Potential sensory/perceptual alterations related to impaired mentation or motor function secondary to hyperchloremic metabolic acidosis with hypokalemia (can occur secondary to reabsorption of Na^+ and Cl^- from the urine in the ileal segment, which results in compensatory loss of K^+ and HCO_3^-)

Desired outcome: Patient verbalizes orientation to person, place, and time (within patient's normal range) and has a regular HR.

1. For patients with ileal conduits, assess for indicators of hypokalemia and metabolic acidosis, including nausea and changes in LOC (from sleepy to combative), muscle tone (convulsions to flaccidity), and HR.
2. If patient is confused or exhibits signs of motor dysfunction, keep the bed in the lowest position and raise the siderails. Notify MD of significant findings.
3. Encourage oral intake as directed, and assess for the need for IV management. MD may prescribe IV fluids with potassium supplements.
4. If patient is hypokalemic and allowed to eat, encourage foods high in potassium, such as bananas, cantaloupes, and apricots. See Table 11-4, p. 555, for a list of foods that are high in potassium.
5. Encourage patient to ambulate by the second or third day after surgery. Mobility will help prevent urinary stasis, which increases the risk of electrolyte problems.
6. For more information, see "Metabolic Acidosis" p. 573, and "Hypokalemia," p. 555.

Potential for impaired skin integrity related to maceration from urine on the skin or sensitivity to the appliance material

Desired outcome: Patient's peristomal skin remains intact.

1. For patient with significant allergy history, patch-test the skin for a 24-hour period, at least 24 hours before ostomy surgery to assess for allergies to the different tapes that might be used on the postoperative appliance. If erythema, swelling, itching, weeping, or other indicators of tape allergy occur, document the type of tape that caused the reaction and note on the cover of the chart "Allergic to _____tape."
2. Inspect the integrity of the peristomal skin with each pouch change and question the patient about the presence of itching or burning, which can signal leakage. Change the pouch routinely (per agency or surgeon preference) or immediately if leakage is suspected.
3. Assess for inflamed hair follicles (folliculitis) or a reaction to the tape. Report the presence of a rash to the MD, since this often occurs with a yeast infection and will require topical medication.
4. When changing the pouch, measure the stoma with a measuring guide and ensure that the opening of the skin barrier is cut to the exact size of the stoma to protect the peristomal skin. Protect the skin from maceration caused by pooling of urine on the skin:
   □ *For a patient using a 2-piece system or pouch with a barrier:* Size the barrier to fit snugly around the stoma. If using a barrier and attaching an adhesive pouch, size the barrier to fit snugly around the stoma and size the pouch to "clear" the stoma by at least ⅛ inch.
   □ *For a patient using a 1-piece "adhesive-only" pouch:* If the pouch has an antireflux valve, size the pouch to clear the stoma and any peristomal creases so that the pouch adheres to a flat, dry surface. An antireflux valve prevents "pooling" of urine on the skin. If the pouch does not have an antireflux valve, size the pouch so that it clears the stoma by ⅛ inch in order to prevent stomal trauma, while minimizing the amount of exposed skin. Use a copolymer film sealant wipe on peristomal skin before applying adhesive-only pouch. This will provide a moisture barrier and reduce epidermal trauma when the pouch is removed.
5. Wash the peristomal skin with water or a special cleansing solution marketed by ostomy supply companies. Dry the skin thoroughly before applying the skin barrier and pouch.
6. When changing the pouch, instruct the patient to hold a gauze pad on (but not in) the stoma to absorb the urine and keep the skin dry.

7. After applying the pouch, connect it to the bedside drainage system if the patient is on bed rest. When the patient is no longer on bed rest, empty the pouch when it is ⅓-½ full by opening the spigot at the bottom of the pouch and draining the urine into the patient's measuring container. Do not allow the pouch to become too full as this could break the seal of the appliance with the patient's skin. Instruct the patient accordingly.

8. Change the incisional dressing as often as it becomes wet, using sterile technique.

9. Teach patient to treat peristomal skin irritation following hospital discharge in the following ways:
   □ Dry the skin with a hair dryer on a "cool" setting.
   □ Dust the peristomal skin with an absorptive powder (e.g., Karaya or Stomahesive).
   □ If desired, blot the skin with water or a sealant wipe to "seal" in the powder.
   □ Notify MD or ET nurse of any severe or nonresponsive skin problems.

Potential for impaired tissue integrity related to stomal ischemia/necrosis

Desired outcome: Patient's stoma remains pink or bright red and shiny.

1. Inspect the stoma at least q8h and as indicated. The stoma of an ileal conduit will be edematous and should be pink or red in color with a shiny appearance. A stoma that is dusky or cyanotic in color is indicative of insufficient blood supply and impending necrosis and must be reported to the MD immediately.

2. Also assess the degree of swelling, and inform the patient that the stoma will shrink considerably over the first 6-8 weeks, and less significantly over the next year. For patients with ileal conduit, evaluate stomal height and plan care accordingly (see **Potential for impaired skin integrity,** above). The stoma formed by a cutaneous ureterostomy is usually flush with the skin and pink to white in color.

Alteration in the pattern of urinary elimination: Disruption in normal function secondary to postoperative use of ureteral stents, catheters, or drains and actual urinary diversion surgery

Desired outcome: Patient's urinary output is ≥30 ml/hr and the urine is clear, amber-colored, and with normal, characteristic odor.

1. Monitor color, clarity, and volume of urine output *via* stoma, stents, and/or catheter.
   □ *Ureterostomy:* Urine drainage *via* stoma and/or ureteral stents.
   □ *Intestinal conduit:* Urine drainage *via* stoma. The patient also may have ureteral stents and/or conduit catheter/stent in the early postoperative period to stabilize the ureterointestinal anastomoses and maintain drainage from the conduit during early postoperative edema.
   □ *Continent urinary diversions:* The Koch urostomy usually has a reservoir catheter and also may have ureteral stents. The Indiana (ileocecal) reservoir usually has ureteral stents exiting from the stoma through which the majority of the urine drains, and may have a reservoir catheter exiting from a stab wound, which serves as an overflow catheter.

2. Monitor for evidence of anastomotic breakdown/intraabdominal urine leakage, which may occur in an individual with intestinal conduit or continent diversion: decreasing urinary output from stoma or stents, flank pain, increasing abdominal girth, and increasing drainage from Penrose drains.

3. Monitor functioning of the ureteral stents, which protrude from the stoma under the pouch. These stents maintain the patency of the ureters and assist in the healing of the anastomosis. Right stents usually are cut at a 90-degree angle, while left stents are cut at a 45-degree angle. Each usually produces approximately the same amount of urine, although the amount produced by each is not important as long as each drains adequately and total drainage from all sources equals ≥30 ml/hr. Urine should be pink for the first 24 hours and become amber colored by the third postoperative day. Absent or lessening amounts of urine may indicate a blocked stent or problems with the ureter. **Note:** Stents may become blocked with mucus. As long as urine is draining adequately around the stent and the volume of output is adequate, this is not a problem.

4. Monitor functioning of the catheters. In the Koch continent urinary diversion, a Medina catheter is placed in the reservoir to prevent distention and promote healing of the suture lines. This new reservoir exudes large amounts of mucus, necessitating irrigation of the catheter with 30-50 ml of normal saline, which is instilled gently and allowed to empty *via* gravity. Expect the output to include pink or light red urine with mucus and small red clots for the first 24 hours. Urine should become amber colored with occasional clots in 3 postoperative days. Mucus production will continue but should decrease in volume.

5. Monitor functioning of the drains. Any urinary diversion may have Penrose drains in place to maintain integrity of the ureterointestinal anastomosis. Excessive lymph fluid and urine can be removed *via* these drains without putting pressure on the suture lines. Drainage from the Penrose drain may be light red to pink in color for the first 24 hours and then lighten to amber color and decrease in amount. In a continent urinary diversion, an increase in drainage after amounts have been low might signal reservoir leakage. Notify MD if this occurs.

6. Monitor I&O, and record the total amount of urine output from the urinary diversion for the first 24 hours postoperatively. Differentiate and record separately amounts from all drains, stents, and catheters. Notify MD of an output less than 60 ml during a 2-hour period, because in the presence of adequate intake this can indicate a ureteral obstruction, a leak in the urinary diversion, or impending renal failure. Assess for other indicators of ureteral obstruction: flank pain, nausea, vomiting, and anuria.

7. Monitor drainage from Foley catheter or urethral drain (if present). Patients who have had a cystectomy may have a urethral drain, while those with a cystectomy will have a Foley catheter in place. Note color, consistency, and volume of drainage, which may be red or pink with mucus. Report sudden increase (which would occur with hemorrhage) or decrease (which can signal blockage that can lead to infection). Report significant findings to MD.

8. Advise patient that after removal of urethral catheter or drain, mucus drainage will continue from the urethral meatus for several months.

9. To keep the urinary tract well irrigated, encourage an intake of at least 2-3 L/day in the nonrestricted patient.

Potential for infection related to vulnerability secondary to surgical procedure and risk of ascending bacteriuria with urinary diversion

Desired outcome: Patient is free of infection as evidenced by normothermia and WBC count $\leq 11,000\ \mu l$.

1. Monitor the patient's temperature q4h during the first 24-48 hours after surgery. Notify MD of fever spikes.

2. Inspect the dressing frequently following surgery. Infection is most likely to become evident after the first 72 hours. Assess for the presence of purulent drainage on the dressing and notify MD accordingly. Change the dressing when it becomes wet, using sterile technique. Use extra care to prevent disruption of the drains.

3. Note the condition of the incision. Be alert to indicators of infection, including erythema, tenderness, local warmth, puffiness, and purulent drainage.

4. Monitor and record the character of the urine at least q8h. Mucus particles are normal in the urine of patients with ileal conduits and continent urinary diversions because of the nature of the bowel segment used. Cloudy urine, however, is abnormal and can signal an infection. The urine should be yellow or pink tinged during the first 24-48 hours after surgery. Assess for other indicators of UTI including flank pain, chills, and fever.

5. Note the position of the stoma to the incision. If they are close together, apply the pouch first to avoid the overlap of the pouch with the suture line, which can increase the risk of infection. If necessary, cut the pouch down on one side, or place it at an angle to avoid contact with drainage, which may loosen the adhesive. To help prevent contamination and cross-contamination, wash your hands before and after caring for the patient.

6. Patients with cystectomies may have an indwelling urethral catheter to drain serosan-

guineous fluid from the peritoneal cavity. **Caution:** Do not irrigate this catheter because irrigation can result in peritonitis.

7. Encourage a fluid intake of at least 2-3 L/day as this helps flush urine through the urinary tract, preventing stasis.

Potential fluid volume deficit related to abnormal blood loss secondary to surgical procedure

Desired outcomes: Patient is normovolemic as evidenced by balanced I&O; urinary output ≥ 30 ml/hr; and BP, HR, and RR within patient's baseline range. Urine becomes amber-colored after 2-3 postoperative days.

1. Monitor I&O and note the amount and character of the urine output at least q4h. Initially the urinary output will be blood tinged, clearing within 2-3 days. The amount of urinary output should be normal (≥ 30 ml/hr for 2 consecutive hours).
2. Be alert to the presence of gross hematuria, along with decreasing BP, tachycardia, and tachypnea, which can signal hemorrhage.
3. Report significant findings to the MD.

Knowledge deficit: Self-care regarding urinary diversion

Desired outcome: Patient or significant other demonstrates proper care of stoma and urinary diversion before hospital discharge.

1. Assess patient's or significant other's readiness to participate in self-care.
2. Involve ET nurse in patient teaching if available.
3. Assist patient with organizing the equipment and materials that are needed to accomplish home care. Usually the patient is discharged with disposable pouching systems. The majority of these patients remain in disposable systems for the long term. Those who will use reusable systems usually are not fitted for 6-8 weeks following surgery.
4. Teach patient how to remove and reapply pouch, how to empty it, and how to use gravity drainage system at night, including procedures for rinsing and cleansing the drainage system.
5. Teach patient the signs and symptoms of UTI, peristomal skin breakdown, and the appropriate therapeutic responses, including maintenance of an acidic urine (if not contraindicated), techniques for checking urine pH, and importance of adequate fluid intake.
6. Teach patient with continent diversion the technique for reservoir catheter irrigation.
7. Emphasize the importance of follow-up visits, particularly for those patients with continent urinary diversions, who will be taught how to catheterize the reservoir and use a small dressing over the stoma rather than an appliance.
8. Provide patient with a list of ostomy groups and ET nurses in the area for referral and assistance.
9. Provide patient with enough equipment and materials for the first week following hospital discharge.

See "Fecal Diversions" in Chapter 6 for **Body image disturbance,** p. 368. See the appendix for nursing diagnoses and interventions for the care of preoperative and postoperative patients, p. 637, and for patients with cancer and other life-disrupting illnesses, p. 659.

PATIENT-FAMILY TEACHING AND DISCHARGE PLANNING

Provide patient and significant others with verbal and written information for the following:

1. Medications, including drug name, dosage, schedule, precautions, and potential side effects.
2. Indicators that necessitate medical intervention: fever, chills, nausea, vomiting, abdominal pain and distention, cloudy urine, incisional pain or redness, peristomal skin irritation, or abnormal changes in stoma shape or color from the normal bright and shiny red.

3. Community resources, including local United Ostomy Association, the American Cancer Society, and an ET nurse in the area, if appropriate.
4. Maintenance of fluid intake at least 2-3 L/day to maintain adequate kidney function.
5. Monitoring of urine pH, which should be checked weekly. Urine pH should remain at 6.0 or less. Individuals with urinary diversions have a higher incidence of UTIs than the general public, so it is important to keep their urinary pH acidic. If it is above 6.0, advise patient to increase fluid intake and with MD approval, to increase vitamin C intake to 500-1,000 mg/day, which will increase urine acidity.
6. Care of stoma and application of urostomy appliances. The patient should be proficient in the application technique before hospital discharge.
7. Care of urostomy appliances. Remind patient that proper cleansing will reduce the risk of bacterial growth, which would contaminate the urine and increase the risk of UTI.
8. Importance of follow-up care with MD and ET. Confirm date and time of next appointment.

SELECTED REFERENCES

Bennet C: Surgical treatment for urinary incontinence, Top Geriatr Rehab 3(2):42-47, 1988.

Brink C: Evaluation of urinary incontinence, Top Geriatr Rehab 3(2):1-29, 1988.

Colling J: Educating nurses to care for the incontinent patient, Nurs Clin North Am 23(1):279-289, 1988.

Diokno A: The cause of urinary incontinence, Top Geriatr Rehab 3(2):13-20, 1988.

Eliopoulos C: A guide to nursing of the aging, Baltimore, 1987, Williams & Wilkins Co.

Eschbach JW and Adamson JW: Recombinant human erythropoietin: implications for nephrology, Am J Kidney Dis 11 (3):203-209, 1988.

Goodship TH and Mitch WE: Nutritional approaches to preserving renal function, Adv Intern Med 33:337-356, 1988.

Gray M: Treatment modalities for bladder cancer, Semin Oncol Nurs 2(4):260-264, 1986.

Greig B: Intervention of the ET nurse with the continent urinary Kock pouch patient, J Enterostomal Ther 13:226-231, 1986.

Henderson J: A pubococcygeal exercise program for simple urinary stress incontinence: applicability to the female client with multiple sclerosis, J Neurosci Nurs 20(3):185-188, 1988.

Jirovec M et al: Nursing assessment in the inpatient geriatric population, Nurs Clin North Am 23(1):219-230, 1988.

Lawrence RM: Current therapy of urinary tract infections and pyelonephritis, Semin Nephrol 6(3):241-250, 1986.

Lederer J et al: Care planning pocket guide: a nursing diagnosis approach, ed 2, Redwood City, Calif, 1988, Addison-Wesley Publishing Co.

Lewis S and Collier I: Medical-surgical nursing: assessment and management of clinical problems, ed 2, New York, 1987, McGraw-Hill Book Co.

Linton AL et al: Acute renal failure—a continuing enigma, Renal Failure 10(1):3-7, 1987.

Lonergan E: Aging and the kidney: adjusting treatment to physiologic change, Geriatrics 43(3):27-33, 1988.

Methany N: Renal stones and urinary pH, Am J Nurs 82:1372, 1982.

Noble MJ and Diederich D: Recurrent renal calculi: an update on management, Comp Ther 14(4):40-55, 1988.

Pagana K and Pagana T: Pocket nurse guide to laboratory and diagnostic tests, St Louis, 1986, The CV Mosby Co.

Petillo M: The patient with a urinary stoma: nursing management and patient education, Nurs Clin North Am 22(2):263-279, 1987.

Richard CJ: Comprehensive nephrology nursing, Boston, 1986, Little, Brown & Co.

Richards AB et al: Renal transplantation—nursing management of the recipient, AORN J 41(6):1022-1036, 1985.

Rose BD: Pathophysiology of renal disease, ed 3, New York, 1989, McGraw-Hill Book Co.

Schlueter W and Battle DC: Chronic obstructive nephropathy, Semin Nephrol 8(1):17-28, 1988.

Schrier RW, editor: Renal and electrolyte disorders, ed 3, Boston, 1986, Little, Brown & Co.

Shimp L: Influence of drug therapy on urinary incontinence, Top Geriatr Rehab 3(2):30-41, 1988.

Singer A et al: Postoperative urinary retention: guidelines and an algorithm, Postgrad Med 81(5):154-156, 1987.

Sos TA: Percutaneous transluminal renal angioplasty for the treatment of renovascular hypertension. Hypertension and the kidney: Proceedings of a symposium, 1985, The National Kidney Foundation.

Stewart C: Nephrolithiasis, Emergency Clin North Am 6(3):617-630, 1988.

Turner S: As women age: perspectives on urinary incontinence, Rehab Nurs 13(3):132-135, 1988.

Voith A: Alterations in urinary elimination: concepts, research, and practice, Rehab Nurs 13(3):122-131, 1988.

Watt R: Nursing management of a patient with a urinary diversion, Semin Oncol Nurs 2(4):265-269, 1986.

Watt R: Bladder cancer: etiology and pathophysiology, Semin Oncol Nurs 2(4):256-259, 1986.

Weiskittel PD: Renal-urinary dysfunctions. In Swearingen PL et al: Manual of critical care: applying nursing diagnoses to adult critical illness, St Louis, 1988, The CV Mosby Co.

Wells T: Additional treatments for urinary incontinence, Top Geriatr Rehab 3(2):48-57, 1988.

Wyngaarden JB and Smith LH: Cecil textbook of medicine, ed 8, Philadelphia, 1988, WB Saunders Co.

4
CHAPTER

Neurologic disorders

Section One   INFLAMMATORY DISORDERS OF THE NERVOUS SYSTEM

Inflammation of nervous system tissue results from a wide variety of causes, including bacterial or viral infections, autoimmune processes, or chemical toxins. The inflammatory response may cause increased vascular permeability with exudation of fluids from the vessels, resulting in swelling. Inflammation involving the myelin nerve sheath can cause the destruction or stripping away of the myelin. The resulting demyelinization interferes with the conduction of electric nerve impulses. Inflammation of other brain tissue, such as that which may occur in acute infectious processes, usually results in swelling, which in turn can cause increased intracranial pressure (ICP) and the potential for brain herniation.

Multiple sclerosis

Multiple sclerosis (MS) is an inflammatory disorder causing scattered and sporadic demyelinization of the CNS. Myelin permits nerve impulses to travel quickly through the nerve pathways of the CNS. In response to the inflammation the myelin nerve sheaths peel off the axon cylinders. This demyelinization interrupts electric nerve transmission and causes the wide variety of symptoms associated with MS. If the myelin regenerates, electric nerve impulse transmission may be restored. Symptoms will decrease or disappear (i.e., the patient may go into remission). If the inflammation is severe and causes irreversible destruction of myelin, the involved areas are replaced by dense glial scar tissue that forms areas of sclerotic plaque, which permanently damage the conductive pathways of the CNS. As a disease MS is characterized by remissions and exacerbations with overall long-term progressive decline.

Although the etiology of MS is unknown, autoimmune processes, slow-acting viral infections, and allergic reactions to infectious agents, such as viruses, are suspected causes. MS is more common among people living in cool, temperate climates. It is 12-15 times more common among siblings of individuals who have the disease, suggesting a possible inheritance mechanism. Infection, trauma, and pregnancy are common precipitating factors, as are episodes of fatigue and physical or emotional stress. Heat and fever tend to aggravate symptoms.

ASSESSMENT

Onset of MS can be extremely rapid, causing disability within days, or it can be insidious, with exacerbations and remissions. Seventy percent of MS patients will have prolonged remissions, allowing an active life. Signs and symptoms vary widely, depending on the site and extent of demyelinization, and they can change from day to day. Usually, early symptoms are mild.

Damage to motor nerve tracts: Weakness, paralysis, and spasticity. Fatigue is common. Diplopia may occur secondary to ocular muscle involvement.

Damage to cerebellar or brain stem regions: Intention tremor, nystagmus, or other tremors; incoordination, ataxia; weakness of facial and throat muscles resulting in difficulty chewing, dysphagia, and dysarthria.

Damage to sensory nerve tracts: Decreased perception of pain, touch, and temperature; paresthesias, such as numbness and tingling; decrease or loss of proprioception; and decrease or loss of vibratory sense. Optic neuritis may cause partial or total loss of vision.

Damage to cerebral cortex (especially frontal lobes): Mood swings, inappropriate affect, euphoria, apathy, irritability, depression, and hyperexcitability.

Damage to motor and sensory control centers: Urinary frequency, urgency, or retention; urinary and fecal incontinence; constipation.

Sacral cord lesions: Impotence; diminished sensations that result in inhibited sexual response.

Physical assessment: Ophthalmoscopic inspection may reveal temporal pallor of optic disks. Reflex assessment may show increased DTRs and diminished abdominal skin and cremasteric reflexes.

DIAGNOSTIC TESTS

Note: MS is sometimes called the "great masquerader." Diagnostic testing is often done to exclude disorders with similar symptoms. The diagnosis of MS usually will be made after other neurologic disorders have been ruled out, when the patient has experienced two or more exacerbations of neurologic symptoms, and when the patient has two or more areas of demyelinization or plaque formation throughout the CNS, as demonstrated by diagnostic tests, such as the MRI and evoked potential studies, or by the patient's clinical symptoms.

1. *MRI:* To reveal presence of plaques and demyelinization in the CNS. See "Brain Tumors," p. 214, for patient care considerations.
2. *Evoked potential studies:* May be abnormal due to interference of nerve transmission from demyelinization or plaque formation. Stimulation of a sensory organ, such as the eye or ear, or of a peripheral nerve triggers a measurable electrical response (evoked potential) along the visual, auditory, and somatosensory nerve pathways. Measuring these evoked potentials enables evaluation of the integrity of these nerve pathways. In MS evoked potentials may be slow or absent.
3. *CT scan:* To demonstrate presence of plaques and rule out mass lesions. See "Brain Tumors," p. 250, for patient care considerations.
4. *Lumbar puncture and CSF analysis:* To evaluate oligoclonal IgG, protein, gamma globulin levels, and myelin basic protein, any of which may be elevated in the presence of MS. Increased gamma globulin levels indicate hyperactivity of the immune system due to chronic demyelinization. Detecting oligoclonal bands of immunoglobulin requires examination of the CSF gamma globulin by electrophoresis. During acute MS attacks, destruction of the myelin sheath will release myelin basic protein into the CSF. (See "Bacterial Meningitis," p. 168, for patient care.)
5. *EEG:* Abnormal in a third of patients with MS. (See "Seizure Disorders," p. 242, for patient care.)

MEDICAL MANAGEMENT AND SURGICAL INTERVENTIONS

1. Bed rest: During acute exacerbation.
2. Pharmacotherapy
   - □ *Antiinflammatory agents:* For example, prednisone, dexamethasone, and ACTH may be prescribed during an exacerbation in an attempt to reduce symptoms by decreasing inflammation and associated edema of the myelin, thereby hastening onset of remission.
   - □ *Antispasmodics and muscle relaxants (e.g., baclofen or dantrolene sodium):* May be given to decrease spasticity.
   - □ *Smooth muscle relaxants (e.g., propantheline bromide):* To decrease urinary frequency and urgency.
   - □ *Smooth muscle stimulants (e.g., bethanechol chloride):* May be given to help prevent urinary retention.
   - □ *Tranquilizers (e.g., diazepam):* May be given for both its anxiety-reducing and muscle relaxant effects.
3. Physical medicine: Physical therapy, occupational therapy, and assistive devices or braces may be prescribed so that patient can maintain mobility and independence with ADL. Muscle-strengthening and conditioning exercises and gait training are also frequently indicated.
4. ROM exercises: To maintain or increase joint function and prevent contractures.

5. Counseling or psychotherapy: To help patient and significant others adapt to the disability and deal with emotions and feelings that are either a direct or indirect result of the disease process.
6. Treatment of complications: Complications, such as respiratory or urinary tract infection, may require treatment with antibiotics or other measures.
7. Surgical interventions: To treat complications, such as contractures, spasticity, decreased mobility, and pain. Interventions may include tendotomy, myotomy, peripheral neurectomy, rhizotomy, or stereotaxic thalamotomy.
8. Controversial therapies
   □ *Immunosuppressive drug therapy:* Agents, such as cyclophosphamide (Cytoxan, see p. 664) and azathioprine (Imuran, see p. 126), may slow and stabilize progressive MS.
   □ *Total lymphoid irradiation:* To suppress the body's immune system and slow progression of MS by reducing the immunoinflammatory response that leads to demyelinization of the nerve sheaths. For more information about radiation therapy, see "Caring for Patients with Cancer and Other Life-Disrupting Illnesses," p. 674.
   □ *Interferon drug therapy:* Appears to reduce the exacerbation rate and stabilize the patient's overall clinical status. The mechanism of beneficial effect is unknown but probably related to the drug's ability to enhance the body's immune system rather than its antiviral action (see p. 672 for more information).
   □ *Plasmapheresis:* To reduce the patient's antibodies to CNS tissue by removing the plasma portion of the blood, which contains circulating antibodies. This therapy involves a complete plasma exchange. The RBCs, WBCs, and platelets are returned to the body. Plasmapheresis is a 2-8 hour procedure, usually involving several exchanges, that provides short-term improvement only. Patients are at risk for the following complications with this procedure: fluid volume deficit, hypotension, hypokalemia, hypocalcemia, cardiac dysrhythmias, clotting disorders, phlebitis, and infection.

NURSING DIAGNOSES AND INTERVENTIONS

Knowledge deficit: Factors that aggravate and exacerbate MS symptoms

Desired outcome: Patient verbalizes knowledge of factors that exacerbate, prevent, or ameliorate symptoms of MS.

1. Inform patient that heat, both external (hot weather, bath) and internal (fever), tends to aggravate weakness and other symptoms of MS.
2. Teach preventive measures, such as avoiding hot baths and using acetaminophen or aspirin to reduce fever, if present.
3. Because infection often precedes exacerbations, caution patient to avoid exposure to persons known to have infections of any kind.
4. Teach the indicators of common infections and the importance of seeking prompt medical treatment should they occur. For example, the MS patient is susceptible to urinary tract infection (UTI) because of urinary retention. Due to the disease process the patient may not feel any pain with urination. Teach the patient to monitor for increased frequency, urgency, or incontinence and to check the urine for changes in odor or the presence of cloudiness. Instruct patients to check their body temperature periodically for fever. Signals that a UTI has reached the kidneys include chills and flank pain.
5. Teach patient the relationship between stress and fatigue to the exacerbations. Encourage patients to get sufficient rest and reduce factors causing stress in their lives. See **Health-seeking behaviors:** Relaxation technique effective for stress reduction, p. 49.
6. As appropriate, explain to the patient that pregnancy may precipitate exacerbations. Provide information regarding birth control measures to female patients who desire counseling.

Knowledge deficit: Precautions and potential side effects of prescribed medications

Desired outcome: Patient verbalizes accurate information regarding the prescribed medications.

1. Provide patient with verbal instructions and written handouts that describe the name, purpose, dosage, and schedule of the prescribed medications.
2. For patients taking prednisone or dexamethasone, provide additional instructions for the following:
   □ Common side effects: fluid retention, hypertension, gastric ulcers, stomach upset, weakness, and mood changes.
   □ Importance of monitoring weight and BP for evidence of fluid retention; taking the medication with food, milk, or buffering agents to help prevent gastric irritation; avoiding aspirin, indomethacin, caffeine, or other GI irritants while taking this medication; and tapering rather than abruptly stopping the drug when it is discontinued. Advise patient to report symptoms of potassium deficiency, such as anorexia, nausea, and muscle weakness, and to eat foods high in potassium (see Table 11-4, p. 555).
3. If the patient is taking baclofen or dantrolene, provide instructions for the following:
   □ Common side effects: drowsiness, dizziness, weakness, fatigue, and nausea. In addition, dantrolene can cause diarrhea, hepatitis, and photosensitivity.
   □ Importance of taking the medication with food, milk, or a buffering agent to reduce gastric upset or nausea. Explain that although drowsiness is usually transient, patient should avoid activities that require alertness until their effect on the CNS is known. Patients on dantrolene should monitor for and report occurrence of fever, jaundice, dark urine, clay-colored stools, and itching (all of which signal hepatitis) or severe diarrhea; avoid exposure to the sun; and use sunscreens if exposure is unavoidable.
4. If bethanechol chloride has been prescribed, provide instructions for the following:
   □ Common side effects: hypotension, diarrhea, abdominal cramps, urinary urgency, and bronchoconstriction.
   □ Importance of taking the drug on an empty stomach to avoid nausea and vomiting; notifying MD if lightheadedness occurs, as this can signal hypotension; and seeking medical attention if an asthmatic attack occurs. Caution patient to make position changes slowly and in stages to prevent fainting due to orthostatic hypotension.
5. If the patient is taking propantheline bromide, provide instructions for the following:
   □ Common side effects: dryness of the mouth, blurred vision, constipation, palpitations, tachycardia, decreased sweating, and urinary retention or overflow incontinence.
   □ Measures that relieve constipation; measures for remaining cool in hot or humid weather, as heat stroke is more likely to develop while on the medication; importance of notifying MD immediately if urinary retention or overflow incontinence occurs. In addition, if the patient can chew and swallow effectively, explain that sugarless gum, hard candy, or artificial saliva products may reduce mouth dryness.

Chronic pain and spasms related to motor and sensory nerve tract damage

Desired outcomes: Patient's subjective evaluation of pain and spasms improves, as documented by a pain scale.

1. Because heat tends to aggravate MS symptoms, maintain a comfortable room temperature. Advise patient to keep environment cool in warm weather and avoid hot baths.
2. To reduce muscle tightness and spasms, provide passive, assisted, or active ROM q2h. Teach these exercises to patient and significant others.
3. For other interventions, see **Pain,** p. 254, in "General Care of Patients with Neurologic Disorders."

For patients who are experiencing renal-urinary dysfunction, see related discussions in Chapter 3, "Renal-Urinary Disorders." See "Spinal Cord Injury" for **Potential for dis-**

use syndrome related to inactivity or spasticity, p. 202. See "General Care of Patients with Neurologic Disorders" for the following: **Potential for trauma** related to unsteady gait, p. 248; **Sensory/perceptual alterations** related to impaired pain, touch, and temperature sensations, p. 249; **Potential for impaired tissue integrity** related to risk of corneal irritation/abrasions, p. 249; **Alteration in nutrition:** Less than body requirements, p. 249; **Potential fluid volume deficit** related to decreased intake, p. 250; **Potential ineffective airway clearance** related to coughing and swallowing deficits, p. 251; **Self-care deficit:** Inability to perform ADL, p. 252; **Impaired verbal communication** related to dysarthria, p. 252; **Constipation** related to inability to chew and swallow high-roughage foods, side effects of medications, and immobility, p. 252; and **Sensory/perceptual alterations** related to visual disturbances, p. 254. For patients who are immobile, see related nursing diagnoses in "Pressure Ulcer," p. 630, and "Caring for Patients on Prolonged Bed Rest," p. 651. Also see "Caring for Patients with Cancer and Other Life-Disrupting Illnesses," p. 659, as appropriate.

PATIENT-FAMILY TEACHING AND DISCHARGE PLANNING

The patient with MS may have a wide variety of symptoms that cause disability, ranging from mild to severe. Provide patient and significant others with verbal and written information for the following, as appropriate:

1. Remission/exacerbation aspects of the disease process. Explain the effects of demyelinization on sensory and motor function and factors that aggravate symptoms.
2. Referrals to community resources, such as local and national MS society chapters, public health nurse, visiting nurse association, community support groups, social workers, psychological therapists, vocational rehabilitation agencies, home health agencies, extended and skilled care facilities, and financial counseling. The National Multiple Sclerosis Society is located at 205 East 42nd Street, New York, NY 10017, (800)-624-8236.
3. Safety measures relative to decreased sensation, visual disturbances, and motor deficits.
4. Medications, including drug name, purpose, dosage, frequency, precautions, and potential side effects.
5. Exercises that promote muscle strength and mobility; measures for preventing contractures and skin breakdown; transfer techniques and proper body mechanics; use of assistive devices and other measures to minimize neurologic deficits.
6. Measures for relieving pain, muscle spasms, or other discomfort.
7. Indications of constipation, urinary retention, or UTI; implementation of bowel and bladder training programs; self-catheterization technique or care of indwelling urinary catheters.
8. Indications of URI; implementation of measures that help prevent regurgitation, aspiration, and respiratory infection.
9. Dietary adjustments that may be appropriate for neurologic deficit (e.g., soft, semisolid foods for patients with chewing difficulties or a high-fiber diet for patients experiencing constipation).
10. Importance of follow-up care, including visits to MD, PT, and OT, as well as speech, sexual, or psychological counseling.

Guillain-Barré syndrome

Guillain-Barré syndrome (G-BS) is a rapidly progressing polyneuritis of unknown etiology. An inflammatory process causes lymphocytes to enter the perivascular spaces and destroy the myelin sheath covering the peripheral or cranial nerves. Because posterior (sensory) and anterior (motor) nerve roots can be affected because of this segmental demyelinization, the individual may experience both sensory and motor losses. In about 25% of cases, motor weakness progresses to total paralysis, a life-threatening situation. Respiratory insufficiency may occur in as many as half the individuals affected. Remyelinization and return of complete function usually occur, but it may take months to years for a full recovery. Motor recovery may begin within a few weeks of the onset of symptoms. Residual neurologic deficits tend to be mild motor or reflex alterations in the feet or legs.

G-BS may follow a febrile illness, such as URI or gastroenteritis, a rabies or flu vaccination, lupus erythematosus, and Hodgkin's disease or other malignant process. While the exact cause of G-BS is unknown, it is believed to be an autoimmune response to a viral infection.

ASSESSMENT

Weakness is the most common indicator. Typically, numbness and weakness begin in the legs and ascend upward, progressing to the arms and facial nerves within 1-3 days. Peak severity usually occurs within 10-14 days of onset.

Anterior (motor) nerve root involvement: Weakness or flaccid paralysis. Weakness or paralysis of respiratory muscles can be life threatening. There is a loss of reflexes, muscle tension, and tone, but muscle atrophy usually does not occur.

Autonomic nervous system involvement: Sinus tachycardia, bradycardia, hypertension, hypotension, cardiac dysrhythmias, facial flushing, diaphoresis, inability to perspire, loss of sphincter control, urinary retention, adynamic ileus, and increased pulmonary secretions may occur. Autonomic nervous system involvement may occur unexpectedly and can be life threatening.

Cranial nerve involvement: Inability to chew, swallow, speak, or close the eyes.

Posterior (sensory) nerve root involvement: Paresthesias, such as numbness and tingling, which usually are minor compared to the degree of motor loss. Ascending sensory loss often precedes motor loss. The patient may experience some muscle cramping discomfort but usually does not have severe pain.

Physical assessment: Symmetrical motor weakness, impaired position and vibration sense, hypoactive or absent DTRs, hypotonia in affected muscles, and decreased ventilatory capacity.

DIAGNOSTIC TESTS

Diagnostic tests are performed to rule out other diseases, such as acute poliomyelitis.
1. CBC: Will show presence of leukocytosis early in illness.
2. EMG: Reveals slowed nerve conduction velocities soon after paralysis appears. Findings occur due to segmental demyelinization. Denervation potentials appear later.
3. Lumbar puncture and CSF analysis: Usually show an elevated protein (especially IgG) without an increase in cell count. Although CSF pressure usually is normal, in severe disease it may be elevated. (See "Bacterial Meningitis," p. 161, for patient care.)

MEDICAL MANAGEMENT

The patient is likely to be in ICU when the neurologic deficit is progressing and is at risk for respiratory failure and autonomic dysfunction.
1. Respiratory support: Serial vital capacity measurements and ABG analysis to monitor for respiratory muscle weakness or paralysis. Endotracheal tube, tracheostomy, or mechanical ventilation is used as necessary.
2. Pharmacotherapy: May include a 1-week trial with glucocorticosteroids, such as prednisone or ACTH, to determine whether the symptoms decrease. In the absence of marked improvement, it is discontinued.
3. Exercise and activity: Activity other than passive ROM is restricted during the acute phase. After the patient stabilizes, active ROM or active assistive ROM is implemented, and a physical therapy and rehabilitation program is initiated. Occupational therapy and assistive devices or braces are employed so that patient can maintain mobility and independence with ADL. Muscle-strengthening exercises, conditioning exercises, and gait training are also frequently prescribed.

4. Antiembolism hose: To prevent thrombophlebitis in the legs.
5. Nutritional support: A high-fiber diet may be prescribed to help prevent constipation. If the patient cannot chew or swallow effectively because of cranial nerve involvement, NG or parenteral feedings may be initiated.
6. Management of acute autonomic dysfunction: Short-acting antihypertensive agents for hypertension; intravascular volume expanders or vasopressors for hypotension; cardiac monitoring of dysrhythmias; NG suctioning and parenteral fluids for adynamic ileus; and catheterization and medications for urinary retention.
7. Plasmapheresis: To reduce the patient's antibodies to peripheral and cranial nerve tissue by removing the plasma portion of the blood, which contains the circulating antibodies. Plasmapheresis involves a complete plasma exchange; the RBCs, WBCs, and platelets are returned to the body. If performed within 2 weeks of the onset of symptoms, removal of these auto-antibodies appears to lessen the duration and severity of the disease. Plasmapheresis is a 2-8 hour procedure and the patient may have to undergo several exchanges. The patient is at risk for the following complications during this procedure: fluid volume deficit, hypotension, hypokalemia, hypocalcemia, cardiac dysrhythmias, clotting disorders, phlebitis, and infection.
8. Treatment of complications: For example, antibiotic therapy for aspiration pneumonia or anticoagulant therapy for deep vein thrombosis (DVT) or emboli.
9. Controversial therapies: Immunosuppressive drug therapy with agents such as cyclophosphamide (Cytoxan) (see p. 664) and azathioprine (Imuran) (see p. 126) may slow and stabilize disease progression, probably by suppressing the immunoinflammatory response that leads to demyelinization of the peripheral nerve sheath.

NURSING DIAGNOSES AND INTERVENTIONS

Alteration in nutrition: Less than body requirements related to decreased intake secondary to NPO status with adynamic ileus

Desired outcome: Patient has adequate nutrition as evidenced by stable weight. **Note:** Patients with adynamic ileus generally require NG suctioning to decompress the stomach. Because these patients are unable to take foods orally, parenteral nutrition may be required. (See "Providing Nutritional Support," p. 611, for a discussion of parenteral nutrition.) For other interventions, see **Alteration in nutrition** in "General Care of Patients with Neurologic Disorders," p. 249.

Potential for ineffective breathing pattern related to neuromuscular weakness or paralysis of the facial, throat, and respiratory muscles

Desired outcome: Patient's respiratory rate is 12-20 breaths/min with normal depth and pattern (eupnea), Pao_2 is ≥ 80 mm Hg, vital capacity is ≥ 1 L, and tidal volume is $\geq 75\%$ of predicted value.

1. Test for ascending loss of sensation by touching patient lightly with a pin or fingers at frequent intervals (qh or more frequently initially). Assess from the level of the iliac crest upward toward the shoulders. Measure the highest level at which decreased sensation occurs. Decreased sensation frequently precedes motor weakness, so if it ascends to the level of the T-8 dermatome, anticipate that intercostal muscles (used with respirations) will soon be impaired. Also monitor for upper arm and shoulder weakness, which precede respiratory failure, by checking patient for the presence of arm drift and the ability to shrug the shoulders. Arm drift is detected in the following way: have the patient hold both arms out in front of the body, level with the shoulders and with the palms up. Instruct patient to close the eyes while holding this position. Weakness is present if one arm pronates or drifts down or out from its original position. Alert MD to significant findings.
2. Observe patient for changes in LOC and orientation, which may signal reduced oxygenation to the brain. Monitor patient's respiratory rate and rhythm. Watch for accessory muscle use, dyspnea, and loss of abdominal breathing. Alert MD to significant findings.
3. Monitor effectiveness of breathing by checking vital capacity results on pulmonary

function tests. If the vital capacity is <1 L or if the patient exhibits signs of hypoxia, such as tachycardia, increasing restlessness, mental dullness, or cyanosis, report findings immediately to MD. Monitor ABG levels to detect hypoxia or hypercapnia.

4. The patient may require tracheostomy, endotracheal intubation, or mechanical ventilation to support respiratory function. Prepare patient emotionally for such procedures or for the eventual transfer to ICU or transition care unit for closer monitoring.
5. For other interventions, see **Potential ineffective airway clearance** in "General Care of Patients with Neurologic Disorders," p. 251.

Fear related to threat to biologic integrity

Desired outcome: Patient verbalizes known sources of fear and the attainment of increased psychologic and physical comfort.

1. For the patient in whom the neurologic deficit is still progressing, arrange for a transfer to a room close to the nurses' station to help alleviate the fear of being suddenly incapacitated and helpless.
2. Be sure that patient's call light is within easy reach. Frequently assess patient's ability to use it.
3. Provide continuity of patient care through assignment of staff and use of care plan.
4. Perform assessments at frequent intervals, in a calm and reassuring manner.
5. For other interventions, see **Fear** in "Caring for Patients with Cancer and Other Life-Disrupting Illnesses," p. 692.

For patients with urinary incontinence, retention, neurogenic bladder, or UTI, see related discussions in Chapter 3, "Renal-Urinary Disorders." See "General Care of Patients with Neurologic Disorders" for the following: **Potential for trauma** related to unsteady gait. p. 248; **Sensory/perceptual alterations** related to impaired pain, touch, and temperature sensations, p. 249; **Potential for impaired tissue integrity** related to risk of corneal irritation/abrasions, p. 249; **Potential fluid volume deficit** related to decreased intake, p. 250; **Self-care deficit**, p. 251; **Impaired verbal communication** related to dysarthria, p. 252; **Constipation,** p. 252; and **Sensory/perceptual alterations** related to visual disturbance, p. 254. For patients who are immobile, see related nursing diagnoses in "Pressure Ulcers," p. 630, and "Caring for Patients on Prolonged Bed Rest," p. 651. Also see "Caring for Patients with Cancer and Other Life-Disrupting Illnesses," p. 690, for psychosocial nursing diagnoses as appropriate.

PATIENT-FAMILY TEACHING AND DISCHARGE PLANNING

Most patients with G-BS eventually recover fully. Because the recovery period can be prolonged, the patient often goes home with some degree of neurologic deficit. Discharge planning and teaching will vary according to the degree of disability. Provide patient and significant others with verbal and written information for the following as appropriate:

1. The disease process, expected improvement, and importance of continuing in the rehabilitation or physical therapy program to promote as full a recovery as possible.
2. Referrals to community resources, such as public health nurse, visiting nurse association, community support groups, social workers, psychologic therapy, home health agencies, and extended and skilled care facilities.
3. Safety measures relative to the decreased sensorimotor deficit.
4. Exercises that promote muscle strength and mobility; measures for preventing contractures and skin breakdown; transfer techniques and proper body mechanics; and use of assistive devices.
5. Indications of constipation, urinary retention, or UTI; and, if appropriate, care of indwelling catheters or self-catheterization technique.
6. Indications of URI; measures for preventing regurgitation, aspiration, and respiratory infection.
7. Medications, including drug name, purpose, dosage, schedule, precautions, and potential side effects.

Bacterial meningitis

Bacterial meningitis is an infection that results in inflammation of the meningeal membranes covering the brain and spinal cord. Bacteria in the subarachnoid space multiply and cause an inflammatory reaction of the pia and arachnoid meninges. Purulent exudate is produced and the inflammation and infection spread quickly through the CSF that circulates around the brain and spinal cord. Bacteria and exudate can create vascular congestion, plugging the arachnoid villi. This obstruction of CSF flow and decreased reabsorption of CSF can lead to increased intracranial pressure, brain herniation, and death.
　　Meningitis generally is transmitted in one of four ways: *via* airborne droplets or contact with oral secretions from infected individuals; from direct contamination (e.g., from a penetrating skull wound, lumbar puncture, ventricular shunt, or surgical procedure); *via* the bloodstream (e.g., pneumonia, endocarditis); or from direct contact with an infectious process that invades the meningeal membranes, such as that which can occur with osteomyelitis, sinusitis, otitis media, mastoiditis, or brain abscess. *Haemophilus influenzae* is the leading infecting agent of bacterial meningitis. Meningococcal meningitis caused by *Neisseria meningitidis* is the next leading cause, followed by pneumococcal meningitis, caused by *Streptococcus pneumoniae*. Any bacteria can cause a meningitis and some, such as that caused by *Staphylococcus aureus*, can be difficult to treat due to their resistance to antibiotic therapy. The prognosis is good if the disorder is recognized early and antibiotic treatment is initiated promptly. However, if left untreated, the mortality rate is 70%-100%.

ASSESSMENT

Infection: Fever, chills, malaise.

IICP (increased intracranial pressure) and herniation: Severe headache, decreased LOC (irritability, drowsiness, stupor, coma), nausea and vomiting, a dropping Glasgow Coma Scale score (see p. 207). VS changes (increased BP, decreased HR, widening pulse pressure), changes in respiratory pattern, decreased pupillary reaction to light, pupillary dilatation or inequality.

Meningeal irritation: Back stiffness and pain, nuchal rigidity.

Other: Generalized seizures and photophobia; joint pain (in the presence of *H. influenzae.)*

Physical assessment

☐ A positive Brudzinski's sign may be elicited due to meningeal irritation: When the neck is passively flexed forward, both legs flex involuntarily at the hip and knee.
☐ A positive Kernig's sign also may be found: When the thigh is flexed, the individual is unable to extend the leg completely without pain.
　　In the presence of meningococcal meningitis, a pink macular rash, petechiae, ecchymoses, purpura, and increased DTRs may occur.

DIAGNOSTIC TESTS

1. <u>Lumbar puncture, CSF analysis, and Gram stain and culture:</u> To identify causative organism. Glucose is generally decreased and protein is usually increased. Typically, the CSF will be cloudy or milky due to increased WBCs, and the CSF pressure will be increased owing to the inflammation and exudate, causing an obstruction in outflow of CSF from the arachnoid villi. This test, in the presence of IICP, can cause brain herniation.
　　☐ *Positioning:* Assist patient into a side-lying position with chin tucked into the chest and knees drawn up to the abdomen. This position curves the spine and widens the intervertebral space for easier insertion of the spinal needle.
　　☐ *During the test:* Instruct patient to lie very still. Place your hands behind patient's knees and neck and pull gently to help maintain proper position. Assess for an elevated pulse, paleness, or clammy skin. Notify MD of significant findings.

☐ *After the test:* Minimize risk of headache by having patient lie flat for the amount of time prescribed by MD. Encourage turning from side to side. If prescribed, elevate HOB slightly. Encourage fluids and provide analgesics as prescribed. Monitor puncture site for redness, swelling, and drainage. Be alert to indicators of meningitis, including fever, nuchal rigidity, and irritability. If CSF pressure is elevated, check neurologic status and VS at frequent intervals for signs of brain herniation (decreased LOC; pupillary changes, such as dilatation, inequality, or decreased reaction; irregular respirations; and hemiparesis).

2. *Culture and sensitivity testing of blood, urine, and other body secretions.* To identify infective organism and determine appropriate antibiotic.
3. *Counterimmunoelectrophoresis (CIE):* For detection of bacterial antigens of pneumococci, meningococci, and *H. influenzae* in the CSF, blood, and urine.
4. *Sinus, skull, and chest x-rays:* Taken after treatment is started to rule out sinusitis, pneumonia, and cranial osteomyelitis.
5. *Radioimmunoassay (RIA), latex particle agglutination (LPA), or enzyme-linked immunosorbent assay (ELISA):* To detect microbial antigens in the CSF to identify the causative organism.
6. *CT scan with contrast:* To rule out hydrocephalus and detect exudate in the CSF spaces. See "Brain Tumors," p. 215, for patient care considerations.

MEDICAL MANAGEMENT

1. Respiratory precautions: Patients with *Neisseria meningitidis, H. influenzae,* or in whom the causative organism is in doubt require observation of special respiratory isolation precautions for at least 24 hours from initiation of the appropriate antibiotic therapy. The patient should be placed in a private room. Infection may be spread by contact with airborne droplets or oral secretions. Masks should be used, along with adherence to body fluid precautions.
2. Parenteral antibiotics: Because treatment cannot be delayed until the results of the culture are returned, high doses are started immediately, based on Gram stain results. The antibiotic must penetrate the blood-brain barrier into the CSF. Adjustments in therapy can be made after CIE and culture and sensitivity test results are in. Antibiotics may include the following: penicillin G, ampicillin, nafcillin, oxacillin, chloramphenicol, gentamicin, kanamycin, or vancomycin.
3. Prophylactic antibiotic treatment of significant others and close contacts: Rifampin is administered.
4. Other pharmacotherapy
   ☐ *Osmotic diuretics (e.g., mannitol):* To decrease cerebral edema.
   ☐ *Antiepilepsy drugs (e.g., diazepam and phenytoin):* To control seizures.
   ☐ *Analgesics (e.g., acetaminophen and codeine):* For headache and other pain.
   ☐ *Antipyretics (e.g., acetaminophen):* For control of fever to reduce cerebral metabolism.
   ☐ *Sedatives and tranquilizers:* To promote rest.
5. Support respirations: *Via* oxygen, suctioning, or intubation as necessary.
6. Bed rest: During acute stage of the disease.
7. Limitation of fluids to two-thirds maintenance (about 1,500 ml): To keep patient underhydrated and reduce cerebral edema and effects of inappropriate ADH secretion.
8. Nutritional support: Enteral or parenteral feedings as required for patients who are stuporous or comatose.
9. Measures to reduce hyperthermia: Tepid sponges or cooling blankets to reduce fever.
10. Antiembolism hose: To prevent thrombophlebitis in the legs from venous stasis.
11. Treatment of complications: Examples include disseminated intravascular coagulation (DIC), syndrome of inappropriate antidiuretic hormone (SIADH), respiratory or heart failure, and septic shock.

NURSING DIAGNOSES AND INTERVENTIONS

Knowledge deficit: Side effects and precautions for the prescribed antibiotics

Desired outcome: Patient and significant others verbalize knowledge of the potential side effects and precautions for the prescribed antibiotics.

1. For significant others and contacts placed on prophylactic rifampin, explain the prescribed dosage and schedule. Rifampin should be taken 1 hour before meals for maximum absorption. Emphasize the importance of taking this drug as a preventive measure against meningitis, and describe potential side effects, such as nausea, vomiting, diarrhea, orange urine, headache, and dizziness. Caution against wearing contact lenses, as the drug will permanently color them orange. In addition, rifampin reduces the effectiveness of oral contraceptives, and it is contraindicated in pregnancy.
2. Instruct significant others and patient's other contacts taking rifampin to report the onset of jaundice (yellow skin or sclera), allergic reactions, and persistence of GI side effects.
3. For other interventions, see **Knowledge deficit:** Adverse side effects from prolonged use of potent antibiotics, p. 447, in "Osteomyelitis."

Knowledge deficit: Rationale and procedure for special respiratory or secretion precautions

Desired outcome: Patient and significant others verbalize knowledge of the rationale for isolation or secretion precautions and comply with the prescribed restrictions and precautionary measures.

Note: Patients with *Neisseria meningitidis, H. influenzae,* or meningitis caused by an unidentified organism will be placed in a private room for at least 24 hours and will require special respiratory isolation precautions from the initiation of appropriate antibiotic therapy. Masks should be worn and body fluid precautions observed.

---

1. For patients with meningitis caused by *H. influenzae* and *Neisseria meningitidis,* explain the method of disease transmission *via* airborne droplets and oral secretions and the rationale for private room and special precautions.
2. Provide instructions for covering the mouth before coughing/sneezing and proper disposal of the tissue.
3. Instruct patients with specific respiratory precautions to stay in their room. However, if they must leave the room for a procedure or test, explain that a mask must be worn to protect others from contact with airborne droplets.
4. For individuals in contact with the patient with specific respiratory precautions, explain the importance of wearing a surgical mask and performing good handwashing. Gloves should be worn when handling any body fluid, especially oral secretions, which may contain the infectious organism.
5. Reassure patient that special respiratory precautions are temporary and will be discontinued once patient has been on the appropriate antibiotic for 24-48 hours.

See "Head injury" for **Potential for disuse syndrome,** p. 212. See "Seizure Disorders" for **Potential for trauma** related to oral, musculoskeletal, and airway vulnerabilities secondary to seizure activity, p. 244. See "General Care of Patients with Neurologic Disorders" for the following: **Potential for trauma** related to unsteady gait, p. 248; **Sensory/perceptual alterations** related to impaired pain, touch, and temperature sensations, p. 249; **Potential for impaired tissue integrity** related to risk of corneal abrasions/irritation, p. 249; **Alteration in nutrition:** Less than body requirements, p. 249; **Potential fluid volume deficit,** p. 250; **Potential ineffective airway clearance,** p. 251; **Self-care deficit:** Inability to perform ADL, p. 251; **Constipation,** p. 252; **Potential for injury** related to increased ICP, p. 253; and **Pain,** p. 254. For patients who are immobile, see related nursing diagnoses in "Pressure Ulcers," p. 630, and "Caring for Patients on Prolonged Bed Rest," p. 651. In addition, see "Caring for Patients with Cancer and Other Life-Disrupting Illnesses," p. 690, for appropriate psychosocial nursing diagnoses and interventions.

PATIENT-FAMILY TEACHING AND DISCHARGE PLANNING

The extent of teaching and discharge planning will depend on whether or not patient has any residual damage. As appropriate, provide patient and significant others with verbal and written information for the following:

1. Referrals to community resources, such as public health nurse, visiting nurse association, community support groups, social workers, psychologic therapy, vocational rehabilitation agency, home health agencies, and extended and skilled care facilities.
2. Medications, including purpose, dosage, schedule, precautions, and potential side effects.

In addition:

3. For patients with residual neurologic deficits, teach the following as appropriate: exercises that promote muscle strength and mobility; measures for preventing contractures and skin breakdown; transfer techniques and proper body mechanics; safety measures if the patient has decreased pain and sensation or visual disturbances; use of assistive devices; indications of constipation, urinary retention, or UTI; bowel and bladder training programs; self-catheterization technique or care of indwelling catheters; and seizure precautions if indicated.

Encephalitis

Encephalitis is an inflammation of the brain that can cause severe neuronal dysfunction. In response to infection the brain tissue becomes inflamed, leading to cerebral edema. The brain's ganglion cells may degenerate, leaving diffuse nerve cell destruction and necrotic areas. The cerebral edema can be severe, leading to increased ICP, herniation, and death.

Encephalitis usually is caused by a viral infection. It may be the result of an arbovirus infection that is transmitted by an infected mosquito or tick bite. Postinfectious encephalitis occurs after a vaccination or as a complication of other infections, such as measles, chicken pox, and herpes simplex type I virus. The prognosis varies according to the type of infection. Some cases of encephalitis leave few or no residual side effects, and the neurologic symptoms often subside in several weeks. Other types of encephalitis, such as eastern equine encephalitis (an arbovirus infection), can have a high mortality rate (up to 66%), and survivors frequently have severe residual damage. Herpes simplex encephalitis has a mortality rate ranging from 30%-70%, depending on when the antiviral drug therapy is started, and survivors often are left with seizures, aphasia, or severe mental deterioration, such as dementia.

ASSESSMENT

Infection: Fever, chills, malaise.

Increased ICP and brain herniation: Headache; changes in LOC, such as irritability, confusion, and drowsiness, symptoms that can progress to stupor and coma; a falling Glasgow Coma Scale score (see p. 207); nausea and vomiting; VS changes (hypertension, bradycardia, widening pulse pressure); changes in respiratory pattern; and pupillary changes, such as inequality and decreased reaction to light.

Meningeal irritation: Neck stiffness/rigidity; pain.

Focal: Symptoms vary. Patient may have seizures or photophobia, ataxia, and sensorimotor deficits. Eastern equine encephalitis, for example, can destroy major portions of a lobe or hemisphere and leave the individual with hemiplegia, aphasia, blindness, deafness, and/or seizures. Herpes simplex encephalitis has a special affinity for the frontal and temporal lobes of the brain, resulting in alterations in the senses of smell and taste, seizures, aphasia, organic psychosis, and dementia.

DIAGNOSTIC TESTS

1. _Lumbar puncture and CSF analysis:_ May reveal increased CSF pressure, increased WBC and protein levels, and normal glucose. (See "Bacterial Meningitis," p. 161, for patient care.)
2. _CT scan:_ To rule out other neurologic problems.
3. _EEG:_ May show presence of abnormal electrical activity. (See "Seizure Disorder," p. 242, for patient care.)
4. _Brain biopsy:_ May be done to identify the infecting agent. This requires the drilling of burr holes into the skull to obtain a specimen. The specimen then undergoes an immunofluorescent exam and culture to identify the virus present. Usually the test is done only to determine if the encephalitis is caused by a treatable virus infection, such as herpes simplex. If the diagnosis of herpes simplex is fairly certain, based on other clinical evidence, the MD may decide to initiate drug therapy and forego this test.

MEDICAL MANAGEMENT

Except for herpes simplex encephalitis, the treatment is supportive only.

1. Antiviral agent (e.g., vidarabine): For herpes simplex encephalitis. The patient undergoing drug therapy with vidarabine is at risk for fluid volume excess and additional cerebral edema due to the amount of fluid required to dilute this drug. For therapy with vidarabine to be effective, it should be initiated before the patient becomes comatose. Side effects may include tremor, dizziness, hallucinations, anorexia, nausea, vomiting, diarrhea, itching, rash, and anemia. Acyclovir, another antiviral agent, is being investigated in the treatment of herpes simplex encephalitis.
2. Supportive pharmacotherapy
   □ _Antiepilepsy drugs (e.g., phenytoin):_ To treat or prevent seizures.
   □ _Glucocorticosteroids (e.g., dexamethasone):_ To reduce cerebral edema and inflammation.
   □ _Sedatives:_ For restlessness.
   □ _Analgesics and antipyretics (e.g., aspirin and acetaminophen):_ For headache and fever.
3. Fluid and electrolyte management: IV fluids are given to maintain a balanced electrolyte status. Generally, fluids are limited to two-thirds maintenance (about 1,500 ml) to maintain a state of underhydration, which helps reduce cerebral edema.
4. Support of respirations: Via oxygen, suctioning, or intubation.
5. Nutritional support: Enteral or parenteral feedings for stuporous or comatose patients, as needed. A soft or semisolid diet may be prescribed for some patients, depending on their neurologic deficit.
6. Physical medicine: Physical therapy, occupational therapy, and assistive devices or braces may be prescribed so that the patient can maintain mobility and independence with ADL. Muscle-strengthening and conditioning exercises and gait training also may be prescribed.
7. ROM exercises: To maintain or increase joint function and prevent contractures.
8. Speech therapy: To assist the aphasic or dysarthric patient.

NURSING DIAGNOSES AND INTERVENTIONS

See "Alzheimer's Disease" for **Altered thought processes** related to altered sensory reception, transmission, integration, and evaluation, p. 186; and for **Potential for trauma** related to lack of awareness of environmental hazards, p. 184. See "Head Injury" for **Potential for disuse syndrome,** p. 212. See "Cerebrovascular Accident" for **Impaired verbal communication** related to aphasia or dysarthria, p. 237. See "Seizure Disorders" for **Potential for trauma** related to oral, musculoskeletal, and airway vulnerability secondary to seizure activity, p. 244. See "General Care of Patients with Neurologic Disorders" for the following: **Potential for trauma** related to gait unsteadiness, p. 248; **Sensory/perceptual alterations** related to decreased pain, touch, and temperature sensations, p. 249; **Potential for impaired tissue integrity** related to risk of corneal irritation/abrasion, p. 249; **Alteration in nutrition**, p. 249; **Potential fluid volume deficit**, p. 250; **Potential ineffective airway clearance**, p. 251; **Self-care deficit**, p. 251; **Constipation**, p. 252: **Potential for trauma** related to risk of increased ICP, p. 253: and **Pain**, p. 254. For patients who have varying degrees of immobility, see related nursing diagnoses and interventions in "Pressure Ulcers." p. 630, and "Caring for Patients on Prolonged Bed Rest," p. 651. Also see "Caring for Patients with Cancer and Other Life-Disrupting Illnesses," p. 690, for psychosocial nursing diagnoses and interventions as appropriate.

PATIENT-FAMILY TEACHING AND DISCHARGE PLANNING

The amount of teaching and discharge planning will depend on the degree of neurologic deficit. See teaching/discharge planning interventions, Nos. 2-10, in "Multiple Sclerosis," p. 164, as appropriate.

In addition:
1. Teach interventions that increase effective communication in the presence of aphasia or dysarthria. See "Cerebrovascular Accident" for **Impaired verbal communication** related to aphasia or dysarthria, p. 237.
2. Provide instructions regarding seizure precautions, factors that may precipitate seizures, and actions to be taken should they occur. See "Seizure Disorders," p. 239.

Section Two DEGENERATIVE DISORDERS OF THE NERVOUS SYSTEM

The CNS, peripheral nervous system, and autonomic nervous system are responsible for controlling and coordinating the functions of all body systems. With degenerative nerve disorders the function of the nerve cells, dendrites, or axons is progressively altered or decreased. A variety of mechanisms, including outright destruction of the neurons or decreases in neurotransmitter synthesis uptake or release, account for this change in neuronal function.

Parkinsonism

Parkinson's disease is a slowly progressive, degenerative disorder of the CNS affecting the brain centers that regulate movement. For unknown reasons, cell death occurs in the substantia nigra of the midbrain. When healthy, the substantia nigra projects dopaminergic neurons into the corpus striatum and releases the neurotransmitter dopamine in that area. Degeneration of these neurons leads to an abnormally low concentration of dopamine in the basal ganglia. The basal ganglia controls muscle tone and voluntary motor movement *via* a balance between two main neurotransmitters, dopamine and acetycholine. The deficit of dopamine, which has an inhibitory effect, allows the relative excess of acetycholine. The excitatory effect of acetycholine causes overactivity of the basal ganglia, which interferes with normal muscle tone and the control of smooth, purposeful movement, causing the characteristic symptoms of Parkinson's disease: muscle rigidity, tremors, and slowness of movement.

Possible causes include viral encephalitis, neurotoxins, cerebrovascular disease, head injury, phenothiazide use, and exposure to carbon monoxide. Improper synthesis of a synthetic heroin-like component results in the product MPTP, which causes a severe form of Parkinson's disease in those who have taken this illegal IV recreational drug. The vast majority of Parkinson's disease occurs without an apparent or known cause. Approximately 1% of all individuals over age 50 have this disease. Parkinsonism is usually progressive, and death can result from aspiration pneumonia or choking. *Parkinso-*

nian crisis, a medical emergency, is usually precipitated by emotional trauma or failure to take the prescribed medications.

ASSESSMENT

Initially, symptoms are mild and include stiffness or slight hand tremors. They gradually increase and can become disabling. Cardinal features are tremors, rigidity, and bradykinesia. Assessment findings vary in degree and are highly individualized.

Bradykinesia: Slowness, stiffness, and difficulty with initiating movement. The patient may have a masklike, blank facial expression; "unblinking" stare; difficulty chewing and swallowing; drooling due to decreased frequency of swallowing; and a high-pitched, monotone, weak voice. Speech may be slow and slurred. The patient also has loss of automatic associated movements, such as the ability to swing the arms when walking.

Loss of postural reflexes: Causes the typical stooped over, forward leaning, shuffling, propulsive gait with short, rapidly accelerating steps; stumbling; and difficulty maintaining or regaining balance, which makes the individual prone to stumbling and falling.

Increased muscle rigidity: Limb muscles become rigid on passive motion. Typically, this rigidity results in jerky ("cogwheel") motions.

Tremors: Increase when the limb is at rest and stop with voluntary movement and during sleep (nonintention tremor). "Pill-rolling" tremor of the hands and "to and fro" tremor of the head are typical.

Autonomic: Excessive diaphoresis, seborrhea, postural hypotension, decreased libido, hypomotility of the GI tract, and urinary hesitancy.

Other: Dementia commonly is associated with Parkinson's disease. However, not all patients develop impaired intellectual and mental functioning. Some patients may experience akathisia, a condition of motor restlessness in which the individual has a compelling need to walk about constantly.

Physical assessment: Usually a positive blink reflex is elicited by tapping a finger between the patient's eyebrows. Blinking may occur 5-10 times/min instead of the normal 20 times/min. A positive palmomental reflex (contraction of muscles of the chin and corner of mouth) can be elicited by stroking the patient's palm. Diminished postural reflexes are present on neurologic exam; however, there is risk of injury with this test because the patient may quickly lose balance and fall.

Parkinsonian crisis: This sudden and severe increase in bradykinesia, muscle rigidity, and tremors can lead to tachycardia, hyperpnea, hyperpyrexia, and muscle paralysis, causing an inability to swallow or maintain a patent airway.

Oculogyric crisis: Fixation of the eyes in one position, generally upward, sometimes for several hours. This is relatively rare.

DIAGNOSTIC TESTS

Diagnosis usually is made on the basis of physical assessment and characteristic symptoms, and after other neurologic problems have been ruled out.
1. *Urinalysis:* May reveal decreased dopamine level, which supports the diagnosis.
2. *Medication withdrawal:* Long-term therapy with large doses of medications, such as haloperidol or phenothiazines, can produce Parkinson-like symptoms. If caused by these medications, symptoms will disappear when the drug is discontinued.
3. *EEG:* Often shows abnormalities, such as diffuse, nonspecific slowing of theta waves. (See "Seizure Disorders," p. 242, for patient care.)
4. *Lumbar puncture with CSF analysis:* May show decreased levels of dopamine or its metabolite in the CSF. (See "Bacterial Meningitis," p. 161, for patient care.)
5. *Tremor studies:* Serial measurements of functional activity will show decreased performance.

MEDICAL MANAGEMENT

1. **Pharmacotherapy:** See Table 4-1 for a description of the mechanisms, action, and side effects of anti-Parkinson's drugs.
   - *Dopamine replacement (e.g., levodopa or levodopa-carbidopa combination):* Given in increasing amounts until symptoms are reduced or patient's tolerance to side effects is reached. It may be used as initial therapy or later when other medications no longer can control Parkinson's symptoms.
   - *Antiviral agents (e.g., amantadine):* Less effective than levodopa but has less severe side effects. May be used as the initial therapy or as an adjunct to anticholinergics or levodopa.
   - *Dopamine agonist (e.g., bromocriptine):* Administered with a concomitant reduction of dopamine replacement dosage. It may be used to reduce levodopa-induced dyskinesia, such as involuntary movements and the frequency of "on-off" responses.
   - *Anticholinergics (e.g., trihexyphenidyl, cycrimine, procyclidine biperiden, or benztropine mesylate):* They are often used in conjunction with dopamine replacement therapy, although they may be used by themselves if the patient's symptoms are mild or if the patient cannot tolerate levodopa.
   - *Antihistamines (e.g., diphenhydramine, orphenadrine hydrochloride):* Usually given in conjunction with anticholinergic drugs but may be used alone if the patient's symptoms are mild.
   - *Phenothiazine derivative (e.g., ethopropazine):* Generally used in combination with other anti-Parkinson drugs to reduce rigidity, tremors, and spasms.
   - *Laxatives and stool softeners (e.g., docusate sodium):* To prevent constipation.
2. **Physical therapy and exercise program:** Massage; muscle stretching; active/passive ROM, especially on hands and feet; and walking and gait training exercises.
3. **Treatment of complications of dopamine replacement therapy**
   - *Choreiform or involuntary movements (e.g., facial grimacing, tongue protrusion, or restlessness).*
     —Dose reduction or redistribution throughout the day.
     —Drug "holiday": Treatment is somewhat controversial. After temporary withdrawal, levodopa is resumed at a much lower dose. Generally the patient can be maintained for several months to years at this much lower dose, with fewer drug-related adverse side effects and good mobility. This treatment requires hospitalization because during withdrawal the patient may become completely immobile and dependent. Medications are tapered gradually. These individuals often need psychologic support because without the drug's mitigating effects, this may be the first time they will have experienced the full impact and immobility of their disease.
   - *Severe mental status changes.*
     —Dose reduction.
     —Drug holiday.
   - *On-off response:* This is a rapid fluctuation or change in the patient's condition. The individual is "on" one moment, in a state of relative mobility, and "off" the next, in a state of complete or nearly complete immobility. Attacks can occur over a 2-3 minute period of time and may last several hours. Initially the attacks may occur 3-4 hours after anti-Parkinsonism medication is given. Later in the disease they can occur at any time. Etiology is uncertain but appears to be related to fluctuating drug levels in the brain as loss of striatal ability to store dopamine progresses. Usually this response occurs after the patient has been on medication for several years.
     —Titration of the levodopa dose and spacing the doses during the 24-hour day.
     —Combining levodopa with anticholinergic medications, dopamine agonists, or amantadine may be helpful.
     —Use of substained-release forms of levodopa.
     —Drug holiday.

TABLE 4 - 1   Anti-Parkinson drugs

Medication	Mechanism of action	Side effects
Dopamine replacements		
levodopa	Levodopa is the metabolic precursor of dopamine. Levodopa crosses the blood-brain barrier and restores dopamine levels in the extrapyramidal centers in the brain. Before levodopa crosses the blood-brain barrier, much of it is converted into dopamine by the peripheral metabolism (GI tract and liver). This causes many of the drug's side effects	Choreiform and involuntary movements (e.g., facial grimacing, tongue protusion; on-off response; severe depression with possible suicidal overtones; GI bleeding; orthostatic hypotension; blurred vision; anorexia; nausea and vomiting; dry mouth; constipation; urinary retention; confusion; agitation; hallucination)
carbidopa-levodopa	Carbidopa prevents peripheral metabolism of levodopa, thereby increasing the amount of levodopa available for transport to the brain. Carbidopa does not cross the blood-brain barrier and therefore does not affect the metabolism of levodopa in the brain. Carbidopa reduces the amount of levodopa needed	No reactions to carbidopa alone. Adverse reactions are those of levodopa
Antiviral		
amantadine	Mechanism of action not understood. This medication appears to increase the release of dopamine from neuronal storage sites. It has an anticholinergic effect as well	Most side effects are like those of levodopa but are milder and dose-related. They include insomnia, peripheral edema, CHF, depression, nervousness, slurred speech, ataxia, orthostatic hypotension, blurred vision, anorexia, nausea, vomiting, dry mouth, constipation, urinary retention, confusion, irritability, hallucination

Dopamine agonists
bromocriptine
lisuride
pergoline

Have a direct stimulating effect on dopamine receptors, thereby enhancing their activity

Produce less nausea and vomiting than levodopa, but otherwise have similar side effects, including orthostatic hypotension, blurred vision, nausea, vomiting, dry mouth, constipation, urinary retention, confusion, paranoia, insomnia, ataxia, digital vasospasm

Anticholinergics
trihexyphenidyl
cycrimine
procyclidine
biperiden
benztropine mesylate

Reduce the excitatory action of acetacholine on cholinergic neuron receptors. In Parkinson's disease, due to the dopamine deficit, there is an imbalance between dopamine, with its inhibitory action, and acetylcholine, with its excitatory action. Anticholinergics reduce acetylcholine action and work to reestablish this balance

Side effects are dose-related and include decreased sweating, orthostatic hypotension, tachycardia, dry mouth, blurred vision, photophobia, nausea, drowsiness, constipation, urinary retention or overflow incontinence, confusion, mental slowness, insomnia, nervousness, headache

Antihistamines
diphenhydramine
orphenadrine HCl

Have a central cholinergic blocking action. They prolong dopamine action by inhibiting its uptake and storage. They are used in conjunction with anticholinergics

GI effects are fairly minimal. Other side effects include drowsiness, mild hypotension, dry mouth, anorexia, constipation, urinary retention

Phenothiazine derivative
ethopropazine

Has a central cholinergic blocking action. Differs from other phenothiazines in that it is used to control extrapyramidal symptoms. It is used in conjunction with other anti-Parkinson drugs

Depression, drowsiness, hypotension, dizziness, ataxia, blurred vision, nausea, vomiting, dry mouth, constipation

4. **Treatment for Parkinsonian crisis:** This crisis necessitates respiratory and cardiac support. The patient is placed in a quiet, calm environment with subdued lighting. Sodium phenobarbital or sodium amobarbital is given IM or IV.
5. **Counseling or psychotherapy:** To help patient and significant others adapt to the disability and deal with emotions and feelings, such as depression, that are either a direct or indirect result of the disease process or drug therapy.
6. **Diet:** A controlled, low-protein diet may be prescribed if the patient is on dopamine replacement therapy because high protein intake reduces the medication's effectiveness. A high-fiber diet may be given to prevent constipation.
7. **Adrenal transplant:** A new surgery that involves grafting one of the patient's own adrenal medullary glands to the caudate nucleus of the brain. The medullary portion of the adrenal gland produces dopamine for the peripheral nervous system. When grafted, the adrenal medullary may continue to produce dopamine in the CNS, reducing or eliminating Parkinson's disease symptoms and the need for medication. This procedure involves three major surgeries: 1) stereotaxic localization of the caudate nucleus, 2) craniotomy (see "Brain Tumors," p. 215), and 3) laparotomy for adrenalectomy. Prepare the patient for transfer to the ICU following surgery.
8. **Stereotaxic surgery:** Rarely performed now owing to the effectiveness of drug therapy. It involves the use of electrical coagulation, freezing, radioactivity, or ultrasound to destroy portions of the globus pallidus of the ventrolateral nucleus of the thalamus to prevent involuntary movement and help relieve tremors and rigidity of the extremities.

NURSING DIAGNOSES AND INTERVENTIONS

Potential for trauma related to unsteady gait secondary to bradykinesis, tremors, and rigidity

Desired outcome: Patient demonstrates effective ambulatory techniques and preventive measures and remains injury free.

1. During ambulation, encourage patient to deliberately swing the arms to assist with the gait, and raise the feet to help prevent falls. Advise patients to step over an imaginary object or line, which will help them raise their feet higher and increase their stride.
2. Have patient practice movements that are especially difficult (e.g., turning). When turning, teach patient to walk in a wide arc rather than pivot.
3. Teach head and neck exercises to help improve patient's posture. Remind patient repeatedly to maintain an upright posture, especially when walking.
4. Advise patient to stop occasionally to slow down the walking speed. Teach patients to concentrate and listen to their feet as they touch the floor and count the cadence in order to prevent too fast a gait.
5. Remind patient to maintain a wide-based gait.
6. Provide a clear pathway when the patient is walking. Teach patient to avoid crowds, scatter rugs, uneven surfaces, fast turns, narrow doorways, and obstructions.
7. For other interventions, see **Potential for trauma** related to unsteady gait in "General Care of Patients with Neurologic Disorders," p. 248.

Knowledge deficit: Methods for overcoming difficulty with initiating movement

Desired outcome: Patient demonstrates measures that enhance the ability to initiate desired movement.

1. Teach patient that rocking from side to side may help initiate leg movement. Marching in place a few steps before resuming forward motion also may be helpful. If the patient's feet remain "glued" to the floor despite these measures, thinking of something else for a few moments and then trying again may enable movement.
2. To get out of a chair, teach patients to get to the edge of the seat, place their hands on the arm supports, bend forward slightly, move their feet back, and then rhythmically rock in the chair a few times before trying to get up. Advise the patient to sit in

chairs with backs and arms and to purchase elevated toilet seats or sidebars in the bathroom to assist with rising.
3. "Freezing" is variable and can fluctuate with stress or the patient's emotional state. Teach patients and significant others to recognize situations that can cause freezing episodes so that they can anticipate and plan so as to avoid them. Attempting two movements simultaneously, such as trying to change direction quickly while walking, can cause freezing. Distracting environmental, visual, or auditory stimuli also can precipitate a freezing episode. Doorways, narrow passages, or a change in floor color, texture, or slope gives many patients problems.

Knowledge deficit: Side effects of and precautionary measures for taking anti-Parkinson medications

Desired outcome: Patient and significant others verbalize knowledge of the side effects of and necessary precautionary measures for taking anti-Parkinson medications.

Note: Teach patient and significant others to report adverse side effects promptly as many side effects are dose related and can be controlled by an adjustment in the dosage.

Side effects common to most anti-Parkinson medications
1. Teach patient to take medications with meals to decrease the potential for nausea and stomach upset.
2. Advise patients that to counteract orthostatic hypotension, they should make position changes slowly and in stages. Teach patient to dangle legs a few minutes before standing. Antiembolism hose may help some patients. Encourage male patients to urinate from a sitting, rather than standing, position if possible. Report dizziness to MD.
3. To lessen dry mouth and maintain the integrity of the oral mucous membrane, teach patient to use sugarless chewing gum or hard candy, frequent mouth rinses with water, or artificial saliva products.
4. Advise patient to report any urinary hesistancy or incontinence as this may signal urinary retention. Individuals taking anticholinergics may find that voiding prior to taking the medication may relieve this problem. See "Urinary Retention," p. 145, for additional measures.
5. Constipation is a common problem with these medications. For interventions, see **Constipation,** p. 656, in "Caring for Patients on Prolonged Bed Rest."
6. Many of these drugs can cause or aggravate mental status changes, such as confusion, mental slowness or dullness, and even paranoia and hallucinations. Teach patient to report these signs to the MD promptly for possible dosage adjustment.

Side effects specific to levodopa
1. Teach patient to avoid vitamin preparations or fortified cereals that contain pyridoxine (vitamin B_6), which reduces the effectiveness of levodopa. The MD may limit the patient's intake of foods high in pyridoxine, such as wheat germ, whole grain cereals, legumes, and liver.
2. Teach patient that a dietary intake high in protein may interfere with the effectiveness of levodopa. While the diet should meet the Recommended Daily Allowance of protein, the patient should avoid excessive amounts of meat, eggs, dairy products, and legumes.
3. Instruct patient to report muscle twitching or spasmodic winking as these are early signs of overdose. Abnormal involuntary movements, such as facial grimacing and tongue protrusion, signal that an adjustment in dosage may be needed.
4. Explain signs and symptoms of Parkinsonian crisis. Emphasize the need for immediate medical intervention with this crisis. Teach patient that to avoid this crisis, taking levodopa as scheduled and avoiding stopping the medication abruptly are critical.
5. Explain the signs of the "on-off" response (see p. 175) and the importance of seeking medical intervention should they occur.
6. Monitor for behavioral changes. Severe depression with suicidal overtones can be caused by this drug and should be reported immediately.

7. Explain that the patient's urine and sweat may be dark colored owing to this medication.
8. Caution patient to avoid alcohol as it impairs levodopa's effectiveness.
9. Explain the importance of medical follow-up while taking this drug to monitor for such problems as increased intraocular pressure and changes in glucose control.

Side effects specific to amantadine
1. Teach patient that to prevent insomnia from this drug, it may be effective to schedule this drug earlier in the day.
2. Teach patient and significant others to monitor for and report any SOB, peripheral edema, significant weight gain, or change in mental status, as these signs often signal congestive heart failure.
3. Instruct patient not to stop taking this medication abruptly, as doing so may precipitate Parkinsonian crisis.

Side effects specific to dopamine agonists
1. Caution patients about avoiding alcohol, as they will experience less tolerance to it when taking this medication.
2. Bromocriptine can cause digital vasospasm. Teach patient to avoid exposure to the cold and to report the onset of finger or toe pallor.

Side effects specific to anticholinergic medications
1. Teach patient that this medication may decrease perspiration. Explain that patient should avoid strenuous exercise and keep cool during the summer to avoid heat stroke.
2. Teach patient not to abruptly stop taking this medication, as doing so can result in Parkinsonian crisis.

Knowledge deficit: Facial and tongue exercises that enhance verbal communication and help prevent choking

Desired outcome: Patient demonstrates facial and tongue exercises and states the rationale for their use.

1. Explain to patient that special exercises can help strengthen and control facial and tongue muscles, which in turn will improve verbal communication and help prevent choking. Emphasize that routine exercises of the facial and tongue muscles, along with the prescribed medications, may prevent or delay disability.
2. Teach the following exercises and have patient return the demonstration: hold a sound for 5 seconds, sing the scale, read aloud, and extend the tongue and try to touch the chin, nose, and cheek. Encourage patient to practice increasing voice volume.
3. Provide a written handout that lists and describes the above exercises. Encourage patient to perform them hourly while awake.
4. Teach patient the importance of stating feelings verbally, as monotone speech and lack of facial expression impede nonverbal communication.

See "General Care of Patients with Neurologic Disorders" for **Potential for impaired tissue integrity** related to risk of corneal irritation/abrasion, p. 249; **Alteration in nutrition,** p. 249; **Potential fluid volume deficit,** p. 250; **Potential ineffective airway clearance,** p. 251; **Self-care deficit,** p. 251; **Impaired verbal communication** related to aphasia or dysarthria, p. 252; and **Constipation,** p. 252. For patients with varying degrees of immobility, refer to related nursing diagnoses in "Pressure Ulcers," p. 630, and "Caring for Patients on Prolonged Bed Rest," p. 651. Also see "Caring for Patients with Cancer and Other Life-Disrupting Illnesses," p. 690, for psychosocial nursing diagnoses and interventions as appropriate.

PATIENT-FAMILY TEACHING AND DISCHARGE PLANNING

Provide patient and significant others with verbal and written information for the following:

1. Referrals to community resources, such as local and national Parkinson's Society chapters, public health nurse, visiting nurses association, community support groups, social workers, psychologic therapy, vocational rehabilitation agency, home health agencies, and extended and skilled care facilities. Provide the address of The American Parkinson Disease Association: 116 John Street, New York, NY 10038, (212) 732-9550; United Parkinson's Foundation: 360 West Superior Street, Chicago, IL 60610, (312) 664-2344; and Parkinson's Disease Foundation, Inc: 640 West 168th Street, New York, NY, 10032, (212) 923-4700.

2. Related safety measures for patients with bradykinesis, muscle rigidity, and tremors.

3. Emphasis that disability may be prevented or delayed through exercises and medications.

4. Techniques for unlocking a position (see p. 178).

5. Signs and symptoms of Parkinsonian crisis (see p. 174) and the need for immediate medical attention.

6. For other interventions, see the same section in "Multiple Sclerosis," p. 164, interventions, Nos. 3-10.

Alzheimer's disease

Alzheimer's disease is a progressive disorder of the brain characterized by changes and degeneration of the cerebral cortical nerve cells and nerve endings, resulting in abnormal neurofibrillary tangles and neuritic plaques. This process causes irreversible impairment of memory and deterioration of intellectual functions. Although etiology is unknown, aluminum poisoning, viruses, autoimmune disease, genetics, and neurotransmitter deficiency are possible causes, of which the last two are considered the most probable. The neurotransmitters that appear to be deficient are acetylcholine, somatostatin, substance P, and norepinephrine. The primary risk factor for Alzheimer's disease is age. Onset is insidious, and it can strike individuals as young as 40 years of age. The disease progresses to total disability and eventually results in death from such problems as infection or aspiration, usually within 3-15 years.

ASSESSMENT

The appearance and severity of signs and symptoms vary from individual to individual. Alzheimer's disease is characterized by progressive memory failure, intellectual deterioration, and personality change. It is classified into four stages: early, middle, late, and terminal, depending on the patient's degree of impairment. Initial indicators are mild, and it may take several years before a definite diagnosis can be made. Often a diagnosis is not made until the middle stage. By the late stage, memory and intellectual ability are absent. The terminal stage finds the individual in both a mental and physical vegetative condition.

Memory: Initially, memory loss is slight, usually consisting of inability to retain recently acquired information. The individual may lose things and forget dates. The individual also may forget how to use common objects and tools, while retaining the power and coordination necessary for performing these activities. Long-term memory eventually is lost. The individual becomes lost in the home or other familiar surroundings. Gradually he or she loses the ability to recognize or name common objects and familiar people, including members of the immediate family.

Cognitive process: The individual demonstrates increasing inability to think through problems, poor decision-making ability, shortened attention span, lack of insight, inability to perform arithmetic calculations, and loss of reading and writing capabilities. Gradually the ability to manage familiar activities, such as shopping or cooking, fails. The individual will become hesitant and reluctant to carry out minor and familiar tasks. As the ability to reason and abstract declines, the individual fails to recognize unsafe behaviors, resulting in a potential for injury. Hallucinations often occur owing to misperception of the environment. There is increasing difficulty following even simple two- or three-step instructions. Eventually there is a total loss of intellectual ability and comprehension and an inability to participate in any activities. In the last stages, there may be instinctual and emotional awareness of family voices, touching, or presence, but there is no intellectual or conscious awareness or interaction with the environment.

Personality changes: The realization that memory and intellect are deteriorating may result in depression, frustration, bitterness, anxiety, and apathy. Difficulty with tasks that are beyond the individual's capacity leads to easy frustration. As insight declines, depression becomes less of a problem. There is often emotional lability, panic, fear, bewilderment, and perplexity. As awareness of the environment declines, apathy may become more prominent. Symptoms of paranoia, delusion, agitation, and hallucination may appear, resulting in suspiciousness and accusing others of stealing things that have been misplaced. Previous psychotic traits are exaggerated. As the ability to communicate lessens and the world becomes more frightening, the potential for violence and agitation increases. The patient may have catastrophic reactions and emotional outbursts when faced with a complex task.

Social behavior: Decreased ability to handle social interaction, loss of social graces, loss of inhibitions, helplessness, dependency.

Communication patterns: Difficulty finding words, loss of spontaneity in speech, inability to express thoughts, incoherent speech. The individual gradually loses all language ability and becomes unable to communicate other than with such behavior as yelling, noisiness, or striking out. Eventually, this limited ability may be lost and he or she may be able only to grunt or express pain by grimacing.

Sleep pattern: Restlessness, pacing, wandering occur. Sleep/wake cycles are maintained but generally there is decreased need for sleep. Nocturnal awakenings and reversals of normal sleep patterns are common. Toward the final stages, the individual often sleeps excessively.

Self-care: Progressive neglect of routine tasks and personal hygiene; weight loss owing to refusal to eat and lack of awareness of the importance of nutrition; increasing inability to dress, bathe, toilet, and feed self or recognize where to urinate or defecate. Eventually the individual becomes totally dependent on others for all self-care activities.

Mobility/posture: Stooped and shuffling gait, progressive balance and coordination problems, falling, inability to walk and use arms, hands, and legs for purposeful movement. The individual becomes bedridden. Joint contractures and muscle rigidity are common in the final stages.

Other: In the last stages of the disease, myoclonus and seizures can occur. Spontaneous involuntary movement occurs, but the ability to open the eyes and track is maintained. Brain stem reflexes are present, and grasping, snout (evidenced by tapping the nose, which results in a marked facial grimace), and sucking reflexes can be elicited. Control of sphincter muscles is gone and the individual may be incontinent of stool and urine. Chewing and swallowing incoordination develop and death usually occurs due to aspiration pneumonia.

DIAGNOSTIC TESTS

Many disorders that can cause a progressive dementia syndrome (e.g., head injuries, brain tumors, depression, arteriosclerosis, drug toxicity, and alcoholism) need to be ruled out. This is especially important because some dementias are reversible.
1. *Mental status examination:* To test orientation, memory, calculation, abstraction, judgment, and mood.
2. *Neurologic examination:* Indicators that may signal Alzheimer's disease include release signs, such as snout, grasp, and sucking reflexes; olfactory deficits; impaired

stereognosis (inability to recognize the touch or smell of a familiar object when placed in the hand); short-stepped, bradykinetic gait; tremor; and abnormalities on cerebellar testing.

3. *Positron emission tomography (PET):* May show lower cerebral cortex metabolic rates for glucose, even in the early stages of the disease. (See "Brain Tumor," p. 215, for patient considerations.)

4. *CT scan:* May reveal brain atrophy and symmetrical, bilateral ventricular enlargement and also helps rule out other neurologic problems, particularly mass lesions. (See "Brain Tumor," p. 215, for patient considerations.)

5. *MRI:* Because of its ability to detect both biochemical and anatomic changes, this test may identify Alzheimer's disease at a very early stage. (See "Brain Tumor," p. 214, for patient considerations.)

6. *EEG:* May reveal generalized, slowed brainwave activity, which supports the diagnosis. (See "Seizure Disorders," p. 242, for patient care.)

7. *In addition:* The following tests may be performed to rule out other causes of dementia: skull and chest x-rays, lumbar puncture, serum tests, urinalysis, arteriograms, drug screen, and brain scan.

MEDICAL MANAGEMENT

Generally, treatment is supportive only. No recognized treatment or cure exists at this time.

1. **Pharmacotherapy:** Medications, if prescribed, are used to treat symptoms or behavioral manifestations. These include:

Early stage

☐ *Ergoloid mesylate:* Only drug shown to be effective in improving cognitive performance in early stages of dementia. However, its effect is only temporary and declines as the disease advances. Side effects include postural hypotension, transient nausea, and GI disturbances.

☐ *Tricyclic or other antidepressants (e.g., desipramine and trazodone):* To relieve depression and elevate mood. Side effects include drowsiness, dizziness, orthostatic hypotension, urinary retention, and lowered seizure threshold.

☐ *Experimental drugs:* May be used to improve cognitive function on a temporary basis, and include nafronyl and anticholinesterase medications, such as physostigmine and tetrahydroaminoacridine (THA).

Middle stage

☐ *Antipsychotic agents (e.g., haloperidol):* Used for combative or extremely agitated patients.

☐ *Tranquilizers or sedatives (e.g., chloral hydrate, diphenhydramine, triazolam, and oxazepam):* Used to control hyperactivity, restlessness, and sleep disturbances.

Late stage

☐ *Antiepilepsy drugs (e.g., phenytoin):* To control seizures.

☐ *Laxatives and stool softeners (e.g., psyllium, docusate):* For constipation.

Terminal stage

☐ *Oral morphine:* Small doses may be given for patients who have developed hypersensitivity to touch or restlessness.

☐ *Atropine or scopolamine:* May be given to decrease respiratory secretions and the need for frequent, uncomfortable suctioning.

2. **Diet:** A high-fiber diet may be given to prevent constipation. For restless, hyperactive patients, a high-calorie diet or supplements may be prescribed. Caffeine is avoided owing to its stimulating effect. While vitamin and lecithin treatments have not been proven effective in treating Alzheimer's disease, they are relatively harmless and the family may find some consolation in their use.

3. **Counseling or psychotherapy:** Counseling focus generally is on the significant others to

help them deal with the depression, grief, guilt, and emotions caused by the patient's progressive disability and behavior. In all but the early stages, Alzheimer patients quickly lose the insight and intellectual ability that would make counseling beneficial to them.

NURSING DIAGNOSES AND INTERVENTIONS

Potential for trauma related to lack of awareness of environmental hazards secondary to cognitive deficit

Desired outcomes: Patient is asymptomatic of physical trauma. Significant others identify and plan to eliminate or control potentially dangerous factors in the patient's home environment.

1. Orient patient to new surroundings. Reorient as needed. Keep necessary items including water, telephone, and call light within easy reach. Assess patient's ability to use these items. Keep siderails up and the bed in its lowest position.
2. Maintain an uncluttered environment to minimize the risk of tripping. Ensure adequate lighting to help prevent falls in the dark.
3. Prevent exposure to hot food or equipment, such as hot pads, which can burn the skin. Discourage use of heating pads. Check temperature of heating device and bath water before patient is exposed to them.
4. Encourage patient to use low-heeled, nonskid shoes for walking. Teach the use of wide-based gait to give unsteady patients a broader base of support. Assess patient for the presence of ataxia, and assist with walking as necessary. Canes and walkers may be too complicated for patients with Alzheimer's disease.
5. Request that significant others assist with watching restless patients. Provide attendant care if necessary. Avoid restraining patient because this usually increases agitation. If restraints are unavoidable, reassure patient that he or she is not being punished, that you are trying to help him or her regain control, and the restraints will be removed when the staff is certain he or she will not cause self-injury.
6. Check patient at frequent intervals. If necessary, move patient closer to the nursing station or seat patient in a chair at the nursing station.
7. Watch for nonverbal clues of pain or distress, such as restlessness, wincing, wrinkled brow, cautious breathing, rapid or shallow breathing, poor appetite, or crying. Report significant findings.
   Suggestions for home safety:
8. Encourage significant others to evaluate the home environment carefully for potential safety hazards. Caution them to remove harmful objects (e.g., matches and scissors) from the bedside and store medications and chemicals in locked cabinets to prevent accidental ingestion. Remove plants that are toxic and toiletries, as patient may attempt to eat these. The temperature of the home hot water heater should be turned down to prevent accidental scalding. Remind significant others to check the house carefully before leaving because the patient may leave the stove on or water running.
9. Advise significant others to keep the patient's home environment simple and familiar. Rearranging furniture can increase the patient's confusion and potential for falls.
10. If the patient tends to wander, encourage significant others to have an identification bracelet made. Locks on doors to keep patient inside may be necessary but shouldn't require a key, since this may hamper escape in the case of a fire.
11. Caution significant others that patients who are disoriented should be allowed to smoke only while being observed. Advise them to get a smoke detector and take control of matches.
12. Advise significant others that when the patient is no longer able to drive safely, the state automobile licensing bureau should be informed of the need for retesting. This will take the burden of restriction off the family. Suggest that significant others hide car keys or disable the car if necessary to prevent patient from driving.

Alteration in nutrition: Less than body requirements related to decreased intake secondary to cognitive and motor deficit; and increased nutritional needs secondary to constant pacing and restlessness

Desired outcome: Patient maintains body weight.

1. Because patient may not eat food that does not look familiar or is on hospital plates, request that significant others assist with menu planning or bring in meals and dishes the patient will recognize.
2. When patient is no longer able to handle a fork, knife, and spoon, supply finger foods.
3. For the patient who is in constant motion, provide a diet that is high in calories unless contraindicated.
4. Try to limit the number of foods on the plate, as too many foods can be overwhelming for patient.
5. For other interventions, see **Alteration in nutrition** in "General Care for Patients with Neurologic Disorders," p. 249.

Alteration in pattern of urinary elimination related to urinating in inappropriate places or incontinence secondary to cognitive deficit

Desired outcome: Patient urinates in the toilet stool (commode).

1. Make sure patient knows location of bathroom. Take patient to the bathroom q1-2h; restrict fluids in the evenings to minimize the risk of enuresis.
2. Identify bathroom door with a picture of a toilet stool to help patient locate the bathroom.
3. Assess for restlessness, which can signal the need to void.
4. As appropriate, provide disposable underpants. Male patients may be able to accept condom catheters to help manage incontinence.
5. Incontinence may signal a urinary tract infection. Investigate the cause of the incontinence to see if it is treatable.

Bowel incontinence or defecating in inappropriate places related to inability to find bathroom; or decreased awareness of or loss of sphincter control secondary to cognitive deficit

Desired outcome: Patient has no or fewer episodes of incontinence.

1. Show patient location of bathroom. Identify the bathroom door with a picture of a toilet stool to help patient locate the bathroom.
2. Assess patient's normal bowel habits. Take patient to the bathroom at the time of day patient normally has a bowel movement (e.g., following meals).
3. Evaluate patient for nonverbal indications of the need to eliminate wastes, such as restlessness, picking at clothes, facial expressions or grunting sounds indicative of bearing down, or the passing of flatus.
4. As appropriate, provide disposable underpants.
5. After bowel elimination, assess patient for cleanliness of perianal area in order to maintain skin integrity. The patient may forget to wipe the perianal area or clean the area only partially.
6. For other suggestions, see **Constipation,** p. 656, in "Caring for Patients on Prolonged Bed Rest."

Self-care deficit: Inability to perform ADL related to memory loss and coordination problems secondary to cognitive and motor deficits

Desired outcome: Patient's physical needs are met by staff, patient, or significant others.

1. Provide care for the totally dependent patient, and assist those who are not totally dependent. Allow ample time to perform activities, encouraging patient's independence. Ask patient to perform only one task at a time. Do not hurry patient. Involve significant others with care activities if they are comfortable with doing so.

2. Place a stool in the shower if sitting will enhance self-care.
3. To facilitate dressing and undressing, encourage significant others or patient to buy shoes without laces and clothing that is loose fitting or has snaps or Velcro closures.
4. Provide a commode chair or elevated toilet seat as needed.
5. If the patient becomes combative or agitated, postpone ADL and try again a short time later. The patient may forget the reason for the resistance and allow completion of ADL at a later time.

Altered thought processes related to impaired sensory reception, transmission, integration, and evaluation secondary to degeneration of intellectual functioning

Desired outcome: Patient verbalizes orientation to person, place, time, and situation and interacts appropriately with the environment.

1. Monitor for and record short-term memory deficit. At frequent intervals, orient patient to reality, time, and place in the following ways: call patient by name; keep clocks and calendars in the room; inform patient of the day and time; correct patient gently; minimize disturbing noise; ensure adequate lighting to prevent shadow formation; request that significant others bring in familiar objects and family pictures; speak with patient about his or her interests, both present and past; allow patient to reminisce; ensure that staff members show name tags and identify themselves; explain upcoming events; and set up regular schedules for hygiene, eating, and waste elimination.
2. Approach patient in a calm, relaxed, nonthreatening, and friendly manner. Treat patient with dignity and respect. Remain calm and patient when having to repeat questions. Be nonjudgmental and objective, even when confronted with unacceptable or inappropriate behaviors.
3. Keep patient's personal belongings where they can be used and seen.
4. Evaluate patient's cognitive impairment for any relation to medication usage, such as sedatives or tranquilizers. If found, inform MD.
5. Provide a quiet, calm environment. Simple rooms that are not overdecorated are best. If the public address system can be turned off in the patient's room, it is advisable to do so to prevent patient stimulation and misinterpretation of sound.
6. Provide stimulation the patient can handle. Soft music may be fine, while television might be too overwhelming as the images change quickly and may be misperceived.
7. Limit visitors as appropriate, as crowds and complex social interaction often are beyond the patient's tolerance and ability.
8. If patient becomes agitated, reduce environmental stimuli. Use a soft, reassuring voice and gentle touch. Avoid quick, unexpected movements.

Impaired verbal communication related to aphasia and altered sensory reception, transmission, and integration secondary to cognitive deficits

Desired outcome: Patient communicates needs to staff, follows instructions, and answers questions.

1. Provide a supportive and relaxed environment for those patients who are unable to form words or sentences or who are unable to speak clearly or appropriately. Acknowledge patient's frustration regarding the inability to communicate. Maintain a calm, positive attitude; eliminate distracting noises. Observe for nonverbal communication cues, such as gestures. Anticipate patient's needs.
2. Explain activities in short, easily understood sentences. Point to objects or use demonstration if possible. When giving directions, be sure tasks have been broken into small, understandable units, using simple terms. Ask patient to perform only one task at a time. Give patient time to accomplish one task before progressing to the next.
3. Be sure that you have the patient's attention. Repeat patient's name or gently touch patient to get his or her attention. Speak slowly and calmly, using a clear, low-pitched voice. Use simple words and sentences, but speak as though patient understands you. Ask only one question at a time, and formulate questions that can be

answered by "yes" or "no." Wait for a response. If patient does not respond, repeat the question again, exactly as before, to help patient mentally process the question.

Anxiety related to actual or perceived threats or changes (e.g., from bewildering hospital environment and multiple tests and procedures) secondary to degeneration of intellectual functioning

Desired outcome: Patient's anxiety is absent or reduced as evidenced by HR ≤100 bpm, RR ≤20 breaths/min with normal depth and pattern, and an absence or decrease in irritability and restlessness.

1. Remain calm with patient. Use slow, deliberate gestures. Patients with Alzheimer's disease frequently mirror the emotions of others. Use a low, soothing voice and a gentle touch. The tone of voice is often more important that the actual words used.
2. Provide time for patient to verbalize feelings of fear, concern, and anxiety. Patients with Alzheimer's disease often have trouble finding the correct words and may not be capable of stringing more than a few words together. Provide calm, realistic assurance, and stay with patient during periods of acute anxiety.
3. To help reduce anxiety and establish ongoing rapport, provide patient with a consistent caregiver.
4. Patients who still have reading capability may find reassurance with notes or lists of names, phone numbers, or activities (e.g., the phone numbers of significant others or a note reminder of the reason they are in the hospital), which may reassure them that they are not lost or abandoned.
5. Permit patient to hoard inanimate objects, as this appears to provide some individuals with a sense of security.

Potential for violence related to irritability, frustration, and disorientation secondary to degeneration of cognitive thinking

Desired outcome: Patient demonstrates control of his or her behavior with absence of violence.

1. Monitor patient for signs of increasing anxiety (e.g., inability to verbalize feelings, suspiciousness of others, fear of others or self, irritability, and agitation), which can precede a violent act.
2. Encourage verbalization of feelings rather than suppression, as frustration can lead to violence.
3. Try to identify what is immediately distressing to patient and attempt to remedy it. Respond to the emotion. Respond to the patient's questions in simple, concrete replies that are meaningful and relate directly to the patient's questions, frustrations, or anger. Do not confront patient and become authoritarian. If the situation cannot be remedied by calming the patient, use distraction and try to defuse the situation.
4. Remain calm and keep gestures slow and deliberate. Keep your hands where they can be seen. Approach patient slowly in a relaxed and open manner. Some patients may respond positively to gentle touch.
5. Reduce environmental stimuli.
6. Do not give routine care when patient is upset or agitated. Leave and return when the patient is more approachable. Use the patient's forgetfulness to your advantage.
7. If patient is upset or agitated, avoid turning your back on patient. Think of escape routes for yourself, and be alert to potential weapons patient may use. Get help; protect yourself.

Sleep pattern disturbance related to restlessness and disorientation secondary to cognitive deficits

Desired outcome: Patient sleeps at least 6 hours per night, or an amount of time appropriate for the patient.

1. Space activities so that patient does not get excessively tired, requiring a daytime nap.

2. Prevent patients from falling asleep during the day through such measures as periodic short walks, planned activities, and keeping them upright as much as possible. **Note:** If patient does nap during the day but also sleeps well at night, there is no need to impose a specific sleep schedule.
3. Patients who nap should do so in an easy chair, if possible, rather than in bed. The easy chair may serve as a cue that their sleep is just a nap.
4. Administer tranquilizers and sedatives as prescribed to facilitate sleeping.

Altered family processes related to illness of family member

Desired outcome: Significant others verbalize knowledge of measures that will assist with coping for the care of the patient after hospital discharge.

1. Encourage significant others to interpret patient's behavior as a reflection of the disease process rather than a willful act. Advise them that generally another illness, surgery, or disease process will exaggerate the patient's disorientation. However, once these problems are corrected, the patient usually returns to his or her previous cognitive level.
2. Encourage patient's major caregiver to have other significant others or hired help take care of patient regularly so that he or she can have scheduled respites. A neighbor looking in or a home-health aide on a part-time, overnight, or live-in basis is another option. Local day care programs also are useful. If the patient is a veteran, he or she may be eligible for some respite programs offered by the Veterans Administration. Advise caregiver that some home health agencies or day care programs have sliding payment scales for their services.
3. If significant other is unaccustomed to handling finances, refer him or her to a place in which assistance with financial management is given. Often, patients with Alzheimer's disease lose the ability to manage finances and balance checkbooks and may "give away" money inappropriately. Eventually, the patient's checkbook and credit cards will have to be taken away.
4. Encourage early financial planning and suggest professional financial counseling. Families should locate and identify the patient's various assets, sources of income, and liabilities and make arrangements for their security and daily management.
5. Encourage early family legal planning and consultation. This is especially important because an individual must have mental capacity and competence to sign documents. Legal planning may involve wills, intervivos trusts, subpayee assignment for Social Security, traditional and durable power of attorney, guardianship, and conservatorship, among other plans. Advise family that some free legal services are available to the elderly in most areas.
6. Explain to significant others that if patient refuses medication or is unable to swallow pills, obtaining a liquid form of the drug or crushing the pills and mixing them with soft food may help.
7. Some individuals with this disease go through a phase in which, due to increased motor activity and lessening social inhibitions, they have increased sexual demands. This may result in sexual encounters with people other than their significant other. Be sure family is aware that this is a symptom of the disease process. Furthermore, the patient eventually will lose the ability to be intimate and tender. Sex will become a mindless act. Mates may feel rejected, frustrated, humiliated, or repulsed. Suggest that professional counseling be obtained to assist the patient's spouse or loved one with dealing with these feelings. Suggest that the use of gentle dissuasion or distraction may be effective with these patients.
8. Encourage professional counseling and support in order for significant others to work through such feelings as anger, guilt, embarrassment, and depression and to develop effective coping strategies and mechanisms. Each new and subtle loss of patient function brings another round of grieving. Decisions regarding institutionalization and the extent of health care measures to be given also are emotionally difficult.

9. Encourage participation in local or national support groups, such as Alzheimer's Disease and Related Disorders Association (ADRDA): 360 North Michigan Avenue, Chicago, IL 60601.
10. For other interventions, see **Alteration in family processes** in "Caring for Patients with Cancer and Other Life-Disrupting Illnesses," p. 699.

See "General Care of Patients with Neuologic Problems" for **Potential fluid volume deficit,** p. 250, and **Potential ineffective airway clearance,** p. 251. For patients experiencing varying degrees of immobility, see related nursing diagnoses in "Pressure Ulcers," p. 630, and "Caring for Patients on Prolonged Bed Rest," p. 651. Also see "Caring for Patients with Cancer and Other Life-Disrupting Illnesses," p. 690, for psychosocial nursing diagnoses as appropriate.

PATIENT-FAMILY TEACHING AND DISCHARGE PLANNING

The degree and scope of discharge teaching and planning will depend on the severity of the patient's condition. Provide patient and significant others with verbal and written information for the following as appropriate:

1. Referrals to community resources, local and national Alzheimer's disease chapters, public health nurse, visiting nurses association, community support groups, social workers, psychologic therapy, home health agencies, and extended and skilled care facilities.
2. Safety measures for preventing injury relative to cognitive deficits.
3. Measures that assist in reorienting and communicating with patient in view of cognitive deficits.
4. Importance of scheduled respites and involvement in support groups for significant others.
5. Medications, including drug name, purpose, dosage, frequency, precautions, and potential side effects.
6. Exercises that promote muscle strength and mobility; measures for preventing contractures and skin breakdown; transfer techniques and proper body mechanics; and use of assistive devices, if appropriate.
7. Techniques for dealing with incontinence; indications of constipation or infection; implementation of bowel and bladder training programs; and indwelling catheter care, if appropriate.
8. Indications of URI and measures that prevent regurgitation, aspiration, and infection.
9. Techniques for encouraging adequate food and fluid intake and performance of ADL.
10. Importance of seeking financial and legal counseling.

Section Three   TRAUMATIC DISORDERS OF THE NERVOUS SYSTEM

Intervertebral disk disease (herniated nucleus pulposus)

The intervertebral disk is a semifluid-filled fibrous capsule that facilitates movement of the spine and acts as a shock absorber. The ability of the disk to withstand stressors is not unlimited and diminishes with aging. Pressure on the disk eventually may force elastic material from the center of the disk, called the nucleus pulposus, to break or herniate through the fibrous rim of the disk. The rupture or bulging of an intervertebral disk causes its typical symptoms by pressing on and irritating the spinal nerve roots or spinal cord itself. Herniated nucleus pulposus usually is the result of injury or a series of insults to the vertebral column from lifting or twisting. When the disk ruptures without a known discrete injury, it is believed to be caused by degenerative changes. Deterioration can occur suddenly, or it may happen gradually, with symptoms occurring months or years after the initial injury. Almost all herniated disks occur in the lumbar spine, with 90% of the problems occurring at L-4–L-5 and L-5–S-1. Cervical disk problems most frequently occur at C-5–C-6 and C-6–C-7 and generally are caused by degenerative changes or trauma, such as whiplash or hyperextension.

ASSESSMENT

General indicators: Onset can be sudden, with intense unilateral pain, or with pain that is dull, diffuse, deep, and aching. Symptoms vary according to the level of injury and nerves involved. Usually, pain is increased with sneezing, coughing, straining, and other activities that increase intraabdominal or intrathoracic pressure. Immediate medical attention is essential if there is any paralysis, extreme sensory loss, or altered bowel or bladder function.

Cervical disk disease: Pain or numbness in the upper extremities, shoulders, thorax, occipital area, or back of the head or neck. Pain can radiate down the forearms and into the hands and fingers. Usually, the neck has restricted mobility, and there can be cervical muscle spasm as well. The patient may have upper extremity muscle weakness with diminished biceps or triceps reflex.

Lumbar disk disease: Pain in the lumbosacral area with possible radiculopathy (sciatica) to the buttock, down the posterior surface of the thigh and calf, and to the lateral border of the foot. Frequently, there is altered mobility, as evidenced by decreased ability to stand upright, listing to one side, asymmetrical gait, limited ability to flex forward, and restricted side movement caused by pain and muscle spasms. The individual walks cautiously, bearing little weight on the affected side, and often finds sitting or climbing stairs particularly painful. Reflex muscle spasms can cause bulging of the back with concomitant flattening of the lumbar curve and possible scoliosis at the level of the affected disk. Usually, there is depression of the patellar and Achilles tendon reflexes.

Physical assessment: Possible findings include depressed reflexes, muscle atrophy, paresthesias (described as "pins and needles"), or anesthesia (numbness) in the dermatome of the involved nerves. The following tests are two of several that are performed to confirm the presence of lumbar disk disease:

☐ *Straight leg raise test:* Examiner extends and raises patient's leg. The test is positive if patient has pain on the posterior aspect of the leg.
☐ *Sciatic nerve test:* Examiner extends and raises patient's leg until pain is elicited and then lowers the leg to a comfortable level. The examiner then dorsiflexes the foot to stretch the sciatic nerve. If this causes pain, the test is positive for sciatic nerve involvement.

DIAGNOSTIC TESTS

1. *MRI:* May reveal that the disk is impinging on the spinal cord or nerve root or related pathology, such as tumors or spondylosis (see "Brain Tumor," p. 214, for patient care considerations).
2. *CT of the spine:* May reveal disk protrusion/prolapse or related pathology, such as tumors, spondylosis, or spinal stenosis. (See "Brain Tumors," p. 215, for patient care.)
3. *Myelogram:* May show characteristic deformity and filling defect or related pathology, such as tumors, spondylolisthesis, spondylosis, spinal stenosis, or Paget's disease. (See "Spinal Cord Injury," p. 219, for patient care.)
4. *X-ray of the spine:* May show narrowing of the vertebral interspaces in affected areas, loss of spine curvature, and spondylosis (formation of bone spurs around vertebral joints).
5. *Electromyelogram:* May show denervation patterns of specific nerve roots to indicate the level and site of injury.

MEDICAL MANAGEMENT AND SURGICAL INTERVENTIONS

1. **Bed rest:** To limit motion of vertebral column, relieve nerve root compression, and enhance shrinkage of the disk.
2. **Bedboards under the mattress:** To support normal spine curvature and minimize spinal flexion.
3. **Orthotics (e.g., splints, braces, girdles, and cervical collars):** To limit motion of the vertebral column. Generally, long term use of braces is discouraged because it prohibits development of necessary musculature. If braces are used, patient is weaned quickly so that adequate musculature can be developed to support the back.
4. **Pelvic/cervical skin traction:** To reduce muscle spasm and distract vertebral bodies to reduce bulging or rupture of the disk. **Note:** There is some controversy regarding whether traction actually provides any therapeutic benefit. However, some individuals find that it increases comfort.
5. **Pelvic traction girdle:** Device used in an attempt to widen the intervertebral space. The patient pulls the side handles in an axial direction to flex the pelvis. Alternatively, the handles can be attached to weights.
6. **Other therapeutic modalities:** Include thermotherapy, massage, diathermy/ultrasound electrotherapy, and stress reduction techniques.
7. **Physical therapy and a graded exercise program:** To strengthen the legs, back, and abdominal muscles. It is initiated once acute symptoms subside.
8. **Local injection of anesthetic or cortisone into paraspinal or paravertebral regions and epidural or subarachnoid spaces:** To reduce pain and muscle spasms and increase function.
9. **Antiembolism hose:** To prevent thrombophlebitis while the patient is on bed rest. Hose should be worn until the amount of time out of bed ambulating is equal to the amount of time spent in bed.
10. **Pharmacotherapy**
    - □ *Analgesics (e.g., aspirin, acetaminophen, and narcotics):* Administer sufficient medication to achieve pain relief or adequate pain reduction. Narcotics generally are used for acute pain episodes. Due to the potential for abuse, individuals with chronic back pain are discharged with nonnarcotic analgesia.
    - □ *Muscle relaxants (e.g., carisoprodol, methocarbamol, and diazepam):* To reduce muscle spasm.
    - □ *Corticosteroids (e.g., dexamethasone):* May be given for a short period of time to reduce cord edema, if present.
    - □ *Nonsteroidal antiinflammatory agents:* See Table 8-1 in "Musculoskeletal Disorders," p. 432, for names and usual dosage.
    - □ *Stool softeners or laxatives (e.g., docusate):* To prevent constipation or straining that would be painful.
11. **Chemonucleolysis:** Injection of enzymes (chymopapain, collagenase) directly into the disk has been used to dissolve fibrocartilage or collagen materials of the nucleus pulposus in an attempt to relieve pressure on the spinal cord or nerve roots. Chemonucleolysis provides pain relief in 50%-80% of patients but may take up to 3 months to do so. Fluoroscopy is used to confirm proper position of the needle. Because of the 1% incidence of allergic reaction and potential for severe anaphylaxis, chymopapain is injected in the operating room with an anesthesiologist or nurse anesthetist in attendance. Additional complications include nerve root injury and transverse myelitis.
    - □ *Before the procedure:* Evaluate for patient allergies to iodine, papaya, fruit, or products that may contain papaya derivatives, such as meat tenderizer, beer, dental powder, digestive aids, and contact lens cleansers. Report any possible papaya or iodine allergies to MD. Document baseline distal neurologic status carefully, especially motor or sensory deficits of the legs and feet. Give any preoperative IM medication in a site other than the patient's affected area so as not to confuse the patient's disk pathology with injection site pain. As appropriate, inform patient that back stiffness, soreness, pain, or spasm may occur after the procedure.
    - □ *After the procedure:* Maintain bed rest as prescribed (usually from several hours

to up to 24 hours postprocedure). Monitor distal neurologic status with VS and report any changes, such as numbness or weakness, from preprocedure baseline findings, which may signal nerve root injury. Be alert to signs of a delayed reaction to chymopapain, such as urticaria, itching, hypotension, stuffy nose, wheezing, and respiratory distress, which can progress quickly to laryngeal edema, laryngospasm, bronchospasm, and cardiac arrest if the patient is not treated promptly. In addition, monitor for bowel and bladder dysfunction, such as nausea, vomiting, and urinary retention, which are other potential complications of this procedure. Alert MD if patient does not have bowel sounds, has abdominal distention, or does not void within 8 hours of the procedure. The patient also may develop acute transverse myelitis several days postprocedure, with paraplegia and paraparesis.

12. **Diskectomy with laminectomy:** An incision is made, allowing removal of part of the vertebra (laminectomy) so that the herniated portion of the disk can be removed (diskectomy). If multiple intervertebral disk spaces are explored, a drain may be present when the patient returns to the room.

□ Monitor VS and perform neurovascular checks including color, capillary refill, pulse, warmth, muscle power, movement, and sensation. Compare to baseline neurologic assessment and report significant findings. Inspect dressing for excess drainage. Report any oozing. Bleeding usually is minimal. Serous drainage should be checked with a glucose reagent strip. The presence of glucose is a signal of CSF leakage.

□ Follow MD directions for activity restriction. The patient may be required to lie supine for several hours postoperatively to reduce wound hematoma formation. The laminectomy patient may be allowed to have the HOB raised to 20-25 degrees to facilitate eating and bedpan use. Use only the logroll method for turning the patient.

□ Monitor for bowel and bladder dysfunction indicating paralytic ileus or urinary retention, both of which are potential complications of this procedure. If patient does not have bowel sounds, has abdominal distention, or has not voided within 8 hours of the surgery, notify MD. Give prescribed antiemetics since nausea and vomiting are not uncommon. Fever may occur the first few days postoperatively but does not necessarily signal an infection. Assess for other indicators of infection, such as heat, erythema, or swelling at the wound site. Muscle spasms tend to occur on the third or fourth postoperative day. Additional complications include CSF leakage with possible fistula formation, meningitis, hematoma at the operative site, nerve root injury causing wrist or foot drop, arachnoiditis, and postural deformity.

13. **Microdiskectomy:** The herniated portion of the disk and small parts of the lamina are removed, using microsurgical techniques. This surgery results in less tissue damage, less pain, fewer spasms, and increased postoperative spinal stability. Patients often are out of bed the first day and may be discharged in 2-3 days.

14. **Percutaneous lumbar disk removal:** Degenerated disk material is aspirated through a cannula that has been placed into the intervertebral disk via fluoroscopy. This procedure cannot be used on patients with L-5–S-1 disk disease or if the disk has extruded into the spinal cord. This is a less invasive method of relieving pain from herniated disks. The procedure is done under local anesthetic and may be performed on an outpatient basis. Complications include back spasm or transient syncope.

15. **Spinal fusion:** May be indicated for patients with recurrent low back pain, spondylolisthesis, or subluxation of the vertebra. Bone chips are taken from the iliac crest or tibia and placed between the vertebrae in the prepared area of the unstable spine to fuse and stabilize the area. Internal fixation may be necessary to provide added stability until the fusion has healed fully.

□ Care of the fusion patient is similar to that of the laminectomy patient (see section above). The fusion patient loses more blood during the operation than a laminectomy patient and may have slight bloody oozing postoperatively. Monitor for signs of hypovolemia. Usually the patient is kept flat and is often kept on bed rest longer than for a simple laminectomy. In order to keep the operative site immobile so that the graft can heal and not dislodge, the patient usually will have a brace or corset for support, which is worn for 3 or more months.

☐ Monitor patients undergoing anterior cervical fusion for difficulty with swallowing or managing secretions, which can occur because of postoperative edema and hematoma formation secondary to retraction of the trachea and esophagus during surgery. Hoarseness also can occur secondary to nerve irritation. Complaints of excessive pressure in the neck or severe, uncontrolled incisional pain may signal excessive bleeding. Report significant findings to MD.

NURSING DIAGNOSES AND INTERVENTIONS

Health-seeking behaviors: Proper body mechanics and other measures that prevent back injury

Desired outcome: Patient verbalizes knowledge of measures that prevent back injury and demonstrates proper body mechanics.

1. Teach patient proper body mechanics: Stand and sit straight with the chin and head up and the pelvis and back straight; bend at the knees and hips rather than at the waist, keeping the back straight; when carrying objects, hold them close to the body, avoiding twisting when lifting. Have patient demonstrate proper body mechanics, if possible, before hospital discharge.
2. Teach patient about the following measures for keeping the body in alignment: sit close to the pedals when driving a car, and use a seat belt and firm back rest to support the back; support the feet on a footstool when sitting so that the knees are at hip level or higher; obtain a firm mattress or bedboard; use a flat pillow when sleeping to avoid strain on the neck, arms, and shoulders; sleep in a side-lying position with the knees bent or in a supine position with the knees and legs supported on pillows; avoid sleeping in a prone position; avoid reaching or stretching to pick up objects.
3. Encourage patient to perform the following measures for relieving pressure on the back: reduce to a proper weight for age, height, and sex; continue the exercise program prescribed by MD for strengthening abdominal, thoracic, and back muscles; use the thoracic and abdominal muscles when lifting to keep a significant portion of the weight off the vertebral disks.
4. Teach patient the rationale and procedure for Williams flexion exercises, which are performed while lying down on the floor with the knees flexed.
   ☐ *Pelvic tilt:* To strengthen the abdominal muscles. Stomach and buttock muscles are tightened and the pelvis is tilted with the lower spine kept flat against the floor.
   ☐ *Knee-to-chest raise:* To help make a stiff back limber. Each knee is individually raised to the chest, returned to the starting position, and then both knees are raised simultaneously to the chest.
   ☐ *Nose-to-knee touch:* To stretch hip muscles and strengthen abdominal muscles. Raise the knee to the chest, and then pull the knee to the chest with the hands. Raise the head and try to touch the nose to the knee. Keep the lower back flat on the floor.
   ☐ *Half situps:* To strengthen abdomen and back. Slowly raise the head and neck to the top of the chest. Reach both hands forward to knees and hold for a count of five. Repeat, keeping lower back flat on the floor.
5. Instruct patient to wear supportive shoes with a moderate heel height for walking.
6. Teach patient the following technique for sitting up at the bedside from a supine position: Logroll to the side, and then rise to a sitting position by pushing against the mattress with the hands while swinging the legs over the side of the bed. Instruct patient to maintain alignment of the back during the procedure.
7. Caution patient that pain is the signal to stop or change an activity or position.
8. Teach patient the following indicators that necessitate medical attention: increased sensory loss, increased motor loss/weakness, and loss of bowel and bladder function.

Knowledge deficit: Pain control measures

Desired outcome: Patient verbalizes knowledge of pain control measures and demonstrates ability to initiate these measures when appropriate.

1. Teach patient about the physiologic mechanisms of pain.
2. Instruct patient about methods of controlling pain and their individual applications. Methods include distraction, use of counterirritants, massage, TENS, behavior modification, relaxation techniques, hypnosis, music therapy, imagery, biofeedback, and diathermy. In addition, suggest the application of local heat or cold massage to painful areas. The latter can be achieved by freezing water in a paper cup, tearing off the top of the cup to expose the ice, and massaging in a circular motion, using the remaining portion of the cup as a handle.
3. Suggest that patient use a stool to rest the affected leg when standing.
4. Advise patient to sit in a straight-back chair that is high enough to get out of easily. Elevated toilet seats also may be useful. Straddling a straight-back chair and resting the arms on the chair back is comfortable for many individuals.
5. Encourage use of a firm mattress to support normal spinal curvature and extra pillows as needed for positioning. Some patients find normal bed height too low and use blocks to raise the bed to a more comfortable height.
6. Instruct patient on bed rest to roll rather than lift off the bedpan. The patient may find a fracture bedpan more comfortable than a regular bedpan.
7. Caution patient to avoid sudden twisting or turning movements. Explain the importance of logrolling when moving from side to side.
8. Advise patient to avoid factors that enhance spasms, such as staying in one position too long, fatigue, chilling, and anxiety.
9. Suggest positions of comfort, such as lying on the side with the knees bent or lying supine with the knees supported on pillows. Teach patient to avoid prolonged periods of sitting, since doing so stresses the back.
10. Inform patient that applying a heating pad to the back 15-30 minutes before getting out of bed in the morning will help allay stiffness and discomfort. Heating pads should be used only for short intervals and only if patient's temperature sensations are intact. Remind patient to place a towel or cloth between heating pad and skin to prevent burns.

Knowledge deficit: Surgical procedure, preoperative routine, and postoperative regimen

Desired outcomes: Patient verbalizes knowledge of the surgical procedure, preoperative routine, and postoperative regimen. Patient demonstrates activities and exercises correctly.

1. Assess patient's knowledge of the surgical procedure, preoperative routine, and postoperative regimen. Provide ample time for instruction and clarification.
2. Teach patient the technique for deep breathing, which will be performed immediately after surgery (coughing may be contraindicated in the immediate postoperative period to prevent disruption of the fusion or surgical repair).
3. Explain that VS and neurologic status will be evaluated at frequent intervals after the surgery. Teach patient the following indicators of impairment, which necessitate immediate attention by the health care staff: paresthesias, weakness, paralysis, radiculopathy, and changes in bowel or bladder function.
4. Inform patient that postoperative pain often is caused by nerve root irritation and edema. Spasms are common on the third or fourth postoperative day and should not discourage patient regarding his or her progress.
5. Teach patient the following logrolling technique for turning: position a pillow between the legs, cross the arms across the chest while turning, and contract the long back muscles to maintain the shoulders and pelvis in straight alignment. Explain that initially, patient will be assisted in this procedure.
6. Teach patient the following technique for getting out of bed: Logroll to the side, splint the back, and rise to a sitting position by pushing against the mattress while swinging the legs over the side of the bed. While in the hospital with an electric bed, the HOB may be raised to facilitate a sitting position.
7. Explain that antiembolism hose will be applied after surgery to prevent thrombus formation. Teach techniques for ankle circling and calf pumping to promote venous circulation in the legs.

8. Advise patient that in the postoperative period, sitting for limited, prescribed periods of time will be permitted in a straight-back chair. Teach patient not to sit for long periods of time on the edge of the mattress, since it does not provide enough support.
9. If patient is scheduled for a cervical laminectomy, explain that a cervical collar will be worn postoperatively. Teach these patients not to pull with their arms on things such as siderails.
10. Instruct patient in use of braces or corsets, if prescribed. Braces should be applied while in bed. Wearing underwear under the brace will help protect the skin from irritation.

Potential for impaired swallowing related to postoperative edema or hematoma formation secondary to anterior cervical fusion

Desired outcome: Patient regains uncompromised swallowing ability as evidenced by normal breath sounds and absence of adventitious breath sounds.

1. As a part of the preoperative teaching, instruct patient in the potential for difficulty with swallowing following anterior cervical fusion. Caution patient of the need to report promptly any significant postoperative difficulty with swallowing.
2. Begin the postoperative diet with clear fluids and progress to more solid foods only after patient demonstrates ability to ingest fluids adequately.
3. To minimize the risk of aspiration, position patient in Fowler's position, or semi-Fowler's position at minimum, when initiating fluid intake.
4. For patients at risk for aspiration, keep suction and oxygen equipment nearby.
5. Also see **Potential ineffective airway clearance,** p. 251, in "General Care for Patients with Neurologic Disorders."

Potential for impaired skin and tissue integrity related to irritation or pressure secondary to cervical or pelvic traction

Desired outcome: Patient's skin remains clear and unbroken; the tissue blanches.

1. *Pelvic traction:* Ensure that patient is positioned correctly with the HOB elevated 30 degrees and the knees flexed 10-20 degrees. Be especially alert to the condition of the skin at the iliac crests, coccyx, and intergluteal fold. Inspect and massage erythemic areas at least q4h. If the area is reddened and does not blanch, massage should be limited to the area around the reddened area to prevent additional tissue damage. Notify MD of significant findings.
2. *Cervical traction:* Maintain bed in low-Fowler's position, and keep a small rolled towel under patient's shoulders to enhance hyperextension. Apply cornstarch to skin that is in contact with the halter. Check the chin, ears, and occipital areas for the presence of erythema or irritation. Inspect and massage erythemic areas at least q4h.
3. Maintain alignment between the patient's body and the weights to keep the traction forces even.

For surgical patients, see the appendix, "Caring for Preoperative and Postoperative Patients," p. 637, for related nursing diagnoses and interventions. For patients experiencing varying degrees of immobility, see "Pressure Ulcers," p. 630, and "Caring for Patients on Prolonged Bed Rest," p. 651.

PATIENT-FAMILY TEACHING AND DISCHARGE PLANNING

Provide patient and significant others with verbal and written information for the following:
1. Prescribed exercise regimen, including rationale for each exercise, technique for performing the exercise, number of repetitions of each, and frequency of the exercise periods. If possible, ensure that patient demonstrates understanding of the exercise regimen and proper body mechanics before hospital discharge.
2. Indicators of postoperative wound infection, which necessitate medical attention. These include swelling, discharge, persistent redness, local warmth, fever, and pain.

3. Use and care of a brace or immobilizer, if appropriate.
4. Medications, including name, rationale, dosage, schedule, precautions, and potential side effects.
5. Anticonstipation routine, which should be initiated during hospitalization.
6. Pain control measures.
7. Telephone number of a resource person, should questions arise after hospital discharge.
8. Postsurgical activity restrictions as directed by MD. These may include the following: driving and riding in a car, sexual activity, lifting and carrying, tub bathing, going up and down steps, and the amount of time spent in or out of bed.
9. Signs and symptoms of worsening neurologic function and the importance of notifying MD immediately if they develop. These include numbness, weakness, paralysis, or bowel and bladder dysfunction.

Spinal cord injury

The spinal cord injuries (SCIs) discussed in this section are caused by vertebral fractures or dislocations that sever, lacerate, or compress the spinal cord and interrupt neuronal function and transmission of nerve impulses. Blood supply to the spinal cord also may be interrupted. The spinal cord swells in response to injury, and this, along with hemorrhage, can cause additional compression, ischemia, and compromised function. Neurologic deficits resulting from compression may be reversible if the resulting edema and ischemia do not lead to spinal cord degeneration and necrosis. Common causes of injury include motor vehicle accidents, diving or other sporting accidents, falls, and gunshot wounds. Spinal cord injuries are classified in a number of different ways according to type (open, closed), etiology, site (level of spinal cord involved), mechanism of injury (compression, hyperflexion, hyperextension, rotational, penetrating), stability, and degree of spinal cord function loss (complete, incomplete).

Prognosis: Any evidence of voluntary motor function, sensory function, or sacral sensation below the level of injury is indicative of an incomplete SCI, with the potential for partial or complete recovery. After an acute injury, the spinal cord usually goes into a condition called spinal shock, in which there can be total loss of spinal cord function below the level of injury. During spinal shock there is no reflex activity. Resolution of spinal shock with return of reflexes usually occurs within 6 weeks. If there is no evidence of returning motor function after local reflexes have returned, the spinal cord is considered irreversibly damaged. Generally, SCI does not cause immediate death unless it is at C-1 through C-3, which results in respiratory muscle paralysis. Individuals who survive these injuries require a ventilator for the rest of their lives. If the injury occurs at C-4, respiratory difficulties may result in death, although some individuals who have survived the initial injury have been successfully weaned from the ventilator. Injuries below C-4 also can be life-threatening because of ascending cord edema, which can cause respiratory muscle paralysis. Immediately after injury, common complications that require treatment include hypotension (systolic BP <80 mm Hg), bradycardia, paralytic ileus, urinary retention, pneumonia, and stress ulcers. Other long-term, life-threatening, potential complications of SCI include autonomic dysreflexia, decubitus ulcers, pneumonia, sepsis, urinary calculi, and UTI.

ASSESSMENT

Acute indicators: Loss of sensation, weakness, or paralysis below the level of the injury; localized pain or tenderness over the site of injury; headache; hypothermia or hyperthermia; and alterations in bowel and bladder function.

Cervical injury: Possible alterations in LOC, weakness or paralysis in all four extremities (quadriparesis or quadriplegia), paralysis of respiratory muscles, or signs of respiratory problems, such as flaring nostrils and use of accessory muscles for respirations. Any cervical injury can result in a low body temperature (to 96° F), slowed pulse rate (<60 bpm) caused by vagal stimulation of the heart, hypotension (systolic BP <80 mm Hg) caused by vasodilation, and decreased peristalsis.

Thoracic and lumbar injuries: Paraparesis/paraplegia or altered sensation in the legs; hand and arm involvement in upper thoracic injuries.

Acute spinal shock: Can last from 2 days to 6 months but usually resolves in 1-6 weeks. Indicators depend on the severity of the injury and include total loss of spinal cord function, loss of skin sensation, flaccid paralysis or absence of reflexes below the level of injury, paralytic ileus and constipation secondary to atonic bowel, bladder distention secondary to atonic bladder, low/falling BP secondary to loss of vasomotor tone and decreased venous return, and anhidrosis (absence of sweating) below level of injury. Resolution of spinal shock is indicated by the return of the bulbocavernosus reflex in men (slight muscle contraction when the glans penis is squeezed or the urinary catheter is pulled) and the anal reflex (puckering of the anus on digital exam or gentle scratching around the anus).

Chronic indicators: As spinal shock resolves, muscle tone, reflexes, and some function may return, depending on severity and level of injury. The return of reflexes usually results in muscle spasticity. Chronic autonomic dysfunction may be manifested as fever; mild hypotension; anhidrosis; and alterations in bowel, bladder, and sexual function. Injuries below L-1 or L-2 may result in permanent flaccid paralysis.

Upper motor neuron (UMN) involvement: UMN describes nerve cell bodies that originate in high levels of the CNS and transmit impulses from the brain down the spinal cord. Injury will interrupt this impulse transmission, causing muscle or organ dysfunction below the level of injury. However, since the injury does not interrupt reflex arcs coming from those muscles or organs to the spinal cord, hypertonic reflexes, clonus paralysis, and spastic paralysis are seen. The patient will have a positive Babinski reflex.

Lower motor neuron (LMN) involvement: LMNs are anterior horn cell bodies that originate in the spinal cord. LMNs transmit nerve impulses to muscles and organs and are involved in reflex arcs that control involuntary responses. Damage to LMNs will abolish voluntary and reflex responses of muscles and organs, resulting in flaccid paralysis, hypotonia, atrophy, and muscle fibrillations and fasciculations. The patient will have an absent Babinski reflex. The spinal cord ends at the L-1–L-2 level. Below that level a bundle of nerve roots from the spinal cord fills the spinal canal and is called the cauda equina. Injuries below L-1–L-2 may result in flaccid paralysis owing to interrupted reflex arc activity.

Bowel and bladder dysfunction: With a spastic (UMN) bladder, although there is loss of conscious sensation, bladder contractions do occur, permitting reflex emptying. Similarly, return of reflexes to the bowel permits reflex evacuation. The bowel and bladder with intact reflexes, even though the patient is incontinent, are generally considered "trainable" with reflex stimulation techniques and increased intraabdominal pressure. A flaccid (LMN) bladder will distend and periodically overflow. This bladder often cannot be trained to empty completely. Intermittent catheterization is usually indicated and the patient may be a candidate for urinary diversion.

Autonomic dysreflexia (AD): For patients with injuries at or above T-6, the uninhibited autonomic reflex response to stimuli can be life-threatening as reflex activity returns. Signs and symptoms include gross hypertension (up to 240-300/150 mm Hg), pounding headache, blurred vision, bradycardia, nausea, and nasal congestion. Above the level of the injury, flushing and sweating may occur. Below the level of injury there is often piloerection (goose bumps) and skin pallor, which signal vasoconstriction. Seizures, subarachnoid hemorrhage, cerebrovascular accident (CVA), or retinal hemorrhage may occur.

Physical assessment

Acute (spinal shock): Absence of DTRs below level of injury; absence of cremasteric reflex (scratching or light stroking of the inner thigh for male patients causes the testicle on that side to elevate) for T-12 and L-1 injuries; absence of penile or anal sphincter reflex.

Chronic: Generally, increased DTRs occur if the spinal cord lesion is of the UMN type.

DIAGNOSTIC TESTS

1. *X-ray of spine:* To delineate fracture, deformity, or displacement of vertebrae, as well as soft tissue masses, such as hematomas.
2. *CT scan:* To reveal changes in the spinal cord, vertebrae, and soft tissue surrounding the spine. See "Brain Tumor," p. 215, for patient care.
3. *Myelography:* Shows blockage or disruption of the spinal canal and is used if other diagnostic exams are inconclusive. Radiopaque dye is injected into the subarachnoid space of the spine using a lumbar or cervical puncture.
   - □ *General pretest guidelines:* Assess for sensitivity to iodine, shellfish, and contrast medium; keep patient NPO, if indicated, for the prescribed amount of time. Document patient's distal neurologic status as a baseline for later comparison.
   - □ *Posttest guidelines:* Keep patient flat for 6-8 hours if oil-based contrast dye, such as isophendylate, was used. For water-soluble dyes, such as metrizamide, keep HOB elevated to 60 degrees and do not allow patient to lie flat for 8 hours to minimize irritation to cranial nerves and cranial structures. Monitor distal neurologic status with VS for 24 hours. Report any increased deficit from pretest status. Headache, nausea, and vomiting are frequent after effects of this test. Keep the patient well hydrated to promote replacement of the CSF lost during this test. Seizures may occur if the contrast agent metrizamide was used. Check puncture site for signs of infection.
4. *MRI:* Reveals changes in the spinal cord and surrounding soft tissue. See "Brain Tumor," p. 214, for patient care.
5. *ABG/pulmonary function tests:* To assess effectiveness of respirations and detect the need for oxygen or mechanical ventilation.
6. *Cystometry:* To assess capacity and function of the bladder.
7. *Pulmonary fluoroscopy:* To evaluate the degree of diaphragm movement in individuals with high cervical injuries.
8. *Evoked potential studies:* To help locate the level of spinal cord lesion by evaluating the integrity of the nervous system's anatomic pathways and connections. Stimulation of a peripheral nerve triggers a discrete electrical response along a neurologic pathway to the brain. This response or lack of same to stimulation is measured in this test.

MEDICAL MANAGEMENT AND SURGICAL INTERVENTIONS

Acute care

1. Immobilization of injury site: See No. 7 within this list.
2. Bed rest on a firm surface: For example, Roto Rest Kinetic Treatment Table.
3. Pharmacotherapy
   - □ *Antiinflammatory agents and corticosteroids (e.g., dexamethasone):* To reduce cord edema after the initial injury and minimize ascending cord edema. Use is controversial.
   - □ *Osmotic diuretics (e.g., mannitol):* Sometimes used for 10 days to reduce cord edema after the initial injury and minimize ascending cord edema.
   - □ *Analgesics and sedatives:* To decrease pain and anxiety.
   - □ *Antacids; histamine H_2 receptor antagonists (e.g., ranitidine):* To prevent gastric ulceration, which may occur owing to increased production of gastric secretions with SCI.
   - □ *Anticoagulants (e.g., heparin or warfarin):* To prevent thrombophlebitis and reduce the potential for pulmonary emboli.
   - □ *Stool softeners (e.g., docusate sodium), laxatives (e.g., bisacodyl), and suppositories:* To begin bowel retraining program and prevent fecal impaction. **Note:** Suppositories are avoided or used with caution in individuals at risk for autonomic dysreflexia (AD).
   - □ *Vasopressors:* To treat hypotension in the immediate postinjury stage caused by loss of vasomotor tone. Typically, patient will be in ICU during this stage.
4. Aggressive respiratory therapy: For all patients with SCIs. Patient with injuries above

C-5 are intubated and put on a ventilator. IPPB and chest physiotherapy are used to prevent and treat atelectasis.

5. **Nasogastric decompression during spinal shock phase:** To prevent aspiration of gastric contents and treat paralytic ileus.

6. **Bladder decompression during spinal shock phase:** Either intermittent catheterization or continuous drainage.

7. **Surgery/immobilization:** May include traction, fusion, laminectomy, and closed or open reduction of fractures. The surgical goal is to immobilize the spine and, if indicated, decompress the spinal cord to help prevent additional neurologic deficit. If indicated, bone fragments are removed and the spine is surgically fused within 5-10 days of the injury.

   □ *Cervical spine:* Immobilized with devices such as Crutchfield tongs, Vinke Gardner Wells tongs, or halo traction.

   □ *Thoracic spine:* May be immobilized with a surgical corset, plaster Minerva jacket, plastic body jacket, Harrington rods, or spinal fusion.

   □ *Lumbar spine injuries:* Usually treated with closed reduction and hyperextension or extension with traction techniques, followed by immobilization in a plastic jacket or spica cast. If these interventions are unsuccessful or if neurologic symptoms occur, a laminectomy is usually performed.

   □ *Sacral (cauda equina) fracture:* Usually treated with a laminectomy and spinal fusion.

8. **Physical and occupational therapy:** Passive ROM is started on all joints. After the injury is stabilized, an aggressive rehabilitation program is initiated, including muscle-strengthening exercises; conditioning exercises; a sitting program; massage; and instruction in adaptive devices, equipment, and transfer techniques as appropriate. Patients with sacral injuries have the potential to walk and should be instructed in the use of braces, crutches, or a cane as appropriate.

9. **Antiembolism hose:** To prevent thrombophlebitis and reduce the effects of orthostatic hypotension.

10. **Counseling and psychotherapy:** To help patient and significant others adjust to the disability.

11. **Controversial treatments**

    □ *Endorphin blocking agents:* Used immediately postinjury to prevent the hypotensive action of endorphins that may contribute to cord ischemia.

    ·□ *Hyperbaric oxygen therapy:* Used immediately postinjury to attempt to prevent ischemic cord destruction.

    □ *Spinal cord cooling:* Used immediately postinjury to reduce edema, thus improving cord circulation. A small pad through which cool saline solution circulates is placed on the epidural layer of the cord for several hours postinjury. A major complication is infection caused by exposure of the cord during cooling.

Chronic care

1. **Pharmacotherapy**

   □ *Muscle relaxants (e.g., diazepam).*

   □ *Antispasmodics (e.g., baclofen and dantrolene):* To decrease spasms. Common side effects include drowsiness, dizziness, weakness, fatigue, and nausea. In addition, dantrolene may cause diarrhea, hepatitis (monitor patient for fever and jaundice), and photosensitivity. Baclofen may lower an individual's seizure threshold. Both drugs may be taken with meals to prevent stomach upset. Patients should avoid alcohol when on these medications owing to the additive CNS depressant effects.

   □ *Antibiotics:* To prevent bladder infection.

   □ *Stool softeners (e.g., docusate sodium), laxatives (e.g., bisacodyl), and suppositories:* To maintain a bowel program that prevents fecal impaction and minimizes incontinence. **Note:** Suppositories are avoided or used with caution in individuals at risk for AD.

2. **Dietary management:** Limiting milk and other dairy products to minimize the risk of renal calculi, and promoting juices (e.g., cranberry, plum, and prune) that leave an

acid ash in the urine and decrease urinary pH, thus reducing the potential for infection. Vitamin C also may be used to acidify the urine. An adequate diet also should include high roughage and fiber to promote soft stools. If not contraindicated, fluids are encouraged to promote adequate hydration.

3. **Management of AD:** AD is a medical emergency that can occur for patients with SCIs at or above level T-6. The noxious stimulus (e.g., a distended bladder) must be found and alleviated as quickly as possible. The following may be administered during crisis to control hypertension: vasodilators, such as hydralazine or nitroprusside; hypotensive nondiuretic thiazides, such as diazoxide; adrenergic blockers, such as IV phentolamine; and ganglionic blocking agents, such as reserpine or guanethidine. Tetracaine or lidocaine may be instilled into the bladder to reduce bladder excitability. (For nursing interventions, see **Potential for dysreflexia,** below.)

4. Surgical interventions

   ☐ *Diaphragm pacer insertion:* This is a phrenic nerve stimulator that may allow selected ventilatory patients to be off the respirator for short periods of time. Electrodes are implanted over the phrenic nerve and when activated, cause the diaphragm to contract, generating a breath.

   ☐ *Intrathecal baclofen:* A programmable pump is implanted to deliver a continuous dose of baclofen into the sheath of the spinal canal to control spasticity.

   ☐ *Tenotomies, myotomies, muscle transplants, peripheral neurectomies, and rhizotomy:* These are some of the surgical approaches that may be used to treat spasticity that cannot be managed by medications or more conservative measures, such as stretching or ROM.

NURSING DIAGNOSES AND INTERVENTIONS

Potential for dysreflexia related to untoward response to noxious stimuli for individuals with SCI at or above T-6

Desired outcome: Patient is asymptomatic of AD as evidenced by BP within patient's baseline range, HR 60-100 bpm, and absence of headache and other clinical indicators of AD.

1. Monitor for indicators of AD, including hypertension (as high as 240-300/150 mm Hg), pounding headache, bradycardia, blurred vision, nausea, nasal congestion, flushing and sweating above the level of injury, and piloerection (goose bumps) or pallor below the level of injury.
2. If AD is suspected, raise HOB immediately or assist patient into a sitting position to lower the BP.
3. Call for someone to notify MD; stay with patient and try to find and ameliorate the noxious stimulus. Speed is essential. Monitor BP q3-5min during the hypertensive episode. Remain calm and supportive of patient and significant others.
4. Assess the following sites for causes, and implement measures for removing the noxious stimulus:

Bladder: Potential causes include distention, UTI, calculus and other obstructions, infection, bladder spasms, catheterization, and bladder irrigations done too quickly or with too cold a liquid.

   ☐ *Do not* perform the Credé maneuver for a distended bladder.
   ☐ If the bladder is distended, catheterize patient using anesthetic jelly and notify MD stat.
   ☐ If a catheter is already in place, check the tubing for kinks and lower the drainage bag. For obstruction, such as sediment in the tubing, irrigate the catheter as indicated, using no more than 30 ml of normal saline. If catheter patency is uncertain, recatheterize patient using anesthetic jelly.
   ☐ If the bladder is not distended, check for signs of UTI and/or urinary calculi, including cloudy urine, hematuria, and positive lab or x-ray results.

Bowel: Potential causes include constipation, impaction, insertion of suppository or enema, and rectal exam.

☐ *Do not* attempt rectal examination without first anesthetizing the rectal sphincter with anesthetic jelly.

☐ Use large amounts of anesthetic jelly in the anus and rectum before disimpacting patient to remove the potential stimulus.

Skin: Possible causes include pressure, infection, injury, heat, or cold.

☐ For male patients, check for a pressure source on the penis or testicles, and remove the pressure, if present.

☐ Check the skin surface below level of injury. Monitor for the presence of a pressure area or sore, infection, laceration, rash, ingrown toenail, or infected area. If indicated, apply a topical anesthetic.

☐ Observe for and remove the source of heat or cold (e.g., ice pack or heating pad).

5. Administer antihypertensive agents as prescribed.

6. On resolution of the crisis, answer patient's and significant others' questions regarding AD. Discuss signs and symptoms, treatment, and methods of prevention.

Note: Prevention is the best way of dealing with AD. A good bowel regimen and skin integrity program are key factors in preventing the noxious stimuli that constipation or pressure areas may cause. Loosen clothing, bedsheets, constricting bands, and turn patient off side to relieve other possible sources of pressure. Keep the bed free of sharp objects and wrinkles. Adhere to turning schedules. Measures should be instituted to reduce the potential for UTI and urinary calculi, and the patient should be taught self-inspection of skin and urinary catheter and the importance of using anesthetic jelly for catheterization and disimpaction.

Constipation or fecal impaction related to immobility and decreased peristalsis, atonic bowel, and loss of sensation and voluntary sphincter control secondary to sensorimotor deficit

Desired outcome: Patient has bowel movements that are soft and formed every 2-3 days or within patient's preinjury pattern.

1. During acute phase of spinal shock, assess patient's bowel function by auscultating for bowel sounds, inspecting for the presence of abdominal distention, and monitoring for nausea and vomiting and fecal impaction. Notify MD of significant findings. In the presence of fecal impaction, gentle manual removal or a small cleansing enema may be prescribed. Because the atonic intestine distends easily, administer small-volume enemas only. Avoid long-term use of enemas.

2. Once bowel activity returns, teach patient to attempt bowel movement 30 minutes after a meal or warm drink. This will allow patient's gastrocolic and duodenocolic mass peristalsis reflexes to assist with evacuation. Increasing intraabdominal pressure by bearing down or applying manual pressure to the abdomen also will help promote bowel evacuation. A prescribed, medicated suppository also may be used if necessary. If allowed, provide a bedside commode rather than a bedpan.

3. For patients with injuries at T-6 or above, promote use of stool softeners and high-fiber diet. Use suppositories and enemas *only* when essential and with extreme caution because they can precipitate AD. Use anesthetic jelly liberally when performing a rectal exam or inserting a suppository or enema.

4. For patients with hand mobility (who are not at risk for AD), teach the technique for digital stimulation of the anus to promote reflex bowel evacuation and suppository insertion.

5. For other interventions, see **Constipation** in "Caring for Patients on Prolonged Bed Rest," p. 656.

Potential for ineffective airway clearance related to neuromuscular paralysis/weakness or restriction of chest expansion secondary to halo vest traction

Desired outcome: Patient has a clear airway as evidenced by RR 12-20 breaths/min with normal depth and pattern (eupnea) and absence of adventitious breath sounds.

1. Monitor ventilation capability by checking vital capacity, tidal volume, and pulmonary function tests. If vital capacity is less than 1 liter or if patient exhibits signs of hypoxia (Pao_2 <80 mm Hg, tachycardia, increased restlessness, mental dullness, cyanosis), notify MD immediately.

2. If indicated, prepare patient for a tracheostomy, endotracheal intubation, and/or mechanical ventilation to support respiratory function. If appropriate, arrange for a transfer to ICU for continuous monitoring.

3. If patient is wearing halo vest traction, assess respiratory status at least q4h. Ensure that the vest is not restricting chest expansion. Teach the use of incentive spirometry. Be alert to the following indicators of pulmonary embolus: SOB, hemoptysis, tachycardia, and diminished breath sounds. Pain may or may not be present with pulmonary emboli, depending on the level of SCI.

4. If the patient's cough is ineffective, implement the following technique known as "quad coughing": place the palm of the hand under the patient's diaphragm (below the xiphoid process and above the navel). As the patient exhales, push up to assist in producing a more forceful cough.

5. For additional interventions, see **Potential ineffective airway clearance,** p. 251, in "General Care of Patients with Neurologic Disorders."

Potential for disuse syndrome related to inactivity or spasticity secondary to SCI

Desired outcomes: Following stabilization of the injury, patient exhibits complete ROM of all joints and a functional grasp. Patient demonstrates measures that enhance mobility, reduce spasms, and prevent complications.

1. Once the injury is stabilized, assist patient with position changes. For example, a prone position, if not contraindicated, will help prevent sacral decubiti and hip contractures. Assist patient into this position on a regularly-scheduled basis.

2. For patients with spasticity, use hand splints or cones to assist with maintaining a functional grasp.

3. To help prevent foot contractures for patients with spasticity, it may be helpful to fit patient with splints or high-top tennis shoes that are cut off at the toes so that each shoe ends just proximal to the metatarsal head. These shoes will help keep the feet dorsiflexed yet prevent the contact of the balls of the feet with a hard surface, which can cause spasticity. Avoid footboards for these patients because the hard surface may trigger spasticity and promote plantarflexion.

4. Teach patients with spasticity proper positioning, ROM, and sustained stretching exercises. Steady, continuous, directional stretching once or twice a day is especially important as it may decrease the amount of spasticity for several hours. Cooling and icing techniques, heat, vibration therapy, and TENS of the spastic muscles also may be helpful.

5. Because tactile stimulation may trigger spasms, touch by caregivers should be limited. When touch is necessary, do it in a firm, gentle, and steady manner.

6. For additional interventions, see **Potential for disuse syndrome** in "Caring for Patients on Prolonged Bed Rest," p. 653, in the appendix.

Potential for injury related to lack of access for external cardiac compression, incorrect neck position, irritation of cranial nerves, and impaired lateral vision secondary to presence of halo vest traction

Desired outcome: Patient exhibits no adverse changes in motor, sensory, or cranial nerve function.

1. Ensure that an open-end wrench is taped to the halo vest so that if external cardiac compression is needed the bolts can be released and the vest removed promptly.

2. Assess position of the patient's neck to the body. Alert MD to the presence of flexion or hyperextension. Assess any difficulty with swallowing, as this may signal improper position of the neck and chin. Keep a torque screwdriver in a secure place so that MD can readily adjust tension on bars to return the patient's neck position to neutral.

3. Evaluate degree of sensation and movement of the upper extremities, and assess cranial nerve function. Changes in cranial nerve function can occur if the cranial pins

compress or irritate a nerve. Notify MD of sudden changes in motor, sensory, or cranial nerve function (e.g., weakness, paresthesias, ptosis, and difficulty chewing or swallowing).
4. Assess pins, bolts, and vest structure for looseness. Clicking sounds may signal a loose pin. Never use the superstructure of the halo traction in turning or moving patient. Notify MD if pins or vest become loose or dislodged. Stabilize patient's head as necessary.
5. Avoid loosening a buckle without MD's directive to do so. Buckle holes should be marked so that they are always cinched correctly to the appropriate snugness.
6. If patient is ambulatory, teach him or her how to survey the environment while walking by either using a mirror or turning the eyes to their extreme lateral positions. Explain that patient will need to adjust his or her balance owing to the additional weight of the halo vest.

Potential for impaired skin and tissue integrity related to irritation and pressure secondary to presence of halo vest traction

Desired outcome: Patient's skin is clear and unbroken; underlying and surrounding tissue blanches appropriately.

1. Inspect the skin around the vest edges for redness and other signs of irritation. Massage these areas routinely to promote circulation and help prevent breakdown.
2. Investigate complaints of discomfort or uncomfortable fit. Pad the vest as needed until it can be properly adjusted or trimmed by MD. Protect the vest from moisture and soiling. Be alert to foul odor from the cast openings, which can signal pressure necrosis beneath the vest.
3. Instruct/assist patient with changing body positions q2h.
4. Skin care should include cleansing with soap and warm water. Avoid use of lotion and powder, which can cake under the vest. Rub unbroken skin with alcohol to toughen the skin. Replace soiled linens promptly. Patient's perspiration may be dried with a hair blower on a cool setting.
5. If a rash appears, the patient may be allergic to the vest's lining. A synthetic liner or knitted body stockinette may correct this problem.
6. In the event of skin breakdown, keep patient's skin cleansed, dried, and covered with a transparent dressing. Notify MD and orthotist accordingly, as skin breakdown requires a brace adjustment.
7. Place rubber corks over the tips of the halo device to prevent lacerations from sharp edges.

Note: For a discussion of pin care, see "Fractures," p. 454, for **Knowledge deficit:** Function of external fixation, pin care, and signs and symptoms of pin site infection.

Urinary retention or reflex incontinence related to spasticity or flaccidity secondary to SCI

Desired outcome: Patient has urinary output without incontinence.

General guidelines for individuals with bladder dysfunction

1. Initially, patient will have an indwelling urinary catheter or scheduled intermittent catheterizations. If intermittent catheterization is used and episodes of incontinence occur or more than 500 ml urine is obtained, catheterize the patient more often.
2. Teach patient and significant others the procedure for intermittent catheterization, care of indwelling catheters, and indicators of UTI.
3. Habit/bladder scheduling program consists of gradually increasing the time between catheterizations or periodically clamping indwelling catheters. The goal is a gradual increase in bladder tone. When the bladder can hold 300-400 ml of urine, measures to stimulate voiding are attempted.
4. Make sure patient takes fluids at even intervals throughout the day. Restrict fluids prior to bedtime to prevent nighttime incontinence.

Individuals with SCI above T-12 will have upper motor neuron lesions causing a spastic bladder. The spinal reflex arc is intact and the bladder has tone and will periodically empty on its own, resulting in reflex incontinence.

1. Explain to these patients that eventually they may be able to empty the bladder automatically and˙may not require catheterization.
2. Teach patient techniques that stimulate the voiding reflex, such as tapping the suprapubic area with the fingers, pulling the pubic hair, or digitally stretching the anal sphincter (contraindicated in individuals with lesions T-6 or above due to potential for AD).

Individuals with SCI below T-12 will have lower motor neuron lesions causing a flaccid bladder. The spinal reflex arc is disturbed, the bladder has no tone, and it will distend until it overfills, causing overflow incontinence.

1. Explain that occasionally these patients may be able to empty their bladders manually well enough that catheterization may not be necessary. Checking residual urine volume will determine this.
2. Teach patient bladder emptying techniques, such as straining or the Valsalva maneuver to increase intraabdominal pressure and the Credé maneuver. If the Credé maneuver is prescribed teach patient the following technique: place the ulnar surface of the hand horizontally along the umbilicus; while bearing down with the abdominal muscles, press the hand downward and toward the bladder in a kneading motion until urination is initiated; continue 30 seconds or until urination ceases.

Note: See related discussions in Chapter 3 under "Urinary Incontinence," p. 140, "Urinary Retention," p. 145, and "Neurogenic Bladder," p. 147.

Decreased cardiac output related to relative hypovolemia secondary to decreased vasomotor tone due to SCI

Desired outcome: Patient has adequate cardiac output as evidenced by systolic BP ≥ 90 mm Hg and orientation to person, place, and time.

1. Monitor patient for indicators of decreased cardiac output, such as hypotension (drop in systolic BP >20 mm Hg from baseline or systolic BP <90 mm Hg), lightheadedness, dizziness, fainting, and confusion.
2. Implement measures that will prevent episodes of decreased cardiac output due to postural hypotension.
   □ Perform ROM exercises q2h to prevent venous pooling.
   □ Prevent patient's legs from crossing, especially when in a dependent position.
   □ In addition to antiembolic hose patients with SCI at higher levels, especially above T-6, may require abdominal binders because these individuals are prone to more severe hypotensive reactions, even with minor changes, such as raising the HOB.
   □ Work with the physical therapist on implementing a gradual sitting program that will help patient progress from a supine to upright position. The goal is to increase the patient's ability and tolerance to sit upright, while avoiding adverse effects, such as hypertension, dizziness, and fainting.
   □ For additional information, see **Potential alteration in tissue perfusion:** Cerebral in "Caring for Patients on Prolonged Bed Rest," p. 656.

Potential alteration in tissue perfusion: Peripheral and cardiopulmonary, related to risk of thrombophlebitis and pulmonary emboli formation secondary to venous stasis occurring with immobility and decreased vasomotor tone

Desired outcome: Patient is asymptomatic of thrombophlebitis and pulmonary emboli as evidenced by absence of heat, erythema, and swelling in calves and thighs; HR ≤ 100 bpm, RR ≤ 20 breaths/min with normal depth and pattern (eupnea), and $Pao_2 \geq 80$ mm Hg.

1. Monitor for indicators of thrombophlebitis: erythema, warmth, and swelling in the calves or thighs. Measure and monitor for increased circumference of the calves and

thighs. The patient may or may not have pain or tenderness, depending on the level of SCI. Notify MD of significant findings.

2. Monitor for indicators of pulmonary emboli: tachycardia, SOB, hemoptysis, decrease in Pao_2, and decreased or adventitious breath sounds. Pain may or may not be present, depending on the level of injury. Notify MD of significant findings.

3. For other interventions, see the same nursing diagnosis in "Caring for Patients on Prolonged Bed Rest," p. 655.

Altered patterns of sexuality related to loss of aspects of sexual functioning secondary to SCI

Desired outcome: Patient discusses concerns about sexuality, verbalizes knowledge of alternative methods of sexual expression, and over time expresses acceptance of changes in sexual functioning.

1. Evaluate your own feelings about sexuality. Refer patient to someone (e.g., knowledgeable staff member, professional sexual therapy counselor) who can address patient's sexual concerns if you are uncomfortable discussing these issues with the patient.

2. Provide a supportive environment that gives the patient permission to have and express sexual concerns. Sexuality can be discussed as it relates to an erection that occurs during a bath or objective findings noted during a physical assessment. Elicit patient's knowledge, concerns, and questions. Expect acting out behavior related to the patient's sexuality. This is a normal response to the patient's anxiety regarding his or her sexual response and prognosis.

3. Provide limited information about normal sexual response and changes caused by SCI. Sexual functioning may be different but still possible with SCI. The general rule for men is the higher the lesion, the greater the chance of retaining the ability to have an erection but with less chance to ejaculate. For example, 25% of male SCI patients can attain erections permitting coitus but less than 10% of paraplegics (SCIs resulting in paralysis of the lower limbs) are able to ejaculate. Women may have problems with lubrication and transient loss of ovulation. Ovulation usually returns, and women can become pregnant and deliver vaginally. Uterine contractions of labor in women with SCI lesion T-6 or above, however, may cause AD.

4. Sexual activity may seem impossible to the SCI patient. Specific suggestions that may provide gratification include the following: oral-genital sex, digital stimulation, cuddling, and massage. Remind patient always to empty the bladder and bowels (if necessary) prior to a sexual encounter. For men, indwelling catheters can be folded back along the penis and held in place with a condom. For women, taping the catheter to the abdomen and leaving it in place works well. Explain that water-soluble lubricants are useful, if needed. Adductor spasms in women may pose a barrier, but can be overcome if a rear entry is acceptable.

5. It is not expected that nurses will be able to answer all the patient's concerns and questions. If this is the case, acknowledge the patient's concerns and refer to someone with more expertise.

6. For additional interventions, see the same nursing diagnosis in "Caring for Patients on Prolonged Bed Rest," p. 658.

See "Multiple Sclerosis" for **Knowledge deficit:** Precautions and potential side effects of prescribed medications, p. 162. See "General Care for Patients with Neurologic Disorders" for the following: **Potential for trauma** related to unsteady gait, p. 248; **Sensory/perceptual alterations** related to impaired pain, touch, and temperature sensations, p. 249; **Alteration in nutrition:** Less than body requirements, p. 249; **Potential fluid volume deficit,** p. 250; **Self-care deficit,** p. 251; and **Pain** and spasms, p. 254. Also see "Peptic Ulcer," p. 322, for related nursing diagnoses and interventions. For patients with varying degrees of immobility, see related nursing diagnoses and interventions in "Pressure Ulcers," p. 630, and "Caring for Patients on Prolonged Bed Rest," p. 651. For individuals undergoing surgery, see "Caring for Preoperative and Postoperative Patients," p. 637. For psychosocial nursing diagnoses, see "Caring for Patients with Cancer and Other Life-Disrupting Illnesses," p. 690, as appropriate.

PATIENT-FAMILY TEACHING AND DISCHARGE PLANNING

Provide patient and significant others with verbal and written information for the following:

1. Referrals to community resources, such as public health nurse, visiting nurses association, community support groups, social workers, psychologic therapy, vocational rehabilitation agency, home health agencies, and extended and skilled care facilities. As appropriate, provide the following addresses: Information Center for Individuals with Disabilities, 20 Park Plaza, Suite 330, Boston, MA 02116; National Spinal Cord Injury Association, 369 Elliot Street, Newton Upper Falls, MA 02164; Spinal Cord Injury Hotline, (800) 638-1733; and American Spinal Injury Association, 250 East Superior, Room 619, Chicago, IL 60611.
2. Safety measures relative to decreased sensation and motor deficits and the symptoms, preventive measures, and interventions for AD.
3. What patient can expect if transferred to a rehabilitation center.
4. Techniques and devices for performing ADL, including bathing, grooming, turning, feeding, and other self-care activities to patient's maximum potential.
5. Indicators of urinary calculi and dietary measures to prevent their formation (see p. 131).
6. For additional information, see teaching/discharge planning interventions Nos. 4-10, in "Multiple Sclerosis," p. 164.

Head injury

Head injuries can cause varying degrees of damage to the skull and brain tissue. Primary injuries that result from head injury occur at the time of impact and include skull fracture, concussion, contusion, scalp laceration, brain tissue laceration, and tear or rupture of cerebral vessels. Problems that arise soon after the primary injury and are the result of that injury include hemorrhage and hematoma formation from the tear or rupture of vessels, ischemia from interrupted blood flow, cerebral swelling and edema, infection, and increased intracranial pressure or herniation, any of which can interrupt neuronal function. These secondary injuries or events increase the extent of initial injury and result in poorer recovery and higher risk of death. Cervical neck injuries are commonly associated with head injuries. Due to the potential for spinal cord injury, all head injured patients should be assumed to have cervical neck injury until it is conclusively ruled out by cervical spine x-ray.

Most head injuries result from a direct impact to the head. Depending on the force and angle of impact, the brain may suffer injury directly under the point of impact, in the region opposite the point of impact owing to brain rebound action within the skull, or tissue tearing or shearing owing to the rotational action of the brain within the cranial vault. Common causes include motor vehicle accidents, falls, and sports-related injuries, such as those occurring in football or boxing. Acts of violence often result in missile or implement head injuries, such as gunshot or stab wounds.

ASSESSMENT

The Glasgow Coma Scale standardizes observations for objective assessment of a patient's LOC (see Table 4-2). This or some other objective scale should be used to prevent confusion with terminology and to detect changes or trends quickly in the patient's LOC.

Concussion: Mild head injury in which there is temporary, reversible neurologic impairment typically involving loss of consciousness and possible amnesia of the event. There is no visible damage to brain structure on CT or MRI examination. After the concussion, the patient may have headache, dizziness, nausea, lethargy, and irritability. Although full recovery usually occurs in a few days, a postconcussion syndrome with headaches, dizziness, irritability, emotional lability, lethargy, and decreased judgment, concentration, and memory abilities may continue for several weeks or months.

TABLE 4-2 Glasgow Coma Scale

Response	Rating	
Best eye opening response (Record "C" if eyes closed due to swelling.)	Spontaneously	4
	To speech	3
	To pain	2
	No response	1
Best motor response (Record best upper limb response to painful stimuli.)	Obeys verbal command	6
	Localizes pain	5
	Flexion—withdrawal	4
	Flexion—abnormal	3
	Extension—abnormal	2
	No response	1
Best verbal response (Record "E" if endotracheal tube in place or "T" if tracheostomy tube is in place.)	Conversation—oriented ×3	5
	Conversation—confused	4
	Speech—inappropriate	3
	Sounds—incomprehensible	2
	No response	1
Total score:	15 = normal	
	13-15 = minor head injury	
	9-12 = moderate head injury	
	3-8 = severe head injury	
	≤7 = coma	
	3 = deep coma or brain death	

Diffuse axonal injury: A diffuse brain injury caused by stretching and tearing of the neuronal projections owing to a shearing type injury. No distinct focal lesion, such as infarction, ischemia, contusion, or intracerebral bleeding, is noted, but the patient has an immediate and prolonged unconsciousness of at least 6 hours' duration. CT scan may show small hemorrhagic areas in the corpus callosum, cerebral edema, and small midline ventricles. The injury may be quite mild with full recovery, or in severe cases the individual may be comatose for months, die, or be left in a vegetative state.

Contusion: Bruising of the brain tissue, which produces a longer-lasting neurologic deficit than concussion. The size and severity of bruising vary widely, and the bruise is usually visible on CT scan. Traumatic amnesia often occurs, causing loss of memory not only of the trauma, but also of events occurring prior to the incident. Loss of consciousness is common, and it is generally more prolonged than that with concussion. Changes in behavior, such as agitation or confusion, can last for several hours to days. Headache, nausea, lethargy, motor paralysis, paresis, and possibly seizures can occur as well. Depending on the extent of damage, there is the potential for either full recovery or permanent neurologic deficit, such as seizures, paralysis, paresis, or coma and death.

Brain laceration: Actual tearing of the cortical surface of the brain results in direct mechanical disruption of neural function, causing focal deficits. Blood vessel tearing causes hemorrhage, resulting in contusion, edema, or hematoma formation. Seizures often occur as well. Brain lacerations usually result from depressed skull fractures, penetrating injuries, missile or implement injuries, or rotational shearing injury within the skull. Contusions and lacerations often are found together. The consequences of a laceration usually are more serious than those with a contusion owing to the increased severity of trauma. Assessment findings are similar to those with contusion but generally are more pronounced.

Skull fracture: Can be *closed* (simple) or *open* (compound), depending on whether the scalp is torn, thereby exposing the skull to the outside environment. Skull fractures are further classified as *linear* (hairline), *comminuted* (fragmented, splintered), or *depressed* (pushed inward toward the brain tissue). A blow forceful enough to break the skull is capable of causing significant brain tissue damage, and therefore, close observation is essential. With a penetrating wound or basilar fracture (see below), there is the potential for meningitis, encephalitis, brain abscess, cellulitis, or osteomyelitis.

☐ *Basilar fracture:* Fractures of the base of the skull do not show up easily on skull/cervical x-rays. Indicators include blood from the nose, throat, ears; serous or serosanguineous drainage from the nose (rhinorrhea), throat, ears (otorrhea), eyes; Battle's sign (bruising noted behind the ear); "Raccoon's eyes" (bruising around the eyes in the absence of eye injury); and bleeding behind the tympanum (eardrum) noted on otoscopic exam. Glucose in serous drainage signals the presence of CSF. CSF leakage indicates a tear in the dura, making the patient particularly susceptible to meningitis.

☐ *Temporal fractures:* May result in deafness or facial paralysis.

☐ *Occipital fractures:* May cause visual field and gait disturbances.

☐ *Sphenoidal fractures:* May disrupt the optic nerve, possibly causing blindness.

Rupture of cerebral blood vessels

☐ *Epidural (extradural) hematoma or hemorrhage:* Usually, bleeding between the dura mater (outer meninges) and skull causes hematoma formation. This creates pressure on the underlying brain and produces a local mass effect, causing increased intracranial pressure and shifting of tissue that leads to brain stem compression and herniation. Indicators are primarily those of IICP: altered LOC, headache, vomiting, unilateral pupil dilatation (on same side as the lesion), and possibly hemiparesis. Typically, the patient loses consciousness for a short period of time immediately after injury, regains consciousness, and has a lucid period lasting a few hours or 1-2 days; however, because arterial bleeding causes a rapid rise in ICP, a rapid decrease in LOC often ensues. These patients are at high risk for brain stem herniation. A unilateral dilated fixed pupil is a sign of impending herniation and is a neurosurgical emergency. The patient should not be left alone as respiratory arrest may occur at any time.

☐ *Subdural hematoma or hemorrhage:* Accumulation of venous blood between dura mater (outer meninges) and arachnoid membrane (middle meninges) that is not reabsorbed. Hematoma formation creates pressure on the underlying brain and produces a local mass effect, causing increased intracranial pressure and shifting of tissue, leading to brainstem compression and herniation. This type of hematoma is classified as acute, subacute, or chronic depending on how quickly indicators arise. In acute subdural hematomas, indicators appear within 24 hours, resulting from focal neurologic deficit (hemiparesis, pupillary dilatation) and IICP (headache, decreased LOC). When indicators occur 2-10 days later, the hematoma is considered subacute. When indicators occur several weeks or more later, it is considered chronic. Early indicators can include headache, progressive personality changes, decreased intellectual functioning, and drowsiness. Later indicators may include unilateral weakness or paralysis and loss of consciousness.

☐ *Intracerebral hemorrhage:* Arterial or venous bleeding into the white matter of the brain. Signs of increased ICP may develop early if the bleeding causes a rapidly expanding space-occupying lesion. If the bleeding is slower, signs of increased ICP can take 36-72 hours to develop. Indicators depend on location of the hematoma and can include altered LOC, headache, aphasia, hemiparesis, hemiplegia, hemisensory deficits, and loss of consciousness.

☐ *Subarachnoid hemorrhage:* Bleeding into the subarachnoid space below the arachnoid membrane (middle meninges) and above the pia mater (inner meninges next to brain). The patient often has a severe headache. Other general indicators include vomiting, restlessness, seizures, and loss of consciousness. Signs of meningeal irritation include nuchal rigidity and a positive Kernig's and Brudzinski's (see p. 168) signs. This patient may be a candidate for a shunt because of hemorrhagic interference with CSF circulation.

Indicators of increased intracranial pressure (IICP)

☐ *Early indicators:* Alteration in LOC ranging from irritability, restlessness, and confusion to lethargy; possible onset or worsening of headache; beginning pupillary dysfunction, such as sluggishness; visual disturbances, such as diplopia or blurred vision; onset or increase in sensorimotor changes or deficits, such as weakness; onset or worsening of nausea.

☐ *Late indicators:* Continued deterioration of LOC leading to stupor and coma; projectile vomiting; hemiplegia; posturing; alterations in VS (typically increased systolic BP, widening pulse pressure, decreased pulse rate); respiratory irregularities, such as Cheyne-Stokes breathing; pupillary changes, such as inequality, dilatation, and nonreactivity to light; papilledema; and impaired brain stem reflexes (corneal, gag, swallowing).

Note: Late indicators of IICP usually signal impending or occurring brain stem herniation. Signs generally are related to brain stem compression and disruption of cranial nerves and vital centers.

Brain herniation: Brain herniation occurs when IICP causes displacement of brain tissue from one cranial compartment to another. See late indicators of IICP, above, for signs of impending or initial herniation. In the presence of actual brain herniation, the patient is in a deep coma, pupils become fixed and dilated bilaterally, posturing may progress to bilateral flaccidity, brain stem reflexes generally are lost, and respirations and VS deteriorate and may cease.

DIAGNOSTIC TESTS

1. *Skull and cervical spine x-rays:* To locate skull and neck fractures. If the fracture crosses the groove of the meningeal artery, epidural hematoma is likely to be found. Because of the close association between head injuries and spinal or vertebral injuries, cervical immobilization is essential until cervical x-rays rule out fracture and potential SCI.
2. *CT scan:* To identify type, location, and extent of injury, such as accumulation of blood or a shift of midline structure caused by IICP. See "Brain Tumor," p. 215, for patient care.
3. *MRI:* To identify the type, location, and extent of injury. Although not usually performed in unstable patients, this test may be used for follow-up. See "Brain Tumor," p. 214, for patient care.
4. *EEG:* May reveal abnormal electrical activity indicating neuronal damage due to ischemia or hemorrhage. EEG may be used to establish brain death in conjunction with other tests. See "Seizure Disorders," p. 242, for patient care.
5. *Evoked response potentials:* Used to evaluate the integrity of the brain's anatomic pathways and connections. Stimulation of a sense organ, such as an ear, triggers a discrete electrical response (i.e., evoked potential) along a neurologic pathway to the brain. Measurement of the brain's response or lack of response to stimulation also aids in predicting neurologic outcome.
6. *Cerebral angiography:* To reveal presence of a hematoma and status of blood vessels secondary to rupture or compression. See "Cerebral Aneurysm," p. 222, for patient care.
7. *Brain scan:* To identify hematoma with chronic subdural hematoma. Generally, it is not done for more acute disorders because of the lengthy uptake time of the radioactive isotope. See "Brain Tumor," p. 215, for patient care.

MEDICAL MANAGEMENT AND SURGICAL INTERVENTIONS

1. Maintenance of airway, respirations, and therapeutic oxygen levels: Oxygen delivery, airway maintenance, intubation, and ventilation to prevent hypoxia. Hyperventilation may be necessary to reduce $Paco_2$ levels and promote cerebral vasoconstriction, which will reduce ICP.

2. **Monitoring of VS/neurologic status:** Baseline assessment is established and patient is monitored frequently for changes.
3. **Bed rest with HOB elevated** (or as prescribed): To promote venous drainage and help reduce cerebral congestion and edema.
4. **Fluids and electrolytes:** NPO status for 8-24 hours (or longer if patient is unresponsive). Fluids are limited to decrease cerebral edema. I&O are measured carefully, and the patient usually has an indwelling catheter. Supplementation of electrolytes is done in response to laboratory results. Hypotonic IV solutions, such as D_5W, are contraindicated because they increase cerebral edema.
5. **Gastrointestinal decompression:** Initially the patient may have an NG tube for gastric decompression to prevent vomiting and aspiration.
6. **Nutritional support:** Total parenteral nutrition, intralipids, tube feedings, or progressive diet, depending on patient's LOC, ability to swallow, and GI tract functioning.
7. **Treatment of secondary complications:** For example, cerebral edema, IICP, syndrome of inappropriate ADH (SIADH) disseminated intravascular coagulation (DIC), adult respiratory distress syndrome (ARDS), and diabetes insipidus.
8. **Pharmacotherapy:** Narcotics and other medications that alter mentation generally are avoided.
   - □ *Antiepilepsy drugs (e.g., phenytoin, phenobarbital, IV diazepam):* Prophylaxis for seizures with or following penetrating wounds.
   - □ *Glucocorticosteroids (e.g., dexamethasone):* To decrease cerebral edema. There is some controversy regarding effectiveness of glucocorticoids in reducing cerebral edema.
   - □ *Osmotic diuretics (e.g., mannitol) and loop diuretics (e.g., furosemide):* To decrease cerebral edema.
   - □ *Antibiotics and tetanus prophylaxis:* In the presence of penetrating wounds and basilar fractures.
   - □ *Antipyretics (e.g., acetaminophen):* For fever so that patient's metabolic needs are not increased.
   - □ *Analgesics (e.g., acetaminophen):* For pain.
   - □ *Mild sedatives (e.g., chloral hydrate or diphenhydramine):* For restlessness.
   - □ *Blood pressure medications:* To control hypertension and hypotension so that optimal cerebral blood flow is maintained and cerebral edema is reduced.
   - □ *Antacids and H_2 histamine receptor antagonists (e.g., ranitidine):* To reduce gastric acidity and prevent gastric ulcer formation.
   - □ *Stool softeners and laxatives (e.g., docusate sodium):* To prevent constipation and straining at stool, which would increase ICP.
   - □ *Tranquilizers (e.g., chlorpromazine):* To control shivering, which can increase ICP.
   - □ *Skeletal muscle relaxants (e.g., pancuronium):* To decrease the skeletal muscle tension that is seen with abnormal flexion and extension posturing, which can increase ICP. This therapy requires transfer of patient to ICU for intubation and ventilation.
   - □ *Barbiturate coma therapy:* To reduce cerebral metabolic rate during uncontrolled intracranial hypertension. This therapy requires transfer of patient to ICU for intubation and ventilation.
9. **Hypothermia:** If indicated, a hypothermia blanket is used to reduce body temperature to 30.5°-32° C (87°-90° F) and thereby minimize metabolic needs.
10. **Antiembolism hose:** To prevent thrombophlebitis and pulmonary emboli.
11. **Surgical procedures**
    - □ *Suturing:* To repair superficial laceration or dural tears.
    - □ *Craniotomy:* To remove bone fragment or elevate depressed fractures. (See "Brain Tumor," p. 215, for patient care.)
    - □ *Craniotomy or trephination ("burr" holes):* To evacuate hematomas, control hemorrhage, remove foreign objects, or debride necrotic tissue.
    - □ *Cranioplasty:* To repair traumatic or surgical defects in the skull.
    - □ *Ventricular puncture:* To remove excess CSF.
    - □ *Ventricular shunt:* To provide drainage of CSF and reduce ICP. See "Brain Tumors," p. 216, for patient care.

☐ *Placement of ICP monitoring device:* To provide accurate and continual monitoring of patient's ICP. This necessitates transfer of patient to ICU.

NURSING DIAGNOSES AND INTERVENTIONS

Knowledge deficit: Caretaker's responsibilities for observing the patient who is sent home with a concussion

Desired outcome: Caretaker verbalizes knowledge of the observation regimen and returns the patient to the hospital if neurologic deficits are noted.

If patient goes home for observation, provide caretaker with verbal and written instructions for the following:
1. Avoid giving patient anything stronger than acetaminophen to relieve headache. Aspirin is usually contraindicated because it can prolong bleeding, if it occurs.
2. Assess patient at least qh for the first 24 hours as follows: Awaken patient; ask patient's name and location and caretaker's name; monitor for twitching or seizure activity. Return patient to the hospital immediately if he or she becomes increasingly difficult to awaken; cannot answer questions appropriately; cannot answer at all; develops slurred speech; develops twitching or seizures; develops or reports worsening headache or nausea/vomiting; has visual disturbances, such as diplopia; develops weakness, numbness, or has difficulty walking; has clear or bloody drainage from the nose or ear; or develops a stiff neck.
3. Ensure that patient rests and eats lightly for the first day or so after the concussion or until he or she feels well.
4. Inform patient and significant others that some individuals may have a postconcussion syndrome in which they continue to have headaches, dizziness, or lethargy for several weeks or months after a concussion. Additional symptoms patient may experience include sleep disturbance, difficulty concentrating, poor memory, irritability, emotional lability, and difficulty with judgment or abstract thinking. Explain the importance of reporting these problems to the MD.

Potential for infection related to increased susceptibility secondary to basilar skull fractures, penetrating or open head injuries, or surgical wounds

Desired outcomes: Patient is asymptomatic of infection as evidenced by normothermia, stable or improving LOC, and absence of headache, photophobia, or neck stiffness. Patient verbalizes knowledge of the signs and symptoms of infection and the importance of reporting them promptly.

1. Monitor injury site or surgical wounds for indicators of infection, such as persistent erythema, warmth, pain, hardness, and purulent drainage. Notify MD of significant findings.
2. Be alert to indicators of meningitis (p. 168) or encephalitis (p. 171), which can occur after a penetrating, open head injury, or cerebral surgical wound.
3. When examining scalp lacerations and assessing for foreign bodies or palpable fractures, wear sterile gloves and follow aseptic technique. Cleanse the area gently, and cover scalp wounds with sterile dressings.
4. If the patient has a clear or bloody drainage from the nose, throat, or ears, notify MD of findings and assume that the patient has a dural tear with CSF leakage until proven otherwise. Inspect the dressing and pillow cases for the presence of a halo ring, which may indicate CSF drainage. Clear drainage may be tested with a glucose reagent strip. The presence of glucose in the drainage signals that leakage is CSF rather than mucus or saliva.
5. If CSF leakage occurs, do not clean the ears or nose unless prescribed by MD. Place a sterile pad over the affected ear or under the nose to catch drainage, but do not pack them. Position patient so that fluids can drain. Change dressings when they become damp using aseptic technique.
6. To prevent introduction of bacteria into the nervous system in the presence of CSF leakage or possible basilar fracture, avoid nasal suction. Instruct patient to avoid nose blowing, sneezing, or sniffing in of nasal drainage.

7. If the patient is intubated, the tube for gastric decompression may be placed orally rather than nasally. If the gastric tube is placed nasally, the MD usually performs the intubation. Check placement of the tube, preferably by x-ray, before applying suction. NG tubes have been known to enter the fracture site and curl up into the patient's cranial vault during insertion attempts. Visually check the back of the patient's throat for the NG tube to help confirm placement.
8. Individuals with basilar skull fractures generally will be kept flat in bed on complete bed rest. This position will help decrease pressure and the amount of CSF draining from a dural tear. Patients will be placed on antibiotics to prevent infection and observed for healing and sealing of the dural tear within 7-10 days.
9. Teach patient to report promptly any indicators of infection.

Potential for disuse syndrome related to prolonged inactivity secondary to sensorimotor deficits and decreased LOC

Desired outcome: Patient exhibits full ROM of all joints.

1. For patients at risk of IICP, perform passive ROM exercises rather than allow active or assisted ROM exercises, which can increase intraabdominal or intrathoracic pressure, and hence, ICP. For the same reason, avoid using the prone position.
2. Once the risk of IICP is no longer significant, additional measures to enhance mobility and strength may be implemented. For discussion, see **Potential for activity intolerance,** p. 651, and **Potential for disuse syndrome,** p. 653, in "Caring for Patients on Prolonged Bed Rest."

Pain related to headaches secondary to head injury

Desired outcome: Patient's subjective evaluation of pain improves, as documented by a pain scale.

1. Monitor and document the duration and character of the patient's pain, rating it on a scale of 0 (no discomfort) to 10.
2. Administer analgesics as prescribed. Patients with head injuries generally do not have much pain, and the pain is usually relieved by analgesics, such as acetaminophen. Sometimes codeine is prescribed, but as a rule, other narcotics are contraindicated because they can mask neurologic indicators of IICP and cause respiratory depression.
3. For other interventions, see **Pain,** p. 254, in "General Care of Patients with Neurologic Disorders."

If the patient has bladder dysfunction, see Renal-Urinary Disorders for related discussions. **Caution:** The Credé maneuver and other measures that can increase intraabdominal and intrathoracic pressure are contraindicated for patients who are at risk of IICP. See "Alzheimer's Disease" for **Altered thought processes,** p. 186. See "Cerebrovascular Accident" for **Impaired verbal communication** related to aphasia or dysarthria, p. 237. See "Seizure Disorders" for **Potential for trauma** related to oral, musculoskeletal, and airway vulnerability secondary to seizure activity, p. 244. See "General Care of Patients with Neurologic Disorders" for the following: **Potential for trauma** related to gait unsteadiness, p. 248; **Potential for impaired tissue integrity** related to risk of corneal irritation/abrasion, p. 249; **Alteration in nutrition,** p. 249; **Potential fluid volume deficit,** p. 250; **Potential ineffective airway clearance,** p. 251; **Self-care deficit,** p. 251; **Constipation,** p. 252; **Potential for injury** related to risk of IICP, p. 253; and **Sensory/perceptual alterations** related to visual disturbances, p. 254. For patients undergoing surgical procedures, see "Caring for Preoperative and Postoperative Patients," p. 637. For patients with varying degrees of immobility, see related nursing diagnoses in "Pressure Ulcers," p. 630, and "Caring for Patients on Prolonged Bed Rest," p. 651. Also see "Caring for Patients with Cancer and Other Life-Disrupting Illnesses," p. 690, for appropriate psychosocial nursing diagnoses and interventions.

PATIENT-FAMILY TEACHING AND DISCHARGE PLANNING

The head-injured patient can have varying degrees of neurologic deficit, ranging from mild to severe. As indicated by the patient's condition and prognosis, provide patient and significant others with verbal and written information for the following:

1. Referrals to community resources, such as cognitive retraining specialist, head injury rehabilitation centers, visiting nurses association, community support groups, social workers, psychologic therapy, vocational rehabilitation agency, home health agencies, and extended and skilled care facilities. In addition, provide the following address: National Head Injury Foundation, 18 A Vernon Street, Framingham, MA 01701.
2. Safety measures related to decreased sensation, visual disturbances, motor deficits, and seizure activity.
3. For other information, see teaching/discharge planning interventions, Nos. 4-10, in "Multiple Sclerosis," p. 164.

Section Four NERVOUS SYSTEM TUMORS

Brain tumors

The abnormal and uncontrolled cell growth of neoplastic or benign tumors can have a wide variety of effects on the brain. Most significant is the disruption of neuronal function caused by infiltration of the tissue, compression of brain tissue and blood vessels, or obstruction of normal flow of CSF. The increase in ICP from tumor growth and other factors, such as cerebral edema, will cause brain structures to shift, eventually leading to brain herniation and death. *Primary brain tumors,* composed of nervous system tissue, rarely metastasize outside the CNS. It is not uncommon, however, for primary brain tumors to metastasize to other parts of the CNS. *Secondary brain tumors* arise from cells that have metastasized from other parts of the body, such as the lung, breast, and skin. Although benign tumors tend to be more treatable than neoplastic tumors, they are considered as serious because they are equally capable of destroying adjacent nerves through compression and increasing ICP, which in turn compromises vital centers.

Tumor classification: Generally, brain tumors are classified according to their cell of origin.

□ *Gliomas:* Comprise 45% of all brain tumors and arise from brain connective tissue. Generally, they are infiltrative and often cannot be removed totally by surgery. As a group, gliomas usually are considered neoplastic.
  – Astrocytomas: The most common glioma, astrocytomas are graded from I-IV, with grade I cytologically (but not necessarily biologically) benign, and grade IV the most malignant. Glioblastoma multiforme is a grade III-IV astrocytoma and is considered the most common and highly malignant glioma. It comprises 20% of all brain tumors, generally is found in the cerebral hemisphere, and may metastasize to other parts of the CNS.
  – Oligodendrogliomas: Are the next most common gliomas and arise out of cells involved in the process of myelination. Generally, they are slow-growing tumors, which often are cytologically (but not necessarily biologically) benign.
  – Medulloblastomas: This relatively rare glioma is highly malignant and found primarily in children.
  – Ependymomas: This glioma arises out of the cells that line the cavities of the CNS, such as the ventricles. These rare tumors are quite invasive and primarily are found in children and young adults.
□ *Meningiomas:* Originate from pia or arachnoid membranes, comprise around 15% of all brain tumors, and, while technically benign, can invade the skull and cause brain tissue compression.
□ *Schwannomas (e.g., acoustic neuroma):* Account for about 10% of brain tumors, affect the craniospinal nerve sheath, and are slow growing. While these tumors are cy-

tologically benign, they may not be diagnosed until they are large in size and compressing sensitive brain stem centers.

□ *Pituitary tumors:* See "Pituitary Tumors," p. 284.

□ *Secondary (metastatic) tumors:* Most often occur in the cerebrum, may be multiple because of the "seeding" effect, and resemble the primary neoplasm histologically. Lung and breast carcinomas are the lesions that most frequently result in metastases to the brain.

ASSESSMENT

Onset of signs and symptoms usually is insidious.

General indicators: Headache, nausea, projectile vomiting, lethargy, forgetfulness, disorientation, personality changes, and seizure activity.

Focal symptoms

□ *Frontal lobe:* Personality/mood changes, impaired judgment, weakness or paralysis (usually unilateral), apraxia, aphasia.

□ *Parietal lobe:* Visual field deficit, sensory disturbance, impaired position sense, and perceptual problems, such as altered stereognosis and dyslexia.

□ *Temporal lobe:* Auditory changes, tinnitus, visual field deficit, sensory aphasia, impaired memory, personality changes, psychomotor seizures.

□ *Occipital lobe:* Seizures, visual agnosia, visual field deficit.

□ *Cerebellar:* Tremors, nystagmus, incoordination, loss of balance, gait disturbances, nuchal headache.

□ *Ventricular or hypothalamic:* Diabetes insipidus, weight gain, somnolence, headache, disturbance of temperature regulation.

□ *Cranial nerve:* Sense of smell alterations, ptosis, diplopia, alterations in ocular movement, drooping of facial muscles on the same side as the tumor, difficulty swallowing, loss of cough/gag reflex, loss of corneal reflex, protrusion of the tongue toward the side of the tumor.

□ *Schwannoma:* Unilateral hearing loss with or without tinnitus, stiff neck. Other symptoms may include decreased facial sensation, facial muscle weakness or paralysis on same side as the hearing loss, and diplopia. Late symptoms include ataxia and arm coordination problems secondary to brain stem and cerebellar compression.

Indicators of IICP: See discussion in "Head Injury," p. 209.

Indicators of brain stem herniation: See discussion in "Head Injury," p. 209.

Physical assessment: Ophthalmoscopic examination may reveal papilledema if ICP is increased; visual field exam may reveal impairment, such as hemianopia (blindness in part of the field of vision); and audiometry or vestibular function studies may show abnormalities as well.

DIAGNOSTIC TESTS

Diagnostic tests are done to rule out vascular etiology, such as hemorrhage, abscess, and trauma, as well as diagnose a brain tumor. Any one or a combination of the following tests may be performed.

1. *MRI:* May reveal presence of tumor, tissue shift, and hydrocephalus. This diagnostic tool, because of its ability to detect biochemical changes, can help diagnose tumors at an early stage.

   □ The MRI cannot be used on critically ill or unstable patients because it is impossible to monitor cardiac rhythm and VS inside the scanner.

   □ Individuals with internal items, such as pacemakers, surgical aneurysm clips, prosthetic heart valves, or umbrella filters for emboli, are ineligible for MRI. The MRI can deactivate pacemakers, and the strong magnetic field can move metal aneurysm clips and valve and umbrella filters within the body, putting the patient at obvious risk.

□ Assess patients for their ability to cope with confined spaces and lie motionless throughout the 15-90 minute test. The MD may prescribe a sedative. Patients should void prior to the test. They will need to remove such items as jewelry, hair clips, clothing with metal fasteners, and glasses before entering the scanner.

2. *CT scan:* May detect tumor mass, tissue shift, and hydrocephalus. Serial screens may be done to track the tumor's response to therapy.
   □ If contrast agents are not used, there are no known complications from CT scans. Food and fluid restrictions are unnecessary.
   □ If a contrast agent is to be used, the patient should be asked about allergies to iodine or iodine-containing substances, such as shellfish.
   □ When a contrast agent is used, food and fluids may be restricted 4 hours prior to the test.
   □ The patient may experience nausea and vomiting or headache from the contrast agent.

3. *X-rays of the skull and spinal cord:* May reveal tumors that contain calcium or cause bony erosion.

4. *Positron emission tomography (PET):* May distinguish tumor tissue from normal brain tissue by identifying abnormal metabolic activity of the tumor tissue.
   □ *Pretest:* Alcohol, caffeine, and tobacco may be restricted for 24 hours prior to the test to prevent skewing of test results. Since the test is based on tissue glucose metabolism, the patient should eat a meal 3-4 hours prior to the test. Physicians may give special instructions regarding the diabetic patient's insulin prior to the PET test since insulin will alter glucose metabolism and hence, the test results. Generally, the diabetic individual will be allowed to take insulin before the pretest meal.
   □ *During the test:* Evaluate the patient for the ability to stay still during the 60-90 minute test and for excessive anxiety. Tranquilizers alter glucose metabolism and cannot be administered.

5. *EEG:* May localize abnormal brain wave activity, which may suggest tumor growth. (See "Seizure Disorders," p. 239, for patient care.)

6. *Brain scan:* May demonstrate presence of a space-occupying lesion *via* uptake of radioisotope. This test is helpful in localizing certain tumors, such as meningiomas.

7. *Echoencephalography of the cranium:* May show shift of brain structure, which may signal a tumor. This test generally has been replaced by the CT scan.

8. *Cerebral angiography:* May show abnormal perfusion patterns, which suggest tumor location. Also may reveal alterations in the position of vessels caused by the tumor, and may even outline the tumor *via* its circulation. The test may be performed preoperatively in order to plan surgical strategy. (See "Cerebral Aneurysm," p. 221, for patient care.)

9. *Lumbar puncture and CSF analysis:* May be performed in the absence of any indicators of IICP. CSF may be clear to bloody; protein values and WBC count may be increased; glucose values may be decreased; and cytology may reveal the presence of cancer cells. This test usually is done when there is concern about the possibility of an infectious process. (See "Bacterial Meningitis," p. 161, for patient care.)

10. *Lesion biopsy:* Identifies pathologic cells and confirms diagnosis.

MEDICAL MANAGEMENT AND SURGICAL INTERVENTIONS

The mode of treatment depends on the tumor's histologic type, anatomic location, and sensitivity to radiation. Treatment usually includes surgery, often in combination with radiation or chemotherapy. Immunotherapy also is being evaluated as a treatment modality. The location and accessibility of the tumor determine whether or not surgery can be performed. Tumors of the brain stem, medulla, pons, and corpus callosum tend to be inaccessible.

1. Craniotomy: Surgical opening into the skull. The dura and bone flap may be left open postoperatively to accommodate cerebral edema and prevent compression. Preoperatively, patients generally are started on corticosteroids (dexamethasone) and antiseptic shampoos. They also may be started on an antiepilepsy drug. A good baseline

neurologic assessment should be documented preoperatively to serve as a basis of comparison for postoperative neurologic checks. Typically, the patient is in ICU immediately after surgery, where the following interventions are performed:

☐ Respiratory and airway support, which may include oxygen, intubation, or ventilation.

☐ Frequent VS and neurologic assessment to monitor for changes and trends.

☐ Assessment of the dressing for the presence of abnormal bleeding or CSF leakage. Document drainage, amount, color, and odor. CSF drainage on dressings and bedsheets typically produces a lighter "halo" ring around darker drainage. Nonsanguineous drainage is tested with a glucose reagent stick, which is positive in the presence of CSF. Sterile technique is maintained to prevent wound infection and meningitis.

☐ If surgery was performed with the patient in Fowler's position, a 30-35 degree angle is usually maintained as prescribed.

☐ Patients with supratentorial craniotomies are maintained with HOB elevated to 30 degrees or as prescribed. They can be turned but must be kept off the operative site. The head and neck should be kept in good alignment.

☐ Patients with infratentorial craniotomies for cerebellar or brain stem tumors are usually kept flat and off their backs for 48 hours. To prevent pressure areas with subsequent skin breakdown, the patient is logrolled q2h to the side with the head kept in alignment. Pressure is kept off the operative site.

☐ Oral temperatures are avoided because of the patient's decreased cognitive function. Rectal temperature is taken q2-4h, and the staff is alert to the presence of hyperthermia. A temperature of 38.9° C (102° F) is considered a dangerous level, and the patient is sponged with tepid water and/or placed on a hypothermia blanket if this occurs.

☐ Usually the patient is kept NPO for the first 36-48 hours because of the risk of vomiting and choking. Fluids are generally restricted to reduce cerbral edema. Usually, an indwelling catheter is inserted to allow more accurate monitoring of urine output.

☐ In the presence of periorbital edema, petroleum jelly and cold compresses are lightly applied around patient's eyes. Maximum swelling usually occurs withing 24-48 hours of surgery.

☐ Measures are taken to reduce IICP (see **Potential for injury** related to IICP in "General Care of Patients with Neurologic Disorders," p. 253.) Precautions are taken for seizures (see **Potential for trauma** related to oral, musculoskeletal, and airway vulnerability secondary to seizure activity, p. 244, in "Seizure Disorders").

2. **Surgical techniques:** Laser neurosurgery has been proven useful in certain types of tumor removal, such as meningiomas. *Laser neurosurgery* tends to be more precise than conventional dissection, resulting in less tissue damage and postoperative swelling. New *stereotaxic neurosurgery* techniques using the CT scan and computer processing of stereoactive data enable the precise guidance of a surgical probe to the tumor. Some deep tumors now can be removed or debulked without extensive damage to surrounding brain tissue.

3. **Transsphenoidal hypophysectomy:** For pituitary tumors (see "Pituitary Tumors," p. 285).

4. **Ventricular shunt for ventricular drainage:** May be done to allow drainage of CSF. Shunt types vary but can extend from the lateral ventricle of the brain to one of the following: subarachnoid space of the spinal canal, right atrium of the heart, a large vein, or the peritoneal cavity. This procedure is usually performed if the brain tumor is inoperable and obstructs the flow of CSF. After the shunt procedure, the patient should be kept off the insertion site to prevent pressure on the shunt mechanism. Head and neck should be kept in good body alignment to prevent kinking or compressing of the shunt catheter. If the shunt has a valve for controlling CSF drainage or reflux, pump the valve according to MD instructions to ensure proper functioning. If the valve is working properly, you will be able to feel it emptying and refilling.

5. Supportive pharmacotherapy
   □ *Antiepilepsy agents:* If indicated.
   □ *Diuretics:* To decrease cerebral edema and ICP.
   □ *Corticosteroids (e.g., dexamethasone):* To reduce cerebral edema.
   □ *Antacids and H₂ receptor antagonists:* To prevent/treat stress ulcers.
   □ *Analgesics:* For headaches.
6. **Radiation therapy:** Frequently begun as soon as the surgical incision has healed. It can be localized or include the entire brain and part of the spinal cord, depending on the type, location, and extent of the tumor. Radiation can cause inflammation of the brain, which in turn increases ICP and neurologic symptoms. With inoperable tumors, radiation therapy often becomes the primary modality. Under investigation is the placement of radionuclide seeds into the tumors of patients with recurrent malignant gliomas. Placement of the seeds requires either a stereotaxic procedure or a craniotomy. After placement, radiation precautions will need to be observed. The individual with radioactive implants in the brain wears a lead shield or helmet to protect others from the radiation. The lead shield should remain in place at all times except when the head dressing is changed. When the patient's shield is removed, the caregiver should wear a lead apron. For more information about radiation therapy, see section "Caring for Patients with Cancer and Other Life-Disrupting Illnesses," p. 659.
7. **Chemotherapy:** Nitrosourea agents, such as carmustine (BCNU), lomustine (CCNU), and methyl-CCNU, cross the blood-brain barrier and because of this are particularly useful for patients with brain tumors. Generally, chemotherapy is used only as an adjunct to surgery and radiation therapy. Chemotherapy on some tumors is used only after tumor regrowth or when the tumor is not sensitive to radiation therapy. Intraarterial, intrathecal, and intraventricular delivery of chemotherapeutic agents to the brain is being investigated in the hopes of getting higher drug doses to the tumor, while limiting the degree of systemic side effects. See section "Caring for Patients with Cancer and Other Life-Disrupting Illnesses," p. 659, for more information about chemotherapy.

Depending on the presence and severity of neurologic deficits, the patient also may need the following:
8. **Respiratory support and intubation:** To maintain the airway and supply oxygen as needed.
9. **Fluid and nutritional support:** The patient may require high-calorie, high-protein supplements and enteral feedings or parenteral nutrition because of swallowing/chewing deficits or side effects of radiation and chemotherapy, and IV fluids to prevent dehydration. See "Providing Nutritional Support," p. 611, for more information.
10. **Physical medicine:** For example, PT, OT, and assistive devices or braces, so that the patient can maintain mobility and independence with ADL. Muscle-strengthening exercises, conditioning exercises, and gait training are also frequently prescribed.
11. **ROM exercises:** To maintain or increase joint function and prevent contractures. While the patient is at risk for IICP, the exercises are passive only. Once the risk for IICP is minimized, active or active-assistive ROM is employed.
12. **Treatment of secondary complications:** For example, cerebral edema, IICP, syndrome of inappropriate antidiuretic hormone (SIADH), and diabetes insipidus.

NURSING DIAGNOSES AND INTERVENTIONS

See "Alzheimer's Disease" for **Altered thought processes,** p. 186. See "Head Injury" for **Potential for disuse syndrome,** p. 212. See "Cerebrovascular Accident" for **Impaired verbal communication** related to aphasia or dysarthria, p. 237. See "Seizure Disorders" for **Potential for trauma** related to oral, musculoskeletal, and airway vulnerability secondary to seizure activity, p. 244. See "General Care for Patients with Neurologic Disorders" for **Potential for trauma** related to unsteady gait, p. 248; **Potential impaired tissue integrity** related to corneal irritation/abrasion, p. 249; **Alteration** in nutrition, p. 249; **Potential fluid volume deficit,** p. 250; **Potential ineffective airway clearance,** p. 251; **Self-care deficit,** p. 251; **Constipation,** p. 252; **Potential for injury** related to IICP, p. 253; **Sensory/perceptual alterations** related to visual disturbances, p. 254; and **Pain,** p. 254. For patients with varying degrees of immobility, see related nursing diagnoses in "Pressure Ulcer," p. 630, and "Caring for Patients on Prolonged Bed Rest," p. 651. Also see "Caring for Preoperative and Postoperative Patients," p. 637, and "Caring for Patients with Cancer and Other Life-Disrupting Illnesses," p. 659, as appropriate.

PATIENT-FAMILY TEACHING AND DISCHARGE PLANNING

Provide patient and significant others with verbal and written information for the following as appropriate:

1. Safety measures specific to sensory deficits, motor deficits, incoordination, cognitive deficits, and seizures.
2. Measures to promote communication in the presence of aphasia.
3. Appropriate referrals to community resources, such as public health nurse, visiting nurses association, community support groups, social workers, psychologic therapy, vocational rehabilitation agency, home health agencies, and extended and skilled care facilities. In addition, provide the address for the American Cancer Society, 777 Third Avenue, New York, NY 10017. In addition, the Association for Brain Tumor Research, 6232 N. Pulaski Road, Suite 400, Chicago, IL 60646, also has set up local support groups and will try to assist brain tumor patients and their families.
4. Care of postoperative or postprocedure wounds and indicators of infection.
5. Potential side effects and precautions for patients undergoing radiation therapy.
6. Medications, including drug name, purpose, dosage, frequency, precautions, and potential side effects, especially for chemotherapeutic agents.
7. Exercises that promote muscle strength and mobility, measures for preventing contractures and skin breakdown, transfer techniques and proper body mechanics, use of assistive devices.
8. Measures for relieving pain, nausea, or other discomfort.
9. Indications of constipation, urinary retention, or UTI; implementation of bowel and bladder training programs; and if appropriate, care of indwelling catheters.
10. Indications of URI and measures to prevent regurgitation, aspiration, and respiratory infection.
11. Importance of follow-up care, including MD visits, PT, OT, speech therapy, psychologic counseling, and laboratory monitoring for side effects of radiation/chemotherapy.
12. First aid measures for seizures.
13. Causes of IICP and measures to prevent it.
14. Care of ventricular shunt, if present. Include specific instructions for shunt care and information regarding how to identify shunt infection or malfunction and steps to take should they occur.

Spinal cord tumors

The majority of spinal cord tumors interrupt neuronal function and nerve impulse transmission by compressing the spinal cord, its roots, or its blood supply, and eventually causing cord degeneration. Spinal cord tumors can occur anywhere along the length of the spinal cord, and, if untreated, lead to paralysis and sensory deficits. *Intramedullary tumors* occur within the cord itself and are fairly rare. *Extramedullary tumors* occur outside the spinal cord and are further classified as intradural or extradural. *Intradural tumors,* such as meningiomas and schwannomas, arise from the membrane covering the spinal cord and nerve roots and account for the majority of all primary spinal cord tumors. Intradermal tumors occur in the space between the cord and the dura. *Extradural tumors* usually are secondary (metastatic) tumors that have been "seeded" from other sites in the body, such as the prostate, bone marrow, lymph tissue, breast, or lungs. They occur in the epidural space or in the vertebrae that surround the spinal cord and related tissue.

ASSESSMENT

Indicators vary according to tumor site.

Motor involvement: Weakness or paralysis of one or more body parts with the potential for spasticity below the level of the tumor. If the tumor interrupts the spinal cord reflex arc (e.g., a tumor at the level of the cauda equina), decreased or loss of reflexes, flaccidity, muscle atrophy, and fasciculations can occur.

Sensory involvement: Decreased sensation to pain, touch, and temperature with potential loss of position and vibration sense.

Pain: Neck or back pain that persists despite bed rest is most severe over the tumor site and potentially radiates around the trunk or down the affected side because of nerve root irritation. The spinal processes can be quite tender to the touch. Pain often is aggravated by straining, coughing, and sneezing.

Bladder and bowel dysfunction: Initially, the patient may have difficulty starting a stream or may empty the bladder incompletely. The patient may have a spastic bladder, causing urinary retention; a flaccid bladder, causing incontinence; and bowel incontinence from loss of control. The patient also may be constipated.

Physical assessment: Depending on location of the tumor, patient may exhibit increased or decreased/absent DTRs.

DIAGNOSTIC TESTS

1. *X-ray:* May show changes in vertebrae, such as destruction and collapse of bony matrix.
2. *MRI:* To show tumor location and the presence of cord compression. Because it can detect biochemical abnormalities, it may detect the tumor at a very early stage. MRI is of particular value in evaluating high cervical lesions, where the presence of bone makes the CT scan less effective. (See "Brain Tumors," p. 214, for patient care.)
3. *Spinal CT scan:* To reveal tumor location and presence of cord compression. (See "Brain Tumors," p. 215, for patient care.)
4. *Bone scan:* Shows increased radioactive tracer uptake where there is metastatic invasion of the vertebrae causing increased osteoblastic activity. **Note:** Check for pregnancy in appropriate patients, and notify MD accordingly. After procedure, patient should drink several glasses of water to facilitate clearance of free-circulating isotope.
5. *Lumbar puncture and CSF analysis:* May show malignant cells in CSF. With partial blockage, there may be slightly increased levels of protein and a yellow tinge to the fluid; with complete blockage, there are definite increases in protein and the fluid is yellow. (See "Bacterial Meningitis," p. 161, for patient care.)
   □ *Queckenstedt's test:* Performed by compressing the jugular vein for 10 seconds during the LP. Normally, a rise in CSF pressure occurs. For patients in whom a tumor is partially blocking the spinal cord above the level of the LP, the test may cause a sluggish rise in CSF. With complete blockage, there will be no rise in CSF pressure.
6. *Myelography:* Shows level at which the tumor is located if the spinal canal is not totally obstructed. This procedure can be dangerous because withdrawal of CSF may cause increased compression of the cord by the tumor. (See "Spinal Cord Injury," p. 198, for preprocedure and postprocedure care.)
7. *Tissue biopsy:* Confirms presence of a tumor.

MEDICAL MANAGEMENT AND SURGICAL INTERVENTIONS

1. **Bed rest:** For patients with cancer that has invaded the bony vertebral body. Body weight alone can cause vertebral collapse, resulting in possible cord laceration or compression.
2. **Pharmacotherapy**
   □ *Steroids:* To decrease compression caused by cord edema.
   □ *Hormone therapy:* For hormone-mediated metastatic tumor.
   □ *Analgesics:* For pain.
3. **TENS:** Battery-operated device that delivers electrical impulses to the body to relieve pain.
4. **Surgery:** May include a laminectomy or decompression or excision of primary tumors. Microsurgery techniques and the use of spinal cord-evoked potentials (see p. 198) during surgery has helped surgeons protect cord function. Generally, surgery is not indicated for metastatic tumors. Emergency surgical decompression of the spinal cord may save function in instances of sudden onset of partial paralysis. (See "Intervertebral disk disease," p. 192, for care of patient with a laminectomy.)
5. **Radiation therapy:** May be performed preoperatively and postoperatively to reduce tumor mass and symptoms and help prevent recurrence. Radiation therapy is the primary treatment modality for secondary metastatic tumors and those tumors that cannot be removed totally. Cord inflammation and edema caused by radiation therapy can result in an increase in the neurologic deficit.
6. **Physical medicine:** May include PT, OT, and assistive devices or braces so that patient can maintain mobility and independence with ADL. Muscle-strengthening exercises, conditioning exercises, and gait training are also frequently prescribed.
7. **ROM exercises:** To maintain or increase joint function and prevent contractures.

NURSING DIAGNOSES AND INTERVENTIONS

Pain (acute or chronic) related to tissue compression secondary to tumor growth

Desired outcome: Patient's subjective evaluation of pain improves, as documented by a pain scale.

1. Assess patient's degree and character of pain, using a pain scale. Rate pain from 0 (no pain) to 10.
2. Advise patient that moving slowly with good body alignment may help minimize pain.
3. Suggest that keeping knees and hips slightly flexed when in bed will help reduce pain by preventing full extension of the spinal cord.
4. Inform patient that sneezing and straining can cause pain.
5. For other interventions, see **Pain** in "General Care of Patients with Neurologic Disorders," p. 254.

If patient has bladder dysfunction, see related discussions in "Renal-Urinary Disorders," pp. 102-157. See "Spinal Cord Injury," p. 200, for nursing diagnoses and interventions related to the care of patients with disorders of the spinal cord. See "Pressure Ulcers," p. 630, and "Caring for Patients on Prolonged Bed Rest," p. 651, for nursing diagnoses and interventions for patients who are immobile. See "Caring for Patients with Cancer and Other Life-Disrupting Illnesses," p. 659, for additional nursing diagnoses and inteventions.

PATIENT-FAMILY TEACHING AND DISCHARGE PLANNING

Provide patient and significant others with verbal and written information for the following, as appropriate:
1. Safety measures relative to sensorimotor deficits.

2. For more information, see teaching/discharge planning interventions, Nos. 3-11, in "Brain Tumor," p. 218.

Section Five VASCULAR DISORDERS OF THE NERVOUS SYSTEM

Cerebral aneurysm

An aneurysm is a localized weakness and dilatation of an artery. With cerebral aneurysms, this dilatation generally takes one of two forms: *fusiform,* in which the entire circumference of a vessel section is dilated; or *saccular,* in which there is dilatation of the side of a vessel. Saccular aneurysms, also called "berry" aneurysms, are the most common. Depending on their size and location, unruptured aneurysms can produce neurologic symptoms by compressing brain tissue or cranial nerves. Usually, however, the aneurysm causes no symptoms until it ruptures. When this occurs, hemorrhage into the subarachnoid space produces adequate circulation of CSF, which increases ICP. In addition, interruption of blood flow to the areas supplied by the ruptured artery can cause brain ischemia and possibly, infarction. Hemorrhage sometimes occurs directly into the intracranial tissue, causing direct neuronal damage. The patient may experience permanent neurologic deficits, depending on the size and site of the bleed and development of any complications.

Aneurysm can be caused by a congenital defect in the arterial wall, degenerative processes, such as hypertension or atherosclerosis, or vessel trauma. Prognosis depends on the site and size of the ruptured aneurysm, but 45%-50% of affected individuals die immediately.

Common causes of death for individuals who survive the initial rupture include IICP, rebleeding, and vasospasm of the blood vessels. The patient is at the greatest risk of rebleeding within the first 24-48 hours following the initial rupture. Rebleeding, however, is a significant risk for the first 2 weeks because of the body's normal process of clot lysis at the rupture site. Approximately 20% of patients will rebleed within 2 weeks. Nearly two-thirds of patients experiencing rebleeding will die. Rebleeding may occur up to 6 months after the initial rupture.

The patient also is at risk of experiencing cerebral vasospasm, which decreases cerebral blood flow, leading to cerebral ischemia. The cerebral ischemia can increase the patient's neurologic deficits and may cause cerebral infarct and death. Vasospasm seems to be directly related to the amount of blood present in the subarachnoid space after rupture. Vasospasm usually starts within 3-4 days after the subarachnoid hemorrhage, peaks between 7-10 days, and usually resolves in about 3 weeks.

Following rupture, 20%-25% of patients may develop acute or chronic hydrocephalus. The presence of blood in the subarachnoid space appears to damage the arachnoid villi and decrease or prevent CSF reabsorption. This will increase ICP, leading to possible brain herniation. Other complications the patient may be at risk for are diabetes insipidus (see p. 280) and SIADH owing to pituitary gland or hypothalamus compression or damage.

ASSESSMENT

Indicators vary, depending on the site and amount of bleeding.

Signs and symptoms

☐ *Prodromal (as the aneurysm enlarges but before it ruptures):* Periodic headaches, transitory weakness, numbness, tingling on one side, and transitory speech disturbances.

☐ *Acute (with leakage and rupture):* Sudden and severe headache, nausea and/or vomiting, and neck stiffness are among the most common symptoms.

IICP and herniation: Sudden, severe headache; nausea and vomiting; changes or alteration in LOC ranging from confusion, irritability, and restlessness to coma; a falling score on the Glasgow Coma Scale (see p. 207); pupillary dilatation and changes in their size and reaction to light; VS changes, such as increasing BP with widening pulse pressure and decreased pulse rate; irregular respiratory pattern.

Meningeal irritation (caused by blood in the subarachnoid space): Neck stiffness; neck, back, and leg pain; fever; photophobia; seizures.

Cranial nerve irritation/compression: Blurred vision and other visual disturbances, ptosis, inability to rotate the eyes, difficulty with swallowing or speaking, tinnitus.

Focal symptoms: Sensory loss, motor weakness, or paralysis on one side of the body.

Physical assessment: Positive Kernig's and Brudzinski's signs confirm presence of meningeal irritation. (See description with "Bacterial Meningitis," p. 168.)

Grading: Individuals with ruptured aneurysms are often graded according to the severity of the bleeding or injury:

□ *Grade 1:* Patient alert with no neurologic deficit; slight neck stiffness; minimal headache, if present.
□ *Grade 2:* Patient alert with mild to severe headache; presence of stiff neck; may have minimal neurologic deficit, such as third cranial nerve palsies.
□ *Grade 3:* Patient drowsy or confused; presence of stiff neck; may have mild focal neurologic deficits.
□ *Grade 4:* Patient stuporous, semi-comatose; presence of stiff neck; may have neurologic deficits, such as hemiparesis.
□ *Grade 5:* Patient comatose and posturing.

DIAGNOSTIC TESTS

1. *CT scan:* To reveal presence of aneurysm and the site, size, and amount of bleeding from the subarachnoid or intracerebral hemorrhage. The scan also may reveal the presence of hydrocephalus. (See "Brain Tumors," p. 215, for patient care.)
2. *Cerebral angiography:* To pinpoint site, structure, and size of aneurysm and presence of vasospasm. This test provides the definitive diagnosis of aneurysm. Before the test, keep patient NPO for 8-10 hours, or as prescribed; and assess for and notify MD of allergies to iodine, shellfish, or radiopaque dyes. Inform patients they will feel a warm or burning sensation when the dye is administered. If prescribed, shave the proposed site. If the femoral approach is to be used, check pedal pulses prior to the test and mark their location. If the carotid approach is to be used, measure, mark, and record the patient's neck circumference (bleeding, hematoma formation, or thrombus obstruction of the artery can occur following the test). Document baseline neurologic assessments for postprocedure comparison. After the test follow these guidelines:
   □ Maintain patient on strict bed rest for 6-24 hours, followed by a specified period of "bathroom privileges only."
   □ If bleeding occurs, apply manual pressure until it has ceased, and then apply a pressure dressing to prevent further bleeding. Notify MD, and reinstate frequent monitoring of VS and puncture site.
   □ Monitor VS at frequent intervals, as prescribed, and evaluate the patient for changes in neurologic status, such as altered LOC, and for indicators of reactions to the dye, such as respiratory distress, hypotension, hives, and itching. Notify MD of any adverse reactions.
   □ If the femoral approach was used, keep leg straight for the prescribed amount of time (usually 6-12 hours) to minimize risk of bleeding. Patients will need to use bedpan and eat on their side during this time period. At frequent intervals, assess pedal pulses and temperature, color, and tactile sensation of the leg. Notify MD of loss or weakening of pulses, numbness, tingling, cooling, pallor, or cyanotic feet, which can occur with thrombus formation or obstruction of the artery.

□ If brachial approach was used, immobilize arm 6-12 hours or as prescribed. Check radial pulses frequently, and be alert to loss or weakening of pulses; numbness; tingling; or coolness, pallor, cyanosis in the hand. If these occur, notify MD because they are indicative of thrombus formation and obstruction of the artery. Do not measure BP in affected arm; post a sign over patient's bed to alert other staff members.

□ If the carotid artery was the puncture site, check for tracheal displacement, an increase in neck circumference, difficulty with swallowing or breathing, weakness, numbness, confusion, or neurologic deficits, any of which can occur with bleeding, hematoma formation, or thrombus obstruction in the artery. Notify MD of significant findings.

3. _MRI:_ Can reveal presence of even small amounts of blood or small aneurysms that are not visualized with the CT scan or angiography. (See "Brain Tumors," p. 214, for patient care.)

4. _Lumbar puncture and CSF analysis:_ May reveal presence of bloody CSF, increased CSF pressure, and increased protein. Blood in the CSF indicates a subarachnoid hemorrhage has occurred. This procedure is contraindicated for patients with increased ICP. (See "Bacterial Meningitis," p. 161, for patient care.)

5. _Skull x-ray:_ May reveal calcification in the wall of a large aneurysm.

MEDICAL MANAGEMENT AND SURGICAL INTERVENTIONS

1. Respiratory support: Airway maintenance, intubation, and ventilation as necessary. ABG values are often monitored for evidence of hypoxia. If indicated, oxygen is administered to prevent hypoxia and carbon dioxide retention, which can cause vasodilatation of the cerebral arteries and cerebral edema.

2. Activity restrictions: Strict bed rest in a quiet, dark room; limitation of visitors; restriction of ADL. Although active ROM is occasionally permitted, even the alert patient is usually limited to passive ROM. Restraints are avoided because they can result in IICP if the patient struggles against them.

3. Elevation of HOB: To 30 degrees or as prescribed to reduce cerebral congestion.

4. Pharmacotherapy

□ _Antifibrinolytic agent (e.g., aminocaproic acid):_ To decrease the risk of rebleeding at the site of aneurysm by delaying the body's lysis of the blood clot. Use of this drug is controversial because, while it reduces the risk of rebleeding, it appears to increase the risk of vasospasm. If used, generally a loading dose of 5 grams in 50 ml D_5W is given over an hour; 24-30 grams in 500 ml D_5W is given by constant IV infusion for 10 days. This is followed by 3 grams orally q2h for 21 days or until surgical repair is performed. Rapid IV infusion may cause hypotension, bradycardia, or dysrhythmias. Side effects include phlebitis at the insertion site (IV route) and nausea and diarrhea (oral route). Other side effects include headache, tinnitus, dizziness, fatigue, and generalized thrombosis.

□ _Corticosteroids (e.g., dexamethasone):_ To help decrease cerebral edema and ICP. Antacids and histamine H_2 antagonists may be given concurrently in order to inhibit gastric secretions and reduce GI trace irritation.

□ _Antihypertensives (e.g., hydralazine):_ If indicated, to treat underlying hypertension.

□ _Laxatives and stool softeners (e.g., docusate sodium):_ To prevent straining with bowel movements.

□ _Sedatives/tranquilizers (e.g., phenobarbital):_ To reduce stress and restlessness and promote rest.

□ _Osmotic diuretics (e.g., mannitol):_ To reduce cerebral edema.

□ _Loop diuretics (e.g., furosemide [Lasix]):_ Being used by some physicians because it appears to decrease cerebral edema without causing the increase in intracranial blood volume that occurs with mannitol.

□ _Antiepilepsy drugs (e.g., phenytoin or phenobarbital):_ To control or prevent seizures.

□ _Antipyretics (e.g., acetaminophen):_ To control fever, which increases the brain's metabolic activity. Aspirin is avoided because it prevents platelet adhesion.

☐ *Analgesics (e.g., acetaminophen and codeine):* To manage pain. Aspirin is contraindicated because it prevents platelet adhesion.

5. Fluid limitation: Generally, fluids are limited to 1,500-1,800 ml/day to keep patient slightly underhydrated and reduce cerebral congestion and ICP.

6. Nutrition: Coffee and other stimulants are restricted. Very hot and very cold liquids also may be restricted. A high-fiber diet may be prescribed to prevent constipation. For patients with dysphagia, enteral or parenteral feedings may be necessary. A low-sodium, low-cholesterol diet is often prescribed to control hypertension and atherosclerosis.

7. Antiembolism hose: To help prevent thrombophlebitis and deep-vein thrombosis.

8. Avoiding rectal stimulation: Rectal suppositories, thermometers, enemas, and digital examinations are contraindicated because they can stimulate a Valsalva-type maneuver in the patient, causing increased intrathoracic pressure and ICP, resulting in rupture or rebleeding

9. ICU monitoring: May be necessary, particularly if the patient develops cerebral vasospasm or IICP. In ICU, a cannula, if indicated, may be inserted into the ventricle to monitor ICP and provide ventricular drainage.

10. Surgical management: The patient's surgical candidacy depends on LOC, extent of neurologic deficit, nature and location of the aneurysm, and presence of vasospasm. The timing of the surgery is based on the patient's status and surgeon's preference. Usually, surgery is performed within 3-14 days of the initial bleed. Surgery is not performed in the presence of vasospasm. Repair of a cerebral aneurysm requires a craniotomy, so the patient will be in ICU during the immediate postoperative period. Patients graded 1-2 are the best surgical candidates. In order to isolate the aneurysm and prevent rebleeding, the aneurysm is repaired by clipping, ligating, coagulating, wrapping the aneurysm neck with muscle, or encasing the aneurysmal sac in plastic or surgical gauze. For internal carotid artery aneurysms, and sometimes for other inaccessible aneurysms, a carotid artery clamp may be used to reduce blood flow and blood pressure. After surgery, the carotid artery clamp is tightened slowly over several days, which allows time for collateral circulation to take over in the brain. (For information on postoperative care, see craniotomy discussion, p. 216, in "Brain Tumors.")

11. Ventricular shunt for ventricular drainage: Performed to allow drainage of CSF in patients who develop hydrocephalus after a subarachnoid hemorrhage. (See discussion of ventricular shunt in "Brain Tumors," p. 216.)

12. Experimental treatments for cerebral vasospasm: There is no completely effective treatment for cerebral vasospasm. The following are experimental and some necessitate ICU monitoring:

☐ *Craniotomy:* Done within 48 hours to remove any blood clot that may aggravate vasospasm.

☐ *Hemodilution:* The patient is kept well hydrated with IV fluids or volume expanders to decrease blood viscosity in order to improve cerebral blood flow through narrowed arteries.

☐ *Hypervolemic-hypertensive therapy:* Usually only performed following aneurysm repair to increase blood volume and arterial pressure in order to reduce the ischemia and resulting neurologic deficits during vasospasm.

☐ *Theophylline:* To increase cerebral perfusion through smooth muscle dilatation.

☐ *Isoproterenol:* To increase cerebral perfusion through smooth muscle dilatation and increased cardiac output.

☐ *Plasma protein fraction, colloids, or whole blood:* To increase cerebral perfusion by expanding volume and increasing BP.

☐ *Nitroprusside sodium:* To dilate cerebral vessels by relaxing smooth muscle.

☐ *Nifedipine:* A calcium channel blocker used to cause vasodilatation.

☐ *Barbiturate coma:* To decrease cerebral metabolic needs so that injury will be minimized until vasospasm subsides and cerebral blood flow improves.

NURSING DIAGNOSES AND INTERVENTIONS

The following relate primarily to the patient whose aneurysm is graded 1-3. If the patient's aneurysm is graded 4 or 5, see nursing diagnoses in "Cerebrovascular Accident," p. 235, for patient care.

Knowledge deficit: Aneurysms and the potential for rebleeding, rupture, or vasospasm

Desired outcome: Patient verbalizes knowledge of the potential for rebleeding or vasospasm, measures to prevent their occurrence, and the symptoms to report to the health care staff should they occur.

1. Assess patient for sensorimotor deficits, such as decreased or absent vision, impaired temperature and pain sensation, unsteady gait, weakness, or paralysis. Document baseline neurologic and physical assessments so that changes in patient status are detected promptly. Teach patient and significant others these indicators, and explain the importance of reporting them to the staff promptly should they occur.
2. Teach patient the importance of maintaining strict bed rest and reducing activity level to avoid rebleeding or rupture. Explain that the number and frequency of visitors, as well as other stimuli, such as television and radio, will be limited. Teach patient measures that will prevent a sudden increase in ICP, such as opening the mouth when sneezing and exhaling when being moved in bed. Caution patient to avoid straining with bowel movements.
3. Teach patient and significant others the indicators of cerebral vasospasm, which can lead to ischemia and infarction. These include visual disturbances, numbness, weakness, slurred speech, seizures, confusion, and drowsiness. Instruct patient and significant others to alert the staff immediately should they occur. At this time there is no completely effective treatment for vasospasm.

Knowledge deficit: Effects of aminocaproic acid drug therapy

Desired outcome: Patient verbalizes knowledge of the side effects of aminocaproic therapy, the measures to prevent complications from the drug therapy, and signs and symptoms that should be reported immediately to health care staff should they occur.

1. Teach patients on aminocaproic acid therapy the indicators of pulmonary embolus, including SOB, chest pain (especially that which increases with inspiration), and blood-tinged sputum, as well as indicators of deep-vein thrombosis, such as calf pain or tenderness and increased heat, swelling, or redness of the leg. Stress the importance of notifying staff immediately should they occur.
2. Alert patient to the potential for loose stools, frequent stools (more than 3/day), cramps, and weakness with aminocaproic therapy. Instruct patient to report these problems promptly, because if the diarrhea is a side effect of oral aminocaproic therapy, MD may switch patient to IV medication.
3. Inform patients that because the drug may cause postural hypotension, they should make position changes very slowly and in stages. Faintness or dizziness should be reported promptly.
4. Instruct patient to report any muscle weakness, muscle pain, sweating, fever, or myeloglobinuria (reddish-brown urine), as these may be signs of myopathy caused by this drug therapy.
5. Teach patient to report nausea, tinnitus, or fatigue, which are other side effects of aminocaproic drug therapy.

Potential for ineffective airway clearance related to imposed inactivity secondary to the risk of aneurysm rupture or rebleeding

Desired outcomes: Patient's airways and lungs remain clear to auscultation. Secretions are thin and clear and the patient remains normothermic.

1. Assess patient for increased work of breathing or a change in the rate or depth of respirations. Auscultate lung fields for breath sounds, noting presence of crackles

(rales), rhonchi, and diminished or adventitious sounds. Assess for fever, purulent sputum, and cyanosis, and monitor patient's ABG values for evidence of hypoxemia (Pao_2 <80 mm Hg) or hypercapnia ($Paco_2$ >45 mm Hg). Notify MD of significant findings.

2. Encourage patient to breath deeply and change positions q2h to help expand the lungs. Instruct patient to avoid coughing or sneezing, as these activities increase intraabdominal and intrathoracic pressures, which in turn increase ICP and the risk of aneurysm rupture. Explain that if sneezing is unavoidable, it should be done with an open mouth.
3. Maintain patient on oxygen as prescribed.
4. Assist patient with using incentive spirometry, if prescribed.

Potential for disuse syndrome related to imposed activity restrictions secondary to risk of aneurysm rupture or rebleeding

Desired outcome: Patient exhibits complete ROM and maintains muscle mass.

1. To maintain joint mobility, perform passive ROM exercises during the period of activity restriction. Even if the patient feels well enough to perform assisted or active ROM, these activities are contraindicated because they increase ICP and the risk of rupture or rebleeding. Explain to patient the rationale for activity limitation.
2. Maintain joint alignment, and provide support to the joints and extremities with pillows, trochanter rolls, sand bags, and other positioning devices.
3. When the patient is no longer on bed rest and activity restrictions, additional strengthening and conditioning exercises may be necessary to counteract the effects of prolonged bed rest. In addition, the patient may have residual neurologic deficits that necessitate gait training or the use of assistive devices to promote mobility. Obtain a PT/OT referral as appropriate. For additional interventions, see **Potential for disuse syndrome** in "Caring for Patients on Prolonged Bed Rest," p. 653.

Self-care deficit: Inability to perform ADL related to imposed activity restrictions secondary to risk of aneurysm rupture or rebleeding

Desired outcome: Patient's care activities are completed for him or her during the period of strict bed rest.

1. During the period of strict bed rest and activity restrictions, perform care activities, even for patients who do not exhibit signs of neurologic deficit.
2. If patient has bathroom privileges, provide a commode as appropriate, and assist patient with transferring as necessary.

See "Seizure Disorders" for **Potential for trauma** related to oral, musculoskeletal, and airway vulnerability secondary to seizure activity, p. 244. See "General Care of Patients with Neurologic Disorders" for **Potential fluid volume deficit**, p. 250; **Constipation**, p. 252; **Potential for injury** related to IICP, p. 253; and **Pain**, p. 254. For patients with varying degrees of immobility, see "Pressure Ulcers," p. 630, and "Caring for Patients on Prolonged Bed Rest," p. 651. For surgical patients, see "Caring for Preoperative and Postoperative Patients," p. 637. Also see "Caring for Patients with Cancer and Other Life-Disrupting Illnesses," p. 690, as appropriate for psychosocial interventions.

PATIENT-FAMILY TEACHING AND DISCHARGE PLANNING

Provide patient and significant others with verbal and written information for the following:

1. Wound care and indicators of wound infection for patients who have undergone surgery.
2. Importance of avoiding strenuous physical activity. Check with MD regarding activity restrictions/limitations; instruct patient accordingly.
3. Low-sodium (see Table 11-3, p. 550), low-cholesterol (see Table 2-2, p. 48) diet if prescribed to control hypertension and artherosclerosis.

4. Medications, including drug name, rationale, schedule, dosage, precautions, and potential side effects.
5. Signs and symptoms of rupture and rebleeding, for which the patient is at risk for 6 months after the initial bleed.
6. Care of the ventricular shunt, if present. Instructions should include indicators of shunt infection and steps to take in the event of shunt infection or malfunction.

In addition:
7. See the teaching/discharge planning section in "Cerebrovascular Accident," p. 239, for additional interventions for patients who have residual neurologic deficits.

Cerebrovascular accident

A cerebrovascular accident (CVA) is the sudden disruption of oxygen supply to the nerve cells, generally caused by obstruction or rupture in one or more of the blood vessels that supply the brain. *Ischemic CVA* has three main mechanisms: thrombosis, embolism, and systemic hypoperfusion. Thrombosis or embolism results in a blockage of blood supply to the brain tissue. The resulting ischemia, if prolonged, causes brain tissue necrosis (infarction) as well as cerebral edema and IICP. A transient ischemic attack (TIA), which is a temporary (less than 24 hours) neurologic deficit that resolves completely without permanent damage, may precede a permanent ischemic CVA by hours, days, months, or years. Ischemic stroke due to systemic hypoperfusion usually is the result of decreased cerebral blood flow owing to circulatory failure. Circulatory failure results from too little blood, too low a blood pressure, or failure of the heart to pump blood adequately. Hypoxia from any cause also can produce this syndrome. *Hemorrhagic CVA* causes neural tissue destruction because of the infiltration and accumulation of blood. Ischemia and infarction may occur distal to the hemorrhage due to interrupted blood supply. Although a cerebral hemorrhage usually results from hypertension or an aneurysm, trauma also can cause hemorrhagic CVA. Bleeding may occur in the brain tissue itself, causing an intracerebral hemorrhage, or into the subarachnoid space (see "Cerebral Aneurysm," p. 221, for discussion of subarachnoid hemorrhage). CVA is the third most common cause of death and the most common cause of neurologic disability. Half the survivors are left permanently disabled or experience another CVA.

ASSESSMENT

General findings: Classically, symptoms appear on the side of the body opposite that of the damaged site. For example, a CVA in the left hemisphere of the brain will produce symptoms in the right arm and leg. However, when the CVA affects the cranial nerves, the symptoms of cranial nerve deficit will appear on the same side as the site of injury. Similarly, an obstruction of an anterior cerebral artery can produce bilateral symptoms, as will severe bleeding or multiple emboli. Hemiplegia is fairly common. Initially, the patient usually has flaccid paralysis. As spinal cord depression resolves, more normal tone is seen and hyperactive reflexes occur.

Signs and symptoms: Vary with the size and site of injury and may improve in 2-3 days as the cerebral edema decreases. Changes in mentation including apathy, irritability, disorientation, memory loss, withdrawal, drowsiness, stupor, or coma; bowel and bladder incontinence; numbness or loss of sensation; weakness or paralysis of part or one side of the body; aphasia; headache; neck stiffness and rigidity; vomiting; seizures; dizziness or syncope; and fever may occur.

☐ *Cranial nerve involvement:* Visual disturbances including diplopia, blindness, hemianopia; inequality or fixation of the pupils; nystagmus; tinnitus; difficulty chewing and swallowing.

Physical assessment: Papilledema, arteriosclerotic retinal changes, or hemorrhagic retinal areas on ophthalmic exam. Hyperactive DTRs, decreased superficial reflexes, and positive Babinski's sign also may be present. To check for Babinski's response, stroke the lateral aspect of the sole of the foot (from the heel to the ball of the foot) with a hard

T A B L E   4 - 3   Selected hemispheric-related problems associated with CVA

Deficit	Comments	Suggestions

I. Dominant (left) hemisphere damage
A. Impaired verbal communication

Deficit	Comments	Suggestions
1. Aphasia: partial or complete inability to use or comprehend language and symbols	Aphasia is not the result of impaired hearing or intelligence	Treat patient as an adult. It is not necessary to raise your voice unless patient is indeed deaf. Be respectful
	There are many different types of aphasia. The patient generally has a combination of types, which vary in severity	Describe patient's aphasia symptoms, using simple terms and specific examples. Communicate simply; ask questions that have yes or no answers. Progress to more complex statements as indicated
☐ Word deafness: may not recognize or comprehend spoken word (as if a foreign language were being spoken). This is also called sensory, receptive, or Wernicke's aphasia	Patient is frequently good at responding to nonverbal cues, such as gestures and facial expressions	When evaluating patient for aphasia, be aware that patient may be responding to nonverbal cues and may understand less than you think. Use gestures, nonverbal cues, and pantomime to enhance day-to-day communication. Give short, simple directions, and repeat as needed to ensure understanding
☐ Difficulty expressing words, naming objects. This is also called motor, expressive, or Broca's aphasia	Patient may use gestures, groans, swearing, nonsense words. Patient has difficulty with symbols and their meaning, not with the muscles used in speaking. Patient knows what (s)he wants to say but cannot say it. May mix appropriate/	Give patient practice in verbal expression by encouraging him/her to repeat words after you. Listen and respond to patient's communication efforts; otherwise patient may give up. Give practice in receiving word images by pointing to an object and clearly stat-

TABLE 4-3 Selected hemispheric-related problems associated with CVA—cont'd

Deficit	Comments	Suggestions
	inappropriate words or have problems finding words	ing its name. Watch signals patient gives you
☐ Loss of ability to monitor verbal output	Patient may not produce sensible language, but may think s(he) is making sense. Patient will not understand why no one understands or responds appropriately	Avoid labeling patient "belligerent" or "confused" when the problem is aphasia and frustration
☐ Nonrecognition of number symbols or relationships	Impaired ability to do math, calculations Difficulty understanding time concept, telling time	Avoid instructing patient to "wait 5 minutes," as this may not be meaningful
B. Sensory/perceptual alterations	Patient has a better grasp of the "general" scope than of specifics (i.e., can see the forest but not the trees)	
1. Perceptions/ reactions	Can be slow, cautious, or disorganized when approaching an unfamiliar problem	Provide frequent, accurate, and immediate feedback on performance
☐ Impaired ability to think logically, reason (deduction/ induction), and make decisions		Give step-by-step instructions Keep questions simple initially
☐ Poor abstract thinking		Keep conversation on concrete level (use "water" instead of the term "fluid," "leg" instead of "limb")
☐ Short attention span		Keep messages short
2. Impaired contralateral sensory interpretation/ association	Inability to recognize items by touch	Give patient item to feel and name it (e.g., give patient a washcloth and name it as such)

Continued.

TABLE 4-3 Selected hemispheric-related problems associated with CVA—cont'd

Deficit	Comments	Suggestions
3. Visual field deficits	Sees only a portion of normal visual field	Instruct patient to make a conscious effort to scan the rest of the environment by turning head from side to side
	May also have visual "neglect," but this does not happen as often as with right hemisphere damage	Approach patient on unaffected side. Place commonly used items on unaffected side. Check toward end of meal to be sure patient has eaten from both sides of the plate

II. Nondominant (right) hemisphere damage
A. Impaired verbal communication:

1. Copious speech	When speaking, patient may use excessive detail, with irrelevant information. Gets off on a tangent	Bring patient back to the subject by saying, "Let's come back to what we were talking about"

B. Sensory/perceptual alterations

1. Perceptions/ reactions	Denial of disability or loss of abilities; overestimation of abilities; tends to be impulsive and too quick with movements. May lack motivation	Encourage patient to slow down
		Encourage patient to check each step or task as completed
	Unawareness of deficits; impaired judgment	Patient may need to be restrained from attempting unsafe activities
	Patient may be able to describe a task in detail but cannot necessarily perform it	Have patient return demonstrated skills
		Patient may be able to be "talked through" a task step-by-step
		Patient may be able to talk self through a task with verbal cues; encourage this

TABLE 4-3 Selected hemispheric-related problems associated with CVA—cont'd

Deficit	Comments	Suggestions
	Generally retains ability to think logically; sees specifics rather than global picture (i.e., can see the trees, but not the forest)	
☐ Literal association	If, for example, you say you ate the "lion's share," patient may take it literally and think there was a lion at the meal	Be careful what you say, as it may be taken literally
☐ Impaired ability to make subtle distinctions	The distinction between a fork and a spoon may be too subtle	
2. Impaired ability to recognize, associate, or interpret sounds	May not recognize voice qualities, animal noises, musical pieces, types of instruments	If for example, the sound of a cat appears on television, verbally state that it is the sound a cat makes, and point to the cat on the screen
3. Visual-spatial misperception; difficulty comprehending spatial relationships	May underestimate distances and bump into doors. May confuse the inside and outside of an object, such as an article of clothing. May lose place when reading or adding up numbers, and thus never complete the task	
4. Difficulty recognizing and associating familiar objects, environments, or faces	May not recognize dangerous or hazardous objects. Purpose of object is unknown to the patient	May need assistance eating as will not know purpose of silverware; monitor the environment for safety hazards and remove unsafe objects, such as scissors from the bedside

Continued.

T A B L E 4 - 3   Selected hemispheric-related problems associated
with CVA—cont'd

Deficit	Comments	Suggestions
Inability to orient self in space	May not know if (s)he is sitting, standing, or leaning	
5. Misperception of own body and body parts	Potential for self-care deficits May not perceive foot as being a part of the body	Needs to be taught to make a conscious effort to keep track of body parts, for example, by watching feet very carefully while walking
6. Impaired contralateral sensory interpretation/ association: Impaired ability to recognize objects by means of hearing, vision, touch	Patient has difficulty with visual cues	Keep environment simple to reduce sensory overload and enable patient to concentrate on visual cues Remove distracting stimuli
7. Visual field deficit	May only see a portion of normal visual field	See "Visual field deficit" in "Dominant (Left) Hemisphere Damage," p. 230
8. Often has problems with "neglect": auditory/visual field and involved body part		See nursing diagnosis **Unilateral neglect,** p. 235
9. Impaired conceptualization of motor movement pattern	*Apraxia:* inability to perform purposeful movement in the absence of paresis, paralysis, ataxia, and sensory dysfunction, resulting in difficulty making voluntary muscle movements needed for speech, eating, or dressing	

NOTE: Problems will vary, depending on the portion of the brain that has been damaged, as well the severity and type of injury.

object. Dorsiflexion of the great toe with fanning of the other toes is a positive sign. A positive Kernig's or Brudzinski's sign (see "Bacterial Meningitis," p. 168) is indicative of meningeal irritation.

History of: TIAs; hypertension; atherosclerosis; high serum cholesterol or triglycerides; diabetes mellitus; gout; smoking; cardiac valve diseases, such as those that may result from rheumatic fever, valve prosthesis, and atrial fibrillation; cardiac surgery; blood dyscrasias; anticoagulant therapy; neck vessel trauma; oral contraceptive use; family predisposition for arteriovenous malformation (AVM); aneurysm; or previous CVA.

DIAGNOSTIC TESTS

The CT scan or MRI is the test most likely to be obtained for every patient with a suspected stroke. However, technologic advances have provided numerous diagnostic tests for CVA. The selection, sequence, and urgency of these tests will be determined by the patient's history and symptoms. For example, the patient who has a TIA will have a different set or sequence of tests than the patient who is in coma.

1. *CT scan:* To reveal site of infarction, hematoma, and shift of brain structures. CT scan is of particular value in identifying blood released during hemorrhagic strokes. (See "Brain Tumors," p. 215, for patient care.)

2. *MRI:* To reveal site of infarction, hematoma, shift of brain structure, and cerebral edema. MRI is of particular value in identifying ischemic strokes early on. (See "Brain Tumors," p. 214, for patient care.)

3. *Phonoangiography/Doppler ultrasonography:* May identify presence of bruits if there is a partial occlusion of the carotid blood vessels.

4. *Oculoplethysmography:* To obtain indirect measurement of carotid blood flow.

5. *Transcranial Doppler ultrasound:* A noninvasive test that provides information about pressure and flow in the intracranial arteries.

6. *PET:* To provide information on cerebral metabolism and blood flow characteristics. This test is useful in identifying ischemic stroke. (See "Brain Tumors," p. 215, for patient care.)

7. *EEG:* To show abnormal nerve impulse transmission, which will help locate the lesion and/or indicate the amount of brain wave activity present. (See "Seizure Disorders," p. 242, for patient care.)

8. *Brain scan:* Reveals ischemic areas; however, results may not be positive until 2 weeks after the CVA.

9. *Lumbar puncture and CSF analysis:* May reveal increase in CSF pressure; clear to bloody CSF, depending on the type of stroke; and presence of infection or other nonvascular cause for bleeding. CSF glutamic oxaloacetic transaminase (GOT) will be increased for 10 days postinjury. Blood in the CSF signals that a subarachnoid hemorrhage has occurred. (See patient care in "Bacterial Meningitis," p. 161.)

10. *Cerebral angiography:* To pinpoint site of rupture or occlusion and identify collateral blood circulation, aneurysms, or AVM. (See "Cerebral Aneurysm," p. 122, for patient care.)

11. *Digital subtractive angiography (DSA):* To visualize cerebral blood flow and detect vascular abnormalities, such as stenosis, aneurysm, and hematomas. In this test, contast medium is injected into a vein or artery to visualize cerebral circulation. This test is considered a safer procedure than angiography. If the contrast medium is injected into a vein, it carries no risk of embolus and can be performed on an outpatient basis. However, intravenous injection requires more contrast medium than intraarterial injection, putting the patient with impaired kidney function at greater risk.

Preprocedure

□ Patient must be evaluated for the ability to cooperate and lie still during the 30-60 minute procedure. Patients will be expected to lie still and hold their breath on command.

□ Patient must have good cardiac output in order to disperse the dye.

☐ Assess for and notify MD of patient allergies to iodine, shellfish, or radiopaque dyes.
☐ Food and fluid usually are withheld 3-4 hours prior to the test. Sometimes, clear liquids are allowed.
☐ Advise patients they may feel a warm sensation with the dye injection.

Postprocedure

☐ Encourage large amounts of fluid, if not contraindicated, to promote dye excretion by the kidneys.
☐ If an arterial route was used for injection, follow postprocedure guidelines with angiography in "Cerebral Aneurysm," p. 222.

MEDICAL MANAGEMENT AND SURGICAL INTERVENTIONS

1. **Respiratory support:** Maintenance of airway and delivery of oxygen, as needed. IPPB and chest physiotherapy also may be prescribed.
2. **IV fluids:** To maintain fluid and electrolyte balance.
3. **Bed rest during acute stage:** Activity level is increased as patient's condition improves.
4. **Diet:** NPO status if swallow and gag reflexes are diminished or if patient has decreased LOC. A low-sodium and/or low-fat, low-cholesterol diet may be prescribed to minimize other risk factors. Diet may consist of fluids and pureed, soft, or chopped foods, or tube feedings, depending on patient's LOC and ability to chew and swallow.
5. **Pharmacotherapy**
   ☐ *Anticoagulants:* May be used for patients with thrombotic CVAs. Medications include heparin sodium and warfarin sodium to help prevent further thrombosis. If the stroke or neurologic deficit is in evolution (still progressing), anticoagulants may be useful for 24-72 hours. Once the stroke is completed and neurologic status is stable, anticoagulants are no longer useful. Anticoagulants are contraindicated with hemorrhagic CVA.
   ☐ *Antihypertensive agents:* To control high BP.
   ☐ *Antiplatelet medications (e.g., aspirin in conjunction with dipyridamole):* To prevent platelet aggregation that may lead to thrombus formation. Patients with TIAs or those at risk for additional thrombotic strokes may be started on this therapy to prevent future ischemic strokes from thrombosis. **Note:** These medications should not be used in the presence of hemorrhagic CVA.
   ☐ *Vasopressors:* To treat low BP.
   ☐ *Corticosteroids (e.g., dexamethasone) and osmotic diuretics (e.g., mannitol):* To prevent or reduce cerebral edema.
   ☐ *Cimetidine or antacids:* To reduce the risk of GI hemorrhage from gastric ulcer caused by stress or corticosteroid therapy.
   ☐ *Antiepilepsy drugs (e.g., phenytoin or phenobarbital):* To control and prevent seizures.
   ☐ *Sedatives/tranquilizers:* To promote rest. These are used cautiously to avoid further impairment of neurologic function.
   ☐ *Analgesics (e.g., acetaminophen):* To control headache. If CVA is hemorrhagic, aspirin is avoided because it can cause an increase in bleeding.
   ☐ *Stool softeners:* To prevent straining, which can result in IICP.
6. **Physical medicine:** May include PT, OT, and assistive devices or braces so that patient can maintain mobility and independence with ADL. Muscle-strengthening exercises, conditioning exercises, swallowing facilitation exercises, and gait training are also frequently prescribed.
7. **ROM:** To maintain or increase joint function and prevent contractures. Exercises may include passive ROM, active ROM, or active-assistive ROM. Passive ROM is started immediately for all joints.
8. **Speech therapy:** For aphasic and dysarthric patients.
9. **Antiembolism hose:** To help prevent thrombophlebitis and deep-vein thrombosis.

Typically, patients are placed in ICU in the immediate postoperative period for the following surgeries:

10. **Carotid endarterectomy:** Surgical removal of plaque in the obstructed artery to increase blood supply to the brain.

Postoperative assessments should include the following:

□ At least every hour, assess VS and neurologic status, especially of cranial nerves. Note and document patient's ability to swallow, move the tongue, smile, and speak. Monitor for facial drooping, tongue deviation, hoarseness, dysphagia, or loss of facial sensation. Stretching of cranial nerves during surgery is not uncommon and may cause temporary deficit, but all significant findings should be reported to the surgeon. Monitor for the presence of hypertension, which if not controlled, can lead to cerebral infarction.

□ Palpate superficial temporal and facial pulses to evaluate patency of the external carotid artery.

□ Check neck for edema, hematomas, or bleeding as these may lead to airway compromise.

11. **Cerebral artery bypass surgery:** Anastomosis of an extracranial vessel to an intracranial vessel in order to increase blood flow to the brain. The patient typically has an occlusion in the internal carotid artery, which is not accessible through the neck. Most commonly, the superficial temporal artery is anastomosed to the middle cerebral artery in order to provide collateral circulation to the area distal to the stenosis.

Postoperative assessments/interventions should include the following:

□ Assess VS and neurologic status at least qh. Be alert to any neurologic deficit, especially differences on either side of the body or face. Blood pressure must be monitored and kept within MD-prescribed limits to prevent loss of the graft.

□ To prevent impaired circulation to the temporal area, position patient away from operative side. Elevate HOB 30 degrees or as prescribed. Maintain good head, neck, and body alignment to prevent neck flexion or hyperextension. It is critical that there be no pressure on the graft site. Dressings should not be tight or constricting. Nasal cannulas or the elastic bands found on oxygen masks should be taped to the face so that they do not become a constricting band around the graft site. Patients with eyeglasses are not allowed to wear them unless the earpiece on the operative side is removed. These precautions with eyeglasses and other constricting gear often are in effect for up to 3 months following surgery.

□ Ensure that patient maintains bed rest for 24-48 hours.

□ Assess graft patency by palpating or using a Doppler probe on the temporal pulse.

□ Monitor for indicators of IICP. Check head dressing for drainage. Be aware that the scalp may swell. Be alert to patient complaints of burning, which can occur with ischemia. (For additional interventions, see **Potential for injury** related to IICP" in "General Care for Patients with Neurologic Disorders, p. 253.)

12. **Craniotomy:** May be performed for evacuation of a hematoma, repair of a ruptured aneurysm, or application of arterial clips or plastic spray to the involved vessel to prevent further rupture. Craniotomy also may be performed in order to do an embolectomy. This is a controversial procedure. If done, it must be performed within 6-12 hours of the occlusion. (See "Brain Tumor," p. 215, for patient care.)

NURSING DIAGNOSES AND INTERVENTIONS

Unilateral neglect: Disturbed perceptual ability secondary to neurologic insult

Desired outcome: Patient scans environment, responding to stimuli on the affected side.

1. Assess patient's ability to recognize objects to the right or left of his or her visual midline; perceive body parts as his or her own; perceive pain, touch, and temperature sensations; judge distances; orient self to changes in the environment; differentiate left from right; maintain posture sense; and identify objects by sight, hearing, or touch. Document specific deficits.
2. Neglect of the affected side occurs more often with right hemisphere injury. Neglect cannot be totally accounted for on the basis of loss of physical senses. For example, both ears are used in hearing, but with auditory neglect, patient may ignore conversation or noises that occur on the affected side. Assess patient for neglect of the affected side as follows:
   □ *Visual neglect:* Patient does not turn his or her head to see all parts of an object (e.g., he or she may read only half of a page or eat from only one side of the plate). When the patient exhibits signs of visual neglect, continue to place objects necessary for ADL on the unaffected side and approach patient from that side, but gradually increase stimuli on the affected side. For example, while communicating with patient, physically move across her or his visual boundary and stand on that side in order to bring the patient's attention to the neglected side. Encourage patient to turn his or her head and scan the environment. As another example, place patient's food on the neglected side and encourage patient to look to the neglected side and name the food prior to the meal.
   □ *Self-neglect:* Patient does not perceive his or her arm or leg as being a part of the body. For example, when combing or brushing the hair, patient attends to only one (the unaffected) side of the head. Encourage patients to touch their affected sides and make a conscious effort to care for neglected body parts and check them for proper position to ensure against contractures and skin breakdown. To enhance patient's self-recognition, periodically refer to the patient's body parts on the neglected side. When patient is in bed or up in a chair, provide safety measures, such as bedrails and restraints, to prevent patient from attempting to get up, which can occur because of unawareness of the affected side. Teach patient to use unaffected arm to perform ROM exercises on the affected side. Integrate patient's neglected arm into activities. Position the arm on the bedside table, where patient can see it.
   □ *Auditory neglect:* Patient ignores individuals who approach and speak from his or her affected side, but communicates with those who approach or speak from the unaffected side. To stimulate patient's attention to the affected side, move across the auditory boundary while speaking and continue speaking from the patient's neglected side to bring patient's attention to that area.
3. Arrange the environment to maximize performance of ADL by keeping necessary objects on patient's unaffected side. Perform activities on the unaffected side unless you are specifically attempting to stimulate the neglected side. After attempting to stimulate the neglected side, return to patient's unaffected side for activities and communication.

Impaired physical mobility related to alterations in the upper or lower limbs secondary to weakness, hemiparesis, or hemiplegia occurring with CVA

Desired outcome: Patient and significant others demonstrate techniques that enhance ambulating and transferring.

1. Teach patient methods for turning and moving, using the stronger extremity to move the weaker extremity.
2. Encourage patient to make a conscious attempt to look at the extremities and check their position before moving. Remind patient to make a conscious effort to lift and then extend the foot when ambulating.
3. Instruct patient with impaired sense of balance to compensate by leaning toward the stronger side. (The tendency is to lean toward the weaker or paralyzed side.) As necessary, remind patient to keep body weight forward over the feet when standing.
4. Protect impaired arms with a sling to support the arm and shoulder when the patient is up to help maintain anatomic position.
5. Use the Bobarth principle when incorporating patient mobility teaching.

Note: Incorporate the help of other staff members, as necessary, when helping patient with these movements.

☐ The goal is to restore patient's normal bilateral function. Encourage patient to practice normal movement patterns and to establish and maintain correct positioning and posture. Incorporate the patient's affected side into bearing the patient's weight. Use verbal, visual, and tactile stimulation to guide patient in the correct movements.

☐ To bridge (lift hips up) from a supine position: Teach patient to bend knees with feet flat on the bed, stabilize the affected foot by placing the unaffected foot on top of it, and tighten the muscles in the gluteus to lift the hips. Stand on patient's affected side and assist patient by placing hand on patient's knee. Apply downward pressure on the knee while helping to lift the affected hip with your other hand.

☐ To roll in bed: Teach patient to clasp hands together and stretch them upward, bend knees, and turn head to look in the direction of the turn. Explain that the upper body will move first and the lower body will follow. When the patient swings the extended arms toward the side to which he or she will roll, the shoulder and upper torso will turn. The knees should be allowed to follow.

☐ To scoot up in bed: Teach patient to move hips to the side or up in bed using the bridge technique (see above). Explain that it takes two separate movements to scoot up and that the hips and upper body will move at different times. To move the upper body, teach patient to clasp hands together and reach forward while lifting the head. Assist this movement by placing your hand under the patient's scapula to help move the patient's trunk upward.

☐ Correct positioning: When in bed, have patient lie on the affected side as much as possible to help stretch the trunk and counteract abnormal posture. Keep the affected side slightly anterior in its relationship to the rest of the body in each side-lying position, with the head maintained in a neutral position. When the patient is sitting in a chair, ensure that the feet are flat on the floor. Make sure that the hips are well back into the seat. Support the affected arm, ideally on a table.

☐ To adjust a seated position: Stand in front of the patient's affected side. With patient's feet flat on the floor, have patient clasp both hands and reach toward the floor. This action will move the head and trunk forward over the feet and lift the hips from the chair. Assist patient by blocking patient's affected foot with one of your own feet. Reach over patient's back and move patient's hips toward the rear of the seat.

☐ For transferring from bed to chair: Position chair at an angle to the bed and close to the patient's affected side. Stand in front of patient's affected side. Ensure that patient's feet are flat on the floor, with the feet directly under or slightly behind the plane of the knees. Instruct patient to clasp both hands and reach forward, which will bring patient's head and trunk forward over the knees and lift the hips from the bed. Assist patient by leaning over patient's back and moving patient's hips. To accomplish this action, rock backward and shift your weight to your back foot to help leverage the patient upward. Pivot patient's hips toward the chair and lower patient gently to the chair. The patient should maintain a partial standing position. Transferring patients in the direction of their weaker, affected side will improve their weightbearing and muscle tone on that side, which will prepare them for subsequent standing and walking.

Impaired verbal communication related to aphasia or dysarthria secondary to cerebrovascular insult

Desired outcome: Patient demonstrates self-expression and two-way communication.

1. Evaluate the nature and severity of the patient's aphasia. When doing so, avoid giving nonverbal cues. Assess patient's ability to point or look toward a specific object, follow simple directions, understand yes/no questions, understand complex questions, repeat both simple and complex words, repeat sentences, name objects that are shown, demonstrate or relate the purpose or action of the object, fulfill written requests, write requests, and read. Document this assessment, using it as the basis for a communication plan.

2. One example of an intervention in a communication plan for a patient who has difficulty expressing words is to provide practice by having patient repeat words after you. See Table 4-3 for additional information.

3. Obtain a referral to a speech therapist/pathologist as needed. Provide therapist with a list of words that would enhance patient's independence and/or care. In addition, ask for tips that will help improve communication with patient.

4. Communicate with patient as much as possible. General principles include the following: speak slowly and clearly; give patient time to process your communication and answer; keep messages short and simple; stay with one clearly defined subject; avoid questions with multiple choices; phrase questions so that they can be answered "yes" or "no"; and use the same words each time you repeat a statement or question. If patient does not understand after repetition, try different words. Use gestures and facial expressions liberally to supplement and reinforce your message.

5. When helping patients regain use of symbolic language, start with nouns first, and then progress to verbs, pronouns, adjectives.

6. Dysarthria can complicate aphasia. Encourage patient to perform exercises that will increase the ability to control facial muscles and tongue. This includes holding a sound for five seconds, singing the scale, reading aloud, and extending the tongue and trying to touch the chin, nose, or cheek. Encourage patient to exaggerate pronunciation and speak slowly. Teach patient to organize thoughts before speaking and use short sentences and simple words.

7. Provide a supportive and relaxed environment for those patients who are unable to form words or sentences, or who are unable to speak clearly or appropriately. If patient makes an error, do not criticize patient's effort, but rather compliment it by saying "that was a good try." Do not react negatively to patient's emotional displays. Address and acknowledge patient's frustration over the inability to communicate. Maintain a calm and positive attitude. If you do not understand the patient, say so. Ask patient to repeat unclear words, ask for more clues, ask patient to use another word, or have patient point to the object. Observe for nonverbal cues and anticipate patient's needs.

8. For additional interventions for patients with dysarthria, see **Impaired verbal communication** related to dysarthria in "General Care of Patients with Neurologic Disorders," p. 252.

See "Pulmonary Embolus" in "Respiratory Disorders" for **Potential for injury** related to increased risk of bleeding secondary to anticoagulant therapy, p. 16. See "Renal-Urinary Disorders" for a discussion of disorders specific to patient's bladder condition. **Caution:** The Credé maneuver and other interventions that increase intrathoracic or intraabdominal pressure are contraindicated until the risk of IICP is no longer a factor. See "Alzheimer's Disease" for **Altered thought processes,** p. 186. See "Head Injury" for **Potential for disuse syndrome** related to prolonged inactivity, p. 212. See "Seizure Disorders" for **Potential for trauma** related to oral, musculoskeletal, and airway vulnerability secondary to seizure activity, p. 244. See "General Care of Patients with Neurologic Disorders" for the following: **Potential for trauma** related to unsteady gait, p. 248; **Potential impaired tissue integrity** related to risk of corneal irritation/abrasion, p. 249; **Alteration in nutrition:** Less than body requirements, p. 249; **Potential fluid volume deficit,** p. 250; **Potential for ineffective airway clearance,** p. 251; **Self-care deficit,** p. 251; **Constipation,** p. 252; **Potential for injury** related to IICP, p. 253; and **Sensory/perceptual alterations** related to visual disturbances, p. 254. See "Pressure Ulcer," p. 630, and "Caring for Patients on Prolonged Bed Rest," p. 651, for nursing diagnoses and interventions related to immobility. Adjust interventions accordingly if patient has IICP or is at risk for this problem. See "Caring for Patients with Cancer and Other Life-Disrupting Illnesses," p. 690, for appropriate psychosocial nursing diagnoses.

PATIENT-FAMILY TEACHING AND DISCHARGE PLANNING

Provide patient and significant others with verbal and written information for the following:
1. Importance of minimizing or treating the following risk factors: diabetes mellitus, hypertension, high cholesterol, high sodium intake, obesity, inactivity, smoking, prolonged bed rest, and stressful lifestyle.
2. Interventions that increase effective communication in the presence of aphasia or dysarthria.
3. Referrals to the following as appropriate: public health nurse, visiting nurses association, psychologic therapy, vocational rehabilitation agency, home health agencies, and extended and skilled care facilities.
4. For other information, see teaching/discharge interventions, Nos. 3-10, in "Multiple Sclerosis," p. 164.

Section Six SEIZURE DISORDERS

Seizures result from an abnormal, uncontrolled, electrical discharge from the neurons of the cerebral cortex in response to a stimulus. If the activity is localized in one portion of the brain, the individual will have a partial seizure, but when it is widespread and diffuse, a generalized seizure occurs. Symptoms vary widely, depending on the involved area of the cerebral cortex.

Seizure threshold refers to the amount of stimulation needed to cause the neural activity. Although anyone can have a seizure if the stimulus is sufficient, the seizure threshold is lowered in some individuals and this may result in spontaneous seizures. Potential causes for lowered seizure threshold include congenital defects; head injury, particularly that from a penetrating wound; intracranial tumors; infections, such as meningitis or encephalitis; exposure to toxins, such as lead; hypoxia; and metabolic and endocrine disorders, such as hypoglycemia, hypocalcemia, uremia, hypoparathyroidism, and excessive hydration. Phenothiazine, tricyclic antidepressants, and alcohol usage increase the risk of seizure due to lowering of the seizure threshold. For susceptible individuals, "triggers" may include physical stimulation, such as loud music or bright, flashing lights; lack of sleep or food; fatigue; emotional tension or stress; menses or pregnancy; and excessive drug/alcohol use.

Although a seizure itself generally is not fatal, individuals can be injured by hitting their head or breaking bones if they lose consciousness and fall to the ground. Instances of prolonged and repeated generalized seizures, *status epilepticus,* can be life threatening because exhaustion, anoxia, respiratory arrest, and cardiovascular collapse can occur.

ASSESSMENT

There is a great variety of seizures (see Table 4-4), but the following are the most serious or common:

Generalized tonic-clonic (grand mal): Possible prodomal phase of increased irritability, tension, or mood changes preceding the seizure by hours or days. Patient may experience the presence of an aura (a sensory warning, such as a sound, odor, or a flash of light) immediately preceding the seizure by seconds or minutes. The seizure usually does not last more than 2-6 minutes and includes the following phases:

☐ *Tonic (rigid/contracted):* Often lasts only 15 seconds, usually subsiding in less than a minute. Symptoms include loss of consciousness, clenched jaws (potential for tongue to be bitten), apnea (may hear cry as air is forced out of the lungs), and cyanosis. The patient may be incontinent and the pupils may dilate and become nonreactive to light.
☐ *Clonic (rhythmic contraction and relaxation of the extremities and muscles):* May subside in 30 seconds but can last 2-5 minutes. The eyes roll upward and excessive

T A B L E 4 - 4 International classification of epileptic seizures

Classification	Seizure type	Involvement/amplification

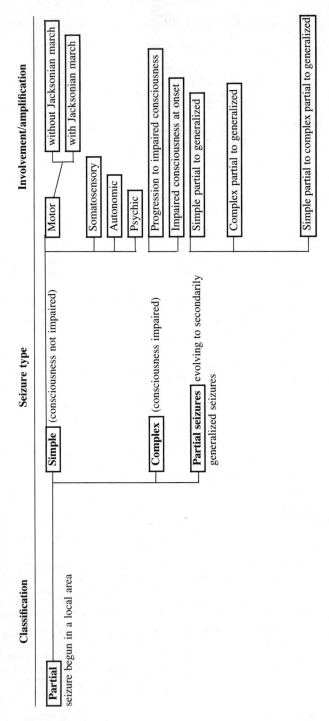

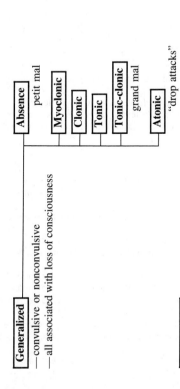

Generalized
—convulsive or nonconvulsive
—all associated with loss of consciousness

Absence
petit mal

Myoclonic

Clonic

Tonic

Tonic-clonic
grand mal

Atonic
"drop attacks"

Unclassified
(cannot be classified due to inadequate or incomplete data)

Adapted from Commission on Classification and Terminology of the International League Against Epilepsy, 1981.

salivation results in foaming at the mouth. During this phase, the potential is greatest for biting the tongue.

□ *Stupor:* May last 5 minutes. The individual is limp and unresponsive. The pupils begin to react to light and return to their normal size.

□ *Postictal:* Patient may be sleepy, semiconscious, confused, unable to speak clearly, uncoordinated, have a headache, complain of muscle aches, and have no recollection of the seizure event.

Generalized absence (petit mal): Patient has momentary loss of awareness with an abrupt cessation of voluntary muscle activity. The patient may appear to be daydreaming with a vacant stare. Patient may experience facial, eyelid, or hand twitching. The individual resumes previous activity when the seizure ends. There is usually no memory of the seizure, and the patient may have difficulty reorienting after the seizure event. This type of seizure can last 1-10 seconds and may occur up to 100 times a day.

Generalized myoclonic: Sudden, very brief contraction or jerking of muscles or muscle groups. The individual may have a very brief, momentary loss of consciousness with some postictal confusion.

Partial simple motor (focal motor seizures): An irritative focus located in the motor cortex of the frontal lobe causes clonic movement in a particular part of the body, such as the hands or face. If the seizure activity spreads or marches in an orderly fashion to adjacent areas (e.g., the hands to the arms to the shoulder), the seizure is termed a focal motor seizure with Jacksonian march. The seizure usually lasts several seconds to minutes.

Partial complex seizure (psychomotor): Generally lasts from 1-4 minutes. Usually there is loss of consciousness and a postictal state of confusion lasting several minutes. However, the individual does not fall to the ground. The patient is able to interact with the environment, exhibits purposeful but inappropriate movements or behavior, and has no memory of the event. The individual will perform such automatisms as lip sucking, chewing, facial grimacing, picking, or swallowing movements. These patients may experience and remember various sensory or emotional hallucinations or sensations that occur immediately prior to the seizure, such as smells, ringing or hissing sounds, or feelings of déjà vu, fear, or pleasure.

Status epilepticus: State of continuous or rapidly recurring seizures in which the individual does not completely recover baseline neurologic functioning between seizures. Individuals who suddenly stop taking their antiepilepsy medication are likely to develop this condition. This is a medical emergency, resulting in potential complications, such as cerebral anoxia and edema, aspiration, hyperthermia, and exhaustion. Death may result.

DIAGNOSTIC TESTS

Because a variety of problems can precipitate seizures, testing may be extensive. Common tests include the following:

1. *Serum electrolytes:* To rule out metabolic causes, such as hypoglycemia or hypocalcemia.
2. *EEG—both sleeping and awake:* May reveal abnormal patterns of electrical activity, particularly with such stimuli as flashing lights or hyperventilation. Telemetry EEGs also may be performed.
   □ *Before the test:* As directed, withhold antiepilepsy medications, sedatives, and tranquilizers for 24-48 hours. Alert EEG staff to drugs the patient is taking, and provide a normal diet to prevent hypoglycemia. If a sleep EEG is prescribed, keep patient awake the night before the test.
   □ *After the test:* Check with MD regarding reinstatement of medications. If needed, provide hairwashing or acetone swabs to remove the paste used for attaching the electrodes.
3. *Positron emission tomography (PET):* May find areas of cerebral glucose hypome-

tabolism, which correlate with the irritative seizure-causing focus. This test is useful in partial seizures. See "Brain Tumor," p. 215, for patient care.

4. *MRI:* May show structural lesions causing partial seizures; also may reveal a space-occupying lesion, such as a tumor or hematoma. See "Brain Tumor," p. 214, for patient care.
5. *CT scan:* May reveal presence of a space-occupying lesion, such as a tumor or hematoma. See "Brain Tumor," p. 215, for patient care.
6. *Skull x-rays:* To reveal fractures, tumors, calcifications, or congenital anomalies (pineal shift, ventricular deformity).
7. *Lumbar puncture and CSF analysis:* To rule out IICP or infection, such as meningitis, as the source of the seizures. See "Bacterial Meningitis," p. 161, for patient care.

MEDICAL MANAGEMENT AND SURGICAL INTERVENTIONS

1. Antiepilepsy drugs: To help prevent seizure activity.
   □ *Hydantoin derivatives (e.g., phenytoin, mephenytoin, or ethotoin):* For tonic-clonic, partial simple, and partial complex seizures.
   □ *Carbamazepine:* For tonic-clonic, partial simple, and partial complex seizures.
   □ *Valproic acid:* For absence, tonic-clonic, and mixed seizures types.
   □ *Succinimide derivatives (e.g., ethosuximide):* For absence seizures.
   □ *Barbiturate derivatives (e.g., phenobarbital or primidone):* May be used in conjunction with one of antiepilepsy drugs above or as monotherapy for tonic-clonic or partial seizures.
2. Treatment of underlying causes: Such as metabolic disorder or infectious process.
3. Nutrition: A balanced diet spaced evenly throughout the day is recommended to avoid hypoglycemia, which may trigger seizures. Patients are advised to avoid caffeine and alcohol products and to prevent overhydration, which also can precipitate seizure activity.
4. Counseling or psychotherapy: For patients with poor self-concept or coping difficulties related to the diagnosis.
5. Surgery: For medically intractable seizures in an attempt to excise as much of known epileptogenic areas as possible without causing new or increased neurologic deficits. Temporal lobectomy or corpus callostomy may be done for seizure control. Brain tumors or hematomas may be removed or evacuated if they are the source of the seizure activity. All of these procedures require a craniotomy (see "Brain Tumor," p. 215).
6. Management of status epilepticus
   □ *Maintenance of patent airway:* Oxygen therapy, oral airway, suctioning, and intubation as needed to prevent airway collapse and hypoxia.
   □ *Assessment of serum glucose and administration of IV glucose:* If indicated, to reverse hypoglycemia.
   □ *Serum drug screens:* To assess serum antiepilepsy drug level and determine the presence of alcohol or other drugs that may be causing the seizures.
   □ *Slow administration of IV diazepam, 2 mg/min.* **Note:** Monitor for signs of respiratory depression and hypotension.
   □ *Administration of IV phenytoin:* If diazepam is unsuccessful.

Note: Do not mix phenytoin with other medications and most IV fluids; give it slowly, undiluted, IV push, at no more than 50 mg/min. It should be given only with normal saline IV fluids as it will precipitate in the presence of D_5W. Monitor for hypotension, apnea, and cardiac dysrhythmias.

   □ *Administration of IV phenobarbital:* If diazepam and phenytoin are unsuccessful. **Note:** Monitor for signs of respiratory depression.
   □ *Administration of thiamine:* If alcohol withdrawal occurs or is suspected.
   □ *Administration of glucocorticosteroids (e.g., dexamethasone):* To relieve cerebral edema.

□ *Administration of paraldehyde:* May be given if other medications are unsuccessful. **Note:** Because the solution reacts negatively with plastic, use a glass syringe for IM and IV routes or a rubber catheter if it is given *via* retention enema.

□ *Intubation and general anesthesia with large doses of short-acting barbiturate or neuromuscular blocking agent:* For severe cases. Neuromuscular blocking agents may stop the movement but will not stop brain activity.

□ *Search for the underlying cause:* May include a wide variety of diagnostic tests (see diagnostic test section, above). Patients in status epilepticus typically are transferred to ICU

NURSING DIAGNOSES AND INTERVENTIONS

Potential for trauma related to oral, musculoskeletal, and airway vulnerability secondary to seizure activity

Desired outcome: Patient exhibits no signs of oral or musculoskeletal trauma or airway compromise following the seizure. Significant others verbalize knowledge of actions that are necessary during seizure activity.

Seizure precautions
1. Pad siderails with blankets or pillows. Keep siderails up and the bed in its lowest position when the patient is in bed.
2. Tape a soft rubber oral airway to the bedside. Keep suction equipment readily available.
3. Avoid using glass or other breakable oral thermometers when taking patient's temperature.
4. Caution patients to lie down and push the call button if they experience a prodromal or aural warning.
5. Do not allow unsupervised smoking.

During the seizure
1. Remain with patient. Observe for, record, and report type, duration, and characteristics of seizure activity and any postseizure response.
2. Prevent or break the fall, and ease patient to the floor if the seizure occurs while patient is out of bed. Keep patient in bed if the seizure occurs while he or she is there.
3. If the patient's jaws are clenched, do not force an object between the teeth as this can break teeth or lacerate oral mucous membranes. If able to do so safely and without damage to oral tissue, insert an airway. Tongue depressors should not be used as they may splinter. A rolled washcloth may be used as an alternative. Never put your fingers in the patient's mouth.
4. Protect patient's head from injury during seizure activity. A towel folded flat may be used to cushion the head from striking the ground. Be sure the head's position does not occlude the airway. Remove objects from the environment that the patient may strike. Pad the floors to protect the patient's extremities.
5. Do not restrain patient, but rather, guide the patient's movements gently to prevent injury.
6. Roll patient into a side-lying position to promote drainage of secretions and maintain a patent airway. Provide oxygen and suction as needed.
7. Loosen tight clothing.
8. Maintain patient's privacy.
9. Administer antiepilepsy drugs as prescribed.

Following the seizure
1. Reassure and reorient patient after the seizure. Ask patient if an aura preceded the seizure activity; record this information.
2. Provide significant others with verbal and written information for the above interventions.

Knowledge deficit: Life-threatening environmental factors and preventive measures for seizures

Desired outcomes: Patient verbalizes accurate information regarding measures that may prevent seizures and environmental factors that can be life-threatening in the presence of seizures. Patient exhibits health care measures that reflect this knowledge.

1. Assess patient's knowledge of measures that can prevent seizures and environmental hazards that can be life-threatening in the presence of seizure activity. Provide or clarify information as indicated.
2. Advise patient to check into state regulations regarding automobile operation. Most states require 1-3 years of being seizure-free before an individual can obtain driver's license.
3. Caution patient to refrain from operating heavy or dangerous equipment, swimming, and possibly even tub bathing until he or she is seizure-free for the amount of time specified by MD. Teach patient never to swim alone, regardless of the amount of time he or she has been seizure-free. Caution patient to swim only in shallow water to make rescue easier in the event of a seizure.
4. Advise patient to turn the temperature of hot water heaters down to prevent scalding should a seizure occur in the shower.
5. Advise patient that some activities, such as climbing or bicycle riding, require careful risk-benefit evaluation.
6. Encourage vocational assessment and counseling. The patient's epilepsy may place others at risk in some occupations, such as bus driver or airline pilot.
7. Advise female patients that seizure activity may change (increase or decrease) during pregnancy. Tonic-clonic seizures have caused fetal death. Antiepilepsy drugs are associated with birth defects. However, 90% of women have normal pregnancies and normal children. Provide birth control information if requested.
8. Teach patient that use of stimulants (e.g., caffeine) and depressants (e.g., alcohol) should be avoided. Withdrawal from stimulants and depressants can increase the likelihood of seizures.
9. Teach patient that getting adequate amounts of rest, avoiding physical and emotional stress, and maintaining a nutritious diet may help prevent seizure activity. If such stimuli as flashing lights appear to trigger seizures, advise patient to avoid environments that are likely to have these stimuli.
10. Encourage patient to wear a Medic-Alert bracelet or similar identification.

Knowledge deficit: Purpose, precautions, and side effects of antiepilepsy medications

Desired outcome: Patient verbalizes accurate information regarding the prescribed antiepilepsy medication.

1. Stress the importance of taking the prescribed medication regularly and on schedule and not discontinuing the medication without MD guidance. Explain that missing a scheduled dose can precipitate a seizure several days later. Stress that abrupt withdrawal of any antiepilepsy medication can precipitate seizures and that discontinuing these medications is the most common cause of status epilepticus. Assist patients with finding methods that will help them remember to take the medication and monitor their drug supply to avoid running out.
2. Reinforce prescribed drug dosage instructions.
3. Stress the importance of informing MD of side effects and keeping appointments for periodic lab work, which determines whether blood levels are therapeutic and assesses for side effects. See Table 4-5 for common side effects and precautions.
4. Explain that antiepilepsy medications may make people drowsy. Advise patient to avoid activities that require alertness until his or her CNS response to the medication has been determined.
5. Caution patients who are taking phenytoin that there are two types of this drug. Dilantin Kapseal is absorbed more slowly and is longer acting. It is important not to confuse this extended-release phenytoin with prompt-release phenytoin. Doing so may cause dangerous underdosage or overdosage. Generic phenytoin should not be substituted for Dilantin Kapseal.

TABLE 4 - 5 Common antiepilepsy drugs

Name	Side effects	Precautions
phenytoin (Dilantin)	Drowsiness, ataxia, diplopia, gingival hypertrophy, nystagmus, nausea, vomiting, increased body hair, rash, or blood dyscrasias	Ensure frequent oral hygiene, gum massage, and gentle flossing. Take drug with food or large amounts of liquid to decrease gastric upset. Periodic blood counts are necessary. Call MD if rash or jaundice appears. Vitamin K may be given to pregnant women 1 month before and during delivery to prevent neonatal hemorrhage. If prescribed, supplement with vitamins K and D and folic acid
carbamazepine (Tegretol)	Blood dyscrasias, ataxia, rash, nystagmus, diplopia, nausea, vomiting, liver damage, drowsiness, and dizziness	Check CBC frequently. Patient should report fever, mouth ulcers, sore throat, bruising, or bleeding immediately. Take drug with food. Liver and renal function tests should be performed periodically. Report jaundice to MD
phenobarbital (Luminal)	Drowsiness, lethargy, dizziness, nausea, vomiting, constipation, ataxia, and depression	Do not stop abruptly as this may cause withdrawal seizures. Avoid alcohol, which would potentiate CNS depressant effects. Vitamin D supplements usually are advised. Take with foods to prevent stomach upset. Vitamin K usually is given to pregnant women 1 month before and during labor to prevent neonatal hemorrhage

T A B L E   4 - 5   Common antiepilepsy drugs—cont'd

Name	Side effects	Precautions
primidone (Mysoline)	Drowsiness, emotional changes including depression, irritability, ataxia, decreased muscle coordination, nausea, vomiting, impotence	Do not stop abruptly as it may cause withdrawal seizures. Take with food or large amounts of fluid. See information above with phenobarbital regarding alcohol avoidance and vitamin K
ethosuximide (Zarontin)	Gastric distress, nausea, vomiting, dizziness, drowsiness, aplastic anemia, vaginal bleeding	Take with food or large amounts of fluid. Follow-up lab studies are important for detecting anemia. Patient should report fever, mouth ulcers, sore throat, bruising, and bleeding immediately
valproic acid (Depakote)	Sedation, dizziness, nausea/vomiting, anorexia, liver damage, transient alopecia, ataxia	Do not chew as it may irritate mucous membranes. Take with food to prevent gastric upset. Patient should report any bleeding or bruising immediately and monitor liver function studies through periodic lab tests. This drug may produce false-positive test for ketones in the urine

6. Instruct patient to notify MD if a significant weight gain or weight loss occurs because it may necessitate a change in dosage or scheduling.
7. Teach patient to avoid alcoholic beverages or OTC medications containing alcohol. Chronic alcohol use stimulates the body to metabolize phenytoin more quickly, thereby lowering the seizure threshold owing to the decreased plasma phenytoin levels.

Noncompliance with the therapy related to denial of the illness or perceived negative consequences of the treatment regimen secondary to social stigma, negative side effects of antiepilepsy medications, or difficulty with making necessary lifestyle changes

Desired outcome: Patient verbalizes knowledge of the disease process and treatment plan, acknowledges consequences of continued noncompliant behavior, and follows the agreed-on plan of care.

1. Assess patient's understanding of the disease process, medical management, and treatment plan. Explain or clarify information as indicated.
2. Assess for causes of noncompliance, such as medication side effects or difficulty with making significant lifestyle changes or with following the medication schedule.
3. Evaluate patient's perception of his or her vulnerability to the disease process, and be alert to signs of denial of the illness. In addition, evaluate patient's perception of the effectiveness or noneffectiveness of treatment.
4. Determine if a value, cultural, or spiritual conflict is causing noncompliance.
5. Assess patient's support systems. Determine whether the presence of a family disruption pattern (whether or not it is caused by the patient's illness), is making compliance difficult and "not worth it."
6. Once the reason for noncompliance is found, intervene accordingly to ensure compliance. If it appears that a change in the medical treatment plan (e.g., in scheduling medications) may promote compliance, discuss this with MD. Provide patient with information regarding interventions that can minimize the drug side effects. (See Table 4-5, p. 246.) Encourage involvement with support systems, such as local epilepsy centers and national organizations.

See "Caring for Patients with Cancer and Other Life-Disrupting Illnesses" in the appendix for **Body image disturbance**, p. 696, **Ineffective individual coping**, p. 693, and **Alteration in family processes**, p. 699.

PATIENT-FAMILY TEACHING AND DISCHARGE PLANNING

Provide patient and significant others with verbal and written information for the following:
1. Reinforcement of knowledge of the disease process, pathophysiology, symptoms, and the precipitating or aggravating factors.
2. Medications, including purpose, dosage, schedule, and potential side effects. See Table 4-5, "Common Antiepilepsy Drugs."
3. Importance of follow-up care and keeping medical appointments. Stress that use of antiepilepsy drugs necessitates periodic monitoring of blood levels to ensure therapeutic medication levels and assessment for side effects.
4. Environmental factors that can be life-threatening in the presence of seizures and measures that may help prevent seizures. Review state and local laws that apply to individuals with seizure disorders.
5. Employment or vocational counseling as needed.
6. Risks of antiepilepsy drugs during pregnancy. Provide birth control information or genetic counseling referral as requested.

In addition:
7. Provide the following address as appropriate: Epilepsy Foundation of America, 4351 Garden City Drive, Suite 406, Landover, MD 20785, (301)-459-3700.

Section Seven   GENERAL CARE OF PATIENTS WITH NEUROLOGIC DISORDERS

NURSING DIAGNOSES AND INTERVENTIONS

Potential for trauma related to unsteady gait secondary to sensorimotor deficit

Desired outcomes: Patient is free of trauma caused by gait unsteadiness. Patient demonstrates proficiency with assistive devices, if appropriate.

1. Evaluate patient's gait, and assess for motor deficit, such as weakness or paralysis. Document baseline neurologic and physical assessments so that changes in status can be detected promptly.

2. To minimize the risk of injury, assist patient as needed when unsteady gait, weakness, or paralysis is noted.
3. Orient patient to new surroundings. Keep necessary items (including water, telephone, and call light) within easy reach of patient. Assess patient's ability to use these items. The patient who is very weak or partially paralyzed may require a tap bell instead of a call light.
4. Maintain an uncluttered environment to minimize the risk of tripping. Ensure adequate lighting at night (e.g., a night light) to help prevent falls in the dark. In addition, keep siderails up and the bed in its lowest position.
5. For unsteady, weak, or partially paralyzed patient, encourage use of low-heel, nonskid shoes for walking. Teach the use of a wide-based gait to provide a broader base of support. Teach, reinforce, and encourage use of canes, walkers, and crutches to provide patient with added stability. Teach exercises that strengthen arm and shoulder muscles for using walkers and crutches. Teach patients in wheelchairs how and when to lock and unlock the wheels.
6. Review with patient and significant others potential safety needs at home, such as safety appliances (wall, bath, and toilet rails; elevated toilet seat). Loose rugs should be removed to prevent slipping and falling. Temperatures on hot water heaters should be turned down to prevent scalding in the event of a fall in the shower or tub.
7. Seek a referral to a physical therapist as appropriate.

Sensory/perceptual alterations related to impaired pain, touch, and temperature sensations secondary to sensory deficit or decreased LOC

Desired outcome: Patient is asymptomatic of trauma caused by impaired pain, touch, and temperature sensations.

1. Assess patient for indicators of sensory deficits, such as decreased or absent vision and impaired temperature and pain sensation. Document baseline neurologic and physical assessments so that changes in status can be detected promptly.
2. Protect patient from exposure to hot food or equipment that can burn the skin. Avoid use of heating pads.
3. Always check the temperature of heating devices and bath water before patient is exposed to them. Teach patient and significant others about these precautions.
4. Inspect patient's skin daily for evidence of irritation. Teach coherent patient to perform self-inspection daily, and provide a mirror for inspecting posterior aspects of the body.

Potential for impaired tissue integrity related to risk of corneal irritation/abrasion secondary to diminished blink reflex or inability to close the eyes

Desired outcome: Patient's corneas remain clear and intact.

1. Normally, blinking occurs every 5-6 seconds. If patient has a diminished blink reflex and/or is stuporous or comatose, assess the eyes for irritation or the presence of foreign objects. Instill prescribed eye drops or ointment to prevent corneal irritation. Instruct coherent patients to make a conscious effort to blink the eyes several times a minute to help prevent corneal irritation.
2. For patient who is unable to close the eyes completely, apply an eyeshield or tape the eyes shut.

Alteration in nutrition: Less than body requirements related to decreased intake secondary to chewing and swallowing deficits, fatigue, weakness, paresis, paralysis, visual neglect, or decreased LOC

Desired outcome: Patient maintains baseline weight.

1. For patient with chewing or swallowing difficulties, assess alertness, ability to cough, and swallow and gag reflexes before all meals. Keep suction equipment at the bedside if indicated. If patient cannot chew or swallow effectively or safely, enteral or parenteral nutrition may be necessary. Alert MD to your findings.
2. For patient who has only slight difficulty chewing or swallowing, request soft, semisolid, or chopped foods. Although a pureed diet may be needed eventually,

this type of food can be unappealing to many people and may have a negative impact on patient's self-concept.

3. To help patient focus on swallowing, reduce other stimuli in the room (e.g., turn off the TV or radio).

4. Teach patient to break down the act of swallowing, which will help prevent choking or the fear of choking: Place food on the tongue, use tongue to transfer food so it is directly under the teeth on the unaffected side of the mouth, chew the food thoroughly, hold the breath, and then swallow.

5. Evaluate patient's food preferences and offer small, frequent servings. Plan mealtimes for periods during which the patient is rested; use a warming tray or microwave oven to keep the food warm and appetizing until the patient is able to eat.

6. Encourage liquid nutritional supplements and try different methods of making them more palatable. For example, making a milkshake, serving it over ice, or diluting with carbonated beverages may appeal to some tastes.

7. Cut up foods, unwrap silverware, and otherwise "set up" the food tray so that patients with a weak or paralyzed arm can manage the tray one-handed.

8. For patient with "visual neglect," place food within patient's unaffected visual field and return during the meal to make sure she or he has eaten from both sides of the plate. Turn the plate around so that any remaining food is in patient's visual field.

9. Feed or assist very weak or paralyzed patients. If not contraindicated, position patient in a chair or elevate HOB as high as possible. Ensure that patient's head is flexed slightly forward to close the airway. Begin with small amounts of food. Do not hurry patient. Be sure that each bite is completely swallowed before giving another.

10. If appropriate, provide assistive devices, such as built-up utensil handles, broad-handled spoons, spill-proof cups, sectionalized plates, and other devices that promote self-feeding and independence.

11. Provide materials for oral hygiene after meals to minimize risk of aspiration of food particles. Good oral hygiene will also help maintain integrity of the mucous membranes to minimize risk of stomatitis, which may prevent adequate oral intake. Provide oral care for patients unable to do so for themselves.

12. Weigh patient regularly (at least weekly) to assess for loss/gain. If indicated, notify MD of the potential need for high-protein/high-calorie supplements.

13. For the weak, debilitated, or partially paralyzed patient, assess support systems, such as family or friends who can assist patient with meals. Consider referral to an organization that will deliver a daily meal to patient's home.

14. If appropriate for patient's diagnosis (e.g., multiple sclerosis) consider referral to a speech pathologist for exercises that enhance the ability to swallow.

Potential fluid volume deficit related to decreased intake secondary to dysphagia, weakness, paresis, paralysis, or decreased LOC

Desired outcome: Patient is normovolemic as evidenced by balanced I&O, stable weight, good skin turgor, moist mucous membranes, BP within patient's normal range, HR ≤100 bpm, normothermia, and urinary output ≥30 ml/hr.

1. Monitor I&O to assess for fluid volume imbalance; ensure that weight is measured daily if patient is at risk for sudden fluid shifts or imbalances. Patients with neurologic deficits may have great difficulty attaining adequate intake of fluids. Alert MD to a significant I&O imbalance, which may signal the need for enteral or IV therapy to prevent dehydration.

2. Assess for and teach patient the indicators of dehydration, including thirst, poor skin turgor, decreased BP, increased pulse rate, dry skin and mucous membranes, increased body temperature, and decreased urinary output.

3. Evaluate patient's fluid preferences and offer fluids q1-2h. For nonrestricted patients, encourage a fluid intake of at least 2-3 L/day.

4. If not contraindicated, assist patient into high-Fowler's position to facilitate oral fluid intake. Instruct patient to flex the head slightly forward, which closes the airway and helps prevent aspiration. Teach patient with hemiparalysis or hemiparesis to tilt the head toward the unaffected side to facilitate intake.

5. If patient has difficulty swallowing, provide nectars and other thick fluids, which are better tolerated than thin fluids. Instruct patient to sip rather than gulp fluids.
6. For patients at risk for IICP, maintain fluid restrictions.

Potential ineffective airway clearance related to coughing and swallowing deficits secondary to facial and throat muscle weakness or decreasing LOC

Desired outcome: Patient's airway is clear as evidenced by RR 12-20 breaths/min with normal depth and pattern (eupnea), normal color, normal breath sounds, normothermia, and absence of adventitious breath sounds.

1. Monitor patient for the presence of dyspnea, pallor, restlessness, diaphoresis, and a change in the rate or depth of respirations. Auscultate lung fields for breath sounds. Note the presence of crackles (rales), rhonchi, or wheezes, and diminished or adventitious breath sounds. Assess effectiveness of patient's cough and the quality, amount, and color of the sputum. Measure body temperature q4h. Often, a low-grade fever (100° F or less) is indicative of the need for aggressive pulmonary hygiene.
2. Teach patient to deep breathe and cough, and assist with repositioning at least q2h. **Caution:** Instruct patients at risk for IICP not to cough, as it increases intraabdominal and intrathoracic pressure, which in turn increase ICP. Explain that if sneezing is unavoidable, it should be done with an open mouth to minimize the increase in ICP.
3. Assess swallow and gag reflexes. If poor or absent, withhold oral fluids and foods, and inform MD of the possible need for IV therapy or enteral or parenteral nutrition.
4. Keep HOB elevated after meals or assist patient into a right side-lying position to minimize the potential for regurgitation and aspiration. Provide oral hygiene after meals to prevent aspiration of food particles.
5. Assist with prescribed postural drainage (for patients *not* at risk for IICP), chest physiotherapy, and IPPB. Provide incentive spirometry as indicated.
6. Keep oxygen and suction apparatus available as indicated.

Self-care deficit: Inability to perform ADL related to spasticity, tremors, weakness, paresis, paralysis, or decreasing LOC secondary to sensorimotor deficits

Desired outcome: Patient performs care activities independently and demonstrates the ability to use adaptive devices for successful completion of ADL. (Totally dependent patients express satisfaction with activities that are completed for them.)

1. Assess patient's ability to perform ADL.
2. As appropriate, demonstrate use of adaptive devices, such as long- or broad-handled combs, brushes, and eating utensils; nonspill cups; and stabilized plates, all of which may assist the patient with maintaining independence of care. For self-care interventions for oral hygiene, see the same nursing diagnosis in "Stomatitis," p. 315, in "Gastrointestinal Disorders."
3. To facilitate dressing and undressing, encourage patient or significant others to buy shoes without laces and loose-fitting clothing or clothing with snaps or Velcro closures.
4. Place a stool in the shower if sitting down will enhance self-care with bathing. Provide a commode chair or elevated toilet seat if it will facilitate self-care with elimination. Teach self-transfer techniques that will enable patient to get to the commode or toilet.
5. Some individuals may have difficulty with perineal care after elimination. For many patients with limited hand or arm mobility, a long-handled reacher that can hold tissues or washcloth may help patient maintain independence with perineal care.
6. For patient with hemiparesis or hemiparalysis, teach use of the stronger or unaffected hand and arm for dressing, eating, bathing, and grooming.
7. Obtain a referral to an OT if indicated.
8. Provide care to the totally dependent patient and assist those who are not totally dependent. Do not hurry patient. Involve significant others with care activities if they are comfortable with doing so.
9. If indicated, teach patient self-catheterization, or teach the technique to the care-

giver. Provide instructions for catheter care if patient is to be discharged with an indwelling catheter.

Impaired verbal communication related to dysarthria secondary to facial/throat muscle weakness, intubation, or tracheostomy

Desired outcome: Patient communicates effectively, either verbally or nonverbally.

1. If appropriate, obtain referral to a speech therapist/pathologist for assisting patient with strengthening muscles used in speech.
2. Provide a supportive and relaxed environment for those patients who are unable to form words or sentences or who are unable to speak clearly or appropriately. Acknowledge patient's frustration over the inability to communicate. Maintain a calm, positive attitude. Ask patient to repeat unclear words. Observe for nonverbal cues; watch patient's lips closely. Do not interrupt. Anticipate needs and phrase questions to allow simple answers, such as yes or no.
3. Provide alternative methods of communication if patient is unable to speak, for example, a language board, flash cards, or a system that uses eyeblinks, bell signal taps, or gestures, such as hand signals and head nods. Document method of communication used.
4. If patient's voice is very weak and difficult to hear, reduce environmental noise to enhance listener's ability to hear words. Suggest that patient take a deep breath before speaking; provide a voice amplifier if appropriate for patient. Encourage patients to organize thoughts and plan what they will say before speaking. Encourage patients to express ideas in short phrases or sentences, exaggerate pronunciation, and use facial expressions.
5. If patient has swallowing difficulties that result in the accumulation of saliva, suction the mouth to promote clearer speech.
6. For patients with muscle rigidity or spasm, massage the facial and neck muscles prior to a communication effort.
7. If patient has a tracheostomy, ensure that a tap bell is within reach. It may be necessary to place the bell on the pillow near the patient's head so that patient can activate the device with head movement. Reassure tracheostomy patient that the inability to speak is only temporary.

Constipation related to inability to chew and swallow a high-roughage diet, side effects of medications, and immobility

Desired outcome: Patient passes soft, formed stools and maintains his or her normal bowel pattern.

1. Although a high-roughage diet is ideal for the patient who is immobilized or on prolonged bed rest, the individual with chewing and swallowing difficulties may be unable to consume such a diet. For these patients, encourage use of natural fiber laxatives such as psyllium (e.g., Metamucil).
2. A bowel elimination program may include the following elements: setting a regular time of day for attempting a bowel movement, preferably 30 minutes after eating a meal; using a medicated suppository 15-30 minutes before a scheduled attempt; bearing down by contracting the abdominal muscles or applying manual pressure to the abdomen to help increase intraabdominal pressure; and drinking 4 oz of prune juice nightly. **Caution:** SCI patients with involvement at T-6 and above should employ *extreme* caution if use of an enema or suppository is unavoidable, because either can precipitate life-threatening autonomic dysreflexia (AD). Liberal application of anesthetic jelly into the rectum should precede their use. In addition, instruct patient at risk of IICP not to bear down with bowel movements because this action can cause increased intraabdominal pressure, which in turn increases ICP.
3. If indicated by patient's diagnosis (e.g., multiple sclerosis), provide instructions for digital stimulation of the anus to promote reflex bowel evacuation. **Caution:** This intervention is contraindicated for SCI patients with involvement at T-6 or above because it can precipitate life-threatening AD.
4. For other interventions, see **Constipation**, p. 656, in "Caring for Patients on Prolonged Bed Rest."

Potential for injury related to risk of increased intracranial pressure (IICP) and herniation secondary to positional factors, increased intrathoracic or intraabdominal pressure, fluid volume excess, hyperthermia, or discomfort

Desired outcome: Patient is asymptomatic of IICP and herniation as evidenced by stable or improving Glasgow Coma Scale score; stable or improving sensorimotor functioning; BP within patient's normal range; HR 60-100 bpm; pulse pressure 30-40 mm Hg (the difference between the systolic and diastolic BPs); orientation to person, place, and time; normal vision; bilaterally equal and normoreactive pupils; RR 12-20 breaths/min with normal depth and pattern (eupnea); normal gag, corneal, and swallowing reflexes; and absence of headache, nausea, nuchal rigidity, posturing, and seizure activity.

1. Monitor for and report any of the following indicators of IICP or impending/occurring herniation:
   □ *Early indicators of IICP:* Declining Glasgow Coma Scale score (see p. 207), alterations in LOC ranging from irritability, restlessness, and confusion to lethargy; possible onset of or worsening of headache; beginning pupillary dysfunction, such as sluggishness; visual disturbances, such as diplopia or blurred vision; onset of or increase in sensorimotor changes or deficits, such as weakness; onset of or worsening of nausea.
   □ *Late indicators of IICP* (which usually signal impending or occurring brain stem herniation): Continuing decline in Glasgow Coma Scale score (see p. 207); continued deterioration in LOC leading to stupor and coma; projectile vomiting; hemiplegia; posturing; widening pulse pressure, decreased HR, and increased systolic BP; Cheyne-Stokes breathing or other respiratory irregularity; pupillary changes, such as inequality, dilatation, and nonreactivity to light; papilledema; and impaired brain stem reflexes (corneal, gag, swallowing).
   □ *Brain herniation:* Deep coma, fixed and dilated pupils (first unilateral and then bilateral), posturing progressing to bilateral flaccidity, and continuing deterioration in VS and respirations.
2. If changes occur, prepare for possible transfer of patient to ICU. Insertion of ICP sensors for continuous ICP monitoring, CSF ventricular drainage, intubation, mechanical ventilation, neuromuscular blocking, or barbiturate coma therapy may be necessary.
3. For patients at risk for IICP, prevention of hypoxia and CO_2 retention is essential for preventing vasodilatation of cerebral arteries. Preventive measures include ensuring a patent airway, delivering oxygen as prescribed, hyperventilating ("sighing" or bagging) patient before suctioning, and limiting suction to 10-15 seconds. Reduce $Paco_2$ *via* hyperventilation by instructing conscious patients to take deep breaths on their own or by providing manual or machine hyperventilation when patient is intubated or has a tracheostomy.
4. Promote venous blood return to the heart to reduce cerebral congestion by keeping HOB elevated at 15-30 degrees (unless otherwise directed); maintaining head-and-neck alignment to avoid hyperextension, flexion, or turning; ensuring that tracheostomy and endotracheostomy ties or oxygen tubing does not compress the jugular vein; and avoiding Trendelenburg position for any reason. Ensure that pillows under the patient's head are flat so that the head is in a neutral rather than flexed position.
5. Take precautions against increased intraabdominal and intrathoracic pressure in the following ways: teach patient to exhale when turning; provide passive ROM exercises rather than allow active or assistive exercises; administer prescribed stool softeners or laxatives to prevent straining at stool; avoid enemas and suppositories because they can cause straining; instruct patient not to move self in bed as it requires a pushing movement; assist patient with sitting up and turning; instruct patient to avoid coughing and sneezing, or if unavoidable, to do so with an open mouth; instruct patient to avoid hip flexion (increases intraabdominal pressure); do not place patient in a prone position; and avoid using restraints (straining against them increases ICP). In addition, rather than have patient perform the Valsalva maneuver to prevent an air embolism during insertion of central venous catheter, MD should use a syringe to aspirate air from the catheter lumen.

6. Help reduce cerebral congestion by enforcing fluid limitations as prescribed, typically to <1,500 ml/day. Keep accurate I&O records. When administering additional IV fluids, for example with IV drugs, avoid using D_5W because its hypotonicity can increase cerebral edema.

7. Because fever increases metabolic requirements and aggravates hypoxia, help maintain patient's body temperature within normal limits by giving prescribed antipyretics, keeping patient's trunk warm to prevent shivering, and administering tepid sponge baths or hypothermia blanket to reduce fever. If prescribed, administer chlorpromazine to prevent shivering, which would increase ICP.

8. Administer prescribed osmotic and loop diuretics to reduce cerebral edema and produce a state of dehydration. Administer glucocorticosteroids to reduce edema and inflammation. Administer BP medications as prescribed to keep BP within prescribed limits that will promote optimal cerebral blood flow without increasing cerebral edema. Because pain can increase BP and consequently increase ICP, administer prescribed analgesics promptly and as necessary. Barbiturates and narcotics are usually contraindicated because of the potential for masking the signs of IICP and causing respiratory depression.

9. Administer antiepilepsy drugs as prescribed to prevent or control seizures, which would increase cerebral metabolism, hypoxia, and CO_2 retention, thereby increasing cerebral edema and ICP.

10. Monitor bladder drainage tubes for obstruction or kinks, as a distended bladder can increase ICP.

11. Provide a quiet and soothing environment. Control noise and other environmental stimuli. Avoid jarring the bed. Try to avoid situations in which the patient may become emotionally upset. Limit visitors as necessary.

12. Because multiple procedures and nursing care activities can increase ICP by increasing discomfort and anxiety, individualize care to ensure optimal spacing of activities. Rousing patients from sleep has been shown to increase ICP. Plan activities and treatments accordingly so that patient can sleep undisturbed as often as possible.

Sensory/perceptual alterations related to visual disturbance secondary to diplopia

Desired outcome: Patient verbalizes that his or her vision has improved.

1. Assess patient for the presence of diplopia.
2. If patient has diplopia, provide an eye patch or eyeglasses with a frosted lens. Alternate the eye patch q4h.

Pain related to spasms, headache, and photophobia secondary to neurologic dysfunction

Desired outcome: Patient's subjective evaluation of discomfort improves, as documented by a pain scale.

1. Assess duration and intensity of patient's pain or spasms. Devise a pain scale with patient, documenting discomfort on a scale of 0 (no discomfort) to 10. Administer analgesics and antispasmodics as prescribed; document effectiveness of the medication, using the pain scale. Teach patient and significant others the importance of timing the pain medication so that is it taken before the pain becomes too severe and prior to major moves.

2. Instruct patient and significant others in the use of nonpharmacologic pain management techniques, such as repositioning; backrubs, massage, and tactile distraction; auditory distraction, such as soothing music; guided imagery; relaxation tapes and techniques; biofeedback; and a TENS device, as appropriate. See **Health-seeking behaviors:** Relaxation technique effective for stress reduction, p. 49.

3. Teach patient about the relationship between anxiety and pain as well as other factors that enhance pain and spasms (e.g., staying in one position for too long, fatigue, and chilling).

4. If patient has photophobia, provide a quiet and dark environment. Close the door and curtains; avoid artificial lights whenever possible.

SELECTED REFERENCES

Adams RD and Victor M: Principles of neurology, ed 3, New York, 1985, McGraw-Hill Book Co.

Berry P and Ward-Smith PA: Adrenal medullary transplant as a treatment for Parkinson's disease: perioperative considerations, J Neurosci Nurs 20(6):356-361, 1988.

Brewer K and Sperling MR: Neurosurgical treatment of intractable epilepsy, J Neurosci Nurs 20(6):366-371, 1988.

Browner CM et al: Halo immobilization brace care: an innovative approach, J Neurosci Nurs 19(1):24-39, 1987.

Caplan LR: Stroke, Clinical Symposia 40(4):1-32, 1988.

Day LJ et al: Orthopaedics. In Way LW et al: Current surgical diagnosis and treatment, ed 8, San Mateo, Calif and Norwalk, Conn, 1988, Appleton & Lange.

Dejong RN et al: 1988 yearbook of neurology and neurosurgery, Chicago, 1988, Yearbook Medical Publishers, Inc.

Delgado JM and Billo JM: Care of the patient with Parkinson's disease: surgical and nursing interventions: J Neurosci Nurs 20(3):142-150, 1988.

Ferguson JM: Helping an MS patient live a better life, RN 50(12):22-27, 1987.

Gary R et al: Stroke—how to contain the damage, RN 49(5):36-41, 1986.

Gary R et al: Stroke—how to start the long road back, RN 49(6):49-55, 1986.

Goddard LR: Sexuality and spinal cord injury, J Neurosci Nurs 20(4):240-243, 1988.

Govoni LE and Hayes JE: Drugs and nursing implications, ed 6, Norwalk, Conn and San Mateo, Calif, 1988, Appleton and Lange.

Hall GR: Alterations in thought processes, J Gerontol Nurs 14(3):30-37, 1988.

Hartshorn JC: Decreasing side effects of anticonvulsants, Dimens Crit Care 5(1):30-40, 1986.

Hickey JV: The clinical practice of neurological and neurosurgical nursing, ed 2, Philadelphia, 1986, JB Lippincott Co.

Huff FJ et al: The neurologic examination in patients with probable Alzheimer's disease, Arch Neurol 44(9):929-932, 1987.

Koch F and Poisson C: Targeting cerebral tumors, AORNJ 49(3):741-757, 1989.

Komblith PL et al: Neurologic oncology, Philadelphia, 1987, JB Lippincott Co.

Kramer J: Intervertebral disk diseases: causes, diagnosis, treatment, and prophylaxis, Chicago, 1981, Yearbook Medical Publishers, Inc.

Lannon MC et al: Comprehensive care of the patient with Parkinson's disease, J Neurosci Nurs 18(3):121-131, 1986.

Lederer JR et al: Careplanning pocket guide: a nursing diagnosis approach, ed 2, Redwood City, 1988, Addison-Wesley Publishing Co.

Liddel DB: Anterior cervical discectomy—a basis for planning nursing care, J Neurosci Nurs 18(1):29-35, 1986.

McCash AM: Meeting the challenge of craniotomy care, RN 48(6):26-35, 1985.

McCormick KB: Pregnancy and epilepsy: nursing implications, J Neurosci Nurs 19(2):66-74, 1987.

Metcalf JA: Acute phase management of persons with spinal cord injury: a nursing diagnosis perspective, Nurs Clin North Am 21(4):589-610, 1986.

Mims BC: Back surgery: helping your patient get through it, RN 48(5):27-34, 1985.

Mitchell PH: Intracranial hypertension: influence on nursing care activities, Nurs Clin of North Am 21(4):563-574, 1986.

Mitchell S and Yates RR: Cerebral vasospasm: theoretical causes, medical management, and nursing implications, J Neurosci Nurs 18(6):315-324, 1986.

Nurse Review Series: Neurologic problems, Springhouse, Pa, 1987, Springhouse Corporation.

Passarella P and Gee Z: Starting right after stroke, Am J Nurs 87(6):802-807, 1987.

Passarella P and Lewis N: Nursing application of Bobath principles in stroke care, J Neurosci Nurs 19(2):106-109, 1987.

Pettibone KA: Management of spasticity in spinal cord injury: nursing concerns, J Neurosci Nurs 20(4):217-221, 1988.

Pimental PA: Alterations in communication: biopsychosocial aspects of aphasia, dysarthria, and right hemisphere syndromes in the stroke patient, Nurs Clin North Am 12(2):321-337, 1986.

Prendergast V: Bacterial meningitis update, J Neurosci Nurs 19(2):95-99, 1987.

Reimer M: Head-injured patients, Nursing 89 19(3):34-41, 1989.

Reisberg B: Stages of cognitive decline. Am J Nurs 1984; 84:225-228, 1984.

Santilli N and Seirzant TL: Advances in the treatment of epilepsy, J Neurosci Nurs 19(3):141-155, 1987.

Steinke GW: Stages of Alzheimer's disease, San Jose, Calif, 1987, Respite and Research for Alzheimer's Disease.

Stowe AC and Callanan M: Neurologic dysfunctions. In Swearingen PL et al: Manual of critical care: applying nursing diagnoses to adult critical illness, St Louis, 1988, The CV Mosby Co.

Volicer L et al: Clinical management of Alzheimer's disease, Rockville, Md, 1988, Aspen Publishers, Inc.

Wald ME: Cerebral thrombosis: assessment and nursing management of the acute phase, J Neurosci Nurs 18(1):36-38, 1986.

Weiler K and Buckwalter KC: Care of the demented client, J Gerontol Nurs 14(7):26-30, 1988.

5
CHAPTER

Endocrine disorders

Section One   DISORDERS OF THE THYROID GLAND

The thyroid gland produces three hormones: thyroxine (T_4), triiodothyronine (T_3), and thyrocalcitonin (calcitonin). Secretion of T_3 and T_4 is regulated by the anterior pituitary gland *via* a negative feedback mechanism. When serum T_3 and T_4 levels decrease, thyroid-stimulating hormone (TSH) is released by the anterior pituitary. This stimulates the thyroid gland to secrete more hormones until normal levels are reached. T_3 and T_4 affect all body systems by regulating overall body metabolism, energy production, and fluid and electrolyte balance and controlling tissue use of fats, proteins, and carbohydrates. Calcitonin inhibits mobilization of calcium from bone and reduces blood calcium levels.

Hyperthyroidism

Hyperthyroidism is a clinical syndrome caused by excessive circulating thyroid hormone. Because thyroid activity affects all body systems, excessive thyroid hormone exaggerates normal body functions and produces a hypermetabolic state. Family history of hyperthyroidism is a significant factor for development of this disorder. Hyperthyroidism also can be caused by nodular toxic goiters in which one or more thyroid adenomas hyperfunction autonomously.

Graves' disease (diffuse toxic goiter) accounts for approximately 85% of reported cases of hyperthyroidism. It is characterized by spontaneous exacerbations and remissions that appear to be unaffected by therapy. The cause of Graves' disease is unknown, but recent advances in diagnostic techniques have isolated an immunoglobulin known as "long-acting thyroid stimulator" (LATS) in a majority of patients with this disorder, suggesting that Graves' disease is an autoimmune response.

The most severe form of hyperthyroidism is *thyrotoxic crisis* or *thyroid storm*, which results from a sudden surge of large amounts of thyroid hormones into the bloodstream, causing an even greater increase in body metabolism. This is a *medical emergency*. Precipitating factors include infection, trauma, and emotional stress, all of which place greater demands on body metabolism. Thyrotoxic crisis also can occur following subtotal thyroidectomy because of manipulation of the gland during surgery. Despite vigorous treatment, thyroid storm causes death in approximately 20% of affected patients.

ASSESSMENT

Signs and symptoms: Oligomenorrhea or amenorrhea; increased appetite with weight loss; diarrhea or frequent defecation; increased perspiration, especially on the palms of the hands; hyperglycemia; and generalized muscle weakness. In addition, heat intolerance, anxiety, excitability, restlessness, tremors, insomnia, and atrial fibrillation with congestive heart failure (CHF) are sometimes noted.

Physical assessment: Tachycardia with irregular, bounding pulse; increased respirations; elevated temperature; enlargement of the thyroid gland 2-4 times greater than normal; bruit with auscultation over gland; atrophy of skeletal muscles; enlargement of the thymus and lymph nodes; hyperreflexia; and gynecomastia in males. In addition, these patients are usually thin and hyperkinetic with warm, moist skin and fine, silky hair that will not curl. A rare but positive diagnostic sign is the presence of Plummer's nails, in which the distal portion of the nail separates from the nailbed. Patients with Graves' disease may have exophthalmos and pretibial myxedema (nonpitting thickening of the skin over the front distal third of the leg).

Thyrotoxic crisis (thyroid storm): Severe tachycardia, high temperature, CNS irritability, and delirium.

DIAGNOSTIC TESTS

1. *Serum thyroxine and triiodothyronine tests:* Will show elevation of free T_3, T_4 in the presence of disease.
2. *TSH test:* Decreased in the presence of disease.
3. *Free thyroxine index (FTI):* Elevated in the presence of disease.
4. *Thyroid scanning:* Uses radionuclear scanning to determine function of thyroid gland and presence of nodules.

MEDICAL MANAGEMENT AND SURGICAL INTERVENTIONS

1. Pharmacotherapy
   □ *Antithyroid agents (thioamides), including propylthiouracil and methimazole:* To prevent the synthesis and release of thyroxine. Results may not be seen for 4-6 weeks until all stored hormone is used up. Patients are continued on thioamides for a period that ranges from six months to several years. The relapse rate after discontinuation of therapy is high and drug reactions can be severe, including skin rash, fever, pharyngitis, granulocytopenia, arthralgia, myalgia, thrombocytopenia, alterations in taste, hair pigment changes, and lymphadenopathy. By far the most severe side effect is agranulocytosis (acute blood dyscrasia in which the WBC count drops to extremely low levels), which occurs in 0.5% of cases.
   □ *Iodides:* May be given in conjunction with thioamides to inhibit thyroid hormone release. Adverse reactions include skin rash and fever. If used as the only drug to inhibit release of thyroid hormone in Graves' disease or multinodular toxic goiter, iodides must be given cautiously because normal inhibiting factors are absent and their administration can actually increase thyroxine production and release, potentially resulting in increased hyperthyroidism and thyroid storm.
   □ *Propranolol (beta-adrenergic blocking agent):* To relieve tachycardia, anxiety, and heat intolerance. Usually it is contraindicated in individuals with CHF, but if the heart failure is specifically caused by hyperthyroidism and especially if the patient demonstrates atrial fibrillation, propranolol given in conjunction with digitalis may be of benefit.
   □ *Radioactive iodide (sodium iodide^{131}I):* Given orally, based on estimated weight of the gland and results of radioactive iodine uptake scan. This drug destroys hyperactive thyroid cells, decreasing the excessive release of thyroid hormones. The major complication is hypothyroidism, which occurs in 80% of patients receiving this type of therapy. Complications from the medication itself are rare, but a sore throat, swelling of the gland, and radiation sickness do occur, as well as transitory hypoparathyroidism, owing to the close proximity of the parathyroid glands.
   □ *Barbiturates and tranquilizers:* To minimize anxiety and promote rest.
   □ *Antidiarrheals:* To decrease peristalsis and increase absorption of nutrients from the GI tract.
2. Diet: High in calories, protein, carbohydrates, and vitamins to restore a normal nutritional state.
3. Subtotal thyroidectomy: Surgical removal of part of the gland. To minimize postoperative complications, the patient is prepared with antithyroid (thioamide) agents for approximately 6 weeks until normal thyroid function is achieved. Nutritional status is maximized and approximately 2 weeks before surgery the patient is started on iodides to decrease vascularity of the gland and make it firmer, which facilitates removal. The most frequent postoperative complication is hemorrhage at the operative site. Damage to the laryngeal nerve occurs in 1%-4% of cases. If this is unilateral, it will cause minimal voice changes, but if it is bilateral, nerve damage can cause upper airway obstruction. Thyroid storm and tetany, owing to damage to the parathyroid glands with resultant hypocalcemia, are rare occurrences.

NURSING DIAGNOSES AND INTERVENTIONS

Alteration in nutrition: Less than body requirements related to increased need secondary to hypermetabolic state

Desired outcomes: Patient has adequate nutrition as evidenced by stable weight. Patient can list the types of foods that are necessary to achieve optimal nutrition.

1. Provide a diet high in calories, protein, carbohydrates, and vitamins. Teach patient about foods that will provide optimal nutrients. To maximize patient's consumption, provide between-meal snacks.
2. Administer vitamin supplements as prescribed, and explain their importance to the patient.

3. Administer prescribed antidiarrheal medications, which increase absorption of nutrients from the GI tract.
4. Weigh patient daily, and report significant losses to MD.

Sleep pattern disturbance related to agitation secondary to accelerated metabolism

Desired outcome: Patient relates the attainment of sufficient rest and sleep.

1. Adjust care activities to patient's tolerance.
2. Provide frequent rest periods of at least 90 minutes duration. If possible, arrange for patient to have bed rest in a quiet, cool room with nonexertional activities, such as reading, watching television, working crossword puzzles, or listening to soothing music.
3. As necessary, assist patient with walking up stairs or other exertional activities.
4. Administer tranquilizers and sedatives as prescribed to promote rest.

Potential for injury related to risk of thyrotoxic crisis (thyroid storm) secondary to emotional stress, trauma, infection, or surgical manipulation of the gland

Desired outcome: Patient is asymptomatic of thyroid storm as evidenced by normothermia, BP >90/60 (or within patient's baseline range), HR <100 bpm, and orientation to person, place, and time.

1. Assess for and report rectal temperature >37.78° C (100° F), as this is often the first sign of impending thyroid storm.
2. In unstable patients, monitor VS q15-30min for evidence of hypotension and increasing tachycardia and fever.
3. Monitor patient for signs of CHF (which occurs as an effect of thyroid storm), including jugular vein distention, crackles (rales), decrease in quality of peripheral pulses, peripheral edema, and hypotension. Immediately report any positive findings to MD, and prepare to transfer patient to ICU if they are noted.
4. Provide a cool, calm, protected environment to minimize emotional stress. Reassure patient and explain all procedures before performing them. Limit the number of visitors.
5. Ensure good handwashing and meticulous, aseptic technique for dressing changes and invasive procedures. Advise visitors who have contracted or been exposed to a communicable disease not to enter patient's room or to wear a surgical mask, if appropriate.

In the presence of thyroid storm:
6. As prescribed, administer acetaminophen to decrease temperature. **Caution:** Aspirin is contraindicated because it releases thyroxine from protein-binding sites and increases free thyroxine levels.
7. Provide cool sponge baths or apply ice packs to patient's axilla and groin areas to decrease fever. If high temperature continues, obtain a prescription for a hypothermia blanket.
8. Administer propylthiouracil as prescribed to prevent further synthesis and release of thyroid hormones.
9. Administer propranolol as prescribed to block sympathetic nervous system effects.
10. Administer IV fluids as prescribed to provide adequate hydration and prevent vascular collapse. Fluid volume deficit may occur due to increased fluid excretion by the kidneys or excessive diaphoresis. Carefully monitor I&O qh to prevent fluid overload or inadequate fluid replacement. Decreasing output with normal specific gravity may indicate decreased cardiac output, while decreasing output with increased specific gravity can signal dehydration.
11. Administer sodium iodide as prescribed, 1 hour *after* administering propylthiouracil. **Caution:** If given before propylthiouracil, sodium iodide can exacerbate symptoms in susceptible individuals.
12. Administer small doses of insulin as prescribed to control hyperglycemia. Hyperglycemia can occur as an effect of thyroid storm due to the hypermetabolic state.
13. Because oxygen demands are increased as the metabolism increases, administer prescribed supplemental oxygen as necessary.

Anxiety related to untoward response to sympathetic nervous system stimulation

Desired outcomes: Patient and significant others verbalize knowledge of the causes of the patient's behavior. Patient is free of harmful anxiety as evidenced by a HR <100 bpm, RR 12-20 breaths min with normal depth and pattern (eupnea), and absence of or decrease in irritability and restlessness.

1. Assess for signs of anxiety; administer tranquilizers and sedatives as prescribed.
2. Provide a quiet, stress-free environment away from loud noises or excessive activity.
3. Limit number of visitors and the amount of time they spend with patient. Advise significant others to avoid discussing stressful topics and refrain from arguing with the patient.
4. Administer propranolol as prescribed to reduce symptoms of anxiety, tachycardia, and heat intolerance.
5. Reassure patient that anxiety symptoms are related to the disease process, and that treatment decreases their severity.
6. Inform significant others that the patient's behavior is physiologic (a result of CNS irritability) and should not be taken personally.

Potential for impaired tissue integrity: Corneal damage secondary to exophthalmos

Desired outcome: Patient's corneas remain moist and intact.

1. Teach patient to wear dark glasses to protect the cornea.
2. Administer eyedrops as prescribed to supplement lubrication and decrease sympathetic nervous system stimulation, which can cause lid retraction.
3. If appropriate, apply eye shields or tape the eyes shut at bedtime.
4. Administer thioamides as prescribed to maintain normal metabolic state and halt progression of exophthalmos.

Body image disturbance related to exophthalmos or surgical scar

Desired outome: Patient verbalizes measures for disguising exophthalmos or surgical scar and relates the attainment of self-acceptance.

1. Encourage patient to communicate feelings of frustration.
2. Advise patient to wear dark glasses to disguise exophthalmos.
3. Suggest that patient wear customized jewelery, high-necked clothing, such as turtlenecks, or loose-fitting scarves, to disguise the scar.
4. Suggest that after the incision has healed, patient use makeup colored in his or her skin tone to decrease visibility of the scar.
5. Caution patient that creams are contraindicated until the incision has healed completely, and even then there is little evidence that they minimize scarring. Patients are advised by some MDs to increase vitamin C intake to up to 1 g/day to promote healing. Some surgeons also advise against direct sunlight to the operative site for 6-12 months to avoid hyperpigmentation of the incision. Instruct patient accordingly.

Knowledge deficit: Potential for side effects from iodides or from taking or stopping thioamides abruptly

Desired outcome: Patient verbalizes knowledge of the potential side effects of prescribed medications, signs and symptoms of hypothyroidism and hyperthyroidism, and the importance of following the prescribed medical regimen.

1. Explain the importance of taking antithyroid medications daily, in divided doses, and at regular intervals as prescribed.
2. Teach patient the indicators of hypothyroidism (see p. 263), which may occur because of too high a dose of the medications, and the signs and symptoms that necessitate medical attention, including cold intolerance, fatigue, lethargy, and peripheral or periorbital edema.
3. Teach patient the side effects of thioamides and the symptoms that necessitate medical attention, including the appearance of a rash, fever, or pharyngitis, which can occur in the presence of agranulocytosis.
4. Alert patients taking iodides to signs of worsening hyperthyroidism, including high temperature, severe tachycardia, and CNS irritability with delirium.

Pain related to surgical procedure

Desired outcome: Patient's subjective evaluation of pain improves, as documented by a pain scale.

1. Document the degree and character of the patient's pain, including precipitating events. Devise a pain scale with the patient, rating the pain on a scale of 0 (no pain) to 10.
2. Inform patient that clasping the hands behind the neck when moving will minimize stress on the incision.
3. After MD has removed surgical clips and drain, teach patient to perform gentle ROM exercises for the neck.
4. For other interventions, see the same nursing diagnosis in "Caring for Preoperative and Postoperative Patients," p. 638.

Potential for impaired swallowing related to edema or laryngeal nerve damage secondary to surgical procedure

Desired outcome: Patient reports swallowing with minimal difficulty, has minimal or absent hoarseness, and is asymptomatic of respiratory dysfunction as evidenced by RR 12-20 breaths/min with normal depth and pattern (eupnea) and absence of inspiratory stridor.

1. Monitor respiratory status for signs of edema (dyspnea, choking, inspiratory stridor, inability to swallow). Also assess patient's voice. Although slight hoarseness is normal following surgery, hoarseness that persists is indicative of laryngeal nerve damage and should be reported to MD promptly. If bilateral nerve damage has occurred, upper airway obstruction can occur.
2. Elevate HOB 30-45 degrees to minimize edema and incisional stress. Support patient's head with flat or cervical pillows so that it is in a neutral position with the neck (does not flex or hyperextend).
3. Keep tracheostomy set and oxygen equipment at bedside at all times. Suction upper airway as needed, using gentle suction to avoid stimulating laryngospasm.
4. To minimize pain and anxiety and enhance patient's ability to swallow, administer analgesics promptly and as prescribed.

See the appendix for nursing diagnoses and interventions for the care of preoperative and postoperative patients, p. 637.

PATIENT-FAMILY TEACHING AND DISCHARGE PLANNING

Provide patient and significant others with verbal and written information for the following:

1. Diet high in calories, protein, carbohydrates, and vitamins. Inform patient that as a normal metabolic state is attained, the diet may change.
2. Medications, including drug name, purpose, dosage, schedule, precautions, and potential side effects.
3. Changes that can occur as a result of therapy, including weight gain, normalized bowel function, increased strength of skeletal muscles, and a return to normal activity levels.
4. Importance of continued and frequent medical follow-up; confirm date and time of next appointment.
5. Indicators that necessitate medical attention, including fever, rash, or sore throat (side effects of thioamides), and symptoms of hypothyroidism (see p. 263) or worsening hyperthyroidism.
6. For patients receiving radioactive iodine, the importance of not holding children to the chest for 72 hours following therapy, as they are more susceptible to the effects of radiation. Explain that there is negligible risk for adults.
7. Importance of avoiding physical and emotional stress early in the recuperative stage and maximizing coping mechanisms for dealing with stress. See **Health-seeking behaviors:** Relaxation technique effective for stress reduction, p. 49.

Hypothyroidism

Hypothyroidism is a condition in which there is an inadequate amount of circulating thyroid hormone, causing a decrease in metabolic rate that affects all body systems.

Primary hypothyroidism accounts for more than 90% of cases of hypothyroidism and is caused by pathologic changes in the thyroid itself. There are several possible causes, including dietary iodine deficiency, thyroiditis, thyroid atrophy or fibrosis of unknown etiology, radiation therapy to the neck (such as with the treatment for hyperthyroidism), surgical removal of all or part of the gland, drugs that suppress thyroid activity including propylthiouracil and iodides, or a genetic dysfunction resulting in the inability to produce and secrete thyroid hormone. *Secondary hypothyroidism* is caused by dysfunction of the anterior pituitary gland, which results in decreased release of TSH. It can be caused by pituitary tumors, postpartum necrosis of the pituitary gland, or hypophysectomy. *Tertiary hypothyroidism* is caused by a hypothalamic deficiency in the release of TRH.

When hypothyroidism is untreated, or when a stressor, such as infection, affects an individual with hypothyroidism, a life-threatening condition known as *myxedema coma* can occur. The clinical picture of myxedema coma is that of exaggerated hypothyroidism, with dangerous hypoventilation, hypothermia, hypotension, and shock. Coma and seizures can occur as well. Myxedema coma usually develops slowly, has a >50% mortality rate, and requires prompt and aggressive treatment.

ASSESSMENT

Signs and symptoms can progress from mild early in onset to life-threatening.

Signs and symptoms: Early fatigue, weight gain, anorexia, constipation, menstrual irregularities, muscle cramps, lethargy, inability to concentrate, hair loss, cold intolerance, and hoarseness. Some usually placid patients may become depressed or extremely agitated.

Physical assessment: Possible presence of goiter, cardiomegaly, bradycardia, hypothermia, peripheral nonpitting edema, and periorbital puffiness. Patients are often obese with cool, dry, yellowish skin. The voice is hoarse and the speech is frequently slurred. The hair is thin, coarse, and brittle; and the tongue is enlarged. Slow mentation and reflexes usually are present.

Myxedema coma: Hypoventilation, hypoglycemia, hyponatremia, stupor, unresponsiveness, hypotension, and shock.

DIAGNOSTIC TESTS

1. *Serum tests:* TSH will be elevated in the presence of primary hypothyroidism and low or normal in other forms of the disease. This is the most significant test for differentiating primary from secondary or tertiary hypothyroidism. Serum T_3 and T_4 will be decreased.
2. *Iodine-131 uptake:* Will be less than 10% in a 24-hour period. In secondary hypothyroidism, uptake increases with administration of exogenous TSH.
3. *Thyroid antibody tests:* Positive in primary hypothyroidism.

MEDICAL MANAGEMENT

1. Oral thyroid hormone: Given early in treatment for primary hypothyroidism. To prevent hyperthyroidism caused by too much exogenous thyroid hormone, patients are started on low doses that are increased gradually, based on serial laboratory tests (T_3 and T_4) and the patient's response to medication. This therapy is continued for the patient's lifetime. For patients with secondary hypothyroidism, thyroid supplements can promote acute symptoms and therefore are contraindicated.
2. Stool softeners: To minimize constipation owing to decreased gastric secretions and peristalsis.

3. Diet: High in roughage and protein to help prevent constipation; restriction of sodium to decrease edema; and reduction in calories to promote weight loss.

Treatment of myxedema coma

1. Intubation and mechanical ventilation: To compensate for decreased ventilatory drive.
2. IV thyroid supplements: Rapid IV administration of thyroid hormone can precipitate hyperadrenocorticism, but this can be avoided by the concomitant administration of IV hydrocortisone.
3. Treatment of hypotension: IV isotonic fluids, such as normal saline and lactated Ringer's solution, are administered. Hypotonic solutions, such as D_5W, are contraindicated because they can decrease serum sodium levels further. Because of altered metabolism, these patients respond poorly to vasopressors.
4. Treatment of hypoglycemia: IV glucose.
5. Treatment of hyponatremia: Either fluids are restricted or hypertonic (3%) saline is administered, or both.
6. Treatment of associated illnesses such as infections.

Caution: Because of alterations in metabolism, patients do not tolerate barbiturates and sedatives, and therefore CNS depressants are contraindicated. Also, external warming measures are contraindicated for hypothermia because they can produce vasodilatation and vascular collapse.

NURSING DIAGNOSES AND INTERVENTIONS

Potential for ineffective breathing pattern related to hypoventilation secondary to decreased ventilatory drive or upper airway obstruction occurring with myxedematous infiltration

Desired outcome: Patient has an effective breathing pattern as evidenced by RR 12-20 breaths/min with normal depth and pattern (eupnea), presence of normal breath sounds over the lung fields, and absence of adventitious sounds

1. Assess rate, depth, and quality of breath sounds and be alert to the presence of adventitious sounds (e.g., from developing pleural effusion) or decreasing or crowing sounds (e.g., from swollen tongue or glottis).
2. Be alert to signs of inadequate ventilation, including changes in respiratory rate or pattern and circumoral or peripheral cyanosis. Immediately report significant findings to MD.
3. Teach patient coughing, deep breathing, and use of incentive spirometer. Suction upper airway prn.
4. For a patient experiencing respiratory distress, be prepared to assist MD with intubation or tracheostomy and maintenance of mechanical ventilatory assistance, or transfer patient to ICU.

Fluid volume excess: Edema related to retention of fluids secondary to decreased metabolic rate and adrenal insufficiency

Desired outcome: Patient becomes normovolemic as evidenced by urinary output ≥ 30 ml/hr, stable weights, nondistended jugular veins, presence of eupnea, and peripheral pulses $\leq 2+$ on a 0-4+ scale.

1. Monitor I&O qh for evidence of decreasing output.
2. Weigh patient at the same time every day, with the same clothing, and using the same scale. Report increasing weight gains to MD.
3. Monitor patient for signs of CHF: jugular vein distention, crackles (rales), SOB, dependent edema of extremities, and decreased peripheral pulses. Report significant findings to MD.
4. Restrict fluid and sodium intake as prescribed. See Table 11-3, p. 550, for foods that are high in sodium.

5. Administer IV fluids using a mechanical controller to prevent accidental fluid overload.

Activity intolerance related to weakness and fatigue secondary to slowed metabolism and decreased cardiac output caused by pericardial effusions, atherosclerosis, and decreased adrenergic stimulation

Desired outcome: Patient exhibits cardiac tolerance to activity as evidenced by HR ≤20 bpm over resting HR, systolic BP ≤20 mm Hg over or under resting systolic BP, warm and dry skin, and absence of crackles, murmurs, and chest pain.

1. Monitor VS and apical pulse at frequent intervals. Be alert to hypotension, slow pulse, dysrhythmias, complaints of chest pain or discomfort, decreasing urine output, and changes in mentation. Promptly report significant changes to MD.
2. Balance activity with adequate rest to decrease workload of the heart.
3. As prescribed, administer IV isotonic solutions, such as normal saline, to help prevent hypotension.
4. To prevent problems of immobility, assist patient with ROM and other in-bed exercises and consult with MD regarding the implementation of exercises that require greater cardiac tolerance. For detail, see the appendix for **Potential for activity intolerance** related to deconditioning secondary to prolonged bed rest, p. 651, and **Potential for disuse syndrome, p. 653.**

Potential for infection related to increased susceptibility secondary to alterations in adrenal function

Desired outcome: Patient is free of infection as evidenced by normothermia, absence of adventitious breath sounds, normal urinary pattern and characteristics, and well-healing wounds.

1. Be alert to early indicators of infection, including fever, erthema, swelling, or discharge from wounds or IV sites; urinary frequency, urgency, dysuria, cloudy or malodorous urine; presence of adventitious sounds on auscultation of lung fields; and changes in color, consistency, and amount of sputum. Notify MD of significant findings.
2. Minimize the risk of UTI by providing meticulous care of indwelling catheters.
3. Use meticulous, sterile technique when performing dressing changes and invasive procedures.
4. Because open sores are sites of ingress for bacteria, provide good skin care to maintain skin integrity and prevent decubitus ulcers.
5. Advise visitors who have contracted or been exposed to a communicable disease not to enter patient's room or to wear surgical mask, if appropriate.

Alteration in nutrition: More than body requirements of calories related to decreased need secondary to slowed metabolism

Desired outcomes: Patient does not experience weight gain. Patient verbalizes understanding of the rationale and measures for the dietary regimen.

1. Provide a diet that is high in protein and low in calories. As prescribed, restrict or limit sodium (see Table 11-3, p. 550) to decrease edema. Teach patient about foods to augment and limit or omit.
2. Provide small, frequent meals of appropriate foods the patient particularly enjoys.
3. Encourage foods that are high in fiber content (e.g., fruits with skins, vegetables, whole grain breads and cereals, nuts) to improve gastric motility and elimination.
4. Administer vitamin supplements as prescribed.

Constipation related to decreased peristalsis secondary to slowed metabolism

Desired outcome: Patient relates the attainment of his or her normal pattern of bowel elimination.

1. Query patient about current bowel function; document changes.
2. Be alert to decreasing bowel sounds and the presence of distention and increases in

abdominal girth, which can occur with ileus or an obstructive process.

3. Encourage patient to maintain a diet with adequate roughage and fluids. Examples of foods high in bulk include fruits with skins, fruit juices, cooked fruits, vegetables, whole grain breads and cereals, and nuts. Ensure that fluid intake is at least 2-3 L/ day.

4. Administer stool softeners and laxatives as prescribed. **Caution:** Suppositories are contraindicated because of the risk of stimulating the vagus nerve, which would further decrease HR and BP.

5. Advise patient to increase the amount of exercise to promote regularity.

Sensory/perceptual alterations related to sensorium changes secondary to cerebral retention of water

Desired outcome: Patient verbalizes orientation to person, place, and time.

1. Monitor patient's mental status at frequent intervals by assessing orientation to person, place, and time. Report increasing lethargy or confusion to MD, as these can signal onset of myxedema coma.

2. Reorient patient frequently. Have a clock and calendar visible and use radio or television for orientation.

3. Clearly explain all procedures to patient before performing them. Allow adequate time for patient to ask questions.

4. If necessary, remind patient to complete ADL, such as bathing and brushing hair.

5. Encourage visitors to discuss topics of special interest to patient to enhance patient's alertness.

6. Administer thyroid replacement hormones as prescribed to increase metabolic rate, which in turn will enhance cerebral blood flow.

Potential for injury related to risk of myxedema coma secondary to inadequate response to treatment of hypothyroidism or stressors such as infection

Desired outcomes: Patient is asymptomatic of myxedema coma as evidenced by HR ≥60 bpm, BP ≥90/60 mm Hg (or within patient's normal range), RR ≥10 breaths/min with normal depth and pattern (eupnea), and orientation to person, place, and time.

1. Monitor VS at frequent intervals and be alert to bradycardia, hypotension, or decrease in RR. Report systolic BP <90 mm Hg, pulse <60 bpm, or RR <10.

2. Monitor patient for signs of hypoxia (circumoral or peripheral cyanosis, decrease in LOC). Immediately report significant findings to MD.

3. Double check medication dosages carefully before administering, especially barbiturates and sedatives, which are not well tolerated by these patients. Observe for signs of toxicity, such as decreased LOC and decreases in BP or ventilatory effort.

4. Monitor serum electrolytes and glucose levels. Be especially alert to decreasing sodium (<130 mEq/L) and glucose (<80 mg/dl).

5. In the presence of myxedema coma, implement the following:
   □ Restrict fluids or administer hypertonic saline as prescribed to correct hyponatremia. Use an infusion control device to maintain accurate infusion rate of IV fluids.
   □ As prescribed, administer IV thyroid replacement hormones with IV hydrocortisone and IV glucose to treat hypoglycemia.
   □ Monitor patient for signs of CHF: jugular vein distention, crackles (rales), SOB, peripheral edema, weakening peripheral pulses, and hypotension. Notify MD of any significant findings.
   □ Prepare to transfer patient to ICU. Keep an oral airway and manual rescusitator at the bedside in the event of seizure, coma, or the need for ventilatory assistance.

PATIENT-FAMILY TEACHING AND DISCHARGE PLANNING

Provide patient and significant others with verbal and written information for the following:

1. Medications, including drug name, purpose, dosage, schedule, precautions, and potential side effects. Remind patient that thioamides, iodides, and lithium are contraindicated because they decrease thyroid activity. Be sure that patient is aware that thyroid replacement medications are to be taken for life.
2. Dietary requirements and restrictions, which may change as hormone replacement therapy takes effect.
3. Expected changes that can occur with hormone replacement therapy: increased energy level, weight loss, and decreased peripheral edema. Neuromuscular problems should improve, as well.
4. Importance of continued, frequent medical follow-up; confirm date and time of next medical appointment.
5. Importance of avoiding physical and emotional stress, and ways for patient to maximize coping mechanisms for dealing with stress. See **Health-seeking behaviors:** Relaxation technique effective for stress reduction, p. 49.
6. Signs and symptoms that necessitate medical attention, including fever or other symptoms of upper respiratory, urinary, or oral infections, and signs and symptoms of hyperthyroidism, which may result from excessive hormone replacement.

Section Two   DISORDERS OF THE PARATHYROID GLANDS

The parathyroid glands regulate serum calcium and phosphorus levels *via* release of parathyroid hormone (PTH). This is accomplished by a negative-feedback mechanism: when serum calcium levels rise, PTH secretion is suppressed. PTH acts on bone to decrease calcium binding, and it stimulates the kidneys to increase resorption of calcium. The parathyroid glands affect serum phosphorus levels in two ways: directly, in that PTH causes increased renal excretion of phosphorus; and indirectly, in that phosphorus and calcium combine readily to form an insoluble salt, and therefore increased serum phosphorus will facilitate this reaction and effectively lower circulating calcium levels. PTH is also involved in the synthesis of a renal enzyme that catalyzes the formation of vitamin D, which in conjunction with PTH, increases absorption of calcium from the GI tract.

Hyperparathyroidism

Hyperparathyroidism is a clinical syndrome in which there is excessive secretion of PTH. *Primary hyperparathyroidism* is caused by pathology of one or more of the parathyroid glands. Approximately 80% of these cases are caused by a benign adenoma of one gland, another 10% by hyperplasia of all four glands, and in rare cases, by carcinoma. In this disorder, excessive PTH acts on the skeletal, renal, and GI systems, and the overall effect is that of increased serum calcium levels and decreased phosphate levels.

Hyperparathyroidism is the second most common cause of hypercalcemia. *Secondary hyperparathyroidism* is usually caused by renal insufficiency, with decreased glomerular filtration. Although calcium and phosphorus are retained because of the lack of renal filtration, the high serum phosphate level depresses calcium concentration because phosphorus combines with calcium ions to form insoluble salts, resulting in hypocalcemia. In turn, the resulting hypocalcemia stimulates the parathyroid glands to release PTH in an effort to increase serum calcium levels. Bone resorption occurs because of increased PTH, but absorption of calcium from the GI tract is depressed because of calcium binding with high-phosphate GI secretions. The overall effect is that of decreased calcium levels and increased phosphate levels. *Tertiary hyperparathyroidism* occurs when secondary hyperparathyroidism progresses to a state in which excessive PTH is released independent of serum calcium levels.

ASSESSMENT

Signs and symptoms: Muscular weakness, fatigue, personality disturbances, emotional lability, constipation, weight loss, renal calculi, nausea, vomiting, anorexia, polyuria, hematuria, drowsiness, stupor, and coma. In addition, the patient may have kidney infections, anemia, arthralgia, pancreatitis, peptic ulcers, and pathologic fractures, as well as heart disease caused by calcium deposits in the tissues.

Physical assessment: Hypotonic muscles, enlarged parathyroid glands, hypertension. If the condition is severe, renal failure also may be present.

DIAGNOSTIC TESTS

1. *Serum calcium:* Elevated in primary hyperparathyroidism and low in secondary hyperparathyroidism. This test usually is repeated at least three times to confirm the diagnosis. Venous blood is drawn in the morning after the patient has been in a fasting state. Because calcium is bound to protein, the test results must be "corrected," based on a simultaneous test for albumin level. Serum calcium will change by 0.8 mg/dl for each 1 G/dl change in albumin level above or below normal. This represents the circulating calcium available for use by body cells and is considered the "true" calcium level.

Note: To avoid venous stasis, which can produce erroneously high results, care must be taken not to apply the tourniquet too tightly or occlude the vessel for longer than necessary.

2. *Serum PTH:* High or inappropriately high for serum calcium levels.
3. *Plasma phosphorus:* Decreased in primary hyperparathyroidism and elevated in secondary hyperparathyroidism.
4. *24-hour urine calcium:* Elevated in primary hyperparathyroidism. This test is often used to rule out other causes of hypercalcemia.
5. *Skeletal x-rays:* Will show diminution of bone mass in virtually all patients with hyperparathyroidism, as well as calcification of articular cartilage. X-rays of the hands will show subperiosteal resorption of the phalanges.
6. *EKG:* May show shortened Q-T interval, which is reflective of hypercalcemia.

MEDICAL MANAGEMENT AND SURGICAL INTERVENTIONS

Surgical treatment for primary hyperparathyroidism: The most effective form of treatment for primary hyperparathyroidism is the surgical removal of one or more of the parathyroid glands (parathyroidectomy). The incision is somewhat wider than with a thyroidectomy, but the surgery is very similar. Only the affected gland(s) is removed, and in cases where all of the parathyroid glands are enlarged, 3½ of the glands are removed. The remaining tissue is enough to provide normal calcium regulation. In addition to the postoperative complications potentially found with a thyroidectomy, abnormalities in serum calcium levels also may be found.

Medical treatment for primary hyperparathyroidism: Reserved for patients who are poor surgical risks or who have only a mild form of the disease. The goals of treatment are to provide adequate hydration and reduce serum calcium levels. **Note:** Calcium levels >14 mg/dl are life-threatening and require vigorous and immediate treatment if the patient is to survive.

1. Promotion of calcium excretion: Done in the absence of CHF or renal insufficiency. This is accomplished by forcing fluids orally or providing IV normal saline for patients who are stuporous or nauseated. Volumes up to 1,000 ml/hr may be given for short periods.
2. Increase in salt intake: Either *via* diet or salt tablets. Because sodium competes with calcium for excretion by the kidneys, increased sodium levels will cause the kidneys to excrete more calcium.

3. **Diet:** Limitation of dietary calcium (e.g., milk, many cheeses, cottage cheese, mustard greens, kale, broccoli) intake to one serving per day.
4. **Pharmacotherapy**
   - ☐ *Diuretics:* To prevent volume overload and maintain brisk diuresis. Loop diuretics (furosemide and ethacrynate sodium) are preferred because they increase urinary calcium excretion. Thiazide diuretics are contraindicated because they decrease calcium excretion.
   - ☐ *Oral phosphate supplements:* To decrease bone resorption of calcium and bind calcium in the intestine to limit calcium absorption. Because they may cause precipitation of insoluble calcium-phosphate complexes in the soft tissues of the kidneys, lungs, and cardiac conductive system, they are given only to patients with low serum phosphate or to those who have normal kidney function. Diarrhea is a common side effect. IV phosphates are avoided except for extreme emergency (calcium >14 mg/dl).
   - ☐ *IM calcitonin:* To decrease bone resorption of calcium and increase renal clearance. This has limited use, however, because it is short acting and patients frequently become resistant.
   - ☐ *IV mithramycin:* To inhibit bone resorption and lower serum and urine calcium levels. This is the drug of choice for treatment of *severe* hypercalcemia because it is more effective and works more rapidly than calcitonin. Effects usually are seen within 2 hours. Side effects include bleeding abnormalities and hypocalcemia.
   - ☐ *Oral steroids:* For their calciuric effect and to decrease calcium absorption in the presence of vitamin D intoxication. To avoid the immunosuppressive effects of these drugs, they are given in as small a dose as it takes to achieve therapeutic effects.
5. **Hemodialysis in a low-calcium bath:** Sometimes prescribed for severe hypercalcemia to remove calcium ions from the plasma.

Treatment for secondary hyperparathyroidism

1. **Reduction of dietary phosphorus:** Helps prevent formation of insoluble salts, thus increasing the available circulating calcium ions. For example, meat, poultry, fish, eggs, cheese, dried beans, and cereals may be limited.
2. **Oral calcium supplements:** To increase serum calcium levels, which will help prevent further release of PTH.
3. **Aluminum-containing antacids (e.g., AlternaGel, Amphojel):** For patients with chronic renal failure to bind phosphorus in the intestine and prevent resorption.
4. **Oral vitamin D supplements:** To correct deficiency.

NURSING DIAGNOSES AND INTERVENTIONS

Activity intolerance related to neuromuscular weakness and joint pain secondary to increased serum calcium and altered phosphate levels

Desired outcome: Patient demonstrates progression to his or her highest level of activity without evidence of weakness or joint pain.

1. Administer analgesics and antiinflammatory agents as prescribed to minimize discomfort and enhance the effectiveness of prescribed or necessary activity. Time exercise/activity to coincide with the peak effectiveness of the medication.
2. Adjust activity to patient's tolerance and provide rest periods at frequent intervals. Discuss the importance of activity with the patient and set realistic short-term and long-term goals in clearly understood, empirical terms (e.g., "Ambulate the length of the ward three times four times a day.")
3. Assist with ambulation as necessary. Provide a walker or cane if appropriate.
4. Request PT and OT consultations for gradually increasing the patient's muscular strength and endurance.

Fluid volume deficit related to abnormal loss secondary to osmotic diuresis, vomiting, or diarrhea caused by oral phosphate supplements

Desired outcome: Patient becomes normovolemic as evidenced by balanced I&O, urinary output ≥30 ml/hr, good skin turgor, moist tongue and mucous membrane, brisk capillary refill (<3 seconds), and BP ≥90/60 mm Hg (or within patient's baseline limits).

1. Monitor and document I&O. Be alert to indications of dehydration, including decreasing urinary output, dry mucous membranes, poor skin turgor, thirst, furrowed tongue.
2. Monitor serum calcium levels. Decreasing levels signal correction of the dehydration. Normal range for calcium is 8.5-10.5 mg/dl.
3. Be alert to the presence of hypotension, which can be further potentiated by oral phosphate supplements.
4. Unless patient has coexisting renal or cardiac disease, encourage oral fluids to 3 L/day.
5. Rehydrate with IV fluids (typically normal saline) if prescribed.
6. Administer prescribed medications (e.g., calcitonin, mithramycin) to decrease hypercalcemia and medications (e.g., loop diuretics, steroids) to increase urinary calcium excretion.

Potential for trauma related to risk of pathologic fractures secondary to bone demineralization

Desired outcome: Patient is asymptomatic of pathologic fractures.

1. Minimize the risk of pathologic fractures from falling by keeping the bed in its lowest position, keeping walkway free of clutter, and assisting patient with ambulation or any strenuous activity. Instruct unstable patient to request help when getting out of bed, promote the use of a cane or walker, and keep call light within patient's reach.
2. Pad the siderails for patients with severe bone pathology.
3. Apply chest or wrist restraints for patients who are severely confused and may attempt to leave the bed, or arrange for significant other to sit with patient.
4. Notify MD of patient complaints of back or chest pain, which may signal vertebral or rib fracture.

Constipation related to decreased peristalsis secondary to increased serum calcium level

Desired outcome: Patient verbalizes knowledge of measures that promote bowel elimination and relates bowel elimination within his or her normal pattern.

1. Inform patient that increasing fluid intake to 3 L/day will help promote bowel elimination.
2. Teach patient to increase dietary fiber by adding dried fruits, whole-grain cereals, nuts, fresh fruits, and vegetables to the diet.
3. Administer stool softeners and laxatives as prescribed.
4. Encourage as much activity as tolerated.

Potential for injury related to risk of hypercalcemia, hypocalcemia, tetany, and thyroid storm secondary to surgical procedure or manipulation of the gland

Desired outcome: Patient is asymptomatic of hypercalcemia, hypocalcemia, tetany, and thyroid storm as evidenced by RR 12-20 breaths/min with normal depth and pattern (eupnea); orientation to person, place, and time; absence of Chvostek's and Trousseau's signs; normal strength and motion in all extremities; HR 60-100 bpm; and normothermia.

1. Be alert to the presence of hypercalcemia, which can be caused by an increased release of PTH secondary to surgical manipulation of the gland. Signs include nausea, vomiting, anorexia, abdominal pain, weakness, thirst, dyspnea, and coma.
2. Monitor patient for numbness and tingling around the mouth, an early sign of hypocalcemia. Also be alert to indicators of tetany: muscle twitching, painful tonic muscle spasms, and grimacing facial spasms. Two tests for assessing for tetany include

Chvostek's and Trousseau's signs. Chvostek's sign is elicited by tapping the face just below the temple where the facial nerve emerges. The sign is positive if twitching occurs along the nose, lip, or side of the face. Trousseau's sign is tested by applying a BP cuff to the arm and inflating it to slightly higher than the systolic BP and leaving it inflated for 1-4 minutes. Carpopedal spasms are indicative of hypocalemia. Report significant findings to MD.

3. Keep IV calcium at the bedside for prescribed treatment of hypocalcemia.
4. Be alert to indicators of thyroid storm, including tachycardia, agitation, and hyperpyrexia. Immediately report the presence of these signs to MD. Although thyroid storm occurs rarely, it can be caused by a sudden release of excessive amounts of thyroid hormone into the bloodstream from manipulation of the gland during surgery.

Pain related to surgical procedure or arthralgia secondary to bone demineralization.

Desired outcome: Patient's subjective evaluation of pain improves, as documented by a pain scale.

1. Monitor patient for pain, noting and documenting intensity, character, and precipitating factors. Devise a pain scale with patient that rates discomfort from 0 (no pain) to 10.
2. Administer analgesics as prescribed and document their effectiveness.
3. Advise patient to notify staff as soon as discomfort occurs so that analgesics can be administered before pain becomes too severe.
4. Administer analgesics 30-60 minutes before scheduled activities, such as turning or ambulation.
5. Teach patient to clasp hands behind the neck during postoperative moving to minimize stress on the incision.
6. Teach gentle ROM exercises for the neck, as well as assisted or active ROM for painful joints.
7. Provide comfort measures, such as a foam mattress and a foot cradle, to minimize pressure on the extremities.
8. Provide backrubs, especially at bedtime, to reduce discomfort from prolonged bed rest and enhance relaxation.

Knowledge deficit: Potential for negative side effects from steroids, phosphate supplements, and mithramycin

Desired outcome: Patient verbalizes knowledge of the side effects of prescribed medications and the importance of notifying MD should they occur.

1. Teach patient the importance of monitoring for side effects of steroids. This includes frequent BP checks for hypertension, assessment for mental changes, daily weight measurement for evidence of weight gain, and blood tests for the presence of hyperglycemia.
2. For patient taking phosphate supplements, explain that diarrhea is a common side effect.
3. Teach patient to be alert to the following side effects of mithramycin: lower-extremity petechiae, which signal thrombocytopenia; jaundice, which signals hepatocellular necrosis; and tetany, which occurs with hypocalcemia. Explain that urinalysis results must be monitored for evidence of proteinuria.
4. Explain the importance of notifying MD promptly should side effects occur.

See "Renal Calculi," p. 110, for nursing diagnoses and interventions for the care of patients with renal calculi. See "Hyperthyroidism" for **Potential for impaired swallowing** related to edema or laryngeal nerve damage, p. 262. Also see "Calcium Imbalance," p. 559, for nursing diagnoses and interventions for the care of patients with hypercalcemia and hypocalcemia. See the appendix p. 637, for the care of preoperative and postoperative patients.

PATIENT-FAMILY TEACHING AND DISCHARGE PLANNING

Provide patient and significant others with verbal and written information for the following:

1. Diet, including the foods to limit or restrict. As appropriate, arrange for a dietary consultation to help patient with meal planning and integration of individual restrictions into family meals.
2. Importance of continued medical follow-up; confirm date and time of next medical appointment.
3. Signs and symptoms of hypocalcemia and hypercalcemia, which necessitate medical attention if they occur.
4. Medications to be taken at home, including drug name, purpose, dosage, schedule, precautions, and potential side effects.
5. If surgery was performed, the indications of wound infection (e.g., erythema, local warmth, swelling, discharge, pain, or fever).

Hypoparathyroidism

Hypoparathyroidism is a condition in which there is decreased production of parathyroid hormone (PTH). Most commonly, this disorder is iatrogenic, caused by damage to or accidental removal of the parathyroid glands during thyroid surgery or radioactive iodine treatment for hyperthyroidism. Damage can be temporary or permanent. If injury occurs in the absence of gland removal, the tissue generally recovers within a period of months and returns to normal function. Familial or autoimmune factors also can be significant in the development of hypoparathyroidism. Because the function of PTH is the regulation of serum calcium levels, symptoms relate to tissue response to hypocalcemia.

ASSESSMENT

Signs and symptoms: Numbness and tingling around the mouth, fingertips, and sometimes in the feet; painful contractions or twitching of skeletal muscles; clonic and tonic spasms; grand mal seizures; laryngeal spasms; carpopedal spasm; nausea; vomiting; dysrhythmias; heart failure; cataracts (from calcium deposits); conjunctivitis; and photophobia.

Physical assessment: Dry, scaly skin with increased pigmentation; thinning of scalp hair; loss of hair in axilla and pubic areas, eyebrows, and eyelashes; brittle fingernails and toenails, which may be deformed with horizontal ridges; and positive Chvostek's and Trousseau's signs.

DIAGNOSTIC TESTS

1. *Serum tests:* Levels of calcium will be decreased; phosphate will be increased; and plasma PTH will be decreased.
2. *Skull and skeletal x-rays:* May show evidence of increased density and calcification of basal ganglia.

MEDICAL MANAGEMENT

1. Calcium supplements: For cases of severe hypocalcemia, given either orally (route of choice) or IV.
2. Parathyroid hormone injections: To replace lost PTH.
3. Vitamin D preparations: To facilitate absorption of calcium from the GI tract.
4. Sedatives (phenobarbital) and magnesium sulfate: To minimize tetany and seizures. Phenytoin may be given to control seizures.
5. Aluminum hydroxide gels (e.g., ALternaGel, Amphojel): To bind phosphorus in the intestines and decrease serum phosphate levels.
6. Diet: High in calcium (1 quart milk/day) and low in phosphorus (limit meat, poultry, fish, eggs, cheese, dried beans, and cereals). If hyperphosphatemia persists, it may

be necessary to restrict dairy products and egg yolks and provide oral calcium supplements. Foods high in oxalate, which binds to calcium, also should be avoided. These include beets, figs, nuts, spinach, black tea, and chocolate.

NURSING DIAGNOSES AND INTERVENTIONS

Activity intolerance related to weakness and fatigue secondary to decreased cardiac contractility

Desired outcome: Patient exhibits cardiac tolerance to activity as evidenced by HR ≤20 bpm over resting HR, systolic BP ≤20 mm Hg over or under resting systolic BP, RR 12-20 breaths/min with normal depth and pattern (eupnea), normal skin color, warm and dry skin, and absence of crackles, murmurs, and chest pain.

1. Monitor patient for indicators of increasing cardiac failure, including hypotension, weak and thready pulse, tachycardia, SOB, pallor, or cyanosis. Report significant findings to MD.
2. Provide adequate rest periods.
3. Administer oral or IV calcium supplements as prescribed.
4. Assist patient with ROM and other in-bed exercises to help prevent complications of inactivity. Consult with MD regarding exercises that require increased cardiac tolerance. For guidelines, see the appendix for **Potential activity intolerance,** p. 651, and **Potential for disuse syndrome,** p. 653.

Potential for injury related to risk of tetany, respiratory distress, and seizures secondary to hypocalcemia

Desired outcome: Patient is asymptomatic of tetany, respiratory distress, and seizures as evidenced by negative Chvostek's and Trousseau's signs; RR 12-20 breaths/min with normal depth and pattern (eupnea); absence of muscle spasms and adventitious breath sounds; and orientation to person, place, and time.

1. Observe for early signs of hypocalcemia, such as tingling around the mouth and in the hands. Be alert to indicators of tetany, including muscle twitching, painful tonic muscle spasms, grimacing facial spasms, and positive Chvostek's and Trousseau's signs (see p. 271). Report significant findings to MD.
2. Monitor for evidence of respiratory distress, including stridor, wheezing, and dyspnea; report significant findings to MD immediately.
3. Monitor serum calcium levels, noting whether levels are increased or decreased. Either extreme will require a change in calcium therapy. Serum calcium levels <7mg/dl or >14 mg/dl (after being "corrected" with albumin level) are life-threatening. If they occur, notify MD immediately.
4. Provide a restful, quiet environment away from loud noises and bright lights.
5. Administer sedatives and anticonvulsant medications as prescribed.
6. Pad siderails and keep them up at all times. Keep an oral airway at the bedside.
7. Keep tracheostomy set, oxygen equipment, and IV calcium at the bedside.
8. Also see "Calcium imbalance," p. 559, for nursing interventions for the care of patients with hypocalcemia and hypercalcemia.

PATIENT-FAMILY TEACHING AND DISCHARGE PLANNING

Provide patient and significant others with verbal and written information for the following:
1. Diet, including foods to increase or limit. As appropriate, arrange for a dietary consultation so that patient's requirements and restrictions can be integrated into family meal planning.
2. Medications, including drug name, purpose, dosage, schedule, precautions, and potential side effects.
3. Signs and symptoms necessitating medical attention, including signs of worsening hypocalcemia (such as tetany) or signs of hypercalcemia, including weakness, fatigue, constipation, polyuria, and renal calculi.

4. Importance of continued medical follow-up; confirm date and time of next appointment.

Section Three DISORDERS OF THE ADRENAL GLANDS

Each of the two adrenal glands is composed of two distinct parts: the adrenal cortex and the medulla. Adrenocortical hormones include glucocorticoids (cortisol is the primary glucocorticoid), which are responsible for regulation of protein, fat, and carbohydrate metabolism and affect the immunologic and inflammatory responses; mineralocorticoids (aldosterone), which affect sodium, potassium, and water metabolism; and androgens, which affect sexual development. These hormones are released in response to serum levels of adrenocorticotropic hormone (ACTH), which functions *via* a negative-feedback mechanism: when serum cortisol levels decrease, ACTH release increases. The medulla secretes the catecholamines epinephrine and norepinephrine, which are released in response to sympathetic nervous system stimulation.

Addison's disease

Addison's disease is a deficiency of adrenocortical hormones following destruction of the adrenal cortex, which can occur suddenly as a result of such stressors as trauma, infection, or surgery. More commonly, however, the process occurs gradually. As many as 80% of reported cases involve an autoimmune factor. *Primary Addison's disease* is a pathology of the adrenal glands themselves; while *secondary Addison's disease* results from impaired functioning of the pituitary gland, which causes decreased levels of ACTH.

Deficiency of glucocorticoids retards the mobilization of tissue protein and inhibits the ability of the liver to store glycogen, causing muscle weakness and hypoglycemia to occur. Wound healing is slowed and these individuals become particularly susceptible to infection. There is a loss of vascular tone in the periphery as well as decreased vascular response to the catecholamines epinephrine and norepinephrine. Decreased secretion of aldosterone causes sodium, chloride, and water loss from the kidneys and increased reabsorption of potassium.

The presence of acute symptoms in response to stressors is called *adrenal* or *Addisonian crisis*. It can be precipitated by any emotional stressor, simple infection, minor surgery, or trauma. Abrupt withdrawal of exogenous steroids also can precipitate a crisis. Unless treated rapidly and aggressively, this condition can lead to death within hours.

ASSESSMENT

Signs and symptoms: Apprehension, headache, nausea, anorexia, abdominal pain, diarrhea, confusion, and restlessness. In addition, individuals may have muscular weakness that becomes progressively worse throughout the day, anorexia, fatigue, weight loss, postural hypotension, and emotional instability.

Physical assessment: Possible presence of cyanosis, fever, pallor, weak pulse, and tachypnea. Often, there is emaciation with dehydration, generalized dark pigmentation of the skin with brown or black freckles, hypotension, and a small heart size.

Addisonian crisis: Headache, nausea, vomiting, fever, intractable abdominal pain, and severe hypotension, which can lead to vascular collapse and shock.

History of: Familial tendency, bilateral adrenalectomy, tuberculosis, any kind of trauma or infection, damage to the pituitary gland.

DIAGNOSTIC TESTS

1. *Blood cortisol levels:* Drawn at 8 AM, 4 PM, and 12 midnight. In normal individuals, blood cortisol levels are highest in the morning and gradually decrease until they

reach their lowest level at 12 midnight. Individuals with Addison's disease do not show this variation.

2. *Other blood studies:* Will reveal elevated potassium; decreased plasma aldosterone, sodium, and chloride levels; and decreased blood sugar. Serum ACTH will be increased in primary Addison's disease and decreased in secondary Addison's disease.

3. *Urine sodium:* Increased because of increased renal excretion.

4. *IM ACTH stimulation test:* Involves drawing a fasting blood sample for blood cortisol levels, giving 25 units of ACTH IM, and drawing blood for cortisol levels after 30 and 60 minutes. If the cortisol level does not rise by at least 10 μg/dl, the test is positive for Addison's disease.

5. *IV ACTH stimulation test:* On the first day, the patient is given 25 units of ACTH IV in 500 ml D_5NS between 8 AM and 4 PM. After the infusion, blood cortisol levels are drawn at 12 midnight, 8 AM, and 4 PM. This procedure is repeated on the second day. If there is no increase in blood cortisol levels, indicating an inability of the adrenal glands to respond to ACTH, the patient has primary Addison's disease. If the cortisol levels show a gradual increase over several days, the patient has secondary Addison's disease.

6. *CT scan or MRI:* May show decrease in adrenal or pituitary size, which is indicative of glandular destruction.

MEDICAL MANAGEMENT AND SURGICAL INTERVENTIONS

1. Pharmacotherapy
   □ *Antibiotics or antituberculosis therapy:* If infection or tuberculosis is the cause.
   □ *Maintenance doses of mineralocorticoids; oral supplementary sodium; and oral corticosteroids:* Exogenous steroids must be increased before and immediately after surgery, during times of stress, or in the presence of infection, because these conditions deplete adrenocortical hormones and place greater demands on body tissue. Patients must take hormone replacements for life.
2. Diet: High in calories, carbohydrates, proteins, and vitamins, and provided in small, frequent feedings to enhance nutritional state for these patients, who tend to be anorexic.

For adrenal crisis

1. Replacement of fluids: To correct severe dehydration. 1-2 L D_5NS is given over a brief period of time (e.g., 2 hours).
2. Hydrocortisone sodium succinate: To replace decreased cortisol. It is given 100 mg IV immediately and then q6h *via* infusion drip.
3. Vasopressors: To maintain adequate BP.
4. Continuous cardiac monitoring: For prompt identification of life-threatening dysrhythmias.

NURSING DIAGNOSES AND INTERVENTIONS

Potential for infection related to lowered resistance secondary to decreased adrenal function

Desired outcome: Patient is free of infection as evidenced by normothermia, WBC count ≤11,000 μl, clear urine, well-healing wounds, negative cultures, and absence of adventitious breath sounds and sore throat.

1. Monitor for and report early signs of infection including fever; leukocytosis; urinary frequency, urgency, and dysuria; cloudy or malodorous urine; persistent erythema, pain, swelling, or purulent discharge from wounds or the IV site; complaints of sore throat and pharyngitis. As directed, culture any drainage. Teach patient these signs and symptoms and the importance of reporting them to MD or staff promptly should they occur.
2. Monitor temperature q2-4h, and report significant elevation to MD.
3. Use meticulous aseptic technique for all invasive procedures or when changing dress-

ings. Ensure meticulous indwelling catheter care to help prevent UTI. Perform stringent handwashing technique before caring for these patients.
4. Caution visitors who have contracted or been exposed to a communicable disease not to enter room (or to wear surgical masks when visiting patient).

Potential for injury related to risk of Addisonian crisis or side effects from the drug therapy used to treat it

Desired outcomes: Patient is asymptomatic of Addisonian crisis as evidenced by normothermia; BP >90/60 mm Hg (or within patient's baseline range); HR <100 bpm; RR 12-20 breaths/min with normal depth and pattern (eupnea); orientation to person, place, and time; and absence of abdominal pain, nausea, vomiting, and headache. Patient is asymptomatic of sodium retention and fluid volume excess as evidenced by stable weight; absence of headache and crackles over the lung fields; and edema <2+ on a 0-4+ scale.

1. Be alert to the following indicators of Addisonian crisis: headache, nausea, vomiting, fever, abdominal pain, and severe hypotension. Be aware that the profound hypotension can lead to vascular collapse and shock.
2. Place patient in a quiet room away from loud noises and excessive activity. Caution staff and visitors not to discuss stress-provoking topics with patient.
3. As prescribed, administer corticosteroids and prophylactic antibiotics, which help prevent Addisonian crisis from occurring.
4. If Addisonian crisis is diagnosed, implement the following:
   □ As prescribed, administer vasopressors to maintain BP and hydrocortisone sodium succinate to replace cortisol.
   □ Administer IV fluids as prescribed to prevent circulatory collapse.
   □ Monitor VS q15min until stable, then as prescribed. Report significant changes in BP, HR, or respiratory rate or pattern to MD.
   □ Administer oxygen as prescribed.
   □ Usually, a continuous cardiac monitor is used if Addisonian crisis is diagnosed. Monitor for signs of hypokalemia (increased PVCs, depressed T waves) or hyperkalemia (peaked T waves).
5. Monitor for and report signs of sodium retention and fluid volume excess (peripheral, pulmonary, and cerebral edema) caused by excessive doses of corticosteroids, sodium, and fluids. Be alert to dependent edema, crackles (rales), weight gain, severe headache, irritability, and confusion. Teach these symptoms to the patient and significant others and stress the importance of reporting them promptly to MD or staff.

Activity intolerance related to fatigue and weakness secondary to decreased cardiac output

Desired outcome: Patient exhibits cardiac tolerance to exercise as evidenced by HR ≤20 bpm over resting HR, systolic BP ≤20 mm Hg over or under resting systolic BP, RR ≤20 breaths/min with normal depth and pattern (eupnea), warm and dry skin, and absence of crackles (rales), murmurs, and chest pain.

1. Monitor VS at frequent intervals. Observe for and report indicators of impending circulatory collapse, such as hypotension, tachycardia, weak and thready pulse, pallor, and cyanosis.
2. Gear activities to patient's tolerance. Provide for frequent rest periods.
3. To prevent complications of immobility, assist patient with ROM and other in-bed exercises. For details, see the appendix for **Potential for activity intolerance,** p. 65, and **Potential for disuse syndrome,** p. 653.

Fluid volume deficit related to abnormal loss secondary to diuresis

Desired outcome: Patient becomes normovolemic as evidenced by balanced I&O, urinary output ≥30 ml/hr, good skin turgor, stable weight, and moist tongue and oral mucous membranes.

1. Monitor I&O and be alert to indicators of fluid volume deficit, including thirst, poor skin turgor, and furrowed tongue.

2. If deficit is noted, encourage oral fluids.
3. Administer maintenance doses of mineralocorticoids as prescribed to promote salt and water retention.
4. If prescribed, administer supplementary sodium to correct hyponatremia. As appropriate, advise patient to add salt to foods or eat foods relatively high in sodium, such as meat, fish, poultry, eggs, and milk. See Table 11-3, p. 550, for a list of foods high in sodium.

If patient experiences Addisonian crisis, see the appendix for nursing diagnoses and interventions for the care of patients with cancer and other life-disrupting illnesses, p. 690.

PATIENT-FAMILY TEACHING AND DISCHARGE PLANNING

Provide patient and significant others with verbal and written information for the following:
1. Medications, including drug name, purpose, dosage, schedule, precautions, and potential side effects. Ensure that patient understands the necessity of lifetime hormone replacement.
2. Diet, for example, foods to increase such as those high in sodium (see Table 11-3, p. 550).
3. Relationship between hormonal levels and stress. Instruct patient to seek medical help during periods of emotional or physical stress so that medication dosages can be adjusted accordingly.
4. Signs and symptoms that necessitate medical attention. These include indicators of excessive adrenal hormones (e.g., weight gain, moon face, dependent edema, headache, weakness, irritability), adrenal insufficiency (e.g., progressive fatigue, nausea, vomiting, weakness, and postural hypotension), and infections (e.g., URI, wound, UTI, and oral).
5. Methods for maximizing coping mechanisms to deal with stress, such as diversional activities and relaxation exercises. Explain the importance of avoiding physical or emotional stress. See **Health-seeking behaviors:** Relaxation technique effective for stress reduction, p. 49.
6. Need for continued medical follow-up.
7. Obtaining a Medic-Alert bracelet and identification card outlining the diagnosis and emergency treatment.

In addition:
8. Prepare an emergency kit, including alcohol sponges and syringes with 100 mg hydrocortisone to be carried and used in the event of Addisonian crisis. Teach technique for IM administration of the medication to patient and significant others.

Cushing's disease

Cushing's disease is a spectrum of symptoms associated with prolonged elevated plasma concentration of adrenal steroids. In normal individuals, the pituitary gland secretes ACTH, which stimulates the adrenal glands to release the adrenal steroid hormones. This is regulated by a negative-feedback mechanism in which increasing levels of plasma cortisol suppress ACTH. In cases of pituitary pathology, this mechanism does not function and the pituitary gland continues to secrete excessive amounts of ACTH, with resultant abnormally high levels of adrenocortical hormone. This accounts for approximately 70% of reported cases and is termed *Cushing's disease. Cushing's syndrome,* on the other hand, is caused by pathology of the adrenal glands themselves, from ectopic ACTH-secreting tumors, or from iatrogenic causes, such as excessive ingestion of cortisol or ACTH.

Actions of excessive glucocorticoid (cortisol) secretion include the following: increased protein catabolism; increased production of glucose and glycogen, with resultant hyperglycemia; a rise in plasma lipid levels, which causes atherosclerotic changes in blood vessels; decreased bone formation and increased bone resorption, with resulting osteoporosis; and inhibition of the inflammatory response to tissue injury. Actions of excessive mineralocorticoid (aldosterone) include the following: sodium and water retention, increased renal excretion of potassium, and increased secretion of angiotensin II, a potent vasoconstrictor.

ASSESSMENT

Signs and symptoms: Weight gain; muscle weakness; kyphosis and back pain; generalized osteoporosis, especially in the vertebrae; pathologic fractures of the long bones; mental and emotional disturbances; easy bruising; arteriosclerotic changes in the heart, brain, and kidney; renal calculi; thirst and polyuria; menstrual changes; and impotence.

Physical assessment: Patients exhibit "central obesity" with pendulous abdomens and thin legs and arms; moon face; fat deposits on the neck and supraclavicular area (buffalo obesity); edema; hypertension; and thin, transparent skin with multiple ecchymoses. Androgen excess is most noticeable in females, as evidenced by changes in menstruation, as well as virilism and hirsutism. Patients frequently have stretch marks with red and purple striae showing through the stretched skin. Patients with Cushing's syndrome have hyperpigmentation of facial skin secondary to ectopic ACTH-secreting tumors.

History of: Excessive exogenous steroid ingestion, pituitary tumor.

DIAGNOSTIC TESTS

1. *Blood cortisol:* Normally, cortisol levels fluctuate throughout the day, with the highest level in the morning and a gradual decline until the lowest level is reached about midnight. Therefore, early-morning samples can be misleading, and several specimens are usually drawn throughout the day. Individuals with Cushing's disease exhibit high cortisol levels in the morning that do not decline as the day progresses.
2. *Serum ACTH:* Measured in the same way as blood cortisol. Results will be abnormally high at least part of the day.
3. *Overnight dexamethasone suppression test:* Will show absence of suppression in individuals with Cushing's syndrome. At exactly 11 PM the patient is given 1 mg of dexamethasone, which is enough to suppress adrenal production of cortisol in patients with normal adrenal function. At the same time, 100 mg of pentobarbital is administered to ensure an unstressed night's sleep. In the morning, a fasting cortisol level is drawn. In individuals with Cushing's syndrome, it will not be suppressed lower than 10 μg/dl. Women using birth control pills should have baseline levels of cortisol drawn before this test so that results can be adjusted to avoid false positives.
4. *Other blood tests:* Will reveal elevated postprandial blood sugar in 80%-90% of patients with Cushing's disease and decreased serum potassium.
5. *24-hour urinary free cortisol:* Will be elevated. Cushing's syndrome is confirmed if the results are elevated in an individual with no cortisol suppression.
6. *High-dose dexamethasone test:* Patient is given 8 mg dexamethasone orally over a 24-hour period. A 24-hour urine analysis for 17-hydroxycorticosteroid (17-OHCS) is obtained, and the results are interpreted as follows:
   □ High ACTH with no 17-OHCS suppression indicates an ectopic source of ACTH production.
   □ Low ACTH with no 17-OHCS suppression indicates an adrenal tumor.
   □ Normal to high ACTH with suppression of 17-OHCS indicates Cushing's disease.
7. *CT scan or MRI:* May show adrenal masses or abnormalities in sella turcica, which are indicative of pituitary dysfunction.

MEDICAL MANAGEMENT AND SURGICAL INTERVENTIONS

1. Adrenocortical inhibitors (e.g., metapyrone, aminoglutethimide, and cyproheptadine): To inhibit production of adrenocortical hormones. Exogenous steroids also may be given in conjunction with the adrenocortical inhibitors to prevent hypocortisolism. Adreno-

cortical inhibitors are used only short-term, however, because increased ACTH production quickly overcomes their effect.

2. **Irradiation of the pituitary gland:** To decrease pituitary production of ACTH. It is used for patients with a mild form of the disease or those who are poor surgical risks.

3. **Diet:** Low in calories and carbohydrates to reduce hyperglycemia. Salt is restricted to reduce BP; and foods high in potassium, including bananas, apricots, figs, dried peaches and prunes, oranges, and tomatoes are given to raise serum potassium levels.

4. **Transsphenoidal hypophysectomy:** May be performed if the pathology involves the pituitary gland. Patients return from this surgery with nasal packing and nasopharyngeal airways in place. Potential complications of this surgery include transient diabetes insipidus and CSF leakage. See "Pituitary Tumors," p. 216, for more information about this procedure.

5. **Adrenalectomy, either bilateral or unilateral:** May be performed, depending on the extent of involvement. Potential complications of this surgery include splenic injury, retroperitoneal hemorrhage, pancreatitis, infection, and wound dehiscence. Hemorrhage, infection, and wound dehiscence are especially prevalent because of abnormal cortisol levels, which can cause thinning of the skin and poor wound healing.

NURSING DIAGNOSES AND INTERVENTIONS

Body image disturbance related to physical changes secondary to increased ACTH production

Desired outcome: Patient relates the attainment of self-acceptance and verbalizes knowledge that symptoms will abate with treatment.

1. Encourage patient to verbalize feelings and frustrations.
2. Reassure patient that symptoms should subside with adequate treatment of the disorder.
3. Assist patient with measures to improve appearance, such as keeping hair well groomed, wearing own gown or pajamas if possible, and performing personal hygiene (e.g., bathing and brushing of teeth). Encourage women to apply makeup and perfume, if appropriate.
4. Provide privacy, if indicated.

Potential for impaired skin integrity related to vulnerability secondary to thinning of skin and fragility of capillaries

Desired outcome: Patient's skin remains clear and intact.

1. Ensure that patient on bed rest turns q2h. Establish and post a turning schedule. Provide gentle massage with lotions to help prevent decubitus ulcers.
2. Place alternating air pressure mattress or other pressure-relief mattress or pad on the bed.
3. Position foot cradle over the bed to prevent pressure areas on lower extremities by keeping bed linen off the feet.
4. To protect the skin of confused patients, pad the siderails of the bed.

See "Hyperparathyroidism" for **Potential for trauma** related to risk of pathologic fractures, p. 270. See "Addison's Disease" for **Potential for infection**, p. 275. See "Pituitary Tumors" for **Potential for injury** related to risk of IICP, CSF leak, and diabetes insipidus secondary to transsphenoidal hypophysectomy), p. 285. Also see the appendix for nursing diagnoses and interventions for the care of preoperative and postoperative patients, p. 637, and care of patients with life-disrupting illnesses, p. 690.

PATIENT-FAMILY TEACHING AND DISCHARGE PLANNING

Provide patient and significant others with verbal and written information for the following:

1. Diet, including foods to increase, such as those high in potassium (see Table 11-4, p.

555), and foods to restrict, including those that are high in sodium (see Table 11-3, p. 550) or carbohydrates. Arrange for a dietary consultation to help patient with meal planning and integration of individual restrictions into family diet.

2. Medications, including drug name, purpose, dosage, schedule, precautions, and potential side effects. Advise patient with bilateral adrenalectomy of the necessity for lifetime hormone replacement therapy.

3. Importance of continued medical follow-up; confirm date and time of next medical appointment.

4. Relationship between hormone levels and stress. Advise patient to seek medical assistance during periods of emotional or physical stress so that medications can be adjusted accordingly. Provide suggestions for patient to maximize coping mechanisms, such as relaxation exercises or diversional activities. See **Health-seeking behaviors:** Relaxation technique effective for stress reduction, p. 49.

5. Indicators of *excessive adrenal hormone:* weight gain, thirst, polyuria, easy bruising, and muscle weakness; or *adrenal insufficiency:* easy fatiguability, weight loss, and abdominal pain, any of which necessitate medical attention.

6. Signs and symptoms of UTI, URI, wound, and oral infections and the importance of seeking medical care should they occur.

7. Importance of wearing a Medic-Alert bracelet and carrying an identification card to describe the disease and the necessary emergency measures.

In addition:

8. For patients with bilateral adrenalectomy, provide an emergency kit with alcohol sponges and syringes filled with 100 mg of hydrocortisone for episodes of acute adrenal insufficiency. Teach patient and significant others the technique for IM administration of the medication for emergency treatment.

Section Four   DISORDERS OF THE PITUITARY GLAND

The pituitary (hypophysis) is composed of two lobes, the anterior pituitary (adenohypophysis) and posterior pituitary (neurohypophysis). The anterior lobe is larger and its secretory activities are controlled by tropic hormones produced by and transmitted from the hypothalamus in response to negative feedback mechanisms. It secretes seven of the nine pituitary hormones. These include (1) adrenocorticotropic hormone (ACTH), which stimulates adrenal cortical growth and secretion of adrenocortical hormones; (2) thyrotropic hormone (TSH), which stimulates thyroid growth and secretion of thyroid hormones; (3) follicle-stimulating hormone (FSH), which stimulates ovulation in females and sperm production in males; (4) luteinizing hormone (LH), called the interstitial cell-stimulating hormone (ICSH) in males, in whom it stimulates production of testosterone, and in females stimulates ovulation and development of ovarian follicles; (5) melanocyte-stimulating hormone (MSH), which causes pigmentation; (6) luteotropic hormone (LTH), also called prolactin, which stimulates secretion of milk in females; and (7) growth hormone (GH) or somatotropic hormone (STH), which accelerates body growth.

Posterior pituitary secretion is regulated by nerve impulses originating in the hypothalamus in response to stimuli from other parts of the body. It produces two hormones: antidiuretic hormone (ADH) or vasopressin, which acts on the renal tubules to increase reabsorption of water; and oxytocin, which stimulates milk "letdown" and contraction of the uterus.

Diabetes insipidus

Diabetes insipidus results from a defect in the release or synthesis of ADH from the hypothalamus, or a defect in renal tubular response to ADH, causing impaired renal conservation of water. The onset usually is insidious, with progressively increasing polydipsia and polyuria, but it can develop rapidly following an injury or infectious disease. Depending on the degree of injury, the condition can be either temporary or permanent.

There are three phases associated with diabetes insipidus. The first phase of polydipsia and polyuria immediately follows the injury and lasts 4-5 days. In the second phase, which lasts about 6 days, the symptoms disappear; and in the third phase, the patient experiences permanent polydipsia and polyuria. The chief danger to these patients is dehydration from the inability to take in adequate fluids to balance the excessive output of urine.

ASSESSMENT

Signs and symptoms: Polydipsia, polyuria with dilute urine.

Physical assessment: Usually within normal limits, however patient may show signs of dehydration if fluid intake is inadequate.

History of: Cranial injury, especially basilar skull fracture; meningitis; primary or metastatic brain tumor; surgery in the pituitary area; cerebral hemorrhage; encephalitis; syphilis; or tuberculosis. Familial incidence is rarely a factor.

DIAGNOSTIC TESTS

1. *Urine osmolality:* Decreased (<50-200 mOsm/kg) in the presence of disease.
2. *Specific gravity:* Decreased (<1.007) in the presence of disease.
3. *Serum osmolality:* Increased ($\geq$300 mOsm/kg) in the presence of disease.
4. *Water deprivation test:* Baseline measurements of body weight, serum and urine osmolalities, and urine specific gravity are obtained. Fluids are not permitted and the above measurements are repeated qh. The test is terminated when urine specific gravity exceeds 1.020 and osmolality exceeds 800 mOsm/kg (normal responses); or when 5% of body weight is lost. The latter is, in itself, an abnormal response and the corresponding urine osmolality will be <400 mOsm/kg, which is diagnostic of diabetes insipidus. Because the most serious side effect of this test is severe dehydration, the test should be performed early in the day so the patient can be more closely monitored. Before a firm diagnosis of diabetes insipidus can be made from an abnormal water deprivation test, it is also necessary to demonstrate that the kidneys can respond to vasopressin (see below).
5. *Vasopressin (exogenous ADH):* Given SC, followed by urine collections q15min for 2 hours. Quantity and specific gravity are then measured. The normal individual will show a concentration of urine, but not as pronounced as that for the person with diabetes insipidus; while a person with kidney disease will have a lesser response to vasopressin. **Note:** One serious side effect of this test is the precipitation of CHF in susceptible individuals.

MEDICAL MANAGEMENT

1. **Administration of exogenous vasopressin (Pitressin):** Replacement therapy for ADH. There are several preparations available, and it is important to read the package insert carefully to ensure proper administration. Potential side effects include hypertension secondary to vasoconstriction, myocardial infarction secondary to constriction of coronary vessels, uterine cramps, and increased peristalsis of the GI tract. See Table 5-1.
2. **Achieving a mild antidiuretic effect:** For example, with chlorpropamide.

NURSING DIAGNOSES AND INTERVENTIONS

Fluid volume deficit related to abnormal loss secondary to polyuria

Desired outcomes: Patient becomes normovolemic as evidenced by stable weight, balanced I&O, good skin turgor, moist tongue and oral mucous membrane, BP >90/60 mm Hg (or within patient's normal range), HR $\leq$100 bpm, and CVP 2-6 mm Hg (or 5-12 cm H_2O).

TABLE 5-1   Vasopressin preparations

Generic name	Brand name	Onset	Duration	Usual Dose	Advantages/disadvantages	Comments
Nasal						
Vasopressin	Pitressin	within 1 hr	4-8 hr	5-10 U bid-tid	Action decreased by nasal congestion/discharge or atrophy of nasal mucosa	Administer by spray, cotton pledget, or dropper
Desmopressin DDAVP acetate	within 1 hr	8-20 hr	0.1-0.4 ml qd in 1-3 doses (10-40 μg)	See above	See above Store in refrigerator at 4° C (39.2° F)	
Lypressin	Diapid	within 1 hr	3-8 hr	7-14 μg qid	See above	See above Store at <40° C (100° F)
Subcutaneous						
Vasopressin	Pitressin	½-1 hr	2-8 hr	0.25-0.5 ml (5-10 U) q3-4h prn increased thirst or increased urine output		
Desmopressin acetate	DDAVP, Stimate	within ½ hr	1 ½-4 hr	0.5 ml-1 ml (2 μg-4 μg) qd in 2 divided doses	Keep refrigerated at 4° C (39.2° F)	

Intramuscular

Vasopressin tannate in oil	Pitressin tannate in oil	within 1-2 hrs	36-48 hr	0.3-1 ml (1.5-5 U) q2-3 days for increased thirst or increased urine output	Longer duration of action/slower absorption than SC route. Response cumulative over 2-3 days	Store at 13-18° C (55-65° F) Shake well before withdrawing from vial. Can warm solution by immersing vial in warm water
Vasopressin tannate	Pitressin	½-1 hr	2-8 hr	0.25-0.5 ml (5-10 U) q3-4h for increased thirst or increased urine output		

Intravenous

Desmopressin acetate	DDAVP	within ½ hr	1 ½-4 hr	0.5-1.0 ml (2-4 µg) qd in 2 divided doses	Not for home use	Keep refrigerated at 4° C (39.2° F). Dilute in 10-50 ml 0.9% NaCl and infuse over 15-30 min

1. Monitor I&O, daily weight, and VS closely. Be alert to evidence of hypovolemia, including weight loss, inadequate fluid intake to balance output, thirst, poor skin turgor, furrowed tongue, hypotension, and tachycardia. If a central line is present, monitor CVP for evidence of hypotension.
2. Provide unrestricted fluids. Keep water pitcher full and within easy reach of patient. Explain the importance of consuming as much fluid as can be tolerated.
3. Administer vasopressin and antidiuretic agents as prescribed.
4. For unconscious patient, administer IV fluids as prescribed. Unless otherwise directed, for every ml of urine output, deliver 1 ml of IV fluid.

Potential for injury related to negative side effects of vasopressin

Desired outcome: Patient is asymptomatic of negative side effects of vasopressin as evidenced by systolic BP ≤20 mm Hg over baseline systolic BP; HR ≤20 bpm over baseline HR; stable weight; absence of chest pain and headache; and orientation to person, place, and time.

1. Monitor VS, especially BP, and report significant changes, such as systolic BP elevated >20 mm Hg over baseline systolic BP or pulse increased >20 bpm over baseline.
2. Be alert to indicators of water intoxication, including changes in LOC, confusion, weight gain, headache, convulsions, and coma. If these develop, stop the medication, restrict fluids, and notify MD. Institute safety measures accordingly.
3. For the older adult or individuals with vascular disease, keep prescribed coronary vasodilators, such as amyl nitrate or nitroglycerine, at the bedside for use should angina occur. Teach patient and significant others how to administer these medications.

PATIENT-FAMILY TEACHING AND DISCHARGE PLANNING

Provide patient and significant others with verbal and written information for the following:
1. Importance of continued medical follow-up; confirm date and time of next appointment.
2. Indicators that necessitate medical attention, for example, signs of dehydration or water intoxication. For more information, see "Fluid Disturbances," p. 546.

Pituitary tumors

Pituitary adenomas account for approximately 10% of intracranial tumors and constitute the most frequent cause of pituitary dysfunction. These tumors are almost always benign and easily treated if discovered early. Ninety percent of pituitary tumors produce no hormones, but if they are allowed to grow, they will compress the rest of the gland, ultimately leading to pituitary destruction with resultant hypopituitarism. This will decrease the levels of all the hormones produced by the pituitary gland. Usually, gonadotropic hormones are suppressed first; and eventually, signs of hypothyroidism (see p. 263) and adrenocortical insufficiency (see "Addison's Disease," p. 274) will appear. Of the remaining 10% of pituitary tumors that do produce hormones, 60% secrete excessive prolactin and 20% secrete excess growth hormone (GH). Another 10% secrete excess ACTH (see "Cushing's Disease," p. 277).

ASSESSMENT

Hypopituitarism: Weakness, easy fatigue, myxedema coma (see "Hypothyroidism," p. 263), or Addisonian crisis (see "Addison's Disease," p. 274). Patients also may have atrophy of external genitalia; amenorrhea and vaginal mucosal atrophy; impotence or loss of libido; minimal perspiration; and lessening of resistance to colds, stress, and infections. Patients often present with extreme pallor; sallow complexion; visual deficits; thinning of eyebrows and hair; dry skin with thin-lined wrinkling of the face; sparse pubic, axillary, and facial hair; hypotension; and orthostatic hypotension.

Excessive GH (acromegaly): Hoarseness, headache, diplopia, hemianopsia (blindness in half the field of vision, either unilateral or bilateral), papilledema, lethargy, amenorrhea, loss of libido, impotence, and weight gain. Patients often present with coarse facial features and enlargement of hands and feet, wide-spaced teeth, thickening of skin and nails, skeletal enlargement (can be 7-8 feet tall) with protusion of the lower jaw, joint deformities, arthritis, and multiple fleshy tumors on the skin, especially the scalp.

Excessive prolactin: Weight gain, fluid retention, irritability, and hirsutism and decrease in vaginal lubrication in females. Males often present with impotence or decreased libido, while females often have galactorrhea and amenorrhea.

Excessive ACTH: See "Cushing's Disease," p. 277.

DIAGNOSTIC TESTS

General

1. *X-ray of skull:* Will show enlarged pituitary gland, thickened skull, and distorted, enlarged pituitary fossa.
2. *CT scan or MRI:* May reveal an abnormality of the sella turcica or extrasellar extension of the tumor.
3. *Skeletal x-rays:* Will show thickening of long bones.
4. *Pneumoencephalogram:* Will reveal extension of pituitary tumor above the sella turcica.
5. *Serum tests (in hyperpituitarism):* Elevated phosphate and postprandial blood glucose will be present.
6. *Urinary calcium (in hyperpituitarism):* Increased secondary to increased production of calcitonin from the thyroid.
7. *GH and basal prolactin:* Increased.

For hypopituitarism

1. *Urinary 17-ketosteroids, 17-hydroxycorticosteroids, and plasma cortisol:* Decreased, but will rise slowly after administration of ACTH. See "Addison's Disease," p. 275.
2. *Urinary and serum gonadotropins:* Decreased.
3. *Plasma testosterone and estradiol:* Decreased.
4. *Serum levels of ACTH, TSH, LH, FSH, and GH:* Decreased.

MEDICAL MANAGEMENT AND SURGICAL INTERVENTIONS

1. Exogenous hormone replacements: As appropriate for syndromes of insufficiency secondary to hypopituitarism.
2. X-ray and heavy-particle radiation therapy: For hormone-secreting tumors. Typically, the response with a return to normal is slow, but tumor progression is halted in most patients. Side effects can include malaise, nausea, serous otitis media, and hypopituitarism. For more information, see "Caring for Patients with Cancer and Other Life-Disruptive Illnesses," p. 659.
3. Transsphenoidal hypophysectomy: Treatment of choice because it offers a more rapid cure with a low morbidity rate. The surgeon makes an incision in the inner aspect of the upper lip and enters the sella turcica through the sphenoid process. Because an opening is created between the nose and upper airway, the patient is at increased risk for postoperative infection, so nasal antibiotics are frequently used preoperatively. In addition, the patient will have two black eyes after surgery. The pituitary is a highly vascularized gland; and therefore, hemorrhage at the operative site is another potential risk. Diabetes insipidus can result from pituitary destruction and removal. For larger tumors, a frontal craniotomy may be necessary. (See "Brain Tumor," p. 215.)

NURSING DIAGNOSES AND INTERVENTIONS

Potential for injury related to risk of IICP, CSF leak, hemorrhage, infection, and diabetes insipidus secondary to transsphenoidal hypophysectomy

Desired outcome: Patient is asymptomatic of complications of transsphenoidal hypophysectomy as evidenced by equal and normoreactive pupils; orientation to person, place, and time; RR 12-20 breaths/min with normal depth and pattern (eupnea); nasal packing drainage negative for glucose and without frank bleeding; urine output ≤200 ml/hr for two consecutive hours or ≤500 ml/hr; urine specific gravity ≥1.007; and stable weight.

1. Be alert to indicators of IICP, such as a change in LOC, sluggish or unequal pupils, and changes in respiratory rate or pattern. Report significant findings to MD.
2. Measure accurate I&O qh for 24 hours and monitor urine specific gravity q1-2h. Report an output >200 ml/hr for 2 consecutive hours or a total of 500 ml/hr. Specific gravity <1.007 is found with diabetes insipidus. Monitor weight daily for evidence of loss. Report significant findings to MD.
3. Inspect nasal packing at frequent intervals for the presence of frank bleeding or CSF leakage. After nasal packing is removed, test *non*sanguineous drainage for the presence of CSF fluid using a glucose reagent strip. If the drainage contains CSF, the test will be positive for the presence of glucose. **Note:** Because the presence of CSF represents a serious breach in the integrity of the cranium, elevate the HOB to minimize the potential for bacteria entering the brain and immediately report any suspicious drainage.
4. Elevate the HOB 30 degrees to decrease ICP and swelling.
5. Explain to patient that coughing, sneezing, and other Valsalva-type maneuvers must be avoided because these actions can stress the operative site and increase ICP, causing CSF leakage. If coughing or sneezing is unavoidable, teach patient to do so with an opened mouth. If indicated, obtain a prescription for a mild cathartic or stool softener to prevent straining with bowel movements.
6. To prevent disturbance in the integrity of the operative site, do not allow patient to brush teeth. Provide mouthwash and Toothette for oral hygiene.

Sexual dysfunction related to physiologic limitations secondary to abnormal hormone levels

Desired outcome: Patient relates the attainment of satisfying sexual activity.

1. Encourage patient to express feelings of anger and frustration and to communicate feelings to significant other.
2. If appropriate, suggest alternatives other than sexual intercourse for pleasuring partner and self.
3. Administer testosterone or estrogens as prescribed.
4. Support MD's referral or suggest referral for psychotherapy related to loss of libido, sterility, impotence, or loss of self-esteem.

See the appendix for nursing diagnoses and interventions for the care of preoperative and postoperative patients, p. 637.

PATIENT-FAMILY TEACHING AND DISCHARGE PLANNING

Provide patient and significant others with verbal and written information for the following:
1. Medications, including drug name, purpose, dosage, schedule, precautions, and potential side effects. Reinforce that following hypophysectomy, patient will be on lifetime hormone replacement therapy.
2. Relationship between hormone levels and stress. Advise patient to seek medical help during times of emotional or physical stress so that dosages of medications can be adjusted accordingly.
3. Measures for maximizing coping mechanisms to deal with stress such as relaxation tapes, meditation, diversional activities. See **Health-seeking behaviors:** Relaxation technique effective for stress reduction, p. 49.
4. Importance of continued medical follow-up; confirm time and date of next appointment.

5. Indicators of *adrenal hormone excess:* weight gain, easy bruising, muscle weakness, moon face, thirst, and polyuria; *adrenal hormone insufficiency:* weight loss, easy fatigue, and abdominal pain; *hypothyroidism:* weight gain, anorexia, apathy, slowed mentation, and cold intolerance; and *hyperthyroidism:* tachycardia, diaphoresis, and heat intolerance. All of these signs and symptoms necessitate medical attention.
6. Importance of obtaining a Medic-Alert bracelet and identification card outlining diagnosis and emergency treatment.

For patients who have had a transsphenoidal hypophysectomy

7. Importance of avoiding bending or straining until after postoperative follow-up and clearance by MD.
8. Not brushing front teeth until the incision is healed (about ten days). Recommend use of mouthwash and gentle use of Toothette instead.
9. Signs and symptoms of infection, which necessitate medical attention: fever, nuchal rigidity, headache, photophobia.

Section Five   DISORDERS OF THE PANCREAS

The pancreas serves both exocrine (nonhormonal) and endocrine functions. The exocrine portion comprises 98% of tissue mass. Its function is the secretion of potent enzymes that act to reduce proteins, fats, and carbohydrates into simpler chemical substances. Pancreatic lipase acts on fats to produce glycerides, fatty acids, and glycerol; pancreatic amylase acts on starch to produce disaccharides. The pancreas also secretes sodium bicarbonate to neutralize the strongly acidic gastric contents as they enter the duodenum. The resultant mixture of acids and bases provides an optimal pH for the activation of pancreatic enzymes.

Pancreatitis

Pancreatitis can involve edema, hemorrhage, or necrosis of the pancreas and its blood supply. It is characterized by varying degrees of pancreatic insufficiency, which results in decreased production of enzymes and bicarbonate and malabsorption of fats and proteins. The digestion of fat is affected most severely. As a result, a high fat content in the bowel stimulates water and electrolyte secretion, which produces diarrhea. The action of bacteria on fecal fat produces flatus, fatty stools (steatorrhea), and abdominal cramps. Autodigestion, the activation of pancreatic enzymes within the pancreas, is the pathologic process in pancreatitis.

Initially, pancreatic ductal flow becomes obstructed, injuring the adjacent acinar cell where pancreatic enzymes are stored. Acinar cell damage causes release of the stored enzymes and the autodigestive process begins. Often, diabetes mellitus occurs as a result of chronic pancreatitis because of damage to the beta cells, which normally produce insulin, with resultant decreased insulin production.

ASSESSMENT

Acute pancreatitis: Sudden onset of severe epigastric pain following a large meal or alcohol intake. The pain radiates to the back and is unrelieved by vomiting. The patient also may have persistent vomiting, extreme malaise, restlessness, cold and sweaty extremities, dehydration, left pleural effusion, adult respiratory distress syndrome (ARDS), and jaundice.

Physical assessment: Diminished or absent bowel sounds, suggesting presence of ileus; crackles (rales) at the lung bases related to persistent hypoventilation associated with splinting and guarding with pain. In addition, edema in and around the pancreas impinges on the diaphragm and prevents full expansion of the lungs with inspiration. Patients also may have low-grade fever of 37.8°-38.9° C (100°-102° F) and an abdominal mass.

Chronic pancreatitis: Constant, dull epigastric pain; steatorrhea resulting from malabsorption of fats and protein; severe weight loss; and onset of symptoms of diabetes mellitus: polydipsia, polyuria, polyphagia. In addition, chemical addiction is often seen because of the chronic pain.

History of: Biliary tract disease, chronic excessive alcohol consumption, duodenal ulcer, coxsackie virus, mumps, hypothermia, and use of estrogen-containing oral contraceptives, glucocorticoids, sulfonamides, chlorothiazides, and azothioprine.

DIAGNOSTIC TESTS

1. *Serum amylase:* When significantly elevated (>500 U/100 ml), rules out acute abdomen conditions, such as cholecystitis, appendicitis, bowel infarction/obstruction, and perforated peptic ulcer, and confirms presence of pancreatitis. These levels return to normal 48-72 hours after the onset of acute symptoms, even though clinical indicators may continue.
2. *Serum lipase:* Levels rise more slowly than serum amylase and persist longer. Both lipase and amylase levels reflect the degree of necrotic pancreatic tissue.
3. *Serum calcium and magnesium:* Levels may be lower than normal. On EKG, hypocalcemia is evidenced by prolonged QT segment with a normal T wave.
4. *CBC:* Elevated WBCs owing to inflammatory process. Polymorphonuclear (PMN) bodies may increase if bacterial peritonitis is present secondary to duodenal rupture.
5. *Urinalysis:* May show presence of glycosuria, which can signal the onset of diabetes mellitus. Elevated urine amylase levels are useful diagnostically when serum levels have dropped off. An elevated specific gravity reflects the presence of dehydration.
6. *Hyperglycemia:* Occurs because of interference with beta-cell function. It is transient with acute pancreatitis but common with chronic pancreatitis, during which diabetes mellitus is likely to develop.
7. *Abdominal x-rays:* May show dilatation of the small or large bowel and presence of pancreatic calcification in chronic pancreatitis.
8. *GI x-rays:* May reveal an edematous pancreatic head that exerts pressure on the duodenum or stomach.
9. *Percutaneous transhepatic cholangiogram (PTHC):* To rule out obstructive versus non-obstructive jaundice.
10. *Endoscopic retrocholangiopancreatography (ERCP):* A combined endoscopic-radiographic tool that is used to study the degree of pancreatic disease *via* assessment of biliary-pancreatic ductal systems. It allows direct visualization of the ampulla of Vater, diagnoses biliary stones and duct stenosis, and distinguishes cancer of the pancreas from pancreatic calculi. This test is also used for patients with bleeding tendencies for whom PTHC is contraindicated; it is not performed until the acute episode has subsided.

MEDICAL MANAGEMENT AND SURGICAL INTERVENTIONS

Medical goals are to reduce stimuli for pancreatic secretion and rehydrate with fluids.

For acute pancreatitis

1. Fluid and electrolyte replacement: To maintain adequate circulating blood volume. For example, protein solutions that do not stimulate the pancreas, such as glucose or free amino acids, and blood volume expanders, such as plasma and albumin.
2. Bed rest: To reduce metabolic demands on the body and thereby minimize need for pancreatic activity.
3. Pharmacotherapy
   □ *Meperidine:* For pain. **Note:** Both morphine and meperidine may cause spasms at the sphincter of Odi. Atropine is often given to prevent this from occurring.
   □ *Broad spectrum antibiotics:* For infection, if present.
   □ *Steroids:* To reduce inflammation.
   □ *Anticholinergics:* To impede impulses that stimulate pancreatic secretions.

4. **NPO status and NG suction:** To decrease stimulus for pancreatic secretions and alleviate pressure in the GI tract.
5. **Rule out underlying factors** (e.g., hyperparathyroidism and hyperlipoproteinemia): Can contribute to the development of pancreatitis.
6. **Surgery:** May be performed for biliary pancreatitis or acute necrotizing hemorrhagic pancreatitis. (See "Surgery" below.)

For chronic pancreatitis

1. **For exacerbations:** See treatment for acute pancreatitis.
2. **Alcohol rehabilitation:** If alcoholism is the cause of pancreatitis.
3. **Long-term pain management:** With analgesics or the lowest effective dose of meperidine.
4. **Oral enzyme supplements** (e.g., pancreatin and pancrelipase): To treat malabsorption.
5. **Diet:** High in carbohydrates and protein and low in fat.
6. **Insulin therapy:** May be required to ensure adequate carbohydrate metabolism if endocrine function is impaired. Lab values of fasting blood sugar and bedside monitoring of blood glucose will reveal abnormalities in blood glucose levels and direct the appropriate insulin therapy. (See "Diabetes Mellitus," p. 296, for more information.)
7. **Surgical interventions:** Often indicated when pancreatitis is due to an obstructive process, such as gallstone formation or cancer. When gallstones are the cause of the pancreatitis, surgical removal of the stone(s) and usually the gallbladder is performed (see "Cholelithiasis/Cholecystitis" in "Gastrointestinal Disorders," p. 391). The surgery is performed when the acute symptoms of pancreatitis have abated or there is no improvement after 48 hours. A common bile duct exploration may be done at the time of surgery to uncover and retrieve all stones. See "Pancreatic Tumors," p. 292, for a discussion of total pancreatectomy or other surgical procedures performed if cancer of the pancreatic head is present.

NURSING DIAGNOSES AND INTERVENTIONS

Fluid volume deficit related to abnormal loss secondary to NG suctioning, vomiting, diaphoresis, or pooling of fluids in the abdomen and retroperitoneum

Desired outcome: Patient becomes normovolemic as evidenced by HR 60-100 bpm, CVP 2-6 mm Hg (5-12 cm H_2O), brisk capillary refill (<3 seconds), peripheral pulses >2+ on a 0-4+ scale, urinary output ≥30 ml/hr, and stable weight and abdominal girth measurements.

1. Monitor VS q2-4h and be alert to falling BP and increasing tachycardia, which can occur with moderate to severe fluid loss.
2. Measure I&O, and if appropriate, CVP q2-4h. Because fluid loss requires immediate replacement to prevent shock and circulatory collapse, be alert to and report I&O imbalances. CVP <2 mm Hg (<5 cm H_2O) can occur with volume-related hypotension.
3. Administer plasma volume expanders as prescribed. For high volumes, use volume control pump to prevent sudden fluid shifts caused by excessive osmotic pressure, which can result in fluid overload.
4. Administer electrolytes (potassium, calcium) as prescribed to prevent cardiac dysrhythmias and tetany.
5. Be alert to indicators of hypocalcemia, such as muscle twitching, tetany, or irritability, which can occur with electrolyte loss.
6. Monitor lab values, such as hematocrit, hemoglobin, calcium, glucose, BUN, and potassium.

Pain related to inflammatory process of the pancreas

Desired outcome: Patient's subjective evaluation of discomfort improves, as documented by a pain scale.

1. Assess for and document the degree and character of the patient's discomfort. Devise a pain scale with the patient, rating the discomfort on a scale of 0 (no pain) to 10.

2. To minimize pancreatic secretions and pain and to maximize needed rest, ensure that patient maintains bed rest.
3. Maintain NPO status to minimize stimulation of pancreatic secretions.
4. Administer analgesics, steroids, and anticholinergics as prescribed; be alert to patient's response to medications, using the pain scale. If analgesia is ineffective, notify MD because patient may require surgical intervention.
5. Assist patient with attaining position of comfort. A supine position with knees flexed often helps to relax abdominal muscles.
6. Emphasize nonpharmacologic pain interventions (e.g., relaxation techniques, distraction, guided imagery, massage). This is especially important for patients who develop chronic pancreatitis and are prone to chemical dependence. See **Health-seeking behaviors:** Relaxation technique effective for stress reduction, p. 49.

Alteration in nutrition: Less than body requirements related to decreased intake secondary to anorexia and dietary restrictions; and increased need secondary to digestive dysfunction

Desired outcomes: Patient maintains baseline body weight and exhibits a positive or balanced nitrogen state on nitrogen studies.

1. When NG tube is removed, provide diet as prescribed, for example, small high-carbohydrate meals at frequent intervals (e.g., 6/day) and adding protein to patient's tolerance. Keep diet bland to minimize pancreatic stimulation, and instruct patient to avoid stimulants that increase enzyme secretion, such as coffee, tea, alcohol, and nicotine.
2. Provide oral hygiene at frequent intervals to enhance appetite and minimize nausea.
3. Monitor blood sugar levels for presence of hyperglycemia and be alert to dysphagia, polydipsia, and polyuria, which occur with diabetes mellitus. These indicators reflect the need for medical evaluation and intervention to ensure proper metabolism of carbohydrates.
4. Weigh patient daily to assess gain or loss. Weight loss may signal the need to change the diet or provide enzyme replacement therapy.
5. Note amount and degree of steatorrhea as an indicator of fat intolerance. As prescribed, administer pancreatic enzyme supplements, which are given before introducing fat into the diet.
6. If prescribed, administer other dietary supplements that support nutrition and caloric intake. These may include products that consist of medium-chain triglycerides (MCTs), such as Isocal or MCT oil. Their advantage is that they do not require pancreatic enzymes for absorption.
7. Avoid administering pancreatin with hot foods or drinks, which will deactivate enzyme activity.
8. To help alleviate the bloating, nausea, and cramps experienced by some patients, provide meals in small feedings throughout the day.

See the appendix for nursing diagnoses and interventions for the care of preoperative and postoperative patients, p. 637.

PATIENT-FAMILY TEACHING AND DISCHARGE PLANNING

Provide patient and significant others with verbal and written information for the following:
1. Cause for current episode of pancreatitis, if known, so that recurrence may be avoided.
2. Alcohol consumption, which can cause or exacerbate chronic pancreatitis.
3. Availability of chemical dependency programs to prevent/treat drug dependence, which is a common occurrence with chronic pancreatitis; or to treat alcoholism. For more information, see "Chemical Dependency," p. 597.
4. Diet: frequent, small meals that are high in carbohydrates and protein. Food should be bland until gradual return to normal diet is prescribed. Remind patient to avoid enzyme stimulants, such as coffee, tea, nicotine, and alcohol.

5. Medications, including drug name, purpose, dosage, schedule, precautions, and potential side effects.
6. Signs and symptoms of diabetes mellitus, including fatigue, weight loss, polydipsia, polyuria, and polyphagia.
7. Necessity of medical follow-up; confirm time and date of next medical appointment.
8. Potential for recurrence of steatorrhea as evidenced by foamy, foul-smelling stools that are high in fat content. Steatorrhea can indicate recurrence of disease process or ineffectiveness of drug therapy and should be reported to MD.
9. Weighing daily at home; importance of reporting weight loss to MD.
10. If surgery was performed, the indicators of wound infection: redness, swelling, discharge, fever, pain, or local warmth.

Pancreatic tumors

Pancreatic tumors, either benign (adenoma) or malignant (carcinoma), can develop anywhere within the pancreas. A tumor that develops at the islet cells is called an insulinoma and is characterized by hypersecretion of insulin. Usually it is treated surgically with a subtotal pancreatectomy. The most frequent site for pancreatic tumors is the pancreatic head, particularly in the region around the ampulla of Vater. These are malignant tumors (adenocarcinomas), for which detection is difficult and the prognosis poor. Because of vague, ill-defined symptoms that appear early in the disease process with pancreatic cancer, metastasis often occurs before a diagnosis can be made.

ASSESSMENT

Signs and symptoms: Progressive, unexplained, rapid weight loss; upper or midabdominal pain that radiates to the back, can be aggravated by eating, and is not related to posture or activity. The patient also may have clay-colored stools, dark urine, pruritus, anorexia, nausea, vomiting, steatorrhea caused by fat and protein malabsorption, bleeding tendency from vitamin K deficiency, malnutrition, and electrolyte disturbances. In addition, diabetes mellitus symptoms often appear as early indicators of the disorder. (See "Diabetes Mellitus," p. 294.)

Physical assessment: Jaundice caused by obstruction of the flow of bile from the liver. The patient also may have generalized weakness and poor skin turgor.

DIAGNOSTIC TESTS

1. *Serum alkaline phosphatase:* Elevated with obstructive bile duct disease.
2. *Serum bilirubin:* Elevated if the pancreatic tumor obstructs the flow of bile from the liver. Levels >3 mg/100 ml will result in jaundice; levels >25 mg/100 ml are common with this condition.
3. *PT:* Prolonged because of vitamin K deficiency. Vitamin K is required for synthesis of prothrombin in the liver, and it is absorbed poorly in the presence of pancreatic insufficiency because it is a fat-soluble vitamin.
4. *GI x-rays:* May show displacement of visceral organs by the enlarged pancreatic tumor.
5. *Percutaneous transhepatic cholangiogram (PTHC):* To determine the level of biliary obstruction and confirm the presence of cholelithiasis.
6. *Endoscopic retrocholangiopancreatography (ERCP):* Permits direct visualization of the ampulla of Vater *via* injection of a radiopaque dye into the pancreatic and biliary ducts. In patients with marked bleeding tendencies, neither ERCP nor PTHC is performed.
7. *5-hour glucose tolerance test:* Helps confirm diagnosis of insulinoma.
8. *CT scan of pancreas:* To delineate pancreatic mass.
9. *Cytologic examination of duodenal contents:* Reveals malignant cells, if present.
10. *Ultrasound:* To rule out presence of cystic lesions and metastases.
11. *Fine-needle aspiration biopsy:* To confirm diagnosis.

SURGICAL INTERVENTIONS

Pancreatic cancer frequently results from metastasis; and even when the pancreas is the primary site, diagnosis and interventions are thwarted by the vague symptomatology and insidious onset of this disease. The medical and surgical approaches will vary depending on the status of the tumor found with the initial exploratory surgery (exploratory laparotomy).

1. **Whipple procedure (pancreatoduodenectomy):** A surgical attempt to cure cancer of the pancreatic head when the tumor is judged to be resectable (e.g., if it has not metastasized and is not interfering with major blood vessels). This extensive surgery involves resection of the head of the pancreas and duodenum and three anastomoses of the following: common bile duct to the jejunum (choledochojejunostomy); the remainder of the pancreas to the jejunum (pancreaticojejunostomy); and the stomach to the jejunum (gastrojejunostomy).

2. **Vagotomy (dividing the vagus nerve branches to the stomach):** May be done in addition to the Whipple procedure to minimize gastric secretions.

3. **Total pancreatectomy:** May be performed for patients with chronic pancreatitis or cancer of the pancreatic head. The location of the surgical incision will vary with the extent of the surgery; however, whether it is vertical or oblique, the incision usually extends high into the abdomen. The patient will have one or two drains, depending on the extensiveness of the surgery. A Penrose drain may exit from the abdomen; a T-tube, sump tube, or portable wound drainage system also may be present. For patients who have undergone a total pancreatectomy, the resultant pancreatic endocrine and exocrine deficiency requires treatment with insulin, pancreatic enzymes, and a diabetic diet that is low in fat.

4. **Palliative measures:** Initiated when the tumor is not resectable (90% of the cases). Although the tumor is left intact, the gallbladder may be anastomosed to the duodenum to permit bile from the liver to bypass the tumor and flow directly into the duodenum. Another approach is the percutaneous biliary drain, which is used for inoperable liver, pancreatic, or bile duct carcinoma. This tube or catheter, which is perforated with holes at the distal end, is inserted percutaneously through the liver, past the obstructed common bile and pancreatic ducts, and into the duodenum. The catheter collects fluid from the surrounding tissues and permits their passage into the duodenum for excretion. It is a palliative measure to prolong life and minimize discomfort. The catheter must be changed q6-8 weeks and flushed qod with small amounts of saline to maintain patency.

5. **Postoperative chemotherapy:** Sometimes used for further palliation after patient has recovered from surgery.

Note: Postoperative prognosis is extremely poor: patients usually survive <1 year, and the 5-year survival rate is 2%.

NURSING DIAGNOSES AND INTERVENTIONS

Potential fluid volume deficit related to loss secondary to postsurgical hemorrhage (due to vascularity of surgical site or multiple anastomosis sites) and risk of fluid shift to third-space (interstitial) compartments

Desired outcome: Patient is normovolemic as evidenced by BP ≥90/60 mm Hg (or within patient's baseline range), HR <100 bpm, RR ≤20 breaths min with normal depth and pattern (eupnea), good skin turgor, brisk capillary refill (<3 seconds), balanced I&O, urinary output ≥30 ml/hr, stable weight, and moist mucous membranes.

1. Monitor BP, pulse, and respirations, and check capillary refill in nail beds at frequent intervals. Tachycardia, hypotension, increased respirations, and slow capillary refill can signal the presence of dehydration and hypovolemia, which can lead to shock. Also be alert to cool, clammy skin, which can occur with hemorrhage, and a low urinary output (<30-40 ml/hr for 2 consecutive hours). Report significant findings to MD.

2. Prevent increased pressure on suture lines by keeping all tubes patent and free of kinks. *Gently* irrigate NG tube with air or saline q4h or as needed. Keep gravity drains dependent to the wound site and secure all connections with tape.
3. Note and document the amount and character of drainage from the tubes. Persistent, bloody drainage in steady or increasing amounts is indicative of active bleeding. Report significant findings to MD.
4. Monitor blood study results, including PT for clotting factor and hematocrit and hemoglobin, which can fall with blood loss. Optimal values are as follows: PT 11-15 seconds, hematocrit 40%-54% (male) and 37%-47% (female), and hemoglobin 14-18 g/dl (male) and 12-16 g/dl (female).
5. Monitor serum protein levels (normal range for random specimen is 2-8 mg/dl) and be alert to weight gain, which may signal interstitial spacing of fluids. Monitor I&O and note occurrence of intake exceeding output. Preoperatively, most of these patients are protein deficient. Low serum protein alters serum colloid osmotic pressure, resulting in fluid shift from intravascular to interstitial compartments (third spacing of body fluids). **Note:** Intravascular fluid loss can occur despite adequate fluid replacement.
6. Monitor lab study results for evidence of electrolyte imbalances, especially potassium and sodium. Normal potassium range is 3.5-5.0 mEq/L and normal sodium range is 137-147 mEq/L.

Potential for impaired skin and tissue integrity related to irritation secondary to wound drainage or pressure on incision

Desired outcome: Patient's skin remains intact with evidence of good wound healing.

1. Promote adequate drainage from drainage tubes to prevent pressure from fluid collection around wound site.
2. Assess and document condition of incision and quality/quantity of wound drainage. Fistula formation is a major complication of the Whipple procedure, so it is important to monitor peri-incisional skin carefully for signs of irritation. If irritation occurs or a fistula does form, cover site with a pectin wafer skin barrier (and stoma pouch for fistula).
3. Keep patient in semi-Fowler's position to minimize pressure on the incision. Use alternating pressure mattress to minimize potential for skin breakdown.
4. When regular diet is resumed after surgery, provide small, frequent meals that are high in protein, vitamins, and calories, and low in fat. Administer pancreatic enzyme replacements and insulin, as prescribed, for patient who has had a total pancreatectomy. These interventions will help ensure optimal tissue repair, as well.
5. For more information, see "Managing Wound Care," p. 624.

Pain related to major abdominal surgery

Desired outcome: Patient's subjective evaluation of discomfort improves, as documented by a pain scale.

1. Assess the degree and quality of the patient's discomfort. Devise a pain scale with the patient, rating discomfort from 0 (no pain) to 10.
2. Because physical dependence on narcotics is of minimal importance in patients who are terminally ill, administer analgesics liberally, but use caution to prevent respiratory depression. Document the degree of pain relief obtained, using the pain scale.
3. Since peritonitis and pancreatitis are potential postoperative complications, note and report patient's failure to respond to analgesics.
4. Because intraabdominal pressure may be a source of the patient's discomfort, ensure proper drainage from tubes.
5. Minimize anxiety, which can compound the intensity of pain, by explaining all procedures, keeping call light within patient's reach, and including significant others in patient care.
6. Augment pharmacologic analgesia with nonpharmacologic interventions: rhythmic breathing, relaxation, massage, distraction, guided imagery. See **Health-seeking behaviors:** Relaxation technique effective for stress reduction, p. 49.

Ineffective breathing patterns related to hypoventilation secondary to respiratory depression with use of narcotics or guarding secondary to painful abdominal incision

Desired outcome: Patient's respiratory rate is 12-20 breaths/min with normal depth and pattern (eupnea).

1. Assess rate and character of respirations q2-4h. Be alert to shallow, rapid, or depressed respirations, which can prevent adequate gas exchange.
2. Teach patient to deep breathe, cough, and use incentive spirometer qh while awake. Use pillows to splint wound and assist patient into semi- to high-Fowler's position for optimal lung expansion. Assist patient with turning and positioning q2h.
3. Administer analgesics at frequent intervals for patient comfort and to ensure optimal coughing and moving. Because narcotics depress the respiratory center, administer the lowest effective doses.
4. Since backed-up fluid in the abdomen creates pressure on the diaphragm, ensure patency of drains.
5. If patient exhibits or reports presence of dyspnea, consult with MD about obtaining ABG valves.

See "Hepatitis" in "Gastrointestinal Disorders," for **Impaired skin integrity** related to pruritus, p. 384, **Body image disturbance** related to presence of jaundice, p. 384, and **Potential for injury** related to increased risk of bleeding secondary to decreased vitamin K absorption, p. 384. See the appendix for nursing diagnoses and interventions for the care of preoperative and postoperative patients, p. 637, and the for the care of patients with cancer and other life-disrupting illnesses, p. 659.

PATIENT-FAMILY TEACHING AND DISCHARGE PLANNING

Provide patient and significant others with verbal and written information for the following:

1. For patients who are diabetic, a review of insulin action, dosage, and administration; diabetic diet; and signs and symptoms of hyperglycemia and hypoglycemia. See "Diabetes Mellitus," p. 294, for more information.
2. Wound care, such as cleansing, dressing changes, and care of drains if patient is discharged with them; indicators of wound infection, such as drainage, warmth along incision line, persistent incisional redness, swelling, fever, and pain.
3. Medications, including drug name, purpose, dosage, schedule, precautions, and potential side effects.
4. Arrangements for community services in home care, such as Visting Nurse Association, or placement in hospice facility.

Section Six   DIABETES MELLITUS

General discussion

Normal cellular metabolism uses glucose as its primary source of energy. Insulin is required to transport glucose molecules into the cell, where it is available for maintenance of cellular functioning. Normally an increase in blood glucose from any source (food intake, glycogen breakdown, gluconeogenesis) stimulates the release of insulin from pancreatic beta cells, facilitating glucose use by body cells and causing blood glucose to return to normal levels (60-120 mg/dl).

Individuals with diabetes mellitus (DM) demonstrate a dysfunction in glucose use, resulting either from a complete (insulin-dependent diabetes mellitus) or relative (noninsulin-dependent diabetes mellitus) lack of insulin. Diabetes mellitus is a chronic metabolic disorder that requires constant, vigilant care to prevent complications. Diabetes mellitus may be precipitated by any of the following factors: genetics, autoimmune defect, obesity, stress, pregnancy, or some medications.

Insulin-dependent diabetes mellitus (IDDM) or juvenile DM: Most commonly develops in childhood or adolescence. Onset is sudden with possible ketoacidosis. IDDM accounts for 10% of cases of diabetes. These individuals lack endogenous insulin because of the absence of beta-cell function and require exogenous insulin to meet the demands of glucose metabolism and normal physiologic function. Individuals with IDDM are totally dependent on insulin for survival.

Noninsulin-dependent diabetes mellitus (NIDDM) or adult-onset diabetes: Most commonly begins after age 40. Normal or above-normal quantities of insulin are present in the body fluids. It is ketosis-resistant because the presence of insulin prevents lipolysis. These individuals may require insulin during times of stress, including surgery, infection, or when diet and oral hypoglycemic medications fail to control hyperglycemia. As many as 90% of individuals with NIDDM are obese at the time of diagnosis. Patients with NIDDM may become insulin-dependent when diet or diet plus oral hypoglycemic medications fail to maintain normoglycemia.

DM affects all body systems. Patient involvement in self-management is crucial for maintaining normoglycemia and delaying long-term complications.

ASSESSMENT

Early indicators

☐ *IDDM:* Fatigue, weakness, nocturnal enuresis, weight loss and the cardinal symptoms of hyperglycemia: polyuria, polydipsia, and polyphagia.
☐ *NIDDM:* Fatigue, polyuria, and polydipsia may be discovered on routine assessment.

Late indicators

☐ *IDDM:* Dehydration, electrolyte imbalance, possible hypovolemic shock, changes in mentation, possible coma, Kussmaul's respirations, acetone breath, weak and rapid pulse, hypotension, hyperglycemia.
☐ *NIDDM:* Marked dehydration, hypovolemic shock, obtundation, shallow respirations, gross hyperglycemia. There is absence of ketosis.

COMPLICATIONS

1. Potential acute complications: *For IDDM* include diabetic ketoacidosis (DKA) and hypoglycemia; *for NIDDM* include hyperosmolar hyperglycemic nonketotic coma (HHNC) and hypoglycemia. These complications are usually preventable. Each is discussed later in this section.
2. Long-term complications: The most important factor in prevention is the maintenance of consistent, stable blood glucose levels within normal physiologic range. The following describe the levels of vascular pathology.
   ☐ *Microangiopathy:* Thickening of the basement membrane of the capillaries. Diabetic microangiopathy is manifested by retinopathy, nephropathy, and neuropathy. It compounds the effects of macroangiopathy.
   ☐ *Macroangiopathy:* Affects the larger vessels of the brain, heart, and lower extremities resulting in cerebrovascular, cardiovascular, and peripheral vascular disease. The risk factors are hyperglycemia, hypertension, hypercholesterolemia, smoking, aging, and extended duration of DM.

DIAGNOSTIC TESTS

1. *Fasting blood sugar (FBS):* A value >140 mg/dl is indicative of glucose intolerance.
2. *Oral glucose tolerance test (OGTT):* When two or more values of glucose are >200 mg/dl for 0-2 hours, glucose intolerance is present. It is sometimes used concurrently with serum insulin values by radioimmunoassay (RIA). The presence of insulin can help distinguish between NIDDM and IDDM.
3. *2-hour PPG:* Can be diagnostic if a standard glucose load (1.75 gm/kg body wt) is

administered with the meal. A blood glucose level of 180 mg/dl or higher in an individual for whom there is no other cause for impaired carbohydrate intolerance is significant.

4. _Urinalysis for glycosuria or ketonuria:_ By itself is a poor diagnostic tool, but it is reflective of the renal threshold for glucose when used in addition to the above tests. Glycosuria is usually present when blood glucose exceeds 170 mg/dl. The renal threshold for glucose is elevated in the elderly. Ketonuria will be present with IDDM in the presence of ketosis.

5. _Glycosylated hemoglobin:_ Measured to assess diabetic control over a preceding 2-3 month period. The larger the percentage of glycosylated hemoglobin, the poorer the diabetic control. Normal range is 4%-7%. Individuals with DM will have values >7%.

MEDICAL INTERVENTIONS

1. Diet: The exchange programs of the American Diabetes and American Dietetic Associations are the most commonly used methods of diet calculation and patient education. Dietary management is individually based on ideal body weight and adjusted to metabolic and activity needs. Typically the patient is put on a fixed ADA diet that is composed of 60% carbohydrates, 20% protein, and 20% fat. The focus on weight reduction for individuals with NIDDM necessitates significant carbohydrate restriction if they are treated by diet alone. When treatment also includes oral hypoglycemic medications or insulin, increased amounts of carbohydrates are required to offset the hypoglycemic effects of these medications. Individuals with IDDM require day-to-day consistency in diet and exercise to prevent hypoglycemia. Typically, three daily meals and an evening snack are prescribed. Some fat and protein should be present in all meals and snacks to slow down the elevation of postprandial blood glucose. Added fiber will slow the digestion of monosaccharides and disaccharides. For both types of diabetes, refined and simple sugars should be avoided. Various artificial sweeteners are used in "diet" products. Some contribute calories, which must be accounted for in a calorie-restricted diet.

2. Oral hypoglycemic medications (sulfonylureas): Used in individuals with NIDDM for whom diet alone cannot control hyperglycemia. Their primary action is to increase insulin production by affecting existing beta-cell function. The most serious side effect is hypoglycemia, particularly with chlorpropamide (Diabenese), which has a 72-hour duration and an average half life of 36 hours. Hypoglycemia involving the oral hypoglycemics can be severe and persistent. Nursing monitoring needs to be diligent. Oral hypoglycemics should be omitted several days before planned surgery. Any condition, situation, or medication that enhances the hypoglycemic effects of these drugs requires close monitoring of blood glucose when symptoms of hypoglycemia arise. Fasting for diagnostic purposes, malnourishment related to illness or nausea and vomiting, and other medication therapy (any of which adds to the hypoglycemic action of the oral hypoglycemics) are common factors in the development of hypoglycemia.

3. Insulin: Examples of short-, intermediate-, and long-acting insulins are shown in Table 5-2.
   □ A split-dose regimen of insulin administration is preferred because it allows for a higher level of blood glucose control. Daily insulin therapy usually consists of administering two-thirds of the total daily intermediate-acting insulin dose in the morning, with the remaining dose given in the evening. A rapid-acting insulin might be added to either or both doses. This regimen precludes the use of the longer-acting insulins, which are rarely used in a single dose because of the risk of nocturnal hypoglycemia.
   □ Multidose therapy permits better control of blood glucose for some individuals. Alteration in the quantity of food and timing of meals is a benefit to the patient who values flexibility. For the self-motivated individual who has control difficulties in spite of multidose therapy, portable insulin pumps can be helpful.
   □ The degree to which bovine and porcine sources of insulin deviate from the protein

T A B L E 5 - 2   Types of insulin

Insulin type		Onset of action (after subcutaneous injection)*	Peak action*
Rapid-acting	Regular	0.5-1 hour	2-3 hours
	Semilente	0.5-1 hour	4-6 hours
	Actrapid	0.5 hour	4 hours
	Humulin	0.5 hour	4 hours
Intermediate-acting	NPH	1-2 hours	8-12 hours
	Lente	1-2 hours	8-12 hours
Long-acting	Ultralente	4-8 hours	16-18 hours

*Action times may vary slightly.

structure of human insulin relates to the extent of their antigenic properties. Biosynthetic and semisynthetic human insulins are less likely to produce allergic responses in susceptible individuals and are used most frequently.

4. **Portable insulin pumps:** Devices that deliver a constant basal rate of insulin throughout the day and night with the capability of delivering a bolus of insulin at mealtime. The needle, which attaches to a syringe *via* a long strip of plastic tubing, remains indwelling in the subcutaneous tissue of the abdomen. Patients program their own pumps to deliver the optimal amount of insulin, based on self-monitoring of blood glucose.

5. **Patient teaching about drugs that potentiate hyperglycemia:** These include estrogens, corticosteroids, thyroid preparations, diuretics, phenytoin, glucagon, and medications that contain sugar, such as cough syrup.

6. **Patient teaching about drugs that potentiate hypoglycemia:** These include salicylates, sulfonamides, methyldopa, anabolic steroids, acetaminophen, ethanol, haloperidol, marijuana. Propranolol masks the signs of and inhibits recovery from hypoglycemia.

7. **Exercise:** As important as diet and insulin in treating DM. It lowers blood glucose levels, helps maintain normal cholesterol levels, and increases circulation. These effects increase the body's ability to metabolize glucose and help reduce the therapeutic dose of insulin in most patients. The exercise program must be consistent and individualized (especially for individuals with IDDM). Patients should be given a complete physical exam and encouraged to incorporate acceptable activities as part of their daily routine.

NURSING DIAGNOSES AND INTERVENTIONS

Alteration in tissue perfusion: Peripheral, cardiopulmonary, renal, cerebral, and gastrointestinal related to impaired circulation and sensation secondary to development and progression of macroangiopathy and microangiopathy

Desired outcomes: Patient complies with the therapeutic regimen and exhibits BP within his or her optimal range. Patient is asymptomatic of injury or complications caused by diabetic retinopathy or peripheral or autonomic neuropathy.

1. Check blood glucose levels before meals and at bedtime. Encourage patient to perform regular home blood glucose monitoring. Urine testing is less reliable and should not be used by patients with reduced renal function.

2. Hypertension is a common complication of diabetes. Careful control of BP is critical in preventing or limiting the development of heart disease, retinopathy, or nephropathy. Check BP q4h. Alert MD to values outside of the patient's normal range. Administer antihypertensive agents as prescribed and document the response.

3. Patients may experience decreased sensation in the extremities because of peripheral neuropathy. Protect patients from injuring themselves with sharp objects or heat. For example, avoid use of heating pads.

    4. Provide a safe environment for patients with diminished eyesight secondary to diabetic retinopathy. Orient patient to the location of items such as water, tissues, glasses, and call light.

    5. Approximately half of all individuals with IDDM develop chronic renal failure (CRF) and end-stage renal disease (ESRD). Monitor patients for changes in renal function, for example, increases in BUN and creatinine and altered urine output. Proteinuria is an early indicator of developing CRF. Individuals with DM with reduced renal function are at significant risk for developing acute renal failure after exposure to contrast media. Observe these patients for indicators of acute renal failure. (See "Acute Renal Failure," p. 116, and "Chronic Renal Failure," p. 121, in Chapter 3 for more information.) Insulin dosages will decrease as renal function decreases. Also be alert to indicators of hypoglycemia. See Table 5-4, p. 305, for clinical indicators and treatment.

    6. Individuals with DM may experience multiple problems secondary to autonomic neuropathy, such as the following:

      ☐ *Orthostatic hypotension:* Assist patients when getting up suddenly or after prolonged recumbency. Check BP while patient is lying down, sitting, and then standing to document presence of orthostatic hypotension. Alert MD to significant findings.

      ☐ *Impaired gastric emptying with nausea, vomiting, and diarrhea:* Administer metoclopramide before meals, if prescribed. Keep a record of all stools. Nausea, vomiting, and anorexia can be indicative of developing uremia in patients with progressive renal failure.

      ☐ *Neurogenic bladder:* Encourage patients to void q3-4h during the day, using manual pressure (Credé maneuver) if necessary. Intermittent catheterization may be necessary in severe cases. Avoid the use of indwelling urinary catheters because of the high risk of infection.

Potential for infection related to increased susceptibility secondary to disease process (e.g., hyperglycemia, neurogenic bladder, poor circulation)

Desired outcome: Patient is asymptomatic of infection as evidenced by normothermia, negative cultures, and WBC <11,000 µl.

Note: Infection is the most common cause of diabetic ketoacidosis (DKA)

---

    1. Monitor temperature q4h. Alert MD to elevations.

    2. Maintain meticulous sterile technique when changing dressings, performing invasive procedure, or manipulating indwelling catheters.

    3. Monitor for indicators of infection: dysuria, urgency, frequency, cloudy and foul-smelling urine; erythema, local warmth, swelling, discharge, and pain from skin

---

T A B L E 5 - 3 Infectious processes necessitating medical intervention

Classification	Indicators
Upper respiratory infection (URI)	Fever, chills, cough productive of sputum, crackles (rales), rhonchi, dyspnea
Urinary tract infection (UTI)	Burning or pain with urination, cloudy or malodorous urine, fever, chills, tachycardia, diaphoresis, nausea, vomiting, abdominal pain
Systemic sepsis	Fever, chills, tachycardia, diaphoresis, nausea, vomiting, hypothermia, (Gram-negative sepsis), flushed skin, hypotension
Localized (IV sites)	Erythema, swelling, purulent drainage, warmth

wounds or lesions; inflamed pharynx and complaints of sore throat and swollen glands; changes in the color, amount, or consistency of sputum; chest pain and SOB; fever; leukocytosis.

4. Consult MD about obtaining cultures for blood, sputum, and urine during temperature spikes or for wounds that produce purulent drainage.

Potential impairment of skin and tissue integrity related to increased susceptibility secondary to peripheral neuropathy and vascular pathology

Desired outcomes: Patient's skin remains intact. Patient verbalizes and demonstrates knowledge of proper foot care.

1. Assess integrity of the skin and evaluate reflexes of the lower extremities by checking knee and ankle DTRs, proprioceptive sensations, and vibration sensation (using a tuning fork on the medial malleolus). If sensations are impaired, anticipate patient's inability to respond appropriately to harmful stimuli. Monitor peripheral pulses, comparing the quality bilaterally. Be alert to pulses $\leq 2+$ on a 0-4+ scale.
2. Use foot cradle on bed, spaceboots for ulcerated heels, elbow protectors, and alternating air pressure mattress to prevent pressure points and promote patient comfort.
3. To alleviate acute discomfort yet prevent hemostasis, minimize patient activities and incorporate progressive passive and active exercises into daily routine. Discourage extended rest periods in the same position.
4. Teach patient the following steps for foot care:
   □ Wash feet daily with mild soap and warm water; check water temperature with water thermometer or elbow.
   □ Inspect feet daily for the presence of erythema or trauma, using mirrors as necessary for adequate visualization.
   □ Alternate between at least two pairs of properly fitted shoes to avoid potential for pressure points that can occur by wearing one pair only.
   □ Prevent infection from moisture or dirt by changing socks or stockings daily and wearing cotton or wool blends.
   □ Prevent ingrown toenails by cutting toenails straight across after softening them during bath.
   □ Do not self-treat corns or calluses; visit podiatrist regularly.
   □ Attend to any foot injury immediately, and seek medical attention to avoid any potential complication.

Knowledge deficit: Proper insulin administration

Desired outcome: Patient verbalizes and demonstrates knowledge of proper insulin administration.

1. Teach patient to check expiration date on insulin vial and to avoid using it if outdated.
2. Explain that intermediate- and long-acting insulins require mixing. Demonstrate rolling the insulin vial between the palms to mix the contents. Caution patient that vigorous shaking produces air bubbles that can interfere with accurate dosage measurement.
3. Explain that insulin should be injected 30 minutes before mealtime.
4. Explain that either making a change in insulin type or withholding a dose of insulin may be required for the following: when fasting for studies or surgery, when not eating because of nausea/vomiting, or when hypoglycemic. Adjustments are always individually based and require clarification with patient's MD.
5. Provide patient with a chart that depicts rotation of the injection sites. Explain that injection sites should be at least 2.5 cm (1 inch) apart.

As appropriate, see "Atherosclerotic Arterial Occlusive Disease" in "Cardiovascular Disorders," p. 85, and "Amputation" in "Musculoskeletal Disorders," p. 465. Also see the appendix for psychosocial nursing diagnoses and interventions for the care of patients with cancer and other life-disrupting illnesses, p. 390.

PATIENT-FAMILY TEACHING AND DISCHARGE PLANNING

Provide patient and significant others with verbal and written information for the following:

1. Importance of carrying a diabetic identification card and wearing Medic-Alert bracelet or necklace.
2. Recognizing warning signs of both hyperglycemia and hypoglycemia and factors that contribute to both conditions. Remind patient that stress from illness or infection can increase insulin requirements (or necessitate insulin therapy for one who is normally controlled with oral hypoglycemics) and that increased exercise will necessitate additional food intake to prevent hypoglycemia when there is no change made in insulin dosage.
3. Home monitoring of blood glucose using commercial kits and daily urine testing for glucose and ketones, which provide ongoing data reflecting the degree of control and may identify necessary changes in diet and medication before severe metabolic changes occur. These tests also provide a means for patient's self-control and psychologic security. Stress the need for careful control of blood glucose as a means of decreasing the risk of or minimizing long-term complications of DM.
4. Importance of daily exercise, good blood glucose control, maintenance of normal body weight, and yearly medical evaluation, including visits to a podiatrist and ophthalmologist.
5. Diet that is low in fat and high in fiber as an effective means of controlling blood fats, especially cholesterol and triglycerides. Stress that diet is the sole method of control for many individuals with NIDDM. The importance of adequate nutrition and controlled calories is essential in maintaining normoglycemia in these diabetics.
6. Necessity for individuals with IDDM to use U-100 syringes with U-100 insulin.
7. Availability of syringe magnifiers that can be used for patients with poor visual acuity. Other products that permit safe and accurate filling of syringes are also available.
8. Necessity of rotating injection sites and injecting insulin at room temperature. Provide a chart showing possible injection sites and describe the system for rotating the sites.
9. Importance of good foot care.
10. Importance of annual eye examinations for early detection and treatment of retinopathy.

In addition

11. Explain the importance of inserting the needle perpendicular to the skin rather than at an angle to ensure deep subcutaneous administration of insulin. Individuals who are very thin, however, may use a 45-degree angle.
12. Assist patient with identifying available resources for ongoing assistance and information including nurses, dietitian, patient's MD, and other individuals with DM in the patient care unit. Other resources include the local chapter of American Diabetes Association (ADA); subscription to ADA Forecast (a publication of ADA); and local library for free access to current materials on diabetes.
13. For any supplemental medications used, patient should be taught the name, purpose, dosage, schedule, precautions, and potential side effects.

Diabetic ketoacidosis

Diabetic ketoacidosis (DKA) is a life-threatening condition resulting from insulin deficiency or an inability of the cells to use available insulin. Because insulin facilitates the use of glucose by body tissues, a deficiency of this hormone leads to decreased cellular uptake of plasma glucose as well as an increased release of glucose from the liver. In addition, increased glucagon is released from the pancreas, promoting the conversion of glycogen to glucose in the liver. The result of these three actions is plasma hyperglycemia with intracellular starvation. Plasma hyperglycemia produces an osmotic diuresis, with concomitant loss of sodium and potassium, and can lead to severe dehydration and hypovolemic shock. Thromboembolism can occur owing to dehydration with increased blood viscosity and platelet aggregation and adhesiveness. Cerebrovascular accident can occur as a result of decreased cerebral perfusion or thromboemboli.

When cells are unable to use glucose, the body is forced to break down fats and protein to produce the energy necessary for cell function. Protein depletion decreases the body's ability to fight disease, while the plasma hyperglycemia encourages bacterial growth, making individuals with DKA extremely susceptible to infection. Fat breakdown increases the amount of plasma ketones and leads to ketoacidosis. In addition, dehydration decreases tissue perfusion, resulting in lactic acidosis. The lowered pH stimulates the respiratory center, producing the deep, rapid respirations known as Kussmaul respirations. The large amount of ketones lends a fruity or acetone odor to the breath. If not treated promptly, the acidosis and dehydration depress consciousness to the point of coma. Left untreated, death may result from hypovolemia or CNS depression.

ASSESSMENT

See Table 5-4, p. 305.

DIAGNOSTIC TESTS

See Table 5-4, p. 305.

MEDICAL MANAGEMENT

1. **Rehydration:** Usually, normal saline or 0.45% saline is administered until plasma glucose falls to between 200-300 mg/dl. After that, dextrose-containing solutions usually are given to prevent rebound hypoglycemia. Initially, IV fluids are administered rapidly (i.e., 200-300 ml/hr).
2. **Rapid-acting insulin:** Usually given IV for rapid action and because poor tissue perfusion caused by dehydration makes SC route less effective. The initial dose may vary between 10-25 units or 0.3 u/kg. Then the patient is maintained on 5-10 units per hour or 0.1 u/kg/hr as a continuous infusion. Dosage is adjusted, based on serial glucose levels.
3. **Restoration of electrolyte balance:** Sodium is replaced with IV normal saline. Potassium must be monitored and replaced carefully because potassium returns to the intracellular compartment following correction of acidosis and the patient is then at risk of becoming hypokalemic. Use of phosphorus replacement is controversial. Recent studies suggest that there is no difference in the outcome of patients who receive phosphorus replacement and those who do not.
4. **IV bicarbonate:** For pH <7.1. Its use is limited because acidosis will be corrected by insulin therapy. Excessive use of sodium bicarbonate can produce alkalosis and respiratory depression.
5. **Insertion of nasogastric tube:** Prevents gastric aspiration, particularly in comatose patients.
6. **Treatment of underlying cause:** For example, infection is treated with appropriate antibiotics.

NURSING DIAGNOSES AND INTERVENTIONS

Fluid volume deficit (with concomitant electrolyte disturbance) related to decreased circulating volume secondary to hyperglycemia and osmotic diuresis

Desired outcomes: Patient becomes normovolemic as evidenced by BP ≥90/60 mm Hg (or within patient's normal range), HR 60-100 bpm, CVP 2-6 mm Hg (5-12 cm H_2O), good skin turgor, moist mucous membranes, balanced I&O, and urinary output ≥30 ml/hr. Serum potassium is 3.5-5.0 mEq/L, serum sodium is 137-147 mEq/L, and serum glucose is 100-150 mg/dl.

1. Monitor VS q15min until stable for 1 hour. Notify MD promptly of the following: HR >120 bpm, BP <90/60 or decreased ≥20 mm Hg from baseline, and CVP <2 mm Hg (or <5 cm H_2O).
2. Monitor patient for physical indicators of dehydration, such as tachycardia, orthostatic hypotension, cyanosis, poor skin turgor, dry mucous membranes, and sunken and soft eyeballs.
3. Measure I&O accurately. Decreasing urinary output may signal diminishing intravascular fluid volume or impending renal failure. Report to MD urine output <30 ml/hr for 2 consecutive hours.
4. Administer IV fluids as prescribed to ensure adequate rehydration. Be alert to indicators of fluid overload, which can occur secondary to the rapid infusion of fluids: jugular vein distention, dyspnea, crackles (rales), CVP >6 mm Hg (>12 cm H_2O).
5. Administer insulin as prescribed to prevent worsening hyperglycemia and correct existing hyperglycemia. Be aware that insulin, when added to IV solutions, may be absorbed by the container and plastic tubing. Before initiating treatment, flush the tubing with 50-100 ml of the insulin-containing IV solution to ensure that maximum absorption by the container and tubing has occurred before patient use.
6. Monitor lab results for abnormalities. With insulin therapy, the serum glucose should decline steadily until it stabilizes between 150-300 mg/dl. A too-rapid return to normal levels may produce fluid shifts and cerebral edema. Notify MD if serum glucose drops to <100 mg/dl and discontinue insulin drip until MD gives further instructions. Serum potassium should decline until it reaches normal. Promptly report to MD serum potassium levels <3.5 mEq/L. Serum sodium levels will increase gradually with appropriate IV saline replacement.
7. Observe for clinical manifestations of electrolyte imbalance as follows:
   □ *Hyperkalemia:* Lethargy, nausea, hyperactive bowel sounds with diarrhea, numbness or tingling in extremities, muscle weakness.
   □ *Hypokalemia:* Muscle weakness, hypotension, anorexia, drowsiness, hypoactive bowel sounds.
   □ *Hyponatremia:* Headache, malaise, muscle weakness, abdominal cramps, nausea, seizures, coma.
   □ *Hypoglycemia:* Headache, impaired mentation, dizziness, nausea, pallor, tremors, agitation, tachycardia, diaphoresis.
   □ *Metabolic acidosis:* Lassitude, nausea, vomiting, Kussmaul's respirations, lethargy progressing to coma.
   □ *Hypophosphatemia:* Muscle weakness, progressive encephalopathy possibly leading to coma.
   □ *Hypomagnesemia:* Anorexia, nausea, vomiting, lethargy, weakness, personality changes, tetany, tremor or muscle fasciculations, seizures, confusion progressing to coma.
   □ *Hypochloremia:* Hypertonicity of muscles, tetany, depressed respirations.
8. To prevent accidental injury caused by altered mentation occurring with cellular dehydration or electrolyte imbalance, institute safety measures, such as padded side rails; bed in lowest position with side rails up when not at patient's side; and bite block, oral airway, and supplemental oxygen at the bedside. Apply soft restraints as necessary to prevent falls. Reorient and reassure patient as needed.

Potential for infection related to susceptibility secondary to protein depletion and hyperglycemia

Desired outcome: Patient is free of infection as evidenced by normothermia, HR ≤100 bpm, BP within patient's normal range, WBC count <11,000 μl, and negative cultures.

1. Monitor patient for evidence of infection (see Table 5-3, p. 298). Monitor lab results for increased WBC count and culture purulent drainage as prescribed.
2. Ensure good handwashing technique when caring for patient.
3. Because patient is at increased risk of bacterial infection, use of invasive lines should be limited. Peripheral IV sites should be rotated q48-72 hours, depending on agency policy. Central lines should be discontinued as soon as feasible, and when in place

should be handled carefully. Schedule dressing changes according to agency policy and inspect the site(s) for signs of local infection, including erythema, swelling, or purulent drainage. Document the presence of any of these indicators and notify MD.

4. Provide good skin care to maintain skin integrity. Use eggcrate mattress on the bed to help prevent skin breakdown. Air circulation beds are recommended for severe skin breakdown.
5. Use meticulous aseptic technique when caring for or inserting indwelling catheters to minimize the risk of bacterial entry *via* these sites. **Note:** Because of the increased risk of infection, limit use of indwelling urethral catheters to patients who are unable to void in a bedpan or when continuous assessment of urine output is essential.
6. To help prevent pulmonary infection, provide incentive spirometry and encourage its use, along with deep-breathing and coughing exercises, qh while patient is awake.

Potential for injury related to confusion, obtundation, coma, or seizures secondary to cerebral edema or dehydration

Desired outcome: Patient verbalizes orientation to person, place, and time; RR is 12-20 breaths/min with normal depth and pattern (eupnea); adventitious breath sounds are absent; normal breath sounds are auscultated over patient's airways; and patient's oral cavity and musculoskeletal system remain intact and free of injury.

1. Reduce the likelihood of falls for confused patients by maintaining bed in lowest position, siderails up at all times, and using soft restraints as necessary.
2. Monitor respiratory status, especially airway patency, at frequent intervals. Keep oral airway, manual resuscitator and mask, and supplemental oxygen at the bedside.
3. Insert NG tube in comatose patients, as prescribed, to decrease the likelihood of aspiration.
4. Elevate HOB to 45 degrees to minimize the risk of aspiration.
5. Initiate seizure precautions. For details, see "Seizure Disorders," p. 239.

Potential alteration in tissue perfusion: Peripheral, related to risk of thromboembolism secondary to increased viscosity of blood, increased platelet aggregation and adhesiveness, and patient immobility

Desired outcomes: Patient has adequate peripheral perfusion as evidenced by peripheral pulses >2+ on a 0-4+ scale; warm skin; brisk capillary refill (<3 seconds); and absence of swelling, bluish discoloration, erythema, and discomfort in the calves and thighs. Hematocrit is 40%-54% (male) or 37%-47% (female) and BUN is ≤20 mg/dl.

1. Monitor hematocrit results. With proper fluid replacement, results should return to normal within 24-48 hours. Assess for a falling BUN value as an indicator of improved tissue perfusion and renal function.
2. Assess peripheral pulses q2-4h. Report any decrease in amplitude or absence of pulse(s) to MD immediately.
3. Be alert to indicators of deep vein thrombosis, such as erythema, pain, tenderness, warmth, swelling, or bluish discoloration or prominence of superficial veins in the extremities, especially the lower extremities. Arterial thrombosis may produce cyanosis with delayed capillary refill, mottling, and coolness of the extremity. Report significant findings to MD immediately.
4. Perform ROM exercises to all extremities q4h to increase blood flow to the tissues.
5. Apply antiembolic hose, ace wraps, or pneumatic alternating pressure stockings to the lower extremities as prescribed to aid in the prevention of thrombosis.

Also see psychosocial nursing diagnoses and interventions in "Caring for Patients with Cancer and Other Life-Disrupting Illnesses, p. 390.

PATIENT-FAMILY TEACHING AND DISCHARGE PLANNING

Patients who are seriously ill often experience heightened anxiety, and at times, denial of the severity of the disease, which blocks learning. Use simple terms and incorporate patient teaching frequently into patient care routines. Give patient and significant others verbal and written instructions for the following:

1. Causes, prevention, and treatment of DKA. As needed, explain the disease process of diabetes mellitus and DKA and the common early symptoms of worsening hyperglycemia including polyuria, polydipsia, polyphagia, dry and flushed skin, and increased irritability. Stress the importance of maintaining regular diet, exercise, and medication regimen for optimal control of serum glucose levels and prevention of adverse physical effects of diabetes mellitus, such as peripheral neuropathies and increased atherosclerosis.

2. Importance of testing urine sugar and acetone or blood glucose levels qid: before meals and at bedtime. Blood glucose >200 mg/dl should be reported to MD so that insulin dose can be increased. As indicated, review testing procedure with patient.

3. Medications, including drug name, dosage, route, and potential side effects. Teach patient that insulin must be taken every day and that lifetime insulin therapy is necessary to achieve control of blood glucose. Explain that insulin is administered 2-4 times a day as prescribed and that it may require adjustment during periods of illness or stress.

4. Indicators of insulin excess (hypoglycemia), such as dizziness, impaired mentation, irritability, pallor, tremors; and indicators of insulin deficiency (hyperglycemia), such as increased polyuria and polydipsia, dry and flushed skin. Teach patient the importance of receiving prompt treatment if any of these indicators occurs.

5. Importance of dietary changes as prescribed by MD. Typically, patient is put on a fixed calorie ADA diet composed of 60% carbohydrates, 20% fats, and 20% proteins. Explain that the fats should be polyunsaturated and the proteins chosen from low-fat sources. Teach patient the importance of eating three meals a day at regularly scheduled times and a bedtime snack.

6. Causes for adjustments in insulin dosage: (1) increased or decreased food intake; (2) any physical (e.g., exercise) or emotional stress. Teach patient that exercise and emotional stress increase release of glucose from the liver, which may increase insulin demand. Instruct patient to monitor blood glucose levels closely during periods of increased emotional stress and periods of increased or decreased exercise and to adjust insulin dose accordingly.

7. Susceptibility to infection: Explain that individuals with diabetes are more susceptible to infection and that preventive measures, such as good hygiene and meticulous, daily foot care, are necessary to prevent infection. Stress the importance of avoiding exposure to communicable diseases and that the following indicators of infection necessitate prompt medical treatment: fever, chills, increased HR, diaphoresis, nausea, and vomiting. In addition, teach patient and significant others to be alert to wounds or cuts that do not heal, burning or pain with urination, and a productive cough.

8. Necessity of continued medical follow-up; confirm time and date of next medical appointment.

9. Procedure for obtaining Medic-Alert bracelet or card identifying patient's diagnosis.

10. Address of American Diabetes Association for acquisition of pamphlets and magazines related to the disease, its complications, and appropriate treatment: American Diabetes Association, Inc, 18 East 48th Street, New York, New York 10017.

Hyperosmolar hyperglycemic nonketotic coma

Hyperosmolar hyperglycemic nonketotic coma (HHNC) is a life-threatening emergency resulting from a relative or actual insulin deficiency that causes severe hyperglycemia. Usually, patients are elderly with undiagnosed or inadequately treated noninsulin dependent diabetes mellitus (NIDDM). Often HHNC is precipitated by a stressor, such as trauma or infection, that increases insulin demand. It is believed that enough insulin is present to prevent lipolysis and the formation of ketone bodies, thereby preventing acidosis, but not enough to prevent hyperglycemia. Without adequate insulin to facilitate use by most body cells, glucose molecules accumulate in the bloodstream, causing serum hyperosmolality with resultant osmotic diuresis and simultaneous loss of electrolytes, most notably potassium, sodium, and phosphate. Patients may lose up to 25% of their total body water. Owing to increasing serum hyperosmolality and extracellular fluid loss, fluids are pulled from individual body cells, causing intracellular dehydration and body cell shrinkage. Neurologic deficits (i.e., slowed mentation, confusion, seizures, or coma) can occur as a result. Although loss of extracellular fluid stimulates aldosterone release, which will help the body retain sodium and prevent further loss of potassium, the aldosterone cannot halt severe dehydration. As extracellular volume decreases, the blood becomes more viscous and flow is impeded. Thomboemboli are common owing to increased blood viscosity, enhanced platelet aggregation and adhesiveness, and immobility. Cardiac workload is increased and may lead to myocardial infarction (MI). Renal blood flow is decreased, potentially resulting in renal impairment or failure. Cerebrovascular accident may result from thromboemboli or decreased cerebral perfusion. These severe complications, in addition to the initial precipitating disorder, contribute to a mortality rate in excess of 50%.

Unlike DKA, in which acidosis produces severe symptoms requiring prompt hospitalization, symptoms of HHNC develop slowly and frequently are nonspecific. The cardinal symptoms of polyuria and polydipsia are the first to appear, but they may be ignored by elderly patients or their families. Neurologic deficits may be mistaken for signs of impending CVA or senility. Owing to the similarity of these symptoms to other disease processes common to this age group, proper diagnosis and treatment may be delayed, allowing progression of pathophysiologic processes.

ASSESSMENT

See Table 5-4, below. **Note:** Because these individuals usually are older than 50 years of age and have preexisting cardiac or pulmonary disorders, assessment parameters often cannot be evaluated based on normal values, but rather on what is normal or optimal for each individual patient. CVP and BP therefore should be evaluated in terms of deviations from the patient's baseline and concurrent clinical status.

TABLE 5-4 Comparisons of DKA, HHNC, and hypoglycemia

	DKA	**HHNC**	Hypoglycemia
Diabetes type	Usually IDDM (type I)	Usually NIDDM (type II)	IDDM or NIDDM
Typical age group	Any age	Usually over 50	Can occur at any age
Signs and symptoms	Polyuria, polydipsia, polyphagia, weakness, orthostatic hypotension, lethargy, changes in LOC, fatigue, nausea, vomiting, abdominal pain	Same as DKA	Changes in mentation, apprehension, erratic behavior, trembling, slurred speech, staggering gait, possible seizure activity
Physical assessment	Dry, flushed skin; poor skin turgor; dry mucous membranes; decreased BP; tachycardia; altered LOC (irritability, lethargy, coma); Kussmaul's respirations; fruity odor to the breath	Same as DKA, but no Kussmaul's respirations or fruity odor to the breath. Instead, patient will have tachypnea with shallow respirations	Tachycardia, cool and clammy skin, pallor

TABLE 5-4   Comparisons of DKA, HHNC, and hypoglycemia—cont'd

	DKA	HHNC	Hypoglycemia
History and risk factors	Undiagnosed IDDM; recent stressors, such as surgery, trauma, infection, MI; insufficient exogenous insulin	Undiagnosed NIDDM; recent stressors, such as surgery, trauma, pancreatitis, MI, infection; high-caloric enteral or parenteral feedings in a compromised patient; use of diabetogenic drugs (e.g., phenytoin, thiazide diuretics, thyroid preparations, mannitol, corticosteroids, sympathomimetics); dialysis; major burns treated with high concentrations of sugar	Vomiting, missing meals, relative excess in insulin, increased exercise, alcohol intake, drug interactions
Monitoring parameters **Diagnostic tests**	*CVP:* <2 mm Hg (<5 cm H$_2$O) *Serum glucose:* 200-800 mg/dl *Serum ketones:* elevated *Urine glucose:* positive *Urine acetone:* positive *Serum osmolality:* 300-350 mOsm/L *Serum pH:* <7.38	*CVP:* >3 mm Hg below patient's baseline 800-2,000 mg/dl normal or slightly elevated positive negative >350 mOsm/L normal or mildly acidotic due to lactic acidosis (pH 7.30-7.42)	N/a <60 mg/dl
	Serum sodium: <137 mEq/L *Serum hematocrit:* elevated due to osmotic diuresis with hemoconcentration *BUN:* elevated >20 mg/dl *Serum creatinine:* >1.5 mg/dl *Serum potassium:* normal or elevated above 5.0 mEq/L initially and then decreased	elevated, normal, or low elevated due to hemoconcentration elevated elevated normal or <3.5 mEq/L	

TABLE 5-4   Comparisons of DKA, HHNC, and hypoglycemia—cont'd

	DKA	HHNC	Hypoglycemia
	Serum phosporus, magnesium, chloride: decreased	decreased	
Onset	Hours to days	Hours to days; can be longer	Minutes to an hour
Mortality rate	<10%	>50% due to age group and complications, such as CVA, thrombosis, pancreatitis	Usually not fatal

DIAGNOSTIC TESTS

1. *Serum osmolality:* Will be >350 mOsm/kg. A quick bedside calculation of serum osmolality can be obtained by using this formula:

$$2(\text{Na} + \text{K}) + \frac{\text{BUN(mg/dl)}}{2.8} + \frac{\text{glucose (mg/dl)}}{18} = \text{mOsm/L}$$

For example: $\text{Na}^+ = 140$; $\text{K}^+ = 4.5$; BUN $= 20$, glucose $= 120$

$$2(140 + 4.5) + \frac{20}{2.8} = \frac{120}{18} = 289 + 7 + 6.7 = 302.7$$

2. See Table 5-4, above, for a discussion of other diagnostic tests.

MEDICAL MANAGEMENT

1. Replacement of electrolytes and extracellular fluid volume: Most often, 0.45% saline or normal saline is used; potassium or phosphate supplements may be added, based on laboratory values. IV fluids will be changed to 5% dextrose in normal saline or 5% dextrose in 0.45% saline to prevent hypoglycemia as blood glucose decreases.
2. Rapid-acting insulin: Usually administered in low doses. Because of poor tissue perfusion in these patients, the IV route is preferred. In the majority of cases, continuous drips are used and titrated, based on serum glucose levels.
3. Insertion of central venous catheter: To assess fluid status on a continuous basis.
4. Treatment of underlying cause: The most frequent cause is infection, which is treated with appropriate antibiotics.

NURSING DIAGNOSES AND INTERVENTIONS

See "Diabetic Ketoacidosis" for the following: **Fluid volume deficit** (with concomitant electrolyte disturbance) related to decreased circulating volume secondary to hyperglycemia and osmotic diuresis, p. 301; **Potential for infection** related to susceptibility secondary to protein depletion and hyperglycemia, p. 302; **Potential for injury** related to confusion, obtundation, coma, or seizures secondary to cerebral edema or dehydration, p. 303; and **Potential alteration in tissue perfusion:** Peripheral related to risk of thromboembolism, p. 303. For psychosocial nursing diagnoses and interventions, see the following as appropriate: "Caring for Patients with Cancer and Other Life-Disrupting Illnesses," p. 390.

PATIENT-FAMILY TEACHING AND DISCHARGE PLANNING

Patients who are seriously ill often experience heightened anxiety, and at times, denial of the severity of the disease that blocks learning. Use simple terms and incorporate patient teaching frequently into patient care routines. Give patient and significant others verbal and written instructions for the following:

1. Causes, prevention, and treatment of HHNC. Allow patient to verbalize fears and feelings about the diagnosis; correct any misconceptions. As needed, explain the disease process of DM and HHNC and the common early symptoms of worsening diabetes, including polyuria, polydipsia, polyphagia, dry and flushed skin, and increased irritability.
2. Importance of testing blood glucose levels qid: before meals and at bedtime. Explain that blood glucose >200 mg/dl should be reported to MD so that insulin dose can be increased. As indicated, review testing procedure with patient.
3. Importance of dietary changes as prescribed by MD. Typically, the individual with NIDDM is obese and will be on a reduced-calorie diet with fixed amounts of carbohydrates, fat, and protein. Explain that the fats should be polyunsaturated and the proteins chosen from low-fat sources. Teach patient the importance of eating three meals a day at regularly scheduled times and a bedtime snack. Explain that increased or decreased food intake will necessitate an adjustment in insulin dosage. Provide a referral to a dietitian as needed.
4. Importance of taking oral hypoglycemic agents as prescribed. In addition, explain that exogenous insulin may be required during periods of physical and emotional stress and that blood glucose levels should be monitored closely during these times.
5. For patient with NIDDM, importance of regular exercise due to benefits in maintaining blood glucose levels by increasing insulin effectiveness and reducing serum triglyceride and cholesterol levels, thus also decreasing the risk of atherosclerosis. Aerobic exercises, such as walking or swimming, are most effective in lowering blood glucose levels.
6. Necessity of preventive measures for infection, such as good hygiene and meticulous, daily foot care. Stress the importance of avoiding exposure to communicable diseases and that the following indicators of infection necessitate prompt medical treatment: fever, chills, tachycardia, diaphoresis, and nausea and vomiting. In addition, teach patient and significant others to be alert to wounds or cuts that do not heal, burning or pain with urination, and cough that is productive of sputum.
7. Procedures for obtaining Medic-Alert bracelet or card identifying patient's diagnosis.
8. Necessity for continued medical follow-up; confirm date and time of next medical appointment.
9. In addition, provide booklets or pamphlets from the American Diabetes Association or pharmaceutical companies about diabetes and appropriate treatment.

Hypoglycemia

Hypoglycemia is a lowering of blood glucose caused by an overdose of insulin, skipping meals, or too much exercise without a concomitant increase in food intake. Unlike DKA and HHNC, hypoglycemia can have a sudden onset, and its course is precipitous if it is left untreated. Typically, hypoglycemia occurs during the time of the peak action of the hypoglycemic medication or at night when the patient is fasting.

The patient usually becomes symptomatic when blood glucose is less than 50 mg/dl or there is a relative significant drop in blood glucose, for example, when an elderly patient's blood glucose drops to 90 mg/dl from 180-200 mg/dl. Alcohol consumption also can cause hypoglycemia because it depletes glycogen stores, resulting in increased insulin levels.

Note: Mentation changes caused by severe hypoglycemia can be indistinguishable from those caused by alcoholic stupor. If hypoglycemic symptoms are misdiagnosed as alcoholic stupor and a hypoglycemic diabetic is left to "sleep it off," death can ensue.

ASSESSMENT

See Table 5-4, p. 305.

NURSING DIAGNOSES AND INTERVENTIONS

Potential for injury related to risk of brain damage or death secondary to hypoglycemia

Desired outcomes: Patient is alert and verbalizes orientation to person, place, and time. Blood glucose levels return to normal.

Caution: Hypoglycemia requires immediate intervention because if it is severe, it can lead to brain damage and death. When in doubt as to the cause of coma in a diabetic patient, draw a stat blood glucose and prepare to administer 50% glucose IV.

1. Administer a fast-acting carbohydrate: 4 ounces orange or apple juice; 2½ tsp sugar; 3 ounces nondiet soda; or 5-7 lifesavers. Notify MD if patient is incoherent, unresponsive, or incapable of taking carbohydrates by mouth. If any of these indicators occur, an IV access is required and you should prepare to administer prescribed 50 ml 50% dextrose by IV push. Consciousness should be restored within 10 minutes.
2. Using an appropriate reagent strip, continue to monitor blood glucose levels q30-60min to identify recurrence of hypoglycemia.
3. Once alert, question patient about recent intake or absence of food. Any situation preventing food intake, such as nausea, vomiting, dislike of hospital food related to cultural preferences, or fasting for a scheduled test, should be determined and addressed immediately.
4. If food intake has been adequate, consult with MD regarding a reduction in patient's daily dose of antihyperglycemic medication.

Note: Sometimes, hypoglycemia leads to rebound hyperglycemia (Somogyi effect). If hypoglycemia goes undetected, the rebound hyperglycemia may be inappropriately treated with increased insulin. Suspect the Somogyi effect if there are wide fluctuations in blood glucose over a few hours. Notify MD if these changes are observed or if the patient is experiencing nocturnal hypoglycemia.

Potential for trauma related to alterations in LOC and risk of seizures secondary to hypoglycemia

Desired outcome: Patient is asymptomatic of trauma caused by seizures or alterations in LOC.

1. Monitor LOC at frequent intervals. Anticipate seizure potential in presence of severe hypoglycemia and have airway, protective padding, and suction equipment at bedside. Keep all siderails up.
2. Notify MD of any seizure activity; do not leave patient unattended if it occurs.
3. Place call light within patient's reach and have patient demonstrate its proper use every shift. Inability to use the call light properly necessitates checking on the patient at least q30min. If necessary, consider moving patient to a room next to the nurses' station for close monitoring.
4. Keep all potentially harmful objects, such as knives, forks, and hot beverages, out of patient's reach.
5. If necessary to prevent patient from wandering and causing self-injury, obtain a prescription for soft restraints. Explain these safety precautions to patient and significant others.
6. For other information, see "Seizure Disorders," p. 239.

Knowledge deficit: Disease process, diagnostic testing, indicators of hypoglycemia, and therapeutic regimen

Desired outcome: Patient verbalizes knowledge of DM, including testing and management, the indicators of hypoglycemia, and the therapeutic regimen.

1. Assess patient's knowledge of DM, including diagnostic testing and management. Provide information or clarify as appropriate.
2. Review the indicators and immediate interventions for hypoglycemia with the patient.
3. Evaluate current diet for adequate nutritional requirements, calorie content, and patient satisfaction. Assist patient with making acceptable and realistic changes. Take into account patient's activity level and need for changes to achieve normoglycemia. Refer patient and significant others to dietitian as needed.
4. Review with patient the onset, peak action, and duration of the hypoglycemic medication. Advise patient to avoid drugs that contribute to hypoglycemia (see p. 297).
5. Stress the importance of testing blood glucose at the time symptoms of hypoglycemia occur.
6. Explain that injection of insulin into a site that is about to be exercised heavily, for example, the thigh of a jogger, will result in quicker absorption of the insulin and possible hypoglycemia.
7. Inform patient that a change in the type of medication may require a change in dosage to prevent hypoglycemia. Caution patient about the need to follow prescription directions precisely.

See "General Discussion," p. 297, for nursing diagnoses and interventions for the care of patients with diabetes mellitus.

PATIENT-FAMILY TEACHING AND DISCHARGE PLANNING

See "General Discussion," p. 300, for the care of patients with diabetes mellitus.

SELECTED REFERENCES

American Hospital Formulary Service: Drug information 88, Bethesda, Md, 1988, American Society of Hospital Pharmacists.

Avioli L: Primary hyperparathyroidism: recognition and management, Hospital Pract 22(9):69-74, 1987.

Butts D: Fluid and electrolyte disorders associated with diabetic ketoacidosis and hyperglycemic hyperosmolar nonketotic coma, Nurs Clin North Am 22(4):827-836, 1987.

Bybee D: Saving lives in parathyroid crises, Emerg Med 19(5):62-65, 71-72, 75-78, 1987.

Bybee D: Saving lives in thyroid crises, Emerg Med 19(6):20-23, 27, 31, 1987.

Contreras L et al: Urinary cortisol in the assessment of pituitary-adrenal function: utility of a 24-hour and spot determinations, J Clin Endocrin and Metab 62(5):965-969, 1986.

Cooper D and Ridgway C: Clinical management of patients with hyperthyroidism, Med Clin North Am 69(5):953-969, 1985.

Fischbach F: A manual of laboratory diagnostic tests, ed 3, Philadelphia, 1988, JB Lippincott Co.

Fuhrman S: Appropriate laboratory testing in the screening and work-up of Cushing's syndrome, Am J Clin Pathol 90(3):345-350, 1988.

Jeffres C: Complications of acute pancreatitis, Crit Care Nurs 9(4):38-48, 1989.

Kershner D: Endocrine dysfunctions. In Swearingen PL et al: Manual of critical care: applying nursing diagnoses to adult critical illness, St Louis, 1988, The CV Mosby Co.

Mampalam T et al: Transsphenoidal microsurgery for Cushing disease: a report of 216 cases, Ann Intern Med 109(6):487-493, 1988.

Melby J: Therapy of Cushing disease: a consensus for pituitary microsurgery, Ann Intern Med 109(6):445-446, 1988.

National Institutes of Health: Diet and exercise in non-insulin dependent diabetes mellitus, Conn Med 51(4):249-253, 1987.

Nicoloff J: Thyroid storm and myxedema coma, Med Clin North Am 69(5):1005-1017, 1985.

Riccardi G and Rivellese A: New indices for selection of carbohydrate foods in the diabetic diet: hopes and limitations, Diabetic Med 4:140-143, 1987.

Sabo C and Michael S: Diabetic ketoacidosis: pathophysiology, nursing diagnosis, and nursing interventions, Focus on Crit Care 16(1):21-28, Feb 1989.

Sabo C and Michael S: Managing DKA and preventing a recurrence, Nursing 89:50-56, 1989.

Sarsany S: Thyroid storm, RN 51(7):46-48, 1988.

Schira M: Steroid-dependent states and adrenal insufficiency: fluid and electrolyte disturbances, Nurs Clin North Am 22(4):837-841, 1987.

Schroeder S et al: Current medical diagnosis and treatment, Norwalk, Conn, and San Mateo, Calif, 1988, Appleton and Lange.

Sherwood L: Diagnosis and management of primary hyperparathyroidism, Hospital Pract 23(3A):9-10, 15, 1988.

Spaulding S and Lippes H: Hyperthyroidism: causes, clinical features, and diagnosis, Med Clin North Am 69(5):937-951, 1985.

Tyrell B et al: An overnight high-dose dexamethasone suppression test for rapid differential diagnosis of Cushing's syndrome, Ann Intern Med 104(2):180-186, 1986.

6
CHAPTER

Gastrointestinal disorders

Section One DISORDERS OF THE MOUTH AND ESOPHAGUS

Stomatitis

Inflammatory and infectious diseases of the mouth are commonly overlooked in the debilitated hospitalized patient. Typically, they occur secondary to systemic disease and infection, nutritional and fluid deficiencies, poorly fitting dentures, neglect of oral hygiene, and as side effects of irritants and drugs. Stomatitis (inflammation of the mouth and mucous membrane) is the term generally applied to a variety of mouth disorders characterized by mucosal cell destruction and disruption of the mucosal lining. It is one of the major side effects of cancer chemotherapy, occurring in over 30% of this population. It also is seen frequently in long-term ICU patients, as well as in individuals with HIV infection.

ASSESSMENT

Signs and symptoms: Oral pain; sensitivity to hot, spicy foods; foul taste; oral bleeding or drainage; fever; xerostomia (dry mouth); difficulty chewing or swallowing; poorly fitting dentures.

Physical assessment: The oral mucosa will appear swollen, red, and ulcerated; the lymph glands may be swollen; and the breath is often foul-smelling. The lips may have cracks, fissures, blisters, ulcers, and lesions; the tongue may appear dry and cracked and contain masses, lesions, or exudate.

DIAGNOSTIC TESTS

In most incidences, diagnosis of the offending organism is made by physical examination. However, the following may be used in selected patients:
1. *Culture:* May be taken of the lesion or drainage to identify the offending organism. The most common organism is *Candida albicans,* followed by herpes simplex virus I.
2. *Platelet count:* Taken if any bleeding is present.

MEDICAL MANAGEMENT

The treatment varies, depending on the type of impairment and its cause.
1. Identification and attempt to control or remove causative factor(s): If appropriate. For example, if poor nutrition is the cause of stomatitis, the goal is to improve nutrition and follow through with other treatments that may be necessary, such as antibiotics.
2. Oral hygiene/mouth irrigations: The accepted mouthwash, in particular for immunosuppressed patients with stomatitis, is sodium bicarbonate with normal saline. A typical solution is made with 500 ml normal saline and 15 ml sodium bicarbonate. Oral hygiene should be repeated 4-5 times a day or even more frequently, depending on the degree of oral mucosal impairment.
3. Pharmacotherapy
   □ *Local/systemic analgesics and local anesthetics:* For relief of pain.
   □ *Topical/systemic steroids:* To reduce inflammation and promote healing.
   □ *Antibiotics, antifungals, and antiviral agents:* To combat infection.
   □ *Vitamins:* To correct deficiencies (e.g., vitamin C to strengthen connective tissue in the gums, and niacin and riboflavin to promote efficient cellular growth).
4. Dietary management: Typically, a diet high in protein to promote wound healing, high in calories for protein sparing, and high in vitamins to correct the specific deficiency. Usually, hot and spicy foods are restricted, and the consistency of the food ranges from liquid to regular, as tolerated. Fluids are encouraged.
5. Cauterization of ulcerations: If required.

6. Dental restoration and repair: If needed.
7. Adequate rest: For optimal tissue repair.

NURSING DIAGNOSES AND INTERVENTIONS

Alterations in oral mucous membrane related to stomatitis

Desired outcomes: Patient demonstrates knowledge of oral hygiene interventions and complies with the therapeutic regimen. Patient's oral mucosal condition improves, as evidenced by intact mucous membrane, moist and intact tongue and lips, and absence of pain and lesions.

1. Inspect the mouth tid for inflammation, lesions, and bleeding. Record observations and report significant findings to MD.
2. Administer analgesics; corticosteroids; anesthetics, such as xylocaine jelly, diphenhydramine (Benadryl), and Maalox (or other antacid); and mouthwashes (described below) as prescribed. Avoid commercial mouthwashes, which are high in alcohol. For mild stomatitis, provide mouth care after every meal and before bedtime. For moderate stomatitis, provide mouth care q4h; for severe stomatitis, provide mouth care q2h or even qh if indicated.
3. Prepare a solution containing 15 ml sodium bicarbonate and 500 ml normal saline. Instruct patient to rinse the mouth with the solution (as often as indicated in No. 1, above) to provide local relief and promote healing.
4. Instruct the patient to brush teeth after meals and at bedtime, using a soft-bristled toothbrush and nonabrasive toothpaste. Patients with severe stomatitis who have dentures should remove them until the oral mucosa has healed. Dietary alterations may be necessary, for example, changing to a full liquid or pureed diet. A dietary or nutritional consultation may be necessary.
5. Advise patient to floss teeth gently qd, using unwaxed floss.
6. Keep the lips moist with emollients, such as lanolin or any nonpetroleum surgical lubrication.
7. Advise patient to avoid irritants, including smoking and foods that are hot, spicy, and rough in texture.
8. Offer ice or popsicles to help anesthetize the mouth.

Self-care deficit: Inability to perform oral hygiene related to sensorimotor deficit or decreased LOC

Desired outcomes: Patient exhibits good oral hygiene. Patient or significant other demonstrates ability to perform oral care.

1. Assess patient's ability to perform mouth care. Identify such performance barriers as sensorimotor or cognitive deficits.
2. If the patient has decreased LOC or is at risk for aspiration, remove dentures and store them in a water-filled denture cup.
3. If the patient cannot perform mouth care, cleanse the teeth, tongue, and mouth at least bid with a soft-bristled toothbrush and nonabrasive toothpaste. If the patient is unconscious or at risk for aspiration, turn the patient into a side-lying position. Swab the mouth and teeth with a gauze pad or Toothette moistened with the mouthwash solution described in No. 2, above, and irrigate the mouth with a syringe. If the patient cannot self-manage the secretions, use only a small amount of liquid at a time, using a suction catheter or Yankeur tonsil suction catheter to remove the secretions. This regimen should be performed at least q4h. As appropriate, teach the procedure to significant others.
4. For patients with physical disabilities, the following toothbrush adaptations can be made:
   □ *For patients with limited hand mobility:* Enlarge the toothbrush handle by covering it with a sponge hair roller or aluminum foil, attaching either with an elastic band; or by attaching a bicycle handle grip with plaster of Paris.

☐ *For patients with limited arm mobility:* Extend the toothbrush handle by overlapping another handle or rod over it and taping them together.

Knowledge deficit: Disease process, treatment, and factors that potentiate bleeding

Desired outcome: Patient verbalizes knowledge of the cause, preventive measures, and treatment of stomatitis and the factors that potentiate bleeding.

1. Describe the causes of the patient's stomatitis, and remind patient that the best treatment is prevention.
2. Explain the importance of meticulous, frequent oral hygiene and periodic dental examinations.
3. Advise patient to avoid irritating foods and substances (e.g., alcohol, tobacco, and hot, spicy, and rough foods).
4. Teach the importance of discontinuing flossing if the platelet count drops below 50,000, or as suggested by MD, and discontinuing brushing if the count drops below 30,000, or per MD instructions, to avoid possible bleeding. Instead, instruct patient to perform oral hygiene using the mouth irrigation technique described in **Alterations in oral mucous membrane** and gently swabbing the mouth, teeth, and lips with a Toothette moistened in the sodium bicarbonate and normal saline solution.

Alteration in nutrition: Less than body requirements related to decreased intake secondary to discomfort with chewing and swallowing

Desired outcome: Patient exhibits optimal nutrition as evidenced by stable weight, serum protein 6-8 g/dl, serum albumin 3.5-5.5 g/dl, and a balanced or positive nitrogen state.

1. Assess the patient's ability to chew and swallow.
2. Monitor I&O. Unless contraindicated, ensure that patient has optimal hydration (at least 2-3 L/day) and a diet that is high in protein, calories, and essential vitamins and minerals. Alert MD if the need for IV or NG tube feedings becomes apparent.
3. Provide any special equipment that will facilitate ingestion, such as straws, nipples, or syringes.
4. If the patient's mouth is very painful, encourage intake of soft foods (e.g., cooked cereals, soups, gelatin, ice cream). Drinks that are high in calories and protein are especially helpful. Consider adding polycose to beverages and powdered milk or protein powder to food preparations.
5. Encourage mouth care after every meal or more frequently to minimize the risk of infection owing to the nonintact oral mucosa.

PATIENT-FAMILY TEACHING AND DISCHARGE PLANNING

Provide patient and significant others with verbal and written information for the following:
1. Essentials of diet, medications, and oral hygiene; adaptations that may be required at home; and the importance of monitoring for changes of LOC, which will necessitate precautions to prevent aspiration during oral hygiene (see **Self-care deficit,** p. 315).
2. Importance of notifying MD if any of the following recur or worsen: oral pain, fever, drainage, continuous bleeding, or inability to eat or drink.
3. Necessity of follow-up care; reconfirm date and time of next medical appointment.
4. Importance of visiting the dentist at least twice a year.

Hiatal hernia and reflux esophagitis

Hiatal hernia is defined as a herniation of a portion of the stomach into the chest through the esophageal hiatus of the diaphragm. Hernias are classified as 1) rolling or esophageal and 2) sliding or direct. When there is an increase in intraabdominal pressure, a portion of the lower esophagus and stomach may rise up into the chest. Causative factors include degenerative changes (aging), trauma, kyphoscoliosis (a curvature of the spine), and surgery. Increased intraabdominal pressure can occur with coughing, straining, bending, vomiting, obesity, pregnancy, trauma, constricting clothing, ascites, and severe physical exertion. Complications of hiatal hernia include pulmonary aspiration of reflux contents, ulceration, hemorrhage, stricture, gastritis, and in severe cases, strangulation of the hernia.

The diagnosis of diaphragmatic hernia is often suspected on the basis of reflux symptoms. However, gastroesophageal reflux disease is not caused by any one abnormality. The multiple factors that determine whether or not reflux esophagitis is present include 1) efficacy of the antireflux mechanism, 2) volume of gastric contents (in the stomach), 3) potency of refluxed material, 4) efficiency of esophageal clearance, and 5) resistance of the esophageal tissue to injury and the ability for tissue reparation. By definition, however, the patient must have several episodes of reflux for reflux disease to be present. Reflux esophagitis is the result of an incompetent lower esophageal sphincter that allows regurgitation of acidic gastric contents into the esophagus.

The most common type of hiatal hernia is the sliding hernia, which accounts for 90% of adult hiatal hernias. It is characterized by the upper portion of the stomach and esophageal junction sliding up into the chest when the individual assumes a supine position, and sliding back into the abdominal cavity when sitting or standing. The incidence of hiatal hernia increases with age. Women and obese individuals are more often affected.

ASSESSMENT

Many individuals are asymptomatic unless esophageal reflux is present.

Signs and symptoms: Reflux esophagitis often occurs 1-4 hours after eating, possibly aggravated by reclining, stress, and increased intraabdominal pressure. Heartburn, belching, regurgitation, vomiting, retrosternal or substernal chest pain (dull, full, heavy), hiccups, mild or occult bleeding found in vomitus or stools, mild anemia, and dysphagia also can occur. The older adult often presents with symptoms of pneumonitis caused by aspiration of reflux contents into the pulmonary system. Peptic stricture of the esophagus is a serious sequela of aggressive reflux esophagitis.

Physical assessment: Auscultation of peristaltic sounds in the chest, presence of palpitations, abdominal distention. **Note:** These findings are not diagnostic, nor are they usually helpful in making the diagnosis.

DIAGNOSTIC TESTS

For most patients with reflux, obtaining a complete history is sufficient for beginning therapy without the necessity of comprehensive diagnostic tests.

1. *Barium swallow:* This is the most specific diagnostic test for revealing hernias and gastroesophageal and diaphragmatic abnormalities. With fluoroscopy, a hiatal hernia will appear as a barium-containing outpouching at the lower end of the esophagus, and gastric barium will move into the esophagus with reflux. Sometimes it is necessary for the patient to be in Trendelenburg's position for the hernia to appear on x-ray.

2. *Chest x-ray:* Will reveal large hernias, which will look like air bubbles in the chest; infiltrates will be seen in the lower lobes of the lungs if aspiration has occurred.

3. *Upper endoscopy and biopsy:* Aid in differentiating between hiatal hernia and gastroesophageal lesion.

4. *Esophageal motility studies:* Identify primary and secondary motor dysfunction before surgical repair of the hernia is performed. Included are manometry, which graphically records swallowing waves; pH probe, which will be low (acidic) in the presence of gastroesophageal reflux; and Bernstein test (acid perfusion), which attempts to reproduce the symptoms of reflux by instilling hydrochloric acid into the esophagus.

5. *Gastric analysis:* To assess for bleeding, which can occur if ulceration is present.

6. *CBC:* May reveal an anemic condition if bleeding ulcers are present.

7. *Stool occult blood test:* Will be positive if bleeding has occurred.

8. *EKG:* To rule out cardiac origin of pain.

MEDICAL MANAGEMENT

Conservative medical management, which is successful in 90% of the cases, is preferred over surgical intervention. The goals are to prevent or reduce gastric reflux caused by increased intraabdominal pressure and increased gastric acid production.

1. Limitation of activities that increase intraabdominal pressure: For example, coughing, bending, straining, and physical exertion.
2. Restriction or limitation of gastric acid stimulants: For example, caffeine and nicotine.
3. Dietary management: Small, frequent meals; bland foods; weight reduction for obese individuals; food restriction 2-3 hours before reclining; refraining from fatty foods, acidic foods, chocolate, and alcohol.
4. Elevation of HOB: Using 4-10 inch blocks to prevent postural reflux at night, depending on the severity of the reflux; the more severe, the higher the blocks.
5. Restriction of tight, waist-constricting clothing.
6. Pharmacotherapy
   □ *Antacids:* To neutralize gastric acid.
   □ *Histamine H_2 receptor blockers:* For example, ranitidine and cimetidine to suppress acid secretion.
   □ *Sucraltate (carafate):* Binds to the esophageal mucosa and acts as a physical barrier that prevents mucosal injury.
   □ *Gastrointestinal stimulators:* For example, metaclopromide to augment gastric emptying and increase lower esophageal sphincter (LES) pressure.
   □ *Selective anticholinergics and selective prokinetics:* For example, pirenzepine and bethanechol to promote gastric motility and prevent reflux.
   □ *Antiemetics, cough suppressants, and stool softeners:* To prevent increased intraabdominal pressure from vomiting, coughing, and straining with bowel movements.
7. Surgery: To restore gastroesophageal integrity and prevent reflux if symptoms do not resolve and complications (obstruction, bleeding, aspiration) occur. The most common procedure is a fundoplication, in which a portion of the upper stomach is wrapped around the distal esophagus and sutured to itself to prevent reflux from recurring. Typically, an abdominal rather than a thoracic approach is used.
8. Postsurgical management: Includes chest physiotherapy to prevent respiratory complications, administration of IV fluids and electrolytes until bowel sounds are present, a gradual increase in diet as tolerated after the return of peristalsis, and in some cases, gastric tubes for decompression and feeding.

NURSING DIAGNOSES AND INTERVENTIONS

Knowledge deficit: Disease process and treatment for hiatal hernia and reflux esophagitis

Desired outcome: Patient verbalizes knowledge of the cause and therapeutic regimen for hiatal hernia and reflux esophagitis.

Note: The cornerstone for many patients with reflux is a change in lifestyle.

1. Assess the patient's knowledge of the disorder, its treatment, and the methods used to prevent symptoms and their complications. Provide instructions as appropriate.
2. Explain the following methods of dietary management: eating a low-fat, high-protein diet; eating small, frequent meals; eating slowly; chewing well to avoid reflux; avoiding extremely hot or cold foods; limiting stimulants of gastric acid, such as alcohol, caffeine, chocolate, spices, fruit juices, and nicotine; and losing weight, if appropriate.
3. Advise the patient to drink water after eating to cleanse the esophagus of residual food, which can be irritating to the esophageal lining.
4. Explain the following alterations in body positions and activities: avoiding the supine position 2-3 hours after eating; sleeping on the right side with the HOB elevated on 4-10 inch blocks to promote gastric emptying; and avoiding bending, coughing, lift-

ing heavy objects, straining with bowel movements, strenuous exercise, and clothing that is too tight around the waist.
5. Stress the importance of the following pharmacologic regimen: antacids after meals; H₂ receptor blocker on a regular basis, even if symptoms are no longer persistent; and sucralfate 3-4 times a day, 1 hour after antacids are taken.

Pain, nausea, and feeling of fullness related to gastroesophageal reflux and increase in intraabdominal pressure

Desired outcome: Patient's subjective evaluation of discomfort improves, as documented by a pain scale.

1. Assess and document the amount and character of the discomfort. Devise a pain scale with patient, rating discomfort from 0 (no discomfort) to 10.
2. Administer medications as prescribed. Document their effectiveness, using the pain scale.
3. Encourage the patient to follow dietary and activity restrictions.
4. If prescribed, insert a nasogastric tube and connect it to suction to reduce pressure on the diaphragm and relieve vomiting.
5. Determine whether a position change would improve symptoms. For example, raise the HOB or have the patient turn from side to side.

For patients with a fundoplication:

Ineffective breathing pattern related to guarding secondary to pain of thoracic incision or chest tube insertion

Desired outcome: Patient's respiratory rate is 12-20 breaths/min with normal depth and pattern (eupnea).

1. If a thoracic rather than an abdominal approach was used, chest tubes may be present. Assess the insertion site and suction apparatus for integrity, patency, function, and character of drainage. **Caution:** Be alert to the following indications of a pneumothorax: dyspnea, cyanosis, sharp chest pain. (See "Pneumothorax/Hemothorax," p. 17, for care of the patient with a chest tube.)
2. Encourage and assist patient with coughing, deep breathing, and turning q2-4h, and note quality of breath sounds, cough, and sputum.
3. Facilitate coughing and deep breathing by teaching patient how to splint incision with hands or pillow.
4. To enhance compliance with the postoperative routine, medicate patient about a half-hour prior to major moves, such as ambulation and turning. Be aware that narcotics will depress respirations.
5. Reassure patient that sutures will not break and tubes will not fall out with coughing and deep breathing.

Potential for injury related to risk of gastrointestinal complications (obstruction, recurring reflux, esophageal tear, or perforation) secondary to surgery

Desired outcomes: Patient is free of gastrointestinal complications, as evidenced by presence of bowel sounds 24-72 hours following surgery; bowel movements 48-72 hours after surgery; a soft and nondistended abdomen; absence of reflux and severe midsternal pain; ease with swallowing and burping; BP, RR, and HR within patient's baseline limits; and normothermia.

1. Assess the abdomen for the presence of distention, tenderness, and bowel sounds; document all findings. Bowel sounds normally reappear within 24-72 hours and bowel movements return within 48-72 hours following surgery.
2. Instruct the patient to report reflux, a symptom that should *not* be present after fundoplication, and which may signal that the surgical wraparound is too loose. Also have the patient alert you to difficulty with swallowing or burping, which may be indicative of a wraparound that is too tight and may lead to obstruction.
3. Patient will have an NG tube after surgery, and often it will remain in place until the esophagus has healed. Assess for patency immediately after surgery qh for 6 hours

and then q2-3h for 24 hours. Generally, the surgeon will prescribe a specific irrigating solution. If a specific irrigating solution has not been prescribed, check for patency by instilling 10 ml normal saline and aspirating the same amount. Do not leave connected to low intermittent suction unless specifically prescribed, as this may lead to ulceration. **Caution:** Do not attempt to replace or manipulate the NG tube because esophageal perforation can occur. It may be necessary to restrain the hands of patients who are uncooperative.

4. Take measures to decrease intraabdominal pressure, which may cause disruption of the suture line: Control nausea and vomiting; prohibit the use of straws, which can cause aerophagia; and introduce food and fluids gradually and in small amounts because the stomach will have a decreased storage capacity. When fluids are allowed, administer them in amounts <60 ml/hr, and be alert to indicators of esophageal tear (see below).

5. An esophageal tear or perforation can be a complication of the surgery. Be alert to and report the following indicators: severe midsternal pain, a drop in BP, and increases in TPR.

6. Teach the patient the signs and symptoms of the potential complications, and stress the importance of reporting them to the staff promptly should they occur.

See "Providing Nutritional Support," p. 622, for nursing diagnoses and interventions for administering NG tube feedings. See the appendix for nursing diagnoses and interventions for the care of preoperative and postoperative patients, p. 637.

PATIENT-FAMILY TEACHING AND DISCHARGE PLANNING

Provide patient and significant others with verbal and written information for the following:
1. Importance of dietary management and activity restrictions (see **Knowledge deficit,** p. 318).
2. Medications, including drug name, dosage, schedule, purpose, precautions, and potential side effects.
3. Indicators that signal recurrence of hernia or reflux (which happens only rarely following surgery): dysphagia, hematemesis, and increased pain.
4. Importance of follow-up care; reconfirm date and time of next medical appointment.
5. Care of incision, including dressing changes. Ensure that the patient can verbalize indicators of infection (e.g., increasing pain, local warmth, fever, purulent drainage, swelling, and foul odor).
6. Procedure for enteral feedings and care of tubes, if appropriate.

Achalasia

Achalasia (cardiospasm) is a chronic, progressive motor disorder that affects the lower two-thirds of the esophagus. It is characterized by ineffective peristalsis, a hypertonic lower esophageal sphincter (LES) that does not relax in response to swallowing, and esophageal dilatation. The exact cause of achalasia is unknown, but evidence indicates there is an impairment in the innervative response of the esophagus to parasympathetic activity. Complications of achalasia include esophagitis with edema and hemorrhage, respiratory complications caused by aspiration of esophageal contents, malnutrition, and a probable predisposition for esophageal carcinoma. On occasion, a gastric carcinoma may mimic achalasia (pseudoachalasia).

ASSESSMENT

As the disease progresses, symptoms increase in severity and frequency.

Signs and symptoms: Dysphagia; halitosis; feeling of fullness in the chest; weight loss; and retrosternal pain during or after meals, which can radiate to the back, neck, and arms. In addition, regurgitation of esophageal contents can occur when the patient is horizontal, and nocturnal choking can occur during the later stages of the disorder.

DIAGNOSTIC TESTS

Barium swallow, esophageal motility studies, and upper endoscopy usually are performed. See "Hiatal Hernia," p. 317 for a description of these tests.

MEDICAL MANAGEMENT AND SURGICAL INTERVENTIONS

Medical management strives toward relieving symptoms caused by the LES obstruction and emptying esophageal contents.

1. **Activity/positional alterations:** The patient is instructed to remain upright after meals, wait 2-4 hours after a meal before lying down, and sleep with the HOB elevated or raised on 4-10 inch blocks. In addition, to help increase hydrostatic pressure and thereby facilitate swallowing, patients are taught to arch their backs, flex their chins toward their chests, and strain (Valsalva maneuver) while swallowing.
2. **Dietary management:** Small, frequent meals are recommended. The patient is taught to eat and drink slowly in a relaxed environment; avoid rough foods and foods that can cause discomfort, such as spices, stimulants, and cold fluids; and drink fluids with meals to enhance movement of food into the stomach.
3. **Pharmacotherapy:** Salicylates and nonsteroidal antiinflammatory agents are contraindicated because they can cause ulceration.
   □ *Antacids:* To reduce the amount of gastric acid and relieve pain. However, reflux esophagitis rarely is a problem because the LES is often closed, preventing any significant reflux.
   □ *Nitrates:* For direct relaxation of the smooth muscle fibers of the LES and improvement of esophageal emptying. Nitrates may cause headaches in a third of the individuals who use them.
   □ *Calcium channel blockers:* Nifedipine and diltiazem also relax the LES muscle.
   □ *Vitamins and iron supplements:* To treat malnutrition and anemia.
4. **Mechanical esophageal dilatation:** Achieved by the insertion of a graduated instrument or inflatable tube into the esophagus. Balloon dilatation with sudden distention of the LES can rupture some muscle fibers and thus facilitate passage of food. This procedure is successful in 60%-80% patients.
5. **Presurgical interventions:** To correct preexisting conditions, such as anemia, malnutrition, and fluid and electrolyte disturbances. Esophageal lavage may be necessary to remove food residue in preparation for surgery or balloon dilatation.
6. **Surgical interventions:** Required in approximately 20%-25% of cases. The most common procedure is an esophagomyotomy or cardiomyotomy, in which an incision is made through the muscle fibers that surround the narrowed area of the esophagus. This enables the mucosa under the muscular layers to expand, enabling food to pass into the stomach unobstructed. Often, an antireflux procedure, such as a fundoplication (see "Hiatal Hernia," p. 318), is performed as well.

NURSING DIAGNOSES AND INTERVENTIONS

Alterations in nutrition: Less than body requirements related to decreased intake secondary to dysphagia or surgery

Desired outcome: Patient exhibits adequate nutrition as evidenced by maintenance of body weight, serum protein 6-8 g/dl, albumin 3.5-5.5 g/dl, and a balanced or positive nitrogen state.

1. Monitor I&O; document weight daily.
2. Administer local anesthetics, analgesics, and other medications (e.g., nifedipine) before meals, as prescribed, to relax the esophagus and aid ingestion.
3. Monitor for and document substances patient can and cannot swallow.
4. Provide oral hygiene before and after meals and at bedtime.
5. During the nonacute phase, provide foods that increase LES pressure, for example, proteins and complex carbohydrates.
6. Restrict or limit (as prescribed) foods and substances that decrease LES pressure,

such as fats and refined carbohydrates, as well as stimulants, such as chocolate, peppermint, alcohol, and tobacco.

7. Restrict or limit (as prescribed) foods that can irritate the esophageal lining, for example, coffee, citrus juices, and tomato juice, as well as all other foods known to cause patient distress.
8. Administer vitamin and iron supplements if prescribed.
9. If advised by MD, have the patient drink water and perform the Valsalva maneuver with swallowing to promote ingestion.

Knowledge deficit: Disease process and therapeutic regimen for achalasia

Desired outcome: Patient verbalizes knowledge of the disease process and therapeutic regimen for achalasia.

1. Assess the patient's knowledge of the disorder, its treatment, and the measures used to prevent symptoms and complications. Provide information as appropriate.
2. Instruct the patient to avoid or limit the intake of foods and substances that decrease LES pressure, irritate the esophageal lining, and cause distress. Provide patient with lists of foods to eat and foods to restrict or limit. See **Alterations in nutrition,** p. 321, for additional information.
3. Advise the patient to avoid smoking and constrictive clothing.
4. Emphasize the importance of increased nutritional intake and the precautions to take while eating. Teach the patient to eat small, frequent meals; chew thoroughly; eat slowly; and dine in a relaxed atmosphere.
5. Instruct the patient to remain upright after meals, wait 2-4 hours after meals before reclining, and sleep with the HOB elevated.
6. Instruct patient to avoid taking salicylates and nonsteroidal antiinflammatory agents, which may result in ulceration and bleeding.
7. If the patient is scheduled for a balloon dilatation, provide only clear liquids the day before the procedure and keep the patient NPO the morning of the procedure.

See the appendix for nursing diagnoses and interventions for the care of preoperative and postoperative patients, p. 637.

PATIENT-FAMILY TEACHING AND DISCHARGE PLANNING

Provide patient and significant others with verbal and written information for the following:
1. Prescribed alterations in dietary patterns.
2. Activity restrictions/alterations.
3. Medications, including drug name, dosage, schedule, purpose, precautions, and potential side effects.
4. Need for follow-up care; confirm date and time of next medical appointment.

Section Two   DISORDERS OF THE STOMACH AND INTESTINES

Peptic ulcers

Peptic ulcer is an erosion of the stomach (gastric ulcer) or duodenum (duodenal ulcer). Most commonly, it is associated with an increase in acidity of the stomach juices or an increased sensitivity of the musocal surfaces to erosion. Erosions can penetrate deeply into the mucosal layers and become a chronic problem; or they can be more superficial and manifest as a more acute problem as a result of severe physiologic or psychologic trauma, infection, or shock (stress ulceration of the stomach or duodenum). Both duodenal and gastric ulcers can occur in association with high-stress lifestyle, smoking, use of irritating drugs, and secondary to other disease states. Ulceration commonly occurs as a part of Zollinger-Ellison syndrome, in which gastrinomas (gastrin-secreting tumors) of the pancreas or other organs develop. Gastric acid hypersecretion and ulceration subsequently occur.

Up to 25% of individuals afflicted with peptic ulcers develop such complications as hemorrhage, gastrointestinal obstruction, perforation and peritonitis, or intractable ulcer. With treatment, ulcer healing usually occurs within 4-6 weeks (gastric ulcers can take up to 12-16 weeks to heal), but there is potential for recurrence in the same or another site.

ASSESSMENT

Signs and symptoms: Postprandial epigastric pain (e.g., burning, gnawing, dull ache). Discomfort occurs more frequently between meals and at night. With duodenal ulcer, eating usually alleviates discomfort; with gastric ulcer, pain often worsens after meals. GI bleeding, if present, is evidenced by hematemesis or melena.

Physical assessment: Tenderness over the involved area of the abdomen. With perforation, there will be severe pain (see "Peritonitis," p. 337, for more information).

History of: Chronic or acute stress; smoking; use of irritating drugs such as caffeine, alcohol, steroids, salicylates, reserpine, indomethacin, nonsteroidal antiinflammatory drugs, or phenylbutazone; disorders of the endocrine glands, pancreas, or liver; and Zollinger-Ellison syndrome.

DIAGNOSTIC TESTS

1. *Barium swallow (upper GI series, small bowel series):* Uses contrast agent (usually barium) to detect abnormalities. Patient should be kept NPO and not smoke for at least 8 hours before the test. Postprocedure care involves administration of prescribed laxatives and enemas to facilitate passage of the barium and prevent constipation and fecal impaction.
2. *Endoscopy:* Allows visualization of the stomach (gastroscopy), duodenum (duodenoscopy), both stomach and duodenum (gastroduodenoscopy), or the esophagus, stomach, and duodenum (esophagogastroduodenoscopy) *via* passage of a lighted, flexible tube. Patient is kept NPO 8-12 hours before the procedure and written consent is required. Prior to the test a sedative is administered to relax the patient, a narcotic analgesic is given to prevent pain, and atropine is administered to decrease GI secretions and prevent aspiration. Local anesthesic may be sprayed into the posterior pharynx to ease passage of the tube and a biopsy may be performed as part of the endoscopy procedure. Postprocedure care involves maintaining NPO status for 2-4 hours, administering throat lozenges or analgesics as prescribed, ensuring return of the gag reflex before allowing the patient to eat (if local anesthetic was used), and monitoring for complications, such as bleeding or perforation (e.g., hematemesis, pain, dyspnea, tachycardia).
3. *Gastric secretion analysis:* Helpful in differentiating gastric ulcer from gastric cancer. If an NG tube is passed, the stomach contents are aspirated and analyzed for the presence of blood and free hydrochloric acid. Achlorhydria (absence of free hydrochloric acid) is suggestive of gastric cancer, while mildly elevated levels suggest gastric ulcer. Excessive elevation of free hydrochloric acid occurs with Zollinger-Ellison syndrome. A tubeless gastric analysis involves administration of a gastric stimulant followed by a resin dye. A urine specimen is obtained 2 hours later and analyzed for the presence of dye. Absence of dye indicates achlorhydria. The patient is kept NPO for at least 8 hours before either test.
4. *CBC:* Reveals a decrease in hemoglobin, hematocrit, and RBCs when acute or chronic blood loss accompanies ulceration.
5. *Stool for occult blood:* Positive if bleeding is present.

MEDICAL MANAGEMENT AND SURGICAL INTERVENTIONS

Conservative management is preferred over surgical intervention, with the therapy aimed at decreasing hyperacidity, healing the ulcer, relieving symptoms, and preventing complications.

1. **Activity as tolerated with adequate rest:** So that tissue repair can occur. The patient who is anemic from bleeding ulcers will require activity limitations and more assistance with ADL owing to fatigue.
2. **Dietary management:** Well-balanced diet with avoidance of foods that are not tolerated. Three meals a day are recommended, with elimination of bedtime snacks. Consumption of coffee and alcohol should be reduced or eliminated. For acute episodes of upper GI hemorrhage, the patient will be NPO and given IV fluid and electrolyte replacement, with foods and fluids introduced orally as bleeding subsides.
3. **Pharmacotherapy (generally short-term and given in combination)**
   □ *Antacids:* Administered PO or through an NG tube to provide symptomatic relief, facilitate ulcer healing, and prevent further ulceration; or they might be administered prophylactically in patients who are especially prone to ulceration. They are administered after meals and at bedtime, or are given periodically *via* NG tube for patients who are intubated and often titrated based on pH of gastric aspirate.
   □ *Histamine H_2 receptor antagonists* (e.g., Tagamet, Zantac, Axid, Pepcid): Administered PO or IV to suppress secretion of gastric acid and facilitate ulcer healing. They also can be used prophylactically for limited periods of time, especially in patients susceptible to stress ulceration. These medications should be administered with meals at least an hour apart from antacids, since antacids can reduce their absorption.
   □ *Sucralfate (Carafate):* An antiulcer agent used to treat duodenal and gastric ulcers. This drug coats the ulcer with a protective barrier so that healing can occur. This drug must be taken qid: before meals and at bedtime. It should not be taken within 30 minutes of antacids since acid facilitates adherence of sucralfate to the ulcer.
   □ *Misoprostol (Cytotec):* Effective in preventing stomach ulcers in individuals taking nonsteroidal antiinflammatory drugs for arthritis.
4. **NG tube with gastric lavage:** For acute, severe GI bleeding to diminish bleeding and prevent accumulation of clotted blood. For this procedure the patient should be in a semi-Fowler's position or higher. A large bore NG tube or an Ewald tube is inserted. Gastric contents are aspirated, followed by the instillation of 100-250 ml room temperature normal saline or tap water, as prescribed, and the contents are then aspirated. The process is repeated until returns are clear or light pink and clot free. Vasopressin may be administered IV or intraarterially to diminish uncontrolled bleeding prior to surgery.
5. **Antacid gavage:** May be prescribed to maintain gastric pH at a level of 4.5 or higher in individuals with an NG tube to facilitate healing, prevent exacerbation, or prevent ulceration in patients at risk. Sixty to ninety ml of antacid (e.g., Maalox, Mylanta, Riopan) is instilled, the tube is clamped for 20-30 minutes, and the stomach contents are aspirated to determine pH. The process is repeated as necessary for pH <4.5.
6. **Surgical interventions:** Indicated for hemorrhage, intractable ulcers, GI obstruction, and perforation. Common surgical procedures include the following, singly or in combination:
   □ *Pyloroplasty:* Enlargement of the pyloric opening to relieve obstruction.
   □ *Vagotomy:* Severing of the branches of the vagus nerve to inhibit gastric acid secretion.
   □ *Subtotal gastrectomy:* Removal of part of the stomach with anastomosis to the duodenum (Billroth I for gastric ulcer) or removal of part of the stomach and the duodenum with anastomosis to the jejunum (Billroth II for duodenal ulcer). Vagotomy may accompany subtotal gastrectomy.
   □ *Total gastrectomy:* Removal of the entire stomach (rarely performed).
7. **Postsurgical care:** Involves temporary GI decompression with NG tube; analgesics for pain; IV fluid and electrolyte replacement; symptomatic relief of dumping syndrome (rapid gastric emptying characterized by abdominal fullness, weakness, diaphoresis, fatigue, tachycardia, palpitations, dizziness) with a low-carbohydrate, high-fat, high-protein diet, small meals without liquids, and supine position after meals; treatment of pernicious anemia (decreased production of intrinsic factor secondary to removal of part of the stomach) with B_{12} injections; and treatment with iron supplements for iron-deficiency anemia (which might occur secondary to loss of blood or iron-absorb-

ing surface in the GI tract). Prevention of hypoventilation and subsequent atelectasis and hypoxemia is especially important in patients who have had abdominal surgery. Deep breathing exercises are imperative (see "Atelectasis," p. 1).

8. **Lifestyle alterations:** Such as smoking cessation, decreased consumption of alcohol, avoidance of irritating drugs, and stress reduction therapies.

See "Obstructive Processes," p. 332, for treatment of GI obstruction secondary to inflammatory edema or scar tissue formation with ulcer healing. See "Peritonitis," p. 337, for care of the patient with peritonitis due to perforation.

NURSING DIAGNOSES AND INTERVENTIONS

Pain related to epigastric discomfort secondary to ulcerative process

Desired outcome: Patient's subjective evaluation of pain improves, as documented by a pain scale.

1. Assess for and document presence of pain, including its severity, character, location, duration, precipitating factors, and methods of relief. Devise a pain scale with patient, rating discomfort on a scale of 0 (no pain) to 10.
2. Administer antacids, histamine H_2-receptor antagonists, or sucralfate as prescribed. Rate the degree of relief obtained using the pain scale.
3. Advise patient to avoid irritating foods and drugs, especially those associated with the symptoms.
4. Advise patient to eat three balanced meals per day and to avoid bedtime snacks.
5. Provide comfort measures, such as distraction, verbal interaction to allow expression of feelings and reduction of anxiety, backrub, and stress reduction techniques. See **Health-seeking behavior:** Relaxation technique effective for stress reduction, p. 49.

Potential for injury related to risk of gastrointestinal complications (bleeding, obstruction, and perforation) secondary to ulcerative process

Desired outcomes: Patient is free of the signs and symptoms of bleeding, obstruction, perforation, and peritonitis as evidenced by negative tests for occult blood, passage of stool and flatus, soft and nondistended abdomen, good appetite, and normothermia. Patient verbalizes knowledge of necessary lifestyle alterations and demonstrates compliance with the medical therapy.

1. Teach the patient the rationale for lifestyle alterations and compliance with medical therapy to prevent exacerbation of the condition. Examples include smoking cessation, stress reduction, avoidance of irritating foods and drugs, and elimination or decreased consumption of alcohol.
2. Assess for indicators of bleeding, including hematemesis, melena, and occult blood in stool. If indicated, administer gastric lavage as prescribed.
3. Monitor patient for indicators of obstruction, including abdominal pain, distention, nausea and vomiting, and the inability to pass stool or flatus. For more information, see "Obstructive Processes," p. 332.
4. Be alert to indicators of perforation and peritonitis, such as abdominal pain, distention and abdominal rigidity, fever, anorexia, nausea, and vomiting. See "Peritonitis," p. 337, for more information.
5. Teach the patient the signs and symptoms of GI complications and the importance of reporting them promptly to the staff or MD should they occur. Notify MD of significant findings.

Pain, abdominal fullness, weakness, and diaphoresis after meals related to postgastrectomy dumping syndrome

Desired outcome: Patient verbalizes preventive measures for discomfort and relates the absence of discomfort following meals.

1. Advise the patient to avoid high-carbohydrate meals, which precipitate an osmotic pull of fluids into the GI tract and contribute to symptoms.
2. Advise the patient to avoid taking liquids with meals and to lie supine after meals to discourage rapid gastric emptying.

See the appendix for nursing diagnoses and interventions for the care of preoperative and postoperative patients, p. 637.

PATIENT-FAMILY TEACHING AND DISCHARGE PLANNING

Provide patient and significant others with verbal and written information for the following:
1. Importance of following the prescribed diet to facilitate ulcer healing, prevent exacerbation or recurrence, or control postsurgical dumping syndrome. If appropriate, arrange a consultation with a dietitian.
2. Medications, including drug name, rationale, dosage, schedule, precautions, and potential side effects.
3. Signs and symptoms of exacerbation, recurrence, and potential complications.
4. Care of the incision line and dressing change technique, as necessary. Teach patient about the signs of wound infection, including persistent redness, swelling, purulent drainage, local warmth, fever, and foul odor.
5. Role of lifestyle alterations in preventing exacerbation or recurrence of ulcer, including smoking cessation, stress reduction (see **Health-seeking behavior:** Relaxation technique effective for stress reduction, p. 49), decreasing or eliminating consumption of alcohol, and avoidance of irritating foods and drugs.
6. Referral to a health care specialist for assistance with stress reduction, as necessary.

Gastric neoplasm

The incidence of cancerous lesions of the stomach has declined in the United States in recent years, although it continues to be a significant problem in Japan, China, Chile, Iceland, and Great Britain. Its incidence has been associated with dietary intake of hypertonic salted, pickled, and smoked foods or other foods containing nitrates that are converted to nitrites, and a history of various disease processes (see "History of," below). Because of the late appearance of the symptoms, detection is often delayed until the disease process is well advanced. Prognosis is grave, especially with late detection. Complications can include bleeding and subsequent anemia, pernicious anemia, GI obstruction, or perforation with peritonitis. Metastases can occur in other GI organs and the lungs, bones, kidneys, brain, skin, uterus, and ovaries.

ASSESSMENT

Signs and symptoms: Epigastric discomfort, anorexia, weight loss, bloating, nausea, and vomiting; weakness, hematemesis, and melena if bleeding is present.

Physical assessment: A mass may be palpated in some patients. Pallor and cachexia also may be present.

History of: Excessive intake of starches, smoked foods, preservatives; chronic gastritis; adenomatous gastric polyps; pernicious anemia; gastric ulcer.

DIAGNOSTIC TESTS

1. *Barium swallow, gastroscopy, and gastric secretion analysis:* See discussion in "Peptic Ulcers," p. 323.
2. *Abdominal ultrasound/CT scan:* To facilitate preoperative staging and identify sites of metastases (see discussion in "Malabsorption," p. 329).
3. *CBC:* Will reveal decreased hgb, hct, and RBCs when acute or chronic blood loss accompanies the neoplastic process.

4. *Biopsy/cytology:* Performed in conjunction with gastroscopy or the insertion of a gastric tube. Postprocedure care involves monitoring for bleeding by noting presence of such signs as hematemesis and melena.

MEDICAL MANAGEMENT AND SURGICAL INTERVENTIONS

1. **Activity as tolerated.** Tolerance may be limited if patient is malnourished or anemic.
2. **Nutritional support:** With oral supplements (e.g., Ensure, Sustacal, Resource Plus), if possible, to maintain patient's weight. With significant weight loss or severe anorexia, parenteral nutrition may be administered (see "Providing Nutritional Support," p. 611). In some cases, patients are NPO if feedings are not tolerated or there are complications, such as bleeding, perforation, or obstruction.
3. **IV fluid replacement:** As necessary, to maintain hydration in patients who cannot tolerate oral feedings or who must remain NPO for long periods of time.
4. **If GI obstruction occurs:** Care of the patient with an obstructive process will apply. See "Obstructive Processes," p. 332.
5. **NG tube with gastric lavage:** For acute, severe GI bleeding. See discussion with "Peptic Ulcer," p. 324.
6. **Blood replacement:** As necessary, if GI bleeding occurs.
7. **Chemotherapy:** Tumor regression occurs in a small percentage of individuals treated with 5-fluorouracil. Combination chemotherapy with 5-fluorouracil, doxorubicin, and mitomycin C is more successful, although the median survival rate is less than 1 year. The success of adjuvant chemotherapy for prevention of metastasis after gastric tumor removal is currently under investigation. For more information, see "Caring for Patients with Cancer and Other Life-Disrupting Illnesses," p. 659.
8. **Radiation:** May be used palliatively to control bleeding or alleviate pain associated with bone metastasis.
9. **Analgesics** to relieve pain; **antiemetics** for symptomatic relief of nausea and vomiting.
10. **Total or subtotal gastrectomy:** Offers the best choice of cure. See description in "Peptic Ulcer," p. 324.

NURSING DIAGNOSES AND INTERVENTIONS

Alteration in nutrition: Less than body requirements related to decreased intake secondary to nausea, vomiting, bloating, and anorexia

Desired outcome: Patient has adequate nutrition as evidenced by stable weight, serum albumin 3.5-5.5 g/dl, and a balanced or positive nitrogen state.

1. Encourage smaller, more frequent feedings in a conducive environment that is free of odors.
2. Determine and offer the patient's diet preferences.
3. Administer prescribed antiemetic agents as indicated, especially before meals to increase the likelihood of eating.
4. Administer prescribed IV fluids and nutrients.
5. Monitor and record daily weight and I&O.
6. For other interventions, see the same nursing diagnosis in "Providing Nutritional Support," p. 622.

Potential fluid volume deficit related to decreased intake secondary to nausea, anorexia, or bloating and loss secondary to vomiting

Desired outcome: Patient is normovolemic as evidenced by good skin turgor, stable weight, moist mucous membranes, urinary output ≥30 ml/hr, HR ≤100 bpm, orthostatic changes in systolic BP <15 mm Hg, and absence of thirst.

1. Ensure precise measurements and documentation of I&O.
2. Assess for indicators of fluid volume deficit: weight loss, poor skin turgor, dry skin and mucous membranes, urinary output <30 ml/hr, tachycardia, orthostatic systolic BP decreases ≥15 mm Hg, and thirst.

3. Encourage patient's preferred fluids at frequent intervals. Fluids at room temperature often are best tolerated.
4. Administer appropriate IV fluids as prescribed.

See "Peptic Ulcer" for **Potential for injury** related to risk of gastrointestinal complications, p. 325, and **Pain,** abdominal fullness, weakness, diaphoresis after meals related to postgastrectomy dumping syndrome, p. 325. See the appendix for nursing diagnoses and interventions for the care of preoperative and postoperative patients, p. 637, and the care of patients with cancer and other life-disrupting illnesses, p. 659.

PATIENT-FAMILY TEACHING AND DISCHARGE PLANNING

Provide patient and significant others with verbal and written information for the following:
1. Measures for symptomatic relief of pain, anorexia, nausea, vomiting, and bloating. Include appropriate use of medications, such as drug name, purpose, dosage, route, schedule, precautions, and potential side effects.
2. Indicators of complications that necessitate medical attention, including bleeding, obstruction, perforation, and exacerbation of the symptoms.
3. Care of incision line and dressing change technique, as necessary. Patient should be able to describe indicators of wound infection, including persistent redness, swelling, pain, purulent drainage, and foul odor.
4. Measures to prevent/alleviate complications of radiation and chemotherapy as necessary.
5. Referral to support person/group as indicated.
6. As appropriate, referrals to visiting nurse association (VNA), community health nurses, and hospice.

Malabsorption/maldigestion

Malabsorption or maldigestion refers to a condition in which a specific nutrient or a variety of nutrients are inadequately digested or absorbed from the GI tract. The causes of malabsorption are varied and can include the following:

Postgastrectomy malabsorption: Frequently seen in individuals following subtotal gastrectomy due to rapid gastric emptying and decreased intestinal transit time.

Inadequate presence of digestive substances in the GI tract: Examples are lactase enzyme deficiency, which is characterized by an inability to digest and absorb lactose, a disaccharide found in milk and dairy products; bile deficiency secondary to liver and gallbladder disease and biliary tract obstruction, which is characterized by inability to digest and absorb fats and fat-soluble vitamins; and pancreatic secretion deficiency secondary to pancreatic insufficiency or obstruction to the flow of pancreatic secretions as seen with pancreatic disorders or cystic fibrosis.

Inadequate absorptive space in the GI tract secondary to GI surgery (especially ileal resection) and characterized by general nutrient malabsorption (short bowel syndrome).

Mucosal lesions that impair absorption: Mucosal changes occur secondary to intestinal invasion of microorganisms endemic to tropical islands (tropical sprue) or ingestion of gluten in the diet (celiac disease, nontropical sprue, gluten-induced enteropathy). Gluten-containing foods include malt, rye, barley, oats, and wheat. With Whipple's disease, which is a rare disorder, a small bowel lipodystrophy occurs, resulting in impaired absorption.

Inflammatory conditions of the GI tract such as ulcerative colitis (see p. 353) and Crohn's disease (see p. 360), which involve significant diarrhea and malabsorption and deficiencies of various nutrients. Inflammation and mucosal ulceration secondary to chemotherapy also can impair digestion and absorption.

Use of drugs that alter intestinal fluids or mucosa (and subsequently affect absorption of specific nutrients). These include antacids, mineral oil, broad-spectrum antibiotics, hypocholesterolemic agents, antiinflammatory agents, oral hypoglycemics, and oral potassium chloride.

Overgrowth of microbes in the GI tract secondary to diverticula (outpouchings) of the small intestine, inadequate gastric acid secretion (e.g., secondary to total/partial gastrectomy), immunologic defects, gastroenteritis, blind loop syndrome, and intestinal obstruction.

Excessive use of enemas or cathartics (nutrients pass too rapidly through the intestinal tract to be absorbed): Complications can include specific or generalized malnutrition, fluid and electrolyte imbalances, and acid-base imbalances, any of which may necessitate hospitalization.

ASSESSMENT

Signs and symptoms: Symptoms will vary, depending on the specific nutrients that are not absorbed. Patient might have unexplained weight loss with muscle atrophy, despite normal or increased appetite; diarrhea; steatorrhea (greasy, pale, foul-smelling stools); bloating; excessive flatus; abdominal cramping; and indicators of specific nutrient deficiencies (e.g., anemia with iron or B_{12} deficiency; tetany and paresthesias with calcium deficiency; bleeding or easy bruising with vitamin K deficiency).

History of: GI surgery; excessive use of enemas or cathartics; diseases that cause diarrhea; immunologic defects; diverticulosis; liver, pancreatic, or gallbladder disease; inflammatory/infectious disorders of the intestinal tract; medications that increase GI motility and cause diarrhea; chemotherapy.

DIAGNOSTIC TESTS

1. *72-hour fecal fat test:* Increased when steatorrhea characterizes malabsorption.
2. *Stool culture:* May be diagnostic of bacterial overgrowth.
3. *Schilling's test:* Analysis of a 24-hour urine specimen collected after ingestion of radioactive B_{12} followed by an IM injection of nonradioactive B_{12} will reveal below-normal levels of B_{12}. Further testing, in which intrinsic factor is administered, will facilitate diagnosis of pernicious anemia from malabsorption or renal disease.
4. *D-xylose tolerance test:* Will show inadequate presence of xylose (an easily absorbed monosaccharide) in a 5-hour collection of urine after oral administration.
5. *Serum tests:* Will show depressed levels of carotene, calcium, magnesium, and other electrolytes and minerals, depending on specific malabsorption problem. In addition, serum albumin, total iron-binding capacity, and transferrin may be decreased owing to protein depletion.
6. *Lactose tolerance test:* Will show failure of fasting blood glucose levels to rise and the presence of abdominal symptoms after ingestion of lactose. These signs are diagnostic of lactase deficiency (lactose intolerance).
7. *Hydrogen breath test:* Will show an increase in hydrogen after ingestion of lactose. Because unabsorbed lactose is converted to hydrogen, this test is diagnostic of lactase deficiency.
8. *Lactulose breath test:* Assesses for presence of bacterial overgrowth. Nonabsorbent lactulose is administered and the breath is tested for hydrogen. With the abnormal presence of bacteria in the proximal intestine, lactulose is hydrolyzed earlier than normal.
9. *Barium swallow:* Facilitates diagnosis of the specific etiology of malabsorption. For a description, see "Peptic Ulcers," p. 323.
10. *Abdominal x-ray:* Facilitates diagnosis of the specific etiology of malabsorption; for example, pancreatic calcifications might be noted, which are suggestive of pancreatic etiology.
11. *Ultrasound of the abdomen:* Facilitates diagnosis of the specific etiology of malabsorption; for example, abnormalities of specific organs (e.g., pancreas, gallbladder,

liver) might be noted. Patient usually is NPO 8-12 hours before the procedure and will be required to lie still in the supine position during the procedure, which lasts 30-60 minutes.

12. *CT scan of the abdomen:* Facilitates diagnosis, especially for pancreatic involvement. Patients are NPO 3-4 hours before the procedure. To minimize flatus, a low-residue diet may be prescribed for 48 hours prior to the testing. Patients should be assessed ahead of time for allergy to iodine (as well as to shellfish if patient is not knowledgeable about iodine allergy). For this procedure an iodine dye is injected, and scanning is done over a period of 1-1½ hours. A warm flushed feeling or burning sensation and nausea may be felt with administration of the dye, and patients are required to hold several deep breaths during scanning. Written consent of the patient is required prior to performing a CT scan. Oral or IV fluids should be adequate to ensure elimination of the dye *via* the kidneys after the procedure.

13. *Endoscopy with or without biopsy:* The small (duodenoscopy) or large (colonoscopy) bowel is visualized through a lighted, flexible tube (endoscope) that is inserted through the mouth (duodenoscopy) or rectum (colonoscopy). The patient is NPO prior to the procedure. Written consent is required. Sedation may be prescribed to relax the patient and atropine may be administered to decrease GI secretions. Specimens of tissue may be taken for biopsy or cytologic evaluation. Hemorrhage is a potential complication after biopsy and VS should be monitored closely.

14. *Endoscopic retrograde cholangiopancreatography (ERCP):* Involves passage of an endoscope into the duodenum to the ampulla of Vater (distal end of the pancreatic and common bile duct drainage system) for visualization. A contrast medium is injected into the scope and x-rays are taken. This test is diagnostic for pancreatic disease. Patient is NPO for 8-12 hours before the test and must be assessed for allergies to iodine (and/or to shellfish) before undergoing the test. Written consent is required. Oral or IV fluids should be adequate to ensure elimination of dye *via* the kidneys after the procedure.

15. *Hormonal stimulation test:* Checks for pancreatic insufficiency. A collecting tube is passed into the duodenum of the NPO patient. IV secretin and/or cholecystokinin is given and the duodenal secretions are collected and analyzed for bicarbonate and trypsin levels, which are decreased with pancreatic insufficiency. Written consent is required.

MEDICAL MANAGEMENT AND SURGICAL INTERVENTIONS

Management will vary, depending on the specific etiology of malabsorption and the nutrient deficiencies that are exhibited.

1. **Activity as tolerated:** Patient may be fatigued and require limited activity as a consequence of diarrhea and malnutrition.
2. **Dietary management:** Will vary, depending on the specific disorder that is precipitating the malabsorption. A *low-residue diet* may be useful for controlling diarrhea. For lactase deficiency, a *low-lactose diet* (avoidance of milk and milk products) is prescribed, and for nontropical sprue, a *gluten-free diet* is prescribed (see Table 6-1). Until specific problems (such as liver or gallbladder disorders) are corrected, dietary intake of fats is avoided. Any specific nutrient deficiencies are corrected. For the seriously malnourished patient, parenteral nutrition may be necessary (see "Providing Nutritional Support," p. 611).
3. **Pharmacotherapy:** Will vary, depending on the specific disorder that has precipitated malabsorption and the specific nutrient deficiencies.
   □ *Mineral, vitamin, and electrolyte supplements:* To correct specific deficiencies.
   □ *Antibiotics:* For treatment of bacterial overgrowth.
   □ *Cholestyramine (an antihyperlipidemic agent):* may be given to control diarrhea when it is associated with ileal resection.
4. **IV fluids and electrolytes:** As necessary to correct imbalances.
5. **Surgical intervention:** May be necessary to correct specific disorders that precipitate malabsorption, such as biliary tract obstruction.

NURSING DIAGNOSES AND INTERVENTIONS

Diarrhea, bloating, excessive flatus, and abdominal cramping related to malabsorption disorder

Desired outcome: Patient is free of discomfort from symptoms of malabsorption, as evidenced by passage of normal stools (soft, semi-formed) and absence of excessive flatus and cramping.

1. Assess and document presence of GI discomfort and symptoms, including the onset and duration of symptoms and the precipitating and palliative factors. Instruct patient to avoid foods associated with symptoms.
2. Teach the patient about the importance of dietary compliance in the treatment for some malabsorptive disorders (see Table 6-1). For example, dietary restriction (e.g., low-lactose diet with lactase intolerance or gluten-free diet with nontropical sprue) may be necessary to prevent symptoms.

Fluid volume deficit related to increased need secondary to impaired absorption or abnormal loss secondary to diarrhea

Desired outcome: Patient is normovolemic as evidenced by good skin turgor, moist mucous membranes, urinary output ≥30 ml/hr, HR ≤100 bpm, orthostatic systolic BP changes <15 mm Hg, and absence of thirst.

1. Assess patient for evidence of fluid volume deficit: weight loss, hypotension, poor skin turgor, dry skin and mucous membranes, and thirst.
2. Ensure precise maintenance and documentation of fluid I&O records.
3. Administer IV fluids and parenteral nutrients appropriately and at prescribed rate.
4. Encourage prescribed dietary compliance for relief of symptomatic diarrhea.

TABLE 6-1 Sample diet plans

Low-residue diet
Encourage intake of enriched/refined breads and cereals; rice and pasta dishes. Avoid fruits, vegetables, whole wheat products (cereals and breads)

Gluten-free diet
Avoid cereals and bakery goods made from wheat, malt, barley, rye, and oats. In addition, avoid the following if they contain any of the above grain products: coffee substitutes, sauces, commercially prepared luncheon meats, gravies, noodles, macaroni, spaghetti, flour tortillas, crackers, cakes, cookies, pastries, puddings, commercial ice cream, and alcoholic beverages

High-residue diet
Encourage intake of fruits, vegetables, large amounts of fluid, whole grain breads and cereals. Avoid highly refined cereals and pasta (for example, white rice, white bread, spaghetti noodles) and ice cream

Use the following (if allowed): rice, corn, eggs, potatoes; breads made from rice flours, cornmeal, soybean flour, gluten-free wheat starch, and potato starch; cereals made from corn or rice (grits, corn meal mush, cooked Cream of Rice, puffed rice, rice flakes); pasta made from corn or rice flour; homemade ice cream; tapioca pudding

5. Administer medications and teach patient self-administration of medications to control diarrhea or treat underlying condition.

Note: For assessment of nutrient deficiencies, see "Providing Nutritional Support," p. 611.

PATIENT-FAMILY TEACHING AND DISCHARGE PLANNING

Provide patient and significant others with verbal and written information for the following:
1. Use of medications (vitamins, antibiotics), including drug name, purpose, dosage, schedule, precautions, and potential side effects.
2. Prescribed dietary replacement of deficient nutrients and dietary management of symptoms, if appropriate.
3. Problems that necessitate medical attention: nutrient deficiencies (see "Providing Nutritional Support," p. 611), hypovolemia (see "Fluid and Electrolyte Disturbances," p. 546), and acid-base imbalances (see p. 563).

Obstructive processes

Obstruction of the GI tract is a condition in which the normal peristaltic transport of GI contents does not take place. Therefore digestion and absorption of foods and fluids and the elimination of wastes are impaired or totally blocked. Furthermore, GI fluids become hypertonic, precipitating osmotic fluid loss from the body into the GI lumen. Subsequently, nutritional and fluid and electrolyte status are compromised and distention occurs. Increased pressure in the GI tract also can result in perforation and peritonitis or necrosis of the GI mucosa. Obstruction can occur anywhere along the GI tract, but most commonly it occurs at the pyloric area of the stomach or in the small bowel owing to adhesions in the ileum. Obstruction can occur as a result of the inflammation and edema that accompany GI disease (peptic ulcers, diverticulitis, colitis, gastroenteritis, trauma); GI surgery with subsequent edema and possible adhesions (gastrectomy, appendectomy, colon resection); growths (polyps, tumors); adynamic (paralytic) ileus secondary to peritoneal insult, such as surgery or peritonitis; or diminished GI motility owing to uremia, diabetes mellitus, or use of narcotics, diuretics, or anticholinergic drugs; volvulus; or incarcerated hernia.

ASSESSMENT

Signs and symptoms: Severe and crampy pain, abdominal distention, vomiting, back pain, restlessness, hiccoughs, eructation, and inability to pass stool or flatus (accompanied by a feeling of "fullness"). Symptoms vary, depending on the type and site of obstruction (see Table 6-2).

Physical assessment: Abdominal distention, abdominal tenderness (with strangulation of the intestine), high-pitched and intermittent bowel sounds above the point of obstruction. Bowel sounds are absent or diminished with paralytic ileus. Patients may have decreased urinary output, poor skin turgor, and dry skin and mucous membranes associated with dehydration owing to pathophysiology of the obstruction. Rectal bleeding may be noted on rectal exam if strangulation or tumor is present.

History of: Abdominal hernia, recent or past abdominal surgery, GI inflammation or perforation secondary to various disease processes, diabetes mellitus, chronic renal failure, or use of narcotics, diuretics, or anticholinergics.

DIAGNOSTIC TESTS

1. *WBC count:* Usually elevated in the presence of strangulation or obstruction secondary to inflammatory process.
2. *X-ray of abdomen:* Will reveal distention of bowel loops with air and fluid proximal

TABLE 6-2 Assessment of patients with obstructive processes

	Small bowel obstruction	Large bowel obstruction	Paralytic ileus
Pain*	Severe, episodic	Moderate, more continuous	Not prominent
Vomiting	Occurs early; may be projectile	Occurs late; feculent (if duodenal valve is incompetent)	Not prominent
Abdominal distention	Occurs late	Pronounced	Present
Passage of stool/flatus	———None, except with partial obstruction of the large——— bowel, "pencil" stools may be passed		

***Note:** With obstruction associated with intestinal strangulation, pain always is severe, vomiting is present, and the abdomen is distended, rigid, and tender.

to the obstruction. The presence of free air under the diaphragm indicates intestinal perforation.

3. *Barium swallow/barium enema:* Facilitates quick assessment to determine presence and location of obstruction. Barium enema (to exclude colon obstruction) should precede barium swallow. Barium will not advance past the site of obstruction. For more information, see "Peptic Ulcer," p. 323.

4. *Aspiration of fecal matter from NG/intestinal tube:* Foul fecal matter is an indication of obstruction.

MEDICAL MANAGEMENT AND SURGICAL INTERVENTIONS

The specific cause of the obstruction must be identified quickly so that the appropriate treatment can be instituted and complications prevented. In the interim, management is supportive and aimed at maintaining nutritional and fluid and electrolyte balance and promoting comfort.

1. **Activity as tolerated:** With paralytic ileus, the patient is encouraged to ambulate to enhance return of peristalsis. With other forms of obstruction, activity may be limited due to pain or complications.

2. **Dietary management:** Patient will be NPO until obstruction is resolved (or bowel sounds are returned in paralytic ileus).

3. **GI decompression:** Accomplished *via* NG or intestinal tube connected to low, intermittent suction. See Table 6-3, below.

4. **IV fluid and electrolyte support:** Lactated Ringer's or isotonic saline solutions (or isotonic dextrose/saline combinations) are commonly prescribed. Volume of IV fluid required often is dependent on the amount of NG or intestinal tube drainage (replacement fluids often prescribed ml for ml). Potassium is added to IV fluids to prevent hypokalemia. TPN may be indicated to meet nutritional needs if obstruction/recovery is prolonged.

5. **Pharmacotherapy:** May include the following:
   □ *Antibiotics:* To prevent infection.
   □ *Analgesics:* For pain relief. However, they can mask symptoms and interfere with diagnosis. Narcotics, such as morphine, can decrease intestinal motility and increase nausea and vomiting.
   □ *Antiemetic agents (e.g., Compazine):* For relief of nausea and vomiting.

6. **Surgical intervention:** Indicated for obstruction that does not subside. In some cases, inflammatory processes subside and obstruction resolves without surgery. Paralytic ileus generally resolves in 2-3 days without any treatment. In most cases, surgery is indicated to identify and relieve the source of obstruction. Exploratory laparatomy is performed when diagnosis is uncertain. When diagnosis is known, the indicated sur-

T A B L E 6 - 3   Gastric/intestinal tubes used in obstructive processes

Tube	Obstructive process	Purpose
NG tube*	Pyloric obstruction, small bowel obstruction, paralytic ileus	Decompresses the GI tract of retained fluids, alleviates abdominal distention, relieves edema in the intestinal wall, prevents vomiting, and promotes comfort
Intestinal tube† (e.g., single-lumen Cantor or Harris tube or double-lumen Miller-Abbott tube)	Small or large bowel obstruction, paralytic ileus	See NG tube, above. Presence of tube may promote return of peristalsis in paralytic ileus. Tube may relieve edema sufficiently enough to relieve obstruction, thereby avoiding need for surgery.

*In some cases, NG and intestinal tubes are used together.
†Long intestinal tubes primarily are indicated when obstruction is partial.

gery is performed, for example, pyloroplasty for pyloric obstruction or bowel resection with or without colostomy for removal of tumor or adhesions.

NURSING DIAGNOSES AND INTERVENTIONS

Pain, nausea and distention related to obstructive process and presence of NG or intestinal tube

Desired outcome: Patient's subjective evaluation of discomfort improves, as documented by a pain scale.

1. Assess the degree of the patient's discomfort. Devise a pain scale with patient, rating discomfort from 0 (no discomfort) to 10.
2. Implement comfort measures to provide pain relief: distraction, backrubs, conversation, relaxation therapy. See **Health-seeking behavior:** Relaxation technique effective for stress reduction, p. 49.
3. Administer prescribed analgesics and antiemetic agents as indicated. Assess and document the degree of relief obtained using the pain scale.
4. Maintain patency and proper functioning of the NG or intestinal tube.
   - ☐ Maintain connection to low, intermittent suction or as prescribed.
   - ☐ Irrigate tube with 30 ml normal saline prn or as prescribed.
   - ☐ Keep NG tube properly positioned in stomach by taping tube to patient's nose.
   - ☐ Advance intestinal tube slowly, 2-3 inches at a time or as prescribed, until it reaches the desired location. Positioning patient in various positions (right side-lying, supine, left side-lying) may facilitate passage of the tube. Do not tape the tube to the patient's skin until it reaches the desired location.
5. Keep HOB elevated 30-45 degrees as permitted, to promote comfort and facilitate respirations. A slightly Trendelenburg, right side-lying position may reduce gas pains in patients with paralytic ileus.
6. Encourage turning in bed and activity as permitted to promote peristalsis.
7. Provide mouth care at frequent intervals. Frequent brushing of teeth and rinsing of the mouth will alleviate dryness. Provide lubricant for lips.
8. Provide mouth rinses at frequent intervals to alleviate pharyngeal discomfort from

tube. Apply water-soluble lubricant to naris to alleviate discomfort. Apply viscous lidocaine solution to naris or back of throat, as prescribed, to alleviate discomfort from the tube.

Fluid volume deficit related to abnormal losses secondary to obstructive process and subsequent vomiting or gastric decompression of large volumes of GI fluids and decreased intake secondary to fluid restrictions

Desired outcome: Patient becomes normovolemic as evidenced by good skin turgor, moist mucous membranes, urinary output $\geq$30 ml/hr, HR $\leq$100 bpm, orthostatic systolic BP changes <15 mm Hg, and absence of thirst.

1. Ensure precise measurement and documentation of fluid I&O. Take special note of the amount and character of GI aspirate (see Table 6-10, p. 377). Check GI aspirate for electrolyte loss or pH as prescribed.
2. Measure abdominal girth q8h.
3. Administer appropriate IV fluids at the prescribed rate. Replace volume of GI fluids aspirated by suction, if prescribed.
4. For other interventions, see the same nursing diagnosis in "Caring for Preoperative and Postoperative Patients," p. 644.

For nursing diagnoses and interventions for the delivery of enteral and parenteral nutrition, see "Providing Nutritional Support," p. 611. If surgery was performed, see "Caring for Preoperative and Postoperative Patients," p. 637.

PATIENT-FAMILY TEACHING AND DISCHARGE PLANNING

Provide patient and significant others with verbal and written information for the following:
1. Specific disease process that precipitated the obstruction and methods to prevent recurrence, such as compliance with prescribed therapies.
2. Symptoms of recurring obstruction to report to MD.
3. Medications, including drug name, purpose, dosage, schedule, precautions, and potential side effects.

Hernia

A hernia is a protrusion of an organ (usually the intestine) through the abdominal wall. Although a hernia can occur secondary to a congenital weakness in the abdominal wall, most commonly it occurs as a consequence of disease, old age, increased abdominal pressure, or disruption of the abdominal wall secondary to trauma or surgery (incisional hernia). Hernias can develop at the umbilicus, inguinal opening (most common), femoral ring, or at a previous surgical or trauma site. They can be precipitated or aggravated by those factors related to an increase in intraabdominal pressure, such as lifting, sneezing, coughing, straining at stool, pregnancy, ascites, and obesity. Potential complications include incarceration (hernia is irreducible in that it cannot be replaced manually in its normal position) with subsequent intestinal obstruction; and strangulation (hernia is incarcerated and blood supply to the bowel is compromised) with subsequent infection or necrosis.

ASSESSMENT

General signs and symptoms: Tenderness and bulging at herniation site; pain with straining.

Obstruction secondary to incarceration: Abdominal pain and distention, nausea, vomiting (may be feculent), hiccoughs, back pain, sensation of constipation, and inability to pass stool or flatus (see "Obstructive Processes," p. 332).

Infection or necrosis secondary to strangulation: Fever and possibly peritonitis (see "Peritonitis," p. 337).

Physical assessment: Bulge with straining will be noted on inspection; palpation of herniation site will reveal a soft and tender mass or bulge. In men, the scrotum should be examined whenever a hernia is diagnosed or suspected because herniation at the inguinal area can cause herniation of bowel into the scrotum. See "Obstructive Processes," p. 332, or "Peritonitis," p. 337, if these complications are present.

DIAGNOSTIC TESTS

1. *X-ray:* May reveal presence of a hernia or incarceration. However, diagnosis is made primarily through physical examination.
2. *WBC count:* Will be elevated in the presence of strangulation.

MEDICAL MANAGEMENT AND SURGICAL INTERVENTIONS

Management is aimed at reduction of the hernia (placement of herniated area back through the abdominal wall) and prevention of strangulation and incarceration.

1. Activity as tolerated: With restriction of stretching and straining, and emphasis on proper body mechanics.
2. Manual reduction: Placement of the herniated area back to its anatomically correct position. The patient is usually placed in Trendelenburg's position and given sedatives/relaxants to facilitate the procedure.
3. Truss (firm support): Might be prescribed for applying pressure to the herniated area to maintain correct anatomic position. A truss is especially important with ambulation and activity.
4. High-residue diet: To prevent constipation and straining with stools.
5. Stool softeners (e.g., Colace, Surfak) and cathartics: May be prescribed to prevent constipation and straining.
6. Antibiotics: Usually prescribed in the presence of strangulation and infection. Also see discussion with "Peritonitis," if peritonitis is present.
7. With incarceration: Care of the patient with an obstructive process will apply (see p. 332).
8. Herniorrhaphy: Surgery performed when the hernia is irreducible by other means, or when strangulation or incarceration occurs. It is performed under general or regional anesthesia. Inguinal hernia repairs often are done with local or spinal anesthesia on an outpatient basis. Hernias in the upper abdomen are often repaired under general anesthesia with hospitalization.

NURSING DIAGNOSES AND INTERVENTIONS

Pain (especially with straining) related to hernia condition or surgical intervention

Desired outcome: Patient's subjective evaluation of discomfort improves, as documented by a pain scale.

1. Assess and document presence of pain: severity, character, location, duration, precipitating factors, and methods of relief. Devise a pain scale with patient, rating discomfort from 0 (no pain) to 10. Report presence of severe, persistent pain, which can signal complications.
2. Advise patient to avoid straining, stretching, coughing, and heavy lifting. Teach patient to splint incision manually or with a pillow during coughing episodes. This is especially important during the early postoperative period and for up to 6 weeks after surgery.
3. Teach patient the use of a truss, if prescribed, and advise its use as much as possible, especially when out of bed. **Note:** Apply truss before patient gets out of bed.
4. Apply or teach patient application of scrotal support or ice packs, which are often prescribed to limit edema and control pain after inguinal hernia repair.
5. Administer prescribed analgesics as indicated, especially before postoperative activities. Use comfort measures as well: distraction, verbal interaction to enhance expressions of feelings and reduction of anxiety, backrubs, and stress reduction techniques,

such as relaxation exercises. Document the degree of relief obtained using the pain scale.

Potential for urinary retention related to pain, trauma, and use of anesthetic secondary to lower abdominal surgery

Desired outcomes: Patient voids without difficulty within 8 hours of surgery. Urine output is ≥100 ml for each voiding and is adequate (approximately 1,500 ml) over a 24-hour period.

1. Assess for and document presence of suprapubic distention or patient verbalizations of inability to void.
2. Monitor urinary output. Document and report frequent voidings of <100 ml at a time.
3. Facilitate voiding by implementing interventions in the section "Urinary Retention," p. 145.

Knowledge deficit: Potential for gastrointestinal complications associated with presence of a hernia and measures that can prevent their occurrence

Desired outcome: Patient verbalizes knowledge of the signs and symptoms of gastrointestinal complications and complies with the prescribed measures for prevention.

1. Teach patient to be alert to and report severe and persistent pain, nausea and vomiting, fever, and abdominal distention, which can herald onset of incarceration or strangulation.
2. Encourage patient to comply with medical regimen: use of a truss or other support and avoidance of straining, stretching, constipation, and heavy lifting.
3. Teach patient to consume a high-residue diet to prevent constipation (see Table 6-1, p. 331). Encourage intake of at least 2-3 L/day of fluids to promote soft consistency of stools.
4. Teach patient proper body mechanics for moving and lifting.

See the appendix for nursing diagnoses and interventions for the care of preoperative and postoperative patients, p. 637. Altered sexual function may occur in men following repair of inguinal hernia owing to decreased blood supply to the testes. See "Nursing diagnoses used in this manual," p. 717, for nursing diagnoses **Body image disturbance, Altered patterns of sexuality,** and **Sexual dysfunction,** as appropriate.

PATIENT-FAMILY TEACHING AND DISCHARGE PLANNING

Provide patient and significant others with verbal and written information for the following:
1. Care of incision and dressing change technique, if appropriate. Teach patient the signs of infection at the incision site, which require medical intervention: fever, persistent redness, swelling, local warmth, tenderness, purulent drainage, and foul odor.
2. Symptoms of hernia recurrence and postsurgical complications.
3. Postsurgical activity limitations as directed: usually heavy lifting (>5 lb) and straining are contraindicated for about 6 weeks.
4. Importance of proper body mechanics to prevent recurrence, especially when lifting and moving.
5. Prevention of constipation and straining with stools, for example, by following a high-residue diet (see Table 6-1, p. 331) and using stool softeners and cathartics when needed.
6. Medications, including drug name, purpose, dosage, schedule, precautions, and potential side effects.

Peritonitis

Peritonitis is the inflammatory response of the peritoneum to offending chemical and bacterial agents invading the peritoneal cavity. The inflammatory process can be local or generalized and acute or chronic, depending on the etiology and pathogenesis of the inflammation. Common causes include intraoperative and abdominal trauma; postoperative leakage into the peritoneal cavity; ischemia; ruptured or inflamed organs; poor aseptic techniques, for example, with peritoneal dialysis; and direct contamination of the bloodstream. The peritoneum responds to invasive agents by attempting to localize the infection, which results in tissue edema, the development of fibrinous exudate, and hypermotility of the intestinal tract. As the disease progresses, paralytic ileus occurs, and intestinal fluid, which then cannot be reabsorbed, leaks into the peritoneal cavity. As a result of the fluid shift, cardiac output and tissue perfusion are reduced, and this leads to impaired cardiac and renal function. If the infection continues, respiratory failure and shock can ensue. Peritonitis is frequently progressive and can be fatal. It is the most common cause of death following abdominal surgery.

ASSESSMENT

Signs and symptoms: Abdominal pain with any movement, nausea, vomiting, fever, malaise, weakness, prostration, hiccoughs, diaphoresis.

Physical assessment: Presence of tachycardia, hypotension, and shallow and rapid respirations caused by abdominal distention and discomfort. Often, the patient assumes a supine position with the knees flexed. On abdominal exam, palpation usually reveals distention, abdominal rigidity with general or localized tenderness, and rebound tenderness. Auscultation findings include hyperactive bowel sounds during the gradual development of the peritonitis and an absence of bowel sounds during later stages if paralytic ileus occurs. Mild ascites may be present, as well.

History of: Abdominal illness, peptic ulcer, ruptured appendix, cholecystitis, trauma, surgery, peritoneal dialysis.

DIAGNOSTIC TESTS

1. *Serum tests:* May reveal the presence of leukocytosis, hemoconcentration, and electrolyte imbalance, particularly hypokalemia. Hypoalbuminemia also can occur.
2. *ABG values:* May reveal the presence of hypoxemia (Pao_2 <80 mm Hg) or acidosis (pH <7.40).
3. *Urinalysis:* Often performed to rule out genitourinary involvement.
4. *Peritoneal aspiration with culture and sensitivity:* May be performed to determine the presence of blood, bacteria, bile, pus, and amylase content and identify the causative organism.
5. *Abdominal x-rays:* May be performed to determine the presence of abnormal levels of fluid and gas, which usually collect in the large and small bowel in the presence of a perforation. "Free air" under the diaphragm also may be visualized.

MEDICAL MANAGEMENT AND SURGICAL INTERVENTIONS

1. Bed rest: With patient in semi- or high-Fowler's position to enhance fluid shift to the lower abdomen, which will reduce pressure on the diaphragm and allow for deeper and easier respirations.
2. NG or intestinal tube: Inserted to reduce or prevent gastrointestinal distention, nausea, and vomiting.
3. IV fluids, electrolyte therapy, and parenteral feedings: To correct fluid, electrolyte, and nutritional disorders. Daily measurements of serum electrolytes and calculations of fluid volume are performed to determine the necessary types of fluids and electrolyte replacement. Plasma, protein, and blood may be administered to correct hypovolemia, hypoproteinemia, and anemia. Patient is NPO during the acute phase, and oral fluids are not resumed until the patient has passed flatus and the gastric tube has been removed. TPN usually is initiated in the early stages to promote nutrition and protein replacement.
4. CVP catheter: May be inserted to monitor circulatory status in the critically ill patient.

CVP values should be maintained at 2-6 mm Hg (5-12 cm H_2O). A pulmonary artery (i.e., Swan-Ganz) catheter may be inserted if the patient develops hypovolemic shock.
5. Parenteral antibiotic therapy.
6. Oxygen: Often prescribed to treat hypoxia.
7. Narcotics and sedatives: To relieve severe pain and discomfort once the diagnosis has been confirmed.
8. Surgical intervention: May be required to remove the source of infection or drain the abscess and accumulated fluids. This can include the removal of an organ, such as the appendix or gallbladder. Drains usually are inserted to remove purulent drainage and excessive fluids. Intestinal decompression may be employed to decrease massive abdominal distention. Intraoperative and postoperative irrigation may be indicated if there has been gross contamination of the peritoneal cavity with bowel contents.
9. Peritoneal lavage: May be used if the patient does not respond to the above interventions and is a surgical risk. Rapid dialysis exchanges may be performed along with antibiotic lavages.

NURSING DIAGNOSES AND INTERVENTIONS

Pain, abdominal distention, and nausea related to the inflammatory process, fever, and tissue damage

Desired outcome: Patient's subjective evaluation of pain improves, as documented by a pain scale.

1. Assess and document the character and severity of the discomfort q1-2h. Devise a pain scale with the patient, rating discomfort on a scale of 0 (no pain) to 10.
2. Once the diagnosis has been made, administer narcotics, analgesics, and sedatives as prescribed to promote comfort and rest. Document the relief obtained, using the pain scale.
3. Keep patient on bed rest to minimize pain, which can be aggravated by activity; provide a restful and quiet environment.
4. Keep patient in a position of comfort, usually semi-Fowler's position.
5. Explain all procedures to patient to help minimize anxiety, which can augment discomfort.
6. Offer mouth care and lip moisturizers at frequent intervals to help relieve discomfort/nausea from continuous or intermittent suction, dehydration, and NPO status.
7. See "Stomatitis," p. 314, for mouth care interventions.

Ineffective breathing pattern related to guarding or decreased depth of respirations secondary to abdominal pain and distention

Desired outcomes: Patient has an effective breathing pattern as evidenced by RR 12-20 breaths/min with normal depth and pattern (eupnea), absence of adventitious breath sounds, Pao_2 ≥80 mm Hg, BP ≥90/60 mm Hg (or within patient's baseline range), HR ≤100 bpm, and patient oriented to person, place, and time.

1. Monitor ABG results and be alert to indicators of hypoxia, including low Pao_2 and to the following clinical signs: hypotension, tachycardia, hyperventilation, restlessness, CNS depression, and possibly cyanosis.
2. Auscultate lung fields to assess ventilation and detect pulmonary complications. Note and document the presence of adventitious breath sounds.
3. Keep patient in semi- or high-Fowler's position to aid respiratory effort; encourage deep breathing to enhance oxygenation.
4. Administer oxygen as prescribed.

Potential for injury related to risk of worsening peritonitis or development of septic shock secondary to inflammatory process

Desired outcome: Patient is asymptomatic of worsening peritonitis or septic shock as evidenced by normothermia, BP ≥90/60 mm Hg (or within patient's normal range), HR

≤100 bpm, presence of eupnea, urinary output ≥30 ml/hr, CVP 2-6 mm Hg (5-12 cm H_2O), decreasing abdominal girth measurements, and minimal tenderness to palpation.

1. Assess the abdomen q1-2h during the acute phase and q4h once the patient is stabilized. Monitor for increasing distention by measuring abdominal girth and auscultate bowel sounds to assess motility. Bowel sounds often are frequent during the beginning phase of peritonitis, but are absent in the presence of paralytic ileus. *Lightly* palpate the abdomen for evidence of increasing rigidity or tenderness, which is indicative of disease progression. If the patient experiences more pain on removal of your hand, rebound tenderness is present. Notify MD of significant findings.
2. If prescribed, insert NG tube and connect it to suction to prevent or decrease distention.
3. Monitor VS at least q2h and more frequently if the patient's condition is unstable. Be alert to signs of septic shock: increased temperature, hypotension, tachycardia, shallow and rapid respirations, urine output <30 ml/hr, and CVP <2 mm Hg (or <5 cm H_2O). In the early (warm) stage of shock, the skin is usually warm, pink, and dry secondary to peripheral venous pooling, and the BP and CVP begin to drop. In the late (cold) stage of shock, the extremities become pale and cool secondary to the decreasing tissue perfusion.
4. Administer antibiotics as prescribed.
5. Monitor the CBC for the presence of leukocytosis, which signals infection, and hemoconcentration (increased hct and hgb), which occurs with a decrease in plasma volume. Normal values are as follows: WBC: 4,500-11,000 µl; Hgb: 14-18 g/dl (male) or 12-16 g/dl (female); and Hct: 40%-54% (male) or 37%-47% (female). With peritonitis, WBC count usually will be greater than 20,000 µl. Notify MD of significant findings.
6. Maintain sterile technique with dressing changes and all invasive procedures.

Alteration in nutrition: Less than body requirements related to loss secondary to vomiting and intestinal suctioning and increased need secondary to NPO status

Desired outcome: Patient has adequate nutrition as evidenced by stable weight, balanced or positive nitrogen state, and serum albumin 3.5-5.5 g/dl.

1. Keep patient NPO as prescribed during acute phase of the disorder. If the patient has an ileus, an NG tube will be inserted to decompress the abdomen. Reintroduce oral fluids gradually once motility has returned, as evidenced by presence of bowel sounds, decreased distention, and passage of flatus.
2. As prescribed, support patient with peripheral parenteral nutrition (PPN) or TPN, depending on the duration of the acute phase (usually by day 3).
3. Administer replacement fluids, electrolytes, and vitamins, as prescribed.

See "Providing Nutritional Support," p. 611, for the care of patients on tube or parenteral feedings. See the appendix for nursing diagnoses and interventions for the care of preoperative and postoperative patients, p. 637. Also see "Caring for Patients on Prolonged Bed Rest" for **Potential for activity intolerance, p. 651**, and **Potential for disuse syndrome, p. 653.**

PATIENT-FAMILY TEACHING AND DISCHARGE PLANNING

Provide patient and significant others with verbal and written information for the following:
1. Medications, including the drug name, dosage, schedule, purpose, precautions, and potential side effects.
2. Activity alterations as prescribed by MD, such as avoiding heavy lifting (>5 lb), resting after periods of fatigue, getting maximum amounts of rest, gradually increasing activities to tolerance.
3. Notifying MD of the following indicators of recurrence: fever, chills, abdominal pain, vomiting, abdominal distention.

4. If patient has undergone surgery, describe indicators of wound infection: fever, pain, chills, incisional swelling, persistent erythema, purulent drainage.
5. Importance of follow-up medical care; confirm date and time of next medical appointment.

Appendicitis

Appendicitis is the most commonly occurring inflammatory lesion of the bowel and one of the most frequent reasons for abdominal surgery. The appendix is a blind, narrow tube that extends from the inferior portion of the cecum and does not serve any useful function. Appendicitis is usually caused by obstruction of the appendiceal lumen by a fecalith (hardened bit of fecal material), inflammation, a foreign body, or a neoplasm. Obstruction prevents drainage of secretions that are produced by epithelial cells in the lumen, thereby increasing intraluminal pressure and compressing mucosal blood vessels. This tension causes impaired viability, which can lead to necrosis and perforation. Inflammation and infection result from normal bacteria invading the devitalized wall. Mild cases of appendicitis can heal spontaneously, but severe inflammation can lead to a ruptured appendix, which can cause local or generalized peritonitis (see "Peritonitis," p. 337).

ASSESSMENT

Signs and symptoms will vary because of differences in anatomy, size, and age.

Early stage: Abdominal pain (either epigastric or umbilical) that may be vague and diffuse; nausea and vomiting; fever; and sensitivity over the appendix area.

Intermediate, "acute" stage: Pain that shifts from epigastrium to RLQ at McBurney's point (approximately 2 inches from the anterior superior iliac spine on a line drawn from the umbilicus) and is aggravated by walking or coughing. The pain may be accompanied by a sensation of constipation ("gas stoppage" sensation). Anorexia, malaise, occasionally diarrhea, and diminished peristalsis also can occur.

On physical assessment, the patient will experience pain in the RLQ elicited by *light* palpation of the abdomen; presence of rebound tenderness; RLQ guarding, rigidity, and muscle spasms; tachycardia; low-grade fever; absent or diminished bowel sounds; and pain elicited with rectal exam. A palpable, tender mass may be felt in the peritoneal pouch if the appendix lies within the pelvis.

Acute appendicitis with perforation: Increasing, generalized pain; and recurrence of vomiting.

On physical assessment, the patient usually will exhibit temperature increases >38.5° C (101.4° F) and generalized abdominal rigidity. Typically, the patient remains rigid with flexed knees. Presence of abscess can result in a tender, palpable mass. The abdomen may be distended.

DIAGNOSTIC TESTS

1. *WBC with differential:* Will reveal presence of leukocytosis and an increase in neutrophils. A shift to the left with more than 75% neutrophils is found in about 90% or more cases.
2. *Urinalysis:* To rule out genitourinary conditions mimicking appendicitis; may reveal microscopic hematuria and pyuria.
3. *Abdominal x-ray:* May reveal presence of a fecalith. If perforation has occurred, the presence of free air will be noted.
4. *IVP:* May be performed to rule out ureteral stone or pyelitis.
5. *Abdominal ultrasound:* May be done to rule out appendicitis or conditions that mimic it, such as Crohn's disease, diverticulitis, or gastroenteritis.
6. *Abdominal CT scan:* May reveal an appendiceal abscess or acute appendicitis.

MEDICAL MANAGEMENT AND SURGICAL INTERVENTIONS

Preoperative care

1. **Bed rest:** For observation.
2. **NPO status:** Parenteral fluids are begun if surgery is imminent.
3. **Pharmacologic therapy:** Narcotics are avoided until diagnosis is certain because they mask clinical signs and symptoms.
   □ *Antibiotics:* To prevent systemic infection.
   □ *Tranquilizing agents:* For sedation.
4. **NG tube:** Inserted for gastric suction and lavage, if needed. **Note:** Cathartics and enemas are contraindicated because they increase peristalsis and can cause perforation.

Surgery:

5. **Appendectomy:** Performed as soon as the diagnosis is confirmed and fluid imbalance and systemic reactions have been controlled. The appendix is removed through an incision made over McBurney's point or through a right paramedial incision. In the presence of abscess, rupture, or peritonitis, an incisional drain is inserted.

Postoperative care:

6. **Activities:** Ambulation begins either the day of surgery or the first postoperative day. The patient may be hospitalized for 3-5 days. Normal activities are resumed 2-3 weeks after surgery.
7. **Diet:** Advances from clear liquids to soft solids during the second through fifth postoperative day; parenteral fluids are continued if required.
8. **Pharmacotherapy**
   □ *Antibiotics:* Continued in the presence of infection.
   □ *Mild laxatives:* Given, if necessary; but enemas continue to be contraindicated during the first few postoperative weeks until adequate healing has occurred and bowel function has been restored.
   □ *Analgesics:* For postoperative pain.

NURSING DIAGNOSES AND INTERVENTIONS

Potential for infection related to risk of rupture, peritonitis, and abscess formation secondary to inflammatory process

Desired outcomes: Patient is free of infection, as evidenced by normothermia, HR <100 bpm, BP >90/60 mm Hg, RR 12-20 breaths/min with normal depth and pattern (eupnea), soft and nondistended abdomen, and bowel sounds 5-34/min in each abdominal quadrant. Patient verbalizes the rationale for not administering enemas or laxatives preoperatively and enemas postoperatively, and demonstrates compliance with the therapeutic regimen.

1. Assess and document quality, location, and duration of pain. Be alert to pain that becomes accentuated and generalized or to the presence of recurrent vomiting, and note whether patient assumes side-lying or supine position with flexed knees. Any of these can signal worsening appendicitis, which can lead to rupture.
2. Monitor VS for elevated temperature, increased pulse rate, hypotension, and shallow/rapid respirations; and assess the abdomen for presence of rigidity, distention, and decreased or absent bowel sounds, any of which can occur with rupture. Report significant findings to MD.
3. Caution patient about the danger of preoperative self-treatment with enemas and laxatives because they increase peristalsis, which increases the risk of perforation. If constipation occurs postoperatively, MD may prescribe hs laxatives/stool softeners after the third day. Remind patient that enemas should be avoided until approved by MD (usually several weeks after surgery).
4. Teach patient about postoperative incisional care, as well as the care of drains if patient is to be discharged with them.
5. Provide instructions about prescribed antibiotics if patient is to be discharged with them.

See "Peritonitis," p. 337, for more information.

Pain and nausea related to the inflammatory process

Desired outcome: Patient's subjective evaluation of pain improves, as documented by a pain scale.

1. Assess and document quality, location, and duration of pain. Devise a pain scale with patient, rating discomfort from 0 (no pain) to 10.
2. Medicate patient with antiemetics, sedatives, and analgesics as prescribed; evaluate and document patient's response using the pain scale.
3. Keep patient NPO before surgery; after surgery, nausea and vomiting usually disappear. If prescribed, insert NG tube for decompression.
4. Teach technique for slow, diaphragmatic breathing to reduce stress and help relax tense muscles.
5. Help position patient for optimal comfort. Many patients find comfort from a side-lying position with the knees bent, while others relate relief when supine with pillows under the knees.

See the appendix for nursing diagnoses and interventions for the care of preoperative and postoperative patients, p. 637.

PATIENT-FAMILY TEACHING AND DISCHARGE PLANNING

Provide patient and significant others with verbal and written information for the following:

1. Medications, including drug name, dosage, purpose, schedule, precautions, and potential side effects.
2. Care of incision, including dressing changes and bathing restrictions, if appropriate.
3. Indicators of infection: fever, chills, incisional pain, redness, swelling, and purulent drainage.
4. Postsurgical activity precautions: avoid lifting heavy objects (>5 lb) for the first 6 weeks or as directed, be alert to and rest after symptoms of fatigue, get maximum rest, gradually increase activities to tolerance.
5. Importance of avoiding enemas for the first few postoperative weeks. Caution patient about the need to check with MD before having an enema.

Hemorrhoids

Traditionally, both internal and external hemorrhoids were believed to be varicosities of the hemorrhoid veins, caused by conditions that precipitate increased intraabdominal pressure or obstruct venous return, for example, pregnancy, chronic constipation, physical exertion, portal hypertension, infiltrating carcinoma, infection, and ulcerative colitis. However, a more current concept is that internal hemorrhoids are normal vascular cushions containing a rich, arteriovenous network. They may be present at birth and can narrow the anal lumen, thereby contributing to continence. These vascular cushions project into the lumen, where they are subjected to downward pressure during defecation. The muscular fibers that anchor the cushions become attenuated, and the hemorrhoids slide, become congested, bleed, and eventually prolapse. Internal hemorrhoids are found proximal to the anal sphincter and are not visible unless they become large enough to protrude through the anus. External hemorrhoids are distal to the anal sphincter and can become thrombosed if the vein ruptures.

ASSESSMENT

Signs and symptoms: Hemorrhoids may be manifested by rectal bleeding (fresh, bright red blood, especially on the toilet paper or surface of the stool), prolapsed tissue, pain in the presence of thrombosis, and pruritus. Chronic blood loss can cause iron deficiency.

Physical assessment: External hemorrhoids are visible as bluish protrusions in the subcutaneous perianal tissue. They appear grapelike on inspection. Internal hemorrhoids may require anoscopy, since they are rarely palpated on digital examination unless they are thrombosed.

Risk factors: Diet low in fiber, obesity, long-term constipation and straining, lifestyle or career that requires constant sitting or standing, portal hypertension, and pregnancy.

DIAGNOSTIC TESTS

1. *Stool occult blood test:* To assess for the presence of blood.
2. *CBC:* To assess for anemia from chronic blood loss.
3. *Anoscopy or flexible sigmoidoscopy:* To confirm the diagnosis and rule out neoplastic or inflammatory disease that may be responsible for the symptoms.
4. *Colonoscopy and barium enema:* May be necessary to exclude other causes of rectal bleeding.

MEDICAL MANAGEMENT AND SURGICAL INTERVENTIONS

1. Regulation of bowel movements: Bulk cathartic, stool softener, high-fiber diet, exercise, augmenting fluid intake, avoiding prolonged sitting.
2. Treatment of pain and itching: Warm or cold compresses and warm sitz baths.
3. Pharmacotherapy: *Topical anesthetics,* such as dibucaine hydrochloride (Nupercainal) ointment, *astringents,* such as witch Hazel (Tucks) pads, and *antiinflammatory preparations,* such as hydrocortisone ointment, to relieve pain and itching and shrink mucous membranes.
4. Manual reduction of prolapsed and strangulated hemorrhoids: Returning hemorrhoid to rectum with a lubricated, gloved finger.
5. Sclerosing agent: Injection into the submucosal tissue surrounding the hemorrhoids to produce an inflammatory response, which leads to tissue shrinkage and fixation of the hemorrhoid. This is a palliative and temporary measure. Usually 5% phenol in vegetable oil is the sclerosing agent.
6. Rubber band ligation: Nonsurgical method of constricting the blood circulation of the hemorrhoid, causing tissue necrosis, separation, and sloughing to occur. Sepsis is a potential complication of this technique if it is done improperly due to the necrosing and sloughing of the tissue. Observation for the following triad of symptoms necessitates prompt medical attention: anal pain, urinary retention, and fever.
7. Incision and drainage: To remove clots from thrombosed hemorrhoids. This is performed on an outpatient basis using a local anesthetic.
8. Newer coagulation techniques: Use of infrared coagulation, bipolar electrode therapy, and direct current electrotherapy of the hemorrhoids. Infrared photocoagulation, for example, is a relatively new procedure, causing fibrosis of the hemorrhoid. There is a very high cost associated with laser therapy and results are similar to those obtained with injections and ligation.
9. Hemorrhoidectomy: Removal by cautery, clamp, or excision of hemorrhoids that do not respond to the above therapies.

NURSING DIAGNOSES AND INTERVENTIONS

Colonic constipation: Diminished frequency of bowel elimination with resultant hard, dry, or painful stools

Desired outcome: Patient reports bowel movements of soft stools without straining or pain.

1. Teach patient about high fiber diet and the need for adequate fluid intake (>2-3 L/ day unless contraindicated).
2. Administer prescribed stool softeners and bulk cathartics. Teach this regimen to the patient.

3. Teach patient about use of such therapeutic measures as sitz baths, warm/cold compresses, topical anesthetics, prescribed antiinflammatory preparations (e.g., hydrocortisone creams or suppositories), astringent pads, exercise, and avoidance of prolonged sitting while attemping to have a bowel movement.
4. Instruct patient to respond to the urge to defecate as quickly as possible to prevent pressure build-up in the rectum.
5. For other interventions, see **Constipation,** in "Caring for Patients on Prolonged Bed Rest," p. 656.

Pain and itching related to hemorrhoidectomy

Desired outcome: Patient's subjective evaluation of discomfort improves, as documented by a pain scale.

1. Monitor patient for the presence of pain. Devise a pain scale with patient, rating discomfort on a scale of 0 (no pain) to 10. Administer topical anesthetics, astringents, and antiinflammatory preparations as prescribed. Rate the degree of relief obtained using the pain scale.
2. Administer cold or warm compresses to rectal area. Provide warm sitz baths 3-4 times a day, or as prescribed. **Caution:** Be alert to hypotension, which can be caused by the dilatation of pelvic blood vessels.
3. Administer narcotics for severe postoperative pain as prescribed.
4. Ensure that the patient takes stool softeners during the early postoperative period in preparation for the first bowel movement.
5. If indicated, position a flotation pad under the buttocks for comfort. Doughnut-shaped cushions are contraindicated because they can increase rather than decrease pressure at the operative site.
6. Provide warm sitz baths after each bowel movement to minimize discomfort and promote healing.

Colonic constipation related to fear of pain with postoperative defecation

Desired outcomes: Patient has bowel movements without straining during the early postoperative period. Patient verbalizes the rationale for the importance of postoperative bowel movements and complies with the therapeutic regimen.

1. Explain to patient that discomfort is common with the first bowel movements after surgery.
2. Administer stool softeners and bulk cathartics as prescribed. Administer analgesic ½ -1 hour before the patient attempts defecation.
3. Encourage ambulation the day of surgery or first postoperative day to enhance peristalsis.
4. In nonrestricted patients encourage fluid intake of at least 2-3 L/day to help soften stools and promote elimination.
5. Document the first bowel movement, which should occur by the third or fourth postoperative day. Stay with the patient or stand just outside the bathroom door because dizziness and fainting are common at this time due to dilatation of the pelvic blood vessels. Record the amount and character of the stool and the patient's response.
6. If the patient avoids having a bowel movement after surgery because of anticipated pain, explain that a normal postsurgical bowel movement will prevent complications, such as constriction of the anal lumen.

Alteration in pattern of urinary elimination: Anuria or dysuria related to local swelling or presence of rectal packing secondary to hemorrhoidectomy

Desired outcome: Patient relates the resumption of the normal pattern of voiding.

1. If patient has difficulty voiding in the early postoperative period because of local swelling or rectal packing, encourage patient to get out of bed to void.
2. Encourage sitz baths or warm showers, which stimulate the voiding reflex.
3. If patient is unable to void, evaluate for the need for urinary catheterization and consult with MD accordingly.

Potential fluid volume deficit related to abnormal blood loss secondary to slipped ligatures

Desired outcome: Patient is normovolemic as evidenced by BP within patient's baseline range, HR ≤100 bpm, RR ≤20 breaths/min with normal depth and pattern (eupnea), and ≤2 saturated dressings/8 hr.

1. Hemorrhage can result from a slipped ligature, yet the bleeding easily can go undetected. Be alert to the presence of pallor, diaphoresis, hypotension, and increasing pulse and respiration rates. Orthostatic hypotension and BP and pulse changes are early signs of hypovolemia. If bleeding does occur, be prepared to assist MD with insertion of a Foley catheter (22-28 F) into the rectum and inflation of the balloon to provide pressure to the bleeding site.
2. Assess for rectal bleeding. After surgery and into the first or second postoperative day, the patient will have rectal packing. Inspect the perianal area for evidence of fresh bleeding. After MD removes the packing, replace the perianal dressing (typically a sanitary napkin) as necessary. Be alert to excess bleeding, as evidenced by >2 saturated pads/8hr. Query patient about the presence of a frequent, unrelieved urge to defecate, which can signal sequestered hemorrhage.
3. Advise patient to avoid straining or sitting on the toilet longer than necessary. Instruct patient to avoid positions that increase pressure, such as prolonged sitting, standing, or squatting.
4. Instruct patient to keep perianal area clean but to avoid vigorous wiping after bowel movement. *Moist* perineal wipes should be used to cleanse the area. Encourage sitz baths after every bowel movement to cleanse the rectal area and relieve local irritation. Be alert to hypotension, which can be caused by dilatation of pelvic blood vessels.
5. As appropriate, advise the patient to abstain from anal intercourse until proper healing has taken place and it is approved by MD.
6. Explain to patient that some bleeding can be expected about 8-12 days postoperatively when the sutures begin to dissolve.
7. Be alert to the potential for sepsis, which is a rare but possible complication of the rubber band ligation technique.

Knowledge deficit: Potential for recurrence of hemorrhoids and measures that help prevent it

Desired outcome: Patient verbalizes knowledge of the potential for recurrence of hemorrhoids and can list preventive measures.

1. Advise patient to use mild, bulk cathartics or stool softeners if constipation recurs and to avoid straining with defecation.
2. Encourage a diet high in fiber content, such as intake of whole grain products (breads, cooked grains, and cereals), apples, peas, and kidney and other dried beans.
3. For nonrestricted patients, explain that a minimum fluid intake of 2-3 L/day is necessary to soften the stool and promote elimination.
4. Encourage daily exercise, which enhances peristalsis and promotes elimination. Advise patient to avoid prolonged standing and sitting.

See the appendix for nursing diagnoses and interventions for the care of preoperative and postoperative patients, p. 637.

PATIENT-FAMILY TEACHING AND DISCHARGE PLANNING

Provide patient and significant others with verbal and written information for the following:
1. Medications, including drug name, dosage, schedule, purpose, precautions, and potential side effects.
2. Importance of avoiding straining and methods for preventing constipation, such as

exercise, diet high in fiber content, augmenting fluid intake, and taking stool softeners or mild, bulk cathartics if necessary.

3. Postoperative activity precautions as directed: avoid fatigue, get maximum rest, and gradually increase activities to tolerance.
4. Awareness that some bleeding can occur about 8-12 days postoperatively, when sutures begin to dissolve.

Section Three   INTESTINAL NEOPLASMS AND INFLAMMATORY PROCESSES

Diverticulosis/diverticulitis

Diverticulosis is acquired small pouches or sacs (diverticula) in the colon formed by the herniation of mucosal and submucosal linings through the muscular layers of the intestine. Although diverticula can be found anywhere in the colon, they are seen most frequently in the sigmoid colon. It is theorized that diverticula develop secondary to a low-residue diet and increased intracolonic pressure, such as that created with straining to have a bowel movement.

Diverticulitis is a complication of diverticulosis. It is an inflammatory process, and it is theorized that it begins with a single diverticulum, usually in the sigmoid colon, and is caused by the irritating presence of trapped fecal material within the diverticulum. When the obstructing fecal plug remains and bacteria proliferate, the inflammation can spread from the thin wall at the apex of the diverticulum to peridiverticular tissue. The resulting inflammation and infection can be localized or be more extensive (as in peritonitis) and life-threatening.

ASSESSMENT

Diverticulosis: Lower GI bleeding or symptoms of irritable bowel syndrome, such as steady or crampy abdominal pain in the LLQ, associated with constipation or diarrhea and increased flatulence. The patient may be asymptomatic.

Diverticulitis: See the above indicators. In addition, fever, nausea, vomiting, and obstipation can be present if obstruction or peritonitis occurs. Fistulas to the bladder, vagina, or skin, and gas or stool elimination from the involved site also may be present.

Physical assessment: Presence of tender, palpable mass, usually in the LLQ; rebound tenderness secondary to infection or abscess formation; abdominal distention, hypoactive or hyperactive bowel sounds; and possibly, absence of stool felt on rectal examination. Tachycardia, hypotension, and shallow respirations can be present if there is severe abdominal discomfort. Often the patient assumes a side-lying position with the knees flexed to relieve pain.

DIAGNOSTIC TESTS

Diverticulosis
1. *Barium enema:* To determine presence and number of diverticula.
2. *CBC:* To determine if anemia is present.
3. *Sigmoidoscopy:* To reveal presence of diverticula and thickening of bowel wall.

Diverticulitis
1. *Abdominal x-rays:* To determine presence of abnormal gas and fluid levels, which collect in the intestine above the affected area of the colon, indicating the presence and degree of bowel obstruction or ileus; and reveal the presence of free air in the peritoneal cavity, signalling noncontainment of diverticular perforation. These films also may show the presence of air in the urinary bladder if a colovesical fistula is present.

2. *CBC with differential:* Usually reveals leukocytosis and an increase in neutrophils, indicating presence of infection.
3. *Blood culture:* May reveal presence of bacteremia in severely ill patients.
4. *Urinalysis:* To rule out bladder involvement; may show presence of red and white cells in the presence of colovesical fistula.
5. *Barium enema:* To support the diagnosis of diverticulitis by demonstrating the presence of barium outside the lumen of the colon or outside of a diverticulum, a fistula or fistulas leading from the colon, or a paracolic mass. This exam should be deferred during the acute phase of illness if perforation is suspected.
6. *CT scan:* To demonstrate diverticula, changes in the wall of the colon that are indicative of diverticulitis, and related abscesses and fistulas. Since this exam is noninvasive, it can be used in acutely ill or septic individuals for whom barium enema studies can be hazardous. Use of this test is limited, however, by its availability and cost.

MEDICAL MANAGEMENT AND SURGICAL INTERVENTIONS

Diverticulosis:

The goal of medical therapy for uncomplicated disease is to relieve symptoms and prevent or postpone complications.
1. High-residue diet: Including fruits and vegetables and the use of wheat bran in the form of 100% bran cereal or 2 tbs/day of unprocessed bran to increase moisture content of the stool, thus softening it to enhance elimination and reduce intracolonic pressure.
2. Pharmacotherapy: Commercial *bulk laxative,* such as psyllium (Metamucil) 1-2 tsp po bid, which can replace bran in the diet.

Diverticulitis:

The goal of medical therapy is to "rest" the bowel, resolve infection and inflammation, and prevent or decrease the severity of complications.
1. Bed rest and NPO status: To promote physical, emotional, and bowel rest.
2. NG suction: To relieve nausea, vomiting, or abdominal distention, if present.
3. Parenteral replacement of fluids, electrolytes, and blood products: As indicated by laboratory test results to maintain intravascular volumes, electrolyte and acid-base balance, urinary output, and caloric intake.
4. Pharmacotherapy
   □ *Parenteral antibiotics:* To limit secondary infection.
   □ *Analgesics:* To relieve pain. Meperidine (Demerol) is the agent of choice. In addition to producing analgesia, it also decreases GI motility and spasm. Pentazocine (Talwin) also reduces sigmoid activity in analgesic doses. It should be used with caution in the older adult since it may cause confusion, disorientation, and hallucinations. The use of morphine and other opiates is contraindicated since they increase intraluminal pressure in the sigmoid colon, thus potentially increasing the risk of perforation.
5. Emergency diverting colostomy with or without resection of the affected bowel segment. This is the therapy of choice for most surgeons. Once inflammation has subsided (after approximately 6 weeks), the affected bowel segment is surgically resected if this was not done with the colostomy. After surgical anastomoses have healed, as documented by x-ray (3-6 weeks later), a third surgery is performed. The colostomy is taken down and the continuity of the GI tract is restored.

NURSING DIAGNOSES AND INTERVENTIONS

For diverticulitis treated by emergency surgical intervention with diverting temporary colostomy: See "Fecal Diversions" for **Bowel incontinence,** p. 367, **Body image disturbance,** p. 368, and **Potential for impaired skin/tissue integrity:** Stoma and peristomal area, p. 366. See the appendix for nursing diagnoses and interventions for the care of preoperative and postoperative patients, p. 637, and for the care of patients with cancer and other life-disrupting illnesses, p. 690.

PATIENT-FAMILY TEACHING AND DISCHARGE PLANNING

Provide patient and significant others with verbal and written information for the following:

1. Medications, including the name, rationale, dosage, schedule, precautions, and potential side effects.
2. Signs and symptoms that necessitate medical attention, including fever; nausea or vomiting; cloudly or malodorous urine; diarrhea or constipation; change in stoma color from the normal bright and shiny red; peristomal skin irritation; and incisional pain, drainage, swelling, or redness.
3. Importance of a normal diet that includes all four food groups (meat, eggs, and fish; fruits and vegetables; milk and cheese; cereal and breads) and drinking adequate fluids (at least 2-3 L/day). Also teach the patient to add fiber to the diet in the form of fruits and vegetables, whole grain cereals, and nuts and with the addition of bran in the form of 100% bran cereal or 2 tbs/day of coarse, unprocessed bran that can be taken with milk or juice or sprinkled over cereal. Because bran initially may cause abdominal distention and excessive flatus, instruct the patient to begin with 1 tbs/day and increase gradually.
4. Gradual resumption of ADL, excluding heavy lifting (>5 lb), pushing, or pulling for 6 weeks to prevent development of incisional herniation.
5. Care of incision, dressing changes, and permission to take baths or showers once sutures/drains are removed.
6. Care of stoma and peristomal skin; use of ostomy skin barriers, pouches, and accessory equipment; and method for obtaining supplies.
7. Referral to community resources, including enterostomal therapy (ET) nurse, home health care agency, and the United Ostomy Association (UOA).
8. Importance of follow-up care with MD or ET nurse; confirm date and time of next appointment.

Colorectal cancer

Colorectal cancer is second only to lung cancer and nonmelanoma skin cancer in the annual number of newly diagnosed cancer cases. Over 90% of colorectal cancers are adenocarcinomas, of which 50% are located in the rectum, 20% in the sigmoid colon, 6% in the descending colon, 8% in the transverse colon, and 16% in the cecum and ascending colon. Many arise from malignant degeneration of benign adenomatous polyps. Metastatic disease occurs through lymph nodes, direct extension to adjacent tissues, and the bloodstream.

The cause of colorectal cancer is unknown, but risk factors include a high-fat, low-fiber diet, age over 40 years, a personal history of colorectal polyps or colorectal carcinoma, a family history of polyposis syndromes (i.e., familial polyposis coli, Gardner's syndrome, Turcot's syndrome, Muir's syndrome, Peutz-Jeghers' syndrome, familial juvenile polyposis from adenomas), first-degree relatives with colorectal cancer, and a personal history of inflammatory bowel disease (i.e., ulcerative colitis, Crohn's disease).

ASSESSMENT

Right colon cancer: Vague, dull abdominal pain. The patient may be asymptomatic.

Physical assessment: Possible presence of a palpable mass in the RLQ, black or dark-red stools, and presence of abdominal distention. The patient also may appear anemic.

Left colon cancer: Increasing abdominal cramping ("gas pains"), change in bowel elimination patterns, decrease in caliber of stools (pencil- or ribbon-shaped stools), constipation, vomiting, obstipation, and acute large bowel obstruction causing progressive increase in abdominal pain. Patient may be asymptomatic.

Physical assessment: Possible absence of stool felt on rectal examination, presence of bright red blood coating the surface of the stool, and abdominal distention.

Rectal cancer: Sensation of incomplete evacuation, tenesmus, and perineal or sacral pain owing to local invasion of surrounding nerves, bladder, or vaginal wall. Pain is a late manifestation. The patient may be asymptomatic.

Physical assessment: Potential presence of palpable mass; bright red blood coating surface of the stool.

History of (for all types of colorectal cancer): Blood on or in stools, change in stool elimination pattern, vague abdominal discomfort or pain.

DIAGNOSTIC TESTS

1. *Occult blood test of three serial stool specimens:* To detect presence of blood associated with tumor mass bleeding.
2. *Proctosigmoidoscopy or colonoscopy:* To examine areas of intestine visually. Because rectal and sigmoid lesions sometimes are difficult to diagnose radiologically, proctosigmoidoscopy should be used to complement air contrast barium enemas (ACBaE). If a neoplasm is detected radiographically or on sigmoidoscopy or if the patient is at high risk because of personal or family history, a full colonoscopic examination should be performed.
3. *Biopsy:* To confirm diagnosis.
4. *Barium enema with air contrast (ACBaE):* To detect colon irregularities suspicious of tumor. ACBaE exams are more accurate than single contrast barium enemas in diagnosing cancers and detecting small neoplastic lesions.
5. *Carcinoembryonic antigen (CEA):* Serum elevation can be indicative of intestinal tumor. CEA is not used as a screening test due to its lack of sensitivity in detecting early colorectal cancer. However, CEA may be useful in preoperative staging and postoperative follow-up to identify early recurrence. Other serologic tumor markers currently are being examined for sensitivity for early detection and diagnosis of colorectal cancer; their effectiveness for screening is still undetermined.

MEDICAL MANAGEMENT AND SURGICAL INTERVENTIONS

1. Surgery: Resection of tumor mass and lymph nodes that drain the area, with reanastomosis of colon. If bowel ends cannot be reanastomosed, a colostomy is created. The exact extent of the colonic resection is determined by the distribution of regional lymph nodes and by the blood supply. The margins of the resection should be at least 5 cm from either side of the tumor. Surgical treatment includes a right hemicolectomy for lesions located in the right colon, left hemicolectomy for lesions located in the left colon, a subtotal or total colectomy for synchronous right- and left-sided lesions, low anterior resection for lesions in the rectosigmoid and upper rectum, and abdominoperineal resection (APR) with colostomy for lesions in the mid-rectum and low rectum. With the recent development of end-to-end stapling devices, APR is being replaced by low anterior resection with reanastomosis for lesions of the mid-rectum and even for low rectal lesions, if a distal margin of at least 2 cm of normal bowel can be resected below the lesion. At present, there appears to be no significant difference in survival and recurrence rates with low anterior resection when compared with APR as long as a 2-5 cm distal margin is preserved.
2. Radiation therapy: To eliminate cancer cells, reduce tumor mass, or decrease pain from advanced disease. As a method of treatment of colorectal cancer, radiation therapy generally is ineffective. It may provide palliation of pelvic pain or rectal or vaginal bleeding secondary to tumor invasion in advanced rectal disease. It is used mainly as an adjuvant therapy to surgery. Preoperatively it is used to reduce tumor mass, converting unresectable large tumors and tumors fixed to pelvic organs to re-

sectable lesions. It also is used preoperatively or postoperatively to decrease local recurrence in patients at high risk (penetration of bowel wall and positive lymph nodes) or in a combined preoperative-postoperative "sandwich" technique.

3. **Chemotherapy:** For advanced disease, usually fluorouracil (5-FU), alone or in combination with other agents to eliminate cancer cells and provide relief from pain with advanced disease. Generally it is used as adjuvant therapy, combined with surgery or with both surgery and radiation therapy. For more information, see section "Caring for Patients with Cancer and Other Life-Disrupting Illnesses," p. 659.

4. **Nutritional management:** May include elemental fluid supplements and/or parenteral nutrition if oral intake is inadequate. For further details, see "Providing Nutritional Support," p. 611.

NURSING DIAGNOSES AND INTERVENTIONS

See "Fecal Diversions" for **Bowel incontinence,** p. 367, **Body image disturbance,** p. 368, **Potential for impaired skin/tissue integrity:** Stoma and peristomal area, p. 366, and **Knowledge deficit:** Colostomy irrigation procedure, p. 369. See the appendix for nursing diagnoses and interventions for the care of preoperative and postoperative patients, p. 637, and the care of patients with cancer and other life-disrupting illnesses, p. 659.

PATIENT-FAMILY TEACHING AND DISCHARGE PLANNING

Provide patient and significant others with verbal and written information for the following:

1. Medications, including drug name, rationale, dosage, schedule, precautions, and potential side effects.
2. Signs and symptoms that necessitate medical attention, including fever, nausea and vomiting, diarrhea, or constipation.
3. If an intestinal stoma is present, the importance of reporting change in stoma color from the normal bright and shiny red; presence of peristomal skin irritation; and incisional pain, drainage, swelling, or redness.
4. Importance of a normal diet that includes all four food groups (meat, eggs, and fish; fruits and vegetables; milk and cheese; cereal and breads) and drinking adequate fluids (at least 2-3 L/day).
5. Enteral or parenteral feeding instructions if patient is to supplement diet or is NPO.
6. Gradual resumption of ADL, excluding heavy lifting (>5 lb), pushing, or pulling for 6 weeks to prevent incisional herniation.
7. Care of incision and perianal wounds, including dressing changes, and bathing once sutures/drains are removed. Sitz baths may be recommended for perianal wound.
8. If stoma is present, care of stoma and peristomal skin; use of ostomy skin barriers, pouches, and accessory equipment; and method for obtaining supplies.
9. Referral to community resources, including home health care agency, American Cancer Society (ACS) and, if appropriate, to enterostomal therapist (ET) nurse and United Ostomy Association (UOA).
10. Importance of follow-up care with MD (or ET nurse if appropriate); confirm date and time of next appointment.
11. Reminders regarding the following recommendations:

    For patients who have had colorectal cancer resections:
    □ Colonoscopy 6-12 months after surgery, followed by yearly colonoscopy for 2 consecutive years; if negative, colonoscopy every 3 years or ACBaE plus proctosigmoidoscopy every 3 years.
    □ Fecal occult blood testing every year.
    □ Serum CEA levels measured at regular intervals (3 times at 6-month intervals, then 5 times at yearly intervals).

    Postpolypectomy patients with malignant polyps:
    □ Colonoscopy within 6 months of polypectomy; if this second exam is negative,

colonoscopy every 2 years. However, if the second exam is positive, colonoscopy at yearly intervals until negative, then colonoscopy at 2-year intervals.
☐ Fecal occult blood testing between colonoscopies.

Polyps/familial polyposis

Of the single, multiple, sessile, and pedunculated polypoid colon tumors, the adenomatous polyp is the most common. The practical significance of these polyps is their tendency to become malignant (see "Colorectal Cancer," p. 349). *Familial polyposis* is characterized by, but distinct from, frequent colon polyp formation. This disorder is also known as multiple familial adenomatosis, adenomatosis coli, and hereditary multiple polyposis. In this disorder the glandular epithelia of the colon and rectum undergo excessive proliferation throughout the mucous membranes, which leads to the formation of sessile or pedunculated polyps. These are soft and red or purplish red in color, vary in size from a few millimeters to several centimeters, and range in number from a few to several thousand. They can be found anywhere along the entire length of the colon, but the rectum is almost always involved. Every individual with untreated familial polyposis will develop cancer, because at some point in time, one or more of these polyps will undergo malignant degeneration. This is a hereditary disease passed from generation to generation as an autosomal dominant trait and it appears most often during late childhood through the early thirties. The incidence of familial polyposis is estimated at approximately 1 in 8,300 births.

ASSESSMENT

Familial polyposis: Mild, early symptoms, such as diarrhea or melena, although many patients remain asymptomatic for years. Once malignant degeneration has begun, these symptoms become more pronounced and there can be intermittent or constant colicky pain. Tenesmus and a frequent urge to defecate also can be present. If blood loss is significant, anemia, weight loss, loss of appetite, and fatigue can occur.

Physical assessment: In the presence of a well-developed malignant growth, a mass can be palpated on abdominal exam. Digital rectal examination may detect presence of polyps.

History of: Familial polyposis, mild colicky abdominal discomfort with or without diarrhea, presence of blood in stools.

DIAGNOSTIC TESTS

1. *Proctosigmoidoscopy or colonoscopy:* For visualization of polyposis.
2. *Biopsy:* To confirm diagnosis. Histopathologically, the criteria for malignant potential are polyp size, histologic type, and degree of dysplasia.
3. *X-ray examination with barium enema and air contrast:* To determine extent of the disease.
4. *CBC:* To detect presence of anemia.

MEDICAL MANAGEMENT AND SURGICAL INTERVENTIONS

Because colorectal cancer is inevitable, appearing approximately 10-15 years after the onset of the polyposis if the colon is not removed, surgical resection is the treatment of choice for familial polyposis. Once the diagnosis has been made, it is not advisable to delay surgery.

1. Proctocolectomy: Surgical cure *via* removal of colon and rectum with continent (Kock) ileostomy, conventional (Brooke) ileostomy, or ileoanal reservoir for fecal diversion (see "Fecal Diversions," p. 365).
2. Colectomy with preservation of rectum and ileorectal anastomosis: After this procedure, follow-up proctoscopies are necessary at frequent intervals to assess the rectum for further evidence of the disease or malignant changes.

3. **Radiation or chemotherapy:** May be indicated as adjuvant therapy or for advanced malignant disease.

NURSING DIAGNOSES AND INTERVENTIONS

See "Fecal Diversions" for **Bowel incontinence,** p. 367, **Body image disturbance,** p. 368, and **Potential for impaired skin/tissue integrity:** Stoma and peristomal area, p. 366. See the appendix for nursing diagnoses and interventions for the care of preoperative and postoperative patients, p. 637, and the care of patients with cancer and other life-disrupting illnesses, p. 690.

PATIENT-FAMILY TEACHING AND DISCHARGE PLANNING

Provide patient and significant others with verbal and written information for the following:
1. Importance of informing all close members of the family that because familial polyposis is inherited, periodic examinations of the rectum and colon are essential.
2. For other guidelines, see this section in "Colorectal Cancer," p. 351.

Ulcerative colitis

Ulcerative colitis is a nonspecific, chronic, inflammatory disease of the mucosa and submucosa of the colon. Generally, the disease begins in the rectum and sigmoid colon, but it can extend proximally and uninterrupted as far as the cecum. In some instances, a few centimeters of distal ileum are affected. This is sometimes referred to as "backwash ileitis," and it occurs in only about 10% of patients with ulcerative colitis involving the entire colon. The etiology of ulcerative colitis is unknown, but theories include infection, allergy, immunologic abnormalities, psychosomatic factors, and heredity. Individuals with ulcerative colitis develop colonic adenocarcinomas at 10 times the rate of the general population.

ASSESSMENT

Signs and symptoms: Bloody diarrhea (the cardinal symptom). The clinical picture can vary, from acute episodes with frequent discharge of watery stools mixed with blood, pus, and mucus accompanied by fever, abdominal pain, rectal urgency, and tenesmus, to loose or frequent stools, to formed stools coated with a little blood. However, nearly two-thirds of patients have cramping abdominal pain and varying degrees of fever, vomiting, anorexia, weight loss, and dehydration. Remissions and exacerbations are common. Extracolonic manifestations also can occur, including polyarthritis, skin lesions (erythema nodosum, pyoderma gangrenosum), liver impairment, and ophthalmic complications (iritis, uveitis). See Tables 6-4 and 6-5.

Physical assessment: With severe disease, the abdomen will be tender, especially in the LLQ; and distention and a tender and spastic anus also may be present. With rectal examination, the mucosa might feel gritty, and the examining gloved finger may be covered with blood, mucus, or pus.

Risk factors: Duration of active disease greater than 10 years, pancolitis, and family history of colonic cancer.

DIAGNOSTIC TESTS

1. *Stool examination:* Reveals the presence of frank or occult blood. Stool cultures and smears rule out bacterial and parasitic disorders. **Note:** Collect specimens *before* barium enema is performed.
2. *Sigmoidoscopy:* Reveals red, granular, hyperemic, and extremely friable mucosa; strips of inflamed mucosa undermined by surrounding ulcerations, which form

T A B L E   6 - 4   Comparison of gross physiologic features of ulcerative colitis and Crohn's disease

Pathologic features	Ulcerative colitis	Crohn's disease
Thickened mesentery	Rare	Common
Enlarged mesenteric lymph nodes	Rare	Common
Shortening of colon	Frequent	Rare
Small bowel involvement	Never	May occur
Serositis	Not present	Common
Thickening of intestinal wall	Rare	Common
Segmental disease	Never	Frequent
Strictures	Never	Frequent
Abdominal wall and internal fistulas	None	Frequent
Cobblestoning of mucosa	Rare	Common
Mucosal ulcerations	Diffuse	Normal mucosa between ulcers
Pseudopolyps	Frequent	Rare

From Broadwell DC & Jackson BS: Principles of ostomy care, St Louis, 1982, The CV Mosby Co.

T A B L E   6 - 5   Comparison of clinical features of inflammatory bowel disease

Clinical features	Ulcerative colitis (mucosal)	Crohn's disease (transmural)
Age	Young to middle age	Young
Sex distribution	Equal	Equal
Diarrhea	Remission	More constant
Tenesmus	Constant	Occurs
Fever (intermittent)	Occurs	Common
Weight loss	Common	Severe
Abdominal cramping pains	Occurs	Severe
Gross bleeding	Common	Infrequent
Fistulas	Rare	Common
Perforation	Common	Rare
Abdominal mass	Rare	Occurs
Anal lesions	Occurs	Common
Toxic megacolon	Common	Occurs
Carcinoma	Common	Occurs
Proctoscopic findings	Rectum involved in most cases	Rectum may be spared
Extracolonic complications: arthralgia, ocular (uveitis), skin disorders (erythema nodosum, pyoderma gangrenosum)	Frequent	Common

From Broadwell DC & Jackson BS: Principles of ostomy care, St Louis, 1982, The CV Mosby Co.

pseudopolyps; and thick exudate composed of blood, pus, and mucus. **Note:** Enemas should not be given before the examination because they can produce hyperemia and edema and may cause exacerbation of the disease.

3. _Colonoscopy:_ Will help determine the extent of the disease and differentiate ulcerative colitis from Crohn's disease. However, colonoscopy usually is unnecessary during diagnostic evaluation of ulcerative colitis because sigmoidoscopy and double-contrast barium enema usually will provide sufficient information for making a correct diagnosis. **Note:** This test may be contraindicated in patients with acute disease because of the risk of perforation or hemorrhage.

4. _Rectal biopsy:_ Will aid in differentiating ulcerative colitis from carcinoma and other inflammatory processes.

5. _Barium enema:_ Reveals mucosal irregularity from fine serrations to ragged ulcerations, narrowing and shortening of the colon, presence of pseudopolyps, loss of haustral markings, and the presence of spasms and irritability. A double-contrast technique may facilitate detection of superficial mucosal lesions. With a double-contrast technique, barium is instilled into the colon as with a conventional barium enema, but the majority of the barium is withdrawn and the colon is inflated with air, which causes a thin coating of barium to line the intestinal wall. **Note:** Irritant cathartics and enemas should not be given before the examination since they produce hyperemia and edema and may cause exacerbation of the disease.

6. _Blood tests:_ Anemia, with hypochromic microcytic red blood indices in severe disease, usually is present due to blood loss, iron deficiency, and bone marrow depression. WBC count may be normal to markedly elevated in severe disease. Sedimentation rate is usually increased according to the severity of illness. Hypoalbuminemia and negative nitrogen state occur in moderately severe to severe disease and result from decreased protein intake, decreased albumin synthesis in the debilitated condition, and increased metabolic needs. Electrolyte imbalance is common; hypokalemia is often present due to colonic losses (diarrhea) and renal losses in patients on high doses of corticosteroids. Bicarbonate may be decreased due to colonic losses and may signal metabolic acidosis.

MEDICAL MANAGEMENT AND SURGICAL INTERVENTIONS

Medical therapy is symptomatic. The goals are to terminate the acute attack, reduce symptoms, and prevent recurrences.

1. **Parenteral replacement of fluids, electrolytes, and blood products:** To maintain acutely ill patient, as indicated by laboratory test results.

2. **Physical and emotional rest:** Including bed rest and limitation of visitors.

3. **Pharmacotherapy**
   □ _Sedatives and tranquilizers:_ To promote rest and reduce anxiety.
   □ _Hydrophilic colloids_ (e.g., kaolin and pectin mixture) and _anticholinergics and antidiarrheal preparations_ (e.g., tinctures of belladonna and opium, diphenoxylate hydrochloride, loperamide, and codeine phosphate): To relieve cramping and diarrhea. **Note:** Opiates and anticholinergics should be administered with extreme caution since they contribute to the development of toxic megacolon.
   □ _Antiinflammatory agents:_ Corticosteroids to reduce mucosal inflammation. Dosage and routes of administration vary with the severity and extent of the disease. In patients with mild disease limited to the rectum and sigmoid colon, rectal instillation of steroids (enema or suppository) may induce or maintain remission. In patients with more extensive (pancolonic) or more active disease, oral corticosteroid therapy with prednisone or prednisolone usually is initiated. In severely ill patients, IV corticosteroids are given. Once clinical remission is achieved, IV and oral corticosteroids are tapered until discontinuation since these medications have not been shown to prolong remission or prevent future exacerbations.
   □ _Sulfasalazine:_ To help maintain remissions. This drug generally is effective in the treatment of mild to moderate attacks of ulcerative colitis and appears to decrease the frequency of subsequent relapse. Sulfasalazine is considered inferior to corticosteroids in the treatment of severe attacks of disease; once remission has been

attained by use of corticosteroid therapy, sulfasalazine appears to be superior to systemic corticosteroids in the maintenance of remission.

When administered orally, sulfasalazine is broken down by colonic bacteria into its two constituents: 5-aminosalicylic acid (5-ASA), which is considered the active therapeutic component, and sulfapyridine, which is the carrier and responsible for the side effects experienced by more than a third of the individuals treated with this therapy. 5-ASA alone, when administered as an enema, has been providing encouraging results for individuals with ulcerative colitis limited to the left colon and is proving more effective than hydrocortisone enemas during initial attacks and for subsequent relapses.

☐ *Immunosuppressive therapy:* To reduce inflammation in patients not responding to steroids and sulfasalazine and who are unwilling or unable to undergo colectomy. Azathioprine has been used alone and in combination with steroids. It may have a steroid-sparing effect, thus enabling steroid dosages to be reduced. When used as standard therapy, it may have little to offer in most cases of ulcerative colitis.

☐ *Antibiotics:* To limit secondary infection. Antibiotics are not indicated in the management of mild to moderate disease since infectious agents generally are not thought to be responsible for ulcerative colitis. In the patient with acute pancolitis or toxic megacolon, broad-spectrum IV antibiotic therapy is recommended since secondary bacterial infection of deeply inflamed colonic mucosa is likely. See Table 6-6, below.

4. **Nutritional management:** Varies with patient's condition. In severely ill patients, TPN

T A B L E 6 - 6   Most common drug therapies for ulcerative colitis and Crohn's disease

Drug	Ulcerative colitis	Crohn's disease
Sulfasalazine	Valuable for mild to moderate disease, definitely helpful in maintaining remissions and in chronic disease	Valuable for acute and chronic disease; perhaps of most value for disease of large bowel
Corticosteroids	Definitely valuable for acute and severe cases; not valuable for maintaining remissions	Definitely valuable for acute and chronic cases; most valuable for disease limited to the ileum
Antidiarrheals	Valuable for symptomatic treatment in chronic cases	Valuable for symptomatic treatment in chronic cases
Antimicrobials	Possibly beneficial in acute cases	Possibly beneficial in acute cases
Immunosuppressives	May have a steroid-sparing effect	May have a steroid-sparing effect
Hyperalimentation	Most often indicated as preparation for surgery; possibly of value in severe, acute phase	May be of value in adjunctive treatment; perhaps of most value in patients with moderately severe disease or acute disease and in children

NOTE: There is no current treatment that will reduce relapse rate.
From Broadwell DC & Jackson BS: Principles of ostomy care, St Louis, 1982, The CV Mosby Co.

along with NPO status is prescribed to replace nutritional deficits while allowing complete bowel rest and improving patient's nutritional status before surgery. For less severely ill patients, low-residue elemental diet provides good nutrition with low fecal volume to allow bowel rest. A bland, high-protein, high-calorie, low-residue diet with vitamin and mineral supplements and excluding raw fruits and vegetables provides good nutrition and decreases diarrhea. Milk and wheat products are restricted to reduce cramping and diarrhea in patients with lactose and gluten intolerances. See Table 6-1, p. 331, for sample diet plans.

5. **Referral to mental health practitioner:** As indicated for supportive psychotherapy for patient who has difficulty dealing with any type of chronic or disabling illness.
6. **Surgical interventions:** Indicated only when the disease is intractable to medical management or when the patient develops a disabling complication. *Total proctocolectomy* cures ulcerative colitis and results in construction of a permanent fecal diversion, such as Brooke ileostomy, continent (Kock pouch) ileostomy, or ileoanal reservoir. See "Fecal Diversions," p. 365, for additional details. *Postoperative management* includes routine chest physiotherapy to prevent respiratory complications; IV fluid and electrolyte replacement or TPN as the patient's condition warrants; NG tube for decompression until bowel sounds are present and the patient is eliminating flatus or stool; gradual resumption of diet as tolerated following NG tube removal and return of bowel function; aseptic incisional care to prevent infection; and fecal diversion care and teaching.

NURSING DIAGNOSES AND INTERVENTIONS

Fluid volume deficit related to abnormal loss secondary to diarrhea and active GI bleeding/hemorrhage

Desired outcomes: Patient is normovolemic as evidenced by balanced I&O, urine output $\geq$30 ml/hr, good skin turgor, moist mucous membranes, stable weight, BP $\geq$90/60 mm Hg (or within patient's normal range), and RR 12-20 breaths/min. Serum potassium is $\geq$3.5 mEq/L, hct is 40%-54% (male) and 37%-47% (female), hgb is 14-18 g/dl (male) and 12-16 g/dl (female), and RBCs are 4.5-6.0 million/μl (male) and 4.0-5.5 million/μl (female).

1. If the patient is acutely ill, maintain parenteral replacement of fluids, electrolytes, and vitamins as prescribed.
2. Administer blood products and iron as prescribed to correct existing anemia and losses due to hemorrhage.
3. Monitor I&O; weigh patient daily; and monitor laboratory values to evaluate fluid, electrolyte, and hematologic status.
4. Monitor frequency and consistency of stool. Assess and record presence of blood, mucus, fat, or undigested food.
5. Monitor patient for indicators of dehydration: thirst, poor skin turgor, dryness of mucous membranes, fever, and concentrated and decreased urinary output.
6. Monitor patient for signs of hemorrhage: hypotension, increased HR and RR, pallor, diaphoresis, and restlessness. Assess stool for quality (e.g., is it grossly bloody and liquid?) and quantity (e.g., is it mostly blood or mostly stool?). Report significant findings to MD.
7. When patient is taking food by mouth, provide bland, high-protein, high-calorie, and low-residue diet, as prescribed. Assess tolerance to diet by determining incidence of cramping, diarrhea, and flatulence.

Potential for infection related to vulnerability secondary to deeply inflamed colonic mucosa and risk of perforation

Desired outcome: Patient is free of infection as evidenced by normothermia; HR 60-100 bpm; RR 12-20 breaths/min with normal depth and pattern (eupnea); normal bowel sounds; absence of abdominal distention, tympany, or rebound tenderness; negative cultures; and orientation to person, place, and time.

Note: Patients with severe ulcerative colitis can have markedly elevated WBCs: >20,000 μl, and occasionally as high as 50,000 μl.

---

1. Monitor patient for fever, chills, increased respiratory and heart rates, diaphoresis, and increased abdominal discomfort, which can occur with perforation of the colon and potentially result in localized abscess or generalized fecal peritonitis and septicemia. **Note:** Systemic therapy with corticosteroids and antibiotics can mask the development of this complication.
2. Report any evidence of sudden abdominal distention associated with the above symptoms, since they can signal toxic megacolon. Factors contributing to the development of this complication include hypokalemia, barium enema examinations, and use of opiates and anticholinergics.
3. If patient has a sudden temperature elevation, culture blood and other sites as prescribed. Monitor culture reports, notifying MD promptly of any positive cultures.
4. Administer antibiotics as prescribed and in a timely fashion.
5. Evaluate patient's orientation and LOC q2-4h.

Pain, abdominal cramping, and nausea related to intestinal inflammatory process

Desired outcome: Patient's subjective evaluation of discomfort improves as documented by a pain scale.

1. Monitor and document characteristics of discomfort, and assess whether it is associated with ingestion of certain foods or medications or with emotional stress. Devise a pain scale with patient, rating discomfort from 0 (no pain) to 10. Eliminate foods that cause cramping and discomfort.
2. As prescribed, maintain patient on NPO or TPN to provide bowel rest.
3. Provide nasal and oral care at frequent intervals to lessen discomfort from NPO status or presence of NG tube.
4. Keep patient's environment quiet and plan nursing care to provide maximum periods of rest.
5. Administer sedatives and tranquilizers as prescribed to promote rest and reduce anxiety.
6. Administer hydrophilic colloids, anticholinergics, and antidiarrheals as prescribed to relieve cramping and diarrhea.
7. Document the degree of relief obtained, rating it according to the pain scale.
8. Observe for intensification of symptoms, which can indicate the presence of complications. Notify MD of significant findings.

Diarrhea related to inflammatory process of the intestines

Desired outcome: Patient's stools are normal in consistency; frequency is lessened.

1. Monitor and record the amount, frequency, and character of patient's stools.
2. Provide covered bedpan, commode, or bathroom that is easily accessible and ready to use at all times.
3. Empty bedpan and commode to control odor and decrease patient anxiety and self-consciousness.
4. Administer hydrophilic colloids, anticholinergics, and antidiarrheals as prescribed to decrease fluidity and number of stools.
5. Administer topical corticosteroid preparations and antibiotics *via* retention enema, as prescribed, to relieve local inflammation. If patient has difficulty retaining the enema for the prescribed amount of time, consult with MD regarding the use of corticosteroid foam, which is easier to retain and administer.
6. Monitor serum electrolytes, particularly potassium, for abnormalities. Alert MD to potassium <3.5 mEq/L.

Potential for impaired skin integrity: Perineal/perianal area related to irritation secondary to persistent diarrhea

Desired outcome: Patient's perineal/perianal skin remains intact with no erythema.

1. Provide materials or assist patient with cleansing and drying of perineal area after each bowel movement.
2. Apply protective skin care products such as skin preparations, gels, or barrier films, *only* to normal, unbroken skin. Petrolatum emollients, moisture barrier ointments, and vanishing creams also can be used to prevent irritation from frequent liquid stools.
3. Administer hydrophilic colloids, anticholingergics, and antidiarrheals as prescribed to decrease fluidity and number of stools.

See "Fecal Diversions" for **Bowel incontinence,** p. 367, **Body image disturbance,** p. 368, and **Potential for impaired skin integrity:** Stoma and peristomal area, p. 366. If surgery is performed, see the appendix for nursing diagnoses and interventions for the care of preoperative and postoperative patients, p. 637, and for the care of patients with cancer and other life-disrupting illnesses, p. 690.

PATIENT-FAMILY TEACHING AND DISCHARGE PLANNING

Provide patient and significant others with verbal and written information for the following:
1. Medications, including name, rationale, dosage, schedule, route of administration, precautions, and potential side effects. **Note:** For patients on high-dose steroid therapy, caution them about abrupt discontinuation of steroids to prevent precipitation of adrenal crisis. Withdrawal symptoms include weakness, lethargy, restlessness, anorexia, nausea, and muscle tenderness. Instruct patient to notify MD if these symptoms occur.
2. Signs and symptoms that necessitate medical attention, including fever, nausea and vomiting, diarrhea or constipation, and any significant change in appearance and frequency of stools, any of which can signal exacerbation of the disease.
3. Dietary management to promote nutritional and fluid maintenance and prevent abdominal cramping, discomfort, and diarrhea.
4. Importance of perineal care after bowel movements.
5. Enteral or parenteral feeding instructions if patient is to supplement diet or is NPO.
6. Referral to community resources, including National Foundation for Ileitis and Colitis.
7. Importance of follow-up medical care, particularly in patients with long-standing disease, since so many of them develop colonic adenocarcinoma.
8. Referral to a mental health specialist if recommended by MD.

In addition, if patient has a fecal diversion:
9. Care of incision, dressing changes, and permission to take baths or showers once sutures/drains are removed.
10. Care of stoma, peristomal/perianal skin, or perineal wound; use of ostomy equipment; and method for obtaining supplies. Sitz baths may be indicated for perineal wound.
11. Medications that are contraindicated (e.g., laxatives) or that may not be well tolerated or absorbed (e.g., antibiotics, enteric-coated tablets, or long-acting tablets).
12. Gradual resumption of ADL, excluding heavy lifting (>5 lb), pushing, or pulling for 6-8 weeks to prevent incisional herniation.
13. Referral to community resources, including home health care agency, enterostomal therapy (ET) nurse, and the local chapter of United Ostomy Association (UOA).
14. Importance of reporting signs and symptoms that require medical attention, such as change in stoma color from the normal bright and shiny red; peristomal or perianal skin irritation; diarrhea; incisional pain, drainage, swelling, or redness; signs and symptoms of fluid and electrolyte imbalance; and signs and symptoms of mechanical or functional obstruction.

Crohn's disease

Crohn's disease, also known as regional enteritis, granulomatous colitis, or transmural colitis, is a chronic inflammatory disease that can involve any part of the GI tract from the mouth to the anus. Usually the disease occurs segmentally, demonstrating discontinuous areas of disease with segments of normal bowel in between. The terminal ileum is the most frequent site of involvement, followed by the colon. The disease affects all layers of the bowel: the mucosa, submucosa, circular and longitudinal muscles, and serosa. A family history of this disease or ulcerative colitis occurs in 15%-20% of affected patients. The cause is unknown, but theories include infection, immunologic factors, environmental factors, and genetic predisposition.

During the past 20 years, the incidence of Crohn's disease has increased dramatically, whereas that of ulcerative colitis has not changed. This rise may reflect increased diagnostic awareness, rather than a real change in frequency in Crohn's disease.

ASSESSMENT

Signs and symptoms: Clinical presentation varies as a direct reflection of the location of the inflammatory process, its extent, severity, and relationship to contiguous structures. Sometimes the onset is abrupt and the patient can appear to have appendicitis, ulcerative colitis, intestinal obstruction, or a fever of obscure origin. Acute symptoms include RLQ pain, tenderness, spasm, flatulence, nausea, fever, and diarrhea. A more typical picture is insidious onset with more persistent but less severe symptoms, such as vague abdominal pain, unexplained anemia, and fever. Diarrhea—liquid, soft, or mushy stools—is the most common symptom. The presence of gross blood is rare. Abdominal pain is a frequent symptom, and it may be colicky or crampy, initiated by meals, centered in the lower abdomen, and relieved by defecation because of the chronic partial obstruction of the small intestine, colon, or both. As the disease progresses, anorexia, malnutrition, weight loss, anemia, lassitude, malaise, and fever can occur in addition to fluid, electrolyte, and metabolic disturbances. See Tables 6-4 and 6-5 for comparisons of ulcerative colitis and Crohn's disease.

Physical assessment: In the early stages the exam is often normal, but might demonstrate mild tenderness in the abdomen over the affected bowel. In more advanced disease, a palpable mass may be present, especially in the RLQ with terminal ileum involvement. Persistent rectal fissure, large ulcers, perirectal abscess, or rectal fistula is the first indication of disease in 15%-25% of patients with small bowel involvement and in 50%-75% of patients with colonic involvement. Rectovaginal, abdominal, and enterovesical fistulas also can occur. Extraintestinal manifestations characteristic of ulcerative colitis do occur, but less frequently (10%-20%).

DIAGNOSTIC TESTS

1. *Stool examination:* Usually reveals the presence of occult blood; frank blood may be noted in stools of patients with colonic involvement or with ulcerations and fistulas of the rectum. A few patients present with bloody diarrhea. Stool cultures and smears rule out bacterial and parasitic disorders. Specimens are also examined for presence of fecal fat.
2. *Sigmoidoscopy:* To evaluate possible colonic involvement and obtain rectal biopsy. The finding of granulomas on mucosal biopsy argues strongly for the diagnosis of Crohn's disease. However, since granulomas are more numerous in the submucosa, suction biopsy of the rectum provides deeper, larger, and less traumatized specimens for a better diagnostic yield than mucosal biopsy obtained through an endoscope.
3. *Colonoscopy:* May help differentiate Crohn's disease from ulcerative colitis. Characteristic patchy inflammation (skip lesions) rules out ulcerative colitis. However, colonoscopy usually does not add useful diagnostic information in the presence of positive findings from sigmoidoscopy or radiologic examination. In patients in whom the diagnosis is unclear and there is a question of malignancy, colonoscopy provides

the means of directly visualizing mucosal changes and obtaining biopsies, brushings, and washings for cytologic examination. Colonoscopy also may assist in planning for surgery by documenting the extent of colonic disease. **Note:** Because of the risk of perforation, this procedure may be contraindicated in patients in acute phases of Crohn's colitis or when deep ulcerations or fistulas are known to be present.

4. *Barium enema and upper GI series with small bowel followthrough:* Contribute to the diagnosis of Crohn's disease. Involvement of only the terminal ileum or segmental involvement of the colon or small intestine is almost always indicative of Crohn's disease. Thickened bowel wall with stricture (string sign) separated by segments of normal bowel, cobblestone appearance, and presence of fistulas and skip lesions are common findings. A double-contrast barium enema technique may increase sensitivity in detecting early or subtle changes. **Note:** Barium enema may be contraindicated in patients with acute phases of Crohn's colitis because of the risk of perforation. Upper GI barium series is contraindicated in patients in whom intestinal obstruction is suspected.

5. *Blood tests:* Are nonspecific for the diagnosis of Crohn's disease, but help determine whether or not the inflammatory process is active and evaluate the patient's overall condition. Anemia may be present and may be a) microcytic owing to iron deficiency from chronic blood loss and bone marrow depression secondary to chronic inflammatory process, or b) megaloblastic, due to folic acid or B_{12} deficiency and usually is seen only in patients with extensive ileitis causing malabsorption. Increased WBC count and sedimentation rate reflect disease activity and inflammation. Hypoalbuminemia corresponds with the disease activity and results from decreased protein intake, extensive malabsorption, and significant enteric loss of protein. Hypokalemia is seen in patients with chronic diarrhea; hypophosphatemia and hypocalcemia are seen in patients with significant malabsorption. Liver function studies may be abnormal secondary to pericholangitis.

6. *Urinalysis and urine culture:* May reveal UTI secondary to enterovesicular fistula.

7. *Tests for malabsorption:* Since patients with active, extensive disease (especially when it involves the small intestine) may develop malabsorption and malnutrition, the following tests are clinically significant: D-xylose tolerance test (for upper jejunal involvement); Schilling's test (for ileal involvement); serum albumin, carotene, calcium, and phosphorus levels; and fecal fat (steatorrhea).

MEDICAL MANAGEMENT AND SURGICAL INTERVENTIONS

The initial treatment is nonoperative, and it is individualized and based on symptomatic relief. Medical treatment is more likely to be successful early in the course of the disease, before permanent structural changes have occurred.

1. **Parenteral replacement of fluids, electrolytes, and blood products:** Maintenance therapy for acute exacerbation as indicated by laboratory test results.

2. **Physical and emotional rest:** Complete bed rest with assistance with ADL during acute phases.

3. **Pharmacotherapy:** It has not been proven that drugs, singly or in combination, can prolong remission and prevent relapse of Crohn's disease.

   □ *Sedatives and tranquilizers:* To promote rest and reduce anxiety.

   □ *Antidiarrheals:* To decrease diarrhea and cramping. Codeine or loperamide often reduces diarrhea with a concomitant decrease in abdominal cramping. Anticholinergics are not recommended because they may mask obstructive symptoms and precipitate toxic megacolon. For these reasons, antidiarrheals should be administered with caution. If a patient does not respond appropriately to standard antidiarrheals and mild sedation, the presence of obstruction, bowel perforation, or abscess formation is suspected.

   □ *Sulfasalazine:* To treat acute exacerbations of colonic and ileocolonic disease. It appears to be more effective in patients with disease limited to the colon than in those with disease limited to the small bowel. Since it has not been shown to prevent recurrence, the goal of management is to discontinue the drug gradually, following remission of active Crohn's colitis (Crohn's disease limited to the colon).

Note: Because sulfasalazine impairs folate absorption, patients receive folic acid supplements during treatment.

☐ *Corticosteroids:* To reduce the active inflammatory response, decrease edema, and control exacerbations. Prednisone is effective in diminishing activity of the disease process, but is more beneficial in patients with small bowel involvement than it is in those with disease limited to the colon. As active disease subsides, prednisone is tapered with the goal of eliminating the drug. However, many Crohn's disease patients become "steroid dependent," meaning they are symptomatic with low-dose therapy (5-15 mg/day) or with total discontinuation of the drug. In some cases of chronic disease, continuous corticosteroid therapy may be necessary.

☐ *Immunosuppressive agents:* To reduce inflammation when corticosteroids have failed, or in combination with corticosteroids to allow dosage reduction of corticosteroids. Because they are toxic agents with serious side effects and owing to lack of consensus about their benefits, immunosuppressives such as azathioprine and 6-mercaptopurine are considered only when persistent severe disease does not respond to standard therapy or when reduction of steroid dosage is required but otherwise unattainable.

☐ *Antibiotics:* To control suppurative complications. Patients with bacterial overgrowth of the small bowel may be treated with broad-spectrum antibiotics. See Table 6-6, p. 356.

4. Nutritional management: A major component of therapy. During acute exacerbations TPN and NPO status can be used to replace nutritional deficits and allow complete bowel rest. Elemental diets that are free of bulk and residue, low in fat, and digested in the upper jejunum provide good nutrition with low fecal volume to allow bowel rest in select patients. Bland diets low in residue, roughage, and fat but high in protein, calories, carbohydrates, and vitamins provide good nutrition and reduce excessive stimulation of the bowel. A diet free of milk, milk products, gas-forming foods, alcohol, and iced beverages reduces cramping and diarrhea. When remission occurs, a less restricted diet can be tailored to the individual patient, excluding foods known to precipitate symptoms. Patients with involvement of the small intestine frequently require supplementation of vitamins and minerals, especially calcium, iron, folate, and magnesium secondary to malabsorption or to compensate for foods excluded from the diet. Patients with extensive ileal disease or resection frequently require vitamin B_{12} replacement and, if bile salt deficiency exists, cholestyramine and medium-chain triglycerides might be needed to control diarrhea and reduce fat malabsorption and steatorrhea.

5. Referral to mental health practitioner for supportive psychotherapy: If indicated, because of the chronic and progressive nature of Crohn's disease.

6. Surgical management: Because surgery is not a cure for Crohn's disease, it is reserved for complications rather than used as a primary form of therapy. Common indications for surgery include bowel obstruction, internal and enterocutaneous fistulas, intraabdominal abscesses, and perianal disease. Conservative resection of the affected bowel segments with restoration of bowel continuity, preserving as much of the intestine as possible, is the preferred surgical approach. If fecal diversion using an ostomy is required, the type of diversion used will depend on the location and amount of intestinal segment(s) to be resected. (For details, see "Fecal Diversions," p. 365.)

NURSING DIAGNOSES AND INTERVENTIONS

Fluid volume deficit related to abnormal loss secondary to diarrhea or GI fistula

Desired outcomes: Patient is normovolemic as evidenced by balanced I&O, urinary output ≥30 ml/hr, BP ≥90/60 mm Hg (or within patient's normal range), RR 12-20 breaths/min, stable weight, good skin turgor, and moist mucous membranes. Serum potassium is 3.5-5.0 mEq/L, serum sodium is 137-147 mEq/L, and serum chloride is 95-108 mEq/L. Patient reports that diarrhea is controlled.

1. Maintain patient on parenteral replacement of fluids, electrolytes, and vitamins as prescribed to promote anabolism and healing.

2. Monitor I&O; weigh patient daily; and monitor laboratory values to evaluate fluid and electrolyte status.
3. Monitor frequency and consistency of stools. Assess for and record presence of blood, mucus, fat, or undigested food.
4. Monitor patient for indicators of dehydration: thirst, poor skin turgor, dryness of mucous membranes, fever, and concentrated and decreased urinary output.
5. When the patient is taking food by mouth, provide bland, high-protein, high-calorie, and low-residue diet, as prescribed. Assess tolerance to diet by determining incidence of cramping, diarrhea, and flatulence. Modify diet plan accordingly.

Potential for infection/injury related to risk of complications secondary to intestinal inflammatory disorder

Desired outcome: Patient is free from infection and intraabdominal injury as evidenced by normothermia, HR 60-100 bpm; RR 12-20 breaths/min; normal bowel sounds; absence of abdominal distention, rigidity, or localized pain and tenderness; absence of nausea and vomiting; negative cultures; and orientation to person, place, and time.

1. Monitor patient for indicators of intestinal obstruction, including abdominal rigidity and increased episodes of nausea and vomiting. **Note:** Contributing factors to the development of this complication include use of opiates and the prolonged use of antidiarrheals.
2. Monitor patient for fever, increased RR and HR, chills, diaphoresis, and increased abdominal discomfort, which can occur with intestinal perforation, abscess or fistula formation, or generalized fecal peritonitis and septicemia. **Note:** Systemic therapy with corticosteroids and antibiotics can mask the development of these complications.
3. Evaluate patient's orientation and LOC q2-4h.
4. If the patient has a sudden temperature elevation, obtain cultures of blood, urine, fistulas, or other possible sources of infection, as prescribed. Abscesses or fistulas to the abdominal wall, bladder, or vagina are common in Crohn's disease, as well as abscesses and fistulas to other loops of small bowel and colon. Monitor culture reports and notify MD promptly of any positive results.
5. If draining fistulas or abscesses are present, change dressings or irrigate tubes or drains as prescribed. Note color, character, and odor of all drainage. Report the presence of foul-smelling or abnormal drainage or the loss of tube/drain patency.
6. Administer antibiotics as prescribed and in a timely manner.
7. Prevent the transmission of potentially infectious organisms by good handwashing technique before and after caring for the patient and by disposing of dressings and drainage according to infection control guidelines.

Pain, abdominal cramping, and nausea related to intestinal inflammatory process

Desired outcome: Patient's subjective evaluation of discomfort improves, as documented by a pain scale.

1. Monitor and document characteristics of discomfort, and assess whether it is associated with ingestion of certain foods or with emotional stress. Devise a pain scale with patient, rating discomfort from 0 (no discomfort) to 10. Eliminate foods that cause cramping and discomfort.
2. As prescribed, keep patient NPO and provide parenteral nutrition to promote bowel rest.
3. Administer antidiarrheals and analgesics as prescribed to reduce abdominal discomfort.
4. Provide nasal and oral care at frequent intervals to lessen discomfort from NPO status and presence of NG tube.
5. Administer antiemetic medications before meals to enhance appetite when nausea is a problem.
6. Document relief obtained using the pain scale.

Diarrhea related to intestinal inflammatory process

Desired outcome: Patient experiences a reduction in frequency of stools and a return to a more normal stool consistency.

1. If the patient is experiencing frequent and urgent passage of loose stools, provide covered bedpan or commode, or be sure the bathroom is easily accessible and ready to use at all times.
2. Empty the bedpan and commode promptly to control odor and decrease patient anxiety and self-consciousness.
3. Administer antidiarrheals as prescribed to decrease fluidity and number of stools.
4. If bile salt deficiency (because of ileal disease or resection) is contributing to diarrhea, administer cholestyramine as prescribed to control diarrhea.
5. Eliminate or decrease fat content in the diet because it can increase diarrhea. Also, restrict foods and beverages that can precipitate diarrhea and cramping, such as raw vegetables and fruits, whole grain cereals, condiments, gas-forming foods, alcohol, iced and carbonated beverages, and, in lactose-intolerant patients, milk and milk products.

Fatigue related to intestinal inflammatory process

Desired outcome: Patient adheres to prescribed rest regimen and sets appropriate goals for self-care as the condition improves.

1. Keep patient's environment quiet to facilitate rest.
2. Because adequate rest is necessary to sustain remission, assist patient with ADL and plan nursing care to provide maximum rest periods.
3. As prescribed, administer sedatives and tranquilizers to promote rest and reduce anxiety.
4. As the patient's physical condition improves, encourage self-care to the greatest extent possible, and assist patient with setting realistic, attainable goals.
5. See **Potential for activity intolerance,** p. 651, and **Potential for disuse syndrome,** p. 653, as appropriate, in the appendix.

If surgery is performed, see "Fecal Diversions" for **Bowel incontinence,** p. 367, **Body image disturbance,** p. 368, and **Potential for impaired skin integrity:** Stoma and peristomal area, p. 366. See the appendix for nursing diagnoses and interventions for the care of preoperative and postoperative patients, p. 637, and the care of patients with cancer and other life-disrupting illnesses, p. 690.

PATIENT-FAMILY TEACHING AND DISCHARGE PLANNING

Provide patient and significant others with verbal and written information for the following:

1. Medications, including name, rationale, dosage, schedule, route of administration, precautions, and potential side effects.
2. Signs and symptoms that necessitate medical attention, including fever, nausea and vomiting, abdominal discomfort, any significant change in appearance and frequency of stools, passage of stool through the vagina, or stool mixed with urine, any of which can signal recurrence or complications of Crohn's disease.
3. Importance of dietary management to promote nutritional and fluid maintenance and prevent abdominal cramping, discomfort, and diarrhea.
4. Importance of perineal/perianal skin care after bowel movements.
5. Importance of balancing activities with rest periods, even during remission, because adequate rest is necessary to sustain remission.
6. Referral to community resources, including National Foundation for Ileitis and Colitis.
7. Importance of follow-up medical care, including supportive psychotherapy, because of the chronic and progressive nature of Crohn's disease.

In addition, if the patient has a fecal diversion:

8. Care of incision, dressing changes, and bathing.

9. Care of stoma and peristomal skin, use of ostomy equipment, and method for obtaining supplies.

10. Gradual resumption of ADL, excluding heavy lifting (>5 lb), pushing, or pulling for 6-8 weeks to prevent incisional herniation.

11. Referral to community resources, including home health care agency, enterostomal therapy (ET) nurse, and local chapter of United Ostomy Association (UOA).

12. Importance of reporting signs and symptoms that require medical attention, such as change in stoma color from the normal bright and shiny red; lesions of stomal mucosa that may indicate recurrence of the disease; peristomal skin irritation; diarrhea or constipation, fever, chills, abdominal pain, distention, nausea, and vomiting; and incisional pain, drainage, swelling, or redness.

Fecal diversions

For a discussion of diverticulitis, see p. 347; colorectal cancer, see p. 349; polyps/familial polyposis, see p. 352; ulcerative colitis, see p. 353; and Crohn's disease, see p. 360.

SURGICAL INTERVENTIONS

It is sometimes necessary to interrupt the continuity of the bowel because of intestinal disease or its complications. The resulting fecal diversion can be located anywhere along the bowel, depending on the location of the diseased or injured portion; and it can be permanent or temporary. The most common sites for fecal diversion are the colon and ileum.

1. **Colostomy:** Created when the surgeon brings a portion of the colon to the abdominal skin surface. An opening in the exteriorized colon permits elimination of flatus and stool through the stoma. The continuity of the colon can be interrupted anywhere along its length.

   ☐ *Transverse colostomy:* This is the most frequently created stoma to divert the fecal stream on a temporary basis. Surgical indications include relief of bowel obstruction before definitive surgery for tumors or diverticulitis and colon perforation secondary to trauma. Stool is usually soft, unformed, and eliminated unpredictably. A temporary colostomy may be double-barrelled, with a proximal stoma through which stool is eliminated and a distal stoma adjacent to the proximal stoma called a mucous fistula. More commonly, a loop colostomy is created with a supporting rod placed beneath it until the exteriorized loop of colon becomes affixed to the skin.

   ☐ *Descending or sigmoid colostomy:* This is usually a permanent fecal diversion. Cancer of the rectum is the most common cause for surgical intervention. Stool is usually formed and some individuals may have stool elimination at predictable times. In a permanent colostomy, the surgeon brings the severed end of the colon to the abdominal skin surface. To mature the stoma, the colon above the skin surface is cuffed back on itself and sutured to the skin so that the mucosal surface of the intestine is exposed.

   ☐ *Cecostomy or ascending colostomy:* Uncommon. The procedure done most often is a temporary diverting stoma, which eliminates unformed soft or liquid stool unpredictably. Surgical intervention is similar to that with transverse colostomies.

2. **Ileostomy**

   ☐ *Conventional (Brooke) ileostomy:* Created by bringing a distal portion of the ileum up and out onto the surface of the skin of the abdominal wall. A permanent ileostomy is matured by the same procedure discussed with a permanent colostomy. Surgical indications include ulcerative colitis, Crohn's disease, and familial polyposis requiring excision of the entire colon and rectum.

□ *Temporary ileostomy:* Usually a loop stoma with a supporting rod in place beneath the loop of the ileum until the exteriorized loop of ileum becomes affixed to the skin. The purpose is to divert the fecal stream away from a more distal anastomosis site or fistula repair site until healing has occurred. Output is usually liquid or pastelike, contains digestive enzymes, and is eliminated continually. A collection pouch is worn over the stoma on the abdomen to collect gas and fecal discharge.

□ *Continent (Kock pouch) ileostomy:* An intraabdominal pouch constructed from approximately 30 cm of distal ileum. A 10 cm portion of ileum is intussuscepted to form an outlet valve from the pouch to the skin of the abdomen, where a stoma is constructed flush with the skin. The intraabdominal pouch is continent for gas and fecal discharge and is emptied approximately qid by inserting a catheter through the stoma. No external pouch is needed and a Band-Aid or small dressing is worn over the stoma to collect mucus. Surgical indications include ulcerative colitis and familial polyposis requiring removal of the colon and rectum. Crohn's disease is generally a contraindication for this procedure because the disease can recur in the pouch, necessitating its removal.

3. **Ileoanal reservoir:** A two-staged surgical procedure developed to preserve fecal continence and avoid the need for a permanent ileostomy. During the first stage following total colectomy and removal of the rectal mucosa, an ileal reservoir is constructed just above the junction of the ileum and anal canal; the ileal outlet from the reservoir is brought down through the cuff of the rectal muscle and anastomosed to the anal canal. The anal sphincter is preserved and the resulting ileal reservoir provides a storage place for feces. A temporary diverting ileostomy is required for 2-3 months to allow healing of the anastomosis. The second stage occurs when the diverting ileostomy is taken down and fecal continuity is restored. Initially, the patient experiences fecal incontinence and 10 or more bowel movements a day. After 3-6 months, the patient experiences a decrease in urgency and frequency with 4-8 bowel movements per day. This procedure is an option for patients requiring colectomy for ulcerative colitis or familial polyposis. It is contraindicated in patients with Crohn's disease and incontinence problems.

NURSING DIAGNOSES AND INTERVENTIONS

Potential for impaired skin/tissue integrity: Stoma and peristomal area, related to erythema, improper appliance, or sensitivity to appliance material

Desired outcome: Patient's stoma and peristomal skin and tissue remain intact.

After colostomy or conventional ileostomy (permanent or temporary):
1. Apply a pectin, methylcellulose-based, solid-form skin barrier around the stoma to protect the peristomal skin from contact with stool, which would cause irritation.
   □ Cut an opening in the skin barrier the exact circumference of the stoma, remove the release paper, and apply the sticky surface directly to the peristomal skin.
   □ Remove the skin barrier and assess the condition of the skin q2-3days. Peristomal skin should look like other abdominal skin. Such changes as erythema, erosion, serous drainage, bleeding, or induration signal the presence of infection, irritation, or sensitivity to materials placed on the skin and should be documented and reported to the MD because topical medication might be required. Irritating materials should be discontinued and other materials substituted. Patch-test the patient's abdominal skin to determine sensitivity to suspected materials.
   □ Because stomas will lose surgically induced edema for some weeks following surgery, the opening in the skin barrier must be recalibrated each time it is changed so that it is always the exact circumference of the stoma to prevent contact of stool with the skin.
2. Apply a two-piece pouch system or a pouch with access cap so that the stoma can be inspected for viability q12-24h. A matured stoma will be red in color with overlying mucus. A nonmatured stoma will be red and moist where the mucous membrane is exposed, but can be a darker, mottled, grayish red with a transparent or translucent film of serosa elsewhere.

3. When removing the skin barrier and pouch for routine care, cleanse the patient's skin with mild soap and water, rinse well, and dry it so that the skin will retain its normal integrity and the skin barrier and pouch materials will adhere well to the skin.
4. To maintain a secure pouch seal, empty the pouch when it is a third to a half full of stool or gas.

After a continent ileostomy (Kock pouch):

1. A catheter is inserted through the stoma and into the pouch and sutured to the peristomal skin. Avoid stress on the suture and monitor for erythema, induration, drainage, or erosion. Report significant findings to MD. As prescribed, maintain catheter on low continuous suction or gravity to prevent stress on the nipple valve, and maintain pouch decompression so that suture lines are allowed to heal without stress or tension.
2. Check the catheter q2h for patency and irrigate with sterile saline (30 ml) to prevent obstruction. Notify MD if unable to instill solution, if there are no returns per suction catheter, or if leakage of irrigating solution or pouch contents appears around the catheter.
3. To prevent peristomal skin irritation, change 4×4 dressing around the stoma q2h or as often as it becomes wet. The drainage will be serosanguineous at first and mixed with mucus. Report presence of frank bleeding to MD.
4. Assess stoma for viability with each dressing change. It should be red in color and wet and shiny with mucus. A stoma that is pale or dark purple to black or dull in appearance can indicate circulatory impairment and should be reported to MD immediately and documented.

After ileoanal reservoir:

1. Perform routine care for diverting ileostomy (see above).
2. After the first stage of the operation, patient may have incontinence of mucus. Maintain perineal/perianal skin integrity by irrigating the mucus out of the reservoir qd with 60 ml water or gently cleanse the area with water and cotton balls. Soap should be avoided because it can cause itching or irritation. Use 4×4 gauze at night to absorb incontinence of mucus.
3. After the second stage of operation (when the ileostomy is taken down), expect the patient to experience frequency and urgency of defecation.
4. Wash perineal/perianal area with water or Domeboro solution, using a squeeze bottle or cotton balls. Do not use toilet paper because it can cause irritation. If desired, dry the area with a hair dryer on a cool setting.
5. Provide sitz baths to increase patient comfort and help clean the perineal/perianal area.
6. Apply protective skin sealants or ointments. Skin sealants should not be used on irritated or eroded skin because of the high alcohol content, which would cause a painful burning sensation.

Bowel incontinence: Disruption of normal function secondary to fecal diversion

Desired outcomes: Patient has bowel sounds and eliminates gas and stool *via* the fecal diversion. Patient verbalizes understanding of measures that will maintain normal elimination pattern and demonstrates care techniques specific to the fecal diversion.

After colostomy and conventional ileostomy (permanent and temporary):

1. Empty stool from the bottom opening of the pouch and assess the quality and quantity of stool to document return of normal bowel function.
2. If the colostomy is not eliminating stool after 3-4 days and bowel sounds have returned, gently insert a gloved, lubricated finger into the stoma to determine presence of stricture at the skin or fascial levels and note presence of any stool within reach of the examining finger. To stimulate elimination of gas and stool, MD might prescribe a colostomy irrigation. (For procedure, see **Knowledge deficit:** Colostomy irrigation procedure, p. 369).

After continent ileostomy (Kock pouch):

1. Monitor I&O, and record color and consistency of output.
2. Expect aspiration of bright red blood or serosanguinous liquid drainage from the Kock pouch during the early postoperative period.
3. As GI function returns after 3-4 days, expect the drainage to change in color from blood-tinged to greenish brown liquid. When ileal output appears, suction is discontinued and the pouch catheter is placed to gravity drainage.
4. As the patient's diet progresses from clear liquids to solid food, the ileal output thickens. Check and irrigate the catheter q2h and as needed to maintain patency. If the patient reports abdominal fullness in the area of the pouch, along with decreased fecal output, check placement and patency of the catheter.
5. When the patient is alert and taking food by mouth, teach catheter irrigation procedure, which should be performed q2h; and demonstrate how to empty the pouch contents through the catheter into the toilet.
6. Before hospital discharge, teach the patient how to remove and reinsert the catheter.

After ileoanal reservoir:

1. Monitor I&O, observing quantity, quality, and consistency of output from diverting ileostomy and reservoir. Monitor patient for elevation of temperature accompanied by perianal pain and discharge of purulent, bloody mucus from drains and anal orifice. Report significant findings to MD.
2. Irrigate drains as prescribed to maintain patency, decrease stress on suture lines, and decrease incidence of infection.
3. After the first stage of the operation, patient might experience incontinence of mucus. Advise patient to wear small pad to avoid soiling of outer garments.
4. After the second stage of the operation, expect incontinence and 15-20 bowel movements per day with urgency when patient is on a clear-liquid diet. Assist patient with perianal care and apply protective skin care products. To decrease incontinence at night, the catheter can be placed in the reservoir and connected to gravity drainage bag.
5. Expect the number of bowel movements to decrease to 6-12/day and the consistency to thicken when the patient is on solid foods.
6. Administer hydrophilic colloids and antidiarrheals as prescribed to decrease frequency and fluidity of stools.
7. Provide diet consultation so that patient will be able to avoid foods that cause liquid stools (spinach, raw fruits, highly seasoned foods, green beans, broccoli) and increase intake of foods that cause thick stools (cheese, ripe bananas, apples, jello, pasta).
8. Reassure patient that frequency and urgency are temporary and that as the reservoir expands and absorbs fluid, bowel movements should become thicker and less frequent.

Body image disturbance related to presence of fecal diversion

Desired outcome: Patient demonstrates actions that reflect beginning acceptance of the fecal diversion and incorporates changes into self-concept as evidenced by acknowledging body changes, viewing the stoma, and participating in the care of the fecal diversion.

1. Expect the following fears, which may be expressed by patients experiencing a fecal diversion: physical, work, and social activities will be curtailed seriously; rejection, isolation, and feelings of uncleanliness will occur; everyone will know about the altered pattern of fecal elimination; and loss of voluntary control might occur (many patients view incontinence as a return to infancy).
2. Encourage patient to discuss feelings and fears; clarify any misconceptions. Involve family members in the discussions because they, too, might have anxieties and misconceptions.
3. Provide a calm and quiet environment for patient and significant others to discuss the surgery. Initiate an open and honest discussion. Monitor carefully for and listen

closely to expressed or nonverbalized needs since each patient will react differently to the surgical procedure.

4. Encourage acceptance of fecal diversion by having patient participate in care. Assure patient that education offers a means of control.

5. Assure patient that physical, social, and work activities will not be affected by the presence of a fecal diversion.

6. Expect the patient to have fears regarding sexual acceptance although usually they are not expressed overtly. Concerns center on: change in body image; fears about odor and the ostomy appliance interfering with intercourse; conception, pregnancy, and discomfort from perianal wound and scar in women; and impotence and failure to ejaculate in men, especially after more radical dissection of the pelvis in the patient with cancer. If you are uncomfortable talking about sexuality with patients, be aware of these potential concerns and arrange for a consultation with someone who can speak openly and honestly about these problems.

7. Consult with patient's surgeon regarding a visit by another ostomate. Patients gain reassurance and build positive attitudes by seeing a healthy, active individual who has undergone the same type of surgery.

Knowledge deficit: Colostomy irrigation procedure

Desired outcome: Patient demonstrates proficiency with the procedure for colostomy irrigation before hospital discharge.

Note: Teach prescribed colostomy irrigation to patient with permanent descending or sigmoid colostomy. Colostomy irrigation is performed qd or qod so that wearing a pouch becomes unnecessary. An appropriate candidate is a patient who has 1-2 formed stools each day at predictable times (same as normal stool elimination pattern before illness). In addition, the patient must be able to manipulate the equipment, remember the technique, and be willing to spend approximately an hour a day performing the procedure. It may take 4-6 weeks for the patient to have stool elimination regulated with irrigation.

Instruct patient in the following steps:

1. Position an irrigating sleeve over the colostomy and hold it in place with an adhesive disk or belt. Place the distal end in the toilet.

2. Fill an enema container with 800-1,000 ml warm water. Flush the tubing with the water to remove air from the tubing. Allow the water to slowly enter the colostomy from the container through tubing that has either a lubricated cone attachment or a shield on a lubricated catheter, which keeps the irrigating water in the colostomy. Hold the cone snugly against the stoma. It should take 3-5 minutes for fluid to enter the colon.

3. After water has entered the colon, advise the patient to wait 30-40 minutes for the water to be eliminated along with the stool in the colon.

4. Remove the irrigation sleeve and cleanse and dry the peristomal area.

5. Apply a small dressing or security pouch over the colostomy between irrigations.

See the appendix for nursing diagnoses and interventions for the care of preoperative and postoperative patients, p. 637, and the care of patients with cancer and other life-disrupting illnesses, p. 659.

PATIENT-FAMILY TEACHING AND DISCHARGE PLANNING

Provide patient and significant others with verbal and written information for the following:

1. Medications, including name, rationale, dosage, schedule, route of administration, precautions, and potential side effects.

2. Importance of dietary management to promote nutritional and fluid maintenance.

3. Care of incision, dressing changes, and permission to take baths or showers once sutures/drains are removed.
4. Care of stoma, peristomal, and perianal skin; use of ostomy equipment; and method for obtaining supplies.
5. Gradual resumption of ADL, excluding heavy lifting (>5 lb), pushing, or pulling for 6-8 weeks to prevent development of incisional herniation.
6. Referral to community resources including home health care agency, enterostomal therapy (ET) nurse, and local chapter of United Ostomy Association (UOA).
7. Importance of follow-up care with MD and ET nurse; confirm date and time of next appointment.
8. Importance of reporting signs and symptoms that require medical attention, such as change in stoma color from the normal bright and shiny red; peristomal or perianal skin irritation; any significant changes in appearance, frequency, and consistency of stools; fever, chills, abdominal pain, or distention; and incisional pain, drainage, swelling, or redness.

Section Four ABDOMINAL TRAUMA

Injury to abdominal contents is related to the nature of the force applied and the consistency of the affected structures. Forces involved are classified as blunt (e.g., those caused by falls, physical assault, motor vehicle collisions, crush injury) or penetrating (e.g., stab, gunshot wounds). Organs are categorized as solid (e.g., liver, spleen, pancreas) or hollow (e.g., stomach, intestine). Blunt abdominal trauma typically results in injury to solid viscera because hollow viscera tend to be more compressible. However, hollow organs may rupture, especially when full, if there is a sudden increase in intraluminal pressure. Usually, injury inflicted by stab wounds follows a more predictable pattern and involves less tissue destruction than injury from gunshot wounds, although stab wounds to major vascular structures and organs can be fatal. Removing penetrating objects can result in additional injury, so attempts at removal are made only in a controlled surgical environment. High-velocity weapons (e.g., rifles) not only cause injury to tissue in the direct path of the missile but to adjacent organs as well because of energy shock waves that surround the missile path. Tissue destruction is not as great with low-velocity pistols. The rate of complications and death increases greatly if injury to multiple abdominal organs is sustained.

Abdominal trauma results in direct injury to organs, blood vessels, and supporting structures. Other pathophysiologic changes associated with abdominal trauma include: (1) fluid shifts related to tissue damage, blood loss, and shock; (2) metabolic changes associated with stress and catecholamine release; (3) coagulation problems associated with massive hemorrhage and multiple transfusions; (4) inflammation, infection, and abscess formation due to release of GI secretions and bacteria into the peritoneum; and (5) nutritional and electrolyte alterations that develop as a consequence of disruption of GI tract integrity. The following is a brief overview of common injuries:

Spleen: The organ most frequently injured following blunt trauma. Massive hemorrhage from splenic injury is common. All efforts are made to repair the spleen since total splenectomy increases the long-term risk of sepsis, especially in children and young adults.

Liver: Because of its size and location, it is the organ most frequently involved in penetrating trauma and often is affected with blunt injury, as well. Control of bleeding and bile drainage are major concerns with hepatic injury.

Lower esophagus and stomach: Occasionally, the lower esophagus is involved in penetrating trauma. Because the stomach is flexible and readily displaced, it is usually not injured with blunt trauma, but may be injured by direct penetration. Any serious injury to the lower esophagus and stomach results in the escape of irritating gastric fluids and the release of free air below the level of the diaphragm.

Pancreas and duodenum: Although traumatic pancreatic or duodenal injury occurs relatively infrequently, it is associated with high morbidity and mortality rates because of the difficulty of detecting these injuries and the likelihood of massive injury to nearby organs. These organs are retroperitoneal and clinical indicators of injury often are not obvious for several hours.

Small intestine and mesentery: These injuries are common and may be caused by penetrating or nonpenetrating forces. Compromised intestinal blood flow with eventual infarction is the consequence of undetected mesenteric damage. Perforations or contusions can result in release of bacteria and intestinal contents into the abdominal cavity, causing serious infection.

Colon: Injury most frequently caused by penetrating forces, although lap belts, direct blows, and other blunt forces cause a small percentage of colonic injuries. Because of the high bacterial content, infection is always a serious concern. Many patients with colon injuries require temporary colostomy (see p. 365).

Major vessels: Injuries to the abdominal aorta and inferior vena cava are most often caused by penetrating trauma but also occur with deceleration injury. Hepatic vein injuries frequently are associated with juxtahepatic vena caval injury and result in rapid hemorrhage. Blood loss after major vascular injury is massive and survival depends on rapid prehospital transport and immediate surgical intervention.

Retroperitoneal: Tears in retroperitoneal vessels associated with pelvic fractures or damage to retroperitoneal organs (pancreas, duodenum, kidney) can cause bleeding into the retroperitoneum. Even though the retroperitoneal space can accommodate up to 4 L of blood, detection of retroperitoneal hematomas is difficult and sophisticated diagnostic techniques may be required.

ASSESSMENT

Signs and symptoms: A wide variation can occur. Mild tenderness to severe abdominal pain may be present, with the pain either localized to the site of injury or diffuse. Blood or fluid collection within the peritoneum causes irritation resulting in involuntary guarding, rigidity, and rebound tenderness. Fluid or air under the diaphragm may cause referred shoulder pain. Kehr's sign (left shoulder pain caused by splenic bleeding) also may be noted, especially when the patient is recumbent. Nausea and vomiting may be present, and the conscious patient who has sustained blood loss often complains of thirst, an early sign of hemorrhagic shock. Symptoms of abdominal injury may be minimal or absent in the patient who is intoxicated or has sustained head or spinal cord injury. **Note:** The absence of signs and symptoms does not exclude the presence of major abdominal injury.

Physical assessment: Abdominal assessment is highly subjective and serial evaluations by the same examiner are strongly recommended in order to detect subtle changes.

☐ *Inspection:* Abrasions and ecchymoses are suggestive of underlying injury. For example, ecchymosis over LUQ suggests splenic rupture; ecchymotic areas on the flank are suggestive of retroperitoneal bleeding; and erythema and ecchymosis across the lower abdomen suggest intestinal injury due to lap belts. Ecchymoses may take hours to days to develop, depending on the rate of blood loss.

☐ *Auscultation:* It is important to auscultate before palpation and percussion, as these maneuvers can stimulate the bowel and confound assessment findings. Bowel sounds are likely to be decreased or absent with abdominal organ injury, intraperitoneal bleeding, or recent surgery. However, the presence of bowel sounds does not exclude significant abdominal injury. Bowel sounds should be auscultated frequently, especially in the first 24-48 hours after injury. Absence of bowel sounds is expected immediately after surgery. Failure to auscultate bowel sounds within 24-48 hours after surgery is suggestive of ileus, possibly caused by continued bleeding, peritonitis, or bowel infarction.

☐ *Palpation:* Tenderness or pain to palpation strongly suggests abdominal injury. Blood or fluid in the abdomen can result in signs and symptoms of peritoneal irritation (see Table 6-7).

T A B L E 6 - 7   Signs and symptoms suggestive of peritoneal irritation

- Generalized abdominal pain or tenderness
- Involuntary guarding of the abdomen
- Abdominal wall rigidity
- Rebound tenderness
- Abdominal pain with movement or coughing
- Decreased or absent bowel sounds

□ *Percussion:* Unusually large areas of dullness may be percussed over ruptured blood-filled organs. For example, a fixed area of dullness in the LUQ suggests a ruptured spleen. Tympany suggests the presence of gas.

Vital signs and hemodynamic measurements: Ventilatory excursion often is diminished because of pain, thoracic injury, or limited diaphragmatic elevation due to abdominal distention. Initial compensatory tachycardia and vasoconstriction secondary to blood loss usually maintain a normal BP until blood loss becomes major. At that point, BP rapidly deteriorates.

History: Details regarding circumstances of the accident and mechanism of injury are invaluable in detecting the possibility of specific injuries. In addition, ascertain time of patient's last meal, previous abdominal surgeries, and use of safety restraints (if appropriate). If possible, determine current medications and allergies, particularly to contrast material, antibiotics, and tetanus toxoid. The history may be difficult to obtain due to alcohol or drug intoxication, head injury, breathing difficulties, or impaired cerebral perfusion. In such cases, family members may be valuable sources of information.

DIAGNOSTIC TESTS

1. *Hct:* Serial levels reflect the amount of blood lost. If drawn immediately after the injury hct may be normal, but serial levels will reveal dramatic decreases during resuscitation and as extravascular fluid mobilizes during the recovery phase.
2. *WBC count:* Leukocytosis is expected immediately after injury. Splenic injuries in particular result in the rapid development of a moderate to high WBC count. A later increase in WBCs or a shift to the left reflects an increase in the number of neutrophils, which signals an inflammatory response and possible intraabdominal infection. In the patient with abdominal trauma, ruptured abdominal viscera must be considered as a potential source of infection.
3. *Platelet count:* Mild thrombocytosis is seen immediately following traumatic injury. After massive hemorrhage, thrombocytopenia may be noted. Platelet transfusion usually is not required unless spontaneous bleeding is present.
4. *Glucose:* Initially elevated due to catecholamine release and insulin resistance associated with major trauma. Glucose metabolism is abnormal following major hepatic resection and patients should be monitored in order to prevent hypoglycemic episodes.
5. *Amylase:* Elevated serum levels are associated with pancreatic or upper small bowel injury, but values may be normal even with severe injury to these organs.
6. *SGOT, SGPT, LDH:* Elevations of these enzymes reflect hepatic dysfunction due to liver ischemia during prolonged hypotensive episodes or direct traumatic damage. Fluctuations in these enzymes during the postoperative period can be used to detect evidence of liver necrosis.
7. *X-rays:* Initially, flat and upright chest x-rays exclude chest injuries (frequently associated with abdominal trauma) and establish a baseline. Subsequent chest x-rays aid in detecting complications, such as atelectasis and pneumonia. In addition, chest, abdominal, and pelvic x-rays may reveal fractures, missiles, free intraperitoneal air, hematoma, or hemorrhage.

8. *Occult blood:* Gastric contents and stool should be tested for blood in the initial and recovery periods because GI bleeding can occur as a result of both direct injury and later complications.

9. *Diagnostic peritoneal lavage (DPL):* Involves insertion of a peritoneal dialysis catheter into the peritoneum to check for intraabdominal bleeding. DPL is indicated for confirmed or suspected blunt abdominal trauma for the following patients: (1) those in whom signs and symptoms of abdominal injury are obscured by intoxication, head or spinal cord trauma, narcotic administration, or unconsciousness; (2) those about to undergo general anesthesia for repair of other injuries (e.g., orthopedic, facial); and (3) any patient with equivocal assessment findings. DPL is unnecessary for patients who have obvious intraabdominal bleeding or other indications for immediate laparotomy (see "Surgical Considerations," below).

10. *CT scan:* Can detect intraperitoneal and retroperitoneal bleeding and free air (associated with rupture of hollow viscera). It is most useful in assessing injury to solid abdominal organs. This procedure also is helpful in detecting abscesses and other complications. **Caution:** Because of the risk of rapid deterioration, patients with recent injuries (24-48 hours) or in unstable condition should be accompanied by a nurse during the 30-minute period it takes to perform CT scan. Appropriate monitoring and resuscitation equipment must be readily available.

11. *Angiography:* Performed selectively with blunt trauma to evaluate injury to spleen, liver, pancreas, duodenum, and retroperitoneal vessels when other diagnostic findings are equivocal. **Caution:** Because of the large amount of contrast material used during this procedure, monitor urine output closely for several hours for a decrease and ensure adequate hydration.

12. Abdominal injuries often are associated with multisystem trauma. Also see diagnostic test discussions in "Pneumothorax/Hemothorax," p. 17, "Head Injury," p. 206, and "Acute Spinal Cord Injury," p. 196.

MEDICAL MANAGEMENT AND SURGICAL INTERVENTIONS

1. Oxygen: Individuals sustaining abdominal trauma are likely to be tachypneic with the potential for poor ventilatory effort. Supplemental oxygen is delivered until patient's ABG values while breathing room air are acceptable.

2. Fluid management: Massive blood loss is frequently associated with abdominal injuries. Restoration and maintenance of adequate volume is essential. Initially, Ringer's lactate or similar balanced salt solution is given. Colloid solutions, such as albumin, are helpful in the postoperative period if the patient is hypoalbuminemic. Typed and cross-matched fresh blood is the optimal fluid for replacement of large blood losses. However, since fresh whole blood is rarely available, a combination of packed cells and fresh frozen plasma is often used. For the hemodynamically stable patient, balanced crystalloid solutions with additional potassium are used until the patient is able to tolerate enteral or oral feedings.

3. Gastric intubation: Gastric tube permits gastric decompression, aids in removal of gastric contents, and prevents accumulation of gas or air in the GI tract. Aspirated contents can be checked for blood to aid in the diagnosis of lower esophageal, gastric, or duodenal injury. The tube usually remains in place until bowel function returns.

4. Urinary drainage: An in-dwelling catheter is inserted soon after admission to obtain a specimen for urinalysis and monitor hourly urine output and aid in the diagnosis of genitourinary trauma.

5. Pharmacotherapy
   □ *Antibiotics:* Abdominal trauma is associated with a high incidence of intraabdominal abscess, sepsis, and wound infection, particularly injury to the terminal ileum and colon. Individuals with suspected intestinal injury are started on parenteral antibiotic therapy immediately. Broad-spectrum antibiotics are continued postoperatively and stopped after several days unless there is evidence of infection.
   □ *Analgesics:* Because narcotics alter the sensorium, making evaluation of the patient's condition difficult, they are seldom used in the early stages of trauma. Narcotic analgesics are used in the immediate postoperative period to relieve pain and

promote ventilatory excursion. They may be delivered intermittently by the nurse or *via* patient-controlled pumps. As the severity of pain lessens, alternate analgesics such as nonsteroidal antiinflammatory medications may be prescribed.

☐ *Tetanus prophylaxis:* Tetanus immune globulin and tetanus toxoid are considered, based on CDC recommendations (see Table 6-8).

6. **Nutrition:** Patients with abdominal trauma have complex nutritional needs owing to the hypermetabolic state associated with major trauma and traumatic or surgical disruption of normal GI function. Often, infection and sepsis contribute to negative nitrogen state and increased metabolic needs. Prompt initiation of parenteral feedings in patients unable to accept enteric feedings and the administration of supplemental calories, proteins, vitamins, and minerals are essential for healing. For more information, see "Providing Nutritional Support," p. 611.

7. **Surgical considerations for penetrating abdominal injuries:** The issue of mandatory surgical exploration versus observation and selective surgery, especially with stab wounds, remains controversial. There is a trend toward observation of patients without obvious injury or peritoneal signs. Indications for laparotomy include one or more of the following: (1) penetrating injury suspected of invading the peritoneum; (2) positive peritoneal signs (see Table 6-7); (3) shock; (4) GI hemorrhage; (5) free air in the peritoneal cavity as seen on x-ray; (6) evisceration; (7) massive hematuria; or (8) positive diagnostic peritoneal lavage. **Note:** Recently injured or preoperative patients should be evaluated for peritoneal signs at hourly intervals by the same professional. Notify surgeon immediately if the patient develops peritoneal signs, evidence of shock, gastric or rectal bleeding, or gross hematuria.

8. **Surgical considerations for nonpenetrating abdominal injuries:** Physical examination usually is reliable in determining the necessity for surgery in alert, cooperative, unintoxicated patients. Additional diagnostic tests such as DPL or CT scan are necessary to evaluate the need for surgery in the patient who is intoxicated, unconscious, or who has sustained head or spinal cord trauma. Immediate laparotomy for blunt abdominal trauma is indicated under the following circumstances: (1) clear signs of peritoneal irritation (see Table 6-7); (2) free air in the peritoneum; (3) hypotension due to suspected abdominal injury or persistent and unexplained hypotension; (4) positive DPL; (5) GI aspirate or rectal smear positive for blood; or (6) other positive diagnostic tests such as CT scan or arteriogram. Carefully evaluated, stable patients with blunt abdominal trauma may be admitted to critical care for observation. These patients should be evaluated in the same manner as that described above in "penetrating trauma." It is important to note that damage to retroperitoneal organs, such as the pancreas and duodenum, may not cause significant signs and symptoms for 6-12

TABLE 6-8   Tetanus prophylaxis in routine wound management—United States, 1985

History of adsorbed tetanus toxoid (doses)	Clean, minor wounds		All other wounds*	
	Td†	TIG	Td†	TIG
Unknown or <three	Yes	No	Yes	Yes
≥ three‡	No§	No	No¶	No

From Centers for Disease Control: Morbidity Mortality Weekly Report 34(27):422, 1985.

*Such as, but not limited to, wounds resulting from missiles, crushing, burns, and frostbite.

†For children under 7 years old; DPT (DT, if pertussis vaccine is contraindicated) is preferred to tetanus toxoid alone. For persons 7 years old and older, Td is preferred to tetanus toxoid alone.

‡If only three doses of *fluid* toxoid have been received, a fourth dose of toxoid, preferably an adsorbed toxoid, should be given.

§Yes, if more than 10 years since last dose.

¶Yes, if more than 5 years since last dose. (More frequent boosters are not needed and can accentuate side effects).

hours or longer. Relatively slow bleeding from abdominal viscera may not be clinically apparent for 12 hours or longer after the initial injury. In addition, the nurse should be aware that complications, such as bowel obstruction, may develop days or weeks after the traumatic event. The need for vigilant observation in the care of these patients cannot be overemphasized.

NURSING DIAGNOSES AND INTERVENTIONS

Fluid volume deficit related to decreased circulating volume secondary to active bleeding; GI drainage through gastric, intestinal, or drainage tubes; diarrhea; or fistulas

Desired outcomes: Circulating volume is restored as evidenced by systolic BP ≥100 mm Hg (or within patient's baseline range), HR 60-100 bpm, CVP 2-6 mm Hg or 5-12 cm H_2O, urinary output ≥30 ml/hr, warm extremities, brisk capillary refill (<3 seconds), and distal pulses >2+ on a 0-4+ scale.

1. In recently injured patients, monitor BP qh, or more frequently in the presence of obvious bleeding or unstable VS. Be alert to increasing diastolic BP and decreasing systolic BP (see Table 6-9 for indicators of fluid volume deficit). Even a small but sudden decrease in systolic BP signals the need to notify MD, especially with the trauma patient in whom the extent of injury is unknown. Most trauma patients are young, and excellent neurovascular compensation results in a near normal BP until there is a large intravascular volume depletion. Routine VS assessment is indicated in the stable postoperative patient.
2. Monitor HR and cardiovascular status qh until the patient's condition is stable. Note and report sudden increases or decreases in HR, especially if associated with indicators of fluid volume deficit (Table 6-9).
3. In the patient with evidence of volume depletion or active blood loss, administer fluids rapidly through one or more large caliber (16 gauge or larger) IV catheters. **Caution:** Evaluate patency of IV catheters frequently during rapid volume resuscitation. Monitor patient closely to avoid fluid volume overload and complications, such as heart failure (see p. 54) and pulmonary edema (see p. 76).
4. Measure CVP q1-4h if indicated. Be alert to low or decreasing values. Report sudden decreases in CVP, especially if associated with other indicators of hypovolemia (Table 6-9).
5. Measure urinary output q4h (or when patient voids). Be alert to decreasing urinary output or to infrequent voidings. Low urine output usually reflects inadequate intravascular volume in the abdominal trauma patient. Before administering diuretics, evaluate patient for evidence of hypovolemia (Table 6-9).
6. Monitor for physical indicators of hypovolemia, including diaphoresis, cool extremities, capillary refill >4 seconds, and absent or decreased strength of distal pulses.
7. Estimate ongoing blood loss. Measure all bloody drainage from tubes or catheters, noting drainage color (e.g., coffee ground, burgundy, bright red). Note the fre-

---

TABLE 6-9 Indicators of fluid volume deficit

Increasing diastolic BP (early)
Decreasing systolic BP (later)
Tachycardia (>100 bpm)
Tachypnea (>20 breaths/min)
Anxiety (early)
Altered/depressed mental status (later)
Delayed capillary refill (>3 seconds)
Cool, pale skin
Low or decreasing central venous pressure (CVP)
Low urinary output (<30 ml/hr)

quency of dressing changes due to saturation with blood to estimate amount of blood loss *via* wound site. Note and report significant increases in the amount of drainage, especially if it is bloody.

Pain related to irritation secondary to intraperitoneal blood or secretions, actual trauma or surgical incision, and manipulation of organs

Desired outcome: Patient's subjective evaluation of pain improves, as documented by a pain scale.

1. Evaluate patient for presence of preoperative and postoperative pain. Devise a pain scale with patient, rating discomfort from 0 (no pain) to 10. Preoperative pain is anticipated and is a vital diagnostic aid. The nature of postoperative pain also can be important. Incisional and some visceral pain can be anticipated, but intense pain or prolonged pain, especially when accompanied by other peritoneal signs (see Table 6-7), can signal bleeding, bowel infarction, infection, or other complications. Recognize that the autonomic nervous system response to pain can complicate assessment of abdominal injury and hypovolemia. For detail, see same nursing diagnosis in the appendix, p. 638.
2. Administer narcotics and other analgesics as prescribed. Avoid administering analgesics preoperatively until the patient has been evaluated thoroughly by a trauma surgeon. Postoperatively, administer prescribed analgesics promptly before the pain becomes severe. Analgesics are helpful in relieving pain as well as aiding in the recovery process by promoting greater ventilatory excursion. Be aware that substance abuse often is involved in traumatic events; victims, therefore, may be drug or alcohol users, with a higher-than-average tolerance to narcotics. These same individuals may suffer symptoms of alcohol or narcotic withdrawal that need recognition and treatment. In addition, recognize that narcotic analgesics can decrease GI motility and may delay return to normal bowel functioning. Document the degree of relief obtained, using the pain scale.
3. Monitor patient-controlled analgesia, if prescribed, and document effectiveness, using the pain scale.
4. Supplement analgesics with nonpharmacologic maneuvers (e.g., positioning, backrubs, distraction) to aid in pain reduction.

Potential for infection related to vulnerability secondary to disruption of the GI tract, particularly of the terminal ileum and colon; traumatically inflicted open wound; multiple in-dwelling catheters and tubes; and compromised immune state due to stress of trauma and blood loss

Desired outcome: Patient is free of infection as evidenced by core or rectal temperature $<37.8°$ C ($100°$ F); HR ≤100 bpm; orientation to person, place, and time; and absence of unusual redness, warmth, or drainage at surgical incisions or wound sites.

1. Monitor VS for evidence of infection, noting temperature increases and associated increases in heart and respiratory rates. Notify surgeon for sudden temperature elevations.
2. Evaluate orientation and LOC q8h. Note mental confusion or deterioration from baseline LOC.
3. Ensure patency of all surgically placed tubes or drains. Irrigate or attach to low-pressure suction as prescribed. Promptly report unrelieved loss of tube patency.
4. Evaluate incisions and wound sites for evidence of infection: unusual redness, warmth, delayed healing, and purulent or unusual drainage.
5. Note amount, color, character, and odor of all drainage. Report the presence of foul-smelling or abnormal drainage. See Table 6-10, p. 377, for a description of the *usual* character of GI drainage. Test drainage for pH and the presence of blood; compare to expected characteristics.
6. Administer antibiotics in a timely fashion. Reschedule parenteral antibiotics if a dose is delayed for more than 1 hour. Recognize that failure to administer antibiotics on schedule may result in inadequate blood levels and treatment failure.

TABLE 6-10   Characteristics of GI drainage

Source	Composition and usual character
Mouth and oropharynx	Saliva; thin, clear, watery; pH 7.0
Stomach	Hydrochloric, gastrin, pepsin, mucus; thin, brownish to greenish; acidic
Pancreas	Enzymes and bicarbonate; thin, watery, yellowish brown; alkaline
Biliary tract	Bile, including bile salts and electrolytes; bright yellow to brownish green
Duodenum	Digestive enzymes, mucus, products of digestion; thin, bright yellow to light brown, may be greenish; alkaline
Jejunum	Enzymes, mucus, products of digestion; brown, watery with particles
Ileum	Enzymes, mucus, digestive products, greater amounts of bacteria; brown, liquid, feculant
Colon	Digestive products, mucus, large amounts of bacteria; brown to dark brown, semiformed to firm stool
Postoperative (GI surgery)	Initially, drainage expected to contain fresh blood; later, drainage mixed with old blood and then approaches normal composition
Infection present	Drainage cloudy, may be thicker than usual; strong or unusual odor, drain site often erythematous and warm

7. As prescribed, administer pneumococcal vaccine in patients with total splenectomy to minimize the risk of postsplenectomy sepsis.
8. Administer tetanus immune globulin and tetanus toxoid as prescribed (see Table 6-8, above).
9. Change dressings as prescribed, using aseptic technique. Prevent cross-contamination from various wounds by changing one dressing at a time.
10. If patient presents with or develops evisceration, do not reinsert tissue or organs. Place a sterile, saline-soaked gauze over the evisceration and cover with a sterile towel until the evisceration can be evaluated by the surgeon.

Ineffective breathing pattern related to limited ventilatory excursion secondary to pain from injury or surgical incision; chemical irritation of blood or bile on pleural tissue; and diaphragmatic elevation due to abdominal distention

Desired outcome: Patient becomes eupneic, with RR ≤20 breaths/min and clear breath sounds.

1. Administer supplemental oxygen as prescribed. Monitor and document the effectiveness.
2. Administer analgesics at dose and frequency that relieves pain and associated impaired chest excursion.
3. For additional interventions, see same nursing diagnosis in the appendix, "Caring for Preoperative and Postoperative Patients," p. 644.

Potential alteration in tissue perfusion: GI tract, related to risk of interruption of blood flow to abdominal viscera from vascular disruption or occlusion or moderate to severe hypovolemia caused by hemorrhage

Desired outcomes: Patient does not develop bowel or organ ischemia as evidenced by normoactive bowel sounds; soft, nondistended abdomen; and return of bowel elimination. Hct remains >30%; SGOT is 5-40 IU/L; SGPT is 5-35 IU/L; LDH is 90-200 ImU/ml; and gastric secretions, drainage, and excretions are negative for occult blood.

1. Auscultate for bowel sounds qh for recently injured patients and q8h during the recovery phase. Report prolonged or sudden absence of bowel sounds during the postoperative period as these signs may signal bowel ischemia or infarction.
2. Evaluate patient for peritoneal signs (see Table 6-7, p. 372), which may present acutely secondary to injury or may not develop until days or weeks later if complications due to slow bleeding or other mechanisms occur.
3. Ensure adequate intravascular volume (see discussion in **Fluid volume deficit,** p. 375).
4. Evaluate laboratory data for evidence of bleeding (e.g., serial hematocrit) or organ ischemia (e.g., SGPT, SGOT, LDH).
5. Document amount and character of GI secretions, drainage, and excretions. Note changes suggestive of bleeding (presence of frank or occult blood), infection (e.g., increased or purulent drainage), or obstruction (e.g., failure to eliminate flatus or stool within 72 hours of surgery).

Impaired skin and tissue integrity related to direct trauma and surgery; hypermetabolic, catabolic posttraumatic state; impaired tissue perfusion; or exposure to irritating GI drainage

Desired outcomes: Patient exhibits wound healing within an acceptable timeframe and there is no evidence of skin breakdown due to GI drainage. Nitrogen studies show a positive nitrogen state.

1. Promptly change all dressings that become soiled with drainage or blood.
2. Protect the skin surrounding tubes, drains, or fistulas, keeping the areas clean and free from drainage. Gastric and intestinal secretions and drainage are irritating and can lead to skin excoriation. If necessary, apply ointments, skin barriers, or drainage bags to protect the surrounding skin. Apply reusable dressing supports such as Montgomery straps to protect the surrounding skin. If available, consult ostomy nurse for complex or involved cases.
3. Inspect wounds, fistulas, and drain sites for signs of irritation, infection, and ischemia.
4. Identify infected and devitalized tissue. Aid in their removal by irrigation, wound packing, or preparing patient for surgical debridement.
5. Ensure adequate protein and calorie intake for tissue healing (see **Alteration in nutrition,** below).
6. For more information, see section "Managing Wound Care," pp. 624-632.

Alteration in nutrition: Less than body requirements related to decreased intake secondary to disruption of GI tract integrity (traumatic or surgical) and increased need secondary to hypermetabolic posttrauma state

Desired outcome: Patient has adequate nutrition as evidenced by maintenance of baseline body weight and positive nitrogen state.

1. Collaborate with MD, dietitian, and pharmacist to estimate patient's metabolic needs, based on type of injury, activity level, and nutritional status prior to injury.
2. Consider patient's specific injuries when planning nutrition. For example, expect patients with hepatic or pancreatic injury to have difficulty with blood sugar regulation. Patients with trauma to the upper GI tract may be fed enterally, but a feeding tube must be placed distal to the injury. Disruption of the GI tract may require feeding gastrostomy or jejunostomy. Patients with major hepatic trauma may have difficulty with protein tolerance.
3. Ensure patency of gastric or intestinal tubes in order to maintain decompression and encourage healing and return of bowel function. Avoid occlusion of the vent side of sump suction tubes, as this may result in vacuum occlusion of the tube. Use caution when irrigating NG or other tubes that have been placed in or near recently sutured organs.

4. Do not start enteral feeding until bowel function returns (i.e., bowel sounds are present, patient experiences hunger).
5. Recognize that narcotics decrease GI motility and may contribute to nausea, vomiting, abdominal distention, and ileus. Consider non-narcotic analgesics, such as nonsteroidal antiinflammatory agents.
6. For more information, see section "Providing Nutritional Support," p. 611.

Potential for posttrauma response related to stress reaction secondary to life-threatening accident or event resulting in trauma

Desired outcome: Patient verbalizes that the psychosocial impact of the event has decreased; cooperates with treatment plan; and does not exhibit signs of severe stress reaction, such as display of inconsistent affect, suicidal or homicidal behavior, or extreme agitation or depression. **Note:** Many victims of major abdominal trauma sustain life-threatening injury. The patient is often aware of the situation and fears death. Even after the physical condition stabilizes, the patient may have a prolonged or severe reaction triggered by the trauma.

1. Evaluate mental status at systematic intervals. Be alert to indicators of severe stress reaction, such as display of affect inconsistent with statements or behavior, suicidal or homicidal statements or actions, extreme agitation or depression, and failure to cooperate with instructions related to care.
2. Consult with specialists, such as psychologist, psychiatric nurse clinician, or pastoral counselor, if patient displays signs of severe stress reaction as described above.
3. Consider organic causes that may contribute to posttraumatic response stress (e.g., severe pain, alcohol intoxication or withdrawal, electrolyte imbalance, metabolic encephalopathy, or impaired cerebral perfusion).
4. For other pyschosocial interventions, see section "Caring for Patients with Cancer and Other Life-Disrupting Illnesses," p. 690.

For more information, see nursing diagnoses and interventions in the following as appropriate: "Fecal Diversions," p. 365; "Caring for Preoperative and Postoperative Patients," p. 637; "Caring for Patients on Prolonged Bed Rest," p. 651; and "Caring for Patients with Cancer and Other Life-Disrupting Illnesses," p. 690.

PATIENT-FAMILY TEACHING AND DISCHARGE PLANNING

Anticipate extended physical and emotional rehabilitation for the patient and significant others. Provide them with verbal and written information for the following:
1. Probable need for emotional care, even for patients who have not required extensive physical rehabilitation. Provide referrals to support groups for trauma patients and family members.
2. Availability of rehabilitation programs, extended care facilities, and home health agencies for patients unable to accomplish self-care on hospital discharge.
3. Availability of rehabilitation programs for substance abuse, as indicated. Immediately following the traumatic event, the patient and family members are very impressionable, making this period an ideal time for the substance abuser to begin to resolve the problem. See "Chemical Dependency," p. 597.
4. Medications, including drug name, purpose, dosage, schedule, precautions, and potential side effects. Encourage patients on antibiotics to take the medications for the prescribed length of time, even though they may be asymptomatic. If patient received tetanus immunization, ensure that he or she receives a wallet-sized card documenting the immunization.
5. Wound and catheter care. Have patient or caregiver describe and demonstrate proper technique prior to hospital discharge.
6. Importance of seeking medical attention if indicators of infection or bowel obstruction occur (e.g., fever, severe or unusual abdominal pain, nausea and vomiting, unusual drainage from wounds or incisions, or a change in bowel habits).
7. Injury prevention. Immediately following a traumatic injury, the patient is especially

likely to respond to injury prevention education. Provide instructions on proper seat-belt applications (across the pelvic girdle rather than across soft tissue of the lower abdomen), safety for infants and children, and other factors suitable for the individuals involved.

Section Five HEPATIC AND BILIARY DISORDERS

The liver lies directly beneath the diaphragm and occupies most of the RUQ of the abdomen. It has many functions, among them the storage of vitamins; synthesis of blood proteins; destruction of wornout red blood cells; removal of toxic substances from the body; and management of the formation and secretion of bile.

The gallbladder, which lies directly beneath the right lobe of the liver, and the hepatic, cystic, and common bile ducts compose the biliary system. The biliary duct system transports bile from the liver to the gallbladder. Bile is concentrated and stored in the gallbladder and released to the small intestine (duodenum), where it facilitates the absorption of fats, fat-soluble vitamins, and certain minerals, and also activates the release of pancreatic enzymes. If an obstructive lesion is present in the biliary ducts, the flow of bile is blocked, resulting in hemoconcentration. When this occurs, a variety of clinical manifestations can surface, including obstructive jaundice, dark-amber urine, and clay-colored stools. Pruritus occurs because of the deposition of bile salts in skin tissue. Steatorrhea and bleeding tendencies result from the inability of the duodenum to absorb fats and fat-soluable vitamins A, D, E, and K. Vitamin K is necessary for adequate clotting of the blood.

Note: Pancreatic problems are discussed in Chapter 5, "Endocrine Disorders," p. 287.

Hepatitis

Viral hepatitis is caused by one of the hepatitis viruses: A, B, non-A or non-B. Although symptomatology is similar, immunologic and epidemiologic characteristics are different (see Table 6-11). When hepatocytes are damaged, necrosis and autolysis can occur, which in turn lead to abnormal liver functioning. Generally, these changes are completely reversible after the acute phase. In some cases, however, massive necrosis can lead to liver failure and death.

Chronic hepatitis is inflammation of the liver for more than 6 months in duration. Although the causes are unclear, it is suspected that it is a consequence of viral hepatitis or that it may be associated with drug reactions. *Alcoholic hepatitis* occurs as the result of tissue necrosis caused by alcohol abuse. Generally, it is a precursor to cirrhosis (see p. 384).

Jaundice may be seen in any patient with decreased hepatic function. It is classified as prehepatic (hemolytic), caused by increased production of bilirubin; hepatic (hepatocellular), which is caused by the dysfunction of the liver cells; or posthepatic (obstructive), caused by an obstruction of the flow of bile out of the liver.

ASSESSMENT

Signs and symptoms: Nausea, vomiting, malaise, anorexia, URI, fatigue, irritability, slight to moderate temperature increases, epigastric discomfort, dark urine, clay-colored stools, pruritus, aversion to smoking.

Acute hepatic failure: Nausea, vomiting, and abdominal pain tend to be more severe. Jaundice is likely to appear earlier and deepen more rapidly. Hepatic coma, sharp rise in temperature, significant leukocytosis, rapid decrease in size of the liver, coffee-ground emesis, GI hemorrhage, purpura, ascites, seizure, shock, oliguria, and azotemia all may be present.

Physical assessment: Presence of jaundice; palpation of lymph nodes and abdomen may reveal lymphadenopathy, hepatomegaly, and splenomegaly.

T A B L E 6 - 1 1 Comparison of characteristics of types of viral hepatitis

	Type A	Type B	Non-A, Non-B
Mode of transmission	Fecal-oral route; large-scale outbreaks caused by contamination of food or water	Percutaneous inoculation (needlestick); usually through blood, but may result from saliva or semen	Usually blood; also semen and saliva
Population affected	More common in children and in overcrowded areas with poor sanitation	All ages. Drug addicts, male homosexuals, sexual partners of infected individuals. Patients and staff in hemodialysis units are at high risk.	All ages. Highest risk in recipients of blood transfusions. Also at risk are drug addicts, hemodialysis patients. Nosocomial spread possible
Diagnosis of acute disease	Anti-hepatitis A virus (IgM) antibody in serum (anti-HAV IgM)	Hepatitis B surface antigen in serum (HBsAg)	When causes of type A and type B are ruled out
Incubation period	2-6 weeks	6 weeks-6 months	6 weeks-6 months
Carrier state	No	Yes	Yes
Chronicity	No	Yes	Yes
Measures for reducing exposure	Handwashing; stool precautions	Handwashing; wearing gloves when handling body fluids and masks when fluids may spatter; using care when discarding needles and syringes; autoclaving all nondisposable items. Patient can never become a blood donor.	Same as for type B
Prophylaxis	Immune globulin (IG) before or within 1-2 weeks after exposure	Hepatitis B immune globulin (HBIG) within 24 hours after exposure and 1 month later. Hepatitis B vaccine recommended for medical and laboratory personnel, male homosexuals, neonates of infected mothers, and sexual partners of chronic HBsAg carriers	Still controversial, but currently a single dose of IG is recommended.

History of: Blood dyscrasias, multiple blood transfusions, alcohol or drug abuse, exposure to hepatotoxic chemicals or medications, travel to third world countries.

DIAGNOSTIC TESTS

1. *Hematologic tests:* Anti-HAV IgM will be present with hepatitis A, as will HBsAg with hepatitis B. There is no identifying marker for non-A, non-B. SGOT (frequently called serum aspartate transaminase, AST) and SGPT initially will be elevated and then drop. Total bilirubin will be elevated and the PT will be prolonged. Differential WBC count will reveal leukocytosis, monocytosis, and atypical lymphocytes; gamma globulin levels will be increased.
2. *Urine tests:* Will reveal elevation of urobilinogen, mild proteinuria, and mild bilirubinuria.
3. *Liver biopsy:* Performed for differential diagnosis.

MEDICAL MANAGEMENT

1. Monitoring of activity level: Bed rest may be indicated when symptoms are severe, with a gradual return to normal activity as symptoms subside.
2. Diet: In general, dietary management consists of giving palatable meals as tolerated without overfeeding. If oral intake is substantially decreased, parenteral or enteral nutrition may be initiated. Sodium or protein restrictions may be indicated in the presence of fluid retention or encephalopathy. All alcoholic beverages are strictly forbidden. Vitamins usually are given and folic acid may be indicated in alcoholic hepatitis.
3. Management of pruritus: Alkaline soaps are restricted; emollients and lipid creams (i.e., Eucerin) are prescribed. Antihistamines and tranquilizers, if used, are administered with caution and in low doses, because they are metabolized by the liver. See Table 6-12, below, which lists hepatotoxic drugs.
4. Pharmacotherapy
   □ *Parenteral vitamin K:* For those patients with prolonged PT.
   □ *Antiemetics:* For patients with nausea.
   □ *Gamma globulin:* Given routinely to all close personal contacts of patients with hepatitis A and to individuals travelling to or residing in endemic regions.
   □ *Hepatitis B hyperimmune globulin:* Recommended for individuals exposed to hepatitis B surface antigen contaminated material.
   □ *Hepatitis B vaccines:* Developed for prevention of hepatitis, they reduce the incidence of hepatitis B by approximately 92%.
   □ *Corticosteroids:* Used in some patients to control symptomatology and reduce abnormal liver function.
5. Restriction of hepatotoxic drugs: See Table 6-12.

NURSING DIAGNOSES AND INTERVENTIONS

Sleep pattern disturbance related to agitation secondary to hepatic dysfunction (faulty absorption, metabolism, and storage of nutrients)

Desired outcome: Patient relates the attainment of increasing amounts of sleep and rest.

1. Provide rest periods of at least 90-minute duration before and after activities and treatments.
2. Keep frequently used objects within easy reach.
3. Promote rest and sleep by decreasing environmental stimuli, providing back massage and relaxation tapes, and speaking with patient in short, simple terms.

Knowledge deficit: Causes of hepatitis and modes of transmission

Desired outcome: Patient verbalizes knowledge of the causes of hepatitis and measures that help prevent transmission.

TABLE 6-12 **Hepatotoxic drugs**

Generic/category name	Common trade names
acetaminophen	Tylenol
acetylsalycilic acid	Aspirin
ampicillin	Omnipen, Polycillin, Pfizerpen A
carbamazepine	Tegretol
carbenicillin	Geopen, Pyopen
chloramphenicol	Chloromycetin
chlorpropamide	Diabinese
chlorpromazine	Thorazine
clindamycin	Cleocin
dantrolene sodium	Dantrium
diazepam	Valium
hydrochlorothiazide	Esidrix
isoniazid	Isotamine
methyldopa	Aldomet
nitrofurantoin macrocrystals	Macrodantin
oral contraceptives	
oxacillin	Bactocill
penicillin	Pen-Vee K, Pfizerpen VK
phenytoin sodium	Dilantin
propylthiouracil (PTU)	Propyl-Thyracil
rifampin	Rifadin
sulfonamides	Bactrim, Septra, Gantrisin
tetracyclines (especially parenteral)	Achromycin

1. Assess patient's knowledge of the disease process and educate as necessary. Make sure patient knows you are not making moral decisions regarding alcohol/drug use or sexual behavior.
2. Teach patient and significant others the importance of good handwashing and wearing gloves if contact with feces is possible.
3. If appropriate, advise patients with hepatitis A that crowded living conditions with poor sanitation should be avoided to prevent recurrence.
4. Remind patients with hepatitis B and non-A, non-B hepatitis that sexual relations should be avoided, as directed by MD. Explain that blood donation is no longer possible.
5. Advise patients with hepatitis B that their sexual partners should receive hepatitis B vaccine.
6. Refer patient to alcohol/drug treatment programs as necessary.
7. See Table 6-11, p. 381, for other information.

Alteration in nutrition: Less than body requirements related to decreased intake secondary to anorexia, nausea, and gastric distress

Desired outcome: Patient exhibits stable weight or weight gain.

1. Take a diet history to determine food preferences.
2. Monitor and record intake.
3. Offer mouth care prior to meals to alleviate unpleasant taste and thereby enhance appetite.
4. Encourage small, frequent feedings and provide emotional support during meals.

5. Obtain prescription for vitamin and mineral supplements, if appropriate.
6. Administer antacids, antiemetics, antidiarrheals, and cathartics as prescribed to minimize gastric distress.
7. Encourage significant others to bring in desirable foods, if permitted.

Impaired skin integrity related to pruritus secondary to hepatic dysfunction

Desired outcome: Patient's skin remains intact.

1. Keep patient's skin moist by using tepid water or emollient baths, avoiding soap, and applying emollient lotions at frequent intervals.
2. Encourage patient not to scratch skin and to keep nails short and smooth. Suggest the use of the knuckles if patient must scratch. Wrap or place gloves on patient's hands (especially comatose patients).
3. To prevent infection, treat any skin lesion promptly.
4. Encourage patient to wear loose, soft clothing; provide soft linens (cotton is best).
5. Keep the environment cool.
6. Change wet linen often.

Body image disturbance related to presence of jaundice

Desired outcome: Patient verbalizes knowledge of measures for enhancing appearance and demonstrates an interest in daily grooming.

1. Encourage patient and significant others to verbalize feelings, concerns.
2. Encourage patient to maintain daily grooming.
3. Explain that wearing yellow and green intensifies yellow skin tone. Suggest wearing bright reds and blues or black instead.
4. Provide privacy as necessary.

Potential for injury related to increased risk of bleeding secondary to decreased vitamin K absorption

Desired outcome: Patient is free of injury and bleeding as evidenced by negative tests for occult blood in the feces and urine, absence of ecchymotic areas, and absence of bleeding at the gums and injection sites.

1. Monitor PT levels daily. Optimally the range will be 10.5-13.5 seconds.
2. Handle patient gently (e.g., when turning or transferring).
3. Minimize IM injections. Rotate sites, and use small-gauge needles. Apply moderate pressure after an injection, but do not massage the site. Administer medications IV or PO when possible.
4. Observe for ecchymotic areas. Inspect the gums and test the urine and feces for the presence of bleeding. Report significant findings to MD.
5. Teach patient to use electric razor and soft-bristled toothbrush.
6. Administer vitamin K as prescribed.

PATIENT-FAMILY TEACHING AND DISCHARGE PLANNING

Provide patient and significant others with verbal and written information for the following:
1. Importance of rest and getting adequate nutrition.
2. Hepatoxic agents, especially OTC drugs.
3. Prescribed medications (e.g., multivitamins), including the name, purpose, dosage, schedule, potential side effects, and precautions.
4. Potential complications, including delayed healing, skin injury, and bleeding tendencies.
5. Referral to alcohol/drug treatment programs as appropriate (see "Chemical Dependency," p. 597).

Cirrhosis

Cirrhosis is a chronic, serious disease in which normal configuration of the liver is changed, resulting in cell death. When new cells are formed, the resulting scarring causes disruption of blood and lymph flow. Although pathologic changes do not occur for many years, structural changes gradually lead to total liver dysfunction. Complications include portal hypertension, ascites, esophageal varices, hemorrhoids, splenomegaly, bleeding tendencies, jaundice, hepatorenal syndrome, and hepatic encephalopathy (hepatic coma).

Alcoholic cirrhosis: Associated with chronic alcohol abuse and accounts for 50% of all cases. The major survival factor is the cessation of alcohol intake. Portal hypertension and liver failure will result if alcohol intake is continued.

Postnecrotic cirrhosis: Associated with history of viral hepatitis or hepatic damage from industrial chemicals; accounts for 20% of all cases. This type appears to predispose the patient to the development of a hepatoma.

Biliary cirrhosis: Associated with posthepatic biliary obstruction and accounts for 15% of all cases.

ASSESSMENT

Signs and symptoms: Weakness, fatigability, weight loss, fever, anorexia, nausea, occasional vomiting, abdominal pain, menstrual abnormalities, impotence, loss of libido, sterility, hematemesis.

Physical assessment: Hepatomegaly, ascites, peripheral edema, and fetor hepaticus (a musty, sweetish odor on the breath). There may be slight changes in personality and behavior, which can progress to coma (a result of hepatic encephalopathy); spider angiomas, testicular atrophy, gynecomastia, pectoral and axillary alopecia (a result of excess in circulating estrogen); splenomegaly; hemorrhoids (a result of portal hypertension complications); spider nevi; palmer erythema; and jaundice.

History of: Exposure to hepatotoxic agents, viral or other types of hepatitis, alcoholism, poor nutrition.

DIAGNOSTIC TESTS

1. *Hemogram:* RBCs will be decreased in hypersplenism and decreased with hemorrhage. WBCs will be decreased with hypersplenism and increased with infection.
2. *Blood chemistry:* Direct and total bilirubin will be elevated and BUN will be decreased with liver failure and increased with GI bleeding. Uric acid will be increased in the presence of alcoholism. Ammonia will be increased in hepatic coma. Creatinine will be increased and serum albumin will be low. Gamma globulin will be increased. **Note:** Keep patient NPO except for water for 8 hours before the drawing of the ammonia level. Notify the lab of all antibiotics taken by patient as these will lower the ammonia level.
3. *Electrolytes:* Sodium will be decreased and potassium will be increased owing to hyperaldosteronism.
4. *Blood enzymes:* SGOT (AST) and SGPT will be elevated. Alkaline phosphatase will rise in the presence of biliary obstruction because it cannot be excreted.
5. *Coagulation:* PT will be prolonged.
6. *Urine tests:* Urine bilirubin will be increased; urobilinogen will be normal or increased.
7. *Liver biopsy:* Provides a microscopic picture of hepatocytes and aids in confirming a diagnosis and etiology. It is contraindicated in patients with clotting abnormalities, in cases of obstructive jaundice, or in the presence of local infection at biopsy site or ascites. **Note:** After the biopsy, monitor VS and check site at frequent intervals. Be alert to presence of respiratory distress and to indicators of peritonitis including severe abdominal pain, nausea, vomiting, rising temperature, tachycardia, pallor, and rigid abdomen. The patient should remain immobile on the right side for several hours. If analgesics are given, they must be nonhepatotoxic and must not affect clotting.
8. *Barium swallow:* Verifies the presence of esophageal or gastric varices. This test is not done if the patient is bleeding acutely. **Note:** Keep patient NPO from 12 mid-

night until completion of the test. Check subsequent stools to determine complete evacuation of barium.

9. *Radiologic studies:* Ultrasound differentiates hemolytic and hepatocellular jaundice from obstructive jaundice (see "Hepatitis," p. 380) and shows hepatomegaly and intrahepatic tumors. CT scan of the liver/spleen is done to evaluate size and location of tumors and to rule out gallbladder disease. Percutaneous transhepatic cholangiography reveals the extent of obstruction *via* contrast dye. Endoscopic retrograde cholangiopancreatography is a fiberoptic technique used to show pancreatic causes of jaundice. Portal angiography is done for patients with suspected portal hypertension. Liver scans enable visualization of the spleen and liver *via* injection of radioisotopes. **Note:** After injection of the dye, the patient may experience nausea, vomiting, and transient elevated temperature.

10. *Esophagoscopy:* A fiberoptic technique used to verify presence of esophageal varices or bleeding. This test is done in the presence of acute bleeding.

11. *EEG:* To evaluate the presence or degree of encephalopathy.

MEDICAL MANAGEMENT AND SURGICAL INTERVENTIONS

1. **Treatment of underlying causes:** For example, exposure to hepatotoxins, use of alcohol, biliary obstruction.

2. **Pharmacotherapy**
   □ *Diuretics:* To reduce edema. If potassium-sparing diuretics are used, teach patient to avoid excessive ingestion of potassium-rich foods (see Table 11-4, p. 555) or salt substitutes.

   □ *Antibiotics:* To control intestinal flora that aggravate encephalopathy.

   □ *Hematinics (iron preparations such as ferrous sulfate):* To control anemia. They are used to replace iron after abnormal blood loss.

   □ *Blood coagulants and vasopressors:* To control bleeding.

   □ *Laxatives and stool softeners:* To prevent straining.

   □ *Antidiarrheals:* As necessary to control diarrhea.

   □ *Antipruritics:* For pruritus.

   □ *Topical anesthetics:* For hemorrhoids.

   □ *Supplemental vitamins and minerals:* Such as folic acid for macrocytic anemia and vitamin K for prolonged PT.

Note: Narcotics and sedatives, which are metabolized by the liver, are contraindicated. Small doses of IV oxazepam (Serax) may be administered if absolutely necessary. See Table 6-12, p. 383, for a list of hepatotoxic drugs.

---

3. **Dietary management:** With fluid retention and ascites, sodium and fluids are restricted. Usually, half the calories are supplied as carbohydrates. Protein is restricted in hepatic coma or precoma because the action of intestinal bacteria on protein increases blood ammonia levels, which causes/worsens the coma state. Parenteral or enteral nutrition is administered in the presence of bleeding or coma.

4. **Bed rest:** In the presence of fever, infection.

5. **Treatment of complications**
   □ *Hemorrhage from esophageal varices:* Usually, a 4-lumen Minnesota sump tube or 3-lumen Sengstaken-Blakemore tube is used for tamponade, and surgical management includes a portocaval shunt (anastomosis of portal vein and vena cava) or a splenorenal shunt (anastomosis of splenic vein and left renal vein). Both shunts divert blood from the portal system to the vena cava.

   Hemorrhage may be controlled temporarily by administering infusions of vasopressin to promote arterial vasoconstriction and lower portal pressure. It may be given systemically or *via* the superior mesenteric artery.

   Injection scleropathy may be performed as a long-term control measure. The patient is sedated and the procedure is performed at the bedside. Sclerosing agents are introduced into the bleeding varices with a fiberoptic endoscope.

   □ *Ascites:* Dietary management may include sodium and fluid restrictions. Diuretics, usually aldosterone antagonists, are often given to minimize fluid collection. If indicated, surgical management includes a peritoneovenous shunt (LeVeen or Denver), which provides a route for reinfusion of ascitic fluid into the venous system. Monitor for these potential complications: cardiac or renal overload (see "Heart Failure," p. 54, "Pulmonary Edema," p. 76, "Hypertension," p. 40), shunt occlusion, disseminated intravascular coagulation (DIC, see p. 414), hemorrhage, infection, and extravasation of ascitic fluid from the incisions. Paracentesis is usually not indicated unless there is severe respiratory distress or discomfort or if it is essential for diagnosis of a tumor or bacterial peritonitis.

- □ *Hepatic encephalopathy (hepatic coma):* Dietary management includes restriction of protein from the diet to decrease blood ammonia levels, giving sweetened fruit juices to provide the necessary carbohydrates for energy, and administering parenteral/enteral nutrition if the patient is comatose. Pharmacologic management includes antibiotics to inhibit intestinal bacteria and magnesium sulfate or enemas to cleanse the intestines after GI bleeding. Lactulose is administered to produce 1-2 soft stools/day, which aids in decreasing blood ammonia levels, and in turn improves mentation. The following drugs are contraindicated: barbiturates and narcotics (because of the liver's inability to detoxify them), potassium-depleting diuretics (aldosterone antagonists are the diuretics of choice since edema is related to inadequate detoxification of aldosterone), and ammonia-containing medications, which would cause/worsen hepatic coma.
- □ *Spontaneous bacterial peritonitis:* Occurs in cirrhotic patients with ascites. Abdominal pain, worsening ascites, fever, and progressive encephalopathy suggest peritonitis. Mortality rate is high. See "Peritonitis," p. 337, for treatment.

NURSING DIAGNOSES AND INTERVENTIONS

Alteration in nutrition: Less than body requirements related to decreased intake secondary to anorexia and nausea; and increased need secondary to malabsorption

Desired outcome: Patient exhibits stable or increasing weight and verbalizes knowledge of foods that are permitted and restricted.

1. Encourage foods that are permitted within patient's dietary restrictions. Remember that sodium and fluids are restricted, and if the ammonia level rises (normal levels are whole blood: 70-200 μg/dl and plasma: 56-150 μg/dl), protein also will be restricted. Explain dietary restrictions to the patient.
2. Monitor I&O; weigh patient daily.
3. Encourage small, frequent meals to ensure adequate nutrition.
4. Encourage significant others to bring in desirable foods as permitted.
5. Have nourishing foods available to patient at night.
6. Administer vitamin and mineral supplements, as prescribed.
7. Administer the following prescribed medications to decrease gastric distress: antacids, antiemetics, antidiarrheals, cathartics.
8. Promote bed rest to reduce metabolic demands on the liver.
9. Provide soft diet if patient has esophageal varices that are not bleeding. Patients with bleeding esophageal varices are NPO.
10. Discuss need for tube feedings with MD if appropriate.

Impaired gas exchange related to decreased diffusion of oxygen secondary to shallow breathing occurring with pressure on the diaphragm caused by ascites; retention of sodium and water associated with pleural effusion; and erythrocytopenia

Desired outcome: Patient has adequate gas exchange as evidenced by $Paco_2$ ≤45 mm Hg, Pao_2 ≥80 mm Hg, O_2 saturation ≥95, and RR 12-20 breaths/min with normal depth and pattern (eupnea).

1. During complaints of dyspnea or orthopnea, assist patient into semi-Fowler's or high-Fowler's position to enhance gas exchange.
2. Administer oxygen as prescribed.

3. Monitor ABG values; notify MD of significant findings.
4. Encourage patient to change positions and deep-breathe at frequent intervals to enhance gas exchange. If secretions are present, ensure that the patient coughs frequently.
5. Notify MD of indicators of respiratory infection, such as spiking temperatures, chills, diaphoresis, and adventitious breath sounds.
6. Obtain baseline abdominal girth measurement, and then measure girth either daily or every shift. Measure around the same circumferential area each time; mark the site with indelible ink.

Potential fluid volume deficit related to increased risk of esophageal bleeding secondary to altered clotting factors and portal hypertension

Desired outcomes: Patient is normovolemic and free of esophageal bleeding as evidenced by BP $\geq$90/60 mm Hg, HR $\leq$100 bpm, warm extremities, distal pulses >2+ on a 0-4+ scale, brisk capillary refill (<3 seconds), and the ability to verbalize orientation to person, place, and time.

1. Monitor VS q4h (or more frequently if VS are outside of patient's baseline values). Be alert to hypotension and increased HR, as well as to physical indicators of hypovolemia and hemorrhage, including cool extremities, capillary refill >4 seconds, decreased amplitude of distal pulses, and decreasing LOC.
2. Teach patient to avoid swallowing foods that are chemically or mechanically irritating (e.g., rough or spicy foods, hot foods, hot liquids, alcohol), and would therefore injure the esophagus.
3. Instruct patient to avoid actions that increase intraabdominothoracic pressure such as coughing, sneezing, lifting, or vomiting.
4. Administer stool softeners, as prescribed, to help prevent patient from straining with defecation.
5. Inspect stools for presence of occult blood, which would signal bleeding within the GI tract; perform stool occult blood test as indicated.
6. As appropriate, instruct patient about alcohol's role in causing esophageal varices.
7. Monitor prothrombin time for abnormality (normal range is 10.5-13.5 seconds) and assess patient for signs of bleeding, such as altered VS, irritability, air hunger, pallor, weakness, melena, and hematemesis.
8. Encourage the intake of foods rich in vitamin K (e.g., spinach, cabbage, cauliflower, liver).
9. As often as possible, avoid invasive procedures, such as injections and rectal temperatures.
10. Monitor the scleropathy patient for evidence of perforation, including increased HR, decreased BP, pallor, weakness, and air hunger. If signs of perforation occur, notify MD immediately, keep the patient NPO, and prepare for gastric suction. Administer antibiotics as prescribed.

Potential sensory/perceptual alterations related to mentation and motor disturbances secondary to hepatic coma occurring with cerebral accumulation of ammonia or GI bleeding

Desired outcome: Patient verbalizes orientation to person, place, and time; interacts appropriately with the environment; and exhibits intact signature.

1. Perform a baseline assessment of patient's personality characteristics and assess patient's LOC and orientation. Enlist the aid of significant others to help determine slight changes in personality or behavior.
2. Have patient demonstrate his or her signature daily. If the writing deteriorates, ammonia levels may be increasing. Be alert to generalized muscle twitching and asterixis (flapping tremor induced by dorsiflexion of wrist and extension of fingers). Report significant findings to MD.
3. Remind patient to avoid protein and foods high in ammonia, such as gelatin, onions, and strong cheeses. The diseased liver is unable to convert ammonia to urea and the buildup of ammonia adds to the progression of hepatic encephalopathy.

4. Observe for indicators of GI bleeding, including melena or hematemesis. GI bleeding can precipitate hepatic coma. Report bleeding to MD promptly and obtain prescription for cleansing enemas.
5. Protect patient against injury that can be precipitated by confused state.

Fluid volume excess: *Extravascular* related to edema and ascites secondary to sequestration of fluids with portal hypertension and hepatocellular failure; and *intravascular* related to retention secondary to sodium and electrolyte disturbances

Desired outcomes: Patient becomes normovolemic as evidenced by stable or decreasing abdominal girth, RR 12-20 breaths/min with normal depth and pattern (eupnea), HR ≤100 bpm, edema ≤1+ on a 0-4+ scale, and absence of crackles. Serum sodium is 137-147 mEq/L and serum potassium is 3.5-5.0 mEq/L.

1. Obtain baseline abdominal girth measurement. Place patient in the supine position and mark abdomen with indelible ink to ensure serial measurements from the same circumferential site. Measure girth daily or every shift as appropriate.
2. Monitor weight and I&O. Output should be equal to or exceed input. Weight loss should not exceed 0.23 kg/day (½ pound). Assess the degree of edema, from 1+ (barely detectable) to 4+ (deep, persistent pitting), and document accordingly.
3. Be alert to clinical indicators of pulmonary edema, including dyspnea, basilar crackles that do not clear with coughing, orthopnea, and tachypnea.
4. Give frequent mouth care and provide ice chips to help minimize thirst.
5. Monitor sodium and potassium values and report abnormalities to MD. Restrict sodium and replace potassium as prescribed.
6. Remind patient to avoid food and nonfood items that contain sodium (e.g., canned soups, processed foods, table salt, antacids, baking soda, and some mouthwashes). For more information, see Table 11-3, p. 550.
7. Elevate extremities to decrease peripheral edema. Apply TED stockings as prescribed.
8. Bear in mind that rapid increases in intravascular volume can precipitate variceal hemorrhage in susceptible patients. Monitor for hemorrhage accordingly (see **Fluid volume deficit,** above).
9. If patient has a LeVeen or Denver shunt, teach the patient to inhale against resistance, using a blow bottle to facilitate the flow of ascitic fluid through the shunt. Inhaling against resistance raises intraperitoneal pressure sufficiently to enable ascitic fluid to flow through the shunt. In addition, provide instructions about the following: importance of lifestyle changes, such as low-sodium diet (see Table 11-3, p. 550), abstinence from alcohol, practicing breathing exercises, obtaining daily weight and abdominal girth measurements, and monitoring I&O and edema.

See "Hepatitis" for **Body image disturbance,** p. 384. Also see "Alcoholism," p. 597, as appropriate.

PATIENT-FAMILY TEACHING AND DISCHARGE PLANNING

Provide patient and significant others with verbal and written information for the following:
1. Medications, including drug name, purpose, dosage, schedule, precautions, and potential side effects.
2. Dietary restrictions, in particular that of sodium (see Table 11-3, p. 550), protein, and ammonia.
3. Potential need for lifestyle changes, including cessation of alcoholic beverages. Stress that alcohol cessation is a major factor in survival of this disease. Include appropriate referrals, for example, to Alcoholics Anonymous, Al-Anon, and Al-Ateen. As appropriate, provide referrals to community nursing support agencies.
4. Awareness of hepatotoxic agents (see Table 6-12, p. 383), especially OTC drugs, including acetaminophen and acetylsalicylic acid.
5. Importance of breathing exercises.

6. Indicators of variceal bleeding/hemorrhage (i.e., vomiting of blood, change in LOC) and the need to inform MD should they occur.

Cholelithiasis and cholecystitis

Cholelithiasis is a condition characterized by the presence of stones in the gallbladder. *Choledocholithiasis* is the term used to describe gallstones in the common bile duct. Gallstones usually are composed of cholesterol (70%) and less commonly of calcium bilirubinate or calcium carbonate. Precipitating factors include disturbances in metabolism, biliary stasis, obstruction, and infection. Gallstones are especially prevalent in women who are multiparous, on estrogen therapy, or who use oral contraceptives. Other risk factors include obesity, dietary intake of fats, sedentary lifestyle, and familial tendencies. The incidence increases with age, and it is estimated that one out of every three persons who reach age 75 have gallstones. Cholelithiasis is frequently seen in such disease states as diabetes mellitus, regional enteritis, and certain blood dyscrasias. Usually, cholelithiasis is asymptomatic until a stone becomes lodged in the cystic tract. If the obstruction is unrelieved, biliary colic and cholecystitis can ensue.

Cholecystitis is most commonly associated with cystic duct obstructions due to impacted gallstones; however, it also may result from stasis, bacterial infection, or ischemia of the gallbladder. Cholecystitis involves acute inflammation of the gallbladder, and is associated with pain, tenderness, and fever. With obstruction, structural changes can occur, such as hypertrophy of the gallbladder and a swelling and thickening of the gallbladder walls. If the edema is prolonged, the walls become scarred and fibrosed, and the constant pressure of bile can lead to mucosal irritation. As a complication of the impaired circulation and edema, pressure ischemia and necrosis can develop, resulting in gangrene or perforation. With chronic cholecystitis, stones almost always are present, and the gallbladder walls are thickened and fibrosed.

ASSESSMENT

Cholelithiasis: History of intolerance to fats and occasional discomfort after eating. As the stone moves through the duct or becomes lodged, a sudden onset of mild, aching pain will occur in the midepigastrium after eating and increase in intensity during a colic attack, potentially radiating to the RUQ and right subscapular region. Nausea, vomiting, tachycardia, and diaphoresis also can occur. Many individuals with gallstones are entirely asymptomatic.

Cholecystitis: History of intolerance to fats and discomfort after eating, including regurgitation, flatulence, belching, epigastric heaviness, indigestion, heartburn, chronic upper abdominal pain, and nausea. Amber-colored urine, clay-colored stools, pruritus, jaundice, steatorrhea, and bleeding tendencies can be present if there is bile obstruction. Symptoms may be vague. An acute attack may last for 7-10 days, but it usually resolves in several hours.

Physical assessment: Cholelithiasis: Palpation of RUQ will reveal a tender abdomen during colic attack. Otherwise, between attacks, the examination is usually normal. *Cholecystitis:* Palpation will elicit tenderness localized behind the inferior margin of the liver. With progressive symptoms, a tender, globular mass may be palpated behind the lower border of the liver. With the patient taking a deep breath, palpation over the RUQ will elicit Murphy's sign (pain and inability to inspire when the examiner's hand comes in contact with the gallbladder).

DIAGNOSTIC TESTS

1. *Radiologic studies:* Abdominal ultrasound is the test of choice. Oral cholangiogram, HIDA and DIDDA, IV cholangiogram, nuclear scans, and percutaneous transhepatic cholangiogram also determine the patency of the gallbladder and biliary or cystic ducts and help to rule out other conditions that mimic cholelithiasis or cholecystitis.

Chest, abdominal, upper GI, and barium enema x-rays are often used to rule out pulmonary or other GI disorders.
2. *EKG:* To rule out cardiac disease.
3. *Ultrasonography of the gallbladder and biliary tract:* To detect gallstones and tumors and help distinguish between intrahepatic and extrahepatic jaundice.
4. *CT scan:* To detect dilated bile ducts and the presence of gallbladder cysts.
5. *Endoscopic retrograde cholangiopancreatography (ERCP):* Visualization and evaluation of the biliary tree to rule out or treat common duct stones.
6. *CBC with differential:* To assess for presence of infection or blood loss.
7. *PT:* To assess for a prolonged clotting time secondary to faulty vitamin K absorption.
8. *Bilirubin tests (serum and urine) and urobilinogen tests (urine and fecal):* To differentiate between hemolytic disorders, hepatocellular disease, and obstructive disease. Usually there is an increase of bilirubin in the plasma and urine with biliary disease.
9. *Serum liver enzyme test:* Liver function test values usually are normal in cholecystitis but often become abnormal in the presence of prolonged cholecystitis or common duct stones.

MEDICAL MANAGEMENT AND SURGICAL INTERVENTIONS

1. Pharmacologic therapy
   □ *Analgesics and antacids:* For pain.
   □ *Antibiotics:* For infection.
   □ *Antiemetics:* For nausea and vomiting.
   □ *Hyperlipidemic agents:* Bind with bile salts in the intestine to facilitate their excretion and may be given to provide relief from pruritus caused by prolonged obstructive jaundice.
2. Chemical dissolution of cholesterol gallstones with a solvent: May be used in patients with a functioning gallbladder and an unobstructed biliary tract. The solvent is infused *via* a T-tube. The most common solvent is methyl-tert-butyl ether (MTBE). An oral preparation of bile salts (e.g., chenodeoxycholic acid [CDCA] or ursodeoxycholic acid [UDCA]) may be administered to dissolve cholesterol stones. Oral preparations are used after MTBE therapy to prevent recurrence of stones.
3. Dietary management: Varies according to the patient's condition. During an acute attack, NPO status with IV fluids may be instituted. With severe nausea and vomiting, an NG tube is inserted and attached to low, intermittent suction. Diet advances to patient's tolerance and small, frequent feedings of a low-fat diet are recommended for both the acute and chronic conditions.
4. Endoscopic retrograde cholangiopancreatography (ERCP): The common bile duct may be cannulated and if a stone is present, an endoscopic sphincterotomy (a technique that cuts the opening of the bile duct) can be performed with stone extraction *via* a snare or balloon catheter.
5. Nonoperative biliary stone removal: One method of stone extraction, which is performed under fluoroscopy in the radiology department. The stone is removed with a basket that is inserted *via* a catheter or T-tube through the sinus tract into the common duct. If this technique is unsuccessful, forceps are used to manipulate the stone. A cholangiogram is done before and after the procedure. If the x-ray is normal after the procedure, the T-tube is removed; if stones are still present, a new T-tube or catheter is inserted and the patient returns the following day for the same procedure. This technique may be ideal for an individual who is not a good surgical candidate.
6. Lithotripsy: Gallstones, like kidney stones, can be fragmented by exposure to extracorporeal shock waves. The stones are broken up into small granules that can be furthered pulverized by dissolution therapy. Currently, clinical trials are underway with this relatively new technique.
7. Surgical interventions: Usually required for relief of long-term symptoms of cholelithiasis and acute cholecystitis. The type of surgery depends on the severity and length of illness and site of obstruction. The following procedures may be performed:
   □ *Cholecystostomy:* Opening and draining the gallbladder of gallstones.

□ *Choledochotomy:* Opening the common bile duct to remove stones.
□ *Choledochoduodenostomy:* Anastomosis of the common bile duct to the duode-num.
□ *Choledochojejunostomy:* Anastomosis of the common bile duct to the jejunum.

8. **Cholecystectomy (removal of the gallbladder):** The most commonly performed proce-dure for biliary disease, which accounts for one-third of all surgical procedures that are performed. A right subcostal incision is made. The stones are removed and a T-tube may be inserted to maintain patency of the common duct and drain bile. The gallbladder is then excised from the liver; the cystic duct, vein, and artery are ligated; and a drain (usually Penrose) is inserted and brought out through a stab wound for drainage of blood, serum, and bile.

NURSING DIAGNOSES AND INTERVENTIONS

Pain, spasms, nausea, and itching related to obstructive or inflammatory process

Desired outcome: Patient's subjective evaluation of discomfort improves, as docu-mented by a pain scale.

1. Monitor patient for the presence of pain or other discomfort. Devise a pain scale with patient, rating discomfort on a scale of 0 (no pain) to 10.
2. Explain to patient that a low-Fowler's position will minimize pressure in the RUQ.
3. Teach patient to avoid fatty and rough/fibrous foods to prevent nausea and spasms.
4. Administer bile salt binding agent (e.g., cholestyramine) as prescribed for itching.
5. Help control itching by providing Alpha-Keri baths and using soft linens on the bed.
6. For other interventions, see **Pain** in "Caring for Preoperative and Postoperative Pa-tients," p. 638.

Potential for injury related to use of T-tube or recurrence of biliary obstruction

Desired outcomes: Patient is asymptomatic of postsurgical perforation as evidenced by <1,000 ml/day of dark brown drainage (with gradual diminishment) and the presence of a soft and nondistended abdomen. Patient is asymptomatic of recurring biliary obstruc-tion as evidenced by normal skin color, brown-colored stools, and straw-colored urine.

1. When the patient returns from surgery, mark the T-tube at the skin line with a nar-row strip of sterile tape to provide a baseline for position assessment.
2. Tape the tube securely to the abdomen with adhesive tape, avoiding any tension on the tube.
3. Note and record the color, amount, odor, and consistency of drainage q2h on the day of surgery and at least every shift thereafter. Initially the drainage will be dark brown with small amounts of blood and can amount to 500-1,000 ml/day. Report greater amounts of blood or drainage to MD. The amount should subside gradually as the swelling diminishes in the common duct and drainage into the duodenum normalizes. Typically, the tube is removed within 6 days of surgery.
4. Be alert to abdominal distention, rigidity, and complaints of diaphragmatic irritation along with a cessation or significant decrease in the amount of drainage. If these oc-cur, notify MD immediately and anticipate tube replacement with a 14 F catheter.
5. When the patient ambulates with a T-tube, attach a small drainage collection con-tainer to the distal end, position it in a robe pocket, and ensure that it is below the level of the common duct to prevent reflux.
6. Monitor the color of the skin, sclera, urine, and stool. If obstruction recurs and bile is forced back into the bloodstream, jaundice will be present, the urine will be am-ber, and the stools will be clay-colored. (Clay color is normal if bile is drained *via* the tubes.) The brown color should return to the stools once bile begins to drain nor-mally into the duodenum.

See "Hepatitis" for **Impaired skin integrity** related to pruritus, p. 384. See "Providing Nutritional Support," p. 622, for nursing diagnoses and interventions for the care of pa-tients with tube feedings. See the appendix for nursing diagnoses and interventions for the care of preoperative and postoperative patients, p. 637.

PATIENT-FAMILY TEACHING AND DISCHARGE PLANNING

Provide patient and significant others with verbal and written information for the following:

1. Notifying MD if the following indicators of recurrent biliary obstruction occur: dark urine, pruritus, jaundice, clay-colored stools. Inform patient that loose stools may occur for several months as the body adjusts to the continuous flow of bile.
2. Medications, including drug name, dosage, schedule, purpose, precautions, and potential side effects.
3. Care of dressings and tubes if patient is discharged with them and monitoring the incision and drain sites for signs of infection, for example, persistent redness, pain, purulent discharge, swelling, and local warmth.
4. Importance of maintaining a diet low in fat and eating frequent, small meals for individuals whose condition has not been treated surgically.
5. Importance of follow-up appointments with MD; reconfirm time and date of next appointment.
6. Avoiding alcoholic beverages during the first 2 postoperative months to minimize the risk of pancreatic involvement.
7. Necessity of postsurgical activity precautions: Avoid lifting heavy objects (>5 lb) for the first 4-6 weeks or as directed, rest after periods of fatigue, get maximum amounts of rest, and gradually increase activities to tolerance.

SELECTED REFERENCES

Broadway DC and Jackson BS: Principles of ostomy care, St Louis, 1982, The CV Mosby Co.

Bryant R: Diverticular disease, J Enterostomal Ther 13:114-117, 1986.

Cardona V et al: Trauma nursing: resuscitation through rehabilitation, Philadelphia, 1988, The WB Saunders Co.

Cargile ND: Buying time when you face a bowel obstruction, RN 40-46, Aug, 1985.

Committee on Trauma: Advanced trauma life support instructor manual, Chicago, 1989, American College of Surgeons.

Decker SI: The life-threatening consequences of a GI bleed, RN 18-27, Oct, 1985.

Doughty DB: Colorectal cancer: etiology and pathophysiology, Semin Oncol 2:235-241, 1986.

Freickert DM: Gastric surgery: your crucial pre- and postop role, RN 24-34, Jan 1987.

Given BA and Simmons SJ: Gastroenterology in clinical nursing, ed 4, St Louis, 1984, The CV Mosby Co.

Greenberger NJ and Isselbacher KJ: Disorders of absorption. In Braunwald E et al: Harrison's principles of internal medicine, ed 11, New York, 1987, McGraw-Hill Book Co.

Haibeck SV: Colorectal cancer, SGA J. 10:208-210, 1988.

Harmon AR: Nursing care of the adult trauma patient, New York, 1985, John Wiley & Sons.

Keen JH: Gastrointestinal dysfunctions. In Swearingen PL et al: Manual of critical care: applying nursing diagnoses to adult critical illness, St Louis, 1988, The CV Mosby Co.

Kneisl CR and Ames SW: Adult health nursing: a biopsychosocial approach, Redwood City, Calif, 1986, Addison-Wesley Publishing Co.

MacDonald WC and Rubin CE: Gastric tumors, gastritis, and other gastric diseases. In Braunwald E et al: Harrison's principles of internal medicine, ed 11, New York, 1987, McGraw-Hill Book Co.

McConnell EA: Meeting the challenge of intestinal obstruction, Nursing 87:34-42, July 1987.

McGuigan JE: Peptic ulcer. In Braunwald E et al: Harrison's principles of internal medicine, ed 11, New York, 1987, McGraw-Hill Book Co.

New ulcer drug interacts less, RN 150, Oct 1988.

Patras AZ, Paice JA, and Lanigan K: Managing GI bleeding: it takes a two-track mind, Nursing 88:68-74, April 1988.

Petillo MH: Enterostomal therapy, Nurs Clin North Am 22:253-356, 1987.

Rodman MJ: Your guide to the newest drugs, RN 61-72, March 1989.

Schroeder SA et al: Current medical diagnosis and treatment, Norwalk, Conn, and San Mateo, Calif, 1988, Appleton & Lange.

Silen W: Acute intestinal obstruction. In Braunwald E et al: Harrison's principles of internal medicine, ed 11, New York, 1987, McGraw-Hill Book Co.

Sleisenger MH and Fordtran JS: Gastrointestinal disease: pathophysiology, diagnosis, and management, Philadelphia, 1989, WB Saunders Co.

Swearingen PL et al: Manual of critical care: applying nursing diagnoses to adult critical illness, St Louis, 1988, The CV Mosby Co.

Trunkey D and Lewis FR editors: Current therapy of trauma, vol 2, Philadelphia, 1986, Decker Publishing Co.

When you suspect intestinal obstruction, Patient Care 72-87, Oct 1984.

Wicks LJ: Treatment modalities for colorectal cancer, Semin Oncol Nurs 2:242-248, 1986.

7

<u>CHAPTER</u>

Hematologic disorders

Section One   DISORDERS OF THE RED BLOOD CELLS

The erythrocyte, or red blood cell (RBC), is the transport mechanism for hemoglobin, which carries oxygen from the heart and lungs to the tissues, exchanges it for carbon dioxide, and then returns to the heart and lungs. RBCs are very flexible and capable of bending, elongating, and squeezing through tiny capillaries. Normal RBCs can travel under high pressure and speed, are extremely active metabolically, and have an average life of 120 days. The bone marrow produces and replaces RBCs every day and can respond to the increased need for RBCs by increasing production. However, with increased production, immature RBCs (reticulocytes) often are released into the circulation; a high level of reticulocytes often aids in the diagnosis of RBC disorders.

Anemia is a common hematopoietic disorder defined as a reduced number of RBCs or a reduced amount of hemoglobin. The general effects of anemia result from a deficiency in the oxygen-carrying mechanism, although some effects are related to varied etiologies and pathogenesis. Three basic types of anemias are discussed in this section; pernicious, hemolytic, and hypoplastic.

395

Pernicious anemia

Vitamin B_{12} is supplied by dietary intake of such foods as liver, milk, and eggs and stored in the liver to be used for maturation of RBCs. Deficiency of this vitamin leads to the development of immature erythrocytes, a chronic condition known as pernicious anemia. Decreased dietary intake of animal products, increased need for this vitamin with pregnancy or a tumor, presence of parasites, or surgery involving the small intestine where the vitamin is absorbed are conditions that can lead to vitamin B_{12} deficiency. The most common condition is the decrease in production by the gastric mucosa of the microprotein *intrinsic factor,* which when combined with vitamin B_{12} facilitates absorption and use of the vitamin by body cells, particularly in the bone marrow, GI tract, and nervous system. Anemias related to vitamin B_{12} are called megaloblastic anemias because they are characterized by RBCs that are large and immature (megaloblasts). Altered production of one bone marrow element usually will cause altered or decreased production of the other elements, including leukocytes and thrombocytes.

ASSESSMENT

Chronic indicators: Brittle nails, smooth tongue, numbness and tingling of the extremities, fatigue, and dysphagia. However, because of slow progression, many patients remain asymptomatic. Anorexia, weight loss, jaundice from destruction of malformed erythrocytes, and gingivitis from absence of vitamin B_{12} also can occur.

Acute indicators: Dyspnea on exertion, irritability, palpitations, and dizziness in the presence of severe deficiency. In addition, because the nervous system is particularly sensitive to the lack of vitamin B_{12}, degenerative changes of the cerebral cortex and spinal cord can occur, seen mainly in the form of paresthesias.

Physical assessment: Presence of oral lesions and gingivitis, tachycardia, unsteady gait, and clumsiness.

DIAGNOSTIC TESTS

1. *Schilling's test:* Patient is given radioactive tagged vitamin B_{12}, then urine concentration of tagged B_{12} is measured. For normal individuals, B_{12} is absorbed and excreted in the urine. In the presence of pernicious anemia, B_{12} is not absorbed and urine levels will be low (<3%).
2. *Trial administration of vitamin B_{12}:* May be given to evaluate the patient's response. In the presence of pernicious anemia, symptoms will be relieved.
3. *Hematologic studies:* Hemoglobin, erythrocytes, leukocytes, and thrombocytes will be decreased.
4. *Bone marrow aspiration:* Will reveal hyperplasia with increased numbers of large-sized megaloblasts.
5. *Gastric analysis:* Will reveal decreased volume of gastric secretions. Atrophic gastritis is characteristic of pernicious anemia.
6. *LDH:* May be increased.

MEDICAL MANAGEMENT

1. Vitamin B_{12} replacement: Dosage will depend on the individual and the response to treatment. For example, 100 mg cyanocobalamin may be given IM qd × 7 days. If improvement occurs, it is given qod × 7 days and then q3-4 days × 2-3 weeks. **Note:** Increasing the dietary intake of vitamin B_{12} will not be effective in individuals with intrinsic factor deficiency.
2. Concurrent treatment of underlying disorder: If present (e.g., gastric mucosal problem).
3. Serial measurements of reticulocytes: To determine effectiveness of treatment.

NURSING DIAGNOSES AND INTERVENTIONS

Fatigue related to diminished energy levels secondary to decreased oxygen-carrying capacity of the blood

Desired outcome: Patient participates in activities, reports the lessening of fatigue, and exhibits physical tolerance to activity as evidenced by RR 12-20 breaths/min with normal depth and pattern (eupnea), HR ≤ 100 bpm, and absence of headache and dizziness.

1. Provide frequent rest periods between care activities, allowing time for at least 90 minutes of undisturbed rest.
2. As patient performs ADL, be alert to indicators of decreased tissue oxygenation, such as dyspnea on exertion, dizziness, palpitations, and headaches.
3. Reassure patient that usually symptoms are relieved and tolerance for activity is increased with therapy.
4. As patient's condition improves, encourage increase in activities to tolerance. Set specific goals with patient, for example, "Today I would like you to try to walk from your room to the nurses' station and back three (or appropriate number, depending on patient's tolerance) times."

Potential for infection related to increased susceptibility secondary to decreased leukocyte production (associated with decrease in all blood elements)

Desired outcome: Patient is free of infection as evidenced by normothermia; RR 12-20 breaths/min with normal depth and pattern (eupnea); absence of adventitious breath sounds; absence of unusual erythema, warmth, or drainage at any wound sites; and the presence of urine that is straw-colored, clear, and of characteristic odor.

1. Maintain strict asepsis when performing invasive procedures. Wash hands well before caring for patient.
2. Teach patient and significant others the technique for effective handwashing.
3. Be alert to the following indicators of respiratory infection and report to MD: cough; changes in the amount, color, and consistency of sputum; increased RR; and presence of crackles (rales), rhonchi, and fever. Teach these indicators to patient and significant others, along with the indicators of wound infection and UTI (see Table 5-3, p. 298).
4. To prevent stasis of secretions in the lung, which can lead to infection, teach patient how to perform effective coughing and deep breathing.

Alteration in nutrition: Less than body requirements related to decreased intake secondary to fatigue, impairment of oral mucosa, or anorexia

Desired outcome: Patient has adequate nutrition as evidenced by maintenance of body weight.

1. If patient is easily fatigued, encourage small, frequent meals.
2. If oral lesions/cracks are present, encourage soft and bland foods. For more information, see "Stomatitis," p. 314, in Chapter 6.
3. For patient with decreased appetite, encourage significant others to bring in patient's favorite foods and stay with patient during meals to encourage eating.

Potential for injury related to risk of sensorimotor deficit secondary to inability to absorb and use vitamin B_{12}

Desired outcome: Patient is asymptomatic of injury caused by sensorimotor deficit.

1. Assess for sensory deficit (i.e., paresthesias) and protect patient from extremes of heat and cold if deficit is noted.
2. Assess patient's orientation to person, place, and time. As needed, orient patient to all activities and surroundings at frequent intervals.
3. Assess muscle strength and motor ability before allowing patient to ambulate unassisted.

4. Teach patient and significant others the signs and symptoms of neurologic deficit and the importance of reporting them to staff or MD promptly. Reassure patient that neurologic deficit usually reverses with therapy.

Diarrhea or constipation related to gastrointestinal mucosal atrophy secondary to reduced hct

Desired outcome: Patient relates the return of normal bowel functioning, as evidenced by soft, formed stools.

1. If the patient is constipated, implement the following:
  ☐ Assist patient with establishing a regular bowel pattern, for example, by increasing fluids (to at least 2-3 L/day) and dietary fiber and initiating a regular exercise program.
  ☐ For other interventions, see **Constipation,** p. 656, in "Caring for Patients on Prolonged Bed Rest" in the appendix.
2. If diarrhea occurs, teach patient to avoid high-roughage foods, administer prescribed antidiarrheal medications, and encourage increased intake of fluids to prevent dehydration.

PATIENT-FAMILY TEACHING AND DISCHARGE PLANNING

Provide patient and significant others with verbal and written information for the following:
1. Necessity of vitamin B_{12} replacement for life, even when symptoms resolve.
2. Technique for administering vitamin B_{12} or arrangement for monthly clinic visits for injection.
3. For injections that will be performed by patient or significant other, the need for a supply of vitamin B_{12}, 22-gauge needles, 3-ml syringes, and alcohol sponges. Teach patient the proper method for disposing of needles and provide an appropriate receptacle for needle and syringe disposal.
4. Importance of regular medical follow-up, including serial monitoring of blood levels.

Hemolytic anemia

Hemolytic anemia is characterized by abnormal or premature destruction of RBCs. Hemolysis can be intrinsic or result from such conditions as infection or radiation. *Sickle cell anemia* is a form of chronic hemolytic anemia characterized by abnormal, crescent-shaped, rigid, and elongated erythrocytes. These "sickle" RBCs interfere with circulation because they cannot get through the microcirculation and are destroyed in the process. Sickle cell anemia can affect almost every body system due to decreased oxygen delivery, decreased circulation caused by occlusion of the vessels by RBCs, and inflammatory process. This disorder occurs when the gene is inherited from both parents (homozygous); a carrier state exists when it is inherited from one parent (heterozygous). Medical treatment has improved the prognosis for this disorder, which is seen predominantly in blacks.

Thalassemia is another type of chronic hemolytic anemia. In this disorder, hemoglobin A is manufactured in less-than-normal amounts, although the hemoglobin itself is of normal morphology. This is an inherited disorder passed on through an autosomal gene. Severity depends on whether the inheritance is heterozygous or homozygous. It occurs most often in individuals of Mediterranean descent (e.g., Greeks and Italians). If the condition is severe *(thalassemia major),* the patient seldom survives to adulthood. Individuals with intermediate and minor forms develop normally and usually can expect a normal life span. *Acquired hemolytic anemia* is usually the result of an abnormal immune response that causes premature destruction of RBCs. Hemolysis can occur as a result of a foreign antigen, such as from a transfusion reaction, or an autoimmune reaction in which the hemolytic agent is intrinsic to the patient's body. Other possible causes include exposure to radiation and ingestion of such drugs as sulfisoxazole (e.g., Gantrisin), phenacetin, and methyldopa (e.g., Aldomet).

Hemolytic crisis: Individuals with chronic hemolytic anemia may do relatively well for a period of time, but many factors can precipitate a hemolytic crisis or acute hemolysis. For example, an individual with mild hemolytic anemia can become severely anemic with an acute infectious process or with any other physiologic or emotional stressor, including surgery, trauma, or emotional upset. Widespread hemolysis causes an acute decrease in oxygen-carrying capacity of the blood, resulting in decreased oxygen delivery to the tissues. Organ congestion from the hemolyzed blood cells occurs, and this affects organ function and precipitates a shock state.

ASSESSMENT

Chronic indicators: Pallor (e.g., conjunctival), fatigue, dyspnea on exertion, and intermittent dizziness, all of which depend on the severity of the anemia. With chronic hemolytic anemia, the individual sometimes will exhibit jaundice, arthritis, renal failure, and skin ulcers because of hemolysis and chronic organ damage.

Acute indicators: Fever, visual blurring, temporary blindness, abdominal pain, back pain, palpitations, SOB, chills, hepatomegaly, headache, lymphadenopathy, splenomegaly, and decreased urinary output (signs and symptoms of hemolytic crisis). Peripheral nerve damage can result in paralysis or paresthesias, vomiting, and chills.

DIAGNOSTIC TESTS

1. *Sickle cell test:* To screen for sickle cell anemia.
2. *Hgb and hct:* Decreased because of RBC destruction.
3. *Serum tests:* LDH will be elevated because of the release of this enzyme when the RBC is destroyed. Bilirubin will be elevated because the liver cannot process the excess that occurs from rapid RBC destruction.
4. *Urine and fecal urobilinogen:* Levels are increased. These are more sensitive indicators of RBC destruction than serum bilirubin levels.
5. *Bone marrow aspiration:* Will reveal erythroid hyperplasia, especially with chronic hemolytic anemia.
6. *Hgb electrophoresis:* Will diagnose hgb AS, a sickle cell trait, and may show sickled hemoglobin.
7. *Reticulocyte count:* Will be elevated because of the rapid destruction of RBCs.

MEDICAL MANAGEMENT

1. Elimination or discontinuation of causative factor: If possible (e.g., chemical, drug, incompatible blood).
2. Volume replacement: For hypovolemic individuals to prevent decreased organ perfusion owing to hemolysis.
3. Oxygen therapy: For patients who are hypoxemic.
4. Supportive therapy of shock state: If it occurs.
5. Transfusion: If circulatory failure or severe anemic anoxia occurs.
6. Erythrocytapheresis (red blood cell exchange): A relatively new procedure that removes abnormal RBCs and infuses healthy RBCs to correct the anemia.

Patient assessment during erythrocytapheresis

  ☐ Monitor for symptom relief following one RBC exchange.
  ☐ Monitor arterial Pao_2 for evidence of improvement, optimally ≥80 mm Hg.
  ☐ Monitor hct. Values ≥30% are necessary to prevent bone marrow stimulation.
7. Corticosteroids: To help stabilize cell membranes and decrease the inflammatory response. Usually 50-100 mg prednisone is given with antacids.
8. Folic acid: To help prevent hemolytic crisis by increasing the production of RBCs in individuals with chronic hemolytic anemias.
9. Splenectomy: To provide relief, depending on the cause of the anemia. The spleen is the site of RBC destruction.

NURSING DIAGNOSES AND INTERVENTIONS

Potential for impaired skin/tissue integrity related to vulnerability secondary to occlusion of the vessels and impaired oxygen transport to the tissues and skin

Desired outcomes: Patient's skin and tissue remain intact.

1. Assess the patient's skin, especially that over bony prominences and extremities, noting changes in integrity, such as erythema, increased warmth, and blisters.
2. Use a bed cradle to keep pressure of bed linen and blankets off patient's skin.
3. Keep extremities warm to promote circulation. Also encourage moderate exercises or ROM to promote circulation. **Caution:** Avoid any activity or exercise if the signs and symptoms of hemolytic crisis are present.
4. Caution patient about the importance of avoiding trauma or injury to the skin and tissues.
5. Apply dry, sterile dressings or dressing materials, such as Op-Site and Tegaderm, to areas of tissue breakdown. Use aseptic technique to help prevent infection. See "Managing Wound Care," p. 624, for more information.

Alteration in tissue perfusion: Renal, related to decreased circulation secondary to hemolytic obstruction

Desired outcome: Patient has adequate renal perfusion as evidenced by balanced I&O and urinary output ≥30 ml/hr.

1. Monitor I&O. Report urine output <30 ml/hr in the presence of adequate intake.
2. In the absence of renal or cardiac failure, encourage fluid intake to maintain adequate glomerular blood flow.
3. Deliver IV fluid as prescribed to maintain fluid balance and renal perfusion.

Alteration in tissue perfusion: Peripheral and cardiopulmonary, related to decreased circulation secondary to inflammatory process and occlusion of blood vessels with RBCs

Desired outcome: Patient has adequate peripheral and cardiopulmonary perfusion as evidenced by systolic BP ≤10 mm Hg lower than baseline systolic BP, peripheral pulses >2+ on a 0-4+ scale, HR <100 bpm, RR 12-20 breaths/min with normal depth and pattern (eupnea), and normal skin color.

1. Assess BP at frequent intervals and report significant drops (>10 mm Hg from baseline systolic readings).
2. Assess amplitude of peripheral pulses as an indicator of peripheral perfusion. Be alert to pulses ≤2+ amplitude.
3. Be alert to signs of cardiac depression, including decreased BP, increased HR, decreased pulse amplitude, dyspnea, and decreased urine output.
4. Assess for and report indicators of hypoxia or respiratory dysfunction, such as increased RR, dyspnea, SOB, and cyanosis.
5. Assist patient with ROM exercises to enhance tissue perfusion as well as increase joint mobility. **Caution:** Exercise should be avoided if any early signs of hemolytic crisis appear because exercise can aggravate hemolysis.
6. Report significant findings to MD.

Potential for injury related to sensorimotor deficit secondary to peripheral nerve hypoxia

Desired outcomes: Patient is asymptomatic of injury caused by neurologic deficit. Visual disturbance, which can signal hemolytic crisis, is detected and reported to MD promptly.

1. Monitor motor strength and coordination, and report changes in peripheral sensation. Protect patient from extremes of heat and cold if impaired sensation is noted.
2. Accompany patient during ambulation; provide physical support as necessary.
3. Assess patient for visual disturbances, reporting immediately the presence of blurred vision or blindness, which are indicators of hemolytic crisis.
4. Teach patient and significant others the indicators of sensorimotor dysfunction, in-

cluding gait unsteadiness, incoordination, parasthesias, and paralysis. Instruct them to report these indicators promptly if they occur.

Knowledge deficit: Factors that precipitate hemolytic crisis and measures that can help prevent it

Desired outcome: Patient verbalizes knowledge of factors that precipitate hemolytic crisis and measures that can help prevent it.

1. Teach patient and significant others the indicators of hemolytic crisis, including jaundice, dyspnea, SOB, joint or abdominal pain, decreasing BP, and increased HR.
2. Explain to patient and significant others that stress and anxiety can precipitate hemolytic crisis. Stress the importance of maintaining a calm environment for the patient.
3. Teach patient stress reduction techniques, such as meditation and relaxation exercises. See **Health-seeking behaviors:** Relaxation technique effective for stress reduction, p. 49.
4. Discuss with significant others the importance of avoiding stressful and emotional topics with patient.
5. Caution patient to avoid physical stress, which also can precipitate a crisis.

Pain related to hemolysis in the joints secondary to hemolytic crisis

Desired outcome: Patient's subjective evaluation of discomfort improves, as documented by a pain scale.

1. Monitor for the presence of pain. Devise a pain scale with the patient, rating the discomfort on a scale of 0 (no pain) to 10. Administer pain medications as prescribed and document effectiveness using the pain scale.
2. Reassure patient that pain will subside when acute hemolytic episode is over.
3. Elevate extremities to enhance comfort.
4. Apply moist heat packs to the joints to increase circulation and decrease pain.
5. Apply elastic stockings or wraps, if prescribed, to support joints and promote circulation.

See "Pernicious Anemia" for **Fatigue,** p. 397, and **Potential for infection,** p. 397.

PATIENT-FAMILY TEACHING AND DISCHARGE PLANNING

Provide patient and significant others with verbal and written information for the following:
1. Side effects of steroids, if prescribed, including weight gain, headache, and increased appetite.
2. Support groups available for sickle cell anemia and thalassemia.
3. Factors that precipitate hemolytic crisis, such as stress and trauma or chemicals and drugs, depending on etiology.
4. Importance of avoiding infectious processes, such as URIs, and getting prompt medical attention should infection occur.
5. Medications, including drug name, purpose, schedule, dosage, precautions, and potential side effects.
6. Importance of medical follow-up.

Hypoplastic (aplastic) anemia

This type of anemia results from inability of erythrocyte-producing organs, specifically the bone marrow, to produce erythrocytes. The causes of hypoplastic anemia are varied but can include use of antineoplastic or antimicrobial agents, infectious process, pregnancy, hepatitis, and radiation. Approximately half of the patients with hypoplastic anemia have had exposure to drugs or chemical agents, while the remaining half have had immunologic disorders. Hypoplastic anemia most often involves pancytopenia, the depression of production of all three bone marrow elements: erythrocytes, platelets, and granulocytes. Usually the onset of hypoplastic anemia is insidious, but it can evolve quickly in some cases. Prognosis usually is poor for these individuals.

ASSESSMENT

Chronic indicators: Weakness, fatigue, pallor, dysphagia, and numbness and tingling of the extremities.

Acute indicators: Fever and infection (because of decreased neutrophils); bleeding (because of thrombocytopenia); and dizziness, dyspnea on exertion, progressive weakness, and oral ulcerations.

History of: Exposure to chemical toxins or radiation; use of antibiotics, such as chloramphenicol.

DIAGNOSTIC TESTS

1. *CBC with differential:* Low levels of hemoglobin, WBCs, and RBCs; however, RBCs usually appear to be normal morphologically.
2. *Platelet count:* Low.
3. *Bleeding time:* Prolonged.
4. *Bone marrow aspiration:* Will reveal hypocellular or hypoplastic tissue with a fatty and fibrous appearance and depression of erythroid elements.
5. *Cultures:* If infection is suspected.

MEDICAL MANAGEMENT

1. Determination of the cause of anemia.
2. Transfusion with packed RBCs or frozen plasma: See Table 7-1.
3. Transfusion with concentrated platelets: To keep platelet count $>20,000/mm^3$. Hemorrhage occurs less frequently when platelet count is above this level (see Table 7-1).
4. Bone marrow transplantation: In this procedure, 500-700 ml of bone marrow are aspirated from the pelvic bones of the donor and then filtered and infused into the patient. The donated marrow must be antigen-compatible and therefore the donor is usually a twin or sibling. The procedure involves significant risk and requires isolation, asepsis, specialized staff, and extensive supportive therapy, such as platelet transfusions and RBC transfusions.
5. Antibiotic therapy: If infection is found.
6. Reverse isolation: If granulocytes count is $<200/mm^3$.
7. Steroid therapy: To stimulate granulocyte production, although results with adults are not always successful.
8. Oxygen: If anemia is severe.
9. Granulocyte transfusion: See Table 7-1. Although rarely used today, the following are indications for use: documented infection, fever unresponsive to antibiotics, WBC $<500/mm3$, and expectations for bone marrow regeneration.
10. Androgen therapy: An attempt to stimulate bone marrow activity.

Note: Because of the potential for antibody formation, all blood products and transfusions are avoided, if possible, if there is any possibility of later bone marrow transplantation.

NURSING DIAGNOSES AND INTERVENTIONS

Potential for infection related to increased susceptibility secondary to decreased leukocyte production

Desired outcome: Patient is free of infection as evidenced by normothermia, HR ≤100 bpm, RR 12-20 breaths/min with normal depth and pattern (eupnea), and absence of erythema, warmth, and drainage at any invasive or wound sites.

TABLE 7-1 Commonly used blood products

Product	Approximate volume	Indications	Precautions/comments
Whole Blood (WB)	500-510 ml (450 WB; 50-60 anticoagulants)	Acute, severe blood loss; hypovolemic shock. Increases both red cell mass and plasma	Must be ABO and Rh compatible. Do not mix with dextrose solutions; always prime tubing with normal saline. Observe for dyspnea, orthopnea, cyanosis, and anxiety as signs of circulatory overload; monitor VS
Packed Red Blood Cells (RBCs)	250 ml	Increases RBC mass and oxygen-carrying capacity of the blood	Must be ABO and Rh compatible. Less immunologic risk than with WB because some donor antibodies are removed. Less volume, reducing risk of fluid overload
Fresh Frozen Plasma (FFP)	250 ml	Treatment of choice for combined coagulation factor deficiencies and factor V and XI deficiencies; alternate treatment for factor VII, VIII, IX, and X deficiencies when concentrates are not available	Must be ABO compatible. Supplies clotting factors. Usual dose is 10-15 ml/kg body weight
Platelet Concentrate	25-50 ml (volumes may vary; usual adult dose is 5-6 U)	Treatment of choice for thrombocytopenia. Also used for leukemia and hypoplastic anemia	Usual dose is 0.1 U/kg body weight to increase platelet count to 25,000. Administer as rapidly as tolerated. ABO compatibility is preferable, but is expensive and usually not practical. Effectiveness is decreased by fever, sepsis, and splenomegaly. Febrile reactions are common. Use special "platelet" tubing and filter

Continued.

TABLE 7-1 Commonly used blood products—cont'd

Product	Approximate volume	Indications	Precautions/comments
Platelet Concentrate by Platelet Pheresis	200 ml, but may vary	Treatment for thrombocytopenic patients who are refractory to random donor platelets	Involves removing donor's venous blood, removing the platelets by differential centrifuge, and returning the blood to donor. Approximately 3-4 liters of whole blood are processed to obtain a therapeutic dose of platelets. Uses special donors who may be human leukocyte antigen (HLA) matched to the patient
Cryoprecipitate (factor VIII)	10-25 ml	Routine treatment for hemophilia (factor VIII deficiency) and fibrinogen deficiency (factor XIII deficiency)	Made from FFP. Infuse immediately upon thawing
AHG (factor VIII) Concentrates	20 ml	Alternative treatment for hemophilia A	Allergic and febrile reactions occur frequently. Administer by syringe or component drip set. Can store at refrigerator temperature, making it convenient for hemophiliacs during travel
Factor II, VII, IX, X Concentrate	20 ml	Treatment of choice for hemophilia B and factor IX deficiencies	Can precipitate clotting. Allergic and febrile reactions occur occasionally. Contraindicated in liver disease

Albumin*	50 (25%) or 250 (5%) ml	Hypovolemic shock, hypoalbuminemia, plasma replacement for burn patients	The 50 ml version is osmotically equal to 5× its volume of plasma, whereas the 250 ml version is equal to its volume of plasma. The drug is used as a volume expander or in hypoalbuminemic states and is commercially available
Plasma* Protein Fraction (PPF)	250 ml (83% albumin with some alpha and beta globulins)	Volume expansion	Commercially available; expensive. Certain lots reported to have caused hypotension, possibly related to vasoactive amines used in preparation
Granulocyte Transfusion (collected from a single apheresis donor)	200 ml, but may vary	Leukemia with granulocytopenia related to treatment	Not a common treatment. Febrile and allergic symptoms are frequent. Must be ABO compatible

*These products carry no risk of disease transmission.

Note: When administering blood products it is important to recognize that most blood products have risk associated with delivery. Risks include transmission of HIV; Non-A, Non-B hepatitis; hepatitis B; cytomegalovirus; and HTLV-I.

1. Perform meticulous handwashing before patient contact.
2. If appropriate, maintain protective/reverse isolation, using gloves, gown, and masks; make sure that visitors do the same. Discourage delivery of plants and flowers to the room.
3. Report any signs of systemic infection (e.g., fever); obtain prescription for blood, wound, and urine cultures as indicated.
4. Monitor for and report any signs of local infection, such as sore throat or reddened or draining wounds. **Note:** With decreased or absent granulocytes, pus may not form. Therefore it is important to look for other signs of infection.
5. Provide oral care at frequent intervals to prevent oral lesions, which may result in bleeding and infection.
6. Provide and encourage adequate perianal hygiene to prevent rectal abscess. Avoid giving medications or taking temperature rectally.
7. Avoid invasive procedures, if possible.
8. Encourage ambulation, deep breathing, turning, and coughing to prevent problems of immobility, which can result in pneumonia and skin breakdown.
9. Arrange for patient to have a private room when possible.
10. Teach patient and significant others signs and symptoms of infection and the importance of notifying staff or MD promptly if they are noted.

Knowledge deficit: Potential for bleeding (caused by low platelet count) and measures that can help prevent it.

Desired outcome: Patient verbalizes knowledge of the potential for bleeding, as well as measures that can prevent it.

1. Teach patient about the potential for bleeding and the importance of monitoring for hematuria, melena, frank bleeding from the mouth, epistaxis, or coughing up of blood and notifying staff promptly should they occur.
2. Teach patient to use an electric razor and soft-bristled toothbrush.
3. Explain the importance of maintaining regularity with bowel movements to prevent straining and potential bleeding.
4. Teach patient to avoid potentially traumatic procedures, such as enemas and rectal temperatures.
5. Caution patient to avoid using aspirin and aspirin products, which decrease platelet aggregation and further increase the potential for bleeding.

Fatigue related to diminished energy level secondary to decreased oxygen-carrying capacity of the blood

Desired outcome: Patient reports decreasing fatigue, verbalizes tolerance to increasing levels of activity, exhibits RR 12-20 breaths/min with normal depth and pattern (eupnea) and HR ≤100 bpm with activity, and denies the presence of dizziness and headaches.

1. Plan frequent rest periods, providing time for periods of undisturbed rest.
2. Administer oxygen as prescribed to augment oxygen delivery to the tissues. Also encourage deep breathing, which increases oxygenation by enhancing gas exchange.
3. Administer blood components (usually RBCs) as prescribed. Double-check typing with a colleague, and monitor for and report signs of transfusion reaction.
4. Encourage gradually increasing activities to tolerance as patient's condition improves. Set mutually agreed–on goals with patient. For example, "Let's plan this morning's activity goals. Do you feel you could walk up and down the hall once, or twice?" (or appropriate amount, depending on patient's tolerance).

Potential for injury related to sensorimotor alterations secondary to tissue hypoxia occurring with decreased production of erythrocytes

Desired outcome: Patient is asymptomatic of injury caused by sensorimotor deficit.

1. Perform neurologic checks and assess patient's orientation as indicators of cerebral perfusion. If signs of decreasing cerebral perfusion occur, establish precautionary measures (e.g., keeping siderails up and the bed in the lowest position) to protect patient from injury. Request restraints, if indicated.

2. Assess sensorimotor status to help evaluate nervous system oxygenation. Be alert to paresthesias, decreased muscle strength, and altered gait.
3. Prevent injury from heat or cold applications for patients with paresthesias.
4. Do not allow patient to ambulate unassisted if muscle or gait alterations are present.
5. Administer oxygen as prescribed.
6. Teach patient deep-breathing exercises, which may increase oxygenation by enhancing gas exchange.
7. Promptly report indicators of a worsening condition to MD.

See "Pernicious Anemia" for **Alteration in nutrition, p. 397.**

PATIENT-FAMILY TEACHING AND DISCHARGE PLANNING

Provide patient and significant others with verbal and written information for the following:
1. Medications, including drug name, purpose, dosage, schedule, precautions, and potential side effects.
2. Indicators of systemic infection, including fever, malaise, fatigue, as well as signs and symptoms of URI, UTI, and wound infection.
3. Importance of avoiding exposure to individuals known to have acute infections; preventing trauma, abrasions, and breakdown of the skin; and maintaining good nutritional intake to enhance resistance to infections.
4. Signs of bleeding/hemorrhage, which necessitate medical attention: melena, hematuria, epistaxis, ecchymosis, and bleeding of gums.
5. Measures to prevent hemorrhage, such as using electric razor and soft-bristled toothbrush and avoiding activities that can traumatize the tissues.
6. Importance of reporting general symptoms of anemia, including fatigue, weakness, and paresthesias.
7. Importance of avoiding aspirin and aspirin products in the presence of a bleeding disorder.

Polycythemia

Polycythemia is a chronic disorder characterized by excessive production of RBCs. As the number of RBCs increases, blood volume, blood viscosity, and hemoglobin concentration increase, causing excessive workload of the heart and congestion of such organ systems as the liver and kidney. *Secondary polycythemia* results from an abnormal increase in erythropoietin production, for example, due to hypoxia that occurs with chronic lung disease, or it can occur inappropriately, such as with renal tumors. *Polycythemia vera* is a primary disorder of unknown etiology, resulting in increased RBC mass, leukocytosis, and slight thrombocytosis. Because of the increased viscosity and decreased microcirculation, mortality rate is high if the condition is left untreated. In addition, there is a potential for this disorder to evolve into other hematopoietic disorders, such as leukemia.

ASSESSMENT

Signs and symptoms: Headache, dizziness, visual disturbances, dyspnea, thrombophlebitis, joint pain, pruritus, night sweats, fatigue, chest pain, and a feeling of "fullness," especially in the head.

Physical assessment: Hypertension, crackles (rales), cyanosis, ruddy complexion, hepatosplenomegaly.

DIAGNOSTIC TESTS

1. _CBC:_ Increased RBC mass (8-12 million/mm^3), hemoglobin, and leukocytes; overproduction of thrombocytes.

2. *Platelet count:* Increased.
3. *Bone marrow aspiration:* Will reveal RBC proliferation.
4. *Uric acid levels:* May be increased because of increased nucleoprotein, an end product of RBC breakdown.

MEDICAL MANAGEMENT

1. Phlebotomy: Blood withdrawn from the vein to decrease blood volume (and decrease hct to 45%). Usually 500 ml is removed every 2-3 days until the hct is 40%-45%. For the older adult, 250-300 ml is removed.
2. Myelosuppressive agents such as radiophosphorus: To inhibit proliferation of RBCs.
3. Alkylating (myelosuppressive) agents (e.g., busulfan and chlorambucil): To decrease bone marrow function.

NURSING DIAGNOSES AND INTERVENTIONS

Potential alteration in tissue perfusion: Cardiopulmonary and cerebral, related to decreased circulation secondary to phlebotomy

Desired outcome: Patient has adequate cardiopulmonary and cerebral perfusion as evidenced by orientation to person, place, and time; HR <100 bpm; BP >90/60 mm Hg (or within patient's baseline range); absence of chest pain; and RR ≤ 20 breaths/min.

1. During procedure, keep patient recumbent to prevent dizziness or hypotension.
2. Assess for tachycardia, hypotension, chest pain, or dizziness during procedure; notify MD of significant findings.
3. After the procedure, assist patient with sitting position for 5-10 minutes before ambulation to prevent orthostatic hypotension. For more information about orthostatic hypotension, see this same nursing diagnosis in the appendix, "Caring for Patients on Prolonged Bed Rest," p. 656.
4. Teach patient about the potential for orthostatic hypotension and the need to use caution when standing for at least 2-3 days after the phlebotomy.

Alteration in nutrition: Less than body requirements related to decreased intake secondary to anorexia associated with feelings of "fullness" (owing to congestion of organ systems)

Desired outcome: Patient maintains body weight.

1. Weigh patient daily for trend.
2. Encourage patient to eat small, frequent meals.
3. Request that significant others bring in patient's favorite foods if they are unavailable in the hospital.
4. Advise patient to avoid spicy foods and to eat mild foods, which are better tolerated.

Pain related to headache, angina, and abdominal and joint discomfort secondary to altered circulation occurring with hyperviscosity of the blood

Desired outcome: Patient's subjective evaluation of discomfort improves, as documented by a pain scale.

1. Assess patient for the presence of headache, angina, abdominal pain, and joint pain. Devise a pain scale with the patient, rating discomfort from 0 (no pain) to 10.
2. In the presence of joint pain, elevate the extremity; apply moist heat to ease discomfort.
3. Administer analgesics as prescribed.
4. Encourage use of nonpharmacologic pain control, such as relaxation and distraction.
5. Document the degree of relief obtained using the pain scale.
6. Be alert to indicators of peripheral thrombosis, such as calf pain and tenderness.
7. Report significant findings to MD.

Alteration in tissue perfusion: Renal, peripheral, and cerebral, related to decreased circulation secondary to hyperviscosity of the blood

Desired outcome: Patient has adequate renal, peripheral, and cerebral perfusion as evidenced by urinary output ≥30 ml/hr, peripheral pulses >2+ on a scale of 0-4+, adequate muscle strength, and orientation to person, place, and time.

1. Monitor I&O; report urine output <30 ml/hr in the presence of adequate intake, which can signal congestion and decreased perfusion.
2. In the absence of signs of cardiac and renal failure, encourage fluid intake to decrease blood viscosity.
3. Monitor peripheral perfusion by palpating peripheral pulses. Be alert to amplitude ≤2+ and coolness in the distal extremities.
4. Encourage patient to exercise and ambulate to tolerance to enhance circulation.
5. Monitor patient for indicators of impending neurologic damage, such as muscle weakness and decreases in sensation and LOC. If these indicators are present, protect patient by assisting with ambulation or raising siderails on the bed, depending on the degree of deficit.
6. Report significant findings to MD.

PATIENT-FAMILY TEACHING AND DISCHARGE PLANNING

Provide patient and significant others with verbal and written information for the following:
1. Need for continued medical follow-up, including potential for phlebotomy q1-3mo.
2. Medications, including drug name, purpose, dosage, schedule, precautions, and potential side effects.
3. Importance of augmenting fluid intake to decrease blood viscosity.
4. Signs and symptoms that necessitate medical attention: angina, muscle weakness, numbness and tingling of extremities, decreased tolerance to activity, and joint pain.
5. Nutrition: importance of maintaining a balanced diet to increase resistance to infection and limiting intake of iron to help minimize abnormal RBC proliferation.

Section Two   DISORDERS OF COAGULATION

The formation of a visible fibrin clot is the conclusion of a complex series of reactions involving different clotting factors in the blood that are identified by Roman numerals I-XIII. All are plasma proteins except factor III (thromboplastin) and factor IV (calcium ion). When a vessel injury occurs, these factors interact to form the end product, a clot. The clots that are formed are eventually dissolved by the fibrinolytic system.

Platelets play a role in coagulation by releasing substances that activate the clotting factors. At the time of vascular injury, platelets migrate to the site and adhere to each other to form a temporary plug to stop the bleeding.

Thrombocytopenia

Thrombocytopenia is a common coagulation disorder that results from a decreased number of platelets. It can be congenital or acquired, and it is classified according to cause. Common causes include deficient formation of thrombocytes, such as occurs with bone marrow disease or destruction; accelerated platelet destruction, loss, or increased use, such as in hemolytic anemia, diffuse intravascular coagulation, or damage by prosthetic heart valves; and abnormal platelet distribution, such as in hypersplenism and hypothermia. Potential triggers include autoimmune disorder, severe vascular injury, and spleen malfunction. In addition, thrombocytopenia can occur as a side effect of certain chemotherapeutic agents and antibiotics. Regardless of the cause or trigger, the disorder affects coagulation and hemostasis. With chemical-induced thrombocytopenia, prognosis is good after withdrawal of the offending drug. Prognosis for other types is dependent on the form of thrombocytopenia and the individual's response to treatment.

Thrombotic thrombocytopenic purpura (TTP) is a very acute, usually fatal disorder. The etiology is presumed to be a result of a missing factor in the plasma or the presence of a platelet stimulating factor. Platelets become sensitized and clump in blood vessels, occluding them. *Idiopathic thrombocytopenic purpura* (ITP) is believed to be an immune disorder, specifically involving antiplatelet IgG, which destroys platelets. The acute form is most often seen in children (2-6 years of age) and may be related to a previous viral infection. The chronic form is seen more often in adults (18-50 years of age) and is of unknown etiology.

ASSESSMENT

Chronic indicators: Long history of mild bleeding or hemorrhagic episodes. Increased bruising, gum bleeding, and petechiae also may be noted.

Acute indicators: Fever, splenomegaly, acute and severe bleeding episodes, weakness, lethargy, malaise, hemorrhage into mucous membranes, gum bleeding, and GI bleeding. Prolonged bleeding can lead to a shock state with tachycardia, SOB, and decreased LOC. Intracranial hemorrhage also can occur. **Note:** With TTP, the individual may exhibit signs associated with platelet thrombus formation and ischemic organs, such as decreased renal function or cerebral dysfunction.

History of: Recent infection; vaccination; use of chlorothiazide, digitalis, quinidine, rifampin, sulfisoxazole, chloramphenicol, phenytoin.

DIAGNOSTIC TESTS

1. *Platelet count:* Can vary from only slightly decreased to nearly absent. Less than 100,000 μl is significantly decreased; <20,000 results in a serious risk of hemorrhage.
2. *CBC:* Low hgb and hct levels because of blood loss; WBC within normal range.
3. *Bleeding time:* Increased owing to decreased platelets.
4. *Bone marrow aspiration:* Will reveal increased number of megakaryocytes (platelet precursors) in the presence of ITP, but may be decreased with certain causes of thrombocytopenia.
5. *Platelet antibody screen:* May be positive. The test generally is not available.

MEDICAL MANAGEMENT AND SURGICAL INTERVENTIONS

1. Treatment of underlying cause or removal of precipitating agent.
2. Platelet transfusion: Unless platelet destruction is the cause of the disorder (see Table 7-1, p. 403).
3. Corticosteroids: To enhance vascular integrity or diminish platelet destruction.
4. Splenectomy: Removal of an organ responsible for platelet destruction. This is considered viable treatment unless patient has acute bleeding, a severe deficiency of platelets, or a cardiac disorder that contraindicates surgery.
5. Plasma exchange: Removes the antibody or immune complex.

NURSING DIAGNOSES AND INTERVENTIONS

Potential for injury related to increased risk of bleeding secondary to decreased platelet count

Desired outcomes: Patient does not exhibit bleeding or bruising. Platelet count is 150,000-400,000 μl, secretions and excretions are negative for blood, BP is >90/60 mm Hg or within patient's baseline range, HR is ≤100 bpm, and RR is 12-20 breaths/min with normal depth and pattern (eupnea).

1. Teach patient to use electric razor and soft-bristled toothbrush.
2. When appropriate, protect patient from injury by keeping siderails up and padding them.
3. When possible, avoid venipuncture. If performed, apply pressure on site for 5-10 minutes or until bleeding stops.
4. Avoid IM injections. If performed, use small-gauge needles when possible.
5. Monitor platelet count daily.

6. Advise patient to avoid straining at stool or coughing, which increases ICP and can result in intracranial hemorrhage. Obtain prescription for stool softeners, if indicated, to prevent constipation. Teach patient anticonstipation routine as described in **Constipation,** p. 656, in "Caring for Patients on Prolonged Bed Rest."
7. Administer corticosteroids as prescribed.
8. Monitor patient for hematuria, melena, epistaxis, hematemesis, or severe ecchymosis. Teach patient to be alert to and report these indicators promptly.
9. Administer platelets (see Table 7-1, p. 403) as prescribed, and be alert to transfusion reaction.
10. Alert MD to significant findings.

Potential alteration in tissue perfusion: Cerebral, peripheral, and renal, related to decreased circulation secondary to occlusion of small vessels owing to thrombotic component (TTP)

Desired outcome: Patient's cerebral, peripheral, and renal perfusion is adequate as evidenced by orientation to person, place, and time; normoreactive pupillary responses; absence of headaches, dizziness, and visual disturbances; peripheral pulses >2+ on a 0-4+ scale; and urine output ≥30 ml/hr.

1. Assess patient for changes in LOC and pupillary responses.
2. Monitor for headaches, dizziness, or visual disturbances.
3. Palpate peripheral pulses. Be alert to pulses ≤2+.
4. Assess urine output. Adequate perfusion is reflected by urine output ≥30 ml/hr for 2 consecutive hours.
5. Monitor I&O. The patient should be well hydrated (2-3 L/day) to increase perfusion of the small vessels.

Pain related to joint discomfort secondary to hemorrhagic episodes or blood extravasation into the tissues

Desired outcome: Patient's subjective evaluation of pain improves, as documented by a pain scale.

1. Monitor patient for the presence of fatigue, malaise, and joint pain. Devise a pain scale with patient, rating discomfort on a scale of 0 (no pain) to 10.
2. Maintain a calm, restful environment; provide periods of undisturbed rest.
3. Elevate legs to minimize joint discomfort in the lower extremities. Support legs with pillows, avoid gatching the bed at the knee, which could occlude popliteal vessels.
4. Use a bed cradle to decrease pressure on the tissues of the lower extremities.
5. Administer analgesics as prescribed. Document relief obtained using the pain scale.
   Caution: Aspirin is contraindicated because of its antiplatelet action.

Potential fluid volume deficit related to abnormal loss secondary to postsplenectomy bleeding/hemorrhage

Desired outcome: Patient is normovolemic as evidenced by BP ≥90/60 mm Hg (or within patient's normal range); HR ≤100 bpm, RR 12-20 breaths/min with normal depth and pattern (eupnea), nondistended abdomen, and absence of frank bleeding.

1. Monitor postoperative VS for changes that may indicate bleeding (e.g., decreasing BP and HR). Be alert to restlessness as well.
2. Inspect abdomen for presence of distention, and question patient about abdominal pain or tenderness, any of which can signal internal bleeding.
3. Inspect operative site for the presence of frank bleeding.
4. Monitor postoperative platelet count. Approximately 60%-70% of postsplenectomy patients have increased platelet counts. Optimal range for these patients is 200,000-300,000 μl.
5. Report significant findings to MD.

If surgery is performed, see nursing diagnoses and interventions in the appendix, "Caring for Preoperative and Postoperative Patients," p. 637.

PATIENT-FAMILY TEACHING AND DISCHARGE PLANNING

Provide patient and significant others with verbal and written information for the following:
1. Importance of preventing trauma, which can cause bleeding.
2. Seeking medical attention for *any* signs of bleeding or infection. Review the signs and symptoms of common infections, such as URI, UTI, and wound infection (see Table 5-3, p. 298). Also teach patient to assess for hematuria, melena, hematemesis, oozing from mucous membranes, and petechiae.
3. Importance of regular medical follow-up for platelet counts.
4. If discharged on corticosteriods, the potential side effects that necessitate medical attention: acne, moon face, buffalo hump, hypertension, gastric upset, weight gain, thinning of arms and legs, edema, and mood changes. Stress the importance of *not* discontinuing steroids unless directed by MD.
5. Other medications, including drug name, dosage, purpose, schedule, precautions, and potential side effects.

Hemophilia

Hemophilia is a type of hereditary bleeding disorder characterized by a deficiency of one or more clotting factors. Classic hemophilia is caused by deficiency of factors VIII (hemophilia A) and IX (hemophilia B). Both types of hemophilia are sex-linked inherited disorders. Individuals affected are usually males, whereas their mothers and sisters are asymptomatic carriers. This disorder also can occur in females if it is inherited from an affected male and a female carrier or if it is due to X chromosome inactivation during embryologic development. Intracranial hemorrhage is the most common cause of death.

ASSESSMENT

Chronic indicators: Bruising after minimal trauma, joint pain.

Acute indicators: Acute bleeding episodes after minimal trauma. Hemarthrosis is the most common and debilitating symptom, causing painful and swollen joints. Large ecchymoses can occur, as well as bleeding from the gums, tongue, GI tract, urinary tract, or from cuts in the skin. Shock can result from severe bleeding.

DIAGNOSTIC TESTS

1. *PTT:* Prolonged.
2. *Bleeding time:* Prolonged.
3. *Platelet count:* Usually normal.
4. *Activated clotting time:* Prolonged.
5. *Assays of factors VIII and IX:* Will reveal low activity.

MEDICAL MANAGEMENT

1. Factor transfusion: For hemophilia B (see Table 7-1, p. 403).
2. Transfusion of fresh frozen plasma: See Table 7-1, p. 403.
3. Cryoprecipitate: For infusion of factor VIII with classic hemophilia A (see Table 7-1, p. 403). **Note:** Commercially-prepared, heat-treated factor VIII is also being used to decrease the risk of disease and contamination. A product called monoclonal antibody derived factor VIII currently is demonstrating no risk of disease transmission. However, its use is limited by cost and availability.
4. Agents such as desmopressin (DDAVP) and aminocaproic acid (Amicar): To enhance intrinsic mechanisms and decrease the need for factor replacement.

NURSING DIAGNOSES AND INTERVENTIONS

Potential for injury related to increased risk of bleeding secondary to clotting factor deficiency

Desired outcome: Patient is free of bleeding as evidenced by systolic BP ≥90 mm Hg (or within patient's baseline range), HR ≤100 bpm, RR 12-20 breaths/min with normal depth and pattern (eupnea), and secretions and excretions negative for blood.

1. Monitor VS for signs of bleeding, including hypotension and increased HR. Also be alert to patient restlessness.
2. Monitor patient for evidence of bleeding, including swollen joints, abdominal pain, hematuria, hematemesis, melena, and epistaxis.
3. If signs of bleeding occur, elevate the affected area if possible, and apply cold compresses and gentle pressure to the site.
4. When indicated, institute measures to minimize the risk of bleeding from trauma, such as keeping siderails up and padded, assisting with ambulation, and limiting invasive procedures if possible.
5. Teach patient to use electric razor and soft-bristled toothbrush.
6. Do not administer aspirin; caution patient about its anticoagulant action.
7. Administer clotting factors as precribed.

Impaired skin/tissue integrity related to vulnerability secondary to decreased blood circulation to the tissues due to bleeding

Desired outcome: Patient's skin and tissue remain intact.

1. Inspect patient's skin at least q4h, being alert to bruising, pressure areas, and swelling.
2. Apply ice or pressure over sites of intradermal bleeding to promote vasoconstriction.
3. Handle patient gently to minimize the risk of tissue trauma.
4. To enhance perfusion to the tissues and joint mobility, assist patient with ROM exercises daily. However, avoid exercise for 48 hours following bleeding episode to prevent recurrence.
5. To promote circulation to the tissues, assist patient with ambulation when it is tolerated.

Pain related to swollen joints (hemarthrosis)

Desired outcome: Patient's subjective evaluation of discomfort improves, as documented by a pain scale.

1. Monitor patient for the presence of joint discomfort. Devise a pain scale with the patient, rating discomfort on a scale of 0 (no pain) to 10.
2. Apply splints or other supportive devices to joints, immobilizing them in slight flexion.
3. Elevate or position pillows under affected joints for comfort.
4. Administer analgesics as prescribed; avoid aspirin because of its anticoagulant action. Document the pain relief achieved using the pain scale.
5. Assist patient with ambulation as needed.
6. As needed, use ice for its topical analgesia and ability to constrict the vessels, which will decrease swelling. **Caution:** Avoid use of warm thermotherapy for these patients, as it will increase swelling.

PATIENT-FAMILY TEACHING AND DISCHARGE PLANNING

Provide patient and significant others with verbal and written information for the following:

1. Importance of avoiding trauma, and necessity of seeking medical attention for any bleeding.
2. Phone numbers to call in the event of emergency.
3. Procedure in the event of bleeding: application of cold compresses and gentle, direct pressure; elevation of affected part if possible; seek medical attention promptly.
4. Importance of notifying MD if dental procedures need to be done.
5. Importance of lifetime medical follow-up and regular factor transfusions.
6. Importance of frequent assessment of joint function to allow rapid identification and treatment of hemophilic arthritis.

In addition

7. In patients for whom factor VIII prophylaxis is used, patient or significant other will require instruction in the IV administration of factor VIII.

Disseminated intravascular coagulation

Disseminated intravascular coagulation (DIC) is an acute coagulation disorder characterized by paradoxical clotting and hemorrhage. The sequence usually progresses by massive clot formation, depletion of the clotting factors, and activation of diffuse fibrinolysis, followed by hemorrhage (see Table 7-2). DIC occurs secondary to widespread coagulation factors in the bloodstream caused by extensive surgery, burns, shock, neoplastic diseases, and abruptio placentae; extensive destruction of blood vessel walls caused by eclampsia, anoxia, and heat stroke; or damage to blood cells caused by hemolysis, sickle cell disease, and transfusion reactions (see Table 7-3, p. 415). Prompt assessment of the disorder can result in a good prognosis. Usually, affected patients are transferred to ICU for careful monitoring and aggressive therapy.

ASSESSMENT

Clinical indicators: Bleeding of abrupt onset; oozing from venipuncture sites or mucosal surfaces; bleeding from surgical sites; and presence of hematuria, blood in the stool, bruising, pallor, or mottled skin. Symptoms of hypoperfusion can occur, including decreased urine output and abnormal behavior.

Risk factors: Infection, burns, trauma, hepatic disease, hypovolemic shock, severe hemolytic reaction, obstetric complications, and hypoxia. See Table 7-3, p. 415.

DIAGNOSTIC TESTS

1. *Serum fibrinogen:* Low because of abnormal consumption of clotting factors in the formation of fibrin clots.
2. *Platelet count:* Will be <250,000 µl because of the platelet's role in clot formation.
3. *Fibrin split products (FSP):* Increased, indicating widespread dissolution of clots. Fibrinolysis produces FSPs as an end product.
4. *PT:* Increased because of depletion of clotting factors.
5. *PTT:* High because of depletion of clotting factors.
6. *Peripheral blood smear:* Will show fragmented RBCs.
7. *Bleeding time:* Prolonged because of decreased platelets.

TABLE 7-2   Overview of DIC syndrome

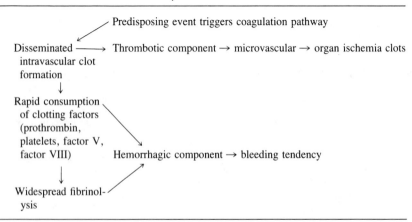

Predisposing event triggers coagulation pathway

Disseminated ⟶ Thrombotic component → microvascular → organ ischemia clots
intravascular clot
formation
↓
Rapid consumption
of clotting factors
(prothrombin,
platelets, factor V,
factor VIII)   Hemorrhagic component → bleeding tendency
↓
Widespread fibrinolysis

MEDICAL MANAGEMENT

1. Identification and treatment of primary disorder: See Table 7-3, below.
2. Anticoagulant therapy: Although this therapy is controversial, heparin may be administered. Heparin interferes with the coagulation process and minimizes consumption of the coagulation factors and activation of the fibrinolytic system. Heparin dose is regulated and determined by the PTT.
3. Compartment replacement of platelets and clotting factors: Replacement of clotting factors by administering fresh frozen plasma, packed RBCs, and platelets may counteract deficiencies. Blood replacement also supports blood volume (see Table 7-1).
4. Epislon-aminocaproic acid (Amicar): Disrupts the fibrinolysis process, and may be administered to stop bleeding.

NURSING DIAGNOSES AND INTERVENTIONS

Alteration in tissue perfusion: Cardiopulmonary, peripheral, renal, and cerebral, related to altered circulation secondary to coagulation/fibrinolysis processes

Desired outcome: Patient has adequate cardiopulmonary, peripheral, renal, and cerebral perfusion as evidenced by BP $\geq$90/60 mm Hg and HR $\leq$100 bpm (or within patient's baseline range); peripheral pulses >2+ on a 0-4+ scale; urinary output $\geq$30 ml/hr; equal and normoreactive pupils; normal motor function; and orientation to person, place, and time.

1. Monitor VS. Be alert to and report decreased BP, increased HR, or decreased amplitude of peripheral pulses, which signal that coagulation is occurring.
2. Monitor I&O; report output <30 ml/hr in the presence of adequate intake, another indicator of the coagulation process.
3. Perform neurologic checks, including orientation, pupil function, and motor response, and assess LOC to evaluate cerebral perfusion. If signs of impaired cerebral perfusion occur, protect patient from injury by instituting such measures as keeping bed in the lowest position and raising siderails.
4. Monitor for hemorrhage from surgical wounds, GI tract, and mucous membranes, which can occur after fibrinolysis.

T A B L E 7 - 3 Clinical conditions that can activate DIC

Obstetric	Liver disease	Tissue damage	Infections
Abruptio placentae	Cirrhosis	Surgery	Viral
Toxemia	Hepatic necrosis	Trauma	Bacterial
Amniotic fluid embolism		Burns	Rickettsial
Septic abortion		Prolonged extracorporeal circulation	Protozoal
Retained dead fetus		Transplant rejection	
		Heat stroke	
Hemolytic processes	**Vascular disorders**	**Miscellaneous**	
Transfusion reaction	Shock	Fat or pulmonary embolism	
Acute hemolysis secondary to infection or immunologic disorder	Aneurysm		
	Giant hemangioma	Snake bite	
		Neoplastic disorder	
		Acute anoxia	
		Necrotizing enterocolitis	

From Miller K. In Swearingen PL et al: Manual of critical care: applying nursing diagnoses to adult critical illness, St Louis, 1988, The CV Mosby Co.

5. Report significant findings to MD; prepare to transfer patient to ICU if condition worsens.

Potential fluid volume deficit related to risk of bleeding secondary to hemorrhagic component of DIC

Desired outcomes: Patient is normovolemic as evidenced by systolic BP ≥90 mm Hg and HR ≤100 bpm (or within patient's normal range), RR 12-20 breaths/min with normal depth and pattern (eupnea), urinary output ≥30 ml/hr, and orientation to person, place, and time. Secretions and excretions are negative for blood; PTT is 30-40 seconds.

1. Monitor VS at frequent intervals, and report significant changes. Be alert to hypotension, tachycardia, and dyspnea, which signal hemorrhage.
2. Monitor coagulation studies, being alert to PTT >40 seconds.
3. Check stool and urine for the presence of blood.
4. Assess puncture sites regularly for oozing or bleeding.
5. Avoid giving IM injections or performing venipunctures for blood drawing.
6. Administer blood products and IV fluids as prescribed.
7. Teach patient to use electric shavers and soft bristled toothbrushes.

Potential for impaired skin/tissue integrity related to decreased circulation secondary to hemorrhage and thrombosis

Desired outcome: Patient's skin and tissue remain intact without bruising or excoriation.

1. Assess patient's skin, noting changes in color, temperature, and sensation, which may signal decreased perfusion and can lead to tissue damage.
2. Eliminate or minimize pressure points by ensuring that the patient turns q2h and using sheepskin on elbows and heels.
3. Keep patient's extremities warm to prevent tissue hypoxia.
4. If patient has areas of breakdown, see interventions in the section "Managing Wound Care," p. 624.

See "Pulmonary Embolus" in "Respiratory Disorders" for **Potential for injury** related to increased risk of bleeding or hemorrhage secondary to anticoagulant therapy, p. 16.

PATIENT-FAMILY TEACHING AND DISCHARGE PLANNING

See patient's primary diagnosis.

Section Three NEOPLASTIC DISORDERS OF THE HEMATOPOIETIC SYSTEM

White blood cells (WBCs), also called leukocytes, are the blood cells responsible both for immunity and the body's response to infectious organisms. Different types of WBCs are classified according to structure, specialized function, and response to dye in the laboratory. The three main classifications of WBCs are granulocytes, lymphocytes, and monocytes, all of which may undergo malignant transformations. The bone marrow has a reserve of approximately 10 times the number of circulating WBCs, which are released into the circulation during an infectious process.

Hodgkin's disease

Hodgkin's disease is a tumor of the lymph tissue. It is distinguished from other lymphomas by the presence of large, variable cells called Reed-Sternberg cells, which proliferate and invade normal lymph tissue throughout the body. Lymph tissue is found in the spleen, liver, bone marrow, lymph nodes, and lymph channels, which connect virtually all tissues. Clinical presentation depends on the degree of malignant cell growth, extent of the invasion, and the tissues that are affected. Hodgkin's disease frequently affects young people, and it can be treated successfully, particularly with early diagnosis and intervention. The etiology of the disorder is unclear, but a hereditary component has been implicated. Although no infectious organism has been identified, infection has been suggested as a potential cause. Long-term survival (20 years) is now possible. *Non-Hodgkin's lymphomas* also can occur, but they tend to affect individuals around the age of 50. This disorder involves an abnormal, malignant lymphocytic invasion of the lymph nodes; however, Reed-Sternberg cells are not involved in the malignancy.

ASSESSMENT

Chronic indicators: Nonspecific symptoms, such as persistent fever, night sweats, malaise, weight loss, and pruritus.

Acute indicators: Worsening of the above symptoms, in addition to unexplained pain in the lymph nodes after drinking alcohol.

Physical assessment: Enlarged (painless) lymph nodes in the cervical area; possible splenomegaly and hepatomegaly.

DIAGNOSTIC TESTS

1. *CBC:* Decreased hgb and hct (confirming anemia); increased, decreased, or normal levels of WBCs.
2. *Platelet count:* May be low.
3. *Lymph node biopsy:* May reveal presence of characteristic Reed-Sternberg cells.
4. *Lymphangiogram:* To determine extent of involvement. Cannulas are inserted into the lymph vessels and contrast medium is injected. Before the procedure, assessment must be made regarding patient allergy to contrast medium.
5. *Biopsy of the bone marrow, lung, liver, pleura, or bone:* May be performed to determine involvement.
6. *Serum alkaline phosphatase:* If elevated, will indicate liver or bone involvement.
7. *ESR:* Will be elevated.
8. *Staging laparotomy with splenectomy and liver biopsy:* To determine extent of the disease and plan of care.
9. *Chest x-ray or abdominal CT scan:* To help determine presence of nodal involvement.

MEDICAL MANAGEMENT

1. Staging: To determine extent of the disease. A simplified description of staging follows (based on Ann Arbor Staging Classification):
   □ *Stage I:* Limited to a single lymph node region or a single extralymphatic organ.
   □ *Stage II:* Involves two or more lymph node regions on the same side of the diaphragm or localized involvement of an extralymphatic organ.
   □ *Stage III:* Involves lymph node regions on both sides of the diaphragm, accompanied by involvement of an extralymphatic region and/or the spleen.
   □ *Stage IV:* Diffuse involvement of one or more extralymphatic region or tissue.
2. Radiation therapy to lymph node regions: For stages I and II.
3. Chemotherapy in combination with radiation: For stages III and IV. One common combination of chemotherapeutic agents includes mechlorethamine hydrochloride (nitrogen mustard), vincristine, prednisone, and procarbazine. For non-Hodgkin's lymphoma, a variety of antineoplastic drugs currently are being used, including cytoxan, vincristine, prednisone, procarbazine, doxorubicin, and bleomycin. For more information, see section "Caring for Patients with Cancer and Other Life-Disrupting Illnesses," p. 659.

NURSING DIAGNOSES AND INTERVENTIONS

See "Pernicious Anemia" for **Fatigue,** p. 397, and **Alteration in nutrition:** Less than body requirements, p. 397. See "Hypoplastic Anemia" for: **Potential for infection,** p.

402. See the appendix for the care of preoperative and postoperative patients, p. 637, and the care of patients with cancer and other life-disrupting illnesses, p. 659.

PATIENT-FAMILY TEACHING AND DISCHARGE PLANNING

Provide patient and significant others with verbal and written information for the following:
1. For patients in stage I or II, the resumption of normal lifestyle with minor adjustments, as prescribed.
2. Continuing radiation or chemotherapy, if prescribed, which is given on an outpatient basis; confirm date and time of next appointment.
3. Signs and symptoms that necessitate medical attention: persistent fever, weight loss, enlarged lymph nodes, malaise, and decreased exercise tolerance.
4. Importance of preventing infection and avoiding exposure to individuals with infection, which is essential because of alterations in WBC count and patient's decreased resistance to infection secondary to therapy. Teach patient the indicators of common infections, such as UTI, URI, and wound infection.
5. Importance of maintaining good nutritional habits to increase resistance to infection.
6. Referral to American Cancer Society and local support groups.
7. Avoiding trauma, which can cause bruising, especially in the presence of thrombocytopenia, which can occur secondary to chemotherapy.
8. If appropriate, measures for assisting patient with ADL.

Acute leukemia

Acute leukemia is an abnormal, malignant proliferation of WBC precursors, also called "blasts." These abnormal cells accumulate in bone marrow, body tissues, and blood vessels and eventually cause malfunction by encroachment, hemorrhage, or infection. In addition, they function inappropriately in response to infection and prevent normal WBC maturation. Moreover, the accumulation of WBCs in the bone marrow alters and decreases the production of RBCs and platelets. The two most common types of acute leukemia are *myelocytic* (arising from the myeloblast, which matures into a neutrophil) and *lymphocytic* (arising from the lymphoblast, which matures into a lymphocyte). Untreated, acute leukemia invariably is fatal, and even with treatment the prognosis varies. Acute lymphocytic leukemia (ALL) most often affects children under 15 years old, while acute myelocytic leukemia (AML) usually affects individuals older than 20 years.

ASSESSMENT

Chronic indicators: Fever, pallor, chills, and weakness, which can be present for days, weeks, or months before acute crisis occurs.

Acute indicators: High fever, diffuse petechiae, ecchymosis, epistaxis, anorexia, nausea, vomiting, headaches, visual disturbances, weakness, feeling of abdominal fullness, lethargy, and seizures.

Physical assessment: Sternal and bone tenderness on palpation, splenomegaly, hepatomegaly, palpable lymph nodes, pallor, papilledema, cranial nerve disorders, and diffuse bleeding of mucous membranes.

DIAGNOSTIC TESTS

1. *CBC:* Hgb will be decreased; WBC value may be low, normal, or elevated, and will include many immature cells.
2. *Bone marrow aspiration:* Will reveal increased numbers of myeloblasts or lymphoblasts.
3. *Platelet count:* Will be decreased.
4. *Uric acid:* Increased secondary to rapid cell destruction.

MEDICAL MANAGEMENT

The goal is the complete remission or reduction in the number of malignant cells and increased number of normal leukocytes by normal hematopoiesis. Secondary management goals are to return the erythrocyte index and thrombocyte count to normal.

1. **Chemotherapy/pharmacotherapy:** Used in combination to produce remission (less than 5% blast cells and no identifiable leukemic cells in the bone marrow). Treatment may be continued for 1½ -2 years after remission occurs. **Note:** For children with ALL, treatment may last up to 3 years.
   □ *For acute lymphocytic leukemia:* Vincristine sulfate and prednisone, asparaginase, and doxorubicin and methotrexate for CNS prophylaxis.
   □ *For acute myelocytic leukemia:* Daunorubicin hydrochloride, cytarabine, and thioguanine.

Note: For lymphocytic leukemias, therapeutic lymphocytapheresis or leukocytapheresis may be performed to decrease tumor load prior to and at the start of chemotherapy. Usually this is performed when the WBC count is >100,000 µl and the individual has signs of decreased circulation.

2. **Transfusion of packed RBCs:** To restore erythrocytes. Leukocyte-poor packed RBCs are preferable to whole blood because febrile reactions to WBCs or platelet antibodies are prevented. Because of possible antibody formation and increased transfusion reactions over time, transfusions are given conservatively, especially in individuals for whom long-term transfusions of platelets and granulocytes are anticipated. Therefore patients may need to tolerate a certain degree of anemia. (See Table 7-1, p. 403.)
3. **Platelet transfusion:** To restore platelet levels to >20,000/mm³. (See Table 7-1, p. 403.)
4. **Bone marrow transplantation:** Available in specialized centers. (See discussion in "Hypoplastic Anemia," p. 402.)

NURSING DIAGNOSES AND INTERVENTIONS

Potential for infection related to increased susceptibility secondary to myelosuppression from disease process or therapy

Desired outcome: Patient is free of infection as evidenced by normothermia, negative cultures, absence of adventitious breath sounds, and the presence of well-healing wounds.

1. Perform meticulous handwashing before caring for patient.
2. Be aware that as the neutrophil count decreases, the risk of infection increases. When the patient becomes neutropenic, perform reverse (protective) isolation using a gown, mask, and gloves; provide a private room.
3. Avoid all invasive procedures (e.g., catheterization) unless absolutely necessary. When such procedures are performed, use strict asepsis.
4. Assist patient with ambulation when possible. Institute turning, coughing, and deep breathing at frequent intervals to help prevent problems of immobility that can result in infection, such as skin breakdown and respiratory dysfunction.
5. Provide oral hygiene and perianal care at frequent intervals.
6. Monitor patient's temperature at frequent intervals. In the presence of any suspected infections, obtain prescription for a culture.
7. Administer antibiotic therapy if prescribed.
8. Deliver transfusion of granulocytes if prescribed.

Potential for injury related to increased risk of bleeding secondary to decreased platelet count

Desired outcomes: Patient is asymptomatic of bleeding as evidenced by BP ≥90/60 mm Hg and HR ≤100 bpm (or within patient's baseline range). Excretions and secretions are negative for blood.

1. Monitor platelet counts. Counts <50,000 dramatically increase the risk of bleeding.
2. Request that patient alert staff to oozing from the gums.
3. Inspect patient's skin, mouth, nose, urine, feces, sputum, emesis, and IV sites for signs for bleeding. Test all excretions for the presence of occult blood.
4. Monitor VS at frequent intervals, and be alert to such signs of bleeding as hypotension and increased HR.
5. Limit invasive procedures to those that are absolutely necessary.
6. Use small-gauge needles when possible. Maintain gentle pressure on injection site until bleeding stops.
7. If bleeding occurs, elevate the affected part, if possible, and apply cold compresses and gentle pressure.
8. Pad side rails to prevent trauma.
9. Administer platelet transfusions as prescribed.
10. Teach patient the signs and symptoms of bleeding and the importance of notifying staff promptly should they occur.
11. Teach patient to use soft-bristled toothbrushes or Toothettes and electric shavers.

Fatigue related to diminished energy level secondary to decreased oxygen-carrying capacity of the blood

Desired outcome: Patient's subjective evaluation of fatigue improves, as documented by a 0-10 scale.

1. Monitor patient's fatigue level, rating it on a scale of 0 (no fatigue) to 10.
2. If prescribed, administer packed RBCs to restore normal erythrocyte level.
3. Assist patient with ADL as necessary.
4. Provide periods of undisturbed rest.
5. Minimize restlessness, which increases oxygen use, by providing frequent comfort measures, such as backrubs.
6. Administer oxygen, if prescribed. Encourage deep-breathing exercises, which may promote oxygenation by enhancing gas exchange.
7. As patient's condition improves, encourage activities to tolerance. Set mutually agreed–on goals, for example, "Can you walk the length of the hall two or three times (or appropriate number, depending on tolerance) this morning?"

Alteration in tissue perfusion: Renal, related to decreased circulation secondary to destruction of RBCs and their precipitation in kidney tubules

Desired outcome: Patient has adequate renal perfusion as evidenced by balanced I&O, urinary output ≥30 ml/hr, and stable weight.

1. Monitor for and report signs of renal insufficiency, including positive fluid balance, weight gain, and urinary output <30 ml/hr in the presence of adequate intake.
2. Maintain adequate hydration of at least 2-3 L/day (unless contraindicated) to enhance urinary flow.
3. Encourage ambulation or in-bed exercises to patient's tolerance to promote renal circulation.
4. Alert MD to significant findings.

See the appendix for nursing diagnoses and interventions for the care of patients with cancer and other life-disrupting illnesses, p. 659.

PATIENT-FAMILY TEACHING AND DISCHARGE PLANNING

Provide patient and significant others with verbal and written information for the following:
1. Importance of avoiding infections and bleeding and measures to prevent same, including the following: Avoid exposure to individuals with infection, maintain good hygiene, avoid situations with high risk of trauma or injury, and report any signs of infection to MD (e.g., fever, chills, and malaise).
2. Side effects of chemotherapy: constipation, alopecia, nausea and vomiting, anorexia,

diarrhea, stomatitis, skin rash, nail changes, hyperpigmentation of the skin, weight gain from steroid use, ecchymosis, and cystitis. For more information, see "Caring for Patients with Cancer and Other Life-Disrupting Illnesses," p. 659.

3. Importance of good nutrition, eating small and frequent meals, consuming 2-3 L/day of fluids (unless contraindicated by cardiac or renal disorder), and using soft-bristled toothbrush and electric razor.

4. Referrals to American Cancer Society, Leukemia Society of America, local support groups, and home care or hospice groups, if appropriate.

Chronic leukemia

Chronic leukemias are characterized by malignant proliferation of abnormal immature WBCs. These abnormal cells eventually infiltrate body tissues and organs and prevent maturation of normal WBCs, thus preventing usual and necessary WBC function. The proliferation of abnormal WBCs in the bone marrow inhibits the formation of other bone marrow elements, including RBCs and platelets. Chronic leukemic cells are a more mature form than is seen in acute leukemias, and they accumulate much more slowly. The two most common types of chronic leukemia are *chronic myelocytic* (involves the myelocyte, precursor of the neutrophil) and *chronic lymphocytic* (involves the lymphocyte). Causes of chronic leukemia are unclear, although chromosomal abnormality is suspected in many cases of myelogenous leukemia. Also implicated are hereditary factors and immunologic defects.

ASSESSMENT

Chronic indicators: Fatigue, anorexia, weight loss, sensation of heaviness in the spleen area, malaise, unexplained low-grade fever, and lymph node enlargement.

Acute indicators: High fever, diffuse petechiae, ecchymosis, epistaxis, anorexia, headaches, visual disturbances, weakness, sensation of abdominal fullness, and lethargy.

DIAGNOSTIC TESTS

1. *CBC with differential:* Elevated WBC; decreased hemoglobin and neutrophils.
2. *Platelet count (thrombocytes):* Low.
3. *Bone marrow aspiration:* Usually identifies abnormal distribution or increased number of cells.

MEDICAL MANAGEMENT AND SURGICAL INTERVENTIONS

For chronic lymphocytic leukemia
1. Chemotherapy: Chlorambucil and prednisone to produce remission.
2. Local irradiation of spleen and lymph nodes: Performed when drug therapy has failed. This procedure frequently is associated with decreasing peripheral leukocyte counts.

For chronic myelocytic leukemia
1. Chemotherapy
   □ *Busulfan and hydroxyurea:* During the stable, chronic phase.
   □ *Daunorubicin, cytarabine, vincristine, prednisone, and thioguanine:* During the acute phase.
2. Splenectomy: May be necessary if the spleen is destroying platelets.

NURSING DIAGNOSES AND INTERVENTIONS

See "Acute Leukemia," p. 419.

Note: Although patients survive longer and the severity of symptoms is less with chronic leukemias, the same principles and nursing interventions apply.

Also see the appendix for nursing diagnoses and interventions for the care of preoperative and postoperative patients, p. 637, (if splenectomy is performed); and for the care of patients with cancer and other life-disrupting illnesses, p. 659.

PATIENT-FAMILY TEACHING AND DISCHARGE PLANNING

See same section in "Acute Leukemia," p. 420.

SELECTED REFERENCES

Consalvo K and Gallagher M: Winning the battle against Hodgkin's disease, RN 49(12):20-25, 1986.

Daenan S et al: Risk of transmission of human immunodeficiency virus (HIV) by heat-treated factor VIII concentrates in patients with severe hemophilia A, Transfusion 27(6):482-484, 1987.

Davoric G: Disseminated intravascular coagulation, Crit Care Nurse 2(6):36-46, 1982.

France-Dawson M: Sickle-cell disease: implications for nursing care, J Adv Nurs 11(6):729-737, 1986.

Griffin JP: Hematology and immunology: concepts for nursing, Norwalk, Conn, 1986, Appleton-Century-Crofts.

Hubner C: Altered clotting. In Carrieri VK et al: Pathophysiological phenomena in nursing, Philadelphia, 1986, WB Saunders Co.

Kinney MR et al, editors: AACN's clinical reference for critical care nursing, ed 2, New York, 1988, McGraw-Hill Book Co.

Lakhani AK: Current management of acute leukemia, Nursing 3(20):755-758, 1987.

Luby CK and Wood PW: Thrombotic thrombocytopenia purpura, Dimens Crit Care Nurs 4(4):209-214, 1985.

Miller K: Hematologic dysfunctions. In Swearingen PL et al: Manual of critical care: applying nursing diagnoses to adult critical illness, St Louis, 1988, The CV Mosby Co.

Peetoom F: Therapeutic cytapheresis. In Westphal RG and Kasprisin DO: Current status of hemapheresis: indications, technology, and complications, Arlington, Va, 1987, American Association of Blood Banks.

Simonson GM: Caring for patients with acute myelocytic leukemia, Am J Nurs 88(3):304-309, 1988.

Westphal RG and Kasprisin DO: Current status of hemapheresis: indications, technology, and complications, Arlington, Va, 1987, American Association of Blood Banks.

8
CHAPTER

Musculoskeletal disorders

Section One   INFLAMMATORY DISORDERS

Arthritis is inflammation of a joint. There are many forms, including osteoarthritis, gouty arthritis, rheumatoid arthritis, Reiter's syndrome, ankylosing spondylitis, systemic lupus erythematosus, and psoriatic arthritis. Osteoarthritis, gouty arthritis, and rheumatoid arthritis are frequently seen in hospitalized patients and therefore are discussed in this section.

Osteoarthritis

Osteoarthritis, also known as degenerative joint disease (DJD), is an extremely prevalent disorder. It is a chronic, progressive disease characterized by increasing pain, deformity, and loss of function. It can be found in any age group, usually following trauma or as a complication of congenital malformation. True joint inflammation seldom is present (except in the distal interphalangeal joints). Hereditary and mechanical factors are suspected to be the primary causes of this process.

Primary osteoarthritis is idiopathic and occurs in the distal interphalangeal (DIP), proximal interphalangeal (PIP), metacarpophalangeal (MCP), and carpometacarpal (CMC) joints of the thumb, hip, knee, first metatarsophalangeal (MTP) joint, and the cervical and lumbosacral spine. *Secondary arthritis* can occur in any joint and usually follows some form of intraarticular injury or extraarticular change that affects joint dynamics. Examples include fractures involving joint surfaces and chronic insults, such as poor posture, obesity, occupational abuse, or a metabolic disease that affects the joint (ochronosis, osteitis deformans, or hyperparathyroidism).

ASSESSMENT

Involvement can range from incidental findings on x-ray to pervasive disease that affects the patient's independence in the performance of ADL.

Signs and symptoms: Onset is insidious, beginning with joint stiffness. It evolves into joint pain, which worsens with activity and is relieved with rest. Signs of local inflammation usually are absent, except occasionally in the DIP, PIP, and CMC joints. There are no systemic signs or symptoms.

Physical assessment: Characteristic findings include limited joint motion, Heberden's nodes (enlargement of the DIP joint), Bouchard's nodes (enlargement of the PIP joint), varus or valgus deformity of the knee, bony enlargement of the joint, and flexion contracture of the knee. Frequently, crepitation is found.

DIAGNOSTIC TESTS

There are no characteristic laboratory studies associated with this disorder.
X-ray studies: May reveal narrowing of the joint space, osteophytosis (bony projections) of the joint margins, bone cysts, sharpened articular margins, and dense subchondral bone.

MEDICAL MANAGEMENT AND SURGICAL INTERVENTIONS

1. **Rest:** The principal therapy for preventing progression. The patient is advised to avoid activities that will stress the joint further. Use of ambulatory assistive devices, splints, or orthotics may be prescribed to allow rest or decreased stress on affected joints, and the patient is instructed in methods that prevent postural strain. Regular rest periods of 30-60 minutes often are advised for patients prone to overworking.
2. **Weight reduction:** For patients for whom excessive weight contributes to the pathology.
3. **Local moist heat:** To decrease stiffness and provide some subjective pain relief. Hydrotherapy with warm water is especially useful in aiding ROM exercises. Patients who cannot afford to purchase a device to supply moist heat may be required to use a

traditional heating pad. Some patients find greater subjective relief from cold packs than from moist heat.

4. **ROM and muscle-strengthening exercises:** May be useful in selected cases to increase joint function and supplement joint strength. Exercises may include passive ROM, active ROM, active-assisted ROM, and isometric and isotonic exercises. The maxim that is followed for the appropriate amount of exercise is that pain that lasts until the next exercise period (or several hours) indicates the exercise was too strenuous.

5. **Intraarticular steroids:** Used by some MDs to provide transient relief of symptoms. However, they do not halt the progression of the disease and run the risk of introducing refractory infections.

6. **Pharmacotherapy:** Includes the use of analgesics and antiinflammatory agents. Analgesics may be necessary to combat the pain associated with DJD. Aspirin, acetaminophen, and the nonsteroidal antiinflammatory agents (see Table 8-1, p. 432) usually are satisfactory, but occasionally narcotic analgesics may be required for short periods following physical therapy or surgical interventions.

7. **Surgical interventions:** Various orthopaedic surgeries may be utilized to correct underlying congenital anomalies or defects created by trauma. Arthroplastic surgery allows damaged joint surfaces to be augmented, repaired, or replaced; while periarticular tissues may be repaired to improve joint strength. Joint replacement has been used to replace most joints, but the greatest success has been found with the hip (see p. 473) and knee (see p. 476) implant arthroplasties. In joints that are chronically infected or not amenable to standard or implant arthroplasties, an arthrodesis (joint fusion) may provide joint stability and permit some function. Arthroscopy may be used to debride osteoarthritic joints of loose bodies, osteophytes, frayed cartilage, and hypertrophied synovium. Valgus osteotomy has been successful in transferring the weightbearing stresses of the proximal tibia from the medial compartment to the usually less diseased lateral compartment.

8. **Splints and orthotic devices:** May be used to supplement joint strength or protect the joint from excessive strain.

9. **Assistive devices:** A great variety have been developed to help patients perform ADL independently, even in cases of significant joint function loss. Examples include stocking helpers, built-up eating utensils, pickup sticks, and raised toilet seats.

NURSING DIAGNOSES AND INTERVENTIONS

Pain related to joint changes and corrective therapy

Desired outcome: Patient's subjective evaluation of pain control improves, as documented by a pain scale.

1. Help patient devise a rating system (e.g., a scale of 0-10) to rate pain and analgesic relief.
2. Administer analgesics and antiinflammatory agents as prescribed and document their effectiveness using the pain scale.
3. Instruct patient in the use of nonpharmacologic methods of pain control, including guided imagery; graduated breathing (as in Lamaze); enhanced relaxation; massage; biofeedback; cutaneous stimulation (*via* a counterirritant, such as oil of wintergreen); transcutaneous electrical nerve stimulation (TENS) device; warm or cool thermotherapy; music therapy; and tactile, auditory, visual, or verbal distractions.
4. Use traditional nursing interventions to counteract the pain, including backrubs, repositioning, and encouraging the patient to verbalize feelings.
5. Incorporate rest, local warmth, and elevation of the affected joints, when possible, to help control discomfort.
6. Advise patient to coordinate the time of peak effectiveness of the antiinflammatory agent with periods of exercise or mandatory use of arthritic joints.
7. Instruct patient in the use of moist heat and hydrotherapy, which will help reduce long-term discomfort.

Knowledge deficit: Use of a heating device

Desired outcome: Patient verbalizes and demonstrates proper use of the heating device.

1. Assess patient's baseline knowledge in the use of a heating device.
2. As appropriate, provide patient with instructions for the proper use of moist or dry heat. Because older individuals may have decreased neuronal function and skin that is more easily traumatized, instruct them in the use of a thermometer (with adequate-size numbers for reading) or a controlled warming device.
3. Caution patient about the potential for increasing his or her tolerance to heat. This can occur when the heat has been used for long periods of time, and may cause the patient to feel the need for a higher degree of heat than that which is safe.

Impaired physical mobility related to adjustment to a new walking gait secondary to the use of an assistive device

Desired outcomes: Patient demonstrates adequate upper body strength for use of an assistive device. Patient demonstrates appropriate use of the assistive device on flat and uneven surfaces.

1. Before ambulation, ensure the necessary strength of the patient's upper extremities for using the assistive device by incorporating the interventions listed in **Potential for disuse syndrome,** p. 653, in the appendix. Triceps strength is especially important for ambulation with crutches or a walker. Having patients push down on the bed as they extend their arms to lift their buttocks off the bed will strengthen the triceps muscles.
2. Provide a thorough discussion with a demonstration to teach the patient how the assistive device is used.
3. When fitting crutches, ensure that the patient is wearing flat-heeled, properly fitting, supportive shoes. With the patient standing and with his or her elbows slightly flexed at 10-30 degrees, be sure that the crutch tops rest 1-1.5 inches (or the width of two fingers) below the axillae. Be aware that complaints of upper extremity paresthesia may be indicative of improperly fitted crutches. Ensure that the crutches have rubber tips to prevent slipping and rubber axillary pads to reduce pressure at the axillae.
4. Once the assistive device is in position, repeat the instructions and then supervise the ambulation. Ambulation should begin in small increments on level ground and eventually progress to all surfaces the patient is expected to encounter after hospital discharge.
5. Ensure that before discharge, the patient is able to demonstrate independence in ambulation with the assistive device on level surfaces and stairs and with getting in and out of a car.

See "Gouty Arthritis" for **Knowledge deficit:** Disease process, medication regimen, and potential drug side effects, p. 428. See "Ligamentous Injuries" for **Knowledge deficit:** Potential for joint weakness and techniques for applying elastic wraps and assessing neurovascular status, p. 436. See "Fractures" for **Knowledge deficit:** Potential for infection, p. 454. See the appendix for nursing diagnoses and interventions for the care of patients on prolonged bed rest, p. 651, and for care of preoperative and postoperative patients (if surgery is performed), p. 637.

PATIENT-FAMILY TEACHING AND DISCHARGE PLANNING

Provide patient and significant others with verbal and written information for the following:
1. Medications, including drug name, dosage, purpose, schedule, precautions, and potential side effects.
2. Importance of systemic rest as well as rest of the affected joints.
3. Weight reduction, if it is appropriate for the patient.
4. Proper use of moist heat.
5. Necessity of ROM and muscle-strengthening exercises.

6. Use of splints or orthotics, including care and cleansing and where to get replacements.
7. Use, care, and replacement of assistive device.
8. If surgery was performed, the precautions related to the procedure, wound care (see "Wounds Closed by Primary Intention," p. 624), indicators of wound infection (i.e., persistent redness, swelling, increasing pain, wound drainage, local warmth, and fever), or complications of surgery.
9. Importance of follow-up care and the date of the next appointment; a phone number to call should any questions arise.

Gouty arthritis

Gout is the most prevalent form of crystal-induced synovitis, which results from an abnormal amount of urates. *Primary gout,* an inherited metabolic disorder, is caused by either excess production or underexcretion of urates. *Secondary gout* results from other conditions in which uric acid is retained or excessively produced, such as lead poisoning, use of thiazide diuretics, chronic renal disease, myeloproliferative disease, hemoglobinopathies, cancer chemotherapy, or multiple myeloma. The pathophysiology involves the formation of tophus (nodular deposition of monosodium urate monohydrate crystals), which causes a pronounced inflammatory response. Tophi may be found in synovial tissues, cartilage, periarticular tissues, tendon, bone, and the kidneys. There appears to be a relationship between rapid fluctuations in the level of serum uric acid and an acute gouty attack. Uric acid renal calculi, nephrosclerosis, and gouty nephritis can accompany this process.

ASSESSMENT

Chronic indicators: Joint changes similar to those of osteoarthritis (see p. 424). Uncontrolled or untreated gout results in a progressive, chronic disorder that causes severe joint deformity and loss of function. Hypertension, uric acid nephrolithiasis, renal failure, and obesity are associated with this process.

Acute indicators: Sudden onset, acute inflammation, and an excruciatingly painful joint that presents with erythema, joint effusion, restricted motion, warmth, and tenderness. Systemic indicators include tachycardia, anorexia, fever, headache, and malaise. Although usually it is monoarticular, polyarticular attacks have been noted with this disorder.

Physical assessment: Tophi may be noted as subcutaneous nodules on the hands, feet, olecranon bursa, prepatellar bursa, and ears. The most commonly affected joint is the metatarsophalangeal joint of the great toe, but the tarsal joints, ankles, and knees also are commonly affected.

History of: Recent surgery, trauma, oral intake high in purines, alcoholic excess, infection, use of diuretics, or severe medical illness (e.g., cerebrovascular accident or myocardial infarction).

DIAGNOSTIC TESTS

1. *Serum tests:* Uric acid frequently is elevated above the normal 7.5 mg/dl during an acute attack unless the patient is taking medications that depress the serum levels of uric acid (large doses of ASA, methyldopa, phenothiazines, x-ray contrast agents, warfarin, sulfinpyrazone, or clofibrate). There also will be leukocytosis and an elevated sedimentation rate.
2. *Joint fluid aspiration:* For examination of wet smears to reveal presence of monosodium urate (MSU) crystals.
3. *Tophus aspiration:* Provides identification of typical monosodium urate crystals.
4. *X-ray:* Will demonstrate no change early in the disease, but with chronic disease there will be radiolucent urate tophi (which look like punched-out areas on the x-ray)

adjacent to soft tissue tophi. During acute attacks there is radiographic evidence of periarticular or intraarticular soft tissue swelling.

MEDICAL MANAGEMENT AND SURGICAL INTERVENTIONS

1. **Pharmacotherapy**
   - ☐ *Colchicine:* Drug of choice during the acute phase. It is believed that it mediates the inflammatory response caused by the urate crystals. Usual dosage is 0.5 mg qh or 1 mg q2h until either the pain is controlled or side effects appear. Side effects include nausea, vomiting, abdominal cramping, and diarrhea. To reduce the incidence of side effects, the initial dose may be given IV. Colchicine is contraindicated in patients with inflammatory bowel disorders, significant hepatic disease, or renal disease.
   - ☐ *Corticosteroids:* May control acute attacks but must be combined with colchicine because discontinuation of the steroid often results in a relapse.
   - ☐ *Nonsteroidal antiinflammatory agents:* May be used for chronic or acute forms of the disease (see Table 8-1, p. 432).
   - ☐ *Analgesics (e.g., acetaminophen with codeine or oxycodone preparations):* To control the pain of gout, which usually is excruciating.
2. **Joint rest:** Mandatory in acute phases and should include complete bed rest with elevation of the inflamed joint. Sometimes, topical cooling (ice applications to the joint) is prescribed to aid in reducing inflammation.
3. **Management between attacks:** May be accomplished with the following:
   - ☐ *Colchicine:* Prophylactic or interim use.
   - ☐ *Uricosuric agents (e.g., probenecid or sulfinpyrazone):* Dosage is determined by the patient's serum uric acid levels. Nonrestricted patients should maintain a fluid intake of at least 2-3 L/day or use an alkalinizing agent, such as sodium bicarbonate, which maintains urinary pH above 6.0 to prevent uric acid calculi. Salicylate drugs are avoided because they antagonize the effects of uricosuric agents.
   - ☐ *Allopurinol, a xanthine oxidase inhibitor:* Lowers serum uric acid, decreases the concentration of uric acid in the urine, and mobilizes the uric acid crystals in tophi. Dosage varies, depending on serum uric acid levels. Because hepatotoxicity and renal calculi can occur, the drug is used cautiously in patients with renal and hepatic disease.
4. **Diet therapy:** Complete restriction of purines (metabolic precursors to uric acid) seldom is prescribed because purines are found in most protein foods, and rigid dietary restriction would be unhealthy; however, visceral meats generally are high in purines and should be avoided. Alcoholic beverage intake should be limited because of its connection with the precipitation of acute attacks.
5. **Surgical intervention:** Gouty tophi are excised when they erode through the skin or cause mechanical impairment. Chronic joint involvement may require surgical procedures discussed in "Osteoarthritis," p. 425.

NURSING DIAGNOSES AND INTERVENTIONS

Knowledge deficit: Disease process, medication regimen, and potential drug side effects

Desired outcome: Patient verbalizes knowledge of the disease process, medication regimen, and potential drug side effects.

1. Assess patient's knowledge of the disease process, medication regimen, and potential side effects of the drugs. As appropriate, teach the pathophysiology of the disease. In addition, when secondary gout is suspected, inform patient about the primary disease causing the gout.
2. Provide thorough instructions for the medication therapy, including rationale, dosage, schedule, precautions, and potential side effects.
3. When initiating colchicine treatment for an acute attack, assess patient carefully for preexisting bowel, liver, or renal disease. Instruct patient to notify the staff promptly when pain has abated or nausea, vomiting, abdominal cramping, or diarrhea occur.

Colchicine dosages are usually decreased or terminated at the onset of any of these indicators.

4. For patients taking uricosuric agents, stress the potential for the development of uric acid renal calculi and the need for at least 2-3 L/day of fluid in nonrestricted patients or the use of an alkaline ash diet or an alkalinizing agent, such as sodium bicarbonate, to ensure that the urine pH remains >6. Instruct these patients in the use of pH test tape to check urine pH.
5. Caution patients taking allopurinol of the potential for renal and hepatic complications.
6. Caution patients taking narcotic analgesics of the potential for altered sensorium, and advise them to avoid using machinery, driving, or performing other activities requiring alertness.

Knowledge deficit: Proper care of inflamed joints

Desired outcomes: Patient verbalizes knowledge of the importance of resting the joint during periods of inflammation and demonstrates elevation of the joint, assisted ROM, and use of thermotherapy.

1. Assess patient's knowledge about care of inflamed joints.
2. As appropriate, teach patient the importance of elevating the inflamed joint with pillows above the level of the heart. Explain the rationale to the patient.
3. Perform passive ROM of the joints bid (or have patient perform assisted ROM).
4. Instruct patient to increase joint ROM as the inflammation subsides, following the process described under the nursing diagnosis **Potential for disuse syndrome,** p. 653, in the appendix.
5. Advise patient to use thermotherapy as prescribed, using care to ensure adequate protection of the involved skin.

Knowledge deficit: Assessments and preventive measures for uric acid renal calculi

Desired outcome: Patient verbalizes knowledge of the assessments and preventive measures for uric acid renal calculi.

1. Assess patient's knowledge of the assessments and preventive measures for uric acid renal calculi.
2. As appropriate, teach patient the indicators of renal calculi (e.g., severe renal colic, costovertebral angle tenderness, chronic UTI, urinary retention, nausea, vomiting, and pain located in the flank, side, lower back, suprapubic area, groin, labia, or scrotum). Instruct patient to alert MD if any of these signs and symptoms occur after hospital discharge.
3. Ensure that patient is knowledgeable about preventive measures, including a fluid intake of at least 2-3 L/day in nonrestricted patients, alkalinating measures to ensure urinary pH >6, and use of pH test tape to monitor urinary pH.

Alteration in nutrition: More than body requirements of purine or alcohol

Desired outcome: Patient demonstrates knowledge of the prescribed dietary regimen by planning three meals a day for 3 successive days.

1. In severe disease forms, it may be necessary to restrict the patient's intake of purine-containing foods. High-purine-content foods include bouillon, broth, consomme, gravy, organ meats, mackerel, yeast, poultry, meats, fish, shellfish, scallops, asparagus, beans, lentils, mushrooms, peas, and spinach. Ensure that the patient receives consultation with verbal instruction in the dietary regimen as well as written instructions to take home.
2. Inform patient that excessive use of alcohol has been known to precipitate gout attacks.

See "Osteoarthritis" for **Pain,** p. 425. See the appendix for nursing diagnoses and interventions for the care of preoperative and postoperative patients, p. 637, and for the care of patients on prolonged bed rest, p. 651.

PATIENT-FAMILY TEACHING AND DISCHARGE PLANNING

Provide patient and significant others with verbal and written information for the following:

1. Pathophysiology of the patient's form of gout.
2. Medications, including drug name, purpose, dosage, schedule, precautions, and potential side effects.
3. Indicators of renal calculi (see "Renal Calculi," p. 110).
4. Diet therapy if appropriate, and the importance of avoiding excessive alcohol consumption.
5. Use of therapeutic local and systemic rest.

Rheumatoid arthritis

Rheumatoid arthritis (RA) is the most common inflammatory arthritis. This systemic disease is characterized by remissions and exacerbations of inflammation of the connective tissue throughout the body. Although many connective tissues have potential for involvement (heart, blood vessels, lungs, spleen, and kidney) and generalized systemic effects may be noted, this discussion centers on the arthritic aspects of this process. RA most commonly affects the synovial joints, but the effects of this disease are highly variable. Recent research into the pathogenesis of RA indicates that the chronic inflammatory reaction in the rheumatoid synovial membrane is the result of active immune response. The originating stimulus of this response is still unknown but it has been speculated to be food allergies; hereditary deficit; or infections by parvovirus, Epstein-Barr virus (EBV), and rubella. The disease onset and progression can be rapid and fulminating or slow and chronic.

The inflammatory process results in chronic synovitis with the formation of pannus, an inflammatory exudate that accumulates over the surface of the synovial membrane, eventually eroding cartilage, bone, ligaments, and tendons. Involvement of connective periarticular tissues results in loss of support structures and leads to characteristic joint changes, which further contribute to the pathology.

ASSESSMENT

Acute indicators: Morning stiffness lasting >30 minutes, symmetrical joint involvement, joint effusion, periarticular edema, pain, local warmth, and erythema. Joint stiffness usually is worsened by stress placed on the joint, and it can follow periods of inactivity as well. Prodromal signs and symptoms may include malaise, weight loss, vague periarticular pain, low-grade fever, and vasomotor disturbances resulting in paresthesias and Raynaud's phenomenon. Sometimes, an acute exacerbation is related to stress, such as infection, surgery, trauma, emotional strain, or the postpartum period.

Chronic indicators: Progressive thickening of the periarticular tissues, subluxation, fibrous ankylosis, atrophy of skin and muscle, severe limitation of ROM with progressive loss of function, joint and muscle contractures, juxtaarticular and generalized osteoporosis, synovial cysts (ganglion on the dorsum of the wrist or Baker's cyst in the popliteal space), tendon rupture, nerve entrapment (carpal or tarsal tunnel syndrome), dryness of the eyes and mucous membranes, and subcutaneous nodules. Some patients develop splenomegaly and enlarged lymph nodes.

DIAGNOSTIC TESTS

1. *Serologic studies:* Many are performed to detect certain macroglobulins that comprise the rheumatoid factor.
   □ *Latex fixation test:* Positive in 75% of the individuals with RA. Higher titers are associated with more severe clinical disease. Because false positives are common, a definite diagnosis cannot be made on this test alone.
   □ *Antinuclear antibodies:* May appear, but titers are lower in RA than in systemic lupus erythematosus.

☐ *ESR:* If elevated, is an indicator of inflammation.

☐ *Gamma globulins, especially IgM and IgG:* If elevated, strongly suggest an autoimmune process as the cause of RA.

☐ *Normocytic hypochromic anemia:* Usually present secondary to long-standing inflammation.

☐ *WBC count:* Usually normal or slightly elevated, but leukopenia can be present, especially in the presence of splenomegaly.

2. *Joint fluid aspiration from the involved joint:* May reveal synovial fluid greater in volume than normal, opaque and cloudy yellow in appearance, glucose level lower than serum level, and elevated WBC and leukocytes in the presence of RA.

3. *X-ray studies of the involved joints:* In the early phases will illustrate soft tissue swelling, erosion of joint surfaces normally covered by articular cartilage, and osteoporosis of adjacent bone. In long-standing disease, the joint will show instability, subluxation, joint space narrowing, bone cyst formation, and concurrent osteoarthritic changes. Special attention is paid to upper cervical vertebrae, where subluxation of C-1 or C-2 can result in life-threatening neurologic complications.

4. *Radionuclide joint scanning:* To identify inflamed synovium in patients with appropriate symptoms.

MEDICAL MANAGEMENT AND SURGICAL INTERVENTIONS

1. Systemic rest: Mandatory throughout all phases of this disease. In exacerbations, bed rest may be required until significant clinical joint findings have decreased for 2 weeks. During this period, proper joint positioning is essential to prevent contractures. Concurrent physical therapy is prescribed to put joints through passive ROM at least once a day. During remissions, the patient should receive 8 hours of sleep each night and 1-2 hours rest at midday. Any increase in symptomatology necessitates increasing the amount of rest.

2. Emotional support: To lessen stress and help patients deal with fear, feelings of helplessness, disability, and the many losses they will incur.

3. Rest of inflamed joints: Imperative. Unstable joints should be splinted or braced to provide support and put through passive ROM at least daily while inflamed. Reduction of inflammation in affected joints is aided by articular rest. Relaxing hip and knee muscles to prevent contractures is best performed by prone positioning for at least 15 minutes tid. Sitting is not an effective method of joint rest and should be avoided for prolonged periods.

4. Joint exercise: Essential to maintain joint function and muscle strength, with the amount increasing as inflammation decreases. A graded exercise program should include the following: passive ROM, active-assisted ROM, active ROM, and resistive ROM with gradually increasing levels of resistance. Isometric exercise is used to maintain muscle strength during active joint inflammation. Any signs of increasing joint inflammation are cause for regression to a less stressful exercise until joint inflammation has again decreased. Inflamed weight-bearing joints should be protected from stress by orthotics and ambulatory adjuncts (cane, crutches, and walker, or a wheel chair if imperative.)

5. Thermotherapy: To relax muscles and reduce pain. Cold therapy is used during inflammatory stages to reduce pain. Moist heat (especially warm tub baths) is useful to exercise stiffened joints, using the heat and buoyancy to aid motion. When submersion is not possible, use of moist warm cloths before exercise will decrease the patient's discomfort. Caution must be employed to avoid thermal injury to atrophied skin over affected joints.

6. Assistive devices: For example, stocking helpers, raised toilet seats, pickup sticks.

7. Antiinflammatory agents: See Table 8-1, p. 432. Aspirin (ASA) is the mainstay of pharmacotherapy in RA. Dosage is determined by the ability to provide adequate symptom relief without toxic reactions. Adult dosages may reach 4-6 grams, producing serum levels of 20-30 mg/dl. Tinnitus and GI upset are prodromal signs of toxicity, indicating a need to reduce dosages until these symptoms clear. GI upset may be decreased by taking ASA with food or antacids or using enteric coated forms. **More**

TABLE 8-1   Nonsteroidal antiinflammatory agents

Generic name	Common brand names	Usual daily dosage (mg)
acetylsalicylic acid	Aspirin	650-1,300 q4h
choline salicylate	Arthropan	650 q4-6h
choline magnesium trisalicylate	Trilisate	1,000-1,250 bid
fenoprofen calcium	Nalfon	300-600 qid
ibuprofen	Motrin, Advil, Nuprin	200-400 qid
indomethacin	Indocin	20-50 tid
magnesium salicylate	Mobidin	600-1,200 tid or qid
meclofenamate sodium	Meclomen	50 tid or qid
mefenamic acid	Ponstel	250 qid
naproxen	Naprosyn	250-375 qid
naproxen sodium	Anaprox	275 q6-8h
oxyphenbutazone	Tandearil	100 tid
piroxicam	Feldene	20 qd
sulindac	Clinoril	150-200 bid
tolmetin sodium	Tolectin	200-400 mg tid
nabumetone	Relafen	1,000 mg qhs
diclofenac sodium	Voltaren	50-75 mg bid

Butazolidin

potent antiinflammatory agents also used in the treatment of RA include the following:
- □ *Antimalarials (chloroquine phosphate, 250 mg/day; or hydroxychloroquine sulfate, 200 mg/day):* Result in long-term control of symptoms for some patients. Side effects include keratitis and retinitis, necessitating periodic ophthalmic examinations for early assessment of complications.
- □ *Chrysotherapy (use of medicinal gold salts):* Benefits up to 60% of patients with RA through an unknown mechanism of action. Contraindications include severe drug allergies, previous gold toxicity, hepatotoxicity, or hematologic pathology. It is administered by weekly injections of increasing dosage (up to 50 mg/week) until clinical results are noted or toxic reactions encountered. A significant antiinflammatory effect often takes several months of therapy. Potential toxic reactions include exfoliative dermatitis, bone marrow depression, stomatitis, and nephritis. Before each injection, the patient should have a urinalysis (for proteinuria and microscopic hematuria) and CBC with differential for hemoglobin, platelet levels, and WBC count. The patient also should be assessed for skin or mucous membrane lesions. Periodic hepatic function tests should be done, and the patient should be advised to avoid direct sunlight.
- □ *Corticosteroids:* To control the symptoms of RA, but they do not substantially alter the progression of the disease. Cessation of the steroid frequently results in exacerbation of symptoms, so steroids usually are used only to carry the patient through a severe flareup or to control concurrent connective tissue disease (e.g., eye lesions or pericarditis). They are used cautiously at the lowest dose possible to control signs of inflammation. Deflazacort is a new corticosteroid with bone-sparing properties for RA patients with significant osteoporosis. Intraarticular steroids may be used on occasion (no more than 4 times a year) for especially troublesome joints.
- □ *Penicillamine:* Used *only after* all other methods have been ineffective in controlling symptoms. Fifty percent of patients taking this drug will develop side effects, including thrombocytopenia, leukopenia, aplastic anemia, nephrotic syndrome,

and immune complex disease (myasthenia gravis). This medication is taken between meals to aid absorption.

8. **Surgical interventions**

☐ *Synovectomy:* To remove the inflamed synovium and prevent pannus formation. This may be performed either by surgical excision or instillation of a radioactive solution to "burn" the synovium.

☐ *Arthroplasty:* To correct periarticular weakness, which in turn will correct subluxation and external stressors on the diseased joint.

☐ *Osteotomy:* To correct disruptive force vectors placed on the joint surfaces or to correct bony malalignments.

☐ *Carpal tunnel release, tarsal tunnel release, ganglionectomy, tendon repair, arthrodesis, and removal of Baker's cyst:* Examples of surgeries performed to correct concurrent connective tissue defects associated with RA.

☐ *Implant arthroplasty:* Significantly increases functional capabilities for selected RA patients. They are used for many joints, but the greatest success has been seen with the hip and knee. The rate of success is dependent on the joint, patient's general condition, stage of disease, and rate of compliance with therapy.

☐ *Arthroscopy:* May be used for diagnosis or treatment. Bodies may be excised, plica (redundant tissue) incised, and cartilage abraded (or "shaved") through an arthroscope.

☐ *Arthrodesis:* Although less often used since the advent of implant arthroplasty, joint fusion allows for a stable, painless joint in severely affected joints with pronouncedly weakened periarticular tissues and muscle atrophy.

9. **Experimental therapies under trial in the United States:** Include additional nonsteroidal antiinflammatory agents, an anthelminitic agent (Levamisole), cyclophosphamide, azathioprine, methotrexate, chlorambucil, plasmapheresis, leukapheresis, and irradiation of the lymph nodes. Experimental surgeries include various new implant designs and joint transplantation.

NURSING DIAGNOSES AND INTERVENTIONS

Fatigue related to pathophysiology of RA and immobility

Desired outcome: Patient verbalizes a decrease in or relief from fatigue.

1. Assess the time the fatigue occurs, its relationship to required activities, and activities that relieve or aggravate the symptoms.
2. Investigate the patient's sleep pattern and intervene as appropriate to ensure adequate rest (see **Sleep pattern disturbance** in "Caring for Patients with Cancer and Other Life-Disrupting Illnesses," p. 691).
3. Assess for dietary and physiologic sources of fatigue and intervene to correct as needed.
4. Determine whether patient's pain is adequately controlled and intervene with pharmacologic and nonpharmacologic treatments as indicated.
5. Assess patient for stress or psychoemotional distress; intervene as necessary or seek assistance from an appropriate clinical specialist in psychiatric nursing.
6. Discuss the rationale for a graded exercise regimen to increase endurance and strength. Encourage patient to set realistic goals and post these goals to facilitate participation of associated health care professionals.
7. Pace activities and intersperse rest periods of at least 90 minutes in duration.
8. Teach patient use of adjunctive and assistive devices.

See "Osteoarthritis" for **Pain,** p. 425, **Knowledge deficit:** Use of heating device, p. 425, and **Impaired physical mobility** related to adjustment to new walking gait, p. 426. See "Gouty Arthritis" for: **Knowledge deficit:** Disease process, medication regimen, and potential drug side effects, p. 428, and **Knowledge deficit:** Proper care of inflamed joints, p. 429. See "Ligamentous Injuries" for **Knowledge deficit:** Need for elevation of the involved extremity, thermotherapy, and exercise, p. 435, **Knowledge deficit:** Care and assessment of the casted extremity, p. 435, and **Knowledge deficit:**

Potential for joint weakness, and the techniques for applying elastic wraps and assessing neurovascular status, p. 436. See "Torn Anterior Cruciate Ligament" for **Potential fluid volume deficit** related to abnormal loss secondary to postsurgical hemorrhage or hematoma, p. 442. See "Fractures" for **Self-care deficit,** p. 452, and **Knowledge deficit: Potential for disuse osteoporosis,** p. 453. See "Amputation" for **Knowledge deficit: Postsurgical exercise regimen,** p. 467. See "Total Hip Arthroplasty" for **Knowledge Deficit: Potential for infection** caused by foreign body reaction to the endoprosthesis, p. 475. See "Intervertebral Disk Disease" in Chapter 4 for **Knowledge deficit:** Pain control measures, p. 193. See the appendix for nursing diagnoses and interventions for the care of preoperative and postoperative patients, p. 637, and the care of patients on prolonged bed rest, p. 651. For psychosocial nursing interventions, see "Caring for Patients with Cancer and Other Life-Disrupting Illnesses," p. 690.

PATIENT-FAMILY TEACHING AND DISCHARGE PLANNING

Provide patient and significant others with verbal and written information for the following:
1. Treatment regimen, including physical therapy, systemic rest, rest of inflamed joints, exercise, and thermotherapy. For more information, see "Ligamentous Injuries" for **Knowledge deficit:** Need for elevation of the involved extremity, use of thermotherapy, and exercises, p. 435.
2. Medications, including drug name, dosage, schedule, precautions, and potential side effects.
3. Potential complications of the disease and therapy and the need to recognize and seek medical attention promptly should they occur.
4. Potential concurrent pathology, such as pericarditis (see p. 58) and ocular lesions, and the need to report them promptly to health care professional.
5. Use and care of splints and orthotics, including return demonstration.
6. Use of adjunctive aids as appropriate, such as pickup sticks, long-handled shoe horn, crutches, walker, and cane, including return demonstration.
7. As necessary, referral to visiting or public health nurses for ongoing care after discharge.
8. Phone numbers to call should questions or concerns arise about therapy or disease after discharge.
9. Treatment and facilities available for these patients, which can be obtained by writing to Arthritis Foundation, 1314 Spring Street NW, Atlanta, Ga 30309.

Section Two   MUSCULAR AND CONNECTIVE TISSUE DISORDERS

Ligamentous injuries

Ligaments are collections of fascial tissues that connect bone to bone, thereby supplementing joint strength. Ligament tears usually result from direct trauma or transmission of a force to the joint. The degree of trauma incurred will vary with the strength of the involved ligament and the force applied. For example, strong ligaments will require more force before tearing than will a ligament weakened by previous injury or disease. Tears either can be longitudinal, transverse, tangential, complete, or partial, or involve avulsion fractures of their origin or insertion.

ASSESSMENT

Signs and symptoms: Localized ecchymosis, edema, tenderness, weakness, pain, joint effusion, limited ROM, or joint instability. A diagnosis is based primarily on consideration of the patient's complaints, the mechanism of the injury, and the physical assessment.

DIAGNOSTIC TESTS

1. *X-ray studies:* Stressing the weakened joint during x-ray exam may reveal an enlarged joint space.
2. *Arthrogram (instillation of a radiopaque dye or radiolucent gas into the joint):* To identify torn or weakened ligaments.
3. *Arthroscopy:* To rule out concurrent intraarticular pathology or trauma.

MEDICAL MANAGEMENT AND SURGICAL INTERVENTIONS

1. Treatment for uncomplicated ligamentous injuries: Rest of the joint, elevation, immobilization, local applications of cold followed by heat, and control of pain. Immobilization usually is accomplished with an elastic wrap, splint, cast, or brace.
2. Surgical repair: For injuries resulting in grossly unstable joints. The surgery involves removal of the nonviable ligament and suture repair or reefing of the stretched ligament, using strong, absorbable suture material. An avulsion injury without fracture may be reinserted onto its bony insertion site by using bone staples or passing a suture through holes drilled into the bony insertion site. Additional procedures may involve use of prosthetic devices to stent, temporarily replace, or augment ligament repairs.
3. ROM and muscle-strengthening exercises: Begun after an appropriate period of immobilization of the injured area (a minimum of 3 weeks).

NURSING DIAGNOSES AND INTERVENTIONS

Knowledge deficit: Need for elevation of the involved extremity, use of thermotherapy, and exercise

Desired outcome: Patient verbalizes understanding of the rationale for treatment and returns a demonstration of the exercise regimen, use of elevation, and use of thermotherapy.

1. Teach patient the pathophysiology of the injury and the concomitant inflammatory response.
2. Instruct patient to keep the injured extremity elevated until edema no longer is a problem (usually 3-7 days). Explain that the involved extremity should be kept above the level of the heart, with each successively distal joint elevated above the level of the preceding joint.
3. Explain that thermotherapy involves the application of ice and warmth. Ice usually is applied for the first 48 hours to prevent excessive edema. Warmth then is applied until the patient is comfortable without it (usually 3-5 days after the injury). Both are contraindicated for patients with peripheral vascular disease, decreased local sensation, coagulation disorders, or similar pathology that increases the potential for thermal injury. Advise the patient to apply thermotherapy with at least two thicknesses of terry cloth to protect the skin from injury. Explain that habituation to heat can cause the patient to apply increasingly warmer applications and that doing so is a potential source of injury.
4. Explain each prescribed exercise in detail, including the rationale. The optimal method is to teach it to the patient, demonstrate it, and then have the patient return the demonstration. Provide written instructions that review the exercise and list the frequency and number of repetitions for each. Include a phone number, should the patient have questions after hospital discharge.

Knowledge deficit: Care and assessment of the casted extremity

Desired outcome: Patient verbalizes understanding of the care of the casted extremity and knowledge of self-assessment of neurovascular status and returns a demonstration of the use of ambulatory aids, exercise, and general cast care.

1. Explain the function the patient's cast is performing.
2. Instruct patient in the rationale and procedure for neurovascular checks of the casted

extremity. Explain that they should be performed q2-4h for the first 2 days, and then qid until the cast is removed. Advise patient to be alert to and promptly report pallor, cyanosis, coolness, decreased pulse or capillary refill, increasing pain, decreasing sensation, and paralysis of the distal portion of the casted limb.

3. Ensure that the patient demonstrates independence in ADL and ambulation before discharge. If ambulatory aids (crutches, walker, cane) are used, make sure their independent use is demonstrated on all surfaces the patient is likely to encounter and that the precautions are understood and verbalized by the patient. Be sure patient will have adequate assistance or is independent in self-care before discharge. If necessary, initiate a referral for home care.

4. Instruct patient to exercise the parts of the extremity that are not immobilized by the cast, for example, wiggling the toes or fingers and putting the most proximal joints through complete ROM unless doing so is contraindicated by the injury or the MD. Isometric exercises for muscles beneath the cast will be prescribed for some patients. When prescribed, provide patient with the rationale and instructions for these exercises, including written instructions that review the information and explain the frequency and number of repetitions of each exercise.

5. Provide patient with a phone number of the appropriate person to call if problems or questions arise after hospital discharge.

6. Instruct patient in the basic components of cast care:

With plaster of Paris cast:

☐ Use plastic bags while showering or in the rain to avoid getting cast wet. Damp cloths can be used on soiled cast surfaces but saturation must be avoided.

☐ Use white shoe polish *sparingly* to cover stains.

☐ Petal the cast edges with tape if edges are rough or cast crumbs are falling into the cast. If the edges continue to irritate the skin, they can be padded with moleskin, sheepskin, or foam rubber. However, continued irritation should be brought to the attention of the MD.

☐ Avoid putting anything beneath the cast, because skin under the cast is more susceptible to injury.

☐ Report any pain, burning, changes in sensation, drainage on the cast, or foul odor because they can indicate the presence of pressure necrosis.

With synthetic cast material:

☐ Immersion in water may be permitted by MD, depending on the materials used, the type of injury, and whether or not surgery was performed. If immersion is permitted, it is necessary to dry the cast thoroughly (using a hair dryer on a cool setting) to prevent skin maceration.

☐ If permitted, dirt or sand can be rinsed from the cast.

☐ Avoid overexercising the casted extremity; perform the exercises within the prescribed range.

☐ Avoid putting anything beneath the cast, because skin under the cast is more susceptible to injury.

☐ Report any pain, burning, changes in sensation, drainage on the cast, or foul odor because they can indicate the presence of pressure necrosis.

Knowledge deficit: Potential for joint weakness, and the techniques for applying external supports and assessing neurovascular status

Desired outcome: Patient verbalizes understanding of the potential for joint weakness and returns a demonstration of applying external supports and self-checking neurovascular status.

1. Advise patient about the potential for joint weakness and the need for limiting or omitting activities that aggravate the condition.

2. If the MD has prescribed elastic wraps, elastic supports, or orthotic devices to supplement joint strength until exercise has compensated for the joint laxity, explain and demonstrate their use and application. Show the patient how to apply elastic wraps

diagonally from the distal to proximal areas with an overlap of two-thirds to one-half of the width of the wrap for each successive layer.
3. Teach patient how to self-check neurovascular status 15 minutes after application and to rewrap the joint if a deficit is found. For detail, see **Knowledge Deficit:** Care and assessment of the casted extremity, p. 435.
4. Ensure that the patient receives two wraps, supports, or orthotic devices to allow for cleaning. Typically, these devices are washed with mild soap and water and allowed to air dry without stretching (or see manufacturer's recommendations).

If surgery was performed, see "Torn Anterior Cruciate Ligament" for **Potential fluid volume deficit** related to abnormal loss secondary to postsurgical hemorrhage or hematoma, p. 442. See the appendix for nursing diagnoses and interventions for the care of preoperative and postoperative patients, p. 637.

PATIENT-FAMILY TEACHING AND DISCHARGE PLANNING

Provide patient and significant others with verbal and written information for the following:
1. Prescribed therapies, such as elevation, thermotherapy, cast care, exercise, and external supports.
2. Potential complications including subluxation/dislocation (see p. 437), wound infection (i.e., local warmth, persistent redness, swelling, wound drainage, foul odor from beneath the cast, sensation of burning from beneath the cast, drainage from the cast, and fever), and neurovascular deficit (see this section), all of which necessitate immediate medical attention.
3. ADL and ambulation: Ensure that patient demonstrates independence before hospital discharge.
4. Medications, including drug name, rationale, dosage, schedule, precautions, and side effects.

Dislocation/Subluxation

A dislocation occurs when the joint surfaces are completely out of contact. A subluxation is an incomplete dislocation in that some of the joint surfaces remain in contact. Most dislocations and subluxations are the result of trauma and can involve significant periarticular damage, including fractures. Some subluxations are associated with pronounced connective tissue disease, such as ulnar deviation of the phalanges and metacarpals, which is seen with severe rheumatoid arthritis.

ASSESSMENT

Signs and symptoms: Vary with the joint involved. Although any joint can dislocate, some joints are more prone than others. One finding common to most forms of dislocation is limb shortening. Usually there is significant pain, ecchymosis, loss of normal bony contour, edema, and loss or limitation of joint ROM. Complications include recurrent dislocation, joint contracture, neurovascular injury, or eventual traumatic arthritis.

DIAGNOSTIC TESTS

1. *X-rays:* Both anterior/posterior and lateral views commonly are used. Occasionally, an oblique view or other special approach is required. Because muscle spasms frequently force the dislocated bones back into normal alignment, it is sometimes necessary to stress the joint to permit visualization of the injury (called a "stress film").
2. *Bone scans:* May demonstrate nondisplaced avulsion fractures, areas of recent excessive stress, or bony insertions of joint ligaments following dislocation.
3. *Arthrogram:* Use of radiopaque dye or radiolucent gas for outlining the joint cavity to visualize injured ligaments, capsule, or intraarticular structures, such as the menisci.

4. *Arthroscopy:* May be used to rule out injury to joint surfaces or intraarticular structures.

MEDICAL MANAGEMENT AND SURGICAL INTERVENTIONS

Interventions vary with the degree of subluxation or dislocation and the joint involved. Many patients are discharged from the hospital with instructions for the use of thermotherapy, elevation, and pain medication.

1. Dislocation of the sternoclavicular joint: Usually reduced manually with local anesthesia. After reduction, the joint is immobilized with a clavicular strap (figure-of-8 bandage) for 2-6 weeks. Occasionally, an open reduction with internal fixation (ORIF) using screws, pins, or wire is necessary to maintain reduction.

2. Uncomplicated subluxation or dislocation of the acromioclavicular (AC) joint: May be immobilized with a clavicular strap or might require ORIF. After satisfactory joint stability has been achieved, the patient is started on a regimen of progressively more rigorous exercise to regain muscle strength and ROM.

3. Dislocation of the shoulder: Reduced with anesthesia or significant sedation and then immobilized in a Velpeau bandage, sling and swathe binder, or spica cast of the shoulder; all of which support the arm while immobilizing the shoulder. Immobilization usually is continued for 3-6 weeks, followed by progressive exercises to regain muscle strength and ROM. Surgical procedures usually include reefing (taking up redundant ligament with sutures) of the articular capsule and transferring or shortening the subcapsular muscle to tighten the periarticular tissues. Also see "Repair of Recurrent Shoulder Dislocation," p. 471.

4. Dislocation of the elbow: Frequently associated with fractures of the humerus, ulna, or radius. The elbow and fractures are carefully reduced, usually with general anesthesia, and the area is immobilized in a posterior splint at approximately 90-degree flexion for 2-4 weeks. ORIF may be required. Because of the area of the injury, these patients are at risk for Volkmann's ischemic contracture (ischemia myositis), and therefore the extremity must be monitored carefully for evidence of neurovascular deficit. (See "Ischemic Myositis," p. 443.) Progressive exercises are used to regain muscle strength and ROM.

5. Dislocation of the radioulnar or radiocarpal joints: Usually reduced using regional anesthesia and then immobilized in a posterior splint or long arm cast for 2-4 weeks. However, an ORIF may be performed. Progressive exercise is used to regain muscle strength and ROM.

6. Dislocation of the finger: Usually reduced with regional or digital block anesthesia. The finger may be immobilized with a metal splint or taped to an adjacent finger, followed by progressive mobilization. Surgery might be performed to reef the stretched periarticular tissues, followed by transfixation of the joint during the healing period, usually 10-14 days.

7. Dislocation of the metacarpophalangeal joint of the thumb: Surgery usually is indicated owing to the importance of this joint for hand grip strength and function. Surgical repair includes suturing torn ligaments, repair of avulsion injuries, and transfixion of the joint with a K-wire to maintain joint stability in slight (15 degree) flexion. A thumb spica cast immobilizes the joint for 4 weeks, followed by an orthoplast splint, which is used intermittently for an additional 4 weeks, during which ROM exercises are instituted gradually.

8. Dislocation of the hip: Usually requires general anesthesia with significant muscle relaxation for reduction. Typically, immobilization is accomplished *via* balanced suspension traction for 3-6 weeks, followed by progressive ambulation, mobilization of the joint, and muscle-strengthening exercises. Open reduction with surgical repair of the torn capsule and ligaments might be required for severe or recurrent dislocations. A fractured acetabulum may require replacement *via* total hip arthroplasty.

9. Dislocation of the patella: Often self-limiting, in that the patella usually reduces itself. Immobilization may be accomplished with a knee immobilizer, posterior splint, cylinder cast, or long leg cast for 10-21 days, followed by progressive mobilization and quadriceps setting exercises. Surgery may be required to reef the periarticular tissues

or reinsert the insertion of the patellar tendon to overcorrect distorted joint vectors that cause recurrent dislocation.
10. **Dislocation of the ankle:** Usually reduced under regional or general anesthesia. The joint is immobilized in a long leg plaster cast for 6-12 weeks. Surgery may be necessary to reef stretched periarticular tissues. Progressive mobilization and exercises are used to regain motion and strength.
11. **Dislocation of the toe:** Usually reduced with regional anesthesia. Often, the toe is immobilized for 3-5 days using an adjacent toe as a splint (taping the toes together).

NURSING DIAGNOSES AND INTERVENTIONS

See "Osteoarthritis" for **Pain,** p. 425, and **Impaired physical mobility** related to adjustment to a new walking gait, p. 426. See "Ligamentous Injury" for **Knowledge deficit:** Need for elevation of the involved extremity, use of thermotherapy, and exercise, p. 435, and **Knowledge deficit:** Care and assessment of the casted extremity, p. 435. See "Fractures" for **Self-care deficit,** p. 452. If surgery was performed, see "Torn Anterior Cruciate Ligament" for **Potential fluid volume deficit** related to abnormal loss secondary to postsurgical hemorrhage or hematoma, p. 442. See "Bunionectomy" for **Potential alteration in tissue perfusion:** Peripheral, related to impaired circulation secondary to compression from circumferential casts or dressings, p. 464. See the appendix for nursing diagnoses and interventions for the care of preoperative and postoperative patients, p. 637, and for the care of patients on prolonged bed rest, p. 651.

PATIENT-FAMILY TEACHING AND DISCHARGE PLANNING

Provide patient and significant others with verbal and written information for the following:
1. Therapy that will be used at home, including thermotherapy, elevation, and exercises (see "Ligamentous Injuries," p. 435), use of immobilization devices, cast care (see p. 435), and medications.
2. Potential complications that should be observed for at home, such as recurrent dislocations, neurovascular deficit (see "Ligamentous Injuries," p. 436), or wound infection (i.e., persistent redness, swelling, fever, local warmth, increasing pain, wound discharge, foul odor from beneath the cast, burning sensation from beneath the cast, and drainage from the cast).
3. Precautions that should be taken at home, including activity limitations (as directed by MD), monitoring for changes in neurovascular status qid, and following the guidelines described for cast, splint, or orthotic care.
4. Medications, including the drug name, rationale, dosage, schedule, precautions, and potential side effects.

Meniscal injuries

Meniscal injuries involve the intraarticular fibrocartilages on the medial or lateral side of the knee's tibial plateau. These halfmoon-shaped cartilages facilitate joint motion, while also absorbing some of the stress placed on the joint. There are a variety of cartilage injuries that can occur, and all involve a tear to varying degrees. Most commonly, a meniscal injury is the result of trauma to the knee or, less frequently, degeneration of the joint secondary to arthritis. Medial meniscus injuries are the most common and usually follow a knee movement involving internal rotation. Injuries to the lateral meniscus are more commonly associated with external rotation that occurs while the knee is partially flexed.

ASSESSMENT

Chronic indicators: Same as those seen with arthritis because arthritis will follow untreated or severe meniscal injuries. There may be weakness and atrophy of the quadriceps muscle group from disuse caused by joint pain.

Acute indicators: Occur after knee trauma that causes joint effusion and limited ROM. If the tear is large enough, it may result in locking, which is the inability to fully extend the joint. Joint pain or pain along the joint margins will occur. It may be possible to delineate point tenderness along the joint margin in the area of the tear.

DIAGNOSTIC TESTS

1. *McMurray's test for a torn medial meniscus:* With the patient's leg fully flexed, the foot externally rotated, and the leg abducted, the examiner's index finger and thumb are positioned along the joint margins of the knee. The knee is then gradually extended. Clicks or pops accompanied by patient complaints of pain as the leg is extended are indicative of a medial meniscal tear. A lateral meniscal tear is tested for by placing the thumb and index finger along the joint margin of the knee with the patient's leg flexed and adducted and the foot internally rotated. Clicks or pops, with patient complaints of pain as the leg is extended, are indicative of lateral meniscus injury.
2. *Apley grinding test:* Performed with the patient prone and the knee flexed at 90 degrees. With one hand, the examiner forces the foot and lower leg down on the femur while rotating the foot internally and externally. The examiner's other hand is positioned to palpate the joint margins as described in McMurray's test. Grinding or crepitus is usually indicative of a meniscal injury.
3. *Arthrogram:* Involves injection of radiopaque dye and radiolucent gas (usually air) into the joint to outline the area of injury and provide diagnosis of a meniscal tear as evidenced by absence of normal contour.
4. *Arthroscopy:* To diagnose and treat meniscal injuries. Under sterile conditions, the arthroscope is introduced into the joint to allow direct visualization of the meniscus. The patient is given local, regional, or general anesthesia for this procedure.

SURGICAL INTERVENTIONS

Arthroscopic surgery: Preferred over the outdated knee arthrotomy for partial menisectomy or suture repair because it is the least traumatic and allows more normal joint function and a more rapid return to normal level of health. The patient usually is discharged the same evening of surgery and placed on weightbearing as tolerated for 5-21 days using some form of external support for the knee, either an elastic wrap or knee immobilizer. Patients with sutured meniscal tears usually are maintained on nonweightbearing for 4-6 weeks, after which they begin a slow progression of partial weightbearing to full weightbearing. Knee exercises (quadriceps setting and leg lifts) are prescribed for regaining muscle strength.

NURSING DIAGNOSES AND INTERVENTIONS

See "Osteoarthritis" for **Pain,** p. 425, and **Impaired physical mobility** related to adjustment to new walking gait, p. 426. See "Ligamentous Injury" for **Knowledge deficit: Need for elevation of the involved extremity, use of thermotherapy, exercise, p. 435.** See "Torn Anterior Cruciate Ligament" for **Potential fluid volume deficit** related to abnormal loss secondary to postsurgical hemorrhage or hematoma, p. 442. See "Bunionectomy" for **Potential alteration in tissue perfusion:** Peripheral, related to impaired circulation secondary to compression from circumferential casts or dressing, p. 464. See also the appendix for the care of preoperative and postoperative patients, p. 637.

PATIENT-FAMILY TEACHING AND DISCHARGE PLANNING

Provide patient and significant others with verbal and written information for the following:
1. Use of elevation, thermotherapy, and exercise (see "Ligamentous Injuries," p. 435) as prescribed.

2. Use of external support devices (elastic wraps or knee immobilizer), including care of the device, care of the skin beneath the device, and monitoring for areas of irritation and neurovascular deficit (see "Ligamentous Injuries," p. 436).
3. Cast care (see p. 435).
4. Prescribed medications, including drug name, rationale, dosage, schedule, precautions, and potential side effects.
5. Indicators of wound infection, which necessitate medical attention: erythema, edema, joint effusion, purulent discharge, local warmth, pain, and fever.
6. Ambulation and use of assistive device. Ensure that patient is independent with ambulation using the assistive device on level surfaces and stairs before hospital discharge (see "Osteoarthritis," p. 426).

Torn anterior cruciate ligament

The anterior cruciate ligament (ACL) prevents excessive forward motion and internal rotation of the tibia. Injury to this ligament can result in strain with microtears, partial tears, complete tears, or avulsion of the tibial or femoral attachments. Stresses that can result in tears include forceful contraction of the quadriceps muscles combined with restricted extension, "clipping" injuries incurred in football, forced pivoting on the knee, or excessive forward motion of the tibia, which can occur when stopping quickly while running.

ASSESSMENT

Acute indicators: Sensation of the knee "giving way," joint effusion, restricted ROM, and joint instability and pain.

Chronic indicators: Untreated tears of the ACL result in gross instability, which eventually can cause osteoarthritis (see Osteoarthritis assessment, p. 424).

DIAGNOSTIC TESTS

1. *Lachman test:* Positive if the ACL is torn. The patient's knee is partially flexed at 10-15 degrees and the foot is planted flat on the examining table. The examiner then pulls the tibia forward while holding the femur stable. Excessive forward movement of the tibia is evidenced by a convex curve of the patellar tendon, and this is indicative of an ACL tear.
2. *Drawer test:* Performed with the knee flexed at 60 degrees and the foot planted flat on the table. The tibia is pulled forward as the femur is stabilized. Excessive forward movement indicates a tear. The test is then repeated with the foot externally rotated 15 degrees to assess concurrent injury of medial joint structures (meniscus or periarticular ligaments). Finally, the test is repeated with the foot internally rotated 30 degrees to assess concurrent lateral joint injury.
3. *Arthrography:* Outlines tears *via* injection of radiopaque dye and radiolucent gas.
4. *Radiography of the knee (including anterior/posterior, lateral, tunnel, and skyline views, with and without stress on the joint):* Evaluates for the presence of abnormal joint contours.
5. *Arthroscopy:* Allows direct visualization of the ACL injury to determine degree of injury and assess need for surgery.

MEDICAL MANAGEMENT AND SURGICAL INTERVENTIONS

The type of therapy is determined by the type of injury, length of time since the original injury, concurrent joint pathology, and the patient's age and functional goals.
1. **Bracing:** To provide primary support for an incompletely torn ACL or to supplement adjunctive joint support structures (posterior oblique ligament, collateral ligaments, lateral capsular ligament, and the menisci). Any of several commercial braces can be used to provide anteroposterior, lateral, and rotational stability of the joint. They

also may be used during joint rehabilitation following surgical intervention. Concurrent physiotherapy is provided to strengthen periarticular structures and muscles.

2. **Primary ACL repair:** Involves direct suturing of the torn ligament *via* an arthrotomy or arthroscopy. The suture is heavy and nonabsorbable and is used in repairing tears that are less than 6 weeks old.

3. **ACL reconstruction:** Involves use of either anatomic grafts or prosthetics. Regardless of the surgical procedure used, an arthrotomy requires prolonged knee immobilization (6-12 weeks in flexion in a long leg cast and/or a splint), followed by extensive physiotherapy and bracing. Physiotherapy is continued until the knee is functionally normal. In addition, many patients return from surgery with a closed wound drainage system consisting of a wound drain, tubing, and a reservoir. Most MDs bring the drainage tubing out through the area using a separate stab wound.

NURSING DIAGNOSES AND INTERVENTIONS

Potential fluid volume deficit related to abnormal loss secondary to postsurgical hemorrhage or hematoma formation

Desired outcome: Patient is asymptomatic of excessive bleeding or hematoma formation as evidenced by BP ≥90/60 mm Hg (or within patient's normal range), HR ≤100 bpm, RR ≤20 breaths/min, balanced I&O, output from drainage device <50 ml/hr, and brisk capillary refill (<3 seconds), peripheral pulses >2+ on a 0-4+ scale, warmth, and normal color in the involved extremity distal to the surgical site.

Note: A hematoma is a collection of extravasated blood within the tissues following surgery (or trauma). During most orthopaedic surgeries, a tourniquet is used to restrict blood flow from the operative field. Sometimes the tourniquet is left inflated until after the dressing or cast has been applied, and therefore major bleeding might not be noted during surgery. Even when the tourniquet is deflated, it is possible that a significant bleeding vessel may be overlooked or that bleeding will begin later during the patient's recovery.

1. When taking VS, monitor drainage from the drainage system as well as that on the dressings or cast. Report output from the drainage system that exceeds 50 ml/hr.

2. Because noting the amount of drainage on the cast does not always provide an accurate assessment of drainage beneath the cast, carefully evaluate the patient's VS, subjective complaints, and neurovascular status.

3. Be alert to and report patient complaints of feelings of warmth beneath the cast or dressing, things "crawling" under the cast, aching, increasing pressure or pain, or coolness distal to the area of surgery, which can occur with hemorrhage or hematoma formation.

4. Monitor for and report VS indicative of shock or hemorrhage, including hypotension and increasing pulse rate.

5. Monitor for pallor, decreased posterior tibial or dorsalis pedis pulses, slowed capillary refill, or coolness of the distal extremity, which can occur with hemorrhage or hematoma formation.

6. If hemorrhage or hematoma formation is suspected, notify MD promptly. If the limb is casted, elevate it above the level of the patient's heart to slow the bleeding. If the limb is not casted, apply an elastic wrap for direct pressure on the site of bleeding.

7. If hemorrhage or hematoma formation is suspected and the patient's VS are indicative of shock but an MD is unavailable, the surgical area should be exposed by windowing the cast or loosening the dressing to allow direct inspection of the area. Direct pressure usually will control hemorrhage; if not, apply a thigh blood pressure cuff over sheet wadding to serve as a tourniquet until the MD arrives for definitive therapy.

See "Intervertebral Disk Disease" for **Knowledge deficit:** Pain control measures, p. 193. See "Osteoarthritis" for **Pain,** p. 425, and **Impaired physical mobility** related to adjustment to new walking gait, p. 426. See "Ligamentous Injury" for **Knowledge def-**

icit: Need for elevation of the involved extremity, use of thermotherapy, and exercise, p. 435, and **Knowledge deficit:** Potential for joint weakness and the techniques for applying elastic wraps and assessing neurovascular status, p. 436. See "Fractures" for **Self-care deficit,** p. 452. See "Bunionectomy" for **Potential alteration in tissue perfusion:** Peripheral, related to impaired circulation secondary to compression from circumferential casts or dressings, p. 464. See the appendix for nursing diagnoses and interventions for the care of preoperative and postoperative patients, p. 637.

PATIENT-FAMILY TEACHING AND DISCHARGE PLANNING

Provide patient and significant others with verbal and written information for the following:
1. Telephone number of appropriate person for patient's questions after hospital discharge.
2. Use of external support devices (elastic wraps, knee immobilizer, or orthosis), including care of the device, care of the skin beneath the device, and monitoring for areas of irritation and neurovascular deficit (see "Ligamentous Injuries," p. 436).
3. Cast care, as described in the nursing diagnosis **Knowledge deficit:** Care and assessment of the casted extremity in "Ligamentous Injuries," p. 435.
4. Prescribed exercise regimen, including the rationale, how it is performed, the number of repetitions, and the frequency.
5. Prescribed medications, including drug name, rationale, dosage, schedule, precautions, and potential side effects.
6. Indicators of wound infection, which necessitate medical attention: erythema, edema, joint effusion, purulent discharge, local warmth, pain, and fever.
7. Ambulation with assistive device, including patient's demonstration of independence on level and uneven ground and stairs (see "Osteoarthritis," p. 426).

Ischemic myositis (compartment syndrome)

Ischemic myositis is a progressive degeneration of muscle that occurs because of a severe interruption in blood flow to an area. Volkmann's ischemic contracture of the forearm and anterior tibial compartment syndrome (ATCS) are associated with this process. Edema within an anatomic compartment (either of the forearm or the anterior tibial compartment) eventually can occlude arterial blood supply and cause ischemic myositis. Similarly, impaired venous return from a compartment can lead to edema, which can impinge on arterial blood supply. Arterial injury, from fracture fragments or the mechanism of injury, with resultant reflex vasospasm, also has been implicated as a potential etiology in this process.

An iatrogenic compartment syndrome can result from any circumferential cast or dressing that adversely affects the circulation of tissues. This syndrome is most commonly seen in trauma or surgery involving the elbow, wrist, knee, or ankle. Additional causes include bleeding disorders (hemophilia), major vascular surgery, thermal injuries (especially circumferential burns or frostbite), snakebites, or infiltration of IV infusions into deep veins. Because muscle tissue requires large amounts of blood to meet the muscle's demands, necrosis will occur within 6-8 hours if the blood supply is inadequate. If not corrected quickly, ischemic myositis can result in a severely contracted, functionally useless, and disfiguring limb distal to the area of injury. Complications of ischemic myositis include infection, renal failure from excessive release of myoglobin, hyperkalemia owing to potassium loss from injured muscle cells, and metabolic acidosis due to loss of built-up lactic acid in injured muscle.

ASSESSMENT

Signs and symptoms: The 5 P's: pain, paresthesia, paralysis, pallor, and pulselessness. The pain is especially diagnostic because it increases in severity, exceeds that expected for the incurred trauma, and might not be controlled by narcotics. Passive movement of the involved distal extremity, especially movement that stretches the muscles of the involved compartment, will result in severe pain. Paresthesias may include sensations of numbness, decreased sensation, or burning. Weakness of involved muscle groups generally precedes frank paralysis. Paralysis can involve pseudoparalysis because of the patient's avoidance of movements that stress the involved compartment, or frank paralysis of muscle that is enervated by injured nerves in the involved compartment. Pallor and pulselessness are associated with lost circulation through the compartment, while slowed capillary refill and impaired venous return can be prodromal signs. Progressive edema may be noted as tenseness or swelling over the length of the compartment.

DIAGNOSTIC TESTS

1. *Compartment pressure:* Can be measured *via* a large-bore catheter that is introduced into the compartment and attached to a saline-primed manometer. Normal tissue pressures are 0-4 mm Hg; sustained pressures >8 mm Hg are considered significantly elevated above normal. Continuous monitoring of high-risk patients may be necessary to warn of impending ischemic myositis.
2. *Arteriogram:* To rule out vasospasm or arterial trauma, which can result in ischemic myositis, especially in patients with supracondylar fractures of the humerus.

MEDICAL MANAGEMENT AND SURGICAL INTERVENTIONS

1. Conservative measures: Used initially when ischemic myositis is suspected. The constriction limiting the swelling (e.g., cast, splint, or circumferential dressing) is loosened down to skin level. However, if a fracture is involved, adequate immobilization should not be compromised. The limb is elevated to enhance venous return, and ice is applied to cause vasoconstriction in the area of the injury and inhibit further edema formation. Often, larger-than-normal levels of narcotics with potentiation such as aspirin, acetaminophen, promethazine (Phenergan), or hydroxyzine (Vistaril) are required for pain control.
2. Fasciotomy: Necessary if conservative measures fail to control the progressive symptoms. This involves the complete removal of the anatomic restrictions in the involved compartment. After several days the fasciotomy is closed primarily or the area is grafted with skin.
3. Surgical repair of a lacerated artery: Performed if the cause is arterial injury. If vasospasm is the suspected cause, some surgeons will expose the involved artery and apply topical papaverine to control the problem; if unsuccessful, resection of the involved artery with reanastomosis frequently is necessary.

NURSING DIAGNOSES AND INTERVENTIONS

Potential for infection related to risk secondary to large skin deficit following fasciotomy and the presence of devitalized muscle tissue

Desired outcome: Patient is asymptomatic of infection as evidenced by normothermia, WBC count ≤ 11,000/µl, negative culture and sensitivity findings, and absence of wound erythema, edema, pain, increased drainage, localized warmth, and other clinical indicators of local infection.

1. Teach patient about the increased potential for infection with this type of wound and that chronic infection and osteomyelitis are late complications following compartment syndrome.
2. Teach patient the indicators of wound infection and the importance of reporting these findings promptly.
3. Monitor VS q4h until the wound is closed or healed. Report temperature elevations >38.3° C (>101° F).
4. Monitor the dressing, cast, or wound for local indicators of infection. Monitor WBC counts and culture and sensitivity reports.
5. Monitor distal neurovascular status (see **Potential alteration in tissue perfusion** in

"Bunionectomy," p. 464) for deficit, which may be indicative of infection or pressure on these structures owing to nearby deep infection.

6. Use stringent, aseptic technique when changing dressings or providing wound care. As indicated, teach aseptic technique to patient prior to hospital discharge.

See "Osteoarthritis" for **Pain,** p. 425. See "Ligamentous Injuries" for **Knowledge deficit:** Need for elevation of the involved extremity, use of thermotherapy, and exercise, p. 435. See "Bunionectomy" for **Potential alteration in tissue perfusion:** Peripheral, related to impaired circulation secondary to compression from circumferential casts or dressings, p. 464. If surgery was performed, see the appendix for nursing diagnoses and interventions for the care of preoperative and postoperative patients, p. 637.

PATIENT-FAMILY TEACHING AND DISCHARGE PLANNING

Provide patient and significant others with verbal and written information for the following:

1. Phone number of appropriate person to call for questions after hospital discharge.
2. Instructions regarding the process of ischemic myositis, use of elevation and ice, and loosening of restrictive dressings.
3. Discharge instructions for patients with fractures (see "Fractures," p. 449).
4. Importance of seeking medical attention promptly if signs and symptoms of wound infection occur.
5. Importance of monitoring for vascular changes for patients who have undergone vascular surgery (exploration or resection). Teach patient to be alert to color changes (pallor, cyanosis, duskiness), coolness, pulselessness, or decreased or absent capillary refill. Caution patient about the importance of reporting these findings rapidly.

Section Three   SKELETAL DISORDERS

Osteomyelitis

Osteomyelitis is an acute or chronic infection involving a bone. *Primary osteomyelitis* is a direct implantation of microorganisms into bone *via* compound fractures, penetrating wounds, or surgery. *Secondary or acute hematogenic osteomyelitis* is an infection of bone that occurs through its own blood supply or from infection from contiguous soft tissues (especially ischemic, diabetic, or neurotrophic ulcers), IV drug abuse, or joints involved with septic arthritis. Although osteomyelitis often remains localized, it can spread through the marrow, cortex, and periosteum. Conditions favoring the development of osteomyelitis include recent bone trauma or areas with low oxygen tension, such as that found in sickle cell anemia. Acute hematogenic osteomyelitis is most frequently caused by *Staphylococcus aureus* (90%-95%), but it also can result from *Escherichia coli, Pseudomonas species, Klebsiella, Enterobacter, Proteus, Streptococcus* (groups A, B, & G), and *Haemophilus influenzae.* Chronic osteomyelitis is comparatively rare and is characterized by persistent, multiple draining sinus tracts.

ASSESSMENT

Acute osteomyelitis: Abrupt onset of pain in the involved area, fever, malaise, and limited motion. Pseudoparalysis is especially indicative of osteomyelitis in children who refuse to move an adjacent joint because of pain.

Chronic osteomyelitis: Bone infection that persists intermittently for years, usually flaring up after minor trauma to the area or lowered systemic resistance. Edema and erythema over the involved bone, weakness, irritability, and generalized signs of sepsis can occur. Sometimes the only symptom is persistent purulent drainage from an old pocket or sinus tract.

History of: Total joint replacement, compound fracture, use of external fixator, vascular insufficiency (e.g., with diabetes mellitus), recurrent UTIs.

DIAGNOSTIC TESTS

1. *CBC:* Will reveal leukocytosis and anemia in the presence of osteomyelitis.
2. *ESR:* Elevated in the presence of osteomyelitis.
3. *Bone biopsy:* Will provide infectious material for accurate culture and sensitivity studies. This study is limited to large bones because of the risk of fracture in small bones.
4. *Blood or sequestrum cultures:* To identify the causative organism. Sequestrum is a piece of necrotic bone that is separated from surrounding bone as a result of osteomyelitis.
5. *X-rays:* May reveal subtle areas of radiolucency (osteonecrosis) and new bone formation. No x-ray changes will be evident until the disease has been active at least 5 days in infants, 8-10 days in children, and 2-3 weeks in adults.
6. *Radioisotope scanning:* Methods include bone scans of technetium-99 and gallium-67 and leukocyte scans of indium-111. These scans may reveal areas of increased vascularity (called "hot spots"), which may be indicative of osteomyelitis. False positive results occur frequently with these tests and they are used cautiously for this reason.
7. *CT and MRI scans:* CT scans may demonstrate bone damage and soft tissue inflammation. MRI will not reveal bone changes, but it is an excellent means for identifying pockets of purulence.

MEDICAL MANAGEMENT AND SURGICAL INTERVENTIONS

1. IV antimicrobial therapy: Continued for at least 6 weeks.
2. Bed rest.
3. Immobilization of affected extremity: With splint, cast, or traction to relieve pain and decrease the potential for pathologic fracture.
4. Blood transfusions: To correct any accompanying anemia.
5. Removal of internal fixation device or endoprosthesis, if present: To help control the infection.
6. Surgical decompression of infected bone: May be followed by primary closure, myocutaneous flaps to cover the denuded bone, or leaving the area open to drain and heal by secondary intention or with secondary closure.
7. Drains: May be inserted into the affected bone to drain the site or act as ingress-egress tubes to funnel topical antibiotics directly into the area of infection.
8. Topical antibiotics: May be used *via* continuous or intermittent infusion and are continued until three successive drain cultures have been negative. As an alternative, acrylic beads with antibiotics may be packed into affected sites for 2-4 weeks, after which the wound is reopened, the beads are removed, and the bone graft is packed in the deficit.
9. Long-term antibiotic therapy: May be continued for 3-6 months.
10. Hyperbaric oxygen: May be used in selected patients with accessible areas of involvement to improve local oxygen supply.
11. Amputation: Although rarely performed, it may be required for extremities in which persistent infection severely limits function.

NURSING DIAGNOSES AND INTERVENTIONS

Potential for infection (for others) related to cross-contamination; (for patient) related to disease chronicity

Desired outcomes: Patient, other patients, and staff are asymptomatic of infection as evidenced by normothermia and WBC count $\leq$ 11,000/μl. Patient verbalizes knowledge of the potential chronicity of the disease and the importance of strict adherence to the prescribed antibiotic therapy.

1. When appropriate for the infecting organism, isolate the patient from other patients, especially those with orthopaedic disorders.
2. Ensure that the patient's drainage system is properly handled and that careful hand-washing is observed between patients to prevent cross-contamination.
3. Teach patient about the disease and potential for chronic infection. Stress the importance of adherence to the prescribed antibiotic therapy.
4. Follow universal infection control precautions (i.e., use of gloves) when performing irrigations, changing dressings, or handling contaminated dressings. Wash hands well between patients.

Knowledge deficit: Adverse side effects from prolonged use of potent antibiotics

Desired outcomes: Patient verbalizes knowledge of potential side effects of antibiotic therapy and precautions that must be taken.

Aminoglycoside antibacterials: Gentamicin sulfate, kanamycin sulfate, neomycin, streptomycin, and tobramycin are used to combat gram-negative organisms. Potential toxic reactions include ototoxicity (exhibited by dizziness, vertigo, tinnitus, and decreased auditory acuity); nephrotoxicity (evidenced by rising BUN and serum creatinine levels from progressive renal tubular necrosis, which can progress to renal failure if untreated); and superimposed infections, which occur because of loss of normal body flora protection against bacterial overgrowth.

1. Teach patient about the potential complications and the need to report symptoms as early as possible.
2. Advise patient that with long-term therapy, a baseline audiogram with weekly audiograms should be performed to identify potential hearing deficit; serum creatinine and BUN should be drawn weekly while patient is on aminoglycosides; and weight should be checked daily to help assess for fluid retention. Monitor I&O during patient's hospitalization to help assess renal function.
3. Advise patient to observe for superimposed infections, especially fungal infections, by assessing for fever, black or furry tongue, nausea, diarrhea, oral monilial growth, or vaginal monilial growth. If a Hickman catheter or similar device is used for antibiotic administration, the infusion site should be closely monitored for indicators of irritation that do not respond to usual treatments with topical antibiotics. During hospitalization, consult with MD about culturing suspicious areas of inflammation.

Penicillins: Ampicillin, carbenicillin, cyclacillin, methacillin, and oxacillin are used to combat organisms that demonstrate sensitivity to them. Potential toxic reactions include anemia, hypersensitivity reactions, and overgrowth of nonsusceptible organisms.

1. Teach patient about the potential complications and the need to report symptoms promptly.
2. Use penicillin cautiously in patients with allergies or such allergic pathologies as asthma, hay fever, or dermatitis. Erythematous, maculopapular rash; urticaria; and anaphylaxis can occur. Caution patient about these potential reactions.
3. Instruct patient to seek medical attention if rash, fever, chills, or signs of infection/inflammation develop.

Cephalosporins: Cefazolin, cephalothin, cephapirin, cephradine, cefoxitin, cefuroxine, cefadroxil, and cefamandole are used in the treatment of susceptible organisms. Potential toxic reactions include overgrowth of nonsusceptible organisms, photosensitivity, increased BUN, hepatotoxicity, and pseudomembranous colitis.

1. Advise patient about the potential complications, which necessitate prompt medical attention.
2. Explain that patients with suspected renal or hepatic disease should have baseline and serial (weekly) serum liver enzymes (LDH, SGOT, SGPT), BUN, and serum creatinine evaluations. I&O should be monitored along with daily weight to determine hydration status. Scleral and skin icterus, as well as darkening of the urine (from increased urobilinogen), should be noted. Persistent diarrhea (>3 liquid stools or liquid stools for >2 days) should be reported promptly to the health care provider.

3. Advise patient to avoid direct sunlight or ultraviolet light sources. Suggest the use of sunscreening agents to help prevent photosensitivity reactions.
4. When oral medications are used, instruct patient to avoid intake with dairy or iron products because they can inhibit absorption from the gut.

Sulfonamides: Sulfadiazine, sulfamethoxazole, sulfapyridine, and sulfisoxazole can cause toxic reactions including disruption of intestinal flora, which results in decreased production of metabolically active vitamin K and hemorrhagic tendencies; agranulocytosis; nephrotoxicity; and crystalluria.

1. Teach patient about the potential complications and the importance of seeking prompt medical attention if they occur.
2. Advise patients on long-term therapy to have baseline BUN and serum creatinine level determination along with weekly levels to rule out nephrotoxicity. Baseline and serial (weekly) granulocyte determinations also should be performed. Agranulocytosis can manifest as lesions of the throat, mucous membranes, GI tract, and skin. Daily weight and I&O evaluation should be watched to help assess hydration status.
3. Teach patient how to monitor for bleeding, especially epistaxis, bleeding gums, hemoptysis, hematemesis, melena, hematuria, prolonged bleeding from wounds, and ecchymosis. During patient's hospitalization, hematest suspicious secretions, or send them to the lab if prescribed, to determine if blood is present. Teach patient to control bleeding with ice, pressure, or elevation and to seek medical assistance promptly if unable to control hemorrhage.
4. Advise patient to consume at least 2-3 L/day of fluids (unless contraindicated by cardiac or renal disease) to prevent crystalluria. Teach the indicators of urinary calculi and the importance of getting medical attention should they occur: hematuria, pyuria, retention, frequency, urgency, and pain in the flank, lower back, perineum, thighs, groin, labia, or scrotum.

Knowledge deficit: Potential for infection and air embolus related to use of Hickman catheter or similar device for long-term intermittent antibiotic therapy

Desired outcome: Patient demonstrates care of the catheter and verbalizes knowledge of the indicators of infection and air embolus.

1. Teach patient how to care for the catheter and monitor the entry site for indicators of infection or inflammation if therapy is to be continued at home. Use sterile technique for dressing changes, following hospital protocol for the procedure, which usually includes defatting the skin with alcohol, applying povidone-iodine, and covering the site with an air-occlusive dressing. Have patient or significant other return the demonstration before hospital discharge. If appropriate, arrange for a visit by a home health care nurse.
2. Caution patient about the importance of keeping the tubing clamped unless he or she is aspirating or injecting solutions into the catheter. Teach patient and significant others to be alert to indicators of air embolism: labored breathing, cyanosis, cough, chest pain, and syncope. Explain that if air embolism is suspected, the patient should be rolled immediately to the left side and placed in Trendelenburg's position while reclamping the catheter.
3. Teach patient the importance of preventing inadvertent puncture or breakage of the tubing and checking for kinks or cracks daily. Explain the necessity of taping all tube junctures to prevent accidental separation and positioning the clamp over tape tabs to minimize stress on the tubing.

See "Intervertebral Disk Disease" for **Knowledge deficit:** Pain control measures, p. 193. See "Osteoarthritis" for **Pain,** p. 425. See "Fractures" for **Self-care deficit,** p. 452. See the appendix for nursing diagnoses and interventions for care of preoperative and postoperative patients, p. 637, the care of patients on prolonged bed rest, p. 651, and the care of patients with cancer and other life-disrupting illnesses, p. 690.

PATIENT-FAMILY TEACHING AND DISCHARGE PLANNING

Provide patient and significant others with verbal and written information for the following:

1. Necessary patient care after hospital discharge, for example, dressing changes, warm soaks, ROM exercises. Involve significant others in patient care during hospitalized period to familiarize them with care activities after discharge.
2. When parenteral antibiotic therapy is to be done at home (usually *via* a Hickman catheter, Portacath, or similar long-term vascular access device), the method of administering medications and care of the device used.
3. Medications, including drug name, route, dosage, purpose, schedule, precautions, and potential side effects.
4. Involving a public health, visiting nurse, or similar home health care service professional to ensure adequate follow-up at home.
5. Indicators of potential complications, such as recurring infection, pathologic fracture, joint contracture, pressure necrosis, and medication reactions or toxic effects.

Fractures

A fracture is a break in the continuity of a bone. It occurs when stress is placed on the bone that exceeds the bone's biologic loading capacity. Most commonly, the stress is the result of trauma. *Pathologic fractures* are the result of decreased biologic loading capacity, so that even normal stress can result in a break.

ASSESSMENT

Chronic indicators: These are rare. Osteoporotic fractures of the vertebral column may be found incidental to an x-ray in an asymptomatic patient or in a patient who complains of back discomfort. Delayed union is a failure of the bone to unite within the normally accepted timeframe for that bone's healing, and a chronic fracture may result. Nonunion is demonstrated by nonalignment and lost function secondary to lost bony rigidity. Pseudoarthrosis is a state in which the fracture fails to heal and a false joint forms at the fracture site. Avascular necrosis occurs when the fracture interrupts the blood supply to a segment of bone, which then eventually necroses. Reflex sympathetic dystrophy is an incompletely understood process that results in pain, reduced function, joint stiffness, and trophic changes in soft tissues and skin following fracture.

Acute indicators: Sudden pain, which usually is associated with trauma or physical stress, such as jogging or strenuous exercise. In pathologic fractures, the patient may describe signs and symptoms associated with the underlying pathology (see "Benign Neoplasms," p. 455, and "Malignant Neoplasms," p. 457).

Physical assessment: Loss of normal bony or limb contours, edema, ecchymosis, limb shortening, decreased ROM of adjacent joints, false motion (movement that occurs outside of a joint), and crepitus, which should not be elicited purposely because of the risk of injury to surrounding soft tissues. Complicated and complex fractures can present with signs and symptoms of perforated viscus, neurovascular deficit, joint effusion, or excessive joint laxity. Compound fractures involve a break in the skin and will demonstrate a wound in the area of suspected fracture or bone may be exposed in the wound.

Note: Any patient with a suspected fracture should be treated as though a fracture is present until it is ruled out. Interventions should include immobilization and elevation of the involved area, application of ice, and careful monitoring of the neurovascular status distal to the injury.

DIAGNOSTIC TESTS

Most fractures are identified easily with standard AP and lateral x-rays. MRI may be useful in evaluating complicated fractures; its usefulness in identifying different bone densities is limited. Occasionally, it is necessary to involve special techniques, such as the mortise view to demonstrate bimalleolar ankle fractures or x-rays through the open mouth to identify fractures of the odontoid process. Bone scans, tomograms, CT scans, stereoscopic films, and arthrograms also can be used. Intraarticular fractures sometimes may be diagnosed with arthroscopy.

MEDICAL MANAGEMENT AND SURGICAL INTERVENTIONS

The choice of treatment varies with the complexity of the fracture, the patient's age and concurrent health problems, and functional goals. The goal of treatment is to provide immobilization of the bone until healing occurs. The length of time for immobilization varies with the type of fracture. The following is a brief overview of common examples of treatment interventions.

1. **Bed rest:** May be all that is required to maintain reduction for simple, uncomplicated fractures, such as those of the posterior elements of the vertebrae and some pelvic fractures.

2. **Traction**
   □ *Cervical fractures:* Skeletal traction *via* Turner, Cone, Vinke, or Crutchfield tongs, which are inserted into the outer plate of the cranial vault. An alternative is the halo vest, which allows the insertion of four pins into the outer plate of the cranium. The pins are attached to a halo device that is connected to four metal posts encompassed within a body jacket, cast, or orthosis. This "four-posted" jacket allows exposure of the head and neck, yet maintains immobilization of the fracture. Cervical collars can be used to provide support for some simple fractures.
   □ *Humeral fractures:* Dunlop's side arm or overhead 90/90 traction.
   □ *Pelvic fractures:* Pelvic sling or pelvic belt may be used for nondisplaced fractures, while skeletal traction with pins in the ilium or femur may be required for displaced fractures.
   □ *Femoral fractures:* Skin traction (Buck's extension, Russell's, or balanced suspension traction) may be applied until skeletal traction can be used or the fracture is internally or externally fixated. Skeletal traction may involve a Steinmann pin or Kirshner wire positioned through the distal femur or proximal tibia. When skeletal traction is used, it is provided in combination with balanced suspension or Russell's traction and is used for 1-4 months.
   □ *Tibial fractures:* Temporary traction can be accomplished with Buck's extension, or for longer periods of time with a pin placed through the distal tibia or calcaneus, augmented with balanced suspension or Russell's traction.

3. **Immobilization devices**
   □ *Uncomplicated, simple fractures of the cervical vertebrae:* Soft or hard cervical collars or a minerva jacket cast for less stable fractures.
   □ *Dorsal and lumbar vertebral fractures:* Plaster of Paris body cast or a variety of orthotic devices.
   □ *Clavicular fractures:* Figure-of-8 dressing, modified Velpeau dressing (a wrap that holds the arm against the thorax with the elbow flexed at 90 or 45 degrees), sling and swathe shoulder immobilizer, clavicular straps.
   □ *Humeral fractures:* Velpeau cast, shoulder spica cast (which abducts or extends the upper arm), or Caldwell's hanging plaster cast, which is a long arm cast with additional layers of plaster of Paris that provide weight to distract fracture fragments and aid in alignment. Patients in Caldwell's casts need to be instructed to allow the cast to be dependent, which will help ensure adequate fracture distraction. A coaptation splint may be used to immobilize midshaft humeral fractures. The coaptation splint consists of a long plaster splint applied over a thick layer of padding, beginning at the medial aspect of the upper arm in the axilla and extending around the elbow and up the outside of the upper arm. An elastic wrap secures the splint. Posterior splints temporarily may immobilize distal shaft fractures. Posterior or coaptation splints accommodate progressive edema, reducing the potential for compartment syndrome (see p. 443). Undisplaced, stable fractures may require immobilization only, with a sling and swathe shoulder immobilizer or functional bracing.

☐ *Ulnar or radial fractures:* Long arm casts for proximal fractures or short arm casts for distal fractures. In the presence of significant edema, a sugar tong splint may be used to provide immobilization while accommodating progressive edema. This is applied over heavy padding and consists of one long plaster splint that extends from the back of the wrist, bends around the elbow, covers the underside of the forearm to the wrist, and is held in place with an elastic wrap. Some fractures are immobilized in a posterior splint for 3-7 days before casting to allow for the edema to subside. Fractures involving both the radius and ulna usually are immobilized in a long arm cast.

☐ *Hand fractures:* Short arm posterior splints until edema subsides, and then a short arm cast can be applied. Some fractures of the hand may be immobilized safely in splints or orthoses. A thumb spica cast may be used for various fractures involving the thumb.

☐ *Pelvic fractures:* Corsets, orthoses, or external fixators.

☐ *Femoral fractures:* Spica cast that extends from the thorax and completely encompasses the affected leg and opposite leg to the midthigh, or a long leg cast, which may be applied instead. After sufficient callus has formed, it may be possible to use a cast brace to allow motion of the knee and weight-bearing stress, which can facilitate bony union in certain fractures.

☐ *Patellar fractures:* Cylinder cast for nondisplaced fractures. Following any knee surgery, the leg is immobilized in a Jones dressing, which includes AP and lateral splints over bulky padding and is held in place with an elastic wrap. Once swelling subsides, a cylinder or long leg cast is applied. A knee immobilizer may provide sufficient immobilization for some stable patellar fractures.

☐ *Tibial fractures:* Cylinder or long leg cast; short leg cast for easily stabilized fractures. Some casts will be converted to walking casts at a later time.

☐ *Fibular shaft fractures:* While some fibular fractures may not require casting, a short leg walking cast is often applied if adequate support is not provided by the tibia.

☐ *Malleolar fractures:* Short leg cast that is converted to a walking cast after callus has formed; long leg cast for nondisplaced bimalleolar fractures. Trimalleolar fractures require open reduction and internal fixation (ORIF) to ensure joint integrity.

☐ *Avulsion fractures of the insertion of the Achilles tendon from the calcaneous:* Often require a long leg cast with the knee flexed at 30 degrees and the ankle slightly plantarflexed to reduce stress on the Achilles tendon.

☐ *Tarsal and metatarsal fractures:* Short leg cast that can be converted to a walking cast; stiff-soled shoe or slipper cast.

☐ *Phalangeal fractures:* Splints made of plaster, metal, or plastic, or the phalanx can be immobilized by taping it to an adjacent phalanx.

4. **Closed reduction:** Allows for manipulation of displaced fragments to their normal anatomic alignment. It can be done under general, regional, local, or hematoma-block anesthesia.

5. **ORIF:** Indicated for fractures that are grossly unstable or for patients who cannot tolerate prolonged bed rest or traction. Internal fixation may be accomplished with screws, pins, wires, plates, bone grafts, methylmethacrylate, or rods. In some fractures in which avascular necrosis is likely or the fracture is severely comminuted, placement of an endoprosthesis may be necessary. Endoprostheses most commonly are used to replace the head of the humerus or femur. Fibrin sealant may be used to aid in the internal fixation of some small fractures, avulsion fractures, and osteochondral fractures, as well as to aid in the internal fixation of bone grafts.

6. **External fixation:** Consists of skeletal pins that penetrate the fracture fragments and are attached to universal joints, which in turn are attached to rods to provide stabilization. These rods form a frame around the fractured limb for immobilization. The external fixator is left in place until sufficient soft tissue repair or bony callous formation allows either application of a cast or complete removal of any form of immobilization. Sometimes the skeletal pins are left in place (after removing the external fixation rods) and incorporated into a cast that immobilizes the limb until the fracture has healed. The external fixator can be used to treat massive open comminuted fractures with extensive soft tissue injury or neurovascular injury in which there is in-

creased risk of infection. It is also the treatment of choice for infected nonunion, segmental bone loss, limb-lengthening procedures, arthrodesis (joint fusion), and multiple trauma with injuries involving other body systems.

7. **Progressive ROM and muscle-strengthening exercises:** Begun after the designated period of immobilization to help the patient regain joint function.

8. **Continuous passive movement (CPM):** A motor-driven device developed to place a joint through repeated extension and flexion. It is used as an adjunctive treatment for femoral condyle and tibial plateau injuries as well as humeral head fractures.

NURSING DIAGNOSES AND INTERVENTIONS

See "Intervertebral Disk Disease" in Chapter 4 for **Knowledge deficit:** Pain-control measures, p. 193. See "Osteoarthritis" for **Pain,** p. 425, and **Impaired physical mobility** related to adjustment to new walking gait, p. 426 (useful for any patient with spinal or lower extremity injuries). See "Rheumatoid Arthritis" for **Fatigue,** p. 433. See "Ligamentous Injuries" for **Knowledge deficit:** Need for elevation of the extremity, use of thermotherapy, and exercise, p. 435 (useful for patients discharged after a recent fracture or surgery), and **Knowledge deficit:** Care and assessment of casted extremity, p. 435 (applies to any patient in a cast). See "Torn Anterior Cruciate Ligament" for **Potential fluid volume deficit** related to abnormal loss secondary to postsurgical hemorrhage or hematoma, p. 442 (for patients with ORIF). See "Bunionectomy" for **Potential alteration in tissue perfusion:** Peripheral, related to impaired circulation secondary to compression by circumferential cast or dressing, p. 464 (relates to iatrogenic compartment syndrome and builds on information provided under "Ischemic Myositis," p. 443). See "Amputation" for **Knowledge deficit:** Postsurgical exercise regimen, p. 467 (applies for any patient begun on exercise therapy). See "Repair of Recurrent Shoulder Dislocation" for **Potential impairment of skin integrity** related to maceration of the axillary skin, p. 472 (useful for any patient with moist areas trapped by a therapeutic device that is necessary to treat a fracture). See "Total Hip Arthroplasty" for **Knowledge deficit:** Potential for and mechanism of THA dislocation, p. 474 (for patients undergoing hemiarthroplasty for replacement of the femoral head), **Knowledge deficit:** Potential for infection caused by foreign body reaction to an endoprosthesis, p. 475 (useful for any patient with an internal fixation device, especially large devices), and **Potential alteration in tissue perfusion,** p. 475 (can be adapted for any patient in traction). See the appendix for nursing diagnoses and interventions for the care of preoperative and postoperative patients, p. 637, and for the care of patients on prolonged bed rest, p. 651.

Specific nursing diagnoses for patients with casts, traction, ORIF, and external fixators:

Self-care deficit: Inability to perform ADL related to physical limitations secondary to cast or surgical procedure (applies to patients with casts, ORIF, and external fixators)

Desired outcome: Patient demonstrates independence with ADL.

1. For patients with insufficient strength to manipulate casted extremities to allow independence in self-care, incorporate a structured exercise regimen that will increase strength and endurance. Direct the regimen toward development of those muscle groups necessary for the patient's activity deficit. See the guidelines described in **Knowledge deficit:** Postsurgical exercise regimen, p. 467, in "Amputation" and **Potential for disuse syndrome** related to inactivity secondary to prolonged bed rest, p. 653, in the appendix.

2. Use assistive devices liberally. These include stocking helpers, Velcro fasteners, enlarged handles on eating utensils, pickup sticks, raised toilet seats, and similar self-help devices.

3. As appropriate, ask social services department of hospital for assistance with funding for purchasing assistive equipment.

4. Because pain control is an essential element in enhancing self-care activities, ensure

that the patient is as comfortable as possible (see **Pain** related to inflammatory process or corrective therapy, p. 425, in "Osteoarthritis" and **Knowledge deficit:** Pain control measures, p. 193, in "Intervertebral Disk Disease").

5. When needed, teach significant others how to assist patient with self-care.
6. If economic assistance is needed for home help, consult with social services for intervention.
7. As appropriate, utilize adaptive clothing (e.g., garments with Velcro fasteners for easy removal and application) that is designed to accommodate the cast.

Potential for impaired skin integrity related to irritation secondary to the presence of a cast (applies to patients with casts and ORIF)

Desired outcomes: Patient denies the presence of discomfort under the cast and exhibits intact skin once the cast is removed. Patient verbalizes knowledge of the indicators of pressure necrosis.

1. When assisting with cast application, ensure that adequate padding is put on the affected extremity before the cast is applied.
2. While the cast is curing (drying), handle it only with the palms of the hands to avoid pressure points caused by finger indentations. Ensure that the cast surface is exposed to facilitate drying.
3. Petal the edges of plaster casts with tape or moleskin to prevent cast crumbs from falling beneath the cast and causing pressure necrosis.
4. Instruct patient never to insert anything between the cast and skin. In the presence of severe itching, advise patient to notify MD, who may prescribe a medication to relieve itching.
5. Teach patient the indicators of pressure necrosis beneath the cast: pain, burning sensation, foul odor from cast opening, or drainage on the cast.

Knowledge deficit: Potential for disuse osteoporosis (appropriate for patient with cast or traction)

Desired outcome: Patient verbalizes knowledge of the process of and measures to prevent disuse osteoporosis.

1. Teach patient about the process of disuse osteoporosis, gearing the explanation to the patient's level of understanding: the immobilized limb has insufficient stress to stimulate osteoblastic (bone building) activity.
2. Instruct patient to report any indicators of pain in the immobilized limb or findings of spontaneous fracture, such as bony deformity, pain, lost function, edema, and ecchymosis.
3. Consult with patient's MD about appropriate alternative methods of bone stress, and teach them to the patient. These can include use of a tilt table, sandbags applied intermittently against the bone, or having patient push against a footboard or perform isometric exercise of the immobilized limb.

Potential alteration in tissue perfusion: Cerebral or cardiopulmonary, related to impaired circulation secondary to fat embolization (applies to patients with multiple trauma, multiple fractures, or surgical repair of fractures)

Desired outcome: Patient has adequate circulation as evidenced by Pao_2 ≥80 mm Hg, HR ≤100 bpm, RR ≤20 breaths/min, normothermia, normal skin color, absence of adventitious breath sounds over the tracheobronchial tree, absence of petechial rash, and orientation to person, place, and time.

1. Ensure strict maintenance of fracture immobilization to help prevent embolization.
2. Carefully monitor patient for the initial 72 hours following injury or surgery for indicators of fat embolism: tachycardia, tachypnea, profuse tracheobronchial secretions, cyanosis, fever, petechial rash (involving the conjunctiva, trunk, neck, and axilla), anxiety, apprehension, progressive mental dysfunction (confusion, disorientation), and the presence of fat globules in the retina of the eye. The hematocrit may drop, serum lipase will rise, and fat may be noted on urinalysis. Frequent ABG levels should be drawn on patients at risk for fat embolus for the first 48 hours follow-

ing injury because early hypoxemia that is indicative of fat embolism is apparent on laboratory measurement only. In addition, a platelet count indicative of thrombocytopenia ($<$150,000 mm^3) is diagnostic of fat embolism.

3. Because fat embolism is a life-threatening emergency, notify MD immediately should any of the above occur. Inform patient and significant others of these potential indicators so that they can notify the staff if they occur.
4. As prescribed, perform respiratory support measures with oxygen and rigorous pulmonary hygiene. Entubation with ventilation using positive end-expiratory pressure (PEEP) may be necessary. As a general rule, all patients with significant trauma and fractures should receive oxygen at 40% concentration *via* mask or nasal prongs until the threat of fat embolism has been ruled out.
5. Administer IV steroids, diuretics, and dextran as prescribed.

Knowledge deficit: Potential for infection related to orthopedic procedure or presence of internal or external device (appropriate for patients with ORIF or external fixators)

Desired outcome: Patient verbalizes knowledge of the potential for infection, lists the indicators that may occur, and relates the significance of reporting them promptly.

1. Advise patient about the potential for infection, which can occur as a result of the surgical procedure.
2. Teach patient the following indicators of infection and the importance of reporting them to a health care professional promptly should they occur: persistent redness, swelling, increasing pain, wound drainage, local warmth, foul odor from beneath the cast, sensation of burning beneath the cast, drainage from the cast, and fever.
3. For patients with internal fixation devices, alert them to the potential for infection for as long as the implant is present. Instruct them to report any of the above indicators promptly.

Knowledge deficit: Potential for refracture owing to vulnerability secondary to presence of internal fixator (applies to patients with ORIF)

Desired outcome: Patient verbalizes knowledge of the potential for refracture and demonstrates adherence to the prescribed regimen for prevention.

1. Advise patient that while the internal fixation device supplements strength of the bone at the fracture site in the early stages of healing, the implant will compromise the bone's strength later. Larger internal fixation devices alter the vectors of stress placed on the bone, changing the normal physiologic balance between osteoblasts and osteoclasts, which results in a bone that is made weaker in the long run by the implant.
2. Be sure the patient verbalizes understanding of this process and demonstrates adherence to the prescribed regimen of limb usage and/or ambulation.
3. Ensure patient is aware that intramedullary nails or rods and large plates probably will be removed within a year.

Knowledge deficit: Function of external fixation, pin care, transport, and signs and symptoms of pin site infection

Desired outcomes: Patient verbalizes knowledge of the rationale for the external fixator and demonstrates ways to adapt his or her lifestyle around the fixator. Patient demonstrates knowledge of pin care and verbalizes knowledge of the indicators of infection at the pin sites.

1. Teach patient the rationale for use of the fixator with his or her type of fracture or injury, emphasizing benefits for the patient.
2. Discuss ways in which the patient can adapt his or her lifestyle to accommodate the fixator (e.g., by wearing adaptive clothing that fits the device).
3. Instruct patient and significant others in pin care as prescribed by MD. Some MDs prescribe daily pin site care with hydrogen peroxide or skin prep solutions such as pHisoHex, alcohol, or povidone-iodine. Some MDs prescribe that buildup of crusts from serous drainage be removed when cleansing pin sites, while others request that the crust be left intact to minimize the risk of infection. If prescribed, teach the pa-

tient how to apply antibacterial ointments and small dressings to the pin site. External fixator pins should be cleansed with alcohol daily. **Note:** Literature supplied with some external fixators cautions against the use of iodine-based mixtures, which may cause corrosion of the device.

4. Instruct patient and significant others not to use the external fixator as a handle or support for the extremity. Teach them to support the extremity with pillows, two hands, slings, and other devices as necessary to prevent excessive stress on the skeletal pins.

5. Teach patient how to monitor the pin sites for indicators of infection, including persistent redness, swelling, drainage, increasing pain, temperature >38.33° C (>101° F), and local warmth, and to be alert to pin migration or "tenting" of the skin on the pin, which can signal movement of the pin or infection. Instruct patient to report significant findings promptly to MD.

6. Advise patient of the need for follow-up care to ensure that the device is functioning properly and maintaining adequate immobilization of the fracture(s).

PATIENT-FAMILY TEACHING AND DISCHARGE PLANNING

Provide patient and significant others with verbal and written information for the following:

1. Medications, including the name, dosage, purpose, schedule, precautions, and potential side effects.

2. Importance of rest, elevation, and use of thermotherapy (see "Ligamentous Injuries," p. 435).

3. Rationale for the individual's therapy after discharge and how that therapy will be accomplished, for example, casting, external fixation, internal fixation.

4. Precautions of therapy
   □ *Casts:* Caring for the cast, monitoring neurovascular status of the distal extremity, watching for evidence of pressure necrosis beneath the cast, performing prescribed exercises, preventing skin maceration, and preventing disuse osteoporosis (also see **Knowledge deficit:** Care and assessment of the casted extremity, p. 435).
   □ *Internal fixation devices:* Caring for the wound, noting signs of wound infection, preventing refracture of the limb, performing prescribed exercises, and monitoring for delayed infection.
   □ *External fixator:* Demonstrating understanding of pin care, knowing when to notify MD of problems with the fixator, performing prescribed exercises, monitoring neurovascular status of the limb, and monitoring pin site for indicators of infection.

5. Ways in which patient can control discomfort (see **Knowledge deficit:** Pain control measures, p. 193, in "Intervertebral Disk Disease").

6. Use of assistive devices and ambulatory aids. Ensure that the patient can perform a return demonstration and is independent with devices and aids before hospital discharge (see "Osteoarthritis," p. 424). If needed, initiate a referral for a home visit early after discharge to ensure patient safety.

7. Materials that are necessary for care at home and agencies that can supply materials.

In addition:

8. For patients who require home help, a collaborative effort between hospital nurses and community care agencies should be made to ensure continuity of care. The appropriate agency should see patient before hospital discharge.

Benign neoplasms

The three most common benign bone tumors are osteochondromas, enchondromas, and giant cell tumors. *Osteochondromas* are the most common, representing 45% of all benign tumors. Usually they are found in the metaphysis (wider portion of the shaft) of the long bones, typically the distal femur or proximal humerus, although they also can occur in a rib or vertebra. Individuals under the age of 20 are most commonly affected. Some osteochondromas are the result of an inheritable autosomal dominant trait that causes concurrent growth retardation and bowing of the long bones. *Enchondromas* (chondromas) are most commonly found in the hand (metacarpals or phalanges) or the proximal humerus. They represent approximately 10% of all diagnosed benign tumors. Although they occur most commonly in people in their thirties, they may be seen at any time. *Giant cell tumors* are found most often around the proximal humerus, distal radius, or the knee (most common) in the area of the fused epiphyseal growth plate in individuals 30-40 years old. Ten percent of these tumors degenerate into malignancy with a potential for metastasis. Giant cell tumors recur 40% of the time.

ASSESSMENT

Osteochondromas: Indicators arise from mechanical irritation of surrounding musculotendinous structures, and include pain upon specific movements of the involved areas or from irritation.

Enchondromas: Local pain. Unless the growth is in an area with little soft tissue, the growth usually is not palpable.

Giant cell tumors: Pain occurs before the mass becomes palpable.

DIAGNOSTIC TESTS

AP and lateral x-rays are most commonly used for preliminary diagnosis. CT scans, tomograms, contrast radiography, and angiograms can be used to clarify the extent of the tumor.

MEDICAL MANAGEMENT AND SURGICAL INTERVENTION

All three types of tumors are best treated with surgical removal. Resection can require allografting, prosthetic replacement, or use of methylmethacrylate to replace resected bone. When removal is impossible, curettage (scraping) of the lesion is usually done. In some giant cell tumors, radiation therapy is used to inhibit recurrence.

NURSING DIAGNOSES AND INTERVENTIONS

Knowledge deficit: Disease process and potential for recurrence (if appropriate)

Desired outcomes: Patient verbalizes understanding of the disease process. Patients with giant cell tumors verbalize understanding of the potential for recurrence, slight chance of malignancy, and increased potential for infection.

1. Provide patient with a clearly understood description of the disease process. Drawings, models, books, and other references should be used to enhance patient's learning.
2. Validate that the patient clearly understands the disease process and does not confuse it with a malignant tumor.
3. Be sure that patients with giant cell tumors are aware of the potential for recurrence and slight potential for degeneration to malignancy, as well as the importance of reporting renewed indicators of tumor to MD. In addition, teach these patients that they are at increased risk for infection and that they should report the following indicators promptly to the MD: persistent erythema, edema, fever, local warmth, wound drainage, and increasing pain.

See "Osteoarthritis" for **Pain,** p. 425. Also see "Fractures," pp. 452-455 for nursing diagnoses as appropriate. See the appendix for nursing diagnoses and interventions for the care of preoperative and postoperative patients, p. 637.

PATIENT-FAMILY TEACHING AND DISCOUNT PLANNING

Provide patient and significant others with verbal and written information for the following:

1. Description of the disease process.
2. For patients having surgery, the indicators of wound infection (swelling, persistent redness, wound drainage, pain, local warmth, and fever) and the necessity of reporting these indicators promptly to MD.
3. For patients with casts and orthotics, the care of the extremity and immobilization device. For more information about casts, see **Knowledge deficit:** Care and assessment of the casted extremity, p. 435.
4. Medications, including the name, dosage, purpose, schedule, precautions, and potential side effects.
5. Post-hospitalization therapy and the importance of follow-up.

Malignant neoplasms

The most common malignant tumors affecting bones are osteogenic sarcoma, primary chondrosarcoma, and myeloma. *Osteogenic sarcoma* is the most common true tumor originating from bone tissue, occurring most frequently in adolescents. It is found (in order of prevalance) in the distal femoral metaphysis, proximal tibial metaphysis, proximal humeral metaphysis, pelvis, and proximal femur. Most osteosarcomas become apparent during the time of a skeletal growth spurt. Less frequently, osteosarcoma is associated with Paget's disease (see p. 461). This tumor is associated with early metastasis to the lung, lymph involvement, and rapid death unless rigorous treatment is begun early in the disease process. The current survival rate following resection and adjunctive chemotherapy is 60%. Children treated with radiation or alkylating agents for other cancers have a greatly increased risk of developing osteosarcoma. *Chondrosarcomas* occur half as frequently as osteogenic sarcomas and usually are seen between ages 50-60. Most of these tumors originate in the pelvic girdle, ribs, or shoulder girth. Resection of all of the tumor results in an excellent 5-year cure rate; however, inadequate resection frequently results in recurrence and late metastasis to the lung. *Myelomas* arise from bone marrow and thus are not truly bone tumors; however, they are the most common malignant tumor that affects the bones. The peak time of onset is the sixth and seventh decades. Myelomas can occur in any bone, although they are seen less frequently in smaller bones. Average survival after diagnosis is 1-2 years.

ASSESSMENT

Osteogenic sarcomas: Pain, tenderness, limited ROM, and swelling near a joint. Night pain usually is more severe. A history of trauma frequently is noted.

Chondrosarcomas: Localized pain, rarely with a demonstrable mass.

Myelomas: Symptoms of anemia as well as weight loss, significant pain, tenderness, backache, or pathologic and spontaneous fracture.

DIAGNOSTIC TESTS

1. *Standard x-rays, CT scans, tomograms, and radioisotope (gallium) uptake tests:* To delineate extent of the disease. *MRI* is useful in delineating the extent of cortical involvement and degree of medullary spread and may prove useful in identifying metastasis.

   For myelomas:
2. *Standard blood and electrolyte tests:* May reveal moderate normocytic anemia and a markedly elevated sedimentation rate. Serum calcium levels, alkaline phosphatase, PTT, and PT usually are elevated.

3. *Bence Jones protein:* Urine will be positive in 40% of patients with myeloma.
4. *Bone marrow aspiration:* May reveal plasma cells with large nuclei and nucleoli.
5. *Immunoelectrophoresis:* Will show an abnormal amount of either IgG or IgA produced by the tumor cells.

MEDICAL MANAGEMENT AND SURGICAL INTERVENTIONS

1. Osteogenic sarcoma: Treated with resection of the tumor, most commonly by amputation. Recent attempts to perform less radical resections (en bloc tumor resection with limb salvage procedures), including therapy with chemotherapeutic agents (especially methotrexate, citrovorum, cyclophosphamide, vincristine, and adriamycin in various combinations), have met with increasing success.
2. Chondrosarcoma: Usually treated with resection, with the degree of resection dependent on the stage of tumor development. Radiotherapy and chemotherapy have not proven to be effective in treating this disease.
3. Multiple myeloma: Requires extensive therapy with radiation and chemotherapy. Radiation is used to control localized bone pain and treat areas with pathologic fractures. Chemotherapy with melphalan, prednisone, and vincristine has been shown to be helpful. Vincristine, doxorubicin, and dexamethasone may be useful in treating the up to 50% refractory cases of myeloma. Occasionally, hypercalcemia requires additional therapy with increased volumes of IV fluids, furosemide, prednisone, or mithramycin. Laminectomy may be required for spinal cord compression caused by vertebral lesions. Pathologic fractures frequently require ORIF. Blood transfusions and potent analgesics are usually required.

NURSING DIAGNOSES AND INTERVENTIONS

See "Intervertebral Disk Disease" for **Knowledge deficit:** Pain control measures, p. 193. See "Osteoarthritis" for **Pain,** p. 425, and **Impaired physical mobility** related to adjustment to new walking gait, p. 426. See "Torn Anterior Cruciate Ligament" for **Potential fluid volume deficit** related to abnormal loss secondary to postsurgical hemorrhage or hematoma, p. 442.

Note: When postoperative casts, use of orthotics, exercises, or similar therapies are prescribed, refer to appropriate nursing diagnoses throughout this chapter. If the patient undergoes amputation, refer to "Amputation," p. 465.

See the appendix for nursing diagnoses and interventions for the care of preoperative and postoperative patients, p. 637, the care of the patient on prolonged bed rest, p. 651, and care of patients with cancer and other life-disrupting illnesses, p. 659.

PATIENT-FAMILY TEACHING AND DISCHARGE PLANNING

Provide patient and significant others with verbal and written information for the following
1. Medications, including the name, rationale, dosage, schedule, precautions, and potential side effects.
2. For surgical patients, the following indicators of wound infection and the importance of notifying MD should they occur: persistent redness, swelling, local warmth, fever, discharge from the wound, or pain. As appropriate, also see "Ligamentous Injuries" for **Knowledge deficit:** Need for elevation of the involved extremity, use of thermotherapy, and exercise, p. 435.
3. For patients with casts, orthotics, prosthetics, ambulatory aids, assistive devices, or similar therapies, instructions for their use, including a return demonstration by patient and a phone number to call should any questions arise after hospital discharge. See "Osteoarthritis" for **Impaired physical mobility** related to adjustment to a new

walking gait, p. 426. See "Ligamentous Injuries" for **Knowledge deficit:** Care and assessment of the casted extremity, p. 435.
4. Referral to hospice or agency that provides home help. This should occur before discharge planning begins to ensure continuity of care between the hospital and home or hospice.

Osteoporosis

Osteoporosis is a condition in which the amount of bony mass decreases, while the size of the bone remains constant, making bone more brittle and more susceptible to fractures. It is a major health problem in the United States, potentially affecting as many as 15-20 million Americans and causing over a million fractures a year in people over the age of 45. The risk of osteoporosis increases with age and is higher in females than in males.

ASSESSMENT

Signs and symptoms: Documented loss of bone density, most commonly found in conjunction with pathologic fractures secondary to osteoporosis. Most fractures occur in the dorsal (thoracic) and lumbar vertebral bodies (usually D-8 through L-2), the neck and intertrochanteric regions of the femur, and the distal radius. Vertebral compression fractures can develop gradually, resulting in loss of height, kyphosis, back discomfort, and constipation. Fractures of the hip result in significant morbidity and mortality.

History and risk factors: Loss of ovarian function (surgical or physiologic menopause), race (non-black, especially Caucasian or Asiatic), family history, nulliparity, preexisting skeletal disease, underweight, inadequate childhood nutrition (lifelong low calcium intake), high caffeine intake, sedentary lifestyle, high alcohol intake, and cigarette smoking. Secondary causes include metastatic disease, drugs (heparin, alcohol, phosphate-binding antacids, corticosteroids, phenytoin, and isoniazid), hyperparathyroidism, immobilization, hypercortisolism, hyperthyroidism, hypogonadism, and connective tissue disease.

DIAGNOSTIC TESTS

1. *Standard AP and lateral x-rays of the spine:* Provide a diagnosis for osteoporotic fractures. Bone density loss is not easily demonstrated by standard radiographs, since 20%-30% of bone density must be lost before it can be noted on x-ray.
2. *Radiogrammetry, photodensitometry, single- and dual-photon absorptiometry, neutron activation, quantitative digital radiography (QDR), and single- and dual-energy computed tomography:* These are examples of some of the sophisticated noninvasive tests that can be used to determine bone density. However, the availability of these tests varies. Bone mass measurement is indicated in individuals who are at risk.

MEDICAL MANAGEMENT AND SURGICAL INTERVENTIONS

1. Oral estrogen: Doses as low as 0.625 mg have been shown to be effective in preventing osteoporosis in postmenopausal women. Use of cyclic estrogen/progesterone also may reduce the risk of endometrial cancer.
2. Calcium intake: Should exceed 1,000-1,500 mg/day for women approaching menopause. Each 8 oz glass of milk provides 275-300 mg of calcium, indicating that an intake of 4-6 glasses/day is ideal. Vegetable calcium sources (e.g., dark green, leafy vegetables; sesame seeds) are also good. For lactose-intolerant patients or those unable to consume dietary calcium, calcium supplementation is prescribed. Some antacids (e.g., Tums) contain calcium and may serve as a calcium supplement. In individuals prone to osteoporosis, lifelong intake of adequate amounts of calcium should be stressed. **Note:** Because smoking and a high-sugar, high-meat diet affect the phos-

phorus-calcium ratio, and therefore calcium utilization, individuals who do not smoke or eat red meat or sugar have a lower calcium requirement.

3. **Vitamin D:** Necessary to allow adequate intestinal absorption and usage of calcium. Adequate dietary vitamin D usually is supplied in vitamin-enriched cereals and milk products. When necessary, the recommended daily intake of this vitamin is 600-800 U twice daily. Because excessive vitamin D is associated with significant toxicity, higher intake is discouraged without clear documentation of need.

4. **Moderate weightbearing exercise:** To stress bones and activate osteoblastic bone formation, because inactivity has been shown to result in disuse osteoporosis. Williams' back exercises, pectoral stretching, isometric abdominal exercises, and walking often are recommended. For older individuals, swimming appears to be the best all-around exercise.

5. **Antiresorptive agents:** To reduce further bone mass loss. The most effective is calcitonin, although its action is not sustained and prolonged therapy has been ineffective in correcting the disease process. Additional antiresorptive agents include androgen and biphosphonates. Fluoride is the only therapeutic agent known to stimulate osteoblastic activity. However, fluoride has not demonstrated the ability to restore the normal architecture of osteoporotic bone.

NURSING DIAGNOSES AND INTERVENTIONS

Health-seeking behavior: Patient requests knowledge regarding prevention of osteoporosis, its treatment, and the importance of choosing and using calcium supplements effectively

Desired outcome: Patient verbalizes knowledge of the disease process and understanding of the most effective calcium supplements and the way in which they are used. **Note:** It is important to begin instructing all individuals at risk for osteoporosis (see section "history and risk factors," p. 459) as early in their lives as possible, owing to the prolonged period of time involved in developing, and thus preventing, this process.

1. Ensure that the MD has recommended or approves use of calcium supplements for the patient. Increased calcium can result in nephrolithiasis in susceptible individuals.
2. Be sure patient is aware of the silent nature of this disorder and realizes that by the time symptoms arise, it is too late for effective treatment.
3. Teach patient that calcium supplements come in many varieties. The most effective form is calcium carbonate, which delivers about 40% calcium. Bonemeal and dolomite should be avoided because they may contain high amounts of lead or other toxic substances.
4. Teach patient that when evaluating supplement labels to look for the amount of elemental calcium available rather than the weight of the total compound. Patient should avoid supplements with added vitamin D since hypervitaminosis of this vitamin is possible.
5. Teach patient not to take calcium and iron supplements simultaneously since iron absorption will be impaired. Calcium also may reduce the absorption of some medications. Similarly, some foods inhibit absorption of calcium (e.g., red meats, spinach, colas, bran, bread, and whole grain cereals). Therefore, calcium should be taken 2 hours before or after other medications or meals.
6. Caution patient to avoid taking more than 500-600 mg of calcium at one time and to spread dosages out over the entire day. Remind patient to drink a full glass of water with each supplement to minimize the risk of developing renal calculi.

Alteration in nutrition: Less than body requirements related to increased need for calcium and vitamin D

Desired outcome: Patient demonstrates intake of adequate amounts of calcium and vitamin D and plans a 3-day menu that provides sufficient intake of both.

1. Ensure that the patient demonstrates understanding of the foods that are high in calcium, including cheese, milk, dark green leafy vegetables, eggs, peanuts, sesame

seeds, and oysters. Provide patient with a list of these foods, including the relative amounts of calcium for each.

2. Teach patient how to plan menus that provide sufficient daily intake of calcium and vitamin D-fortified foods, such as eggs, halibut, herring, fortified dairy products, liver, mackerel, oysters, salmon, and sardines.

3. Provide patient with sample menus that include adequate daily amounts of calcium and vitamin D. Have patient plan a 3-day menu that incorporates these foods.

4. Provide patient with a phone number to call should questions arise after hospital discharge.

See "Amputation" for **Knowledge deficit:** Postsurgical exercise regimen, p. 467.

PATIENT-FAMILY TEACHING AND DISCHARGE PLANNING

Provide patient and significant others with verbal and written information for the following:

1. Medications, including the name, dosage, purpose, schedule, precautions, and potential side effects.

2. Instructions for the prescribed dietary regimen, including the rationale for the diet and foods to include and avoid, if appropriate.

3. Prescribed exercise regimen, including how to perform the exercise, number of repetitions of each, and frequency of exercise periods (see **Knowledge deficit:** Postsurgical exercise regimen, p. 467).

4. Importance of establishing measures for preventing falls in the home (e.g., placing a handrail in the bathtub, avoiding use of throw rugs). Arrange for a home visit for fall prevention as necessary.

5. Importance of reporting to health care provider indicators of pathologic fracture (i.e., deformity, pain, edema, ecchymosis, limb shortening, false motion, decreased ROM, or crepitus). Stress that indicators of vertebral fractures resulting in spinal cord or nerve compression (e.g., paresthesia, weakness, paralysis, or loss of bowel or bladder function) must be reported promptly.

Paget's disease (osteitis deformans)

Paget's disease is an idiopathic process suspected of being caused by a slow viral infection in genetically susceptible individuals. Three to four percent of the population over age 40 have some Pagetic findings, and 20% over age 80 have some Pagetic bone. This disorder results from an aberrant function of osteoclasts (bone-resorbing cells) and osteoblasts (bone-building cells), resulting in bone that is high in mineral content, weaker, of poor quality, grossly deformed, and thickened. Active lesions have increased vascularity and have been attributed to high-output cardiac failure in extensive disease.

ASSESSMENT

Signs and symptoms: Most patients are asymptomatic except for pain at the involved site(s), which can be difficult to differentiate from osteoarthritis or myalgia. Some patients develop pathologic fractures through the Pagetic lesions, or the process can be an incidental finding on x-rays taken to rule out other processes. Cranial enlargement or radiculoneuropathy can result in the following: oculomotor deficits, visual deficits, deafness, dysphagia, dysphasia, headaches, hemifacial paresthesia, or paralysis. Vertebral involvement is evidenced by kyphoscoliosis or stenotic lesions of the spinal cord or nerves, resulting in radiculoneuropathy of these structures. Patients with Paget's disease who are suddenly immobilized may develop hypercalciuria and even hypercalcemia.

DIAGNOSTIC TESTS

1. *Standard x-rays:* May reveal typical mosaic-appearing lesions, osteoporosis circumscripta (an area of radiolucency surrounded by normal bone), protrusio acetabuli

(protrusion of the acetabulum into the pelvis), pseudofractures, microfractures, incomplete transverse fractures, sclerotic bony lesions, invaginated foramen magnum, and pathologic fractures.

2. *Serum tests:* Will reveal an elevated serum alkaline phosphatase, indicating new bone formation.
3. *Urine assay:* Will reveal elevated hydroxyproline, indicating bony lysis.
4. *Bone biopsy:* Can be used to confirm the diagnosis in questionable cases.
5. *Bone scans:* Technetium pyrophosphate may aid in identifying active bone lesions.

MEDICAL MANAGEMENT AND SURGICAL INTERVENTIONS

Because the treatment involves significant risk, it is restricted to patients who have pervasive disease or significant symptoms of involvement in critical areas. Suppressive therapy is restricted to patients with radiculoneuropathy, imminent complications, and highly resorptive lesions, and who are immobilized or require surgery on involved areas.

1. **Nonsteroidal antiinflammatory agents:** May be used to control pain (see Table 8-1, p. 432).
2. **Suppressive therapy:** May include the following:
   - □ *Calcitonin (porcine, human, and salmon):* 50-100 Medical Research Council (MRC) units SC, 3 times a week to as frequently as 200 MRC q12 hours. This hormone inhibits bone resorption while combating parathyroid gland action. Side effects include nausea, a feeling of warmth following injection, and flushing. Salmon calcitonin is the most potent form and may result in allergic reaction with skin manifestations. Calcitonin therapy is expensive and long-term therapy has not been proven to control progression of this disease in all patients.
   - □ *Diphosphonates (etidronate disodium—EHDP):* Daily dosages of 5 mg/kg of body weight. Diphosphonates inhibit calcium deposition in biologic tissues. Side effects include cramps, diarrhea, and nausea. EHDP should be given on an empty stomach for optimal absorption. This medication is contraindicated in patients with new fractures or who are immobilized, and it can increase the risk of pathologic fracture in patients with extensive disease. Because of their adverse effect on normal bone (i.e., spontaneous fractures due to demineralization), diphosphonates are indicated for short-term therapy only.
   - □ *Mithramycin:* A cytotoxic agent given in short courses (10 doses) of 25 μg/kg IV. It is theorized that this medication suppresses the action of osteoclasts in bone resorption. Toxic reactions with mithramycin may be severe, limiting its use only to the most severe cases. Side effects include anorexia, nausea, vomiting; elevated SGOT, BUN, and creatinine; and depressed platelets and leukocytes.
3. **Surgical interventions:** Restricted to repair of pathologic fractures. Surgery on involved bones requires adequate preparation *via* typing and cross-matching of several units of blood, meticulous hemostasis during surgery, and careful monitoring for hemorrhage after surgery.

NURSING DIAGNOSES AND INTERVENTIONS

Knowledge deficit: Potential complications of Paget's disease

Desired outcome: Patient verbalizes knowledge of the disease pathology and awareness of the importance of promptly reporting untoward indicators to the health care provider.

1. Teach patient the disease pathology, including the signs and symptoms of imminent complications, such as renal calculi, significant cranial or spinal radiculoneuropathy (decreased hearing, headache, paresthesia, weakness, paralysis, visual defects, dysphasia, dysphagia, oculomotor weakness); hydrocephalus (headache, pupil inequality, altered LOC); and alterations in gait.
2. Instruct patient to report any indicators of pathologic fracture: pain, deformity, decreased ROM, limb shortening, ecchymosis, edema, false motion, and crepitus.

See "Gouty Arthritis" for **Knowledge deficit:** Assessments and preventive measures for uric acid renal calculi, p. 429. See "Torn Anterior Cruciate Ligament" for **Potential fluid volume deficit** related to abnormal loss secondary to postsurgical hemorrhage or bleeding), p. 442. Also see "Hypercalcemia," p. 561.

PATIENT-FAMILY TEACHING AND DISCHARGE PLANNING

Provide patient and significant others with verbal and written information for the following:
1. Medications, including drug name, purpose, dosage, schedule, potential side effects, and precautions.
2. Signs to monitor for and report while on suppressive therapy, especially ecchymosis, melena, hematoma, and hematuria, as well as indicators of prolonged bleeding, hemorrhage, and superimposed infections.
3. Indicators to monitor for and report related to complications of the disease (see **Knowledge deficit,** p. 462).

Section Four   MUSCULOSKELETAL SURGICAL PROCEDURES

Bunionectomy

Bunionectomy is surgery to correct hallux valgus. Hallux refers to the great toe and valgus means that it is bent outward, away from the midline. The bunion is actually a prominence of the first metatarsal head, resulting from altered joint dynamics as the hallux subluxates laterally into a valgus deformity. Although a bunion can occur because of hereditary intrinsic joint weakness, the most frequent cause is improperly fitting footwear.

ASSESSMENT

Signs and symptoms: Can range from mild valgus deformity to severe valgus deformity with altered gait. In acute conditions, the patient has inflammation of the adventitial bursa, resulting in erythema, local warmth, and tenderness. The patient has great difficulty fitting shoes. X-rays often are used to define bony involvement and displacement of the lateral sesamoid bone.

MEDICAL MANAGEMENT AND SURGICAL INTERVENTIONS

1. Conservative treatment: Begins with appropriately fitted footwear to accommodate the deformity. Night splints may be useful in decreasing discomfort for some patients, although they have not been effective in preventing progression of hallux valgus.
2. Bunionectomy: Performed when the patient has significant pain and alterations in ambulation affecting ADL. Many forms of surgery can be used, but the main elements include removal of the projecting metatarsal head (bunionectomy), excision of the displaced sesamoid bone, release of the adductor hallucis tendon, and tightening of the medial periarticular tissues to prevent recurrence. Transfixion of the repaired joint with a K-wire may be necessary to enhance support, especially if an osteotomy is used in the correction. The tip of the K-wire is left exposed and removed 10-21 days after surgery. Ambulation with appropriate immobilization of the involved foot is begun within 2-5 days of surgery. A short leg cast, slipper cast, or bunion boot is used for immobilization of the great toe.

NURSING DIAGNOSES AND INTERVENTIONS

Pain related to joint changes and corrective therapy

Desired outcome: Patient verbalizes a reduction in discomfort and does not exhibit signs of uncontrolled pain, such as facial grimacing.

1. Patients recovering from bunionectomy often experience a great deal of discomfort. Help patient devise a rating system (e.g., a scale of 0-10) to rate pain and analgesic relief.
2. Administer analgesics and antiinflammatory agents as prescribed and document their effectiveness.
3. Instruct patient in the use of nonpharmacologic methods of pain control, including guided imagery; graduated breathing (as in Lamaze); enhanced relaxation; massage; biofeedback; cutaneous stimulation (*via* a counterirritant such as oil of wintergreen); transcutaneous electrical nerve stimulation (TENS) device; warm or cool thermotherapy; music therapy; and tactile, auditory, visual, or verbal distractions.
4. Use traditional nursing interventions to counteract the pain, including backrubs, repositioning, and encouraging the patient to verbalize feelings.
5. Incorporate rest, local warmth, and elevation of the affected joints, when possible, to help control discomfort.
6. Advise patient to coordinate the time of peak effectiveness of the antiinflammatory agent with periods of exercise or mandatory use of joints.
7. Instruct patient in the use of moist heat and hydrotherapy, which will help reduce long-term discomfort.

Knowledge deficit: Disease process and therapeutic regimen

Desired outcome: Patient verbalizes knowledge of bunion formation, preventive measures, prescribed postoperative immobilization, and potential complications.

1. Assess patient's level of understanding about the disease process and treatment modalities involved.
2. Provide instructions about causes and progression of bunion formation, role of improperly fitting shoes as a cause of bunions, role of surgery in bunion correction, rationale for the postoperative regimen of care, need for immobilization of the surgical area to promote healing and maintain realignment, technique for caring for the casted extremity (or dressed foot), and indicators of wound infection.
3. As appropriate, provide written material for cast care, indicators of wound infection, wound care, neurovascular deficit, and use of appropriate pain medication. For further information on cast care, see the nursing diagnosis **Knowledge deficit:** Care and assessment of the casted extremity, p. 435, in "Ligamentous Injury."

Impaired physical mobility related to immobilization device or nonweightbearing secondary to bunionectomy

Desired outcomes: Patient demonstrates compliance with elevation of the operant extremity above the level of the heart during the early postoperative period. Patient demonstrates use of safety measures while ambulating with the immobilization device.

1. Following surgery, the patient will be permitted bathroom privileges with a walker or crutches, with weightbearing as tolerated. At other times, ensure that the operant extremity is kept elevated higher than the level of the heart to facilitate reduction of postoperative edema. **Note:** Patients with plaster of Paris casts are restricted to non–weight-bearing ambulation until 48 hours after the cast has been applied.
2. The patient will begin ambulation wearing a cast or bunion boot that is worn for 3-6 weeks following surgery. Remind patient that the primary goal of the immobilization device is to maintain position of the great toe. Caution patient to ambulate with care in the device until it becomes an integral part of ambulation. Special care should be exercised on stairs, hills, and uneven surfaces.

Potential for altered tissue perfusion: Peripheral, related to impaired circulation secondary to compression from circumferential cast or dressing

Desired outcomes: Patient has adequate perfusion to the involved extremity as evidenced by normal color, warmth, brisk capillary refill (<3 seconds), distal pulses >2+ on a 0-4+ scale, ability to move the great toe, and absence of numbness or tingling. Patient verbalizes knowledge of the signs of impaired neurovascular status and awareness of the importance of getting prompt treatment should they occur.

1. Assess the operant extremity for the integrity of neurovascular status each time VS are taken (or at least q4h). Impaired neurovascular status requires nursing interventions, such as elevation, loosening of restrictive dressings, or promptly notifying the MD if these measures are ineffective.
2. Ensure that the patient can verbalize the signs and symptoms of impaired neurovascular status and knows to call the MD should they occur after hospital discharge. These include persistent changes in color (pallor, cyanosis, redness), coolness, delayed capillary refill, paresthesias (numbness, tingling), or inability to move distal areas (the great or second toe).

See the appendix for nursing diagnoses and interventions for the care of preoperative and postoperative patients, p. 637.

PATIENT-FAMILY TEACHING AND DISCHARGE PLANNING

Provide patient and significant others with verbal and written information for the following:

1. Technique for ambulation with the casted extremity or bunion boot and use of assistive devices and ambulatory aids (see **Impaired physical mobility** related to adjustment to a new walking gait, p. 426). Be sure the patient demonstrates independence in ADL before hospital discharge. If necessary, arrange for follow-up instruction *via* a home visit.
2. Medications, including name, rationale, dosage, schedule, precautions, and potential side effects.
3. Indicators of wound infection (see "Fractures," p. 454) and impaired neurovascular status (see "Ligamentous Injuries," p. 436) and the importance of notifying MD promptly should they occur.
4. Use of thermotherapy, elevation, and exercise (see "Ligamentous Injuries," p. 436).
5. Phone number to call should patient have questions after hospital discharge.

Amputation

Today, amputation is less frequently required as an orthopaedic surgical intervention than it was before the advent of antibiotics and microsurgery techniques. However, amputation is still required for certain disorders such as atherosclerotic arterial occlusive disease, osteomyelitis, severe trauma, malignant tumors, or congenital anomalies. In the United States, most amputations are performed for advanced atherosclerotic arterial occlusive disease, especially in diabetic patients over age 60 with pronounced peripheral vascular disease, as evidenced by gangrene. When it is possible to increase an individual's function with a prosthesis, amputation is sometimes offered as an optional treatment. The majority of amputations are of the lower extremity.

ASSESSMENT

Signs and symptoms: Patients with advanced atherosclerotic arterial occlusive disease may have gangrene, a chronic stasis ulcer, or an infected wound that fails to heal. The patient usually complains of pain and there can be rubor (a dark red color) when the limb is dependent, as well as atrophy of the skin and subcutaneous tissues.

See "Atherosclerotic Arterial Occlusive Disease," p. 85, in Chapter 2, "Osteomyelitis," p. 445, and "Malignant Neoplasms," p. 457, as appropriate.

DIAGNOSTIC TESTS

1. *Angiography:* Confirms inadequacy of circulation.
2. *CT scan:* Determines the degree of neoplastic or osteomyelitic involvement.
3. *Biopsy:* May be used to confirm presence of osteomyelitis or neoplasm.
4. *Extensive evaluations by occupational therapist for fine motor function and by physical therapist for gross motor function:* To document functional loss and potential for compensation.
5. *Noninvasive vascular testing:* Documents lack of perfusion of blood vessels, using a Doppler ultrasound device and pneumatic cuffs. Use of a Doppler to measure velocity of flow of microcirculation beneath the skin shows promise as another measure.
6. *Xenon (Xe) 133 studies:* Skin clearance of this agent after intradermal injection is determined using a gamma camera and computer. Skin clearance reflects skin blood flow as a measure of the appropriate level of amputation.
7. *Skin fluorescence:* Measuring skin fluorescence with a fluorometer after IV injection of a fluorescein dye is useful in determining blood supply.
8. *Oxymetry:* Transcutaneous determination of Pao_2 aids in determining levels of tissue perfusion. Levels >40 mm Hg usually support tissue healing.
9. *Laboratory tests:* Serum albumin <3.5 g/ml and a total lymphocyte count <1,500 cells/μl forebode significant problems with healing.

MEDICAL MANAGEMENT AND SURGICAL INTERVENTIONS

1. Amputation: The actual procedure used for amputation depends on the area of the limb involved. Generally, the surgical goals are to remove the least amount of tissue possible, provide adequate tissue for a viable myocutaneous flap to create a stump, and ensure adequate provision for a prosthetic device. Large blood vessels are individually identified and suture-ligated. Nerves are stretched and then suture-ligated to allow them to retract back into the residual limb (stump) to prevent trauma when the stump is used. Usually, bone ends are beveled to prevent trauma from sharp edges. Infected limbs are closed loosely to allow adequate drainage until infected tissues have been treated adequately.
2. Postoperative period: Immediately after surgery, a prosthesis may be used to promote wound healing, minimize stump edema, decrease the length of rehabilitation, and prevent postsurgical complications of immobility. A cast is applied over the postoperative dressing, which incorporates a device that allows subsequent attachment of a pylon prosthesis to allow ambulation while the first prosthesis is being made. Early ambulation prevents flexion contractures, allows earlier gait training, improves psychologic state, prevents loss of muscle strength, and increases local circulation to improve wound healing, which subsequently decreases edema and pain. Complications associated with amputations include increased mortality rates (less than 50% of all lower extremity amputees survive 5 years), fractures in the stump following falls, and stump ischemia.

NURSING DIAGNOSES AND INTERVENTIONS

Potential for disuse syndrome related to pain and immobility secondary to amputation of the extremity

Desired outcome: Patient verbalizes understanding of the exercise regimen and performs the exercises independently.

1. Control patient's pain to ensure appropriate movement.
2. After providing elevation for the first 2 days postoperatively, intersperse elevation with periods of ROM to the remaining joints of the involved extremity. **Note:** Both elevation and ROM are performed with MD prescription.
3. Prevent flexion contractures of the knee and hip by assisting the patient with lying prone for an hour tid.
4. Another method for preventing flexion contractures is to teach the patient to perform

exercises that increase the strength of the muscle extensors. Consult with MD regarding prescriptions for the following exercises:

☐ *Above-the-knee amputation:* Have patient attempt to straighten the hip from a flexed position against resistance or perform gluteal-setting exercises.

☐ *Below-the-knee amputation:* Have patient attempt to straighten the knee against resistance or perform hamstring-setting exercises. These patients also should perform the exercises described with above-the-knee amputations.

5. For other interventions, see **Potential for disuse syndrome** related to inactivity secondary to prolonged bed rest, p. 653, in the appendix.

Impaired physical mobility related to altered stance secondary to amputation of the lower limb

Desired outcome: Patient demonstrates use of muscle-tightening technique to enhance mobilization.

1. Inform patients with lower-extremity amputation that difficulty in adjusting to the altered stance may occur as a result of the amputation. Suggest that to prevent an altered stance, patient should tighten the gluteal and abdominal muscles while standing.
2. For other interventions, see **Impaired physical mobility** related to adjustment to a new walking gait with an assistive device, p. 426, in "Osteoarthritis."

Knowledge deficit: Postsurgical exercise regimen

Desired outcome: Patient verbalizes knowledge of the exercise regimen and returns the demonstration independently.

1. To increase adherence to the prescribed exercise regimen, provide patient with an explanation of the rationale for the exercises, method of performing the exercises, and suggestions for adapting these exercises to home use. Most therapeutic programs include ROM and muscle-strengthening exercises.
2. Demonstrate each exercise until the patient is able to return the demonstration independently. Provide patient with written instructions that review each exercise and describe the number of repetitions and number of times a day it should be performed, and a phone number to call should any questions arise after patient is discharged. If necessary, provide for a postdischarge home visit.
3. If additional equipment is required, provide patient with information regarding where it can be purchased and, if necessary, seek financial assistance from social services.

Knowledge deficit: Care of the stump and prosthesis; signs and symptoms of skin irritation or pressure necrosis

Desired outcomes: Patient verbalizes knowledge of the care of the stump and prosthesis and independently returns the demonstration of wrapping the stump. Patient verbalizes knowledge of the indicators of pressure necrosis and irritation from the wrapping device or prosthesis.

Note: A stump that is inappropriately treated will become edematous and more easily prone to injury, which will delay proper fitting of the permanent prosthesis.

---

1. If molding of the stump for eventual prosthetic fitting is prescribed, instruct the patient in the technique for application of an elastic sleeve or wrap: Application of the elastic wrap is begun with a recurrent turn over the distal end of the stump and then diagonal circumferential turns are made, overlapping half to two-thirds of the width of the wrap. Traction applied to the wrap should ensure more pressure on the distal portion of the stump. The elastic device should be snug but not excessively so, since a tight wrap can impede circulation and healing. Rewrapping should be done q4h, combined with careful inspection of the stump. Areas prone to pressure, such as bony prominences or prominent tendons, should be assessed for evidence of excess pressure. Ensure that all tissue is contained by the elastic device. If any tissue is allowed to bulge, proper fitting of the prosthesis will be difficult.

2. Teach patient to monitor the stump for indicators of skin irritation or pressure necrosis caused by the elastic device or prosthesis, including blebs, abrasions, and erythemic or tender areas. Explain that if massage fails to alleviate the problem, the patient should seek the help of the public health nurse or visiting nurse or notify the MD.

3. For areas that are prone to pressure, provide extra padding with sheet wadding, moleskin, or lambswool to prevent irritation.

4. The day after the sutures have been removed (and assuming the incision is dry and intact) instruct the patient to cleanse the stump daily with mild soap and water. Caution against the use of emollients, which can create skin maceration beneath the prosthesis.

5. Advise patient that when molding is no longer necessary (after 1-6 months), he or she will be fitted with a stump sock that will allow air to circulate around the stump.

6. Ensure that patient receives complete instructions in the care of the prosthesis by the prosthetist or knowledgeable nurse.

Potential fluid volume deficit related to abnormal loss secondary to postsurgical hemorrhage

Desired outcomes: Patient is normovolemic as evidenced by BP $\geq$90/60 (or within patient's usual range), HR $\leq$100 bpm, urinary output $\geq$ 30 ml/hr, peripheral pulses >2+ on a 0-4+ scale, brisk capillary refill (<3 seconds), and drainage $\leq$50 ml/hr in a drainage device. Patient verbalizes knowledge of the importance of reporting bleeding promptly to the staff.

1. Inspect the cast (or postoperative dressing) for increasing drainage. If the stump is elevated, inspect dependent areas for evidence of bleeding. Inform patient of the need to report increasing bleeding to staff.

2. If a drain or drainage device is used, document the amount of drainage. Report drainage that exceeds 50 ml/hr.

Pain related to phantom limb sensation

Desired outcome: Patient relates a reduction in phantom limb sensations as documented by a pain scale and does not exhibit signs of uncontrolled pain, such as facial grimacing.

1. Explain to the patient that continued sensations often arise from the amputated part. Although they can be painful, irritating, or simply disconcerting, these sensations usually resolve with time. As appropriate, devise a pain scale with patient, for example, by rating pain on a scale of 0-10.

2. Manage these painful sensations with the interventions discussed in **Pain,** p. 425, in "Osteoarthritis." For this type of pain, counterirritation is especially useful. Other phantom limb sensations may respond to similar tactics such as distraction, relaxation, or use of cutaneous stimulation *via* oil of wintergreen, heat, or massage. Some patients have found TENS especially effective in managing phantom limb sensation.

3. Some MDs advocate vigorous stimulation of the end of the stump to alter the feedback loop of the resected nerve. Advise patient that this can be done by hitting the end of a *well-healed* stump with a rolled towel.

4. Chronic phantom limb sensation may require exploration of the stump to resect a neuroma at the site of the nerve resection. Inform patient that this may be a possibility if phantom limb sensation continues for more than 6 months.

Body image disturbance and altered role performance related to loss of limb

Desired outcome: Patient begins to show adaptation toward loss of the limb and demonstrates role-related responsibilities.

1. Be aware that use of a prosthesis immediately after surgery allows patients to continue to perceive of themselves as ambulatory (and thus "whole") individuals.

2. Gently encourage patient to look at and touch the stump and verbalize feelings about the amputation. It is essential that the nurse and other caregivers show an accepting attitude as well as encourage significant others to accept the patient as he or she now appears.

3. Assist patient with adapting to the loss of the limb, while maintaining a sense of what is perceived as the "normal" self. This may be accomplished by introducing patient to others who have successfully adapted to an amputation similar to that of the patient. In addition, teaching aids, such as audiovisuals, books, pamphlets, and videotapes, can be employed to demonstrate how others have adapted to the amputation.
4. For patients who continue to have difficulty adapting to the amputation, provide a referral to an appropriate resource person, such as a psychologist or psychiatric nurse.

See "Intervertebral Disk Disease" for **Knowledge deficit:** Pain control measures, p. 193. See "Osteoarthritis" for **Pain,** p. 425. See "Fractures" for **Knowledge deficit:** Potential for infection, p. 454. See the appendix for nursing diagnoses and interventions for the care of preoperative and postoperative patients, p. 637, and for the care of patients with cancer and other life-disrupting illnesses, p. 659.

PATIENT-FAMILY TEACHING AND DISCHARGE PLANNING

Provide patient and significant others with verbal and written information for the following:
1. How and where to purchase necessary supplies and equipment for self-care.
2. Care of the stump and prosthesis.
3. Indicators of wound infection, which necessitate medical attention: swelling, persistent redness, discharge, local warmth, systemic fever, and pain.
4. Medications, including name, rationale, dosage, schedule, precautions, and potential side effects.
5. Phone number of a resource person, should questions arise after hospital discharge.
6. Prescribed exercises. Patient should be able to perform them independently before discharge.
7. Referral to appropriate resource person, should maladaptive behaviors associated with grieving or body image disturbance continue.
8. Ambulation with assistive device and prosthesis on level and uneven surfaces and on stairs. Patient should demonstrate independence before hospital discharge. For patients with an upper extremity amputation, independence with ADL should be demonstrated before discharge. If necessary, arrange for a home visit.

Tendon transfer

A tendon transfer involves the transference of the insertion site of a functioning muscle-tendon unit to a new position to change the action of that unit. This allows compensation of a deficit created by congenital defect or paralyzed or severed muscle. Because there is considerable overlap in function, in that multiple muscles can serve one purpose, tendon transfer may allow the patient to regain function without any loss of function.

DIAGNOSTIC TEST

Electromyography: Can be used to ensure adequate muscle function of the units proposed for transfer.

MEDICAL MANAGEMENT AND SURGICAL INTERVENTIONS

1. Surgical procedure: Involves transection of the tendon at an appropriate level, transfer to the new position, and fixation to the appropriate insertion site with permanent sutures, staples, screws, or wire. It also is possible to attach "new" tendon to the resected tendon above the insertion site, using tendon repair suture techniques. Examples of disorders in which tendon transfer procedures are performed include radial

paralysis, congenital talipes equinovarus (a form of clubfoot), and extensive injury to the extensor pollicis longus that limits thumb extension.

2. **Postsurgical immobilization:** The operant area is immobilized in a cast, splint, or orthosis until there has been sufficient healing of the tendon repair (2-6 weeks) or stabilization of the bony insertion (4-12 weeks).

3. **Physical therapy regimen:** After immobilization, the patient is begun on an intense, progressive physical therapy regimen to regain strength in the transferred tendon, retrain new muscle function, and compensate for decreased strength at the site of the transfer. Various orthotics, dynamic splints, and special exercise rigs can be constructed to aid the patient in regaining function.

NURSING DIAGNOSES AND INTERVENTIONS

See "Osteoarthritis" for **Pain,** p. 425, and **Impaired physical mobility** related to adjustment to new walking gait, p. 426. See "Ligamentous Injuries" for **Knowledge deficit:** Care and assessment of the casted extremity, p. 435. See "Torn Anterior Cruciate Ligament" for **Potential fluid volume deficit** related to abnormal loss secondary to postsurgical hemorrhage or hematoma, p. 442. See "Fractures" for **Self-care deficit,** p. 452. See "Bunionectomy" for **Potential alteration in tissue perfusion** related to impaired circulation secondary to compression from circumferential cast or dressing, p. 464. See the appendix for nursing diagnoses and interventions for the care of preoperative and postoperative patients, p. 637, care of the patient on prolonged bed rest, p. 651, and for the care of patients with cancer and other life-disrupting illnesses (psychosocial nursing diagnoses) p. 690.

PATIENT-FAMILY TEACHING AND DISCHARGE PLANNING

Provide patient and significant others with verbal and written information for the following:

1. Use of such therapies as thermotherapy and elevation (see "Ligamentous Injuries," p. 435).

2. Use of external support devices such as elastic wraps, splints, orthoses, or similar items (see "Ligamentous Injuries," p. 436). This should include care of the device, care of the skin beneath the device, monitoring the area for presence of irritation, and monitoring for neurovascular deficit.

3. Cast care instructions, if patient is discharged with a cast (see "Ligamentous Injuries," p. 435).

4. Prescribed exercise regimen, including rationale for the therapy, how it is accomplished, number of repetitions, and frequency of the exercise.

5. Medications, including name, rationale, dosage, schedule, precautions, and potential side effects.

6. Indicators of wound infection, which necessitate medical attention: persistent redness, swelling, wound discharge, local warmth, and increase in pain.

7. Use of ambulatory aid, if patient is discharged with one (see "Osteoarthritis," p. 426). This should include return demonstration of independence with ambulation on level and uneven surfaces and stairs before discharge.

8. Phone number of resource person, should questions arise after patient has been discharged.

Bone grafting

A bone graft procedure refers to the transfer of cancellous or cortical bone from one site to another. The bone can be from the patient (autogenic), another human (homogenic), or another species (heterogenic). Currently, the most successful results are achieved with autogenic grafts, but homogenic grafting is showing increasing promise as a therapeutic resource. Bone grafts can be required to create bony fusion of a joint (arthrodesis), compensate for lost or inadequately developed bone, or correct bony nonunion of fractures. Fibrin sealant has been used to aid in securing bone grafts and controlling bleeding, especially in patients with hemorrhagic disorders.

Current microsurgical techniques permit myocutaneous-bone or muscle-bone grafts that include bone, overlying muscle, and/or skin. These complex grafting procedures allow much greater potential for success of the graft for procedures that are used to rebuild large areas of tissue loss from trauma or necessary surgical resection. The following discussion is limited to traditional, simple autogenic bone grafting procedures.

DIAGNOSTIC TESTS

The need for bone grafts can be documented by the following: AP x-rays, gallium scans (to rule out osteomyelitis), and angiograms to evaluate blood supply when myocutaneous-bone or muscle-bone grafts are to be done.

MEDICAL MANAGEMENT AND SURGICAL INTERVENTIONS

1. **Bone graft procedure:** Most commonly, bone grafts are taken from the anterior or posterior iliac crest. However, bone grafts also can be harvested from the fibula, tibia, or ribs. The graft usually involves resection of a piece of cortical bone that is fashioned to replace the deficit or enhance bony fusion or aid internal fixation. Usually, cancellous bone is taken from the same site and packed in and around the cortical graft to facilitate new bone formation. The donor site frequently oozes blood, so a postoperative drain is often placed.
2. **Postoperative regimen:** Usually, the recipient site requires immobilization (most often with a cast) to prevent dislodging of the graft. Some bone grafts require internal fixation to hold them in place. Closed drainage systems frequently are placed in the donor site.

NURSING DIAGNOSES AND INTERVENTIONS

See "Osteoarthritis" for **Pain,** p. 425, and **Impaired physical mobility** related to adjustment to new walking gait, p. 435. See "Ligamentous Injuries" for **Knowledge deficit:** Care and assessment of the casted extremity, p. 435. See "Torn Anterior Cruciate Ligament" for **Potential fluid volume deficit** related to abnormal loss secondary to postsurgical hemorrhage or hematoma, p. 442. See "Bunionectomy" for **Potential alteration in tissue perfusion** related to impaired circulation secondary to compression from circumferential cast or dressing, p. 464. See the appendix for nursing diagnoses and interventions for the care of preoperative and postoperative patients, p. 637, care of the patient on prolonged bed rest, p. 651, and care of the patient with cancer and other life-disrupting illnesses (psychosocial nursing diagnoses), p. 690.

PATIENT-FAMILY TEACHING AND DISCHARGE PLANNING

See "Tendon Transfer," p. 470.

Repair of recurrent shoulder dislocation

The shoulder is a complex set of joints including the glenohumeral, sternoclavicular, acromioclavicular, and thoracoscapular joints, all of which act in combination to allow function. Of these joints, the glenohumeral joint is most commonly affected by dislocation. Most glenohumeral dislocations originate with trauma. Once periarticular weakness and laxity are established, the shoulder can dislocate with minimal stress during abduction. A shoulder repair is necessary when the patient has significant pain and compromised function.

Note: See "Dislocation/Subluxation," p. 437, for a discussion of assessment, diagnostic tests, and medical management.

SURGICAL INTERVENTIONS

1. **Bristow procedure:** Transfers the short ends of the biceps and coracobrachialis muscular origin sites from the coracoid process to the scapular neck. The new positions allow these muscles to hold the head of the humerus in its anatomic position within the glenoid cavity.
2. **Bankart procedure:** Involves reattaching the anterior joint capsule to the front rim of the glenoid cavity to reduce laxity and prevent anterior dislocation.
3. **Putti-Platt procedure:** Involves reefing (shortening) of the subscapularis tendon to prevent excessive lateral rotation, which can contribute to dislocation.
4. **Postoperative care:** After surgery, the patient usually is placed in a shoulder immobilizer for 3-6 weeks. If the patient has large shoulder muscles, a postoperative drain may be required. After immobilization, a regimen of progressive ROM exercises is begun, first to regain ROM and then to increase muscle strength.

NURSING DIAGNOSES AND INTERVENTIONS

Potential impairment of skin integrity related to risk of maceration of the axillary skin secondary to shoulder immobilization

Desired outcomes: Patient's skin remains clear, dry, and intact. Patient verbalizes knowledge of the established plan of prevention and the signs and symptoms of maceration.

1. Assess patient's axillary skin before surgery to evaluate the potential for maceration, including open wounds, areas of irritation, and excessive perspiration.
2. Teach patient the rationale and interventions used for preventing maceration and the need to report indicators of maceration, such as pain, burning, irritation, and foul odor.
3. Cleanse the axilla well before surgery.
4. Before the shoulder immobilizer is positioned, the operating room nurse will place a cotton (ABD) pad in the axilla. After 2-3 days, remove the pad. Then cleanse, dry thoroughly, and inspect the axilla (as well as possible) without abducting the shoulder. Usually, this can be done by holding a washcloth in the hand and sliding the hand into the axilla. Although talc can be used, its use should be judicious because it can build up and act as a reservoir for moisture. Replace the cotton pad with a new one and document the condition of the skin. If the patient is not allergic, a deodorant pad may be used, instead.

Potential alteration in tissue perfusion: Peripheral, related to impaired circulation to and compression of the musculocutaneous nerve secondary to pressure from the immobilization device

Desired outcomes: Patient has adequate tissue perfusion in the operant arm as evidenced by the ability to contract the biceps muscle, presence of normal sensations along the radial portion of the forearm, and brisk capillary refill (<3 seconds), adequate pulses (>2+ on a 0-4+ scale), normal color, and warmth in the distal extremity. Patient verbalizes knowledge of the signs and symptoms of impaired sensorimotor function and the importance of notifying the staff promptly should they occur.

1. Unless it is contraindicated, encourage flexion and extension of the fingers and wrist to enhance perfusion to the distal tissues.
2. Monitor the wrist and upper arm for evidence of pressure and irritation from the immobilizer. However, be aware that the device must be sufficiently tight to ensure adequate immobilization.

3. With every VS assessment, evaluate upper extremity neurovascular function. Be especially alert to the patient's inability to contract the biceps muscle and to absent or abnormal sensations along the radial portion of the forearm. Notify MD of significant findings.
4. Instruct patient to notify the staff promptly should any alterations in sensory or motor function occur.

See "Osteoarthritis" for **Pain,** p. 425. See "Fractures" for **Self-care deficit,** p. 452. See "Amputation" for **Knowledge deficit:** Postsurgical exercise regimen, p. 467. See the appendix for nursing diagnoses and interventions for the care of preoperative and postoperative patients, p. 637.

PATIENT-FAMILY TEACHING AND DISCHARGE PLANNING

Provide patient and significant others with verbal and written information for the following:
1. Prescribed exercise regimen, including rationale for each exercise, method of performing the exercise, number of repetitions for each, and frequency of the exercise periods (see "Ligamentous Injuries," p. 435). Be sure the patient can return the demonstration independently before hospital discharge.
2. Indicators of wound infection, which necessitate medical attention: swelling, persistent redness, local warmth, fever, and pain.
3. For patients discharged with braces or immobilizers, the use and care of the device and care of the axilla on the operant side.
4. Indicators of neurovascular deficit: decreasing sensation, paresthesias, weakness or paralysis, coolness, pallor, cyanosis, decreased pulses, delayed capillary refill, and increasing pain in the distal extremity.
5. Medications, including name, rationale, dosage, schedule, precautions, and potential side effects.
6. Phone number of a resource person, should questions arise after hospital discharge.

Total hip arthroplasty

Total hip arthroplasty (THA) is surgery involving resection of the hip joint and its replacement with an endoprosthesis. Conditions resulting in the need for a THA include osteoarthritis, rheumatoid arthritis, ankylosing spondylosis (Marie-Strumpell disease), Legg-Calvé-Perthes disease, and severe hip trauma. Usually, THA is restricted to older patients because the duration of the implant life is unknown. However, younger patients with severe disease also undergo this procedure.

The bipolar or universal endoprosthesis is an intermediary step between replacement of just the femoral head and a complete THA. For this device a polyethylene lined metal cup fits over the femoral component. Articulation occurs between the femoral component and the inside of the metal cup and between the outside of the metal cup and the anatomic acetabulum. The advantages of this system are that it reduces wear on the acetabulum and allows ease in converting the joint to a THA later.

THA is performed when the joint has been severely affected by disease, resulting in significant pain and a dysfunctional femoroacetabular articulation. Because it is an irreversible procedure involving the removal of significant amounts of bone, several conditions should be met before the patient is considered a serious candidate. In addition to severe pain and loss of function, conservative therapies need to have been exhausted and the patient should have adhered to past therapeutic regimens and be free of any concurrent infectious process. Complications of THA include recurrent dislocations, loosening of the implant, breakage of the femoral component, disabling pain, and sepsis. Of these, infection is the most serious and eventually may necessitate removal of the prosthesis, with resultant flail joint and severe limb shortening.

DIAGNOSTIC TESTS

1. *Gallium scan and ESR:* May be indicated to rule out concurrent infection.
2. *Scintigraphy:* Can be used to document leg length discrepancy, which can be surgically compensated for by using alternative neck lengths on the femoral prosthesis.

MEDICAL MANAGEMENT AND SURGICAL INTERVENTIONS

1. **Surgical procedure:** Although the actual surgical procedure for THA can be accomplished *via* a variety of approaches, it is most commonly done through a posterior lateral approach. Methylmethacrylate may be used as a grouting agent to hold the endoprosthesis in place, or special prosthetics coated with porous materials, such as ceramics, may be used to allow bony ingrowth to fix the device internally. Once the prosthetic acetabulum is positioned, the femoral canal is reamed to accept the femoral prosthesis. A drain is then inserted into the deeper layers of the wound.
2. **Antibiotics:** Because the potential for infection is increased with the presence of the massive endoprosthesis, the patient is placed on prophylactic antibiotics before, during, and for at least 5 days after surgery. Infection of the THA may require its temporary or permanent removal.
3. **Postsurgical immobilization:** The patient is immobilized in balanced suspension or similar device (A-frame, abduction pillow, or wedge abduction pillow) to prevent internal rotation, adduction, and flexion past 90 degrees, which can cause dislocation of the endoprosthesis. If methylmethacrylate is used, the patient will be more readily mobile (usually within 5 days) because of the immediate fixation of the device. If a porous-coated device is used, it is not immediately fixed in place and the patient may require longer immobilization (several days to several weeks). If the greater trochanter was removed to allow visualization or correct muscle weakness, it will require wiring and further immobilization for at least 3 weeks in balanced suspension or limited weightbearing for several weeks.
4. **Progressive physical therapy:** To regain muscular strength and to ensure the patient has adequate upper extremity strength to allow ambulation with crutches or a walker. During postoperative immobilization, the patient begins muscle-strengthening exercises using balanced suspension (or a similar device). The patient must be reminded to avoid internal rotation, adduction, and flexion of the hip past 90 degrees.

NURSING DIAGNOSES AND INTERVENTIONS

Knowledge deficit: Potential for and mechanism of THA dislocation, preventive measures, positional restrictions, prescribed ambulation regimen, and use of assistive devices

Desired outcome: Patient verbalizes knowledge of the potential for, preventive measures for, and mechanism of THA dislocation and demonstrates the prescribed regimen for ambulation and performance of ADL without experiencing dislocation.

Note: There is a high risk of dislocation until the periarticular tissues scar down around the endoprosthesis. If it occurs once, there is increased potential for recurrence because the periarticular tissues will have been stretched. Dislocation is treated with reduction under anesthesia and immobilization in balanced suspension for 3-6 weeks. Recurrent dislocation may require surgical intervention to tighten periarticular tissues or revise the THA. After 6 weeks, the properly placed THA has significantly decreased potential for dislocation. The following discussion relates to the *posteriolateral approach* for THA surgery. Other approaches require different positional restrictions.

1. During the preoperative period, advise patient about the potential for dislocation.
2. Show patient what the endoprosthesis looks like (using a model or similar implant) and how easily it can be dislocated when positional restrictions are not followed.
3. During the preoperative period, instruct patient in the use of ambulatory aids and ADL-assistive devices that allow independence without violation of positional re-

strictions. Explain the use of devices used to maintain positional restrictions.

4. After surgery, reinforce positional restrictions and activities that involve these restrictions, including pivoting on the affected leg, sitting on a regular-height toilet seat, bending over to tie shoelaces, or crossing the legs.
5. Advise patient about the need for long-handled shoe horn, pickup sticks, stocking helpers, and a raised toilet seat for use after discharge. Provide addresses for stores that retail these items.
6. Be sure the patient verbalizes and demonstrates understanding of the positional restrictions and is able to accomplish ambulation and performance of ADL independently, using the assistive device.

Knowledge deficit: Potential for infection caused by foreign body reaction to the endoprosthesis

Desired outcome: Patient verbalizes knowledge of the ongoing potential for infection, its indicators, and the importance of seeking prompt medical care should they occur.

1. Advise patient that infection potential will be a permanent situation. Because of foreign body reaction and increased blood supply resulting from associated inflammatory response, these patients are at increased risk for hematogenic (blood-borne) infection. Introduce this as a potential complication as part of the informed consent process and review it as part of preoperative teaching.
2. Before hospital discharge, ensure that the patient verbalizes understanding of the indicators of wound, urinary tract, upper respiratory, and dental infections (see discussion p. 476 in "Patient-Family Teaching and Discharge Planning"). Include this information on a written handout that reviews the information and lists a phone number to call should questions arise after hospital discharge.
3. Advise patient to wear a Medic-Alert bracelet and always to request prophylactic antibiotics for procedures that can result in bacterial seeding of the bloodstream, such as minor or major surgery or dental extractions.
4. Advise patient to call MD promptly should indicators of infection of the THA occur. These can include drainage, pain, fever, local warmth, swelling, restricted ROM of the joint, or feelings of pressure in the hip.

Potential alteration in tissue perfusion: Peripheral, related to impaired circulation secondary to compression from traction or abduction device

Desired outcomes: Patient has adequate perfusion to distal tissues as evidenced by warmth, normal color, and the ability to dorsiflex the involved foot, as well as feel sensations upon testing of the peroneal nerve dermatome. Patient verbalizes knowledge of potential neurovascular complications and the importance of reporting indicators of impairment promptly.

1. Because the traction sling or abduction device can press on neurovascular structures, it is imperative that neurovascular status of the leg in traction, especially peroneal nerve function, be assessed along with the VS. The peroneal nerve runs superficially by the neck of the fibula and can be assessed by testing the dermatome of the first web space between the great and second toes and having the patient dorsiflex the foot. Loss of sensation or movement signals impaired peroneal nerve function.
2. Be sure patient is aware of the potential for neurovascular impairment and the importance of reporting alterations in sensations, movements, temperature, and color of the immobilized extremity.
3. Encourage patient to reposition the leg within the restrictions of the sling and positional limitations.
4. Encourage patient to perform prescribed exercises as a means of stimulating circulation in the area.

See "Osteoarthritis" for **Pain,** p. 425, and **Impaired physical mobility** related to adjustment to new walking gait, p. 426. See "Torn Anterior Cruciate Ligament" for **Potential fluid volume fluid deficit** related to abnormal loss secondary to postsurgical hemorrhage or hematoma, p. 442. See "Fractures" for **Self-care deficit,** p. 452, and **Knowledge**

deficit: Potential for infection, p. 456. See "Amputation" for **Knowledge deficit:** Postsurgical exercise regimen, p. 467. See the appendix for nursing diagnoses and interventions for the care of preoperative and postoperative patients, p. 637, care of patients on prolonged bed rest, p. 651, and care of patients with cancer and other life-disrupting illnesses, p. 690.

PATIENT-FAMILY TEACHING AND DISCHARGE PLANNING

Provide patient and significant others with verbal and written information for the following:

1. Prescribed exercise regimen, including rationale for each exercise, number of repetitions for each, and frequency of the exercise periods. Be sure patient independently demonstrates understanding of the exercises and gives a return demonstration before hospital discharge.
2. Indicators of the types of infections, including the following: wound (persistent redness, swelling, discharge, local warmth, restricted hip ROM, feelings of hip pressure, fever, and pain); urinary tract (dysuria, pyuria, fever, malodorous urine, cloudy urine, urgency, frequency, and pain in the suprapubic, flank, groin, scrotal, or labial area); upper respiratory tract (change in color or amount of sputum, fever, cough, sore throat, malaise, fever); and dental (pain, swelling of the jaw, difficulty with mastication, fever). Advise patient to notify MD promptly if any of these indicators occur and to seek prophylactic antibiotics for minor surgical procedures.
3. Use of assistive devices (pickup sticks, stocking helpers, long-handled shoe horns, and raised toilet seat). Ensure that patient demonstrates independence in their use before hospital discharge.
4. Independent ambulation with crutches on level and uneven surfaces (see "Osteoarthritis," p. 426).
5. Getting in a car safely without risking dislocation. The patient should be able to demonstrate this procedure before hospital discharge.
6. Medications, including name, rationale, dosage, schedule, precautions, and potential side effects.
7. Phone number of a resource person should questions arise after hospital discharge.

Total knee arthroplasty

Total knee arthroplasty (TKA) is surgery that involves resection of the knee joint and its replacement with an endoprosthesis. Several pathologic conditions can result in the need for TKA, including osteoarthritis, rheumatoid arthritis, gouty arthritis, hemophilic arthritis, and severe knee trauma. Generally, TKA is restricted to older patients because the life span of the implant is unknown. However, younger patients also undergo this procedure, depending on the severity of the disease, amount of pain, and degree of functional deficit in the femorotibial or femoropatellar articulations. Because this procedure is irreversible and involves the removal of significant amounts of bone from the femur, tibia, and patella, several conditions must be met before the patient is considered a potential candidate. Conservative methods of therapy must have been exhausted and there has to be significant loss of function and pain that severely limit ambulation and ADL. In addition, the patient must have demonstrated adherence with past medical regimens and be free of any concurrent infectious process.

Complications of TKA have resulted in the need for reoperation in up to 15% of these patients. Complications include loosening of the prosthesis, peroneal nerve palsy, delayed wound healing, and infection. Loosening is by far the most common complication and it occurs most frequently in patients with varus deformity, obesity, overactivity, or decreased bone stock (i.e., osteoporosis).

DIAGNOSTIC TESTS

See discussion with "Total Hip Arthroplasty," p. 474. In addition, arthroscopy may be useful in confirming the extent of the pathology to identify the appropriate prosthesis.

MEDICAL MANAGEMENT AND SURGICAL INTERVENTIONS

1. **Surgical procedure:** The approach varies with the type of prosthetic device used. During the procedure a skin flap is created. If the blood supply is compromised during surgery or from postoperative hematoma formation, the flap can necrose and jeopardize the success of the operation; therefore it requires careful monitoring. The implant is internally fixed with methylmethacrylate or bony ingrowth. The wound is sutured closed in layers and a drain is left in place.

2. **Postoperative immobilization:** Usually accomplished with a Jones dressing, which is composed of a bulky padding with anterior, posterior, and lateral plaster splints that are held in place with an elastic wrap. The Jones dressing ensures immobilization, while allowing for edema formation to minimize the risk of iatrogenic compartment syndrome. If the implant is to be held in place with bony ingrowth, the leg may be immobilized within a cast after postoperative edema has subsided.

3. **Ambulation:** If methylmethacrylate was used to internally fix the implant, the patient may be permitted to ambulate without weightbearing within 3-5 days, slowly advancing to weightbearing as tolerated within 10-14 days. ROM of the knee is often done within 5 days under supervision of a physical therapist. For implants held in place with bony ingrowth, ambulation is not begun until after 10-14 days, and weightbearing may be contraindicated for as long as 6-12 weeks. If there is a cast, ROM is not begun until the cast has been removed.

4. **Continuous passive movement (CPM):** Usually advocated for patients who undergo a TKA. The CPM device is applied to the patient's bed and the operant extremity is positioned in a sling in the device. The device then moves the leg through preset limits of ROM in preset timed cycles. Use of CPM allows greater ROM with less pain. (The minimal flexion for a successful TKA is 90-110 degrees.)

NURSING DIAGNOSES AND INTERVENTIONS

Potential for impaired skin integrity related to irritation secondary to presence of CPM device

Desired outcomes: Skin of the affected leg remains intact and nonerythematous. Patient verbalizes knowledge of the importance of reporting indicators of skin irritation promptly while undergoing CPM.

1. Preoperatively, assess the skin on the operant extremity, being alert to areas of irritation or redness.

2. Preoperatively, introduce the patient to the use of the CPM, demonstrating how it will be used postoperatively. Point out areas prone to pressure or irritation from the device. Teach patient the symptoms to report postoperatively: alterations in sensation or discomfort.

3. Postoperatively, ensure correct positioning of the extremity within the CPM device (i.e., neutral position of the leg, with the knee resting over the area flexed by the device).

4. Encourage patient to perform quadricep sets, gluteal sets, and ankle circles to enhance extremity circulation.

5. During VS, or more often if erythema is noted, examine the medial, lateral, and posterior aspects of the extremity in the CPM device for areas of erythema. Also question patient about alterations in sensation or areas of discomfort.

6. Massage or pad areas of excessive pressure as noted by the presence of erythema. Reposition the leg within the confines of the CPM device. Report areas of irritation.

See all nursing diagnoses (except **Knowledge deficit:** Potential for and mechanism of THA dislocation) in "Total Hip Arthroplasty."

PATIENT-FAMILY TEACHING AND DISCHARGE PLANNING

See "Total Hip Arthroplasty," p. 476.

SELECTED REFERENCES

Althoff DG: External fixation of the lower extremity: care considerations. In Hilt N, editor: Assessment and fracture management of the lower extremities, 1984, National Association of Orthopaedic Nurses.

Berger MR: Bunions: an overview, Orthop Nurs 3:17, Sept/Oct 1984.

Buzaid AC and Durie BGM: Management of refractory myeloma: a review, J Clin Oncol 6(5):889-905, 1988.

Carlson DC: Common fractures of the extremities: how to recognize and treat them, Postgrad Med 83(4):311-317, 1988.

Chang WS and Zuckerman JD: Geriatric knee disorders, part II: differential diagnosis and treatment, Geriatrics 43(3):39-54, 1988.

Day LJ et al: Orthopaedics. In Way LW, editor: Current surgical diagnosis and treatment, ed 8, Norwalk, Conn and San Mateo, Calif, 1988, Appleton & Lange.

Dalinka MK, Aronchick JM, and Haddad JG: Paget's disease, Orthop Clin North Am 14:3, Jan 1983.

Eftekhar NS and Nercessian O: Incidence and mechanism of failure of cemented acetabular component in total hip arthroplasty, Orthop Clin North Am 19(3):557-566, 1988.

Farrell J: Helping the new amputee, Orthop Nurs 2:18, May/June 1982.

Freeman DA: Paget's disease of bone, Am J Med Sci 295(2):144-158, 1988.

Friedel HA and Todd PA: Nabumetone: a preliminary review of its pharmacodynamic and pharmacokinetic properties and therapeutic efficacy in rheumatoid diseases, Drugs 35(5):504-524, 1988.

Gamron RB: Taking the pressure out of compartment syndrome, AJN 88(8):1076-1080, 1988.

Gentry LO: Osteomyelitis: options for diagnosis and management, J Antimicrobial Chemother 21(9 suppl C):115-128, 1988.

Hamdy RC: Metabolic bone disease: a review, J Tenn Med Assoc 81(5):293-296, 1988.

Hamerman D: Osteoarthritis, Orthop Rev 17(4):353-360, 1988.

Holden CEA: Simple bone grafts. In Ackroyd CE et al, editors: The severely injured limb, New York, 1983, Churchill-Livingstone.

Huvos AG: Surgical pathology of bone sarcomas, World J Surg 12:284-298, 1988.

Johnson PH: Recurrent subluxation of the shoulder, J Ark Med Soc 84(8):335-337, 1988.

Josefsson PO et al: Surgical versus nonsurgical treatment of ligamentous injuries following dislocation of the elbow joint, JBJS 69A(4):605-608, 1987.

Kalu DN and Masoro EJ: The biology of aging with particular reference to the musculoskeletal system, Clin Geriatr Med 4(2):257-267, 1988.

Koerner ME and Dickinson GR: Arthritis: a look at some of its forms, AJN 83:254, 1983.

Krupski WC et al: Amputation. In Way LW, editor: Current surgical diagnosis and treatment, ed 8, Norwalk, Conn and San Mateo, Calif, 1988, Appleton & Lange.

Lane PL and Lee MM: New synthetic casts: what nurses need to know, Orthop Nurs 1:13, Nov/Dec 1982.

Lapuk S and Woodbury DF: Volkmann's ischemic contracture: a case report, Orthop Rev 17(6):618-624, 1987.

Lawrence W: Concepts in limb-sparing treatment of adult soft tissue sarcomas, Semin Surg Oncol 4:73-77, 1988.

Lindsay R: Management of osteoporosis, Clin Endocrinol Metab 2(1):103-123, 1988.

McDougall R and Keeling CA: Complications of fractures and their healing, Semin Nuclear Med 18(2):113-125, 1988.

Miller MC: Nursing care of the patient with external fixation therapy, Orthop Nurs 2:11-15, Jan/Feb 1983.

Miller RJ: Dislocations and fracture dislocations of the metacarpophalangeal joint of the thumb, Hand Clinics 4(1):45-65, 1988.

Peltier LF: Fat embolism: a perspective, Clin Orthop Related Res 232:263-270, 1988.

Phillips PE: Evidence implicating infectious agents in rheumatoid arthritis and juvenile rheumatoid arthritis, Clin Exp Rheumatol 6(1):87-94, 1988.

Reginato AJ and Schumacher HR: Crystal-associated arthroplasties, Rheumatic Disorders 4(2):295-322, 1988.

Ross DG: Anatomy and assessment of the knee. In National Association of Orthopaedic Nurses, editors: Lower extremity assessment and fracture management, pp 14-21, 1984.

Ross D: Compartment syndrome. In Swearingen PL et al: Manual of critical care: applying nursing diagnoses to adult critical illness, St Louis, 1988, The CV Mosby Co.

Ross DG: Diagnostic overview: Paget's disease, Orthop Nurs 3:41, May/June 1984.

Rutan F: Preprosthetic program for the amputee, Orthop Nurs 2:14, May/June 1982.

Sambrook PN and Reeve J: Bone disease in rheumatoid arthritis, Clin Sci 74:225-230, 1988.

Sandberg R et al: Operative versus nonoperative treatment of recent injuries to the ligaments of the knee, JBJS 69A(8):1120-1126, 1987.

Schlag G and Redl H: Fibrin sealant in orthopedic surgery, Clin Orthop Related Res 227:269-285, 1988.

Shearn MA: Arthritis and musculoskeletal disorders. In Krupp MA et al: Current medical diagnosis and treatment 1987, Norwalk, Conn and San Mateo, Calif, 1987, Appleton & Lange.

Simon MA: Limb salvage for osteosarcoma, JBJS 70A(2):307-310, 1988.

Skogberg K et al: Beta-hemolytic group A, B, C, and G streptococcal septicemia: a clinical study, Scand J Infect Dis 20:119-125, 1988.

Sommerlath K: The prognosis of repaired and intact menisci in unstable knees—a comprehensive study, Arthroscopy: J Arthroscop and Related Surg 4(2):93-95, 1988.

Spickler LL: Knee injuries of the athlete, Orthop Nurs 2:11, Sept/Oct 1983.

Steinbock G and Hetherington VJ: Austin bunionectomy: transposition "V" osteotomy of the first metatarsal for hallus valgus, J Foot Surg 27(3):211-216, 1988.

Steiner ME and Grana WA: The young athlete's knee: recent advances, Clin Sports Med 7(3):527-546, 1988.

Stevenson JC: Osteoporosis: pathogenesis and risk factors, Clin Endocrinol Metab 2(1):87-100, 1988.

Tebbi CK and Gaeta J: Osteosarcoma, Pediatr Ann 17(4):285-300, 1988.

Vince KG and Insall JN: Long-term results of cemented total knee arthroplasty, Orthop Clin North Am 19(3):575-580, 1988.

Ziff M et al: Pathogenic factors in rheumatoid synovitis, Br J Rheumatol 27(suppl II):153-156, 1988.

9
CHAPTER

Reproductive disorders

Section One   SURGERIES AND DISORDERS OF THE BREAST

Breast augmentation

Breast augmentation is the implantation of suitable material into the breast to increase breast size. The decision for surgery is made by the patient, who then seeks a qualified practitioner, usually a plastic surgeon, to perform the surgery.

ASSESSMENT

Clinical indicators: Because the procedure is elective, there are no specific indicators. Frequently, these individuals have had a decrease in breast size following weight loss, or they may have a long-term history of dissatisfaction with the size of their breasts. The patient should not have unrealistic expectations for the surgery, such as saving a marriage or offsetting a problem such as obesity.

Physical assessment: The breasts may be small, or there may be some muscle looseness that causes them to sag. There should be no signs of breast disease, such as nipple discharge and puckering of the skin (see "Malignant Disorders of the Breast," p. 488, for other signs).

SURGICAL INTERVENTION

An inframammary incision is made into the breast, positioned so that the scar will not be evident. An implant, usually polyurethane-covered or a silastic envelope containing silicone gel, is inserted into the submuscular pocket subpectorally or subcutaneously.

NURSING DIAGNOSES AND INTERVENTIONS

Body image disturbance related to small breast size

Desired outcome: Patient expresses positive and realistic reasons for having breast augmentation and is supported in her decision to have this surgery.

1. Review the patient's expectations for the outcome of surgery. The patient should not have unrealistic expectations as evidenced by such statements as, "Surgery will change my life or marriage."
2. Provide support for the patient's decision to have this surgery by spending time with her and allowing her to verbalize fears and concerns.
3. If appropriate, enable the patient to express feelings such as being "self-centered." Be nonjudgmental about her feelings.

Potential for impaired breast feeding related to breast augmentation procedure

Desired outcome: In the preoperative period, patient verbalizes knowledge that breast feeding can be impaired owing to the breast augmentation procedure.

1. Prior to surgery, explain to patient that breast augmentation surgery may impair breast feeding in future pregnancies.
2. As indicated, arrange for a session with a lactation consultant if patient requires more information.

Pain related to surgical procedure

Desired outcomes: Patient's subjective evaluation of pain improves, as documented by a pain scale; patient is pain free 2-3 days after surgery.

1. Assess and document location, quality, and duration of the pain, using a pain scale from 0-10.
2. Medicate the patient with analgesics as prescribed; evaluate and document the response, based on the pain scale.

3. Provide ice packs to decrease swelling in the early postoperative period.
4. Ensure that the patient has a comfortable bra that adequately supports her breasts.
5. Teach the patient relaxation techniques, such as slow, diaphragmatic breathing and guided imagery.
6. Provide distractions, such as television or soothing music.
7. Encourage activity as tolerated.

Knowledge deficit: Incisional site care and the potential for postoperative capsular contracture

Desired outcome: Patient verbalizes knowledge of incisional site care, the potential for capsular contracture, and the procedure for prevention of capsular formation.

1. Instruct patient to cleanse the incisional site after the sutures have been removed, using basic hygiene, such as soap and water. Explain that heavy lotions, medications, or creams should not be used unless specified by MD.
2. In preparation for hospital discharge, instruct patient in self-examination techniques for signs of fibrotic capsular formation, which can be evidenced by displacement of the implant and hardening of the breast.
3. If prescribed, teach the procedure for breast massage to help prevent capsular contraction: Using a gentle rotary motion, squeeze and then flatten the breast. Typically, this is performed either immediately after the surgery or after the wound heals in 2-3 weeks. It is performed for 15 minutes, 4-5 times a day for at least a month. Have the patient demonstrate the procedure on the nonoperative breast if breast massage is contraindicated until after the wound heals.

See the appendix for nursing diagnoses and interventions for the care of preoperative and postoperative patients, p. 637.

PATIENT-FAMILY TEACHING AND DISCHARGE PLANNING

Provide patient and significant others with verbal and written information for the following:
1. Medications, including the drug name, purpose, dosage, schedule, precautions, and potential side effects.
2. Indicators of wound infection, which require follow-up care by health care provider: persistent redness, pain, swelling, and drainage at the incisional area.
3. Care of the incision site, including cleansing and dressing, if indicated.
4. Importance of monthly breast self-examination (BSE). Teach or review the technique as appropriate.
5. Activity restrictions, which may include limited use of the arm for 2 weeks postoperatively and resumption of full activity after 3 weeks.
6. Breast massage, if prescribed as a prophylaxis for capsular contraction.

Breast reconstruction

After a mastectomy, a woman may elect to have breast reconstruction in an attempt to create a breast "mound" in place of the lost breast. Although there is no medical indication for breast reconstruction, psychologic benefits may result. Breast reconstruction usually can be performed at the time of mastectomy. However, when positive axillary nodes are discovered, reconstruction may be delayed for 3 months to avoid the potential for poorer cosmetic results secondary to radiation or chemotherapy. This surgery has become more popular in recent years because the technique continues to improve and patients are becoming more aware of the procedure and its benefits.

ASSESSMENT

Clinical indicators: Scheduled mastectomy or absence of the breast, patient's desire for surgery, adequate tissue present, and absence of progressive disease.

Physical assessment: There should be no evidence of infection, and healing of the mastectomy scar should be complete if a surgical delay was indicated.

MEDICAL MANAGEMENT AND SURGICAL INTERVENTIONS

1. Analgesics and possibly narcotics: To control postsurgical discomfort.
2. IV therapy: To treat dehydration secondary to the surgical intervention.
3. Balanced diet: As tolerated to enhance tissue restoration.
4. Surgical procedure: Varying procedures may be involved, depending on the amount of tissue left at the reconstruction site. When there is sufficient tissue, an implant is placed under the pectoralis and serratus muscles. A tissue expander can be used either as a temporary device for a later, permanent implant or as a permanent implant concurrent with surgery. The tissue expander is injected with saline through a port at intervals to provide gradual enlargement of the site. If a radical mastectomy has been performed, there is usually inadequate soft tissue, muscle, and skin on which to place the implant. It then becomes necessary to graft tissue from other locations, such as the latissimus dorsi flap or rectus abdominis musculocutaneous flap. Latissimus dorsi flap reconstruction involves the transfer of the muscle, skin, and subcutaneous tissue from the back to the mastectomy site. The rectus abdominis musculocutaneous flap involves the transfer of one of the rectus abdominis muscles, as well as overlying skin, subcutaneous fat (lipectomy), and artery to the mastectomy site. With this procedure an implant also may be needed, depending on the amount of tissue available. If a nipple is desired on the reconstructed breast, it can be created from skin of the inner thigh, buttock, labia, or the other nipple.
5. Suction apparatus: Placed in the wound to minimize the chance of hematoma formation.

NURSING DIAGNOSES AND INTERVENTIONS

Knowledge deficit: Surgical procedure, preoperative care, and postoperative regimen

Desired outcome: Patient verbalizes knowledge of the surgical procedure and expected results as well as preoperative care and the postoperative regimen.

1. Consult with the MD to arrange a visit by a woman who has had breast reconstruction surgery to share feelings and demonstrate the cosmetic results.
2. During the preoperative period, explain that after surgery a suction apparatus will be present, which removes blood to minimize the potential for hematoma formation. Usually this is removed when drainage is less than 10-20 ml over 24 hours.
3. Explain that movement and activity may be restricted following surgery, depending on the procedure used. When an implant is placed under ample tissue, recovery is more rapid and hospitalization is usually 1-3 days; while flap reconstruction is more involved and movement and activity may be more restricted. Patients with a latissimus flap reconstruction are usually discharged after 2-5 days, when the drains are removed. A rectus abdominis procedure is more extensive, and because of the lipectomy the patient usually is on bed rest for several days and discharged after a week.
4. Be aware that patients who undergo nipple reconstruction usually are more satisfied with the results; however, they may experience more anxiety during the postrecovery period, and thus require more reassurance.
5. For other interventions, see the same nursing diagnosis in the appendix "Caring for Preoperative and Postoperative Patients," p. 637.

Knowledge deficit: Potential for postoperative fibrotic capsular contraction and the technique for breast massage

Desired outcome: Patient verbalizes knowledge of the potential for fibrotic capsular contraction and demonstrates the technique for breast massage.

1. Explain to the patient that fibrotic capsular contraction is a potential complication of breast reconstruction surgery and that breast massage will minimize the risk of this condition.

2. Teach breast massage by the second or third postoperative day. The procedure involves a gentle rotary motion to squeeze and flatten the breast. Usually it is performed three times a day.

Potential fluid volume deficit related to abnormal blood loss secondary to postsurgical hemorrhage or hematoma formation

Desired outcomes: Patient is normovolemic as evidenced by BP ≥90/60 mm Hg (or within patient's normal range), HR 60-100 bpm, RR ≤20 breaths/min, warm and dry skin, and urinary output ≥30 ml/hr. Drainage in suction apparatus is ≤50 ml/hr initially and <20 ml/hr within 24 hours following surgery. If patient develops a hematoma, it is detected and reported promptly.

1. Monitor patient for clinical indicators of hemorrhage (e.g., drop of systolic BP 10-20 mm Hg below trend, rapid pulse rate, cool and clammy skin, pallor, confusion, and diaphoresis). Report significant findings.
2. Assess for the appearance of a hematoma as evidenced by swelling, pain, and possibly a bluish discoloration of the skin. Report significant findings to the MD.
3. Assess the suction apparatus for patency, and document the amount and character of the drainage. Report drainage that exceeds 50 ml/hr for 2 hours. Reestablish suction as necessary. Usually the suction apparatus is removed when the total drainage is less than 10-20 ml in 24 hours.

Body image disturbance related to body changes before and following breast reconstruction surgery

Desired outcomes: Patient relates realistic expectations before surgery (e.g., that the breast will look normal under clothing) and demonstrates movement toward acceptance of body changes after surgery.

1. Review with patient her expectations for the outcome of surgery.
2. Discuss the emotional responses that women often have following breast reconstruction, such as elation during the early postoperative period followed by depression or confusion.
3. Explain that some of the depression and confusion may be a result of the memory of the mastectomy and fear of cancer. Reassure patient that these feelings are normal and usually disappear after a short time.
4. Provide emotional support by being with the patient when the dressing is first removed. Explain that the reconstructed breast will not look like the other breast at first, but that the molding process will begin during the recovery period and continue for 3-6 months.

See the appendix for nursing diagnoses and interventions for the care of preoperative and postoperative patients, p. 637, and for patients with cancer and other life-disrupting illnesses, p. 659.

PATIENT-FAMILY TEACHING AND DISCHARGE PLANNING

Provide patient and significant others with verbal and written information for the following:
1. Care of the incision, including applying a gauze dressing until the sutures are removed on about the seventh day. After the sutures are removed, micropore tape strips usually are placed over the incision until healing has taken place, and are replaced when they loosen. Instruct patient to notify MD if signs of infection, including persistent redness, pain, swelling, or drainage, appear at the incision site.
2. Taking showers, which usually are permitted after the suction catheter is removed. If present, the dressing should be removed from the operative site and replaced after bathing.
3. Activity restriction for the first 4-6 weeks or as directed, including strenuous exercise, contact sports, excessive stretching, and heavy lifting (>5 lb).

4. Importance of avoiding putting pressure on the chest wall for 4-6 weeks. For example, patient should use superior position during coitus.
5. Importance of breast massage 3 times a day for the first year after surgery. Explain that it takes 3-6 months for the reconstructed breast to appear natural in contour.
6. Importance of not wearing a bra for three months to allow for unrestricted movement of the implant.
7. Necessity of applying prescribed lotion to the nipple daily if a nipple transplant was performed.
8. Importance of monthly breast self-examination (BSE) of both breasts. Teach or review the procedure as appropriate.
9. Medications, including drug name, purpose, dosage, schedule, precautions, and potential side effects.

Benign breast disease

The most common breast masses are those caused by fibrocystic disease, fibroadenomas, and intraductal papilloma; all are evaluated for potential malignancy.

Fibrocystic condition: Can either be a simple cyst(s) caused by normal changes in the lining of the duct and the secretion of fluid, or a premalignant condition caused by hyperplasia of the cells. Fibrocystic condition is the most common breast lesion in women. It is found most often in the age group of 35-45, increases with advancing age, and rarely is found after menopause, except in women receiving estrogen replacement therapy (ERT).

Fibroadenomas: Solid masses that may occur from age 15 to 60, with peak occurrence at 21-25 years.

Intraductal papilloma: A benign condition of the ductal system of the breast. It occurs infrequently and is found most often in women 35-45 years of age.

ASSESSMENT

Signs and symptoms: The patient palpates a mass in 80% of the cases. Often with fibrocystic condition there are bilateral, multiple masses that are painful and tender. They may change in size relative to the menstrual cycle and are most evident just before menstruation. The masses are firm, mobile, and smooth or regular in shape.

Fibroadenomas are painless masses that are usually unilateral. The mass itself is mobile, solid, firm, well circumscribed, and often spherical, but it can be lobulated or dumbbell-shaped.

The most frequent symptom of intraductal papilloma is serosanguineous or serous nipple discharge. Usually there is no mass.

Physical assessment: With fibrocystic condition, masses usually can be palpated in the upper outer quadrants of the breasts. Fibroadenomas are usually 2-2.5 cm in diameter. An intraductal papilloma often involves a 1 cm area that circumvents the nipple; discharge also may be found.

History of: Benign breast masses. There is potential for recurrence of both cysts and fibroadenomas.

DIAGNOSTIC TESTS

1. *Mammography:* A roentgenographic test used to identify cancerous masses, which appear as small densities with stippled calcifications. There is a slight risk of false-positive and false-negative results.
2. *Xeroradiography:* A noninvasive test that uses a lesser radiation dose than mammography; however, there is a higher risk of false-positive or false-negative results.
3. *Thermography:* Presents a picture of normal and abnormal temperatures in the breast. Malignant masses are warmer because of increased vascularity in the area.

Again, there is the risk of false-positive and false-negative results. Thermography is not as accurate as mammography and cannot be substituted for it.

4. *Ultrasound mammography:* Uses sound waves to delineate the internal pattern of the breast. It is used when cysts and enlarged ducts are suspected. It is 98% accurate in diagnosing cysts and enlarged ducts only.

5. *MRI:* Technique that uses the interaction between magnetism and radio waves (without ionizing radiation) to show the structure of the breasts. It can image breast cancers that are large and palpable; however, it cannot detect microcalcifications indicative of cancers.

6. *Needle aspiration biopsy:* Involves aspirating the contents of the mass *via* a fine (22 g) needle. The aspirate is then placed on a slide for Papanicolaou evaluation.

7. *Incisional biopsy:* Involves the surgical removal of part of the mass for histologic evaluation.

8. *Excisional biopsy:* Involves the removal of the entire mass as well as marginal breast tissue. This procedure results in the most accurate diagnosis.

MEDICAL MANAGEMENT AND SURGICAL INTERVENTIONS

1. **Diet:** For fibrocystic condition, the promotion of nutritious foods and the elimination of methylxanthine substances, such as coffee, tea, and chocolate, may decrease the pain and size of the cysts. Vitamin E therapy may be helpful in some patients to reduce the incidence of recurrent cysts. A low sodium diet in the luteal phase may relieve symptoms by decreasing edema. It is theorized that a diet low in fat and high in fiber helps prevent breast cancer.

2. **Pharmacologic therapy:** Treatment for fibrocystic condition may involve low dose estrogen oral contraceptives to suppress the ovulation cycle, and thus minimize cyst formation. Danazol and promocriptine also may be used. Recurrence is possible 6-12 months after cessation of therapy.

3. **Stress reduction and smoking cessation:** May help relieve or decrease the symptoms of fibrocystic condition.

4. **Excisional biopsy:** Not only useful in diagnosis, it removes the breast mass as well.

5. **Wedge resection of the breast:** Resection of the lobe that is involved in the intraductal papilloma.

NURSING DIAGNOSES AND INTERVENTIONS

Fear related to the possibility of cancer, change in body image, surgical or diagnostic procedure, and pain

Desired outcome: Patient discusses fears and demonstrates increasing psychologic comfort, as evidenced by HR ≤100 bpm, RR ≤20 breaths/min with normal depth and pattern (eupnea), and BP within patient's normal range.

1. Reassure patient that >90% of breast masses are benign.

2. Explain the diagnostic, preoperative, and postoperative procedures as necessary.

3. If appropriate, inform patient that a local anesthetic might be used during the biopsy and that sensations of pulling and probing may be felt.

4. Provide support by allowing time for verbalization of feelings; answer patient's questions.

5. If patient is at high risk of malignancy, see **Fear** in "Malignant Disorders of the Breast," p. 490.

Pain related to surgical biopsy

Desired outcomes: Patient's subjective evaluation of pain improves, as documented by a pain scale; patient is pain free within 1 week following surgery.

1. Assess and document the location, quality, and duration of the pain. Use a pain scale with a range of 0-10 to help patient evaluate the pain intensity.

2. Medicate with the prescribed analgesics; evaluate and document the patient's response, using the pain scale.

3. To help decrease swelling, apply a wrapped ice pack to the involved breast.
4. Ensure that the patient has a comfortable bra that supports the breast adequately.

See the appendix for nursing diagnoses and interventions for the care of preoperative and postoperative patients, p. 637.

PATIENT-FAMILY TEACHING AND DISCHARGE PLANNING

Provide patient and significant others with verbal and written information for the following:
1. Medications, including the drug name, purpose, dosage, schedule, precautions, and potential side effects.
2. Indicators of wound infection, which require followup by health care provider: persistent redness, pain, swelling, and discharge at the operative site.
3. Care of the incision site, including cleansing. After sutures are removed, soap and water should be used for gentle cleansing.
4. Resumption of daily activities to patient's tolerance.
5. Diet as tolerated, with suggestion to eliminate methylxanthine products if fibrocystic condition is diagnosed.
6. Scheduled date for the completed pathology report, or an explanation of the diagnosis, if already available.
7. Importance of BSE. Teach the procedure to patients who do not know it; reinforce and review the technique for those patients who practice it monthly.

Malignant disorders of the breast

Breast cancer is one of the three most common types of breast disease, second only to fibrocystic condition in occurrence. In the United States, it is the most frequently occurring type of reproductive cancer in females. Breast cancer usually is diagnosed in women between the ages of 40 and 70 years, with 54 the median age. However, in the last few years there has been an increase in newly diagnosed cases in women in their twenties and thirties.

The histopathology of breast tumors involves the progression of the tumor from a local preinvasive disease state to invasive malignancy. The changes that occur in the breast are due primarily to hyperplasia of the epithelium. Although carcinoma in situ is usually noninvasive, it too can develop into invasive carcinoma. The differentiation between noninvasive and invasive cancer requires extensive examination of tissue cells obtained during excisional biopsy.

ASSESSMENT

Signs and symptoms: The earliest indicator is a palpable mass. Signs of advanced disease include nipple retraction, change in breast contour, nipple discharge, redness or heat of the breast, palpable lymph glands, dimpling of the skin of the breast, and *peau d'orange* or orange peel appearance of the breast. Ulceration also may be a sign of advanced disease.

Physical assessment: Palpable mass, which usually is located in the upper outer quadrant of the breast. Usually the mass is painless, unilateral, irregular in shape, poorly delineated, and nonmobile. There may be signs of edema, venous engorgement, and abnormal contours.

Risk factors: Previous breast cancer in the contralateral breast; family history of cancer and breast cancer, especially a mother or sister, particularly if the family member was affected at an early age or had bilateral disease; being over age 50; postmenopausal weight gain; early age at menarche (11 or younger); late age of menopause (after 52 years); nulliparity or late age at first full-term delivery (over 30). In addition, it is theorized that exposure to carcinogens and a high-fat diet are other factors in the development of breast cancer.

DIAGNOSTIC TESTS

The most specific test for detection of breast disease is the excisional breast biopsy (see "Benign Breast Disease," p. 487). Mammography may detect breast masses in patients who do not have a palpable mass. However, there is the risk of false-negative and false-positive results. The American Cancer Society recommends a baseline mammogram for women ages 35-40, and a mammogram every 1-2 years for women 40-49 and annually for women over age 50.

MEDICAL MANAGEMENT AND SURGICAL INTERVENTIONS

1. **Staging of the tumor:** Provides a method to formulate the prognosis and treatment plan. The size of the tumor, the appearance of the cancer in the axillary nodes, the histopathologic examination, and the presence of distant metastases determine the degree of staging (see Table 9-1).
2. **Radiation therapy:** Can be used either in metastatic disease or in the treatment of early breast cancer. In early breast cancer, the tumor is excised along with some of the adjacent tissue, followed by external radiation or radioactive implants.
3. **Radical mastectomy or Halstead procedure:** The most extensive surgical procedure. It involves the removal of the breast, nipple and areola, axillary lymph nodes, and the pectoralis minor and major muscles.
4. **Modified radical mastectomy:** Removal of the breast tissue, nipple and areola, the tumor and surrounding skin, the axillary lymph nodes, and possibly the pectoralis minor muscle.

T A B L E 9 - 1 Cancer staging

Stage A

Absence of skin edema, ulceration, or solid fixation of the tumor to chest wall; axillary nodes negative.

Stage B

Same as A, except involvement of axillary nodes occurs, with <2.5 cm transverse diameter; nodes are not fixed to overlying skin or to deeper axillary structures.

Stage C

Presence of any one of the following five signs of advanced cancer:
1. Edema less than a third of the breast skin.
2. Ulceration of the breast skin.
3. Tumor solidly fixed to the chest wall.
4. Axillary node involvement (2.5 cm or more in transverse diameter).
5. Axillary nodes fixed to overlying skin or deeper structures.

Stage D

More advanced cancer than stage C:
1. Any two or more of the signs described under stage C.
2. Edema of more than a third of the breast skin.
3. Satellite skin nodules.
4. Inflammatory carcinoma.
5. Supraclavicular lymph node involvement.
6. Parasternal tumor.
7. Edema of the involved arm.
8. Metastases to other sites.

Based on Columbia Clinical Classification and Staging

5. Total mastectomy or simple mastectomy: Involves the removal of the breast, but the lymph nodes are left intact.
6. Partial mastectomy (lumpectomy, tylectomy, or segmental resection): Refers to the excision of the tumor and a small amount of tissue surrounding it. Axillary nodal dissection is usually done.
7. Quadrectomy: Removal of the entire quadrant of the breast where the tumor is located. Axillary nodal dissection is usually done.
8. Chemotherapy: Includes either the use of a single agent or a combination of agents. This management pattern is used either as an adjunct to surgery, or in advanced disease when metastases have occurred or positive lymph nodes have been identified. The use of cytotoxic drugs has been found to be more effective when used in combination. These combinations include the following:
   □ *Cyclophosphamide, doxorubicin, and fluorouracil:* First line therapy for adjuvant treatment or for metastatic disease. It is used monthly for a year.
   □ *Cyclophosphamide, methotrexate, and fluorouracil:* Used in metastatic or recurrent disease.
9. Hormonal therapy: The hormone used depends on whether the tumor is estrogen-receptor-positive or estrogen-receptor-"poor", and it is also used in advanced disease as adjuvant therapy for stage II breast disease. Some of these hormonal agents include:
   □ *Tamoxifen citrate:* An antiestrogen used in estrogen-receptor-positive tumors.
   □ *Megase:* For relapse of the disease if a previous response to tamoxifen had occurred.

NURSING DIAGNOSES AND INTERVENTIONS

Fear related to the possibility of cancer and its treatment

Desired outcome: Patient expresses fears and anxieties and exhibits increasing psychologic comfort as evidenced by BP within patient's normal range, RR ≤20 breaths/min with normal depth and pattern (eupnea), and HR ≤100 bpm.

1. Assess the patient's understanding of the potential diagnosis and treatment plan; clarify and explain as appropriate.
2. Provide time for patient to express feelings and fears.
3. Evaluate the patient's emotional status, and explore with the patient what her breasts mean to her. The breast may represent nurturance, sexuality, femininity, and desirability.
4. Assess your own feelings about the diagnosis of cancer and the psychologic meaning of the breast. Your attitudes may be reflected in the patient's care, and therefore a positive attitude is essential for optimal patient support.
5. Provide a nonthreatening, relaxed atmosphere for the patient and significant others by using therapeutic communication techniques, such as open-ended questions and reflection.

Ineffective individual coping related to grief or stress secondary to diagnosis of breast cancer

Desired outcomes: Patient demonstrates comfort with expressing her feelings, identifies positive coping patterns (e.g., using support systems, planning daily activities), and accepts the support of others.

1. Assist patient with identifying and developing a support system.
2. Provide support to patient's significant other. Refer significant other to a support group for spouses.
3. If an extensive mastectomy was performed, recognize the signs of grief, such as denial, anger, withdrawal, or inappropriate affect. Provide emotional support, and describe the stages of grief to the patient and significant others. Provide explanations to significant others, who may misunderstand the meaning of the patient's behavior or actions.
4. Consult with the surgeon regarding a visit by a woman who has had a diagnosis sim-

ilar to that of the patient. "Reach to Recovery" volunteers from the American Cancer Society are trained to share their experiences with breast cancer patients.

5. See "Caring for the Patient with Cancer and Other Life-Disrupting Illnesses," p. 690, in the appendix for this and other pyschosocial nursing diagnoses and interventions.

Potential for disuse syndrome related to physical alterations in the upper extremity secondary to mastectomy

Desired outcomes: Upon recovery, patient has full ROM of the upper extremity. Patient verbalizes knowledge of the importance and rationale for upper extremity movements and exercises.

1. Consult with the surgeon prior to the mastectomy to determine the type of surgery anticipated. With the surgeon, develop an individualized exercise plan specific to the patient's needs, which can be implemented as soon as the patient returns from the recovery room.
2. Encourage finger, wrist, and elbow movement to aid circulation and help minimize edema as soon as the patient returns to her room.
3. Encourage progressive exercise by having patient use the affected arm for personal hygiene and ADL the morning after surgery. Other exercises (clasping the hands behind the head and "walking" the fingers up the wall) should be added as soon as the patient is ready. Once the sutures have been removed (usually around the second postoperative week), patient should begin exercises that will enhance external rotation and abduction of the shoulder. Before hospital discharge, the patient should be able to achieve maximum shoulder flexion by touching her fingertips together behind her back. With the surgeon's consent, a "Reach for Recovery" volunteer can visit and provide patient with verbal instructions and written handouts for these exercises.
4. Assist patient with ambulation until her gait is normal. Encourage correct posture with the back straight and shoulders back.
5. To minimize the risk of lymphedema and infection, avoid giving injections, measuring BP, or taking blood samples from the affected arm. Remind the patient about her lowered resistance to infection and the importance of promptly treating any breaks in the skin. To help prevent infection after hospital discharge, advise patient to treat minor injuries with soap and water and to notify her health care provider if signs of infection occur.
6. Advise patient to wear a Medic-Alert bracelet that cautions against injections and tests in the involved arm.
7. To protect the hand and arm from injury, advise the patient to wear a protective glove when gardening or doing chores that require exposure to harsh chemicals, such as cleaning fluids. Explain that cutting cuticles should be avoided and that lotion should be used to keep the skin soft.

Pain related to the surgical procedure

Desired outcomes: Patient's subjective evaluation of pain improves, as documented by a pain scale; patient relates that pain is relieved with IM narcotics for the first 48 hours after surgery and with oral medications for the following 4 weeks, with pain decreasing daily.

1. Assess and document the location, quality, and duration of the pain, rating it with the patient on a scale of 0-10.
2. Medicate patient with the prescribed analgesics before the pain becomes too severe. Evaluate and document the response by again rating the pain on a scale of 0-10.
3. Reassure patient that phantom breast sensations are normal.
4. Provide a comfortable in-bed position, and support the affected arm with pillows.
5. Encourage movement of the fingers on the affected arm to increase circulation. Inform the patient that although progressive exercise will cause some discomfort, it will aid in the mobility of the affected arm and enhance recovery.
6. Reassure the patient that exercise movements will be adapted to her level of tolerance.

7. If appropriate, instruct the patient in relaxation techniques and use of guided imagery.
8. Provide distraction, such as television, radio, or books.
9. Use touch to help relieve tension, for example, by giving a gentle massage.

Body image disturbance related to loss of a breast

Desired outcome: Patient demonstrates movement toward acceptance of the loss of her breast.

1. Recognize that loss of a breast is perceived in different ways by different women. It is frequently more traumatic for the young adult.
2. Provide emotional support by being with the patient when the surgical dressing is removed.
3. As appropriate, explain that sexual dysfunction often occurs after mastectomy and that it can be minimized with resumption of sexual relations as soon as the pain has decreased. Assure patient that relations that were positive before surgery usually remain positive. However, be aware that sexual relationships that were weak before the surgery may not tolerate the added stress.
4. Recognize the need for a supportive person, such as a "Reach for Recovery" volunteer who has experienced the same procedure. Consult with the MD regarding a visit by this individual, if indicated. Support systems also should be made available to significant others.
5. If reconstruction is to be delayed, provide the patient with a breast prosthesis after surgery to help her feel "normal." A temporary prosthesis, made of nylon and filled with dacron fluff, can be worn until the incision heals. Provide the patient with information about where to get a breast prosthesis. The American Cancer Society has lists of distributors and types of prostheses available.
6. Be aware that use of touch often enhances the patient's self-concept.
7. Provide information and answer questions about breast reconstruction (see p. 483).

Potential for altered parenting related to use of radiation therapy and chemotherapy in association with breast malignancy

Desired outcome: The patient of childbearing age verbalizes accurate information about pregnancy and parenthood following breast cancer and its treatment.

Note: Reproductive counselling should take into account the patient's age, stage of disease, type of cancer treatment, and pretreatment fertility status.

---

1. Explain that childbearing should be delayed for approximately 2 years following cancer diagnosis and treatment. This will enable the physician to better evaluate the course of the disease and allow time for the effects of treatment modalities, such as chemotherapy and radiation, to abate.
2. Explain to the patient that she can breastfeed with either breast following chemotherapy, but that after radiation therapy she should use the nonirradiated breast only.
3. Explore adoption as an alternative for the infertile couple.
4. As indicated, discuss issues of parental death and single parenthood with patient and significant other. See appropriate nursing diagnoses and interventions in the appendix "Caring for Patients with Cancer and Other Life-Disrupting Illnesses," p. 659.

See the appendix for nursing diagnoses and interventions for the care of preoperative and postoperative patients, p. 637 and for patients with cancer and other life-disrupting illnesses, p. 659.

PATIENT-FAMILY TEACHING AND DISCHARGE PLANNING

Provide patient and significant others with verbal and written information for the following:
1. Medications, including drug name, purpose, dosage, schedule, precautions, and potential side effects.

2. Type and dates of follow-up treatment.
3. Resumption of sexual activity, which usually can occur as soon as pain is diminished.
4. Care of the incision site, including cleansing. Explain the components of good hygiene.
5. Progressive exercise regimen, which should be continued at home. Advise patient to stop the exercise movement if a pulling sensation or pain is felt.
6. Informing health care professionals to avoid measuring BP or giving injections in the affected arm.
7. Indicators of infection (e.g., fever, erythema, local warmth, skin discoloration) and the importance of reporting them to health care professional.
8. Permanent breast prosthesis, including distributors and types available.
9. Name and telephone number of a support person who can be called during the first postoperative year. An ideal individual is a "Reach for Recovery" volunteer.
10. Importance of performing monthly BSE. In addition, as a part of the BSE, teach patient to palpate the scar, sweep down the chest wall, and palpate the axillary, supraclavicular, and subclavian lymph nodes to assess for lumps. Also teach patient that skin changes, such as rashes and erythema, are suggestive of recurrence and should be reported promptly.

Section Two   NEOPLASMS OF THE FEMALE PELVIS

Cancers of the cervix and ovaries are frequently occurring reproductive cancers in women. 1988 statistics of the American Cancer Society estimate 47,000 new cases of uterine cancer (13,000 of invasive cervical cancer and 34,000 of endometrial cancer) and 19,000 new cases of ovarian cancer. Women of all ages can develop cancer of these structures, although it is most often found in individuals between ages 40 and 60.

Cancer of the cervix

Although the cause of cervical cancer is unknown, the following risk factors have been associated with this disease: early age of first coitus, multiple sexual partners, sexually transmitted diseases (especially herpesvirus infection and condyloma acuminatum), and family history. The two types of cervical cancer are squamous cell, which is the most common, and adenocarcinoma. *Preinvasive* describes cancerous cells that are limited to the cervix, while *invasive* refers to cancer that is present in the cervix, in other pelvic structures, and possibly in the lymphatic system as well. Preinvasive cancer of the cervix typically is found in women aged 30-40, while invasive cancer usually appears between the ages of 40 and 50. Treatment of preinvasive cancer has a greater success rate.

ASSESSMENT

Preinvasive: Patient asymptomatic; Pap smear abnormal.

Invasive: Abnormal vaginal bleeding; persistent, watery vaginal discharge; postcoital pain and bleeding; abnormal Pap smear.

DIAGNOSTIC TESTS

1. *Pap smear:* Cells are collected from the endocervix and squamocolumnar junction on the cervix with an applicator, placed on a slide, fixed, and sent to the lab for analysis. Pap smear results may be reported as follows:
   □ Normal or atypical benign.
   □ Cervical intraepithelial neoplasia (CIN)
   —Grade 1: Mild dysplasia.
   —Grade 2: Moderate to severe dysplasia.
   —Grade 3: Severe dysplasia and carcinoma in situ.
   □ Invasive squamous cell carcinoma.

☐ Adenocarcinoma.
☐ Atypical cells present; repeat to rule out.
☐ Specimen insufficient for diagnosis.

2. *Colposcopy:* Procedure providing a three-dimensional view of the cervix and allowing for cervical staining with an iodine solution (Schiller's test). Cells that do not absorb the stain are considered abnormal and are sent to the lab for further examination. This procedure takes approximately 20 minutes.

3. *Conization biopsy:* Surgical procedure performed under general anesthesia in which a cone-shaped area of the cervix is biopsied for lab analysis to determine the extent of the malignancy.

4. *CT scanning and MRI:* Radiologic detection techniques used to determine the degree and extent of the pathologic process within the pelvis and the spread of the disease outside the pelvis.

5. *Chest x-ray:* May reveal presence of metastasis to the lungs.

6. *Staging of the disease:* The following parameters are used, based on clinical classification of the International Federation of Gynecology and Obstetrics:
   ☐ *Stage O:* Carcinoma in situ; preinvasive.
   ☐ *Stage I:* Cancer cells in the cervix only.
   Stage IA: Cervical cancer with <3 mm spread.
   Stage IB: Cervical cancer with definite invasive areas.
   ☐ *Stage II:* Cancer involving cervix and vagina but not the pelvic wall.
   Stage IIA: No involvement of uterine tissue.
   Stage IIB: Involvement of uterine tissue.
   ☐ *Stage III:* Involvement of the pelvic wall or lower third of the vagina.
   Stage IIIA: No extension onto the pelvic wall.
   Stage IIIB: Extension onto pelvic wall and/or kidney secondary to hydronephrosis (obstructed flow of urine to kidney producing kidney atrophy).
   ☐ *Stage IV:* Cancer in bladder, rectum, and other organs of the pelvis.
   Stage IVA: Metastasis to rectum, bladder.
   Stage IVB: Metastasis to distant organs.

Note: Metastasis to lymph nodes occurs in 15% of stage I and up to 60% in stage IV.

MEDICAL MANAGEMENT AND SURGICAL INTERVENTIONS

Therapies will vary, depending on the type and extent of the lesion.

Preinvasive:

1. **Laser therapy:** Precise destruction of small lesions without destruction of normal tissue.

Invasive:

1. **External radiation therapy:** The best treatment for invasive cancer of the cervix; all stages of cancer are treated with this therapy, which is performed on an outpatient basis in the nuclear medicine department. Dosage and length of treatment is determined by MD specializing in nuclear medicine.

2. **Radium implants:** Used to destroy cervical cancer graded stage II-IV. While the patient is anesthetized, an applicator is positioned into the cervix through the vagina and its position is confirmed by x-ray. After the patient returns to her room, the radiologist inserts a radioactive isotope and leaves it in place for 1-3 days. During this time the patient is in a private room and remains in isolation.

   A combination of external radiation and implants gives the best therapeutic results. While the implant is in place, the patient is kept on strict bed rest, has an indwelling catheter, is on a low-residue diet, and is given analgesia (usually non-narcotic) and diphenoxylate hydrochloride with atropine sulfate (Lomotil) or paregoric to control diarrhea, which often occurs. After the implant has been removed, the patient is allowed to ambulate.

3. **Radical hysterectomy:** May be performed for young women to preserve tissue health. It involves the removal of the uterus, fallopian tubes, ovaries, upper third of the vagina, and parametrium on each side, as well as pelvic lymph node dissection. The patient usually returns to her room with an indwelling catheter.

NURSING DIAGNOSES AND INTERVENTIONS

Pain related to surgery or radiation implant

Desired outcome: Patient's subjective evaluation of pain improves, as documented by a pain scale.

1. Provide back rubs, which are especially helpful for patients who were in the lithotomy position during surgery. Massage the shoulders and upper back for patients with radium implants, who are not allowed position changes.
2. For other interventions, see same nursing diagnosis in "Caring for Preoperative and Postoperative Patients," in the appendix, p. 638.

Potential fluid volume deficit related to abnormal blood loss secondary to operative, postoperative, or postimplant bleeding

Desired outcomes: Patient is normovolemic as evidenced by BP ≥90/60 mm Hg (or within patient's usual range), HR 60-100 bpm, urinary output ≥30 ml/hr, RR ≤20 breaths/min with normal depth and pattern (eupnea), skin dry and of normal color, soft and nondistended abdomen, hct ≥37%, and hgb ≥12 g/dl. Patient and significant others verbalize knowledge of the signs and symptoms of excessive bleeding and are aware of the need to alert staff promptly if they are noted.

1. Monitor VS q2-4h during the first 24 hours. Be alert to indicators of hemorrhage and impending shock: hypotension, increased pulse and respirations, pallor, and diaphoresis.
2. Assess postoperative bleeding q2-4h by noting amount and quality of drainage on dressings and perineal pads if abdominal approach was used, or on perineal pads alone if vaginal approach was used. Normally, the patient's postoperative bleeding is minimal. It should be dark in color (or serosanguineous if an abdominal hysterectomy was performed). If an implant is in place, check for vaginal bleeding, a sign that erosion is occurring.
3. Inspect the abdomen for distention and assess patient for presence of severe abdominal pain; both are indicators of internal bleeding.
4. Review CBC values for evidence of bleeding: decreases in hgb and hct. Notify MD of significant findings.
5. Inform patient and significant others about the signs of excessive bleeding and the need to alert staff immediately should they occur.

Potential alteration in pattern of urinary elimination related to inadequate intake or obstruction of indwelling catheter

Desired outcome: Patient demonstrates a balanced I&O, with urinary output ≥30 ml/hr.

1. Monitor I&O and document every shift. Notify MD if urinary output falls below 30 ml/hr over 2 hours in the presence of an adequate intake. Along with low back pain, this can be indicative of ureteral ligation during surgery.
2. Ensure patency of the indwelling catheter.
3. Administer oral or parenteral fluids as prescribed. Ensure totals of 2-3 L/day in nonrestricted patients.
4. Assess for bladder distention by inspecting the suprapubic area and percussing or palpating the bladder. **Caution:** For patients with radiation implants, bladder distention can result in radiation burns to the bladder.

Grieving related to actual or perceived loss or changes in body image, body function, or role performance secondary to diagnosis of cancer

Desired outcome: Patient and significant other(s) express grief, explain the meaning of the loss, and communicate concerns with each other. The patient completes self-care activities as her condition improves.

1. Anticipate patient's concern about loss of uterus, presence of cancer and the potential for recurrence, and "loss of womanhood." Provide emotional support and an unhurried atmosphere for patient and significant others to ask questions and express concerns, frustrations, and fears.
2. Recognize the covert signs of grief that can accompany self-concept disturbances: anger, withdrawal, demanding behavior, or inappropriate affect. Give support to significant others who might misinterpret patient's coping mechanisms.
3. To enhance patient's sense of control over her situation, encourage her to perform ADL and begin self-care as soon as her condition warrants.
4. Provide materials by such organizations as the American Cancer Society and arrange for a contact person (role model) from such an organization, if appropriate.

See the appendix for nursing diagnoses and interventions for the care of preoperative and postoperative patients, p. 637, and for patients with cancer and other life-disrupting illnesses, p. 659.

PATIENT-FAMILY TEACHING AND DISCHARGE PLANNING

For patients who have had radium implants:

Provide verbal and written information for the following:
1. Necessity of notifying MD if the following problems occur: vaginal bleeding, rectal bleeding, foul-smelling vaginal discharge, abdominal pain or distention, hematuria.
2. Resumption of sexual intercourse, typically 6 weeks after surgery or as directed by MD.
3. Medications, including drug name, dosage, purpose, schedule, precautions, and potential side effects.
4. Need for follow-up care; confirm date and time of next medical appointment if known.
5. Patient is *not* radioactive once the implant has been removed.

For patients who have had a hysterectomy:
1. Necessity of notifying MD if the following indicators of infection occur: incisional swelling, redness, purulent drainage, vaginal bleeding, abdominal pain.
2. Care of the incision.
3. Restriction of activities as directed, such as heavy lifting (>5 lb) and sexual intercourse. Advise patient to get maximum amounts of rest and avoid fatigue.
4. Medications, including drug name, dosage, purpose, schedule, precautions, and potential side effects.
5. Need for follow-up care; confirm date and time of next MD appointment if known.

Ovarian tumors

There are numerous types of ovarian tumors, both benign and malignant. They include solid tumors and cysts of various cell types and can occur in females of all ages. The most common enlargements arise from the normal follicular apparatus of the ovary (i.e., follicle and corpus luteum cysts) and hyperplasias, such as polycystic ovaries. The most common benign neoplasms are the cystadenomas, which comprise 55% of the tumors. *Malignant ovarian tumors* rarely are diagnosed early because the patient tends to be asymptomatic. Because their detection usually occurs during an advanced stage, survival rate is low. Therefore, this is the most lethal type of gynecologic cancer. The average age range of occurrence for malignant lesions is 50-59. Both environmental and genetic factors may contribute to their development.

ASSESSMENT

Benign ovarian tumors: Depending on the type, common symptoms include abdominal enlargement and complaints of abdominal fullness.

Solid ovarian tumors: Abdominal enlargement and pressure; pelvic pressure and discomfort.

Signs and symptoms for both classifications: Amenorrhea, postmenopausal vaginal bleeding and other menstrual irregularities; urinary frequency and urgency; GI complaints, such as nausea, anorexia, and constipation.

Physical assessment: Abdominal distention; an enlarged ovary, which is highly suspicious in prepubertal and postmenopausal women.

DIAGNOSTIC TESTS

1. *Abdominal x-ray:* To reveal presence of an ovarian tumor.
2. *Ultrasound of the abdomen:* May reveal an ovarian mass.
3. *Laparoscopy:* Use of a laparoscope, an instrument with a telescope and light source, to visualize the pelvic organs through an incision made near the umbilicus. This procedure is done under general or regional anesthesia, usually on an outpatient basis.
4. *Cytologic examination of the pelvic washings/ascites:* May show presence of malignant cancerous cells.
5. *Staging of ovarian tumors* (dependent on surgical exploration): The following parameters are used, based on clinical classification of the International Federation of Gynecology and Obstetrics:
   □ *Stage I:* Tumor limited to the ovaries.
   Stage IA: Growth limited to one ovary; no ascites.
   Stage IB: Tumors limited to both ovaries; no ascites.
   □ *Stage II:* Tumors involving one or both ovaries with presence of malignant cells in pelvic organs.
   Stage IIA: Involvement of uterus or fallopian tubes with presence of malignant cells.
   Stage IIB: Presence of malignant cells in other pelvic tissues.
   Stage IIC: Tumors IIA or IIB with ascites or positive peritoneal washings.
   □ *Stage III:* Tumors involving one or both ovaries with metastasis outside the pelvis or positive retroperitoneal nodes. Tumor limited to retroperitoneal lymph nodes. Malignant cells found in small bowel omentum.
   □ *Stage IV:* Tumors involving one or both ovaries with metastasis to distant organs.

MEDICAL MANAGEMENT AND SURGICAL INTERVENTIONS

1. Wedge resection: Surgical procedure in which a benign tumor is removed, leaving normal ovarian tissue. It is done under anesthesia, using an abdominal approach.
2. Salpingo-oophorectomy: Removal of the ovary and fallopian tube on the affected side. It is performed under anesthesia, using an abdominal approach. This procedure is used for solid tumors of the ovary and stage IA ovarian cancer, with a biopsy of the contralateral ovary.
3. Total hysterectomy and bilateral salpingo-oophorectomy: Along with omental biopsy for ovarian cancer, it is performed if both ovaries are affected. If the disease has invaded other abdominal organs, **radiation therapy** is also used. Postoperative care includes adequate hydration and pain management; prophylactic antibiotics, depending on the extent of the surgical procedure and the risk of infection; and ambulation, usually the first evening after surgery.
4. Cytoreductive surgery: Involves removal of as much tumor as possible in order to increase the effectiveness of radiation and chemotherapy, which are more successful when the residual tumor is minimized.
5. Chemotherapy: Used for improving survival rates when the disease has spread to dis-

tant organs. Chemotherapeutic medications are used in combination and may include doxorubicin, cisplantin, melphalen, and cyclophosphamide.

NURSING DIAGNOSES AND INTERVENTIONS

See "Cancer of the Cervix" for **Pain** p. 495, **Potential fluid volume deficit** (blood loss), p. 495, **Alteration in pattern of urinary elimination,** p. 495, and **Grieving,** p. 495. See the appendix for nursing diagnoses and interventions for the care of preoperative and postoperative patients, p. 637, and patients with cancer and other life-disrupting illnesses, p. 659.

PATIENT-FAMILY TEACHING AND DISCHARGE PLANNING

Provide patient and significant others with verbal and written information for the following:

1. Medications, including drug name, dosage, schedule, purpose, precautions, and potential side effects.
2. Importance of reporting indicators of infection (depending on the surgery) to the MD: fever, vaginal bleeding and discharge, abdominal pain and distention, and incisional redness, purulent drainage, local warmth, and swelling.
3. Activity restrictions related to heavy lifting (>5 lb), exercise, sexual intercourse, or housework, as directed by MD.
4. Necessity of follow-up appointments; confirm date and time of next appointments for MD, radiation therapy, and chemotherapy.

Endometrial cancer

Endometrial (uterine) cancer typically occurs in postmenopausal women between the ages of 50 and 70. It is a slow-growing cancer that can take up to 10 years to metastasize. Risk factors for developing uterine cancer include obesity, nulliparity, late menopause (after age 52), hypertension, diabetes mellitus, unopposed menopausal estrogen therapy (i.e., giving estrogens without progestins), and polycystic ovary disease. The tumor can be found in any location within the uterus, either as a focal lesion or diffuse condition. The invasive stages of uterine cancer can involve spread to the vagina, pelvic lymph nodes, ovaries, and through the vascular system to the lungs and liver. Recurrence most frequently is seen in the vagina. When an early diagnosis is made, the prognosis is good, with successful treatment occurring in 80%-90% of the cases. *Adenocarcinoma* is the most common endometrial cancer.

ASSESSMENT

Signs and symptoms: Uterine bleeding in the postmenopausal woman; heavy and prolonged menses and intermenstrual spotting in the premenopausal woman.

Physical assessment: Presence of a palpable uterine mass, uterine polyps; obvious increase in uterine size in advanced disease.

DIAGNOSTIC TESTS

1. *Dilatation and curettage (D&C):* Surgical procedure in which the cervical opening is widened by a dilating instrument and the uterine lining is scraped with a curette to obtain a specimen for examination.
2. *Endometrial biopsy:* Office procedure in which a specimen is obtained from the endometrial surface for biopsy.
3. *Hysteroscopy:* Examination *via* an endoscope, which enters the uterus through the vagina, allowing visualization, biopsy, and photography with a camera. The patient is anesthetized with a pericervical block. This procedure can be used for diagnosis and staging.

4. *Chest x-ray:* To detect metastasis to the lungs.
5. *IVP:* To rule out spread of disease to other organs.
6. *CT scanning:* To direct needle biopsy of suspicious nodes.
7. *Staging of the disease.* The following parameters are used, based on clinical classification of the International Federation of Gynecology and Obstetrics.
   □ *Stage 0:* Carcinoma in situ. Histologic findings suggestive of malignancy.
   □ *Stage I:* Carcinoma confined to the corpus of the uterus.
      Stage IA: Length of the uterine cavity is ≤8 cm from the external os to the upper point of the uterus.
      Stage IB: Length of the uterine cavity is >8 cm.

   Subgroup as to histologic type of adenocarcinoma:
   —*Grade 1:* Highly differentiated adenomatous carcinoma.
   —*Grade 2:* Differentiated adenomatous carcinoma, with partly solid areas.
   —*Grade 3:* Predominately solid or entirely undifferentiated carcinoma.
   □ *Stage II:* Cancer involving the corpus and cervix but not extending beyond the uterus.
   □ *Stage III:* Cancer extending beyond the uterus but confined to the true pelvis.
   □ *Stage IV:* Cancer extending outside the true pelvis or obviously involving the mucosa of the bladder or rectum.

MEDICAL MANAGEMENT AND SURGICAL INTERVENTIONS

1. Total hysterectomy with bilateral salpingo-oophorectomy, with cytologic examination of peritoneal washings: Performed in patients who have a well-defined stage I tumor without cervical involvement. The uterus, cervix, fallopian tubes, ovaries, and a part of the vaginal cuff are removed.
2. Radical hysterectomy with para-aortic lymphadenectomy: Performed for patients with Stage I, Grades 2 and 3; and Stage II uterine cancer.
3. Radiation therapy: If an implant is used, the applicator is positioned in the uterus through the vagina while the patient is anesthetized. After the patient returns to her room, the radioisotope is placed in the applicator by a radiologist. External radiation of the uterus and pelvic nodes is performed on an outpatient basis for a period of time that is determined by the radiologist. When surgery and radiation therapy are used in combination, radiation therapy is done preoperatively (usually about 6 weeks before) to destroy cancer cells in the pericervical lymphatics and inhibit recurrence. This treatment is used for select Stage I, Grades 2 and 3; and Stage II and Stage III cancers.
4. Chemotherapy: Used for advanced and recurrent disease. Chemotherapeutic drugs include cyclophosphamide, hexamethylmelamine, adriamycin, and cisplatin. Combinations of drugs and the dosage and length of treatment are determined by the patient's response to treatment and the severity of recurrence.
5. Hormone therapy: Used for recurrent and advanced endometrial cancers. It produces remission in 30% of the cases. Medroxyprogesterone (Depo-Provera) is a progestin that can be used. Tamoxifen also is used. These therapies are more effective when the tumor has a large number of progesterone receptors.

NURSING DIAGNOSES AND INTERVENTIONS

See "Cancer of the Cervix," p. 495.

PATIENT-FAMILY TEACHING AND DISCHARGE PLANNING

See "Cancer of the Cervix," p. 496.

Section Three DISORDERS OF THE FEMALE PELVIS

Endometriosis is often seen in younger women, while cystocele, rectocele, and uterine prolapse more often are associated with women who are postmenopausal. These conditions occur when there is misplacement of structures or tissue within the female pelvis.

Endometriosis

Endometriosis is a condition in which endometrial tissue is present outside of the uterus. Typically it is found on the ovaries or in the peritoneal cul-de-sac. It also might be found in the vagina, vulva, uterosacral ligaments, or bowel. In extreme cases it is found in the lungs, bones, and other organs of the body. Endometriosis is considered a benign disease; it most often occurs in nulliparous women 30-40 years of age and in those who have had their first child at a later age. Its cause is unknown but it is theorized that a combination of factors play a role, for example, the tissue travelling up the fallopian tubes and into the perineum during the menstrual cycle, during surgical procedures (e.g., cesarean section) the tissue becoming implanted and growing at the surgical site, or the influence of irritation, inflammation, and hormonal alteration on tissue formation.

ASSESSMENT

Signs and symptoms: Dysmenorrhea 5-7 days before and 2-3 days after menses, hypermenorrhea (prolonged, excessive, and/or frequent menses), infertility, painful defecation during menses, sacral backache, and dyspareunia. Patient may be asymptomatic.

Physical assessment: Presence of a tender, fixed, rectoverted uterus. Palpation of the peritoneal cul-de-sac and ovaries may reveal presence of nodules or masses with extensive disease. Nodularity and tenderness of the uterosacral ligaments is common. The pelvic exam is performed several days before the menstrual cycle.

DIAGNOSTIC TESTS

1. *Laparoscopy:* Confirms presence of endometriosis at pelvic organs by passing a lighted instrument through an incision made near the umbilicus.
2. *Culdoscopy:* Also confirms the presence of endometriosis by passing a lighted instrument through the vagina to visualize the pelvic organs.

MEDICAL MANAGEMENT AND SURGICAL INTERVENTIONS

1. Encourage pregnancy in women wishing to have children: Pregnancy softens and atrophies the diseased areas as a result of hormone production. Pregnancy (or pseudopregnancy) stops the spread of endometriosis, and in some cases remission occurs following delivery.
2. Pharmacotherapy: *Danazol* (400 mg bid) is an androgen given to suppress ovulation and, hence, endometriosis. Progestin-estrogen treatment may improve symptoms but will not cure the disease.
3. Surgical procedures: Determined by the patient's age and desire to have children, and by extent of the disease. They are performed if medical treatment is unsuccessful.
   □ *For women without extensive disease who wish to have children, one of the following is performed:* Laser therapy or cauterization of endometrial implants, uterine suspension, lysis of adhesions, or removal of endometrial implants. These procedures are usually performed *via* an abdominal approach or through a laparoscope, although uterine suspension also can be performed by a vaginal approach.
   □ *For women who are not menopausal but do not wish to have children:* A hysterectomy may be performed, leaving the ovaries intact so that normal hormonal balance is maintained.
   □ *When there is extensive disease:* A total hysterectomy with bilateral salpingo-oophorectomy is performed. The ovaries are removed because they are hormone-carrying organs that influence the development and progression of the disease.

NURSING DIAGNOSES AND INTERVENTIONS

See "Cancer of the Cervix" for **Pain,** p. 495, **Potential fluid volume deficit** (blood loss), p. 495, and **Alteration in pattern of urinary elimination,** p. 495. See the appendix for nursing diagnoses and interventions for the care of preoperative and postoperative patients, p. 637.

PATIENT-FAMILY TEACHING AND DISCHARGE PLANNING

See "Ovarian Tumors," p. 498.

Cystocele

A cystocele is the bulging of the posterior bladder wall into the vagina. It is caused by constitutionally poor tissue or the stretching and tearing of the pelvic connective tissue during childbirth. Most often it occurs as a result of the delivery of a very large baby or after several deliveries. Symptoms usually do not appear until menopausal or postmenopausal age. A rectocele also might be present (see "Rectocele," p. 502).

ASSESSMENT

Signs and symptoms: Sensation of vaginal fullness or of bearing down, inability to empty bladder after voiding, urinary frequency, dysuria, stress incontinence, incontinence resulting from urgency, and recurrent cystitis.

Physical assessment: Manual pelvic exam will reveal a soft mass that bulges into the anterior vagina. The mass increases in size with coughing or straining.

DIAGNOSTIC TESTS

1. *Urine culture and sensitivity:* May reveal presence of bladder infection.
2. *Urodynamic evaluation:* Involves the study of the flow of urine from the bladder through the urethra to differentiate stress urinary incontinence from urgency incontinence. A combination of tests is used, including voiding flow rate, urethra pressure profile, urethroscopy, and cystometrogram.

MEDICAL MANAGEMENT AND SURGICAL INTERVENTIONS

1. Urinary catheterization: To empty a distended bladder. This is an emergency measure rather than a permanent correction.
2. Antibiotics: Given if urinary retention results in an infection.
3. Estrogen therapy: Conjugated estrogen (Premarin), sometimes given in small doses daily for three weeks each month in postmenopausal women to maintain hormonal levels. A lack of hormones results in weakness of the anterior vaginal wall, which allows the development of a cystocele.
4. Kegel isometric exercises: To help with bladder control (see p. 144).
5. Anterior colporrhaphy: Surgical procedure *via* vaginal approach to suspend the bladder. It involves separating the anterior vaginal wall from the bladder and urethra, suturing the bladder wall to reduce herniation, and excising the thinned vaginal wall. If both a cystocele and rectocele (see "Rectocele," p. 502) are present, an anterior and posterior colporrhaphy (A&P repair) is performed.
6. Pessary: Used as an internal support for some patients (see discussion in "Uterine Prolapse," p. 504). A Smith-Hodge device often is used if a cystocele exists.

NURSING DIAGNOSES AND INTERVENTIONS

See "Urinary Incontinence" in Chapter 3 for nursing diagnoses related to incontinence, p. 142. See "Cancer of the Cervix" for **Potential fluid volume deficit** (blood loss), p. 495. See the appendix for nursing diagnoses and interventions for the care of preoperative and postoperative patients, p. 637.

PATIENT-FAMILY TEACHING AND DISCHARGE PLANNING

Provide patient and significant others with verbal and written information for the following:

1. Medications, including drug name, purpose, dosage, schedule, precautions, and potential side effects.
2. Activity limitations during the first 6 weeks or as directed, including no heavy lifting (>5 lb) or strenuous exercises.
3. Abstinence from sexual intercourse for 6 weeks or as prescribed if vaginal surgery was performed. Discuss alternate methods of sexual expression.
4. Notifying MD for the following indicators of infection: fever; persistent pain; purulent, foul-smelling drainage.
5. Importance of follow-up appointments; confirm date and time of next appointment if known.

Rectocele

A rectocele is a rectovaginal hernia that develops when the connective tissue between the rectum and vagina is weakened and attenuated during childbirth. If there is straining with defecation or the patient is obese, the condition is aggrevated and progresses. The symptoms of this condition often do not become apparent until the woman is 35-40 years old.

ASSESSMENT

Signs and symptoms: Continuous urge to have a bowel movement, sensation of rectal and vaginal fullness, constipation (digital pressure must be applied vaginally to facilitate defecation), incontinence of flatus or feces, and the presence of hemorrhoids or fecal impaction.

Physical assessment: A nontender fullness can be felt by depressing the perineum as the patient strains; manual rectal examination will reveal the presence of a rectocele.

DIAGNOSTIC TEST

<u>Barium enema:</u> Will reveal the presence of a rectocele. As the hernia increases in size the wall of the anterior rectum tends to be pushed into the vagina.

MEDICAL MANAGEMENT AND SURGICAL INTERVENTIONS

1. Promote bowel elimination: With laxatives, stool softeners, and a high-fiber diet. If not contraindicated, walking is encouraged as a means of exercise to promote elimination.
2. Posterior colporrhaphy: This surgical procedure separates the posterior vaginal wall from the rectum and reduces the rectal herniation. If both a cystocele and rectocele are present, an anterior and posterior colporrhaphy (A&P repair) is performed. (See "Cystocele," p. 501.)

Nursing diagnoses and interventions

Colonic constipation related to restriction against straining, low-residue diet, or pain with defecation secondary to surgical procedure

Desired outcomes: After the early postoperative period, patient relates the presence of bowel movements within her normal pattern and with minimal discomfort. Patient verbalizes knowledge of the rationale for alerting staff before and after bowel movements and for not straining during defecation.

1. Assess patient for the presence of constipation; administer stool softeners or mild laxatives as prescribed.
2. The patient will be on a low-residue diet during the early postoperative period to minimize the potential for disruption of the surgical site. As indicated after the early postoperative period, consult with the MD regarding the introduction of high-residue foods to promote bowel movements.
3. Instruct patient not to strain when having a bowel movement, as this can disrupt the surgical repair.
4. Advise patient that defecation may be painful and to alert staff as soon as the urge to defecate is felt so that she can be medicated prior to the bowel movement.
5. Avoid the use of enemas or rectal tubes, which can disrupt the surgical repair.
6. Provide sitz baths as a comfort measure after bowel movements.
7. Request that the patient notify staff after each bowel movement; document accordingly.

See "Cancer of the Cervix" for **Potential fluid volume deficit** (blood loss), p. 495. See the appendix for nursing diagnoses and interventions for the care of preoperative and postoperative patients, p. 637.

PATIENT-FAMILY TEACHING AND DISCHARGE PLANNING

Provide patient and significant others with verbal and written information for the following:

1. Medications, including drug name, purpose, dosage, schedule, precautions, and potential side effects.
2. Limitation of activities during the first 6 weeks as directed by MD, including heavy lifting (>5 lb) and strenuous exercising. Abstinence from sexual intercourse is usually recommended for 6 weeks. Discuss alternate forms of sexual expression with patient. Advise patient that initially coitus may be painful.
3. Indicators of infection: abdominal or rectal pain, foul-smelling vaginal discharge, and fever.
4. Importance of follow-up care; confirm date and time of next medical appointment if known.

Uterine prolapse

A uterine prolapse is a bulging of the uterus through the pelvic floor into the vagina. It results from an injury to the cardinal and uterosacral ligaments that can occur with childbirth, surgical trauma, or atrophy of the supportive tissue during menopause. A prolapse also can develop as a result of uterine tumors, diabetic neuropathy, neurologic injury to the sacral nerves, obesity, or ascites. A prolapse will progress unless surgically repaired.

A prolapse is graded in the following way:
  □ *Grade I:* Cervix remains within the vagina; the uterus partially descends into the vagina (first degree prolapse).
  □ *Grade II:* Cervix protrudes through the entrance to the vagina. This is second degree prolapse.

☐ *Grade III:* Entire uterus protrudes through the entrance of the vagina and the vagina is inverted. This is a third degree prolapse or procidentia, which occurs most frequently in postmenopausal, multiparous women and often along with a rectocele, cystocele, and enterocele (a hernia containing a loop of small intestine or the sigmoid colon that bulges into the upper posterior vagina).

ASSESSMENT

Signs and symptoms: Complaints of heaviness in the pelvis, low backache, "dragging" sensation in the inguinal region, and involuntary loss of urine with coughing or sneezing.

Physical assessment: Pelvic examination is performed with the patient either standing or supine. As patient bears down, a firm mass can be palpated in the lower vagina. This exam also can confirm diagnosis of a rectocele and cystocele, if present.

MEDICAL MANAGEMENT AND SURGICAL INTERVENTIONS

1. Placement of a vaginal pessary: A rubber device that is inserted into the vagina to support the pelvic structures. It may be used if there is first or second degree prolapse or if surgery is contraindicated or unwanted by patient.
2. Estrogen suppositories: To maintain tone of the pelvic floor.
3. Antibiotics: If patient has a urinary tract infection.
4. High-fiber diet: To aid in bowel elimination.
5. Vaginal hysterectomy: To correct uterine prolapse. For severe prolapse with rectocele and cystocele, a hysterectomy with an anterior/posterior colporrhaphy is performed.

NURSING DIAGNOSES AND INTERVENTIONS

See "Cancer of the Cervix" for **Potential fluid volume deficit** (blood loss), p. 495, and **Grieving** (if a hysterectomy is performed), p. 495. See "Rectocele" for **Colonic constipation**, p. 503. See the appendix for nursing diagnoses and interventions for the care of preoperative and postoperative patients, p. 637.

PATIENT-FAMILY TEACHING AND DISCHARGE PLANNING

See "Rectocele," p. 503.

Section Four   INTERRUPTION OF PREGNANCY

The following conditions or surgical procedures involve women of childbearing age and can result in continued problems with childbearing or sterilization.

Spontaneous abortion

A spontaneous abortion, or miscarriage, occurs in approximately 15% of pregnancies. It is the expulsion of the products of conception before the 24th week of gestation and it is classified in the following ways:

Threatened abortion: Vaginal bleeding and cramping during the first half of the pregnancy. There is no tissue loss and the cervix is closed. Either the symptoms disappear or an abortion occurs.

Inevitable abortion: Vaginal bleeding, cramping, rupture of membranes, and dilatation and effacement of the cervix; cannot be halted.

Incomplete abortion: Partial expulsion of products of conception, with continued vaginal bleeding.

Complete abortion: Expulsion of all products of conception, with cessation of vaginal bleeding and pain following expulsion.

Missed abortion: Presence of a dead fetus in the uterus without expulsion.

Recurrent (habitual) abortion: Three or more pregnancies that are spontaneously aborted by the same woman during the first trimester.

There are three primary causes of spontaneous abortion: *fetal*, which includes defective development and faulty implantation of the fertilized ovum; *maternal*, including infection, malnutrition, endocrine abnormalities, and incompetent cervix; and *placental*, which includes abruptio placenta (premature separation of placenta) and incorrect placental implantation.

ASSESSMENT

Signs and symptoms: Vaginal bleeding, cramping, low back pain, signs of pregnancy, no increase in size of uterus, anorexia.

Physical assessment: A pelvic examination will reveal the size of the uterus and show either that products of conception are intact or have been expelled.

DIAGNOSTIC TESTS

1. *CBC:* Will reveal a decrease in hgb and hct. There is a potential for elevation in leukocyte count, which would signal an infection.
2. *Lab examination of products of conception:* To confirm results of pelvic examination.
3. *Ultrasound:* Will confirm the presence of a dead fetus in a missed abortion, as evidenced by absence of fetal heart motion.
4. *Endocrine studies:* Human chorionic gonadotropin (HCG) will be minimal or absent with pregnancy loss.

MEDICAL MANAGEMENT AND SURGICAL INTERVENTIONS

1. Blood or blood products: Administered for excessive blood loss.
2. Parenteral fluid administration: For excessive fluid loss.
3. Analgesics: For pain management.
4. Antibiotics: When indicated, to prevent development of infection.
5. Dilatation and curettage (D&C): Procedure done in the first trimester to remove products of conception. Under general or local anesthesia, the canal of the cervix is dilated to allow a curette to pass through the cervix into the uterus and scrape out any products of conception that remain. A **suction evacuation,** which utilizes a suction apparatus rather than a curette, may be performed instead.
6. IV oxytocin: To induce labor after 12 weeks gestation. Oxytocin contracts the uterus by stimulating the smooth muscles.
7. Cervical cerclage: Performed early in the second trimester to manage an incompetent cervix when patient has a history of repeated second trimester abortions. With this technique, the cervix is reinforced with a suture (using McDonald, Shirodkar, or transabdominal cervicoisthmic cerclage procedure). The suture is released at term (or immediately if labor begins) to allow a vaginal delivery. This procedure is not performed in the presence of membrane rupture, cramping, vaginal bleeding, or a cervical dilatation greater than 3 cm.
8. RhoGAM: an Rh_O (D), immune globulin, which is given to prevent Rh sensitization in Rh-negative women whose partners are Rh-positive.

NURSING DIAGNOSES AND INTERVENTIONS

Potential fluid volume deficit related to abnormal blood loss secondary to abortion or surgical intervention

Desired outcome: Patient is normovolemic, as evidenced by BP ≥90/60 mm Hg, HR 60-100 bpm, urinary output ≥30 ml/hr, RR ≤20 breaths/min with normal pattern and depth (eupnea), warm and dry skin, and orientation to person, place, and time.

1. Assess and document BP, pulse, and respirations at frequent intervals (typically q15min × 4; q30min × 2; q1-2h until stable; and then q4h). Notify MD of significant changes. Be alert to hypotension, changes in LOC, cool and clammy skin, and increasing pulse and respiration rates.
2. Monitor I&O at least q4h. Be alert to decreasing urinary output, which can signal the onset of shock.
3. Administer parenteral fluids, blood, and blood products as prescribed.
4. Inspect perineal pads and note and document the amount and quality of bleeding. If vaginal bleeding increases or there is expulsion of the products of conception, notify MD at once. Save any tissue or clots that are expelled. **Note:** Bleeding is considered excessive if more than two perineal pads are saturated in 1 hour.
5. If prescribed, administer oxytocin to assist with the contraction of the uterus and expulsion of the fetus.
6. After expulsion of the contents of conception has occurred, palpate the uterine fundus to assess its tone. If it feels soft and boggy, provide light massage by rubbing in a circular motion. **Caution:** Avoid massaging a uterus that is well contracted, because this can result in muscle fatigue and uterine relaxation.

Pain related to uterine contractions

Desired outcome: Patient's subjective evaluation of pain improves, as documented by a pain scale.

1. Monitor and document number and duration of contractions. Assess and document the patient's level of pain and response to pain management, using a scale of 0-10.
2. Administer analgesics as prescribed. Provide backrubs, which are especially relaxing.
3. Instruct patient in alternative methods of pain relief, including deep breathing, relaxation techniques, and guided imagery.
4. Assist patient with ADL as appropriate.

Potential for infection related to increased susceptibility secondary to retention of some or all of the products of conception

Desired outcome: Patient is free of infection, as evidenced by normothermia and absence of foul-smelling vaginal discharge and abdominal tenderness.

1. Assess temperature q4h; notify MD if an elevation occurs.
2. Be alert to the presence of foul-smelling vaginal discharge, an indicator of infection.
3. Administer antibiotics as prescribed.
4. Ensure that perineal care is performed after every voiding and bowel movement.

Altered role performance related to fetal loss

Desired outcomes: Patient verbalizes realistic acceptance of change in her role or verbalizes plans for adaptation. Patient communicates with significant others.

1. Provide emotional support for patient and significant others. Provide time and a supportive atmosphere for patient to feel comfortable with expressing feelings and concerns. Do not minimize patient's feelings of loss.
2. Assist patient with identifying concerns, if present, with role performance as a wife or childbearer. Assist patient with developing plans for adaptation. Provide referral for genetic counseling if genetics was a factor in the pregnancy loss.
3. Involve social services if needed.

Grieving related to anticipated or actual fetal loss

Desired outcome: Patient expresses feelings about the loss (actual or potential) and shares her grief with significant others.

1. Assess the stage of grieving patient is experiencing. Be aware that feelings may be complicated by emotions that preceded the actual or impending fetal loss. For example, if the woman experienced joy regarding her pregnancy, her grief may be more than anticipated. Conversely, if the pregnancy was viewed as a negative experience, she may experience feelings of guilt and self-blame.
2. Do not minimize patient's feelings of loss.
3. Assist patient and significant others with acknowledging the loss by taking the time to sit and talk with them.
4. Offer emotional support and encourage the patient and significant others to discuss the loss among themselves, as well.
5. Ensure privacy for the patient and significant others.
6. Refer the patient to community-based parent support group.
7. Provide for pastoral or other supportive care if indicated.
8. Also see psychosocial nursing diagnoses for patients and families in the appendix "Caring for Patients with Cancer and Other Life-Disrupting Illnesses," p. 690.

PATIENT-FAMILY TEACHING AND DISCHARGE PLANNING

Provide patient and significant others with verbal and written information for the following:
1. Medications, including drug name, purpose, dosage, schedule, precautions, and potential side effects.
2. Vaginal bleeding, which should taper gradually during the first 10 days. Advise patient that increasing bleeding is abnormal and necessitates medical attention.
3. Indicators of infection, which necessitate medical attention: temperature 37.78° C (100° F) or greater and foul-smelling vaginal discharge.
4. Activity limitations as directed by MD, including strenuous exercise and sexual intercourse.
5. Importance of follow-up care; confirm date and time of next medical appointment if known.
6. Name and address of community resources.

Ectopic pregnancy

An ectopic pregnancy is an implanted fertile ovum outside the uterus. The most common site is the fallopian tube; it occurs less commonly in the peritoneum, ovary, or cervix. In the fallopian tube, the implanted ovum causes a weakening of the tubal wall, resulting in a rupture that can cause bleeding into the peritoneum, a medical emergency. Factors that predispose toward ectopic pregnancy include pelvic inflammatory disease (PID), IUD usage, prior surgical procedure of the fallopian tube, and previous ectopic pregnancy. These pathologies may interfere with the structure and function of the fallopian tube and cause a delay in the passage of the ovum into the uterus, which can result in ectopic pregnancy. Ectopic pregnancies occur in approximately 1 out of every 72 pregnancies, a nearly threefold increase from 1970 statistics.

ASSESSMENT

Signs and symptoms: Indications of pregnancy (i.e., amenorrhea, nausea, breast enlargement, urinary frequency), uterine bleeding or spotting, abdominal pain. The following acute symptoms may develop prior to and accompanying rupture: mild to moderate vaginal bleeding with unilateral lower abdominal cramping that becomes increasingly sharp and constant, referred shoulder pain caused by irritation of the diaphragm from the pooling of blood in the peritoneum, and a falling hct and hgb. **Caution:** Immediate intervention is necessary to prevent loss of blood, which can lead to shock and death.

Physical assessment: Abdominal palpation may reveal a unilateral lower quadrant tenderness and size and date discrepancy. **Caution:** Pelvic examination is deferred if ectopic pregnancy is suspected.

DIAGNOSTIC TESTS

1. *CBC:* May reveal a decreased hgb and hct and an increased leukocyte count.
2. *Serum or urine HCG:* Usually positive.
3. *Ultrasound:* May identify the location of pregnancy.
4. *Culdocentesis:* May reveal the presence of blood in the peritoneum. In this test, fluid is aspirated from the vaginal cul-de-sac.
5. *Laparoscopy:* Will confirm the presence of ectopic pregnancy and allow immediate treatment.

MEDICAL MANAGEMENT AND SURGICAL INTERVENTIONS

1. Whole blood or packed cells: To replace loss if necessary.
2. Broad spectrum IV antibiotics: May be administered prophylactically.
3. Analgesics/narcotics: For pain management.
4. Laparoscopy: Conservative procedure performed on a stable patient, using an endoscope inserted through a small opening in the abdomen. Often, it is used in conjunction with tubal sparing procedures.
5. Laparotomy with unilateral salpingectomy (removal of the fallopian tube) or salpingo-oophorectomy (removal of the fallopian tube and ovary): Performed if the ectopic pregnancy ruptures. A ruptured ectopic pregnancy is considered a surgical emergency because of the inevitable loss of blood into the peritoneum. The type of surgical procedure used is dependent on the extent of structural involvement.
6. RhoGAM: If indicated, is given to Rh-negative mothers after ectopic pregnancy.

NURSING DIAGNOSES AND INTERVENTIONS

Potential fluid volume deficit related to abnormal loss secondary to bleeding or hemorrhage with ectopic rupture

Desired outcome: Patient is normovolemic, as evidenced by urinary output $\geq$30 ml/hr, BP $\geq$90/60 mm Hg, RR $\leq$20 breaths/min with normal depth and pattern (eupnea), HR $\leq$100 bpm, warm and dry skin, absent or scant vaginal bleeding, hct $\geq$37%, and hgb $\geq$12 g/dl.

1. Assess VS at frequent intervals, noting changes in BP, pulse, and respiratory rate. Be alert to hypotension, increases in pulse and respiratory rates, and cool and clammy skin as indicators of impending shock.
2. Assess the amount and quality of vaginal bleeding. Bright red, frank bleeding, along with abnormal VS should be reported to the MD at once.
3. Review results of CBC, noting values of hgb and hct, which are decreased with blood loss.
4. Infuse parenteral and blood products as prescribed.

See "Spontaneous Abortion" for **Grieving,** p. 507, and **Altered role performance,** p. 506. See the appendix for nursing diagnoses and interventions for the care of preoperative and postoperative patients, p. 637.

PATIENT-FAMILY TEACHING AND DISCHARGE PLANNING

Provide patient and significant others with verbal and written information for the following, depending on the type of surgical procedure:

1. Medications, including drug name, purpose, dosage, schedule, precautions, and potential side effects.
2. Importance of monitoring vaginal drainage, including the amount, color, consistency, and odor; and reporting significant changes to MD.
3. Activity limitations as directed by MD, including strenuous exercise, housework, and sexual intercourse.
4. Indicators of incisional infection, including persistent redness, swelling, warmth, fever, purulent discharge, and incisional/abdominal pain.
5. Importance of follow-up care; confirm time and date of next medical visit if known.

Section Five DISORDERS AND SURGERIES OF THE MALE PELVIS

Benign prostatic hypertrophy

The prostate is an encapsulated gland that surrounds the male urethra below the bladder neck and produces a thin, milky fluid during ejaculation. As a man ages, the prostate gland grows larger. Although the exact cause of the enlargement is unknown, one theory is that hormonal changes affect the estrogen-androgen balance. This noncancerous enlargement is common in men over age 50, and as many as 80% of men over the age of 65 are believed to have symptoms of prostatic enlargement. Treatment is given when symptoms of bladder outlet obstruction appear.

ASSESSMENT

Chronic indicators: Urinary frequency, hesitancy, and dribbling; decreased force of stream; nocturia; hematuria.

Acute indicators/bladder outlet obstruction: Anuria, nausea, vomiting, severe suprapubic pain, constant urgency, flank pain during micturition.

Physical assessment: Bladder distention, "kettle-drum" sound with percussion over the distended bladder. Rectal exam will reveal a smooth, firm, symmetric, and elastic enlargement of the prostate.

DIAGNOSTIC TESTS

1. *Urinalysis* checks for the presence of WBCs, bacteria, and microscopic hematuria; and *urine culture and sensitivity* verifies presence of infection; the results will specify the type of organism and determine the most effective antibiotic.
2. *Hct/hgb:* Results may signal mild anemia from local bleeding.
3. *BUN and creatinine:* To evaluate renal-urinary function. **Note:** BUN can be affected by the patient's hydration status and the results must be evaluated accordingly: fluid volume excess reduces BUN levels, while fluid volume deficit will increase them. Serum creatinine may not be a reliable indicator of renal function in the older adult, owing to decreased muscle mass and decreased glomerular filtration rate; results of this test must be evaluated along with those of urine creatinine clearance, other renal function studies, and the patient's age.
4. *Cystoscopy:* To visualize the prostate gland, estimate its size, and ascertain the presence of any damage to the bladder wall secondary to an enlarged prostate. **Note:** Because patients undergoing cystoscopy are susceptible to septic shock, this procedure is contraindicated in patients with acute UTI because of the danger of introducing gram negative bacteria into the bladder.
5. *Intravenous pyelography (IVP)/excretory urogram:* Evaluates the structure and function of the kidneys, ureters, and bladder, and reveals calculi if they are present. **Note:** Two complications of IVP are allergic reaction to dye and acute renal failure induced by the contrast medium. Exposure to contrast medium might worsen existing

renal insufficiency, especially in elderly, dehydrated, or diabetic patients. Before the study, patients should be queried about allergies to shellfish and iodine or reactions to previous dye studies. After IVP, patients should be monitored for indicators of renal failure.

Note: All urine specimens should be sent to the laboratory immediately after they are obtained, or refrigerated if this is not possible (specimens for urine culture are *not* refrigerated). Urine left at room temperature has a greater potential for bacterial growth, turbidity, and alkaline pH, any of which can distort the test results.

MEDICAL MANAGEMENT AND SURGICAL INTERVENTIONS

1. Catheterization: To relieve urinary retention.
2. Antibiotics and antimicrobial agents: To treat infection, if one is present.
3. Antiandrogen (estrogen) therapy: May be initiated to lower the levels of testosterone if this is the cause of the prostate's enlargement. Occasionally, an orchiectomy is performed for the same purpose. **Note:** The patient will become impotent while on estrogen therapy. However, an orchiectomy will *not* affect the patient's ability to have intercourse.
4. Reduction of prostatic congestion via rectal massage of the prostate gland: This is performed only if there is substantial congestion. Hot sitz baths also are prescribed to relieve congestion.
5. Restriction of rapid intake of fluids: Particularly alcohol, which can result in episodes of acute urinary retention from loss of bladder tone secondary to rapid distention.
6. Prostatectomy: Removal of enlarged prostatic tissue.
   □ *Transurethral resection of the prostate (TURP):* Prostatic tissue is scraped away *via* cystoscopy. This is the most common approach, especially in patients who are poor surgical risks. It is done under spinal anesthesia.
   □ *Suprapubic transvesical prostatectomy/retropubic extravesical prostatectomy:* Prostatic tissue is removed *via* an incision high in the bladder (abdominal approach) or by a low abdominal incision without entry into the bladder. This is indicated for a large prostate ($\geq$40 g) that cannot be removed transurethrally. These approaches may be used if a large bladder diverticula or calculi exist that can be corrected at the time of surgery, in the presence of a severe urethral stricture, and with orthopaedic conditions that contraindicate positioning for other approaches.

NURSING DIAGNOSES AND INTERVENTIONS

Potential for infection (septic shock) related to susceptability secondary to introduction of gram negative bacteria occurring with cystoscopy or TURP

Desired outcome: Patient is free of gram negative infection as evidenced by normothermia, urinary output $\geq$30 ml/hr, RR 12-20 breaths/min, HR and BP within patient's normal range, and orientation to person, place, and time (within patient's normal range).

Note: Accurate assessment of the patient in the early (warm) stage of septic shock greatly improves the prognosis.

---

1. Monitor patient's VS and mentation status at frequent intervals for indicators of the early (warm) stage of septic shock. During the first 24 hours following surgery, be alert to temperatures of 38.3°-40.0° C (101°-104° F), which occur in the presence of infection due to increased metabolic activity and release of pyrogens. Also assess for moderately increased RR and HR and decreased BP. Classic circulatory signs of collapse occur in the late (cold) stage of septic shock, including profoundly decreased BP (due to decreased stroke volume), greatly increased and weakened HR (compensatory mechanism to maintain cardiac output), and decreased RR (owing to respiratory center depression). Mental status changes of inappropriate behavior, personality

changes, restlessness, increasing lethargy, and disorientation may signal hypoxia owing to decreased cerebral perfusion.

2. Monitor patient's skin for flushing and warmth, which are early signs of septic shock due to vasodilatation. In the cold stage of septic shock, skin will become cool and pale owing to sustained vasoconstriction.

3. Monitor patient's urinary output for decrease and for increased concentration (normal specific gravity is 1.010-1.020).

4. Notify MD promptly if septic shock is suspected. Prepare for the following if septic shock is confirmed: IV infusion (e.g., lactated Ringer's or normal saline); oxygen administration; specimens for WBC, arterial blood gas, and electrolyte values; and administration of antibiotics.

5. Teach the indicators of infection and early septic shock to patient and stress the importance of notifying staff promptly should they occur.

Potential fluid volume deficit related to abnormal blood loss secondary to surgical procedure or pressure on the prostatic capsule

Desired outcomes: Patient is normovolemic as evidenced by balanced I&O, HR ≤90 bpm (or within patient's normal range), BP ≥90/60 mm Hg (or within patient's normal range), RR ≤20 breaths/min, and skin that is warm, dry, and of normal color. Patient relates actions that might result in hemorrhage of the prostatic capsule and participates in interventions to prevent them.

1. Upon patient's return from the recovery room, monitor VS q15min for the first 30 minutes; if stable, check q30min for an hour; and then q4h for 24 hours, or per agency policy. Be alert to increasing pulse, decreasing BP, diaphoresis, pallor, and increasing respirations, which can occur with hemorrhage and impending shock.

2. Monitor catheter drainage closely for the first 24 hours. Watch for dark red drainage that does not lighten to reddish-pink or drainage that remains thick in consistency after irrigation, which can signal venous bleeding within the operative site. Drainage should lighten to pink or blood-tinged within 24 hours after surgery.

3. Be alert to bright red, thick drainage at any time, which can occur with arterial bleeding within the operative site.

4. Do not measure temperature rectally or insert rectal tubes or enemas into the rectum. Instruct patient not to strain with bowel movements or sit for long periods of time. Any of these actions can result in pressure on the prostatic capsule and potentially lead to hemorrhage. Obtain prescription for and provide stool softeners or cathartics as necessary.

5. The surgeon may establish traction on the indwelling urethral catheter in the operating room to help prevent bleeding. Maintain the traction for 4-8 hours after surgery, or as directed.

6. Also monitor patient for signs of disseminated intravascular coagulopathy (DIC), which can occur as a result of the release of large amounts of tissue thromboplastins during a TURP. Watch for unusual oozing from all puncture sites. Report significant findings promptly should they occur. For more information, see "Disseminated Intravascular Coagulation," p. 414.

Potential fluid volume excess related to risk of water intoxication secondary to administration of high volumes of irrigating fluid

Desired outcome: Patient is normovolemic as evidenced by balanced I&O (after subtraction of irrigant total from output); orientation to person, place, and time; and electrolyte values within normal range.

1. Monitor and record I&O. To determine the true amount of urinary output, subtract the amount of irrigant from the total output. Report discrepancies, which can signal fluid retention.

2. Monitor the patient's mental and motor status. Assess for the presence of muscle twitching, seizures, and changes in mentation. These are signs of water intoxification and electrolyte imbalance, which can occur within 24 hours of surgery because of the high volumes of fluid that are used in irrigation.

3. Monitor electrolyte values, in particular those of sodium, for evidence of hyponatremia. Normal range for sodium is 137-147 mEq/L.
4. Promptly report indications of fluid overload and electrolyte imbalance to the MD. See "Fluid and Electrolyte Disturbances," p. 546, for more information.

Pain related to bladder spasms

Desired outcome: Patient's subjective evaluation of pain improves, as documented by a pain scale.

1. Assess and document the quality, location, and duration of pain. Devise a pain scale with patient (e.g., using a range of 0-10, with "0" denoting no pain) to evaluate the degree of pain.
2. Medicate the patient with prescribed analgesics, narcotics, and antispasmodics as appropriate; evaluate and document the patient's response by using the pain scale.
3. Provide warm blankets or a heating pad to affected area, or warm baths to increase regional circulation and relax tense muscles.
4. Teach technique for slow, diaphragmatic breathing to relax patient and help ease pain.
5. Provide backrubs and encourage use of other nonpharmacologic methods of pain relief, such as guided imagery, distraction, relaxation tapes, and soothing music. Also see p. 49 for **Health-seeking behavior:** Relaxation technique effective for stress reduction.
6. Monitor for leakage around the catheter, which can signal the presence of bladder spasms.
7. If the patient has spasms, assure him they are normal and can occur because of irritation of the bladder mucosa by the catheter balloon or a clot that results in backup of urine into the bladder with concomitant irritation of the mucosa. Encourage fluid intake, as this will help prevent spasms. If the MD has prescribed catheter irrigation for the removal of clots, follow instructions carefully to prevent discomfort and injury to patient.
8. Monitor for the presence of clots in the tubing. If clots are present for the patient with continuous bladder irrigation, adjust the rate of bladder irrigation to maintain light red urine (with clots). Total output should be greater than the amount of irrigant instilled. If output equals the amount of irrigant or the patient complains that his bladder is full, his catheter may be clogged with clots. If clots inhibit the flow of urine, irrigate the catheter by hand according to agency or MD directive.

Potential for impaired skin integrity related to risk of irritation secondary to wound drainage from suprapubic or retropubic prostatectomy

Desired outcome: Patient's skin remains clear and intact.

1. Monitor incisional dressings frequently during the first 24 hours and change or reinforce as needed. If the incision has been made into the bladder, excoriation can result from prolonged contact of urine with the skin.
2. Use Montgomery straps rather than tape to secure the dressing.
3. If the drainage is copious after drain removal, apply a wound drainage or ostomy pouch with a skin barrier over the incision. Use a pouch with an antireflux valve to prevent contamination from reflux.

Potential for altered pattern of sexuality related to fear of impotence secondary to lack of knowledge of postsurgical sexual function

Desired outcome: Patient discusses concerns about sexuality and relates accurate information regarding sexual function.

1. Assess patient's level of readiness to discuss sexual function; provide opportunities for patient to discuss fears and anxieties.
2. Assure patient who has had a simple prostatectomy that his ability to obtain and maintain an erection is unaltered. Retrograde ejaculation or "dry" ejaculation will oc-

cur in most patients, but this probably will end after a few months. It will not, however, affect his ability to achieve orgasm.
3. Encourage communication between patient and his significant other.
4. Be aware of your own feelings regarding sexuality. If you are uncomfortable discussing sexuality, request that another staff member take responsibility for discussing feelings and concerns with the patient.
5. As indicated, encourage continuation of counseling after hospital discharge. Confer with MD and social services to identify appropriate referral.

Colonic constipation related to postsurgical discomfort or fear of exerting excess pressure on prostatic capsule

Desired outcome: Patient relates the presence of a bowel pattern that is normal for him with minimal pain or straining.

Note: A patient who states that he needs to have a bowel movement during the first 24 hours following surgery probably has clots in the bladder that are creating pressure on the rectum. Assess for the presence of clots (see **Pain,** p. 512) and irrigate the catheter as indicated.

---

1. Document the presence or absence and quality of bowel sounds in all four abdominal quadrants.
2. Gather baseline information on patient's normal bowel pattern and document findings.
3. Unless contraindicated, encourage patient to consume 2-3 L/day postsurgically.
4. Consult with MD and dietitian regarding need for increased fiber in patient's diet.
5. Teach patient to avoid straining when defecating to prevent excess pressure on the prostatic capsule.
6. Consult with MD regarding use of stool softeners for patient during the postoperative period.
7. See **Constipation,** p. 656, in the appendix for more information.

Urge incontinence related to frequency and dribbling of urine secondary to urethral irritation following removal of urethral catheter

Desired outcome: Patient reports increasing periods of time between voidings by the second postoperative day and regains normal pattern of micturition within 4-6 weeks following surgery.

1. Prior to removal of the urethral catheter, explain to the patient that he may void in small amounts for the first 12 hours after catheter removal because of irritation from the catheter.
2. Instruct patient to save urine in a urinal for the first 24 hours after surgery. Inspect each voiding for color and consistency. First urine specimens can be dark red due to the passage of old blood. Each successive specimen should lighten.
3. Note and document the time and amount of each voiding. Initially, the patient may void q15-30min, but the time interval between voidings should increase toward a more normal pattern.
4. Prior to hospital discharge, inform patient that dribbling may occur for the first 4-6 weeks after surgery. This happens as a result of the disturbance of the bladder neck and urethra during prostate removal. As muscles strengthen and healing occurs (the urethra reaches normal size and function), the dribbling stops.
5. Teach patient pubococcygeal (Kegel) exercises (see p. 144) to improve sphincter control.

See "Cancer of the Bladder" in Chapter 3 for **Alteration in pattern of urinary elimination** related to presence of suprapubic catheter, p. 140. See "Prostatic Neoplasm," for **Potential stress incontinence,** p. 519. See the appendix for nursing diagnoses and interventions for the care of preoperative and postoperative patients, p. 637.

PATIENT-FAMILY TEACHING AND DISCHARGE PLANNING

Provide patient and significant others with verbal and written information for the following:

1. Medications, including drug name, purpose, dosage, schedule, precautions, and potential side effects.
2. Indicators of UTI, which necessitate medical attention: cloudy or foul-smelling urine, fever, pain, dysuria.
3. Care of incision, if appropriate, including cleansing, dressing changes, and bathing. Advise patient to be aware of indicators of infection: persistent redness, increased warmth along incision, or purulent drainage.
4. Care of catheters or drains if patient is discharged with them.
5. Daily fluid requirement of at least 2-3 L/day in nonrestricted patients.
6. Importance of increasing dietary fiber or taking stool softeners to soften stools. This will minimize risk of damage to the prostatic capsule by preventing straining with bowel movements.
7. Avoiding the following activities for the period of time prescribed by MD: sitting for long periods of time, heavy lifting (>5 lb), and sexual intercourse.
8. Pubococcygeal (Kegel) exercises to help regain urinary sphincter control for postoperative dribbling. See discussion, p. 144.

Prostatitis

Prostatitis is inflammation of the prostate gland. Acute bacterial prostatitis is the form most frequently seen in the hospital setting. It is caused by the introduction of bacteria into the prostate *via* the bloodstream, urethra, or kidneys. The urethra is the most common avenue for introduction of bacteria, and patients undergoing urethral instrumentation, such as cystoscopy or catheterization, are at increased risk. Statistics show an increased risk of prostatitis with advancing age and increased prostate size.

ASSESSMENT

Signs and symptoms: Urinary urgency and frequency, dysuria, perineal and low back pain, purulent urethral discharge, chills, and moderate to high fever (fever may be absent or low-grade in the older adult). The older adult may present with acute confusion owing to decreased oxygenation of the brain caused by the infection.

Physical assessment: Presence of tender, swollen, hardened prostate gland palpated on rectal exam

DIAGNOSTIC TESTS

1. *WBC count:* To reveal presence of infection ($\geq 11,000\ \mu l$).
2. *Urinalysis and urine culture:* To detect the presence of UTI and identify the offending bacteria.
3. *BUN and creatinine:* Show evidence of renal involvement when the test results are elevated. **Note:** BUN results are affected by hydration status and the results must be interpretted accordingly. Fluid volume excess will reduce the value, while fluid volume deficit will increase the value. In the older adult, serum creatinine may not be a reliable measure of renal function owing to decreased muscle mass and a decreased glomerular filtration rate. Results of this test should be evaluated along with those of urine creatinine clearance, other renal function tests, and the patient's age.
4. *Culture and sensitivity of the prostatic and urethral exudate:* Identifies the causative bacteria and determines the most appropriate antibiotic. **Note:** Prostatic massage to obtain the prostatic exudate is contraindicated in the acute stage of illness as it can lead to bacteremia.

Note: All urine specimens should be sent to the laboratory immediately after they are obtained, or refrigerated if this is not possible (urine culture specimens are *not* refrigerated). Urine left at room temperature has a greater potential for bacterial growth, turbidity, and alkalinity, any of which will distort the test results.

MEDICAL MANAGEMENT AND SURGICAL INTERVENTIONS

1. **Pharmacotherapy** may include the following:
   - ☐ *Antispasmodics:* Such as propantheline bromide or belladonna and opium (B&O) suppositories.
   - ☐ *Stool softeners:* To prevent pressure on the prostatic capsule.
   - ☐ *Antipyretics:* For fever associated with infections.
   - ☐ *Urinary analgesics:* Such as phenazopyridine hydrochloride to alleviate burning with urination.
   - ☐ *Antibiotics:* Often given in combination (e.g., trimethoprimsulfamethoxazole) to control gram negative bacteria. The erythromycins usually are given for gram positive bacteria, and gentamicin or tobramycin sulfate is used for more severe infections. If sepsis is suspected, ampicillin or amoxicillin is given.
2. **Bed rest:** Either strict or with bathroom privileges during the first 24-48 hours to relieve perineal and suprapubic pain.
3. **Intravenous fluids:** For hydration.
4. **Serial urine cultures, urinalysis, and WBC:** To monitor the infection and determine bacterial level.
5. **Sitz baths:** To relax perineal muscles and reduce risk of urinary retention.
6. **Suprapubic drainage system:** For relief of continued urinary retention.
7. **Restriction of sexual intercourse** during the acute phase.

Note: During the acute phase of bacterial infection, urethral instrumentation is contraindicated.

NURSING DIAGNOSES AND INTERVENTIONS

Pain related to dysuria secondary to the infectious process

Desired outcomes: Patient's subjective evaluation of pain improves, as documented by a pain scale. Patient relates a return to his normal voiding pattern within 2 days of treatment.

1. Assess and document the quality, location, and duration of pain. Establish a pain scale with patient (e.g., 0-10, with "0" indicating no pain).
2. Medicate patient as prescribed with analgesics for urinary burning and antispasmodics for spasms. Evaluate relief obtained, based on the pain scale.
3. Provide sitz baths or apply warm blankets or a heating pad to patient's perineum to improve circulation and relax tense muscles.
4. Teach patient the technique for slow, diaphragmatic breathing for pain control.
5. Answer patient's call light promptly.

Potential urinary retention: Anuria, dysuria, or frequency occurring with obstruction associated with prostatitis

Desired outcomes: Patient exhibits balanced I&O, urinary output of ≥30 ml/hr, and urine that is straw-colored with characteristic odor. Patient reports a return to his normal voiding pattern within 2 days of treatment.

1. Patient may have frequency or urgency with urination; record time and amount of each voiding. Be alert to the following: inability to void, no voided urine for ≥8 hours with normal intake, and voiding in small amounts (10-50 ml) at frequent intervals. Assess the character of the urinary output, which should be straw colored with a characteristic urine odor.
2. Assess the patient's abdomen and note any indicators of retention, such as distention, tenderness, or discomfort. Percuss the abdomen for evidence of "kettle-drum" sound.

Because retention can occur secondary to edematous prostatic tissue, notify MD if patient has any of the above indicators of retention, has not voided in >6 hours, or has increased dysuria unrelieved by medication.

3. If retention persists, it may be necessary to prepare patient for percutaneous insertion of a suprapubic catheter by his MD.

Potential sensory/perceptual alterations related to mentation changes secondary to decreased oxygenation in the brain occurring with the infectious process

Desired outcome: Patient verbalizes orientation to person, place, and time (within normal parameters for patient) and repeats instructions given him by health care personnel.

1. Assess patient's mental status on admission and document in behavioral terms. Ask questions that require more than "yes" or "no" answers, that demonstrate patient's ability to remember instructions, and that test orientation to person, place, and time.
2. Obtain baseline information regarding patient's mental status from sources familiar with patient (e.g., patient's family, friends, personnel at nursing home or residential care facilities).
3. If the patient is confused, keep urinal and other necessary items, such as the call light, within reach. Keep the siderails up and the bed in its lowest position.
4. If the patient is acutely confused, attempt to reorient him by keeping a clock and calendar at the bedside and reminding him of the date and place. Check on the patient at least q30min during the time he is acutely confused.
5. If the patient is unable to follow simple instructions or commands, arrange to have a significant other stay with patient. If sitters are unavailable, obtain a prescription for restraints if appropriate. **Caution:** Use restraints cautiously. Patients may become even more agitated with the use of restraints, particularly those used on wrists or arms.
6. If the patient has permanent or severe cognitive impairment, check on him frequently and reorient to baseline mental status as indicated. **Note:** Patients with severe cognitive impairments (e.g., Alzheimer's disease or dementia) also can experience acute confusional states (i.e., delirium) and can be returned to their baseline mental state.
7. Administer medications carefully, particularly in the older adult. Psychotropics, benzodiazapenes, narcotics, sedatives, and anticholinergic medications can cause acute confusion or increase the degree of acute confusion. Consult with pharmacist or patient's MD if in doubt.

See "Cancer of the Bladder" in Chapter 3 for **Altered pattern of urinary elimination** related to obstruction of suprapubic catheter, p. 140.

PATIENT-FAMILY TEACHING AND DISCHARGE PLANNING

Provide patient and significant others with verbal and written information for the following:
1. Medications, including drug name, purpose, dosage, schedule, precautions, and potential side effects.
2. Indicators of urinary tract infection, which necessitate medical attention: cloudy or foul-smelling urine, fever, dysuria.
3. Care of catheters if patient is discharged with them. Assess need for home health services.
4. Avoidance of methylxanthine-containing foods or such fluids as alcohol, coffee, caffeinated colas, tea, chocolate, and spices, which can cause diuresis or increase prostatic secretions.

Prostatic neoplasm

Cancer of the prostate is the most common reproductive cancer in men over age 50 and the second most commonly occurring cancer overall. Because most prostatic neoplasms develop in the posterior portion of the gland, they can be detected in the early stages of development. Therefore, rectal examinations should be a part of every man's regular health check after the age of 40. When detected early, prostatic cancer usually can be treated successfully. Unfortunately, medical treatment often is not sought until the tumor has affected the urinary pattern or caused hip or back pain, recurring cystitis, or urinary obstruction. This symptomatology indicates that metastasis has occurred, which dramatically decreases the survival rate.

ASSESSMENT

Signs and symptoms: (in the later stages of development): Dysuria, dribbling, decreased strength of stream, hesitancy, anuria, hematuria, nocturia, burning with urination, urgency, chills, fever, cloudy and foul-smelling urine, and decreased urinary output.

Physical assessment: Bladder distention; "kettle-drum" sound with percussion over distended bladder. Rectal exam may reveal a large, hard, fixed prostate with irregular nodules.

DIAGNOSTIC TESTS

1. *Urinalysis and urine culture:* To verify or rule out the presence of pus, WBCs, WBC casts, RBCs, and pH >8.0, which would signal infection.
2. *CBC:* Results may reveal presence of marked anemia in the presence of metastatic disease.
3. *BUN and creatinine:* May be elevated if renal function is compromised. **Note:** BUN values are affected by the patient's hydration status and should be evaluated accordingly. Fluid volume excess decreases the value, while fluid volume deficit increases it. In the older adult, decreased muscle mass and a decreased glomerular filtration rate may affect the values of serum creatinine. Therefore, these values must be evaluated along with those of urine creatinine clearance, other renal function studies, and the patient's age.
4. *Serum acid phosphatase:* To monitor disease progress. Values will be elevated if metastasis has occurred. Because prostate tissue is rich in this enzyme, the spread of the disease results in an increase in the amount of acid phosphatase in the blood.
5. *Serum alkaline phosphatase:* Will be elevated if metastasis has spread to the bones.
6. *Prostatic-specific antigen (PSA):* Monitored along with serum acid phosphatase in staging and following the progress of the disease.
7. *IVP/excretory urogram:* Evaluates the structure and function of the kidneys, ureters, and bladder. Other findings may include ureteral obstruction caused by metastasis to the pelvic lymph nodes or direct invasion by the tumor. (See discussion of the complications of IVP on p. 509.)
8. *Biopsy of the prostate*
   □ Transperineal/transrectal needle core biopsy: Performed under general or spinal anesthesia, the biopsy needle is inserted through the perineal skin or *via* the rectum directly into the area that contains the tumor. The sample is aspirated and sent to the lab for analysis.
   □ Transrectal fine needle aspiration: Performed with a local anesthetic, the biopsy needle is passed into the tumor through the rectum. The sample is aspirated and transferred to slides and sent to the lab for analysis.
9. *Transrectal ultrasonography:* To assess the size and shape of the prostate, including tumor growth. This test is especially useful in recognizing and localizing intracapsular prostatic tumors and in monitoring response of the tumor to therapy.

Note: All urine specimens should be sent to the laboratory immediately after they are obtained, or refrigerated if this is not possible (specimens for culture are *not* refrigerated). Urine left at room temperature has a greater potential for bacterial growth, turbidity, and alkalinity, any of which can distort the test results.

MEDICAL MANAGEMENT AND SURGICAL INTERVENTIONS

1. **Staging of the disease** (based on American Urologic System for Staging Prostate Cancer):
   - ☐ *Stage A:* Well differentiated, clinically occult carcinoma, focal.
   - ☐ *Stage A2:* Poorly differentiated, clinically occult carcinoma, multifocal.
   - ☐ *Stage B1:* Tumor involving less than one lobe, palpable.
   - ☐ *Stage B2:* Tumor involving more than one lobe, palpable.
   - ☐ *Stage C:* Extraprostatic extension, including seminal vesicles; symptomatology.
   - ☐ *Stage D1:* Metastases confined to pelvis, including positive pelvic nodes.
   - ☐ *Stage D2:* Distant metastases.

   The patient may exhibit clinical signs of the disease from stage B1. Symptomatology will depend on the path and extent of the tumor, although the patient with D level staging may present with urinary difficulty or back or bone pain only.

2. **External radiation therapy:** Performed both for curative and palliative therapy, depending on the stage of the neoplasm. Treatment occurs over a 6-week period, and patients can expect to remain sexually potent after treatment. This therapy also is used to shrink the tumor, thereby relieving obstruction in the urinary tract.

3. **Interstitial irradiation of the prostate:** Uses gold, chromium, or iodine implantation to destroy the prostate tumor at its origin. It will not, however, affect other areas if metastasis has occurred.

4. **Estrogen therapy:** Might be initiated to reduce plasma testosterone levels, since it is believed that testosterone is involved in the development of prostate cancer. Typically, diethylstilbestrol (DES) is given daily. Estrogen therapy causes 100% impotence during treatment. **Note:** Because DES can cause fluid retention, it must be given cautiously to patients with a history of cardiac disease or renal problems. Estramustine phosphate, a combination of estradiol and nitrogen mustard, might be used if estrogen therapy is ineffective. This drug does not cause impotence and its side effects are few, although patients tend to experience anorexia and nausea.

5. **Chemotherapy:** Might be used either as a curative or palliative measure.

6. **Surgical procedures** might include the following:
   - ☐ *Prostatectomy (transurethral resection of the prostate, TURP):* Prostatic tissue is scraped away *via* cystoscopy. This technique is used when the tumor is in a beginning stage and is well differentiated. For additional information, see "Benign Prostatic Hypertrophy," p. 509.
   - ☐ *Radical prostatectomy* with or without pelvic node dissection: Using either the perineal or retropubic approach, the entire prostate gland is removed along with the seminal vesicles and a portion of the bladder neck. This procedure is done for tumors that are large or not well differentiated. Erectile impotence occurs in 85%-90% of males having this procedure. However, this side effect can be avoided if periprostatic autonomic nerves are spared. Urinary incontinence also occurs in the majority of patients after removal of the indwelling catheter. In a prostatic cancer, all of the prostate and its capsule are removed (as opposed to the TURP, in which the apex of the prostate and its capsule remain). As a result, the following can occur to cause incontinence: 1) the external sphincter can be damaged because of surgical trauma to the bladder neck and prostate capsule, or 2) portions of the bladder neck are removed as are portions of the urethra in an effort to remove all of the cancer. This damage may take up to 6 months to heal, and the incontinence subsides 6 months after surgery in 85%-90% of this patient population.
   - ☐ *Bilateral orchiectomy:* Although rarely done, it may be implemented along with estrogen therapy to depress testosterone production.

NURSING DIAGNOSES AND INTERVENTIONS

Potential sexual dysfunction related to impotence (risk is 85%-90%) secondary to radical prostatectomy

Desired outcome: Patient verbalizes feelings about sexuality within 3 days following surgery.

1. Assess the patient's readiness to discuss his sexual concerns. Encourage verbalization, and as indicated, use facilitative communication techniques, such as open-ended questions, reflective statements, and rephrasing of patient's statements for clarification.
2. Be alert to signs of grief, such as hostility, depression, and demanding behavior, and to signs of denial, such as inappropriate affect or accepting the diagnosis too well.
3. As appropriate, arrange for care givers who have established rapport with the patient to spend time with him and encourage verbalization of his concerns.
4. Be alert to the needs of the patient and significant other for more information regarding sexual functioning.
5. As indicated, inform MD of the patient's need for more information so that counseling can be reinforced.
6. Confer with MD and social services to identify appropriate referrals for counseling following hospital discharge.

Knowledge deficit: Side effects of estrogen therapy or bilateral orchiectomy

Desired outcome: Patient verbalizes knowledge of the extent and duration of body changes prior to hospital discharge.

1. Inform patient of side effects of estrogen therapy and orchiectomy, for example, breast enlargement, breast tenderness, loss of sexual desire, and impotence.
2. For patients on estrogen therapy, provide reassurance that side effects will disappear after therapy has been discontinued.
3. If appropriate, explain to patient that before initiating estrogen therapy, MD may prescribe radiation therapy to the areolae of the breasts to minimize painful gynecomastia. However, this will not decrease other side effects.
4. Assure the patient undergoing orchiectomy that the procedure will not affect his ability to have an erection but that he will not ejaculate.

Potential stress incontinence related to loss of small (≤50 ml) amounts of urine secondary to temporary loss of muscle tone in the urethral sphincter following prostatectomy

Desired outcome: Patient relates understanding of the cause of the temporary incontinence and returns to a normal voiding pattern after 6 months.

1. Explain to patient that there is a potential for urinary incontinence after prostatectomy, but that it should resolve within 6 months. Describe the reason for the incontinence, using such aids as anatomic illustrations.
2. Encourage patient to maintain an adequate fluid intake of at least 2-3 L/day (unless this is contraindicated by an underlying cardiac dysfunction or other disorder). Explain that a dilute urine is less irritating to the prostatic fossa.
3. Instruct patient to avoid fluids that irritate the bladder, such as caffeine-containing drinks. Explain that caffeine has a mild diuresis effect, which would make bladder control even more difficult.
4. Establish a bladder routine with patient prior to hospital discharge (see "Urinary Incontinence," p. 142).
5. Teach patient pubococcygeal (Kegel) exercises to enhance spincter control (see "Urinary Incontinence," p. 144).
6. Remind patient to discuss any problems with incontinence with his MD during follow-up examinations.

See "Benign Prostatic Hypertrophy" for **Potential for infection,** p. 510, **Potential fluid volume deficit** (abnormal blood loss), p. 511, and **Potential impairment of skin integrity,** p. 512. See "Prostatitis" for **Pain,** p. 515. See "Benign Prostatic Hypertrophy" for **Urge incontinence,** p. 513. See the appendix for nursing diagnoses and interventions for the care of preoperative and postoperative patients, p. 637, and patients with cancer and other life-disrupting illnesses, p. 659.

PATIENT-FAMILY TEACHING AND DISCHARGE PLANNING

Provide patient and significant others with verbal and written information for the following:

1. For patients with radical prostatectomy, a referral to a counselor or counseling agency as necessary, and discussion about incontinence following removal of indwelling catheter.
2. See same section in "Benign Prostatic Hypertrophy," p. 514, for more information.

Testicular neoplasm

Cancer of the testes is most often found in men in their 20s and 30s. Usually it is discovered by accident, often after a traumatic injury to the groin for which professional examination is warranted. Self-examination is the best method of early detection of this disorder. It is believed that men with an undescended testicle are at higher risk than the general male population. Individuals who have had surgery at an early age to correct this condition have a higher than normal chance of developing the cancer. However, these men are better able to check for lumps and thickenings in the testis after it has been surgically descended.

The most common testicular tumors are seminomas, which spread slowly through the lymphatic system to the iliac and periaortic nodes. Embryonal tumors, on the other hand, metastasize quickly. Other tumor types include teratocarcinoma, adult teratoma, choriocarcinoma, and Leydig cell. Most testicular cancers are combinations of two forms of cancer, which can make treatment difficult. However, with treatment, prognosis for all forms of this cancer is good.

ASSESSMENT

Signs and symptoms: Lump the size of a pea or thickening of the testis. There may be an aching or heaviness in the testis caused by swelling of the scrotum owing to an accumulation of fluid or blood. Pain usually is not a symptom. In the later stages of the disease, the patient may experience abdominal pain caused by bowel or ureteral obstruction, coughing caused by metastasis to the lungs, weight loss, or anorexia. Breast enlargement may occur because of reduction in testosterone.

Physical assessment: Palpation of symmetrical, firm scrotal mass; presence of supraclavicular or abdominal mass caused by enlargement of lymph nodes in those areas.

DIAGNOSTIC TESTS

1. *Hct/hgb:* Drawn preoperatively to assess for the presence of anemia, which can occur because of metastasis.
2. *Serum liver function tests (ALT/SGPT, LDH, GGTP):* To assess adequacy of liver function for patients needing chemotherapy and for presence of abnormalities, which is indicative of metastasis. Alanine aminotransferase (ALT), known formerly as serum glutamic pyruvic transaminase (SGPT), detects hepatocellular obstruction or liver damage. Lactic dehydrogenase (LDH) becomes elevated with liver disease or malignant tumors. Serum gamma-glutamyl transpeptidase (GGTP) also rises in the presence of liver damage or disease.
3. *Serum renal function tests (creatinine and electrolytes, such as sodium and potassium):* Help determine adequacy of renal function for the patient needing chemotherapy; abnormalities may signal ureteral obstruction.
4. *Serum alpha-fetoprotein (AFP):* Used as a tumor marker and identification of the type of carcinoma. AFP never is elevated in a seminoma, but it will be with nonseminomas. Response to treatment and assessment for recurrence can be evaluated, based on comparison to the baseline value of this test.
5. *Human chorionic gonadotropin (HCG) levels:* Used as a tumor marker and for iden-

tification of the type of carcinoma. Normally, HCG is found in the maternal circulation during pregnancy and is an abnormal finding in the male. However, it is found with most testicular cancers. As with AFP, response to treatment and assessment for recurrence can be evaluated based on comparison to the baseline value of this test.

6. *Chest x-ray:* May show presence of metastasis to the lungs.
7. *IVP/excretory urogram:* May show displacement of the kidney or ureters by masses of carcinomatous lumbar nodes, which cause ureteral stenosis.
8. *Lymphangiograms:* May reveal enlarged iliac and periaortic lymph nodes if disease has spread. In this procedure, contrast medium is injected into the dorsal aspects of the feet to outline the lymphatic vessels. The contrast medium will discolor the patient's urine and stool for 24-48 hours after the procedure. The injection of this substance might be uncomfortable, and the injection site will be tender for a few days.

Note: Two complications of IVP and lymphangiogram are allergic reactions to the dye and contrast-medium-induced acute renal failure. Exposure to contrast medium may worsen existing renal or cardiac insufficiency, especially in the elderly, dehydrated, or diabetic patient. Before the study, query the patient about allergies to shellfish and iodine and reactions to previous dye studies. After the test, monitor patient for indicators of renal failure.

MEDICAL MANAGEMENT AND SURGICAL INTERVENTIONS

1. Radiation therapy: Most commonly used for patients with seminomas, the use of this therapy varies with the type and stage of the cancer. In the absence of metastasis, lymph nodes often are irradiated to prevent microscopic spread of the seminoma. Low dose radiation is used to minimize complications.
2. Chemotherapy: Used if cancer has spread outside of the testicle or retroperitoneal lymph nodes. It is used for radioresistant tumors (choriocarcinoma) with or without surgery. Most types of testicular carcinomas appear to be sensitive to chemotherapy, particularly to cisplatin, vinblastine sulfate, actinomycin D, and bleomycin.
3. Serial AFP and HCG levels: Drawn routinely over a 2-year period. Levels drop toward normal if the neoplasm has been eradicated, and rise if it has not.
4. Staging of the disease: Necessary for guiding treatment and evaluating the prognosis. The following parameters are used, based on the Boden and Gibbs staging system.
   □ *Stage A:* Tumor confined to testis with no clinical or radiologic evidence that it has spread.
   □ *Stage B:* Clinical or radiologic evidence that tumor has spread to lymph nodes distal to the diaphragm. Subcategories B_1, B_2, and B_3 also are used.
   □ *Stage C:* Clinical or radiologic evidence that tumor has spread to lymph nodes superior to the diaphragm (mediastinal and supraclavicular nodes) or beyond the lymphatic system into the viscera.
5. Biopsy: To confirm the presence of malignancy. In the absence of malignancy, the abnormal benign lump is removed but the testicle is left. If the lump proves to be malignant, an orchiectomy is performed to remove the diseased testicle. A small incision is made at the inguinal area on the affected side rather than in the scrotum itself. This permits high ligation of the cord at the inguinal ring to allow for removal of the whole testis, which other approaches do not allow. The patient may return from surgery with an indwelling catheter and incisional drain for removal of excess exudate.
6. Retroperitoneal lymph node dissection or lymphadenectomy: Patients with seminomas undergo a lymphadenectomy only if the disease has spread beyond the scrotal sac and does not respond to irradiation. Patients with nonseminomatous tumors receive lymphadenectomy as part of a treatment regimen that includes orchiectomy, radiotherapy, and chemotherapy. It is performed at the time of the orchiectomy or a few days later. Lymph nodes are removed from the kidney to the inguinal area on the affected side.

NURSING DIAGNOSES AND INTERVENTIONS

Body image disturbance related to actual and perceived changes in sexual functioning secondary to impending orchiectomy

Desired outcome: Patient verbalizes feelings and frustrations regarding the orchiectomy and relates knowledge of realistic rather than perceived changes that will occur.

1. Provide a calm, unhurried atmosphere for the patient and significant others. Use facilitative communication techniques, such as open-ended questions, reflective statements, and rephrasing of patient's statements for clarification.
2. Encourage communication between patient and significant others.
3. Encourage patient to verbalize feelings, fears, and frustrations regarding sexual attractiveness, feared impotence, and infertility. Explain that the *surgery* will not impair fertility or potency; however, his fertility may be compromised during radiation or chemotherapy, and it can last for 2 years.
4. For patient undergoing lymphadenectomy, explain that ejaculatory failure may occur if the sympathetic nerve is damaged but that he will be able to have an erection. Explain that if ejaculatory failure does occur, artificial insemination is a possibility because the semen flows back into the urine, from which it can be extracted, enabling the ovum to become impregnated artificially.
5. If appropriate, explain that a silicone prosthesis may be placed in the scrotum to achieve a normal appearance. Consult with MD regarding the potential for this procedure.
6. For patient undergoing radiation or chemotherapy, explain that he can store sperm in a sperm bank. However, the rate of pregnancy is only 50% by this method because some sperm do not survive the freezing process.

Pain related to scrotal swelling secondary to orchiectomy or lymphadenectomy

Desired outcome: Patient's subjective evaluation of pain improves, as documented by a pain scale.

1. Assess and document the quality, duration, and location of the pain. Ask the patient to rate the pain on a scale of 0-10, with "0" denoting no pain.
2. Administer prescribed analgesics as indicated. Note and document the patient's response, using the pain scale to evaluate the improvement.
3. Adjust the scrotal support as needed to enhance patient comfort. The scrotal support elevates and supports the scrotum to minimize the amount of edema.
4. Apply ice gloves or packs to the scrotum to reduce swelling.
5. Encourage patient to ambulate as soon as he is able. Explain that exercise improves circulation, which reduces swelling and pain.

Potential fluid volume deficit related to risk of abnormal blood loss secondary to the surgical procedure

Desired outcome: Patient remains normovolemic as evidenced by BP ≥90/60 mm Hg (or within patient's normal range), HR ≤90 bpm (or within patient's normal range), balanced I&O, RR ≤20 breaths/min, and warm and dry skin.

1. Monitor the patient's VS q15min for 30 min upon return from the recovery room. Once stable, check q30min for 1 hour and then q4h for 24 hours (or according to hospital protocol).
2. Be alert to increasing pulse rate, decreasing BP, diaphoresis, pallor, and increasing respiratory rate, which signal hemorrhage and impending shock.
3. Monitor I&O. In nonrestricted patients, ensure a fluid intake of at least 2-3 L/day. Immediately after surgery, fluids are IV and then advanced to oral.
4. Measure and document urine, NG, and drainage apparatus output; record output amounts separately. Optimally, drainage amounts will decrease gradually and then cease.
5. Check the dressing at frequent intervals after surgery, and change it when it becomes damp. Document color and amount of drainage. Notify MD if drainage is heavy (sat-

urates dressings within 1 hour after changing), becomes bright red, or forms clots on the dressings, any of which can occur with arterial or venous bleeding.

See the appendix for nursing diagnoses and interventions for the care of preoperative and postoperative patients, p. 637, and patients with cancer and other life-disrupting illnesses, p. 659.

PATIENT-FAMILY TEACHING AND DISCHARGE PLANNING

Provide patient and significant others with verbal and written information for the following:

1. Medications, including drug name, purpose, dosage, schedule, precautions, and potential side effects.
2. Care of incision, including cleansing and dressing changes. Advise patient to be alert to signals of infection, such as fever, persistent redness, swelling, pain, warmth or puffiness along incision, and purulent drainage.
3. Care of drains or catheters if patient is discharged with them.
4. Review of postoperative activity restrictions as directed by MD, such as no heavy lifting (>5 lb), driving, or sexual intercourse for 4-6 weeks.
5. Necessity of continued care, such as radiation therapy, chemotherapy, serial lab work; confirm date and time of next appointment if known.
6. Importance of self-examination of remaining testicle, since it is possible to get unrelated cancer in the remaining testis.

Penile implants

Erectile dysfunction is the inability to achieve or maintain an erection and is one type of problem involved in male sexual dysfunction. The causes of this type of impotence either are physiologic or psychologic. Physiologic factors include neurogenic, hormonal, or arteriovenous disorders, such as radical pelvic surgery, lower motor neuron interruption, diabetes mellitus, Cushing's syndrome, atherosclerosis, and severe arterial disease. Medication, recreational drugs, or alcohol use also can affect the male's ability to achieve or maintain an erection.

Before surgery the patient must meet the following criteria:

☐ *Have desire for sexual intercourse, including penetration.*

☐ *Have penile sensation:* The presence of these two factors increases the potential for gratification after an implant.

☐ *Lack any prostatic or urinary tract problems:* After implantation, endoscopic or transurethral procedures are difficult to perform.

IMPLANTATION PROCEDURES

1. Insertion of rigid or semirigid penile implants: Silicone rods are placed into the corpora cavernosa through an incision at the base of the dorsal surface of the penis. With this procedure the penis stays semirigid but will not be noticeable under clothing or interfere with ADL.
2. Insertion of inflatable penile implant: Two silicone tubes are placed into the corpora cavernosa *via* a suprapubic incision. A reservoir containing a radiopaque fluid is sutured into the abdominal fascia and a bulb is inserted into one scrotal sac. To initiate an erection the man or his partner must squeeze the scrotal bulb, which fills the rods with radiopaque fluid from the reservoir. Compression of the release bulb, which is located in the lower part of the scrotal sac, allows the erection to subside.

NURSING DIAGNOSES AND INTERVENTIONS

Pain related to surgical procedure

Desired outcome: Patient's subjective evaluation of pain improves, as documented by a pain scale.

1. Assess and document quality, location, and duration of pain, using a pain scale ranging from 0-10 ("0" denotes no pain). Immediately after surgery, the pain can be severe and can last for as long as a week. Mild pain might be present for several weeks after that. Medicate the patient with analgesics or narcotics as prescribed and evaluate the relief obtained, based on the pain scale.
2. Apply ice packs or gloves to the area to reduce swelling; but closely monitor patient's reaction as the weight of the ice might increase discomfort.
3. Assist patient with slow, diaphragmatic breathing and other nonpharmacologic pain control methods, such as guided imagery, distraction, relaxation tapes, and backrubs.
4. Medicate the patient about one-half hour before major moves, such as ambulation and when MD first inflates the implant, which is done a few days after surgery and repeated several times a day for about a week.
5. Use a bedcradle or hoop to prevent discomfort caused by weight of bed linens.

Body image disturbance related to presence of the penile implant

Desired outcomes: Patient expresses his feelings regarding the presence of the implant and exhibits a reduction in self-consciousness by participating in care activities that involve the implant. Patient with semirigid implant verbalizes measures for disguising its appearance.

1. Encourage the patient to discuss his feelings, fears, and frustrations regarding the implant.
2. Recognize that impotence threatens a man's self-concept, regardless of the reason for the impotence.
3. Provide a calm and accepting environment by discussing the procedure with patient openly and objectively. Reassure him that this surgery is not unusual or bizarre.
4. Promote acceptance of the implant by encouraging the patient to look at it and assist with dressing changes or other appropriate measures.
5. For patients with semirigid implants, explain that wearing jockey briefs rather than boxer or bikini briefs will better disguise the appearance of the penis.
6. If the patient feels self-conscious with his appearance in street clothes, encourage him to wear loose fitting trousers until he finds clothing that better suits him.
7. Assure patient that he will be able to participate in any sport he chooses and that work will not be affected by the prosthesis.

See the appendix for nursing diagnoses and interventions for the care of preoperative and postoperative patients, p. 637.

PATIENT-FAMILY TEACHING AND DISCHARGE PLANNING

Provide patient and significant other with verbal and written information for the following:
1. Medications, including drug name, purpose, dosage, schedule, precautions, and potential side effects.
2. Infection indicators, which necessitate medical attention: cloudy or foul-smelling urine, fever, and increased pain or swelling in scrotum or penis.
3. Care of incision, including cleansing and dressings. Teach patient to be alert to signals of local infection: persistent redness, pain, fever, increased warmth along incision line, and puffiness.
4. Activity restrictions established by MD, such as limiting sitting for long periods of time, heavy lifting (>5 lb), and strenuous exercise. Sexual activity can be resumed when all pain and edema have subsided, usually after 4-8 weeks.
5. Technique for operating inflatable device.

SELECTED REFERENCES

American Cancer Society: 1988 cancer facts and figures, New York, 1988, American Cancer Society.

Anderson B: Diagnosis of endometrial cancer, Clin Obstet Gynecol 13(4):739-750, 1986.

Azar I: The transurethral prostatectomy syndrome, Curr Rev Post-Anesthesia Care Nurse 9(9):71-76, 1987.

Blackmore C: The impact of orchidectomy upon the sexuality of the man with testicular cancer, Cancer Nurs 11(1):33-40, 1988.

Chodak G et al: Detecting prostate cancer early, Patient Care 21, 69-73, 1987.

Collins K and Hackler R: Complications of penile prostheses in the spinal cord injury population, J Urol 140(5):984-985, 1988.

Crawford E: Diagnosis and treatment of prostatitis, Hospital Practice 20(9):77-80, 1985.

Crow R et al: Indwelling catheterization and related nursing practice, J Adv Nurs 13(4):489-495, 1988.

Danforth D and Scott J: Obstretics and gynecology, ed 5, Philadelphia, 1986, JB Lippincott Co.

Dodd MJ: Patterns of self care in patients with breast cancer, Western J Nurs Res 10(1):7-24, 1988.

Ehlke G: Symptom distress in breast cancer patients receiving chemotherapy in the outpatient setting, Oncol Nurs Forum, 15(3):343-346, 1988.

Eliopoulos C: A guide to the nursing of the aging, Baltimore, 1987, Williams & Wilkins.

Ellerhorst-Ryan JM et al: Evaluating benign breast disease, Nurs Pract 13(9):13-28, 1988.

Friedman EA et al: Gynecological decision making, ed 2, Philadelphia, 1988, BC Decker, Inc.

Gardner C and Webster B: Endometriosis, JOGNN 14(6):10s-20s, 1985.

Haagensen CD: Diseases of the breast, Philadelphia, 1986, WB Saunders Co.

Harrison B: Testicular neoplasms: an overview, J Urol Nurs 7(1):321-328, 1988.

Hassey KM: Pregnancy and parenthood after treatment for breast cancer, Oncol Nurs Forum 15(4):439-443, 1988.

Heinrich-Rynning T: Prostatic cancer treatments and their effects on sexual functioning, Oncol Nurs Forum 14(6):37-41, 1987.

Jensen MD, Bobak IM, and Zalar MK: Maternity and gynecologic care: the nurse and the family, ed 4, St Louis, 1988, The CV Mosby Co.

Kaye K: Impotence: a current understanding and approach, J Enterostomal Ther 14(3):117-124, 1987.

Lederer J et al: Care planning pocket guide: a nursing diagnosis approach, ed 2, Redwood City, Calif, 1988, Addison-Wesley Publishing Co.

Loughlin K and Whitmore W: Managing prostate disorders in middle age and beyond, Geriatrics 42(7):45-56, 1987.

Lowthian P: Beating the blockage, Nurs Times 84(11):63-65, 1988.

Matteson M and McConnell E: Gerontological nursing: concepts and practice, Philadelphia, 1988, WB Saunders Co.

Norhouse LL: Social support in patients' and husbands' adjustment to breast cancer, Nurs Res 37(2):91-95, 1988.

Pagana K and Pagana T: Pocket nurse guide to laboratory and diagnostic tests, St Louis, 1986, The CV Mosby Co.

Sauer M et al: Nonsurgical management of unruptured ectopic pregnancy: an extended clinical trial, Fertil Steril 48(5):752-755, 1987.

Seff SE and Wardell DW: Surgical approaches to female reproductive system dysfunction. In Kneisl CR and Ames SW: Adult health nursing: a biopsychosocial approach, Menlo Park, Calif, 1986, Addison-Wesley Publishing Co.

Wardell DW: Specific disorder of the female reproductive system. In Kneisl CR and Ames SW: Adult health nursing: a biopsychosocial approach, Menlo Park, Calif, 1986, Addison-Wesley Publishing Co.

Wellisch SK et al: The psychologic contribution of nipple addition in breast reconstruction, Plast Reconstr Surg 80(5):699-703.

10
CHAPTER

Sensory disorders

Section One DISORDERS AND SURGERIES OF THE EYE

Corneal ulceration/trauma

Corneal ulceration is a serious ocular disease that causes a "melting away" of the corneal tissue, which occasionally leads to perforation. Potential causes include chemical burns and prolonged exposure to the air in a nonblinking individual (e.g., one who is comatose or has Bell's palsy), but more often it is caused by bacteria, herpesvirus, and in rarer instances, fungal disease. Corneal ulceration almost always results in scarring (opacity) and the development of an irregular surface, which, regardless of the cause, contributes to a decrease in visual acuity.

Corneal trauma is most commonly caused by the following:

1. *Foreign body:* Metallic or nonmetallic objects can become stuck to the corneal surface or become imbedded in the cornea. Small metallic foreign bodies that have great velocity (e.g., hammering nails, steel) can pass through the cornea with little trace in an individual who is not wearing safety glasses. Damage to the lens or anterior segment also may occur. Unless detected promptly by ultrasound or x-ray, the eye can become damaged from the release of ions. Copper foreign bodies, for example, are especially dangerous.
2. *Chemical burns:* Those resulting from industrial accidents are very dangerous since

527

alkali deeply penetrates the tissue, and they often occur bilaterally. Initial indicators can be greatly underestimated at the time of the accident. Inflammatory ulceration with scarring ensue over months, causing decreased vision. Keratoplasty usually is unsuccessful.

3. *Laceration:* This can occur from shattered eyeglasses, for example. Damage to the lens and other parts of the eye is common. Scleral lacerations may be hidden by a subconjunctival hemorrhage. Surgical repair may be necessary.

4. *Contact lens overwear:* An individual whose soft contact lenses are tight-fitting or one who gradually develops a corneal hypersensitivity reaction can develop corneal trauma. For individuals who use extended wear (overnight use) lenses, infection is not an uncommon occurrence.

ASSESSMENT

Signs and symptoms: Presence of a "red" eye for one or more days, progressive decrease in visual acuity. Pain, both a scratchy "surface" discomfort and a more deep, boring pain, especially with blinking, may be present. There may be increased tearing and photophobia.

Physical assessment: Swollen lid, half shut eye, tearing, and discharge that is occasionally purulent. The inflamed conjunctiva with dilated vessels causes the eye to be red. Slit lamp assessment may reveal a small or large infiltrate, often of yellowish-white and fluffy contour, which is suggestive of bacteria. In other cases, the areas within the defect may be grey, which occurs with necrosis. In advanced cases, all the membrane may be melted away in a small area, enabling the clear Descemet's membrane to bulge out. The barrier can rupture and perforate, with a gush of fluid and sudden sharp pain.

DIAGNOSTIC TESTS

1. *Fluoroscein (filter paper or 2% drop):* Identifies defect in the epithelium by defusing into the corneal stroma and staining it bright green. The findings may be enhanced by using a blue light, called cobalt filter.

2. *Rose Bengal (filter paper or 1% drop):* Identifies devitalized cells at the border of the defect by staining them red.

3. *Corneal scrapings, Gram stain, and immediate microscopic exam:* To identify bacterial or fungal ulceration.

4. *Conjunctival culture:* To identify causative organism, if present.

Note: Prompt culturing and administration of antibiotics are extremely important in the presence of bacterial infection. An hour's delay can make a great difference. Topical antibiotics must be started immediately after cultures are obtained. Any antibiotic in any concentration can be used until positive cultures and sensitivities are determined.

MEDICAL MANAGEMENT AND SURGICAL INTERVENTIONS

For corneal trauma

1. Removal of foreign body: If present.
2. Irrigation: For chemical burns. At the scene of the accident the eyes should be irrigated with any nontoxic fluid available. The individual should then proceed to the emergency room, where the eye is irrigated with normal saline until the tears become neutral, as confirmed by litmus paper.
3. Surgical repair: For laceration.
4. Removal of contact lens: For contact lens overwear.

General management

1. Pharmacotherapy
   □ *Topical and systemic antibiotics or antiviral agents:* To treat identified infection, usually after obtaining the results of corneal scrapings or cultures. Broad-spectrum

antibiotics may be given topically and intravenously until culture results are obtained, after which specific antifungals, antibacterials, or antiviral agents are used accordingly.

☐ *Topical steroids:* To treat hypersensitivity reactions.

2. **Pupil dilatation via mydriatrics:** If an increase in intraocular pressure exists.
3. **Pain management:** Warm moist compresses are used for lid swelling. Cycloplegics (atropine, scopolamine) may be used to decrease pain by dilating the pupil, thereby restricting movements of the iris and ciliary body. Systemic analgesics also may be prescribed.
4. **Cleansing and dressings:** The lid margins are cleansed frequently to remove exudate, at minimum before each administration of ophthalmic drops. A tarsorrhaphy (taping or suturing the eyelids shut) is done in nonblinking individuals to provide a moist eye chamber. The patient also will wear a metal shield, especially for impending perforation. In noninfectious conditions, the patient may wear a soft contact lens as a dressing. In the presence of infection, dressings are not used because they can promote bacterial growth. Loose, dry dressings are used for clean abrasions or erosions.
5. **Corneal transplant:** Considered only after medical management has failed and scarring or perforation has occurred. See p. 531.

NURSING DIAGNOSES AND INTERVENTIONS

Knowledge deficit Diagnosis and treatment plan

Desired outcome: Patient verbalizes understanding of the diagnosis and treatment plan.

1. Assess patient's knowledge of the diagnosis and treatment plan, and clarify or provide explanations as necessary.
2. Encourage questions and provide time for patient to ask questions and express fears and anxieties.
3. Explain that the eyes may be patched, taped, or sutured shut as part of the treatment for the corneal diagnosis.
4. Instruct patient not to touch, rub, or squeeze the affected eye(s), which can spread infection and cause further trauma.

Sensory/perceptual alterations related to visual deficit secondary to disease process or presence of eye shield, eye patch, or other measure that distorts or diminishes vision

Desired outcome: Patient verbalizes orientation to person, place, and time and relates the attainment of adequate amounts of sensory stimulation.

1. Orient patient to surroundings.
2. Request that all individuals entering the room identify themselves, state their purpose for being there, and inform patient when they are leaving.
3. Avoid touching patient without first announcing your intent.
4. Encourage patient to listen to radio or television, which will provide sensory stimulation and help prevent boredom.
5. Place all necessary articles within patient's reach. Encourage patient to utilize sense of touch to familiarize self with new objects and their placement.
6. The degree of assistance with meals will depend on the patient's visual deficit. Set up the food tray and orient patient to the food placement (e.g., "The meat is at 12:00.") and temperature.
7. Depth perception is altered with an eye patch and shield. Teach patient to position fingers just inside the rim of glass while filling to avoid overfilling.
8. Do not move furniture without alerting patient.

Potential for infection related to increased susceptibility secondary to surgical procedure

Desired outcome: Patient is free of infection as evidenced by absence of erythema, swelling, purulent discharge, and persistent pain in the affected eye.

1. Change loose dressings and reapply as needed. Often, the MD will change the first dressing postoperatively. After the MD has removed the initial bandage, inspect the

eye for signs of infection, including erythema, swelling, or purulent discharge. Teach patient to alert the staff to the presence of persistent pain.

2. Wash your hands well, and use clean technique for eye care and instillation of ointment or drops.

3. Assist patient with maintaining a dry operative site; help with hygiene activities as needed, depending on patient's visual deficit.

4. Remind patient not to touch or rub the operative eye.

5. For confused patients, request arm restraints to prevent handling of the eye dressing and rubbing of the operative eye.

Note: If contact lenses are prescribed, use aseptic technique for lens insertion. Teach patient or significant other the technique.

Self-care deficit: Inability to perform ADL related to imposed activity restrictions and visual deficit

Desired outcomes: Patient avoids ADL that may be a safety hazard or can cause increased intraocular pressure and resumes independence with ADL as soon as these activities are permitted. Until patient can resume ADL independently, staff or significant others perform these activities for the patient.

1. Review with the patient the activities that are permitted and those that are not. Some ocular conditions necessitate restriction of shaving, shampooing, hair combing, and vigorous tooth brushing. Most ocular conditions, however, restrict only vigorous activity.

2. Assemble patient's toilet articles at the bedside or in the bathroom, and encourage safety and independence within the limits specified by MD.

3. Continue to perform activities for patient that require stooping and bending, such as putting on shoes and socks and washing feet.

Knowledge deficit: Importance of avoiding increased intraocular pressure and activities that can cause it

Desired outcome: Patient verbalizes knowledge of the importance of avoiding increased intraocular pressure and activities that can cause it.

1. Explain that increased intraocular pressure can cause disruption of the operative site, and caution patient about the following:
   □ Avoid straining with bowel movements; request laxative/stool softeners as needed.
   □ Notify staff when nauseated so that antiemetics can be given.
   □ When coughing and sneezing, do so with mouth and eyes open to minimize intraocular pressure.
   □ Avoid heavy lifting, bending, or vigorous activity until approved by MD.

2. Teach patient the importance of maintaining the prescribed position.

3. Instruct patient to notify staff immediately if persistent or sudden, severe pain occurs in the operative eye, as this can signal increased ocular pressure.

Pain related to corneal ulceration/trauma

Desired outcome: Patient's subjective evaluation of pain improves, as documented by a pain scale.

Note: The intensity and duration of the pain essentially is related to the degree of inflammation.

---

1. Monitor patient for presence of pain. Develop a pain scale with the patient, rating pain from 0 (no pain) to 10. Medicate with prescribed medications as indicated and document pain relief obtained, again using the pain scale.

2. Explain that decreasing eye movements will help minimize pain.

3. If prescribed, apply warm, moist compresses to the eyes.

4. Reading can increase pain; encourage use of alternatives, such as talking books, radio, or television, to divert attention away from pain.

5. Instruct patient to inform staff of increased or sudden severe eye pain and gush of fluid, which can signal that perforation has occurred.

Note: In the presence of acute perforation, place a dry sterile dressing lightly over affected eye, have patient get into bed, and notify MD immediately.

Potential for noncompliance related to frustration secondary to frequency of antibiotic administration and lack of knowledge of its importance

Desired outcomes: Patient verbalizes understanding of the importance of frequent antibiotic administration and adheres to the treatment plan. If indicated, patient or significant other returns demonstration of clean technique for administration of the medication.

1. Stress the importance and rationale for the medication, which usually is administered qh.
2. Teach patient or significant other the technique for instillation of eye drops or ointment if the medication is to be continued after hospital discharge.
3. Teach and stress the importance of good handwashing before instillation of the medication.
4. If indicated, teach patient and significant other the signs and symptoms of continuing infection: persistent redness, swelling, purulent drainage, decreased visual acuity, increased pain, fever, and indicators of perforation.

Sleep pattern disturbance related to frequent antibiotic and steroid administrations

Desired outcome: Patient rests undisturbed for 60- to 90-minute intervals, if not contraindicated by ophthalmic medication administration, and expresses satisfaction with the amount of rest and sleep obtained between care activities.

1. Plan all nursing care activities so that they can be performed at the time of medication administration.
2. Provide a quiet environment for the patient to promote rest.
3. Evaluate treatment regimen with MD on a daily basis to determine if medications can be administered less frequently.

PATIENT-FAMILY TEACHING AND DISCHARGE PLANNING

Provide patient and significant others with verbal and written information for the following:

1. Medications, including drug name, route, purpose, dosage, schedule, precautions, potential side effects, and instructions for clean technique for topical administration. Remind patient to notify MD before running out of medications.
2. Importance of avoiding the following: use of OTC eye drugs without MD approval; rubbing, touching, or bumping the involved eye; and use of eye makeup without MD approval.
3. Reporting the following indicators of eye infection to MD: persistent redness, swelling, purulent drainage, fever, and persistent pain.
4. Importance of follow-up care; confirm date and time of next appointment if known.
5. Wearing glasses by day and shield by night for safety purposes.
6. Using dark glasses with mydriatics to minimize photophobia and prevent eye trauma.

Keratoplasty (corneal transplant)

A keratoplasty is a surgical procedure that replaces a diseased cornea with corneal tissue from a human cadaver. Surgical goals include decreasing corneal opacity, increasing corneal transparency, improving visual acuity and visual field, or providing a better cosmetic appearance. Surgical success and improved vision depend on the extent of damage, degree of corneal vascularization, state of the surface epithelium, and the tear film (eye moistening capability).

ASSESSMENT

See "Corneal Ulceration," p. 528.

MEDICAL MANAGEMENT AND SURGICAL INTERVENTIONS

1. **Preoperatively:** Antibiotic drops are administered in several doses. An osmotic agent, such as Ismotic or Osmoglyn, also may be used to soften the globe.
2. **Surgical procedure:** Performed either under general or local anesthesia. A button-sized piece of tissue is removed from the donor cornea and sutured into the recipient cornea with nonabsorbable sutures that are usually left in place for 1 year or more. Grafts are either full thickness (penetrating keratoplasty) or partial thickness (lamellar keratoplasty). Visual acuity will be slow in returning, owing to the long-standing corneal surface irregularity, and the patient may take up to 1 year to attain an acceptable level of vision.

NURSING DIAGNOSES AND INTERVENTIONS

Knowledge deficit: Diagnosis, surgery, precautionary measures, and treatment plan

Desired outcome: Patient verbalizes (and demonstrates, as appropriate) knowledge of the diagnosis, surgical procedure, precautionary measures, and treatment plan.

1. Assess patient's knowledge of the diagnosis, surgery, and treatment plan. Clarify or provide explanations as appropriate. Encourage patient to ask questions; provide time for expression of fears and anxieties.
2. Explain that the surgical eye will be patched after surgery.
3. To minimize the potential for injury or infection, instruct patient not to touch, rub, or tightly squeeze operative eye after surgery.
4. Explain that an eye shield may be worn nightly for 1 month after surgery to protect the eye. Glasses may be worn during the day for the same purpose.
5. Instruct patient or significant other in clean technique for administration of eyedrops or ointment. Stress that good handwashing is necessary to minimize the potential for infection
6. Inform patient that watching TV usually is permitted.
7. Explain that patient can have full bathroom privileges and movement when alert.

Pain related to surgical procedure

Desired outcome: Patient's subjective evaluation of pain improves, as documented by a pain scale.

Note: Moderate discomfort is anticipated for the first 24 hours. A scratchy sensation may be present for several weeks following surgery, and it is usually relieved with mild analgesics, such as acetaminophen.

1. Assess patient for pain. Devise a pain scale with the patient, rating pain on a scale of 0 (no pain) to 10. Medicate with prescribed analgesics as necessary and document pain relief obtained, using the pain scale.
2. Explain that mild discomfort is normal following surgery. Instruct patient to notify staff of increased pain or sudden severe pain, which can signal complications, such as hemorrhage or slipped graft.

See "Corneal Ulceration/Trauma" for **Sensory/perceptual alterations,** p. 529, **Potential for infection,** p. 529, **Self-care deficit,** p. 530, and **Knowledge deficit:** Importance of avoiding increased intraocular pressure and activities that can cause it, p. 530. Also see nursing diagnoses and interventions for the care of preoperative and postoperative patients, p. 637, in the appendix.

PATIENT-FAMILY TEACHING AND DISCHARGE PLANNING

Provide patient and significant others with verbal and written information for the following:

1. Medications, including route, purpose, dosage, schedule, precautions, and potential side effects.
2. Importance of avoiding rubbing, touching, or bumping the eye(s). Confer with the MD regarding limitations for the following: heavy lifting, strenuous activity, sexual activity, and sports, and review these limitations with the patient.
3. Reporting signs of infection to MD, including purulent drainage, pain, persistent redness, fever, and swelling.
4. Need for follow-up care with MD; confirm date and time for removal of sutures, if known.

Vitreous disorders/vitrectomy

The vitreous plays an important role in maintaining the form and transparency of the eye. With age, disease, or trauma it can degenerate and liquify, forming small fluid-filled cavities. As these cavities merge, the vitreous is pushed forward, causing traction on the retina. Ultimately this can lead to a collapsed or detached vitreous, retinal tears, or vitreous hemorrhage. Advancing age, diabetes mellitus, hypertension, and myopia place individuals at higher risk for vitreal degeneration. Indications for a vitrectomy include eye contusion, vitreous loss, hemorrhage, abscess, inflammation, retinal detachment with severe vitreous traction, and global rupture or penetration.

ASSESSMENT

Signs and symptoms: Complaints of floaters (spots, webs, or streaks) caused by vitreous particles, decreased vision, or flashing lights, which result from abnormal vitreous traction that stimulates the photoreceptors.

Physical assessment: Floaters seen with ophthalmoscopy. Slit-lamp observation may reveal retraction, condensation, diabetic shrinkage, or injury. Visual acuity may or may not be affected, depending on the degree of vitreous damage.

DIAGNOSTIC TEST

B-scan ultrasonography: Diagnoses posterior-segment disorders associated with gross vitreous opacification, intraocular foreign bodies, and vitreoretinal relationships.

MEDICAL MANAGEMENT AND SURGICAL INTERVENTIONS

1. Decreased activity and in some cases, bed rest.
2. Laser photocoagulation: Used in the treatment of vitreous hemorrhage when the vasculature can be visualized.
3. Vitrectomy: A small slit is made in the sclera, and a significant amount of damaged vitreous is removed and replaced with a homogenous fluid that resembles vitreous. Abnormal fibrous traction bands and preretinal membranes can be cut to relieve retinal traction. Absorbable sutures are used, and the patient may be given general anesthesia or MIVA (IV sedation with general anesthesia standby).

NURSING DIAGNOSES AND INTERVENTIONS

Knowledge deficit: Diagnosis, surgery, and treatment plan

Desired outcome: Patient verbalizes (and demonstrates, as appropriate) understanding of the diagnosis, surgery, precautions, and treatment plan.

1. Assess patient's knowledge of the diagnosis, surgical procedure, and treatment plan. Clarify and provide explanation as appropriate. Allow time for questions and expression of fears and anxieties.
2. Explain that the operative eye may be patched for several days after surgery.
3. Explain that patient may be restricted to a specified position for several days after surgery. Confirm position with MD. If patient will be restricted to a specific position for 1-3 days, demonstrate deep-breathing exercises to prevent atelectasis and other postoperative respiratory complications, and ROM exercises to the lower extremities, which will help prevent phlebitis and venous stasis.
4. Caution patient that rubbing, touching, or tightly squeezing the eye must be avoided to maintain the integrity of the dressing.
5. Determine activity limitations with the MD regarding lifting, stooping, straining, coughing, sneezing, bending, and sexual activity, and review the limitations with the patient.
6. Explain to patient that postoperative discomfort may be experienced for 24-48 hours after surgery but that analgesics will be available as needed.

See "Corneal Ulceration/Trauma" for **Sensory/perceptual alterations,** p. 529, **Potential for infection,** p. 529, **Self-care deficit,** p. 530 and **Knowledge deficit:** Importance of avoiding increased intraocular pressure and activities that can cause it, p. 530.

PATIENT-FAMILY TEACHING AND DISCHARGE PLANNING

Provide patient and significant others with verbal and written information for the following:
1. Medications, including route, drug name, purpose, dosage, schedule, precautions, and potential side effects. Stress the importance of notifying MD before the medications run out. Teach patient the importance of good handwashing before instilling ophthalmic medications.
2. Importance of reporting indicators of infection (purulent drainage, pain, persistent redness, swelling, fever) to MD.
3. Lid hygiene. Explain that to remove drainage and crust from the lid margins, the patient should moisten a cotton ball with tap water and gently sweep the cotton ball from the inner to outer aspect of the lid, using a new cotton ball with each sweeping motion. Explain that this procedure should continue for as long as the eye secretes drainage (usually 1-2 weeks).
4. Necessity of avoiding rubbing, touching, or bumping the eye. Confirm with MD which if any of the following activities will be restricted or limited and review with the patient accordingly: heavy lifting, strenuous activities, sexual activity, bending, stooping, straining, coughing.
5. Need for follow-up medical care; confirm date and time of next appointment if known.
6. Wearing dark glasses to minimize photophobia and pain when mydriatic eye drops are used.
7. Wearing glasses by day and an eye shield at night to prevent injury, usually for at least 2-4 weeks.

Glaucoma

Glaucoma is a condition in which the intraocular pressure of the aqueous humor is higher than normal, causing atrophy of the optic disk, visual field loss, death of the nerve fibers, and irreversible loss of vision. This increase in pressure within the eye can be caused by excessive aqueous humor production or obstruction in the outflow pathway, preventing aqueous drainage. Glaucoma is usually genetically associated, and it is estimated that 1%-2% of individuals over age 40 have some signs of this disease. Although glaucoma is usually bilateral, it can affect just one eye.

Note: Glaucoma leads to blindness when it is left untreated.

Primary glaucoma: Usually caused by obstruction of the trabecular meshwork. There are two types: *chronic simple glaucoma* (open-angle) and *acute or chronic congestive glaucoma* (closed/narrow-angle). Approximately 95% of individuals with glaucoma have the open-angle type.

Secondary glaucoma: Usually associated with trauma, tumors, surgery, or uveitis.

Congenital glaucoma: Includes juvenile or infantile glaucoma.

ASSESSMENT

Open-angle glaucoma: Primary open-angle glaucoma is a chronic, slowly progressing disorder that is usually asymptomatic until extensive, irreversible loss of the visual field has occurred.

Narrow-angle glaucoma: Patient complains of seeing halos or rainbows, severe and spontaneous eye pain, cloudy or blurred vision, decreased vision with or without pain in darkened environments, headaches, nausea, vomiting, and poor night vision. There is increased intraocular pressure, bloodshot eyes, and midpositioned or dilated pupils. A history of diabetes is common.

Secondary glaucoma: Patient complains of progressive blurring of vision. Typically, there is history of eye trauma, tumors, surgery, uveitis, or use of corticosteroids. Intraocular pressure is increased.

Congenital glaucoma: Rapidly developing myopia, increased intraocular pressure, decreased visual acuity, and increased corneal diameter in infants. The infantile type is usually identified from birth to age 3, while the juvenile type can develop up to age 30.

DIAGNOSTIC TESTS

1. *Tonometry:* Use of a small instrument to measure intraocular pressure or tension in the eye.
2. *Gonioscopy:* Uses a special lens with a special light and microscope to view the trabecular structures and identify width of the drainage area, adhesions, undiagnosed trauma, and tumors. It is done prior to instillation of mydriatic or cycloplegic drug. This test differentiates open-angle from narrow-angle glaucoma.
3. *Fundoscopy:* Used if it is deemed safe after gonioscopy. The pupil is dilated to inspect the optic disk as well as the shape, color, and size of the fundus. This test can identify disk degeneration.
4. *Ophthalmoscopic examination:* Identifies increased cupping of the disk.
5. *Visual field:* A map that is made of the total visual area the eye can see. It identifies blind spots and can be used as a baseline to identify subsequent degeneration. When done manually, it is conducted by a technician who presents stimuli to the patient. When automated, the stimuli are computer generated.
6. *Tonography:* Uses electronic indentation tonometer and recording device to measure how well aqueous humor flows when a known amount of pressure is placed on the eye. A flat tracing indicates a decreased rate of outflow.
7. *Darkened room test:* To differentiate between open-angle and narrow-angle glaucoma. It must be used cautiously as it can precipitate a narrow-angle attack from increased intraocular pressure and severe pain.

MEDICAL MANAGEMENT AND SURGICAL INTERVENTIONS

Medical management is the treatment of choice, and the regimen selected depends on disease etiology. Surgery is performed only when the disease progresses and medical management or laser treatment is ineffective.
1. Open-angle glaucoma: Drug therapy is the primary treatment. If pharmacotherapy is ineffective, then laser trabeculoplasty or filtering surgery (trabeculectomy) is performed to prevent further optic nerve damage and increased visual field loss.
   □ *Miotics, synthetic epinephrine, and beta blockers:* The drugs used in glaucoma therapy reduce intraocular pressure by decreasing resistance to outflow of aqueous

humor by decreasing aqueous production or by transiently reducing the volume of the intraocular fluid. These drugs are taken until they are no longer effective or side effects occur.

☐ *Trabeculectomy:* Building of a new channel for the aqueous humor.

☐ *Surgical iridectomy:* Removal of a portion of the iris *via* a small corneal incision (to improve aqueous drainage) or use of a laser, which bores a fine hole in the iris to provide an artificial channel for the aqueous humor.

2. **Narrow-angle or angle-closure glaucoma:** Laser iridotomy is the treatment of choice for primary angle-closure glaucoma. To avoid bilateral involvement, the unaffected eye also is lasered prophylactically. The following surgeries may be performed:

☐ *Iridectomy:* (See above).

☐ *Laser iridotomy:* Procedure of choice. Light energy from an argon laser allows the passage of aqueous fluid from the posterior chamber into the anterior chamber. This procedure can be performed on an outpatient basis.

☐ *Cyclocryosurgery:* Freezing of the ciliary body with a cryoprobe to reduce secretions.

☐ *Cyclodialysis:* Separation of the ciliary body from the sclera and its blood supply to decrease aqueous production.

3. **Congenital glaucoma:** Treated surgically, usually with a *trabeculectomy* (see above) because the response to pharmacotherapy is usually poor. Primary congenital glaucoma essentially is a surgical problem.

4. **Secondary glaucoma:** Causative factor is identified and eliminated. Either surgery or drug therapy is initiated, depending on the causative factor. Prognosis is often poor. Complications of surgery include retinal detachment, cataract development, hemolytic glaucoma, hemorrhage, decreased visual acuity, and light sensitivity. It must be emphasized to patients that surgery does not eliminate the need for eyedrops, and a lifetime pharmacologic regimen must be maintained.

NURSING DIAGNOSES AND INTERVENTIONS

Knowledge deficit: Diagnosis, surgery, and treatment plan

Desired outcome: Patient verbalizes (and demonstrates, as appropriate) understanding of the diagnosis, surgery, and treatment plan.

1. For primary interventions, see this nursing diagnosis in "Corneal Transplant," p. 532.

2. Explain that patient probably will be able to ambulate within 24 hours after surgery, as soon as anesthetic has worn off.

3. Explain that with laser treatment there will be minimal to no discomfort. Moderate discomfort will be present for 24 hours following surgery. Mild discomfort will be relieved with acetaminophen.

Potential for noncompliance related to frustration secondary to extensiveness of pharmacologic regimen and lack of knowledge of its importance

Desired outcomes: Patient verbalizes understanding of the importance of frequent medication instillation and the consequences of noncompliance, and demonstrates adherence to the prescribed treatment plan. Patient or significant other returns demonstration of medication administration technique.

1. Explain importance of timely administration of medications and the consequences of noncompliance: blindness can occur if the condition is left untreated.

2. Assist patient or significant other with labeling each eyedrop bottle and writing out schedules for administration. This is especially important for patients with minimal visual acuity, for whom all bottles look alike. Color or texture-coding of the bottles may be effective for some patients.

3. Demonstrate technique for administration of eyedrops or ointment. Stress importance of good handwashing to minimize the risk of infection. Have patient or significant other return the demonstration. Be sure patient or significant other is proficient in this technique before hospital discharge.

See "Corneal Ulceration/Trauma" for **Sensory/perceptual alterations,** p. 529, **Potential for infection,** p. 529, **Self-care deficit,** p. 530, and **Knowledge deficit:** Importance of avoiding increased intraocular pressure and activities that can cause it, p. 530. Also see the appendix, p. 637, for nursing diagnoses and interventions for the care of preoperative and postoperative patients.

PATIENT-FAMILY TEACHING AND DISCHARGE PLANNING

Provide patient and significant others with verbal and written information for the following:
1. Necessity of getting intraocular pressure checked at least four times a year.
2. Importance of family members over age 35 to get a complete eye exam every 2 years, including tonometry.
3. Necessity of providing extra lighting in darkened areas and need for extra caution when driving at night.
4. Importance of wearing a Medic-Alert bracelet, identifying patient's glaucoma and eye medication used.
5. Importance of notifying MD if cardiac drugs are prescribed. Systemic absorption of ophthalmic beta-blocking drugs may act synergistically to potentiate the effects of cardiac drugs.
6. See teaching and discharge planning interventions in "Vitreous Disorders and Vitrectomy," p. 534, for other information.

Retinal detachment

A detached retina is the partial or complete separation of the retina from the choroid. The retina is attached to the choroid in two places, at the optic nerve and at the ora serrata near the ciliary body. It is held in place by the gentle pressure of the vitreous body. A detachment is often spontaneous and occurs most frequently in myopia, aphakia, and eye trauma.

Retinal detachment can be categorized into two groups: rhegmatogenous and serous. *Rhegmatogenous detachments* are induced by a tear in the retina that allows fluid (usually supplied by the vitreous) to leak under the retina and separate it from the pigment epithelium. Retinal tears can be caused by trauma or the aging process. *Serous detachments* are caused by a leak in the blood vessels, causing fluid to be trapped between the pigment epithelium and the retina. Serous detachments can be seen in choroidal tumors, serous retinopathy, and inflammatory conditions.

ASSESSMENT

Signs and symptoms: Patient complains of flashing lights and floaters or visual defects, such as blurred or "sooty" vision, unilateral loss of vision, and sensation of a veil over one eye. Usually, redness and pain are not present.

Physical assessment: Visual acuity as measured by a Snellen eye chart, for example, may or may not be decreased, depending on the detachment location. Ophthalmoscopic evaluation will reveal a retina that is hanging in a vitreous-like, grey-white cloud. Crescent-shaped, red-orange tear(s) will be present, and the retina may appear to be bulging. Visual field testing may reveal a defect in the location of the detachment.

MEDICAL MANAGEMENT AND SURGICAL INTERVENTIONS

Management will range from no treatment in such conditions as serous retinopathy to major invasive surgical procedures.
1. **Presurgical regimen:** Prior to surgery the patient may be on bed rest and placed in various positions to promote reattachment. Mydriatics and cycloplegics are often used to dilate the pupil and decrease movement of the intraocular structures. Both eyes may be patched until surgery is performed to prevent eye movement, which could increase the size of detachment.

2. **Surgery:** The surgical goal is to seal the retinal holes or breaks in an attempt to prevent further breaks from occurring and to place the retina in contact with the choroid. One or more of the following procedures are used:

   □ *Photocoagulation:* A laser emits a bright light onto the pigment epithelium, causing coagulation and attachment of the retina. Peripheral tears may not be accessed *via* this therapy. Photocoagulation is used frequently in torn areas that are small or with retinal holes to prevent further detachment.

   □ *Cryotherapy:* A super-cooled metal probe is placed on the conjunctiva near the tear. Scleral inflammation occurs, leading to scar formation and reattachment in approximately 1 week.

   □ *Scleral buckling:* A band resembling a piece of belt is placed around the sclera at the area of detachment, thereby drawing the sclera closer to the retina to facilitate attachment. Many times, cryotherapy or photocoagulation is used in conjunction with this therapy to "weld" the retina to the choroid.

   □ *Diathermy:* Uses heat rather than cold and is similar to cryotherapy but not as widely used.

NURSING DIAGNOSES AND INTERVENTIONS

Knowledge deficit: Diagnosis, surgical procedure, and treatment plan

Desired outcome: Patient verbalizes (and demonstrates, as appropriate) understanding of the diagnosis, surgical procedure, and treatment plan.

1. Assess patient's knowledge of the diagnosis and surgery. Clarify or provide explanation as appropriate. Allow time for patient to ask questions and express fears and anxiety.
2. Explain that after scleral buckling the operative eye may be patched for several days.
3. Explain that mydriatic and cycloplegic drops will be instilled to dilate the pupil, expose the retina, and decrease iris movement.
4. Explain that the patient may be restricted to a specific position for several days after surgery. For example, depending on the location of the detachment, the patient may be prone.
5. To prevent increased intraocular pressure after surgery, the patient may be told not to strain with bowel movements, cough or sneeze (unless done with the mouth and eyes open), or bend. Tell patient to notify staff of constipation, persistent cough, nausea, or need for assistance.
6. Explain that to minimize excessive movements of the eye muscles, shaving, brushing teeth, washing face, and combing hair are contraindicated until approved by MD.
7. Explain to patient that the eyelid may be very swollen and require ice applications to reduce the swelling and promote comfort.
8. Explain that mydriatic drops will be used postoperatively to enable the surgeon to assess status of the retina and that antibiotic drops will be used as a prophylaxis for infection.
9. Discuss with patient that moderate discomfort can be expected during the first 24-48 hours following surgery and that it can be relieved with acetaminophen.
10. If the patient will be on bed rest, demonstrate deep-breathing exercises to help prevent postsurgical pulmonary complications and passive ROM and limb movements, which are used after surgery to help promote venous return. Have patient return the demonstrations. Coughing exercises are contraindicated because they increase intraocular pressure.

Potential for injury related to increased risk of bleeding secondary to hypervascularity of ocular tissue

Desired outcome: Patient is free of ocular bleeding.

1. Inspect the outer dressing for the presence of bleeding. Notify MD of significant findings.
2. Once the initial dressing has been removed by MD, be alert to hyphema (bleeding in the anterior chamber of the eye), which can occur because of the high vascularity of

the tissue. Teach patient to report to staff the presence of sudden severe pain, which can signal occurrence of hyphema.
3. If bleeding occurs, keep patient calm and in the prescribed position. Notify MD promptly.

Potential for impaired skin/tissue integrity related to imposed position restrictions and frequent removal of eye patch

Desired outcome: Patient's skin and tissue remain intact.

1. Because it is imperative that the patient maintain the prescribed position and avoid head and eye movements, provide skin care at frequent intervals to prevent skin and tissue breakdown. Provide special attention to skin and tissue over body prominences, such as heels, ankles, elbows, sacrum, and greater tuberosities.
2. Use a mattress that minimizes tissue pressure, such as an egg crate, Clinitron, or low air loss bed.
3. Frequent eye patch removal can cause skin irritation. Keep the skin under the tape dry to prevent maceration.

See "Corneal Ulceration/Trauma" for **Sensory/perceptual alterations,** p. 529, **Potential for infection,** p. 529, **Self-care deficit,** p. 530, and **Knowledge deficit:** Importance of avoiding increased intraocular pressure and activities that can cause it, p. 530. Also see the appendix for nursing diagnoses and interventions for the care of preoperative and postoperative patients, p. 637.

PATIENT-FAMILY TEACHING AND DISCHARGE PLANNING

Provide patient and significant others with verbal and written information for the following:
1. Medications, including drug name, route, purpose, dosage, schedule, precautions, and potential side effects. Stress the importance of notifying MD before supply runs out. Explain that good handwashing is essential before administering ophthalmic ointments or drops.
2. Recognizing and reporting signs of infection to MD: purulent drainage, pain, persistent redness, swelling, fever.
3. Avoiding rubbing, touching, and bumping the operative eye. Confer with MD regarding which, if any, of the following activities will be restricted and for how long, and review with patient accordingly: contact sports, heavy lifting, straining, bending, sexual activity.
4. Wearing dark glass to minimize photophobia and pain when mydriatics are used.
5. Wearing glasses by day and an eye shield at night to protect the eye, usually for at least 2-4 weeks.
6. Lid hygiene. For discussion, see "Vitreous Disorders/Vitrectomy," p. 534.
7. Need for follow-up care; confirm date and time of next appointment if known.

In addition, explain the following:
8. Floaters also may appear postoperatively and can disappear in weeks or last for years.
9. Continuing light flashes may indicate that complete vitreous traction was not relieved by surgery. Though this does not necessarily indicate unsuccessful surgery, it does necessitate contacting MD.

Enucleation

Enucleation is the surgical removal of an eyeglobe without disturbance of orbital integrity. Because enucleation is a drastic measure that results in blindness in the affected eye, it is not considered until all other possible medical and surgical therapies have been utilized. Indications for enucleation include malignant tumor; a painful, blind, or disfiguring eye; absolute glaucoma; presence of a nonremovable, irritating, foreign substance in the eye; severe infection; unrepaired ruptured globe; and as prophylaxis in sympathetic ophthalmia.

MEDICAL MANAGEMENT AND SURGICAL INTERVENTIONS

1. **Medical treatment:** Removal of foreign body or treatment of tumor, infection, or pain is instituted initially. If treatment is ineffective or severe trauma or disfigurement exists, surgery is performed.
2. **Surgery:** Usually performed under general anesthesia. The goal of surgery is to maintain orbital integrity, and an attempt is made to preserve the muscles and tendons for later insertion of an ocular prosthesis. Once the globe is removed, a temporary artificial globe called a conformer, which is made of teflon or plastic, usually is inserted to maintain orbit shape until a permanent ocular prosthesis can be made.
3. **Fitting and insertion of an ocular prosthesis:** Often delayed until postoperative edema decreases, usually 4-6 weeks after surgery, but it may be longer in cases of severe trauma.

NURSING DIAGNOSES AND INTERVENTIONS

Knowledge deficit: Surgical procedure, postsurgical precautions, and function of the ocular prosthesis

Desired outcomes: Patient verbalizes knowledge of the surgical procedure, postsurgical precautions, and function of the ocular prosthesis.

1. Assess patient's knowledge of the diagnosis, surgery, and treatment plan; explain or clarify information as necessary.
2. Provide time for patient and significant others to express fears and anxieties and ask questions.
3. Inform patient that a pressure dressing will be applied for 2-3 days after surgery.
4. Caution patient that touching and rubbing the orbit or tightly squeezing the eyelid is contraindicated because these actions can cause injury and infection.
5. Explain that some discomfort after surgery is normal but patient should alert staff to the presence of headache or sharp pain on operative side, which can signal complications, such as hemorrhage, infection, or broken sutures.
6. Explain that to minimize intraorbital pressure, patient should not lie on the operative side, but rather maintain the prescribed position (usually supine to 30 degrees elevation of the HOB), and that stooping, bending, lifting heavy objects, straining with bowel movements, and coughing or sneezing with a closed mouth are contraindicated because they may cause bleeding.
7. Inform patient that there is usually no restriction of activities after the first postoperative day.
8. Teach patient the function of the ocular prosthesis and approximate schedule for insertion, if appropriate.
9. Explain the lifetime need for safety glasses to protect the remaining eye.

Pain related to surgical procedure

Desired outcome: Patient's subjective evaluation of pain improves, as documented by a pain scale.

1. Explain to patient that minor discomfort after surgery is normal and that analgesia will be provided as needed.
2. Monitor for the presence of discomfort at frequent intervals. Devise with the patient a pain scale, rating pain from 0 (no pain) to 10. Ask patient to alert staff to severe pain (i.e., >6+ on the rating scale) or headache on enucleated side, which can signal complications such as hemorrhage, broken sutures, or infection.
3. Provide prescribed analgesia as needed. Rate and document the relief of pain obtained, using the pain scale.
4. There may be discomfort from the pressure dressing, which is used to minimize

edema and ensure hemostasis. Provide rationale for this dressing to the patient, and explain that it is used for the first 2-3 postoperative days.

5. Use prescribed antibiotic ointment to decrease discomfort from drying of tissues, which can occur with excessive conjunctival edema. When removing the dressing, confirm that the plastic or teflon conformer is in place.

See "Corneal Ulceration/Trauma" for **Sensory/perceptual alterations,** p. 529, and **Self-care deficit,** p. 530. Also see "Caring for Preoperative and Postoperative Patients," p. 637, and "Caring for Patients with Cancer and Other Life-Disrupting Illnesses," p. 659, in the appendix.

PATIENT-FAMILY TEACHING AND DISCHARGE PLANNING

Provide patient and significant others with verbal and written information for the following:

1. Medications, including drug name, route, purpose, dosage, schedule, precautions, and potential side effects. Stress the importance of good handwashing before administering ophthalmic medications.
2. Necessity of reporting signs of infection to MD: purulent drainage, swelling of orbit, pain, persistent orbital redness, fever.
3. Importance of avoiding rubbing, touching, or bumping orbit or wearing eye makeup without MD approval.
4. Need for follow-up care; confirm date of next appointment with MD and for the ocular prosthesis.
5. Lid hygiene. See discussion in "Vitreous Disorders/Vitrectomy," p. 534.
6. Referral to social worker or mental health nurse clinician as needed.
7. Use of safety glasses to protect the remaining eye.

In addition, once the ocular prosthesis is inserted:
8. Necessity of obtaining Medic-Alert bracelet and card that identifies patient as having ocular prosthesis.

Section Two   OTOSCLEROSIS (OTOSPONGIOSIS)

Otosclerosis is a disease of the bony inner ear in which normal bone is absorbed and replaced by a vascular and spongy bone (hence the name "otospongiosis"). When the disease involves the footplate of the stapes and the stapes become either partially or completely fixed, hearing loss will occur because stapes vibration will be hindered. This is a hereditary disease that starts in adulthood and affects more females than males.

ASSESSMENT

Signs and symptoms: Slow and progressive loss of hearing (more often bilateral), tinnitus, and sometimes an equilibrium disturbance, from mild dizziness to vertigo.

Physical assessment: Usually the eardrums will appear normal, but a pink blush is seen through the drum when the otosclerotic focus is very vascular. Tuning fork testing will suggest a conductive loss (negative Rinne's test). Pure tone audiometry confirms the presence of a conductive hearing loss. Tympanometry may reveal evidence of stiffness in the sound conduction system. A neurosensory component also may be present.

Risk factors: A positive family history of hearing loss may be obtained. Sometimes pregnancy accelerates the disease process.

MEDICAL MANAGEMENT AND SURGICAL INTERVENTIONS

1. **Hearing aid:** Individuals with otosclerosis usually are good candidates for hearing aids.

2. **Surgical interventions:** Surgical treatments for otosclerosis have evolved since the early 1950s from fenestration, to stapes immobilization, to total stapedectomy, to partial stapedectomy, which is performed today. In this procedure, most of the stapes is removed. A hole is made in the fixed footplate (usually by a laser) and a prosthesis is used to link the incus to the inner ear fluids, thus reestablishing a mobile sound conducting mechanism. Surgery may be done under local or general anesthesia. Patients usually are hospitalized for one night following stapedectomy. If an equilibrium disturbance is severe, continued hospitalization will be required.

NURSING DIAGNOSES AND INTERVENTIONS

Knowledge deficit: Surgical procedure, postsurgical regimen, and expected outcomes

Desired outcomes: Patient verbalizes (and demonstrates, as appropriate) knowledge of the surgical procedure, postsurgical regimen, and expected outcomes.

1. Explain upcoming surgical procedure, postsurgical routine, and expected outcomes. Provide time for patient to ask questions and express fears and anxieties.
2. Stress that patient must maintain the position specified by MD both during and after surgery. After surgery the patient usually will be positioned on the nonoperative side.
3. Explain that bed rest probably will be required for around 24 hours and that it may be necessary to remain flat, even for meals, to prevent slipping of the prosthesis.
4. Instruct patient to inform staff of headache, tinnitus, vertigo, vomiting, weakness of facial muscles, or postoperative pain that increases or is sudden and severe. These signs and symptoms can signal infection, hemorrhage, facial nerve encroachment, labyrinthitis, or irritation of the auditory nerve.
5. Explain that patient may have an earplug after surgery to absorb drainage in the operative ear. Caution patient not to remove this plug or get it wet.
6. Instruct patient not to blow nose because air forced into the eustachian tube can disturb the operative site. If blowing the nose is unavoidable, it should be done gently without restricting either nostril, and with the mouth and eyes open to minimize intracranial pressure.
7. Caution patient not to get water in the operative ear for 2 weeks, or as directed.
8. Reassure patient that minimal discomfort will be experienced postoperatively and that analgesics (usually acetaminophen) will be used as needed for the first 24 hours.

Potential for infection related to susceptibility secondary to invasive procedure and nonsterile field

Desired outcome: Patient is free of infection as evidenced by normothermia and absence of pain, headache, drainage, erythema, and swelling in the canal.

1. After the earplug and bandage have been removed, monitor for drainage, erythema, and swelling in the canal; fever; and patient complaints of pain or headache, which can signal the presence of infection.
2. Assist patient with maintaining a dry operative site, which will help prevent infection. Avoid hair washing and showers until approved by MD.
3. Be alert to the following indicators of meningitis, which is a rare but potential complication of this surgery: fever, chills, headache, nuchal rigidity, photophobia, nausea, and vomiting.

Potential for trauma related to risk of falling secondary to equilibrium disturbance

Desired outcome: Patient is free from trauma caused by equilibrium disturbance.

1. Monitor for the presence of mild dizziness, vertigo, tinnitus, or nausea. Advise patient to alert staff to the presence of nausea or vertigo so that appropriate medications can be administered.
2. To prevent falls, keep side rails up when patient is in bed.
3. Instruct patient to seek assistance with ambulation once it is allowed.
4. Instruct patient to maintain sitting position for a few moments before assuming a standing position.

Sensory/perceptual alterations related to auditory deficit secondary to disease process, postoperative earplug, or tissue edema

Desired outcome: Patient relates the ability to understand speaker and expresses satisfaction with sensory input.

1. Inform patient that hearing may be impaired for a few weeks after surgery because of tissue edema, ear packing, and the presence of blood in the inner ear.
2. Teach patient to maximize hearing by using lipreading, hearing aid in the nonoperative ear, or turning better ear toward the speaker.
3. Maintain quiet environment to minimize extraneous sounds during conversations.
4. Speak to patient slowly, in even tones; avoid turning away from patient or covering mouth while speaking.
5. Provide alternative sensory input, such as books or puzzles.

See nursing diagnoses and interventions for the care of preoperative and postoperative patients, p. 637, in the appendix.

PATIENT-FAMILY TEACHING AND DISCHARGE PLANNING

Provide patient and significant others with verbal and written information for the following:
1. Medications, including drug name, purpose, dosage, schedule, route, precautions, and potential side effects.
2. Need for medical follow-up; confirm date and time of next appointment if known. Usually, the inner earplug is removed 7 days after surgery.
3. Reporting the following indicators of ear infection to MD: persistent erythema and swelling of canal, purulent drainage, vertigo, persistent pain, and fever.
4. Avoiding blowing nose or sneezing. If unavoidable, explain that the mouth and eyes should be kept open in the process to minimize pressure buildup.
5. Avoiding changes in air pressure (air travel, diving, riding elevators) for the period of time determined by MD.
6. Avoiding contact with individuals known to have URIs, which can lead to otitis media.
7. Keeping ear dry for the period of time determined by MD.
8. Changing only the *outer* earplug as prescribed, using clean technique.

SELECTED REFERENCES

Bay-Monk H and Steinmetz CG: Nursing care of the eye, San Mateo, Calif and Norwalk, Conn, 1987, Appleton and Lange.

Bickford ME: Patient teaching tools in the ophthalmic unit, J Opthalm Nurs Technol 7(2):50-55, 1988.

Biddle C: Eye drops: more side effects than meet the eye, RN pp. 46-47, June 1986.

Hannley M: Basic principles of auditory assessment, San Diego, 1986, College-Hill Press.

Lent-Wunderlich E: Helping your patient through eye surgery, RN pp. 43-47, June 1986.

Schultz P and Fartin S: Opening new windows with corneal transplant, J Ophthalm Nurs Technol 5(1):4-7, 1986.

Tooke M, Elders J, and Johnson D: Corneal transplant, Am J Nurs 86:685-687, 1986.

11

CHAPTER

Multi-system disorders

Section One FLUID AND ELECTROLYTE DISTURBANCES

The major constituent of the human body is water. The average adult male is approximately 60% water by weight and the average female is 55% water by weight. Typically, body water decreases with both age and increasing body fat. Body water is distributed between two fluid compartments: approximately two-thirds is located within the cells (intracellular fluid—ICF) and the remaining one-third is located outside the cells (extracellular fluid—ECF). The ECF is further divided into interstitial fluid, which surrounds the cells, and intravascular fluid, which is contained within blood vessels. The body gains water through oral intake, fluid therapy, and oxidative metabolism. Water is lost from the body *via* the kidneys, GI tract, skin, and lungs.

In addition to water, body fluids contain two types of dissolved substances: electrolytes and nonelectrolytes. *Electrolytes* are substances that dissociate in solution and will conduct an electrical current. They dissociate into positive and negative ions and are measured by their capacity to combine (millequivalents/liter—mEq/L). *Nonelectrolytes* are substances, such as glucose and urea, that do not dissociate in solution and are measured by weight (milligrams per 100 milliliters—mg/dl). See Table 11-1, p. 542.

Part One FLUID DISTURBANCES

Hypovolemia

Depletion of ECF volume is termed "hypovolemia." Depending on the type of fluid lost, hypovolemia may be accompanied by acid-base, osmolar, or electrolyte imbalances. Severe ECF volume depletion can lead to hypovolemic shock. Prolonged hypovolemia may lead to the development of acute renal failure (see "Acute Renal Failure," p. 116).

ASSESSMENT

Signs and symptoms: Dizziness, weakness, fatigue, syncope, anorexia, nausea, vomiting, thirst, confusion, constipation.

Physical assessment: Decreased BP, especially when standing (orthostatic hypotension); decreased CVP; increased HR; decreased urine output; poor skin turgor; dry, furrowed tongue; sunken eyeballs; flat neck veins; increased temperature; and acute weight loss, except with third spacing (see Table 11-2).

History and risk factors

1. *Abnormal GI losses:* Vomiting, NG suctioning, diarrhea, intestinal drainage.
2. *Abnormal skin losses:* Excessive diaphoresis secondary to fever or exercise; burns.
3. *Abnormal renal losses:* Diuretic therapy, diabetes insipidus, renal disease (polyuric forms), adrenal insufficiency, osmotic diuresis (e.g., uncontrolled diabetes mellitus, postdye study).
4. *Third spacing or plasma-to-interstitial fluid shift:* Peritonitis, intestinal obstruction, burns.
5. *Hemorrhage.*
6. *Altered intake:* Coma, fluid deprivation.

T A B L E 1 1 - 1 Primary constituents of body water compartments (measured in meq/L)*

Substance	Intravascular	Interstitial	Intracellular (skeletal muscle cell)
Na^+	142	145	12
Cl^-	104	117	4.0
HCO_3^-	24	27	12
K^+	4.5	4.4	150
HPO_4^{--}	2.0	2.0	40

*This is a partial list. Other constituents include Ca^{++}, Mg^{++}, and proteins.

T A B L E 1 1 - 2 Weight loss as an indicator of ECF deficit in the adult

Acute weight loss (%)	Severity of deficit
2-5	Mild
5-10	Moderate
10-15	Severe
15-20	Fatal

DIAGNOSTIC TESTS

1. *BUN:* May be elevated due to dehydration, decreased renal perfusion, or decreased renal function.
2. *Hct:* Elevated with dehydration; decreased in the presence of bleeding.
3. *Serum electrolytes:* Variable, depending on type of fluid lost. Hypokalemia often occurs with abnormal GI or renal losses. Hyperkalemia occurs with adrenal insufficiency. Hypernatremia may be seen with increased insensible or sweat losses and diabetes insipidus. Hyponatremia occurs in most types of hypovolemia due to increased thirst and ADH release, which lead to increased water intake and retention, thus diluting the serum sodium. See individual electrolyte imbalances, pp. 551-563.
4. *ABG values:* Metabolic acidosis (pH <7.35 and HCO_3^- <22 meq/L) may occur with lower GI losses, shock, or diabetic ketoacidosis. Metabolic alkalosis (pH >7.45 and HCO_3^- >26 meq/L) may occur with upper GI losses and diuretic therapy.
5. *Urine specific gravity:* Increased due to the kidneys' attempt to save water; may be fixed at approximately 1.010 in the presence of renal disease.
6. *Urine sodium:* Demonstrates the kidneys' ability to conserve sodium in response to an increased aldosterone level. In the absence of renal disease, osmotic diuresis, or diuretic therapy, it should be <20 meq/L.
7. *Serum osmolality:* Variable, depending on the type of fluid lost and the body's ability to compensate with thirst and antidiuretic hormone.

MEDICAL MANAGEMENT

1. Restoration of normal fluid volume and correction of acid-base and electrolyte disturbances. The type of fluid replacement depends on the type of fluid lost and severity of the deficit.

☐ *Dextrose and water solutions:* Provide free water only and will be distributed evenly through both the ICF and ECF.

☐ *Isotonic ("normal") saline:* Expands ECF only; does not enter ICF.

☐ *Blood and albumin:* Expand only the intravascular portion ECF.

☐ *Mixed saline/electrolyte solutions:* Provide additional electrolytes (e.g., potassium and calcium) and a buffer (lactate or acetate).

2. Restoration of tissue perfusion in hypovolemic shock. Treatment includes rapid volume replacement and plasma expanders (e.g., albumin) to prevent capillary stasis and maintain adequate BP. Vasopressors are used only when response to volume replacement is inadequate.

3. Treatment of underlying cause.

NURSING DIAGNOSES AND INTERVENTIONS

Fluid volume deficit related to decreased circulating volume secondary to abnormal loss of ECF or reduced intake

Desired outcome: Patient attains adequate intake of fluid and electrolytes as evidenced by urine output ≥30 ml/hr, stable weight, specific gravity 1.010-1.030, no clinical evidence of hypovolemia (furrowed tongue, etc.), BP within patient's normal range, CVP 5-12 cm H_2O, and HR 60-100 bpm.

1. Monitor I&O qh. Initially, intake should exceed output during therapy. Alert MD to urine output <30 ml/hr for 2 consecutive hours. Measure urine specific gravity q8h. Expect it to decrease with therapy.

2. Monitor VS for evidence of continued hypovolemia. Be alert to decreased BP and CVP and to increased HR.

3. Weigh patient daily. Daily weight is the single most important indicator of fluid status because acute weight changes are indicative of fluid changes. For example, a 2 kg loss of weight equals a 2 L fluid loss. Weigh patient at the same time of day (preferably before breakfast) on a balanced scale, with patient wearing approximately the same clothing. Document type of scale used (i.e., standing, bed, chair).

4. Administer PO and IV fluids as prescribed. Document response to fluid therapy. Monitor for signs and symptoms of fluid overload or too rapid fluid administration: crackles (rales), SOB, tachypnea, tachycardia, increased CVP, neck vein distention, and edema.

5. Monitor patient for hidden fluid losses. For example, measure and document abdominal girth or limb size, if indicated.

6. Notify MD of decreases in hct that may signal bleeding. Remember that hct will decrease in the dehydrated patient as he or she becomes rehydrated. Decreases in hct associated with rehydration may be accompanied by decreases in serum sodium and BUN.

7. Place shock patient in a supine position with the legs elevated to increase venous return. Avoid Trendelenburg, because this position causes abdominal viscera to press on the diaphragm, thereby impairing ventilation.

Alteration in tissue perfusion: Cerebral and peripheral, related to decreased circulation secondary to hypovolemia

Desired outcome: Patient has adequate perfusion as evidenced by alertness, warm and dry skin, BP within patient's normal range, HR ≤100 bpm, brisk capillary refill (<3 seconds), and distal pulses equal and >2+ on a 0-4+ scale.

1. Monitor for signs of decreased cerebral perfusion: vertigo, syncope, confusion, restlessness, anxiety, agitation, excitability, weakness, nausea, and cool and clammy skin. Alert MD to worsening symptoms. Document response to fluid therapy.

2. Protect patients who are confused, dizzy, or weak. Keep side rails up and bed in lowest position with wheels locked. Assist with ambulation. Raise patient to sitting or standing positions slowly. Monitor for indicators of orthostatic hypotension: decreased BP, increased heart rate, dizziness, and diaphoresis. If symptoms occur, return patient to supine position.

3. To avoid unnecessary vasodilatation, treat fevers promptly.
4. Reassure patient and significant others that sensorium changes will improve with therapy.
5. Evaluate capillary refill, noting whether it is brisk (<3 seconds) or delayed (>4 seconds). Notify MD if refill is delayed.
6. Palpate peripheral pulses bilaterally in arms and legs (radial, brachial, dorsalis pedis, and posterior tibial). Use a Doppler if unable to palpate pulses. Rate pulses on a 0-4+ scale. Notify MD if pulses are absent or barely palpable. **Note:** Abnormal pulses also may be caused by a local vascular disorder.

For additional nursing diagnoses, see specific medical disorder, electrolyte imbalance, or acid-base disturbance.

PATIENT-FAMILY TEACHING AND DISCHARGE PLANNING

Give patient and significant others verbal and written instructions for the following:
1. Signs and symptoms of hypovolemia.
2. Importance of maintaining adequate intake, especially in the elderly, who are more likely to develop dehydration.
3. Medications: name, purpose, dosage, frequency, precautions, and potential side effects.

Hypervolemia

Expansion of ECF volume is termed "hypervolemia." It occurs whenever there is (a) excessive retention of sodium and water due to a chronic renal stimulus to save sodium and water; (b) abnormal renal function, with reduced excretion of sodium and water; (c) excessive administration of IV fluids; or (d) interstitial-to-plasma fluid shift. Severe hypervolemia can lead to heart failure and pulmonary edema (see "Heart Failure," p. 54, and "Pulmonary Edema," p. 76), especially in the patient with cardiovascular dysfunction.

ASSESSMENT

Signs and symptoms: SOB, orthopnea.

Physical assessment: Edema, weight gain, increased BP (decreased BP as the heart fails), increased CVP, bounding pulses, ascites, crackles (rales), rhonchi, wheezes, distended neck veins, moist skin, tachycardia, gallop rhythm.

History and risk factors

1. Retention of sodium and water: Heart failure, cirrhosis, nephrotic syndrome, excessive administration of glucocorticosteroids.
2. Abnormal renal function: Acute or chronic renal failure with oliguria.
3. Excessive administration of IV fluids.
4. Interstitial-to-plasma fluid shift (e.g., remobilization of fluid after treatment of burns).

DIAGNOSTIC TESTS

Laboratory findings are variable and usually nonspecific.
1. <u>Hct:</u> Decreased due to hemodilution.
2. <u>BUN:</u> Increased in renal failure.
3. <u>ABG values:</u> May reveal hypoxemia (decreased Pao_2) and alkalosis (increased pH and decreased $Paco_2$) in the presence of pulmonary edema.
4. <u>Serum sodium and serum osmolality:</u> Will be decreased if hypervolemia occurs as a result of excessive retention of water (e.g., in chronic renal failure).

5. *Urine specific gravity:* Decreased if the kidney is attempting to excrete excess volume. May be fixed at 1.010 in acute renal failure.
6. *Chest x-ray:* May reveal signs of pulmonary vascular congestion.

MEDICAL MANAGEMENT

The goal of therapy is to treat the precipitating problem and return ECF to normal. Treatment may include the following:
1. **Restriction of sodium and water.** See Table 11-3 for a list of foods high in sodium.
2. **Diuretics.**
3. **Dialysis or continuous arterial-venous hemofiltration:** In renal failure or life-threatening fluid overload (see "Renal Dialysis," p. 126). **Note:** Also see specific discussions under "Acute Renal Failure," p. 116, "Chronic Renal Failure," p. 121, and "Burns," p. 577.

NURSING DIAGNOSES AND INTERVENTIONS

Fluid volume excess: Edema (peripheral and pulmonary) related to surplus of circulating fluid secondary to expanded ECF volume

Desired outcome: Patient is normovolemic as evidenced by stable weight, absence of edema, BP within patient's normal range, CVP 5-12 cm H_2O, and HR 60-100 bpm.

1. Monitor I&O qh. With the exception of oliguric renal failure, urine output should be >30-60 ml/hr. Measure urine specific gravity q shift. If patient is diuresing, specific gravity should be <1.010-1.020.
2. Observe for and document presence of edema: pretibial, sacral, periorbital; note pitting.
3. Limit sodium intake as prescribed by MD (see Table 11-3). Consider use of salt substitutes. **Note:** Salt substitutes contain potassium and may be contraindicated in patients with renal failure or in patients receiving potassium-sparing diuretics (e.g., spironolactone, triamterene).
4. Limit fluids as prescribed. Offer a portion of allotted fluids as ice chips to minimize patient's thirst. Teach patient and significant others the importance of fluid restriction and how to measure fluid volume.
5. Provide oral hygiene at frequent intervals to keep oral mucous membrane moist and intact.
6. Document response to diuretic therapy. Many diuretics (e.g., furosemide, thiazides) cause hypokalemia. Observe for indicators of hypokalemia (see "Hypokalemia," p. 555). Potassium-sparing diuretics (e.g., spironolactone, triamterene) may cause hyperkalemia. See "Hyperkalemia," p. 557. Notify MD of significant findings.
7. Observe for physical indicators of overcorrection and dangerous volume depletion secondary to therapy: vertigo, weakness, syncope, thirst, confusion, poor skin turgor, flat neck veins, acute weight loss. Monitor VS for signs of volume depletion

---

T A B L E   1 1 - 3   Foods that are high in sodium content

Bacon	Olives
Bouillon	Pickles
Celery	Preserved meat
Cheeses	Salad dressings and prepared sauces
Dried fruits	Sauerkraut
Frozen, canned, or packaged foods	Snack foods (e.g., crackers, chips, pretzels,
Monosodium glutamate (MSG)	salted nuts)
Mustard	Soy sauce

occurring with therapy: decreased BP and increased HR. Alert MD to significant changes or findings.

Impaired gas exchange related to decreased diffusion of oxygen secondary to pulmonary vascular congestion occurring with ECF expansion

Desired outcomes: Patient has adequate gas exchange as evidenced by Pao_2 ≥80 mm Hg, pH ≤7.45, and $Paco_2$ ≥35 mm Hg. Patient does not exhibit crackles, gallops, or other clinical indicators of pulmonary edema. RR is ≤20 breaths/min with normal depth and pattern (eupnea).

1. Acute pulmonary edema is a potentially life-threatening complication of hypervolemia. Monitor patient for indicators of pulmonary edema including air hunger, anxiety, cough with production of frothy sputum, crackles (rales), rhonchi, tachypnea, tachycardia, and gallop rhythm.
2. Monitor ABGs for evidence of hypoxemia (decreased Pao_2) and respiratory alkalosis (increased pH and decreased $Paco_2$). Increased oxygen requirements are indicative of increasing pulmonary vascular congestion.
3. Keep patient in semi-Fowler's or position of comfort to minimize dyspnea. Avoid restrictive clothing.

PATIENT-FAMILY TEACHING AND DISCHARGE PLANNING

Give patient and significant others verbal and written instructions for the following:
1. Signs and symptoms of hypervolemia.
2. Symptoms that necessitate MD notification after hospital discharge: SOB, chest pain, new pulse irregularity.
3. Low-sodium diet, if prescribed; use of salt substitute, and avoiding foods that are high in sodium. See Table 11-3, p. 550.
4. Medications, including name, purpose, dosage, frequency, precautions, and potential side effects; signs and symptoms of hypokalemia if patient is taking diuretics that may cause hypokalemia.
5. Importance of fluid restriction if hypervolemia continues.
6. Importance of measuring weight daily.

Part Two   ELECTROLYTE DISTURBANCES

Sodium imbalance

Sodium plays a vital role in maintaining concentration and volume of ECF. It is the main cation of ECF and the major determinant of ECF osmolality. Under normal conditions, ECF osmolality can be estimated by doubling the serum sodium value. Sodium imbalances usually are associated with parallel changes in osmolality. Sodium also is important in maintaining irritability and conduction of nerve and muscle tissue and in the regulation of acid-base balance.

Sodium concentration is maintained *via* regulation of water intake and excretion. If serum sodium concentration is decreased (hyponatremia), the kidneys respond by excreting water. Conversely, if serum sodium concentration is increased (hypernatremia), serum osmolality increases, stimulating the thirst center and causing an increased release of antidiuretic hormone (ADH) by the posterior pituitary gland. ADH acts on the kidneys to conserve water. Because changes in serum sodium levels typically reflect changes in water balance, gains or losses of total body sodium are not necessarily reflected by the serum sodium level. Normal serum sodium is 137-147 mEq/L.

Hyponatremia

Hyponatremia (serum sodium <137 mEq/L) can occur because of a net gain of water or a loss of sodium-rich fluids that are replaced by water. Clinical indicators and treatment depend on the cause of hyponatremia and whether it is associated with a normal, decreased, or increased ECF volume. For more information, see "Acute Renal Failure," p. 116, "Burns," p. 557, and "Heart Failure," p. 54.

ASSESSMENT

Signs and symptoms:
Note: Neurologic symptoms usually do not occur until the serum sodium level has dropped to approximately 120-125 mEq/L.

Hyponatremia with decreased ECF volume:
Irritability, apprehension, dizziness, personality changes, postural hypotension, dry mucous membranes, cold and clammy skin, tremors, seizures, coma, decreased CVP.

Hyponatremia with normal or increased ECF volume:
Headache, lassitude, apathy, confusion, weakness, edema, weight gain, elevated BP, hyperreflexia, muscle spasms, convulsions, coma, increased CVP.

History and risk factors:

Decreased ECF volume
1. GI losses: Diarrhea, vomiting, fistulas, NG suction.
2. Renal losses: Diuretics, salt-wasting kidney disease, adrenal insufficiency.
3. Skin losses: Burns, wound drainage.

Normal/increased ECF volume
1. Syndrome of inappropriate antidiuretic hormone (SIADH): Excessive production of antidiuretic hormone.
2. Edematous states: Congestive heart failure, cirrhosis, nephrotic syndrome.
3. Excessive administration of hypotonic IV fluids.
4. Oliguric renal failure.

Note: Hyperlipidemia, hyperproteinemia, and hyperglycemia may cause a pseudohyponatremia.

DIAGNOSTIC TESTS

1. *Serum sodium:* Will be <137 mEq/L.
2. *Serum osmolality:* Decreased, except in cases of pseudohyponatremia.
3. *Urine specific gravity:* Decreased in volume expansion and increased with volume depletion. In SIADH, the urine will be inappropriately concentrated.
4. *Urine sodium:* Decreased (usually <20 mEq/L) except in SIADH, salt-wasting kidney disease, and adrenal insufficiency.

MEDICAL MANAGEMENT

The goal of therapy is to get the patient out of immediate danger (i.e., return sodium to >120 mEq/L) and then *gradually* return sodium to a normal level and restore normal ECF volume.

Hyponatremia with reduced ECF volume:
1. Replacement of sodium and fluid losses.
2. Replacement of other electrolyte losses (e.g., potassium, bicarbonate).
3. IV hypertonic saline: If serum sodium is dangerously low or the patient is very symptomatic.

Hyponatremia with expanded ECF volume:
1. Removal or treatment of underlying cause.
2. Diuretics.
3. Water restriction.

NURSING DIAGNOSES AND INTERVENTIONS

Potential fluid volume deficit or excess related to abnormal fluid loss, excessive intake of hypotonic solutions, or abnormal retention of water

Desired outcome: Patient is normovolemic as evidenced by HR 60-100 bpm, RR 12-20 breaths/min with normal depth and pattern (eupnea), BP within patient's normal range, and CVP 5-12 cm H_2O.

1. If patient is receiving hypertonic saline, assess carefully for signs of intravascular fluid overload: tachypnea, tachycardia, SOB, crackles (rales), rhonchi, increased CVP, gallop rhythm, and increased BP.
2. For other interventions, see "Hypovolemia," p. 548, for **Fluid volume deficit;** see "Hypervolemia," p. 550, for **Fluid volume excess.**

Sensory/perceptual alterations related to mentation changes secondary to sodium level <120-125 mEq/L

Desired outcome: Patient verbalizes orientation to person, place, and time.

1. Assess and document LOC, orientation, and neurologic status with each VS check. Reorient patient as necessary. Alert MD to significant changes.
2. Inform patient and significant others that altered sensorium is temporary and will improve with treatment.
3. Keep side rails up and bed in lowest position, with wheels locked.
4. Utilize reality therapy, such as clocks, calendars, and familiar objects; keep these items at the bedside within patient's visual field.
5. If seizures are expected, pad side rails and keep an airway at the bedside.

PATIENT-FAMILY TEACHING AND DISCHARGE PLANNING

Give patient and significant others verbal and written instructions for the following:
1. Medications, including drug name, purpose, dosage, frequency, precautions, and potential side effects. Teach signs and symptoms of hypokalemia if patient is taking diuretics that cause hypokalemia, and provide examples of foods that are high in potassium (see Table 11-4, p. 555).
2. Fluid restriction, if prescribed. Teach patient that a portion of fluid allotment can be taken as ice or Popsicles to minimize thirst.
3. Signs and symptoms of hypervolemia if hyponatremia is related to abnormal fluid gains.

Hypernatremia

Hypernatremia (serum sodium level >147 mEq/L) may occur with water loss or sodium gain. Because sodium is the major determinant of ECF osmolality, hypernatremia always causes hypertonicity. In turn, hypertonicity causes a shift of water out of the cells, which leads to cellular dehydration and increased ECF volume.

ASSESSMENT

Signs and symptoms: Intense thirst, fatigue, restlessness, agitation, seizures, coma. Symptomatic hypernatremia occurs only in individuals who do not have access to water or who have an altered thirst mechanism (e.g., infants, the elderly, those who are comatose).

Physical assessment: Low-grade fever, flushed skin, peripheral and pulmonary edema (sodium gain); postural hypotension (water loss).

History and risk factors

1. *Sodium gain:* IV administration of hypertonic saline or sodium bicarbonate, increased oral intake, primary aldosteronism, saltwater near drowning, such drugs as sodium polystyrene sulfonate (Kayexalate).

2. *Water loss:* Increased diaphoresis, respiratory infection, diabetes insipidus, osmotic diuresis (e.g., hyperglycemia), altered thirst, and decreased availability of water.

DIAGNOSTIC TESTS

1. *Serum sodium:* Will be >147 mEq/L.
2. *Serum osmolality:* Increased due to elevated serum sodium.
3. *Urine specific gravity:* Increased because of the kidneys' attempt to retain water; will be decreased in diabetes insipidus.
4. *See "Diabetes Insipidus," p. 281, for additional diagnostic tests.*

MEDICAL MANAGEMENT

1. **IV or oral water replacement:** For water loss. If sodium is >160 mEq/L, IV D_5W or hypotonic saline is given to replace pure water deficit. See "Diabetes Insipidus," p. 281, for specific treatment.
2. **Diuretics and oral or IV water replacement:** For sodium gain.

Note: Hypernatremia is corrected slowly, over approximately 2 days, to avoid too great a shift of water into brain cells, which could cause cerebral edema.

NURSING DIAGNOSES AND INTERVENTIONS

Sensory/perceptual alterations related to sensorium changes and risk of seizures secondary to cerebral edema occurring with too rapid correction of hypernatremia

Desired outcome: Patient verbalizes orientation to person, place, and time, with HR ≥60 bpm and BP within patient's normal range.

1. Cerebral edema may occur if hypernatremia is corrected too rapidly. Monitor serial serum sodium levels; notify MD of rapid decreases.
2. Assess patient for indicators of cerebral edema: lethargy, headache, nausea, vomiting, increased BP, widening pulse pressure, decreased pulse rate, and seizures.
3. Assess and document LOC, orientation, and neurologic status with each VS check. Reorient patient as necessary. Alert MD to significant changes.
4. Inform patient and significant others that altered sensorium is temporary and will improve with treatment.
5. Keep side rails up and bed in lowest position, with wheels locked.
6. Utilize reality therapy, such as clocks, calendars, and familiar objects; keep these items at the bedside within patient's visual field.
7. If seizures are anticipated, pad side rails and keep an airway at the bedside.

See "Hypovolemia," p. 548, for **Fluid volume deficit** (applicable to hypernatremia caused by water loss); see "Hypervolemia," p. 550, for **Fluid volume excess** (applicable to hypernatremia caused by sodium gain).

PATIENT-FAMILY TEACHING AND DISCHARGE PLANNING

Give patient and significant others verbal and written instructions for the following:
1. Medications, including drug name, purpose, dosage, frequency, precautions, and potential side effects. Teach signs and symptoms of hypokalemia if patient is taking potassium-wasting diuretics and review foods that are high in potassium (see Table 11-4, p. 555).
2. Signs and symptoms of hypovolemia, if hypernatremia is related to abnormal fluid loss.

TABLE 11-4 Foods high in potassium

Apricots	Mushrooms
Artichokes	Nuts
Avocado	Oranges, orange juice
Banana	Peanuts
Cantaloupe	Potatoes
Carrots	Prune juice
Cauliflower	Pumpkin
Chocolate	Spinach
Dried beans, peas	Swiss chard
Dried fruit	Sweet potatoes
Grapefruit	Tomatoes, tomato juice, tomato sauce

Potassium imbalance

Potassium is the primary intracellular cation, and thus it plays a vital role in cell metabolism. It affects the resting potential of nerve and cardiac cells. Abnormal serum potassium levels adversely affect neuromuscular and cardiac function. A relatively small amount of potassium is located within the ECF and is maintained within a narrow range. The vast majority of the body's potassium is located within the cells. Distribution of potassium between ECF and ICF is affected by ECF pH, as well as by several hormones, including insulin, catecholamines, and aldosterone. Acute changes in serum pH are accompanied by reciprocal changes in serum potassium concentration.

The body gains potassium through foods (primarily meats, fruits, and vegetables) and medications. In addition, ECF gains potassium any time there is a breakdown of cells or movement of potassium out of the cell. An elevated serum potassium level usually does not occur unless there is a reduction in renal function. Potassium is lost from the body through the kidneys, GI tract, and skin. Potassium may be lost from ECF because of an intracellular shift. The kidneys are the primary regulators of potassium balance. Normal serum potassium is 3.5-5.0 mEq/L.

Hypokalemia

Hypokalemia occurs because of a loss of potassium from the body or a movement of potassium into the cells. **Note:** Changes in serum potassium levels reflect changes in ECF potassium, not necessarily changes in total body levels.

ASSESSMENT

Signs and symptoms: Fatigue, muscle weakness, leg cramps, soft and flabby muscles, nausea, vomiting, ileus, paresthesias, enhanced digitalis effect.

Physical assessment: Decreased bowel sounds, weak and irregular pulse, decreased reflexes, and decreased muscle tone.

History and risk factors

Reduction in total body potassium

1. Hyperaldosteronism.
2. Diuretics or abnormal urinary losses.
3. Increased GI losses.
4. Increased loss through diaphoresis.

Note: Poor intake may contribute to, but rarely will cause, hypokalemia.

Intracellular shift
1. Increased insulin (e.g., from TPN).
2. Alkalosis.

DIAGNOSTIC TESTS

1. *Serum potassium:* Values will be <3.5 mEq/L.
2. *ABG valves:* May show metabolic alkalosis (increased pH and HCO_3^-) because hypokalemia usually is associated with this condition.
3. *EKG:* ST-segment depression, flattened T wave, presence of U wave, ventricular dysrhythmias. **Note:** Hypokalemia potentiates the effect of digitalis. EKG may reveal signs of digitalis toxicity in spite of a normal serum digitalis level.

MEDICAL MANAGEMENT

1. Treatment of underlying cause.
2. Replacement of potassium, either PO (*via* increased dietary intake or medication) or IV. The usual dose is 40-80 mEq/L each day in divided doses. IV potassium is necessary if hypokalemia is severe or the patient is unable to take potassium orally. IV potassium should not be administered at rates >10-20 mEq/hr or in concentrations >30-40 mEq/L, unless hypokalemia is severe, because this can result in life-threatening hyperkalemia. If potassium is administered *via* a peripheral line, the rate of administration may need to be reduced to prevent irritation of vessels. Patients receiving 10-20 mEq/hr should be on a continuous cardiac monitor. The development of peaked T waves suggests the presence of hyperkalemia and requires immediate MD notification. **Caution:** Potassium is never given by IV push.
3. Potassium-sparing diuretics: May be given in place of oral potassium supplements.

NURSING DIAGNOSES AND INTERVENTIONS

Potential decreased cardiac output related to risk of ventricular dysrhythmias secondary to hypokalemia or too rapid correction of hypokalemia with resulting hyperkalemia

Desired outcomes: EKG shows normal T-wave configuration and absence of ventricular dysrhythmias. Pulse rate and regularity are normal for patient. Serum potassium levels are within normal range (3.5-5.0 mEq/L). **Caution:** Disorders of potassium balance are potentially life threatening. Symptoms are most likely to occur with sudden changes in serum potassium. Notify MD if any signs of potassium imbalance occur.

1. Administer potassium supplement as prescribed. Avoid giving IV potassium chloride at a rate faster than recommended, as this can lead to life-threatening hyperkalemia. **Note:** Do not add potassium chloride to IV solution containers in the hanging position because this can cause layering of the medication. Instead, invert the solution container before adding the medication and mix well.
2. Be aware that IV potassium chloride can cause local irritation of veins and chemical phlebitis. Assess IV insertion site for erythema, heat, or pain. Alert MD to symptoms. Irritation may be relieved by applying an ice bag, giving mild sedation, or numbing insertion site with small amount of local anesthetic. Phlebitis may necessitate changing of IV site. Oral potassium supplements may cause GI irritation. Administer with a full glass of water or fruit juice; encourage patient to sip slowly. Alert MD to symptoms of abdominal pain, distention, nausea, or vomiting. Do not switch potassium supplements without MD prescription.
3. Encourage intake of foods high in potassium (see Table 11-4, p. 555). Salt substitutes may be used as an inexpensive potassium supplement.
4. Monitor I&O qh. Alert MD to urine output <30 ml/hr. Unless severe, symptomatic hypokalemia is present, potassium supplements should not be given if the patient has

an inadequate urine output because hyperkalemia can develop rapidly in patients with oliguria (urine output <15-20 ml/hr).

5. Monitor for the presence of an irregular pulse or a difference between the apical and radial pulse rates.

6. Monitor serum potassium levels carefully, especially in individuals at risk for developing hypokalemia, such as patients taking diuretics or receiving NG suction. Alert MD to abnormal serum potassium levels.

7. Administer potassium cautiously in patients receiving potassium-sparing diuretics (e.g., spironolactone or triamterene) because of the potential for the development of hyperkalemia.

8. Because hypokalemia can potentiate the effects of digitalis, monitor patients receiving digitalis for signs of increased digitalis effect: multifocal or bigeminal PVCs, paroxysmal atrial tachycardia with varying AV block, Wenckebach (type I AV) heart block.

Potential ineffective breathing pattern related to weakness or paralysis of respiratory muscles secondary to *severe* hypokalemia (potassium <2-2.5 mEq/L)

Desired outcome: Patient has effective breathing pattern as evidenced by normal respiratory depth and pattern (eupnea) and rate of 12-20 breaths/min.

1. If patient is exhibiting signs of worsening hypokalemia, be aware that severe hypokalemia can lead to weakness of respiratory muscles, resulting in shallow respirations and eventually to apnea and respiratory arrest. Assess character, rate, and depth of respirations. Alert MD promptly if respirations become rapid and shallow.

2. Keep manual resuscitator at patient's bedside if severe hypokalemia is suspected.

3. Reposition patient q2h to prevent stasis of secretions; suction airway as needed.

PATIENT-FAMILY TEACHING AND DISCHARGE PLANNING

Give patient and significant others verbal and written instructions for the following:

1. Medications, including name, purpose, dosage, frequency, precautions, and potential side effects. Teach patient the importance of taking prescribed potassium supplements if taking diuretics or digitalis. Review the indicators of digitalis toxicity.

2. Indicators of hypokalemia and hyperkalemia.

3. Foods that are high in potassium (see Table 11-4, p. 555); use of salt substitute to supplement potassium, if appropriate.

Hyperkalemia

Hyperkalemia (serum potassium level >5.0 mEq/L) occurs because of an increased intake of potassium, a decreased urinary excretion of potassium, or movement of potassium out of the cells. **Note:** Changes in serum potassium levels reflect changes in ECF potassium, not necessarily changes in total body levels.

ASSESSMENT

Signs and symptoms: Irritability, anxiety, abdominal cramping, diarrhea, weakness (especially of lower extremities), paresthesias.

Physical assessment: Irregular pulse; cardiac standstill may occur at levels >8.5 mEq/L.

History and risk factors

1. *Inappropriately high intake of potassium:* Usually, IV potassium delivery.

2. *Decreased excretion of potassium:* For example, renal disease, use of potassium-sparing diuretics.

3. *Movement of potassium out of the cells:* For example, with acidosis, insulin deficiency, tissue catabolism (e.g., with fever, sepsis, trauma, surgery).

DIAGNOSTIC TESTS

1. *Serum potassium:* Will be >5.0 mEq/L.
2. *ABG valves:* May show metabolic acidosis (decreased pH and HCO_3^-) because hyperkalemia often occurs with acidosis.
3. *Diagnostic EKG:* Progressive changes include tall, thin T waves; prolonged PR interval; ST depression; widened QRS; loss of P wave. Eventually, QRS becomes widened further and cardiac arrest occurs.

MEDICAL MANAGEMENT

The goal is to treat the underlying cause and return the serum potassium level to normal.

Subacute

1. Cation exchange resins (e.g., Kayexalate): Given either orally or *via* retention enema to exchange sodium for potassium in the gut. Kayexalate usually is combined with sorbitol to induce diarrhea and thus increase potassium loss.

Acute

1. IV calcium gluconate: To counteract the neuromuscular and cardiac effects of hyperkalemia. Serum potassium levels will remain elevated.
2. IV glucose and insulin: To shift potassium into the cells. This reduces serum potassium temporarily (approximately 6 hours).
3. Sodium bicarbonate: To shift potassium into the cells. This reduces serum potassium temporarily. **Note:** The effects of calcium, glucose and insulin, and sodium bicarbonate are temporary. Usually, it is necessary to follow these medications with a therapy that removes potassium from the body, for example, dialysis or administration of cation exchange resins.
4. Dialysis: To remove potassium from the body.

NURSING DIAGNOSES AND INTERVENTIONS

Potential decreased cardiac output related to risk of ventricular dysrhythmias secondary to severe hyperkalemia or too rapid correction of hyperkalemia with resulting hypokalemia

Desired outcomes: EKG shows normal configuration and absence of ventricular dysrhythmias. Pulse rate and regularity are normal for patient. Patient does not complain of muscle weakness. **Caution:** Disorders of potassium balance are potentially life threatening. Symptoms most likely will occur if hyperkalemia or hypokalemia develops suddenly. Notify MD if any signs and symptoms of potassium imbalance occur.

1. Monitor I&O. Alert MD to urine output <30 ml/hr. Oliguria increases the risk for developing hyperkalemia.
2. Monitor for indicators of hyperkalemia (e.g., irritability, anxiety, abdominal cramping, diarrhea, weakness of lower extremities, paresthesias, irregular pulse). Also be alert to indicators of hypokalemia (e.g., fatigue, muscle weakness, leg cramps, nausea, vomiting, decreased bowel sounds, paresthesias, weak and irregular pulse) following treatment. Assess for hidden sources of potassium: medications (e.g., potassium penicillin G); banked blood; salt substitute; GI bleeding; or conditions causing increased catabolism, such as infection or trauma.
3. Monitor serum potassium levels, especially in patients at risk of developing hyperkalemia, such as individuals with renal failure. Notify MD of levels above or below normal range.
4. Administer calcium gluconate as prescribed, giving it cautiously in patients receiving digitalis because digitalis toxicity can occur. Do not add calcium gluconate to solutions containing sodium bicarbonate because precipitates may form. For more information about calcium administration, see "Hypocalcemia," p. 559.

5. If administering cation exchange resins by enema, encourage patient to retain the solution for at least 30-60 minutes to ensure therapeutic effects.

PATIENT-FAMILY TEACHING AND DISCHARGE PLANNING

Give patient and significant others verbal and written instructions for the following:
1. Medications, including name, purpose, dosage, frequency, precautions, and potential side effects.
2. Indicators of both hypokalemia and hyperkalemia. Alert patient to the following signs and symptoms that necessitate immediate medical attention: weakness and pulse irregularities.
3. Foods high in potassium, which should be avoided. See Table 11-4, p. 555. Remind patient that salt substitute and "lite" salt also should be avoided.
4. Importance of preventing recurrent hyperkalemia; review potential causes.

Calcium imbalance

Calcium, the body's most abundant ion, primarily is combined with phosphorus to form the mineral salts of the bones and teeth. In addition, calcium exerts a sedative effect on nerve cells and has important intracellular functions, including development of the cardiac action potential and contraction of muscles. Only 1% of the body's calcium is contained within ECF, yet this concentration is regulated carefully by the hormones parathormone and calcitonin.

Approximately half of plasma calcium is free, ionized calcium. The remaining half is bound, primarily to albumin. Only the ionized calcium is physiologically important. The percentage of calcium that is ionized is affected by plasma pH and albumin level. Patients with alkalosis, for example, may show signs of hypocalcemia because of increased calcium binding. Changes in plasma albumin level will affect total serum calcium level without changing the level of free calcium.

Hypocalcemia

Symptomatic hypocalcemia may occur because of a reduction of total body calcium or a reduction of the percentage of calcium that is ionized. Total calcium levels may be decreased due to increased calcium loss, reduced intake secondary to altered intestinal absorption, or altered regulation (e.g., hypoparathyroidism). Elevated phosphorus levels and decreased magnesium levels may precipitate hypocalcemia.

ASSESSMENT

Signs and symptoms: Numbness with tingling of fingers and circumoral region, hyperactive reflexes, muscle cramps, tetany, convulsions. In chronic hypocalcemia, fractures may be present due to bone porosity.

Physical assessment

☐ *Positive Trousseau's sign:* Ischemia-induced carpopedal spasm. It is elicited by applying a BP cuff to the upper arm and inflating it past systolic BP for 2 minutes.
☐ *Positive Chvostek's sign:* Unilateral contraction of facial and eyelid muscles. It is elicited by irritating the facial nerve by percussing the face just in front of the ear.

EKG changes: Prolonged QT interval caused by elongation of ST segment.

History and risk factors

Decreased ionized calcium
1. Alkalosis.
2. Administration of citrated blood. Citrate added to the blood to prevent clotting may bind with calcium, causing hypocalcemia.

3. Hemodilution (e.g., occurring with volume replacement with normal saline after hemorrhage).
   □ *Increased calcium loss in body fluids:* For example, with diuretics.
   □ *Decreased intestinal absorption:* For example, with impaired vitamin D metabolism or after gastrectomy.
   □ *Hypoparathyroidism.*
   □ *Hyperphosphatemia:* For example, in renal failure.
   □ *Hypomagnesemia.*

DIAGNOSTIC TESTS

1. *Total serum calcium level:* Will be <8.5 mg/dl. Serum calcium levels should be evaluated with serum albumin. For every 1.0 g/dl drop in the serum albumin level, there is a 0.8-1.0 mg/dl drop in total calcium level.
2. *Ionized serum calcium:* Will be <4.5 mg/dl.
3. *Parathormone:* Decreased levels occur in hypoparathyroidism; increased levels may occur with other causes of hypocalcemia.
4. *Magnesium and phosphorus levels:* May be checked to identify potential causes of hypocalcemia.

MEDICAL MANAGEMENT

1. Treatment of underlying cause.
2. Calcium replacement: Hypocalcemia is treated with PO or IV calcium. Tetany is treated with 10-20 ml of 10% calcium gluconate IV or a continuous drip of 100 ml of 10% calcium gluconate in 1,000 ml D_5W, infused over at least 4 hours.
3. Vitamin D therapy (e.g., dihydrotachysterol, calcitriol): To increase calcium absorption from the GI tract.
4. Aluminum hydroxide antacids: To reduce elevated phosphorus level prior to treating hypocalcemia.

NURSING DIAGNOSES AND INTERVENTIONS

Potential for trauma related to risk of tetany and seizures secondary to severe hypocalcemia

Desired outcomes: Patient does not exhibit evidence of trauma caused by complications of severe hypocalcemia. Serum calcium levels are within normal range (8.5-10.5 mg/dl).

1. Monitor patient for evidence of worsening hypocalcemia: numbness and tingling of fingers and circumoral region, hyperactive reflexes, and muscle cramps. Notify MD promptly if these symptoms develop because they occur prior to overt tetany. In addition, notify MD if patient has positive Trousseau's or Chvostek's signs, as they also signal latent tetany.
2. Administer IV calcium with caution. IV calcium should not be given faster than 1 ml/min since rapid administration can cause hypotension. Observe IV insertion site for evidence of infiltration because calcium will slough tissue. Concentrated calcium solutions should be administered through a central line. Do not add calcium to solutions containing sodium bicarbonate or sodium phosphate because dangerous precipitates will form.

Note: Digitalis toxicity may develop in patients taking digitalis because calcium potentiates its effects. Monitor patient for signs and symptoms of digitalis toxicity: anorexia, irregular pulse, nausea, and vomiting.

3. For patients with chronic hypocalcemia, administer oral calcium supplements and vitamin D preparations as prescribed. Administer oral calcium 30 minutes before meals or at bedtime for maximal absorption. Administer aluminum hydroxide antacids immediately after meals.

4. Encourage intake of foods high in calcium: milk products, meats, leafy green vegetables.
5. Notify MD if response to calcium therapy is ineffective. Tetany that does not respond to IV calcium may be caused by hypomagnesemia.
6. Keep symptomatic patients on seizure precautions; decrease environmental stimuli.
7. Avoid hyperventilation in patients in whom hypocalcemia is suspected. Metabolic alkalosis may precipitate tetany due to increased calcium binding.

Potential impaired gas exchange related to decreased availability of oxygen secondary to laryngeal spasm occurring with severe hypocalcemia

Desired outcome: Patient exhibits respiratory depth, pattern, and rate (12-20 breaths/min) within normal range and is asymptomatic of laryngeal spasm: laryngeal stridor, dyspnea, or crowing.

1. Assess patient's respiratory rate, character, and rhythm. Be alert to laryngeal stridor, dyspnea, and crowing, which occur with laryngeal spasm, a life-threatening complication of hypocalcemia.
2. Keep an emergency tracheostomy tray at the bedside of symptomatic patients.

PATIENT-FAMILY TEACHING AND DISCHARGE PLANNING

Give patient and significant others verbal and written instructions for the following:
1. Medications, including drug name, purpose, dosage, frequency, precautions, and potential side effects.
2. Indicators of hypercalcemia and hypocalcemia. Review the symptoms that necessitate immediate medical attention: numbness and tingling of fingers and circumoral region and muscle cramps.
3. Foods that are high in calcium.
Note: Many foods that are high in calcium, such as milk products, also are high in phosphorus and may need to be limited in patients with renal failure. In renal failure, a program of phosphorus control and calcium supplementation may be necessary.

Hypercalcemia

Symptomatic hypercalcemia can occur because of an increase in total serum calcium or an increase in the percentage of free, ionized calcium. If hypercalcemia is accompanied by a normal or elevated serum phosphorus level, calcium phosphate crystals may precipitate in the serum and deposit throughout the body. Soft tissue calcifications usually occur when the product (i.e., calcium × phosphorus) of the serum calcium and serum phosphorus exceeds 70 mg/dl.

ASSESSMENT

Signs and symptoms: Lethargy, weakness, anorexia, nausea, vomiting, polyuria, itching, bone pain, fractures, flank pain (secondary to renal calculi), depression, confusion, paresthesias, personality changes, stupor, coma.

EKG findings: Shortening of ST segment and QT interval. PR interval is sometimes prolonged. Ventricular dysrhythmias can occur with severe hypercalcemia.

History and risk factors

1. Increased intake of calcium: For example, excessive administration during cardiopulmonary arrest.
2. Increased intestinal absorption: For example, with vitamin D overdose or hyperparathyroidism.
3. Increased release of calcium from bone: Occurs with hyperparathyroidism, malignancies, prolonged immobilization, Paget's disease.
4. Decreased urinary excretion: For example, renal failure, medications (e.g., thiazide diuretics).
5. Increased ionized calcium: Acidosis.

DIAGNOSTIC TESTS

1. *Total serum calcium level:* Will be greater than 10.5 mg/dl. Serum calcium level should be evaluated with serum albumin level. For every 1.0 g/dl drop in serum albumin level, there will be a 0.8-1.0 mg/dl drop in total calcium.
2. *Ionized calcium:* Will be >5.5 mg/dl.
3. *Parathormone:* Increased levels occur in primary or secondary hyperparathyroidism.
4. *X-ray findings:* May reveal presence of osteoporosis, bone cavitation, or urinary calculi.

MEDICAL MANAGEMENT

1. Treatment of underlying cause: For example, antitumor chemotherapy for malignancy or partial parathyroidectomy for hyperparathyroidism.
2. IV normal saline: Administered rapidly to increase urinary calcium excretion. Furosemide is administered to prevent fluid overload.
3. IV phosphates: To cause a reciprocal drop in serum calcium.
4. Low-calcium diet and cortisone: To reduce intestinal absorption of calcium.
5. Decreased bone resorption: Accomplished *via* increased activity level, indomethacin, or mithramycin.
6. Calcitonin: To reduce bone resorption, increase bone deposition of calcium and phosphorus, and increase urinary calcium and phosphate excretion.
7. Sodium bicarbonate: To treat acidosis and reduce the percentage of calcium that is ionized.

NURSING DIAGNOSES AND INTERVENTIONS

Sensory/perceptual alterations related to motor and sensorium changes secondary to hypercalcemia

Desired outcomes: Patient verbalizes orientation to person, place, and time. Serum calcium levels are within normal range (8.5-10.5 mg/dl).

1. Monitor patient for worsening hypercalcemia. Assess and document LOC; patient's orientation to person, place, and time; and neurologic status with each VS check.
2. Personality changes, hallucinations, paranoia, and memory loss may occur with hypercalcemia. Inform patient and significant others that altered sensorium is temporary and will improve with treatment. Utilize reality therapy: clocks, calendars, and familiar objects; keep them at the bedside within patient's visual field.
3. Hypercalcemia causes neuromuscular depression with poor coordination, weakness, and altered gait. Provide a safe environment. Keep side rails up and bed in lowest position with wheels locked. Assist patient with ambulation if it is allowed.
4. Because hypercalcemia potentiates the effects of digitalis, monitor patient taking digitalis for signs and symptoms of digitalis toxicity: anorexia, nausea, vomiting, irregular pulse.
5. Monitor serum electrolyte values for changes in serum calcium (normal range is 8.5-10.5 mg/dl); potassium (normal range is 3.5-5.0 mEq/L); and phosphorus (normal range is 2.5-4.5 mg/dl) secondary to therapy. Notify MD of abnormal values.
6. Encourage increased mobility to reduce bone resorption. Ideally, patient should be out of bed and up in a chair at least 6 hr/day.

Alteration in pattern of urinary elimination: Dysuria, urgency, frequency, and polyuria secondary to administration of diuretics, calcium stone formation, or changes in renal function occurring with hypercalcemia

Desired outcome: Patient exhibits voiding pattern and urine characteristics that are normal for patient.

1. Hypercalcemia leads to an increase in calcium in the urine, which inhibits the kidneys' ability to concentrate urine. This leads to polyuria and potential volume deple-

tion. Be alert to polyuria. Also monitor for signs of volume depletion when giving diuretics: decreased BP and CVP and increased HR.

2. Monitor I&O qh. Alert MD to unusual changes in urine volume, for example, oliguria alternating with polyuria, which may signal urinary tract obstruction, or continuous polyuria, which may be indicative of nephrogenic diabetes insipidus caused by hypercalcemia.

3. Because hypercalcemia can impair renal function, monitor patient's renal function carefully: urine output, BUN, creatinine. For more information, see "Acute Renal Failure," p. 116.

4. Provide patient with a low-calcium diet and avoid use of calcium-containing medications (e.g., antacids, such as Tums). Encourage intake of fruits (e.g., cranberries, prunes, or plums) that leave an acid ash in the urine, thereby reducing the risk of calcium stone formation.

5. Assess patient for indicators of kidney stone formation: intermittent pain, nausea, vomiting, hematuria.

PATIENT-FAMILY TEACHING AND DISCHARGE PLANNING

Give patient and significant others verbal and written instructions for the following:

1. Medications, including drug name, purpose, dosage, frequency, precautions, and potential side effects.

2. Signs and symptoms of hypercalcemia.

3. Foods and OTC medications (e.g., antacids) that are high in calcium.

4. If stone formation is a concern, foods that leave an acid ash. Review signs and symptoms of nephrolithiasis.

5. After hospital discharge, the importance of increased fluid intake (up to 3 liters in nonrestricted patients) to minimize risk of stone formation.

Section Two   ACID-BASE IMBALANCES

For optimal functioning of the cells, metabolic processes maintain a steady balance between acids and bases. Arterial pH is an indirect measurement of hydrogen ion (H^+) concentration and is a reflection of the balance between carbon dioxide (CO_2), which is regulated by the lungs, and bicarbonate (HCO_3^-), a basic buffer regulated by the kidneys. Normal acid-base ratio is 1:20, representing 1 part CO_2 (potential H_2CO_3) to 20 parts HCO_3^-. If this balance is altered, derangements in pH occur. If extra acids are present or there is a loss of base, acidosis exists. If extra base is present or there is loss of acid, alkalosis is present.

Part One   EVALUATING ACID-BASE BALANCE

Acid-base balance is regulated by several mechanisms that are exceptionally sensitive to minute changes in pH. Usually, the body is able to maintain pH without outside intervention, if not at a normal level, at least in a life-sustaining range.

Buffer system responses

BUFFERS

Buffers are present in all body fluids and act immediately (within 1 second) after an abnormal pH occurs. They combine with excess acid or base to form substances that do not affect pH. Their effect, however, is limited.

1. Bicarbonate: The most important buffer, it is present in the largest quantity in body fluids. It aids in the excretion of H^+ and is generated in the kidneys.

2. Phosphate: Aids in the excretion of H^+ in the renal tubules.

3. Ammonium: The kidneys produce an acidic urine by adding H^+ to ammonia (NH_3) to form ammonium (NH_4^+).
4. Protein: Present in cells, blood, and plasma. Hemoglobin is the most important protein buffer.

RESPIRATORY SYSTEM

The level of ventilation is determined by cerebrospinal fluid pH, which exerts a direct action on the respiratory center in the brain. Acidemia increases alveolar ventilation to four to five times the normal level, while alkalemia decreases alveolar ventilation to 50%-75% of the normal level. The response occurs quickly—within 1-2 minutes, during which time the lungs eliminate or retain carbon dioxide in direct relation to arterial pH. While the respiratory system cannot correct imbalances completely, it is 50%-75% effective.

RENAL SYSTEM

This system regulates acid-base balance by increasing or decreasing bicarbonate concentration in body fluids. This is accomplished through a series of complex reactions that involve H^+ secretion, Na^+ reabsorption, HCO_3^- conservation, and ammonia synthesis for excretion in the urine. Although the kidneys' response to an abnormal pH is slow—several hours to days—healthy kidneys are able to adjust the imbalance to normal because of their ability to excrete large quantities of excess bicarbonate and H^+ from the body.

ARTERIAL BLOOD GAS ANALYSIS

1. pH: Measures H^+ concentration to reflect acid-base status of the blood. Values reflect whether arterial pH is normal (7.40), acidic (<7.40), or alkalotic (>7.40). Because of the ability of compensatory mechanisms to "normalize" the pH, a near-normal value does not exclude the possibility of an acid-base disturbance.
2. $Paco_2$: Partial pressure of carbon dioxide in the arteries. It is the respiratory component of acid-base regulation and is adjusted by changes in the rate and depth of pulmonary ventilation. Hypercapnia ($Paco_2$ >45 mm Hg) signals alveolar hypoventilation and respiratory acidosis. Hyperventilation results in a $Paco_2$ <35 mm Hg and respiratory alkalosis. Respiratory compensation occurs rapidly in metabolic acid-base disturbances. If any abnormality in $Paco_2$ exists, it is important to analyze pH and

---

Normal blood gas values

Blood gas analysis usually is based on arterial sampling. Venous values are given as a reference.

Arterial values	Venous values
pH: 7.35-7.45	pH: 7.36
$Paco_2$: 35-45 mm Hg	Pco_2: 46 mm Hg
Pao_2: 80-95 mm Hg	Po_2: 40 mm Hg
Saturation: 95%-99%	Saturation: 75%
Base excess: + or − 1	
Serum bicarbonate (HCO_3^-): 22-26 mEq/L*	

---

*Although serum bicarbonate is a buffer, it usually is reported as "CO_2 content" or "total CO_2" and not as serum bicarbonate. The serum HCO_3^- concentration usually is obtained separately from ABG analysis and is critical in the determination of acid-base status, although this value may be calculated from $Paco_2$ and pH results *via* the ABG analysis. Values should be obtained with the initial assessment and daily thereafter.

HCO_3^- parameters to determine if the alteration in $Paco_2$ is the result of a primary respiratory disturbance or a compensatory response to a metabolic acid-base abnormality.

3. **Pao_2**: Partial pressure of oxygen in the arteries. It has no primary role in acid-base regulation if it is within normal limits. The presence of hypoxemia with a Pao_2 <60 mm Hg can lead to anaerobic metabolism, resulting in lactic acid production and metabolic acidosis. There is a normal decline in Pao_2 in the aged.
4. **Saturation**: Measures the degree to which hgb is saturated by oxygen. When the Pao_2 falls below 60, there is a large drop in saturation.
5. **HCO_3^-**: Serum bicarbonate is the major renal component of acid-base regulation. It is excreted or regenerated by the kidneys to maintain a normal acid-base environment. Decreased bicarbonate levels (<22 mEq/L) are indicative of metabolic acidosis; elevated bicarbonate levels (>26 mEq/L) reflect metabolic alkalosis—either as a primary metabolic disorder or as a compensatory alteration in response to respiratory acidosis.
6. **Base excess or deficit**: Indicates, in general terms, the amount of blood buffer (hgb and plasma bicarbonate) present. Abnormally high values reflect alkalosis; low values reflect acidosis.

STEP-BY-STEP GUIDE TO ABG ANALYSIS

A systemic step-by-step analysis is critical to the accurate interpretation of ABG values. For further information, see Tables 11-5 and 11-6.

1. **Step one**: Determine if pH is normal. If abnormal, identify whether it is on the acidotic (<7.35) or alkalotic (>7.45) side of normal.
2. **Step two**: Check $Paco_2$ and HCO_3^- to determine which value corresponds to the pH value. For example, if the pH is acidotic, which value most closely reflects acidosis? This determines whether the primary problem is respiratory or metabolic in nature.
3. **Step three**: If both $Paco_2$ and HCO_3^- are abnormal, the value that deviates the most from normal points to the primary disturbance responsible for the altered pH. A mixed metabolic-respiratory disturbance or compensatory elements may be present.
4. **Step four**: Check Pao_2 and oxygen saturation to determine whether they are decreased, normal, or increased. Decreased Pao_2 and O_2 saturation can lead to lactic acidosis and may signal the need for increased concentrations of oxygen. Conversely, high Pao_2 may be indicative of the need to decrease delivered concentrations of oxygen.

Part Two CARING FOR ADULTS WITH ACID-BASE IMBALANCES

Acute respiratory acidosis

Respiratory acidosis (hypercapnia) occurs secondary to alveolar hypoventilation and results in an elevated $Paco_2$. $Paco_2$ derangements are direct reflections of the degree of

TABLE 11-5 **ABG comparisons of acid-base disorders**

		Alkalosis			Acidosis		
		$Paco_2$	pH	HCO_3^-	$Paco_2$	pH	HCO_3^-
Simple	Respiratory	25	7.6	24	50	7.15	25
	Metabolic	44	7.54	36	38↑	7.20↓	15↓
Compensated	Respiratory	25	7.54	21	66	7.37	34
	Metabolic	50	7.42	31	23↓	7.28↓	9
Mixed Disorder		40	7.56	38	50	7.2	20

TABLE 11-6 Quick assessment guide to acid-base imbalances

Acid-base imbalance	pH	$Paco_2$	HCO_3^-	Clinical signs and symptoms	Common causes
Acute respiratory acidosis	Decreased	Increased	No change	Tachycardia, tachypnea, diaphoresis, headache, restlessness leading to lethargy and coma, cyanosis, dysrhythmias, hypotension	Acute respiratory failure, cardiopulmonary disease, drug overdose, chest wall trauma, asphyxiation, CNS trauma/lesions, impaired muscles of respiration
Chronic respiratory acidosis (compensated)	Decreased	Increased	Increased*	Dyspnea and tachypnea with increase in CO_2 retention that exceeds compensatory ability; progression to lethargy, confusion, and coma	COPD, extreme obesity (Pickwickian syndrome), superimposed infection on COPD

Acute respiratory alkalosis	Increased	No change (a decrease will occur if condition has been present for hours, providing that renal function is adequate)	Paresthesias, especially of the fingers; dizziness	Hyperventilation, salicylate poisoning, hypoxia (e.g., with pneumonia, pulmonary edema, pulmonary thromboembolism), gram-negative sepsis, CNS lesion, decreased lung compliance, inappropriate mechanical ventilation
Chronic respiratory alkalosis	Increased	Decreased*	No symptoms	Hepatic failure; CNS lesion
Acute metabolic acidosis	Decreased	Decreased*	Tachypnea leading to Kussmaul respirations, hypotension, cold and clammy skin, coma, and dysrhythmias	Shock, cardiopulmonary arrest (secondary to lactic acid production), ketoacidosis (e.g., diabetes, starvation, alcohol abuse), acute renal failure, ingestion of acids (e.g., salicylates), diarrhea
Chronic metabolic acidosis	Decreased	Decreased (not as much as acute type)*	Fatigue, anorexia, malaise; symptoms may be related to chronic disease process as well as acidosis	Chronic renal failure

Continued.

TABLE 11-6 Quick assessment guide to acid-base imbalances—cont'd

Acid-base imbalance	pH	$Paco_2$	HCO_3^-	Clinical signs and symptoms	Common causes
Acute metabolic alkalosis	Increased	Increased (can be as great as 60)*	Increased	Muscular weakness and hyporeflexia (due to severe hypokalemia), dysrhythmias, apathy, confusion, and stupor	Volume depletion (Cl^- depletion) as a result of vomiting, gastric drainage, diuretic use, posthypercapnia. Hyperadrenocorticism (e.g., Cushing's syndrome), aldosteronism, severe potassium depletion, excessive alkali intake
Chronic metabolic alkalosis	Increased	Increased*	Increased	Usually asymptomatic	Upper GI losses through continuous drainage; correction of hypercapnia if Na^+ and K^+ depletion remains uncorrected

*Compensatory response

ventilatory function or dysfunction. The degree to which the increased $Paco_2$ alters the pH depends on the rapidity of onset and the body's ability to compensate through the blood buffer and renal systems. The acidemia may develop rapidly because of the delay (hours or days) before renal compensation occurs.

ASSESSMENT

Signs and symptoms: Dyspnea; asterixis; restlessness leading to lethargy, confusion, and coma.

Physical assessment: Increased heart and respiratory rates, diaphoresis, and cyanosis (a late sign). Severe hypercapnia may cause cerebral vasodilatation, resulting in increased ICP with papilledema. Another finding may be dilated conjunctival and facial blood vessels.

History and risk factors

1. *Acute respiratory disease:* In *severe* respiratory disease or respiratory fatigue.
2. *Overdose of drugs:* Oversedation with drugs that cause respiratory center depression.
3. *Chest wall trauma:* Flail chest, pneumothorax.
4. *CNS trauma/lesions:* Can lead to depression of respiratory center.
5. *Asphyxiation:* Mechanical obstruction; anaphylaxis.
6. *Impaired respiratory muscles:* Can occur with hypokalemia, hyperkalemia, polio, Guillain-Barré syndrome.
7. *Cardiopulmonary arrest.*
8. *Iatrogenic:* Inappropriate mechanical ventilation (increased dead space, insufficient rate or volume); high Fio_2 in the presence of chronic CO_2 retention.

DIAGNOSTIC TESTS

1. *ABG analysis:* Aids in diagnosis and determination of severity of respiratory acidosis. $Paco_2$ will be >45 mm Hg and pH will be <7.35.
2. *Serum bicarbonate:* HCO_3^- reflects metabolic and base balance. Initially, HCO_3^- values will be normal (22-26 mEq/L) unless a mixed disorder is present.
3. *Serum electrolytes:* Usually not altered; depend on etiology of respiratory acidosis.
4. *Chest x-ray:* Determines presence of underlying respiratory disease.
5. *Drug screen:* Determines presence and quantity of drug if patient is suspected of taking an overdose.

MEDICAL MANAGEMENT

1. Restoration of normal acid-base balance: Accomplished by supporting respiratory function. If $Paco_2$ is >50-60 mm Hg and clinical signs, such as cyanosis and lethargy, are present, the patient usually requires intubation and mechanical ventilation. Generally, use of bicarbonate is avoided because of the risk of alkalosis when the respiratory disturbance has been corrected. Although a life-threatening pH must be corrected to an acceptable level promptly, a normal pH is not the immediate goal.
2. Treatment of underlying disorder.

NURSING DIAGNOSES AND INTERVENTIONS

Nursing diagnoses and interventions are specific to the pathophysiologic process. See appropriate section(s) in this and other chapters for diagnoses such as **Impaired gas exchange, Ineffective airway clearance,** and **Activity intolerance.** A list of nursing diagnoses used in this manual begins on p. 717.

Chronic respiratory acidosis (compensated)

This disorder occurs in chronic pulmonary diseases (e.g., emphysema and especially in chronic bronchitis) in which effective alveolar ventilation is decreased and a ventilation-perfusion mismatch is present. Chronic hypercapnia also can occur with obesity. In patients with a chronic lung disease, a nearly normal pH can be seen if renal function is normal, even if the $Paco_2$ is as high as 60 mm Hg. Chronic compensatory metabolic alkalosis (serum HCO_3^- >26 mEq/L) occurs and maintains an acceptable acid-base environment, which results in compensated respiratory acidosis and a normal or near normal pH. Patients with chronic lung disease can experience acute rises in $Paco_2$ secondary to superimposed disease states such as pneumonia. If the chronic compensatory mechanisms in place (e.g., elevated HCO_3^-) are inadequate to meet the sudden increase in $Paco_2$, decompensation may occur with a resultant decrease in pH.

ASSESSMENT

Signs and symptoms: If the $Paco_2$ does not exceed the body's ability to compensate, no specific findings will be noted. If $Paco_2$ rises rapidly from the patient's baseline level, the following may occur: dyspnea, asterixis, agitation, and insomnia progressing to somnolence and coma.

Physical assessment: Tachypnea, cyanosis. Depending on underlying pathophysiology, edema may be present secondary to right ventricular failure.

History and risk factors

1. *COPD:* Especially predominant in chronic bronchitis.
2. *Extreme obesity:* Pickwickian syndrome.
3. *Exposure to pulmonary toxins:* Occupational risk; pollution.

DIAGNOSTIC TESTS

1. *ABG values:* Although the $Paco_2$ will be elevated (usually in the range of 45-55 mm Hg), the pH will be on the acidic (low) side of normal in patients who are not experiencing acute pulmonary infection. If the $Paco_2$ has increased abruptly from baseline value, a pH lower than expected may be seen.
2. *Serum electrolytes:* Serum bicarbonate (HCO_3^-) is especially helpful in determining the level of metabolic compensation that has occurred (i.e., HCO_3^- increased with a near normal pH if fully compensated). This information is useful in identifying "mixed" acid-base disturbances because the HCO_3^- is expected to be elevated in chronic respiratory acidosis. If the HCO_3^- is normal or low, this could be diagnostic of a second pathologic process concurrent with the first.
3. *Chest x-ray:* Determines extent of underlying pulmonary disease and identifies further pathologic changes that may be responsible for acute exacerbation, for example, pneumonia.
4. *EKG:* Identifies cardiac involvement from COPD. For example, right-sided heart failure is a complication of chronic bronchitis.
5. *Sputum culture:* Determines presence of pathogens causing an acute exacerbation of a chronic pulmonary disease (e.g., pneumonia) present in a patient with COPD.

MEDICAL MANAGEMENT

1. Oxygen therapy: Used cautiously in patients with chronic CO_2 retention for whom hypoxia, rather than hypercapnia, stimulates ventilation. Patient may require intubation and mechanical ventilation for stupor and coma precipitated by oxygen if drive to breathe is eliminated by high concentrations of oxygen.
2. Pharmacotherapy: Bronchodilators and antibiotics, as indicated. Narcotics and sedatives can depress the respiratory center and are avoided unless patient is intubated and mechanically ventilated.
3. IV fluids: Maintain adequate hydration for mobilizing pulmonary secretions.
4. Chest physiotherapy: Aids in expectoration of sputum. Includes postural drainage if

hypersecretions are present. Assess patient closely during this procedure because it may be poorly tolerated, especially the postural drainage component.

NURSING DIAGNOSES AND INTERVENTIONS

Impaired gas exchange related to trapping of CO_2 secondary to pulmonary tissue destruction (appropriate for the patient with COPD)

Desired outcome: ABG values reflect a $Paco_2$ and pH within acceptable range, based on patient's underlying pulmonary disease.

1. Monitor serial ABG results to assess patient's response to therapy. Report significant findings to MD: an increasing $Paco_2$ and a decreasing pH.
2. Assess and document patient's respiratory status: respiratory rate and rhythm, exertional effort, and breath sounds. Compare pretreatment findings to posttreatment (e.g., oxygen therapy, physiotherapy, or medications) findings for evidence of improvement.
3. Assess and document patient's LOC. If $Paco_2$ increases, be alert to subtle, progressive changes in mental status. A common progression is agitation → insomnia → somnolence → coma. To avoid a comatose state secondary to rising CO_2 levels, always evaluate the "arousability" of a patient with elevated $Paco_2$ who appears to be sleeping. Notify MD if patient is difficult to arouse.
4. Ensure appropriate delivery of prescribed oxygen therapy. Assess patient's respiratory status after every change in Fio_2. Patients with chronic CO_2 retention may be very sensitive to increases in Fio_2, resulting in depressed ventilatory drive.
5. Assess for presence of bowel sounds and monitor for gastric distention, which can impede movement of the diaphragm and restrict ventilatory effort further.
6. Encourage use of pursed-lip breathing (inhalation through nose, with slow exhalation through pursed lips), which helps airways to remain open and allows for better air excursion. Optimally, this technique will diminish air entrapment in the lungs and make respiratory effort more efficient.

Acute respiratory alkalosis (hypocapnia)

Respiratory alkalosis occurs as a result of an increase in the rate of alveolar ventilation (alveolar hyperventilation). It is defined as $Paco_2$ <35 mm Hg. Acute alveolar hyperventilation most frequently results from anxiety and is commonly referred to as "hyperventilation syndrome." In addition, numerous physiologic disorders (see "History and risk factors," below) can cause acute hypocapnia, which results in increased pH. To compensate for increased CO_2 loss and the resultant base excess, hydrogen ions are released from tissue buffers, which in turn lowers plasma bicarbonate concentration, modifying the rise in pH to a small degree.

ASSESSMENT

Signs and symptoms: Lightheadedness, anxiety, paresthesias, circumoral numbness. In extreme alkalosis, confusion, tetany, syncope, and seizures may occur.

Physical assessment: Increased rate and depth of respirations.

History and risk factors

1. *Anxiety:* Patient is often unaware of hyperventilation.
2. *Acute hypoxia:* Pulmonary disorders (e.g., pneumonia, pulmonary edema, and pulmonary thromboembolism) that cause hypoxia, which stimulates the ventilatory effort.
3. *Hypermetabolic states:* Fever; sepsis, especially gram-negative induced septicemia.
4. *Salicylate intoxication.*
5. *Excessive mechanical ventilation.*
6. *CNS trauma:* May result in damage to respiratory center.

DIAGNOSTIC TESTS

1. *ABG values:* $Paco_2$ <35 mm Hg and pH >7.45 will be present. A decreased Pao_2, along with the clinical picture (e.g., pneumonia, pulmonary edema, pulmonary embolism, and ARDS), may help diagnose etiology of the respiratory alkalosis.
2. *Serum electrolytes:* Determine presence of metabolic acid-base disorders.
3. *EKG:* Detects cardiac dysrhythmias, which may be present with alkalosis.

MEDICAL MANAGEMENT

1. Treatment of underlying disorder.
2. Reassurance or sedation: If anxiety is the cause of decreased $Paco_2$. If symptoms are severe, it may be necessary for patient to rebreathe CO_2 through an oxygen mask with an attached CO_2 reservoir. If this is not available, the patient can instead breathe into a brown paper bag, which acts as a CO_2 reservoir.
3. Oxygen therapy: If hypoxia is the causative factor.
4. Pharmacotherapy: Sedatives and tranquilizers may be given for anxiety-induced respiratory alkalosis.

NURSING DIAGNOSES AND INTERVENTIONS

Nursing diagnoses and interventions are specific to the pathophysiologic process. See appropriate nursing diagnoses (e.g., **Ineffective breathing pattern** related to hyperventilation) in this and other chapters. A list of nursing diagnoses used in this manual begins on p. 717.

Chronic respiratory alkalosis

This is a state of chronic hypocapnia, which stimulates the renal compensatory response and results in a decrease in plasma bicarbonate. Maximal renal compensatory response requires several days to occur.

ASSESSMENT

Signs and symptoms: Individuals with chronic respiratory alkalosis usually are asymptomatic.

Physical assessment: Increased respiratory rate and depth.

History and risk factors

1. *Cerebral disease:* Tumor, encephalitis.
2. *Chronic hepatic insufficiency.*
3. *Pregnancy.*
4. *Chronic hypoxia:* Adaptation to high altitude; cyanotic heart disease; lung disease resulting in decreased compliance (e.g., fibrosis).

DIAGNOSTIC TESTS

1. *ABG values:* $Paco_2$ will be <35 mm Hg, with a nearly normal pH; Pao_2 may be decreased if hypoxia is the causative factor.
2. *Serum electrolytes:* Probably will be normal, with the exception of plasma bicarbonate (HCO_3^-), which will decrease as renal compensation occurs.
3. *Phosphate levels:* Hypophosphatemia (as low as 0.5 mg/dl) may be seen with intense hyperventilation.

MEDICAL MANAGEMENT

1. Treatment of underlying cause.
2. Oxygen therapy: If hypoxia is present and identified as causative factor in respiratory alkalosis.

NURSING DIAGNOSES AND INTERVENTIONS

Nursing diagnoses and interventions are specific to the pathophysiologic process. See appropriate medical disorders and nursing diagnoses in this and other chapters. A list of nursing diagnoses used in this manual begins on p. 717 in the appendix.

Acute metabolic acidosis

Metabolic acidosis is caused by a primary decrease in plasma bicarbonate, as reflected by a serum bicarbonate of <22 mEq/L with a pH <7.35. The decrease in serum bicarbonate is caused by one of the following mechanisms: (1) increase in the concentration of hydrogen ions in the form of nonvolatile acids (e.g., ketoacidosis associated with diabetes and alcoholism; lactic acidosis); (2) loss of alkali (e.g., severe diarrhea, intestinal malabsorption); or (3) decreased acid excretion by the kidneys (e.g., acute and chronic renal failure). Respiratory compensation occurs rapidly, as manifested by lowering of the $Paco_2$, which may be reduced to as much as 10-15 mm Hg. The most important mechanism for ridding the body of excess H^+ is the increase in acid excretion by the kidneys. However, nonvolatile acids may accumulate more rapidly than they can be neutralized by the body's buffers, compensated for by the respiratory system, or excreted by the kidneys.

ASSESSMENT

Signs and symptoms: Findings vary, depending on underlying disease states and severity of acid-base disturbance. There may be changes in LOC that range from fatigue and confusion to stupor and coma.

Physical assessment: Tachypnea leading to alveolar hyperventilation (Kussmaul's respirations), decreased BP, and cold and clammy skin as acidosis worsens. Shock may ensue.

History and risk factors

1. *Renal disease:* Acute renal failure, renal tubular acidosis.
2. *Ketoacidosis:* Diabetes mellitus, alcoholism, starvation.
3. *Lactic acidosis:* Respiratory or circulatory failure, drugs and toxins, hereditary disorders, septic shock. It can be associated with other disease states, such as leukemia, pancreatitis, bacterial infection, and uncontrolled diabetes mellitus.
4. *Poisonings and drug toxicity:* Salicylates, methanol, ethylene glycol, ammonium chloride.
5. *Loss of alkali:* Draining wounds (e.g., pancreatic fistulas), diarrhea, ureterostomy.

DIAGNOSTIC TESTS

1. *ABG values:* Determine pH (usually <7.35) and degree of respiratory compensation as reflected by $Paco_2$, which usually is <35 mm Hg.
2. *Serum bicarbonate:* Determines presence of metabolic acidosis (HCO_3^- <22 mEq/ L).
3. *Serum electrolytes:* Elevated potassium may be present because of the exchange of intracellular potassium for hydrogen ions in the body's attempt to normalize acid-base environment.
4. *EKG:* Detects dysrhythmias, which may be caused by acidosis or hyperkalemia. Changes seen with hyperkalemia include peaked T waves, depressed ST segment, decreased size of R waves, decreased or absent P waves, widened QRS complex.

MEDICAL MANAGEMENT

1. Sodium bicarbonate ($NaHCO_3$): Indicated when arterial pH is ≤7.2. The usual mode of delivery is IV drip: 2-3 ampules (44.5 mEq/ampule) in 1,000 ml D_5W, although

$NaHCO_3$ frequently is given by IV push in emergencies. Concentration depends on severity of the acidosis and presence of any serum sodium disorders. $NaHCO_3$ must be given cautiously to avoid metabolic alkalosis and pulmonary edema secondary to the sodium load.

2. **Potassium replacement:** Usually hyperkalemia is present, but a potassium deficit can occur. If a potassium deficit exists (K^+ <3.5), it must be corrected before $NaHCO_3$ is administered because when the acidosis is corrected, the potassium shifts back to intracellular spaces. Therefore, this could result in serum hypokalemia with serious consequences, such as cardiac irritability with fatal dysrhythmias and generalized muscle weakness. See "Hypokalemia," p. 555, for more information.

3. **Treatment of underlying disorder**
   □ *Diabetes ketoacidosis:* Insulin and fluids. If acidosis is severe (with a pH of <7.1 or HCO_3^- 6-8 mEq/L), sodium bicarbonate may be necessary.
   □ *Alcoholism-related ketoacidosis:* Glucose and saline.
   □ *Diarrhea:* Usually occurs in association with other fluid and electrolyte disturbances; correction addresses concurrent imbalances.
   □ *Acute renal failure:* Hemodialysis or peritoneal dialysis to maintain an adequate level of plasma bicarbonate.
   □ *Renal tubular acidosis:* May require modest amounts (<100 mEq/day) of bicarbonate.
   □ *Poisoning and drug toxicity:* Treatment depends on drug ingested or infused.
   □ *Lactic acidosis:* Correction of underlying disorder.

NURSING DIAGNOSES AND INTERVENTIONS

Nursing diagnoses and interventions are specific to the pathophysiologic process. In addition to **Alterations in oral mucous membrane** related to mouth breathing (see appendix, p. 717, for this and other nursing diagnoses used in this manual), refer to nursing diagnoses and interventions in the following sections: "Acute Renal Failure," p. 118, "Diabetic Ketoacidosis," p. 301, and "Caring for the Patient with Cancer and Other Life-Disrupting Disorders," p. 690.

Chronic metabolic acidosis

Most often, this condition is seen with chronic renal failure in which the kidneys' ability to excrete acids (endogenous and exogenous) is exceeded by acid production and ingestion. The acidosis usually is mild in the initial stage, with HCO_3^- 18-22 mEq/L and a pH of 7.35. Treatment is indicated when serum bicarbonate levels reach 15 mEq/L. Respiratory compensation does occur, but to a limited degree. A modest decrease in $Paco_2$ will be noted on ABG values.

ASSESSMENT

Signs and symptoms: Usually patient is asymptomatic, although fatigue, malaise, and anorexia may be present in relation to underlying disease.

History and risk factors: Chronic renal failure.

DIAGNOSTIC TESTS

1. *ABG values:* $Paco_2$ will be <35 mm Hg; pH will be <7.35.
2. *Serum bicarbonate:* Will be <22 mEq/L (usually 18-21 mEq/L). With severe acidosis, it will be ≤15 mEq/L.
3. *Serum electrolytes:* Serum calcium level is checked before treatment of acidosis is initiated to prevent tetany induced by hypocalcemia (caused by a decrease in ionized calcium). Serum potassium level should be monitored after acidosis has been corrected to detect hypokalemia, as potassium shifts back into the cells.

MEDICAL MANAGEMENT

1. **Alkalizing agents:** For serum bicarbonate levels <15 mEq/L, oral alkali are administered (sodium bicarbonate or sodium citrate). They are used cautiously to prevent fluid overload and tetany caused by hypocalcemia.
2. **Oral phosphates:** Given if hypophosphatemia is present (not common with chronic renal failure, but may result from overuse of phosphate binders given to treat hyperphosphatemia).
3. **Hemodialysis or peritoneal dialysis:** If indicated by chronic renal failure or other disease processes. See discussion, p. 126.

NURSING DIAGNOSES AND INTERVENTIONS

Nursing diagnoses and interventions are specific to the underlying pathophysiologic process. See renal chapter, p. 102, in particular, and appendix, p. 717, for a list of nursing diagnoses used in this manual.

Acute metabolic alkalosis

This disorder results in an elevated serum bicarbonate level (up to 45-50 mEq/L) as a result of hydrogen ion loss or excess alkali intake. A compensatory increase in $Paco_2$ (up to 50-55 mm Hg) will be seen. Respiratory compensation is limited because of hypoxia, which develops secondary to decreased alveolar ventilation.

ASSESSMENT

Signs and symptoms: Muscular weakness, neuromuscular instability, and hyporeflexia secondary to accompanying hypokalemia. Decrease in GI tract motility may result in an ileus. Severe alkalosis can result in apathy, confusion, and stupor.

History and risk factors

1. *Clinical circumstances associated with volume/chloride depletion:* Vomiting or gastric drainage.
2. *Posthypercapneic alkalosis:* Occurs when chronic CO_2 retention is corrected rapidly.
3. *Excessive alkali intake:* May be iatrogenic from overcorrection of metabolic acidosis (frequently seen during CPR).
4. *Diuretic therapy.*

DIAGNOSTIC TESTS

1. *ABG values:* Determine severity of alkalosis and response to therapy.
2. *Serum bicarbonate:* Values will be elevated to >26 mEq/L.
3. *Serum electrolytes:* Usually, serum potassium will be low (<4.0 mEq/L) as will serum chloride (<95 mEq/L).
4. *EKG:* To assess for dysrhythmias, especially if profound hypokalemia or alkalosis is present.

MEDICAL MANAGEMENT

Management will depend on the underlying disorder. Mild or moderate metabolic alkalosis usually does not require specific therapeutic interventions.

1. **Saline infusion:** Normal saline infusion may correct volume (chloride) deficit in patients with gastric alkalosis secondary to gastric losses. Metabolic alkalosis is difficult to correct if hypovolemia and chloride deficit are not corrected.
2. **Potassium chloride (KCl):** Indicated for patients with low potassium levels. KCl is preferred over other potassium salts because chloride losses can be replaced simultaneously.
3. **Sodium and potassium chloride:** Effective for posthypercapneic alkalosis. If adequate

amounts of chloride and potassium are not available, renal excretion of excess bicarbonate is impaired and metabolic alkalosis continues.

NURSING DIAGNOSES AND INTERVENTIONS

Nursing diagnoses and interventions are specific to the underlying pathophysiologic process. See the renal chapter, p. 102, in particular, and the appendix, p. 717, for a list of nursing diagnoses used in this manual.

Chronic metabolic alkalosis

Chronic metabolic alkalosis results in a pH >7.45. $Paco_2$ will be elevated (>45 mm Hg) to compensate for the loss of H^+ or excess serum HCO_3^-.

ASSESSMENT

Signs and symptoms: Patient may be asymptomatic. With severe potassium depletion and profound alkalosis, patient may experience weakness, neuromuscular instability, and decrease in GI tract motility, which can result in ileus.

History and risk factors

1. *Diuretic use:* Thiazide diuretics cause a loss of chloride, potassium, and hydrogen ions. Massive depletion of potassium stores with loss of up to 1,000 mEq, which is one-third of total body potassium, may occur, causing profound hypokalemia (K^+ ≤ 2.0).
2. *Hyperadrenocorticism:* Cushing's syndrome, primary aldosteronism. This is not a chloride deficit but a chronic loss of potassium, which can lead to total body depletion of potassium with profound hypokalemia (K^+ ≤ 2.0 mEq/L).
3. *Chronic vomiting or chronic GI losses through GI suction.*
4. *Milk alkali syndrome:* An infrequent cause of metabolic alkalosis. Hypercalcemic nephropathy and alkalosis develop secondary to excessive intake of absorbable alkali.

DIAGNOSTIC TESTS

1. <u>ABG values:</u> Determine severity of acid-base imbalance.
2. <u>Serum bicarbonate:</u> Will be >26 mEq/L.
3. <u>Serum electrolytes:</u> Usually, potassium will be profoundly low (may be ≤ 2.0 mEq/L). Chloride may be <95 mEq/L. Magnesium may be <1.5 mEq/L in both renal system abnormalities.
4. <u>EKG:</u> Frequent PVCs or U waves may be present.

MEDICAL MANAGEMENT

The goal is to correct the underlying acid-base disorder *via* the following interventions:
1. Fluid management: If volume depletion exists, normal saline infusions are given.
2. Potassium replacement: If a chloride deficit also is present, potassium chloride is the drug of choice. If a chloride deficit does not exist, other potassium salts are acceptable.
   □ *IV potassium:* If the patient is on a cardiac monitor, up to 20 mEq/hr of potassium chloride is given for serious hypokalemia. Concentrated doses of KCl (>40 mEq/L) require administration through a central venous line because of the potential for blood vessel irritation.
   □ *Oral potassium:* Tastes *very* unpleasant. Most patients can tolerate only 15 mEq per glass, with a maximum daily dose of 60-80 mEq. Slow-release potassium tablets are an acceptable form of KCl. All forms of KCl may be irritating to gastric mucosa.
   □ *Dietary:* Normal diet contains 3g or 75 mEq of potassium, but not in the form of

potassium chloride. Dietary supplementation of potassium is not effective if a concurrent chloride deficit is also present.
3. **Potassium-sparing diuretics:** May be added to treatment if thiazide diuretics are the cause of hypokalemia and metabolic alkalosis.
4. **Identify and correct cause of hyperadrenocorticism.**

NURSING DIAGNOSES AND INTERVENTIONS

Nursing diagnoses and interventions are specific to the underlying pathophysiologic process. See the renal chapter, p. 102, in particular, and the appendix, p. 717, for a list of nursing diagnoses used in this manual.

Section Three   BURNS

The skin is complex and is the largest organ of the body. It protects against infection, prevents loss of body fluids, controls body temperature, functions as an excretory and sensory organ, aids in activating vitamin D, and influences body image. Burns, the most dramatic injury that can occur to skin, are classified according to the causative agent: thermal (scald, contact, flame), electrical, chemical, and radiation. Extent and depth of the burn injury depend on the *intensity* and *duration of exposure* to the offending agent. The American Burn Association (ABA) has developed an injury severity grading system that categorizes burns as minor, moderate, and major (see Table 11-7). The ABA advocates that major burns be treated in a burn center or facility with expertise in burn care. Moderate burns usually require hospitalization, though not necessarily in a burn unit, and minor burns are often treated in the emergency room or on an outpatient basis.

Damage to the skin frequently is defined in terms of partial-thickness and full-thickness injury, which correspond to the various layers of the skin. Partial-thickness injuries are further differentiated into superficial and deep partial-thickness categories. *Superficial partial-thickness injury,* commonly referred to as "first-degree" burn (e.g., sunburn) damages the epidermis, which is composed of keratinized fiber that is replenished continuously from underlying desquamated cells migrating to the superficial layer; forms a protective barrier between host and environment; and heals within 24-72 hours. *Deep partial-thickness injury,* called a "second-degree" burn, involves varying levels of the dermis, which contains structures essential to skin function (e.g., sweat and sebaceous glands, hair follicles, sensory and motor nerves, and capillary network); and heals within 3-35 days, depending on depth, because epidermal elements germinate and migrate until the epidermal surface is restored. *Full-thickness injury,* a "third-degree"

TABLE 11-7 **ABA classification system**

Magnitude of burn injury	Second-degree		Third-degree		Complications, poor risk, fractures, other trauma
	Adult % BSA*	Children % BSA	Adults and children % BSA	Special location†	
Major	>25	>20	>10	+	+
Moderate	15-25	10-20	<10	−	−
Minor	<15	<10	<2	−	−

*BSA: body surface area.
†Special location: Hands, face, eyes, ears, feet, or genitalia.

burn, exposes the poorly vascularized fat layer, which contains adipose tissue, roots of sweat glands, and hair follicles; and destroys all epidermal elements. Wounds <4 cm in diameter are allowed to heal by granulation and migration of healthy epithelium from wound margins; larger wounds are closed *via* skin grafting.

ASSESSMENT

The extent of the burn wound is estimated quickly by use of the "rule of nines." For adults, each body area is assigned a percentage of surface area to establish the degree of involvement: head and neck 9%, each upper extremity 9%, anterior chest 18%, posterior chest 18%, each lower extremity 18%, and the genitalia 1%. For odd-shaped burns, the size of the victim's palm usually equals 1% of the total BSA. A chart that accounts for changes in the size of body parts occurring with growth is recommended for children and is the most accurate method of determining the extent of the burn.

Respiratory system: Singed nasal hairs; burns in perioral area or neck; burns of oral or pharyngeal mucous membranes; change in voice or coughing up of soot; inelastic, constricting, tight eschar of neck or chest; swelling of membranes of nasooropharyngeal passage.
□ *Clinical indicators:* Crackles (rales), rhonchi, stridor, severe hoarseness, hacking cough, labored breathing, dyspnea, tachypnea, and possible altered LOC, depending on degree of hypoxia.
Note: Physical evidence of respiratory compromise may be absent in spite of marked pulmonary injury.
□ *Risk factors:* History of having been burned in a confined area. Patients with preexisting cardiac or respiratory condition and those who are heavy smokers are most susceptible to respiratory complications associated with smoke inhalation.

Cutaneous system: Increased evaporative water loss and hypothermia caused by impaired skin integrity. To determine burn wound severity, see Table 11-8.
Clinical indicators: See Table 11-9, Characteristics of Burn Wound Depth. **Note:** True depth of the burn may not manifest for 24-72 hours post-burn injury.

Cardiovascular system: There will be third spacing of fluids with decreased circulatory volume proportional to extent and depth of injury caused by increased capillary permeability, decreased vascular colloid osmotic pressure, and a deranged capillary hydrostatic pressure. Patient may have complaints of tingling or numbness in extremities, dry mucous membranes, and thirst. In response to the burn insult, there is an increase in catecholamine, cortisol, renin-angiotensin, antidiuretic hormone, and aldosterone production as the body struggles to retain sodium and water.
□ *Clinical indicators:* Edema formation; skin temperature and color changes; decreased or absent peripheral pulses and delayed capillary refill caused by compromised blood flow occurring with circumferential burns of extremities; elevated serum potassium (first 24-36 hours post-burn) secondary to hemolysis of cells; hemoconcentration; decreased hemoglobin; tachycardia; hypotension; and decreased CVP. Hypoproteinuria may be present due to escape of proteins into the interstitial space. In addition, pa-

TABLE 11-8   Factors determining burn severity

Extent	Severity dependent on intensity and duration of exposure
Depth	Severity dependent on intensity and duration of exposure
Age	Patients <2 years old and >60 years of age
Medical history	Preexisting conditions such as heart disease, chronic renal failure
Body part	Special burn areas: hands, face, eyes, ears, feet, and genitalia
Complications	Burns with concomitant trauma (i.e., fractures)

TABLE 11-9 Characteristics of burn wound depth

	Partial-thickness	Full-thickness
Cause	Flash, flame, ultraviolet (sunburn), hot liquid or solid, chemicals, radiation	Flame, hot liquid or solid, chemical, electrical, radiation
Surface appearance	*Superficial:* Dry, no blisters or edema *Deep:* Moist blebs, blisters, edema, oozing of plasma-like fluid	Dry, leathery, eschar; thrombosed blood vessels may be visible
Color	Cherry red to mottled white; will blanch and refill	Ranges from red to khaki-colored; waxy; charred; does not blanch
Sensation	*Superficial:* Very painful to the touch *Deep:* Extremely sensitive to touch, temperature, and air currents	Anesthetic to touch and temperature because of destruction of sensory nerve endings
Healing	3-35 days	Wounds ≥4 cm must be grafted

tient will have dramatically elevated basal metabolic rate with protein catabolism and increased fat mobilization from fatty acids and triglycerides, resulting in decreased body weight. **Note:** The degree of alteration in the laboratory values and clinical indicators will be proportionate to the percentage of BSA burned.
□ *Risk factors:* Patients with renal disease, diabetes, or preexisting cardiac or respiratory conditions may have complications associated with fluid resuscitation therapy.

Gastrointestinal system: Paralytic ileus associated with or resulting in decreased or absent peristalsis (usually resolves within 72 hours post-burn); development of Curling's ulcer (acute ulceration of stomach or duodenum), a life-threatening complication in burn patients, which is associated with a gastric pH <5 and a positive guaiac stain.
□ *Clinical indicators:* Absence of bowel sounds, stools, flatus; nausea and vomiting in the presence of alcohol intoxication.
□ *Risk factors:* History of peptic ulcer or duodenal ulcer disease, steroid use, hypokalemia, or alcohol abuse.

Renal system: As early intravascular dehydration causes hemoconcentration and oliguria, a high myoglobin or hgb load may be reflected by a dark brown "sludgy" urine. Inadequate fluid resuscitation may lead to acute tubular necrosis and acute renal failure.
□ *Clinical indicators:* Urine output <30 ml/hr; dark, amber, "thick" urine; high urine specific gravity; glycosuria secondary to a decreased glucose tolerance and decreased insulin effectiveness.

In addition, assess for the following:

Wound sepsis: Evaluate for increased rapidity of eschar separation, increased amount of exudate, and isolated pockets containing purulent material, which are all suggestive of burn wound sepsis.
□ *Clinical indicators:* Disappearance of well-defined burn margins; presence of edema, discoloration, superficial ulceration of burned skin at wound margin/skin interface. Granulation tissue may become pale and boggy; focal black, dark brown, or violet areas of discoloration in the wound; partial-thickness burn may change from pink or mottled red to full-thickness necrosis (i.e., sloughing of subcutaneous fat layer); ve-

sicular lesions may appear in healing or healed partial-thickness injury; and there may be erythematous, nodular lesions in unburned skin. In addition, there may be hemorrhagic discoloration of subeschar fat, with remaining eschar spongy and poorly demarcated; cellulitis of unburned skin (common with gram-positive invasion); turquoise-colored, sweet-smelling exudate (with *Pseudomonas* infection); changes in LOC (confusion, disorientation, agitation); labile temperature ranging from 35°-40.5° C (95°-105° F), gastric distention, and paralytic ileus.

- ☐ *Risk factors:* Concomitant injuries (e.g., fractures), long-term steroid therapy, immunosuppression, diabetes mellitus, history of cardiopulmonary disease.

DIAGNOSTIC TESTS

1. *Serial ABG values:* Will demonstrate hypoxemia, hypercapnia, and acidosis with smoke inhalation injury (see previous section, pp. 563-577).
2. *Serial pulse oximetry readings:* Will demonstrate a fall in oxygen saturation with inhalation injury, potentially leading to respiratory distress.
3. *Culture and sensitivity studies:* To evaluate sputum, blood, urine, and wound tissue for evidence of infection. Burn wound sepsis is defined as microorganisms 10^5/g burn wound tissue with active invasion of adjacent, viable, unburned skin. Examples of gram-negative organisms that may be found include *Pseudomonas aeruginosa, Klebsiella, Serratia, E. coli, Enterobacter cloacae.* Less frequently, gram-positive organisms *(Staphylococcus* and *Streptococcus)* and fungal organisms *(Candida* and *Aspergillus)* may be present. **Note:** If a burn wound culture is positive for Group A *Streptococcus,* this may signal the need for an epidemiologic investigation. Contact your facility's infection control nurse or epidemiology department for assistance in evaluating such a culture, especially if more than one patient has a positive culture at approximately the same time.
4. *Urine specimen:* For urinalysis and culture and sensitivity studies. Nitrogen is measured with the return of capillary integrity (3-5 days after the burn injury) and mobilization of third-spaced fluids *via* 24-hour urine collection for total nitrogen, urea nitrogen, and amino acid nitrogen. Large amounts of nitrogen are excreted in the urine secondary to long periods of catabolism during the healing of a burn wound.
5. *Baseline blood work*
   - ☐ *Hct:* Increased secondary to fluid shifts out of the intravascular space.
   - ☐ *Hgb:* Decreased secondary to hemolysis.
   - ☐ *Serum sodium:* Decreased secondary to massive fluid shifts into interstitial spaces.
   - ☐ *Serum potassium:* Elevated due to cell lysis.
   - ☐ *BUN:* Elevated secondary to hypovolemic status.
   - ☐ *Total protein:* Decreased secondary to leakage of plasma proteins into interstitial spaces.
   - ☐ *Creatine phosphokinase (CPK):* Evaluated as an index of muscle damage, so it is particularly important in electrical injuries. The higher the CPK, the more extensive the muscle damage.
6. *EKG:* For baseline evaluation of patient's cardiac status and for comparison should changes occur.

Note: The degree of alteration in the laboratory values will be proportionate to the degree and depth of the burn wound.

MEDICAL MANAGEMENT

1. Humidified oxygen therapy: Treats hypoxemia and prevents drying and sloughing of the mucosal lining of the tracheobronchial tree.
2. Bronchodilators and mucolytic agents: Aid in the removal of secretions.
3. Escharotomy (surgical incision through the eschar or fascia): Relieves respiratory distress secondary to circumferential, full-thickness burns of neck and trunk, or in extremities to lessen pressure from underlying edema and restore adequate perfu-

sion. It may be done at the bedside or in the emergency room. Indications for escharotomy include cyanosis of distal unburned skin, delayed capillary filling, progressive neurologic changes (may mimic compartment syndrome), burns of thorax
that restrict respiratory motion, and weak or absent peripheral pulses.

4. **Fluid resuscitation therapy:** IV fluids (usually lactated Ringer's solution or normal saline) are delivered *via* a large-bore catheter at a high rate of flow to maintain urine
output at a minimum of 30-50 ml/hr. Colloids are avoided during the first 24 hours
post-burn because they can increase edema formation during this period of increased
capillary permeability. **Caution:** Avoid inserting IV catheters into a burned extremity.

5. **In-dwelling urinary catheter:** Enables accurate measurement of urine output.

6. **Nasogastric suction:** Allows aspiration of gastric contents secondary to paralytic ileus
in patients with a ≥30% BSA burn or for those who present with alcohol intoxication.

7. **Tetanus-toxoid prophylaxis:** Given IM to combat *Clostridium tetani,* an anaerobic infection.

8. **Morphine sulfate:** Small doses are given IV for comfort. **Note:** With the onset of
spontaneous diuresis, pain medications (most commonly meperidine or morphine
sulfate) may be given orally or IM. Avoid injecting into burned tissue.

9. **Antacid administration:** Maintains gastric pH >5.0 and prevents development of Curling's ulcer.

10. **High-protein/high-calorie diet:** Achieves nitrogen balance for optimal wound healing. Many formulas are available to determine nutritional requirements and are
based on preburn body weight in kilograms, total body surface area (TBSA)
burned, age, sex, and BMR. Patients unable to meet nutritional requirements for
healing *via* the enteral route are started on TPN by a central line. **Note:** Nutritional
deficiencies generally are not apparent initially unless the patient was malnourished
preinjury.

11. **Multivitamin and mineral supplements:** Vitamins A and C and zinc are especially important for promoting wound healing.

12. **IV antibiotics:** As indicated for specific culture and sensitivity findings.

13. **Wound care:** Cleansing, debridement (manual or surgical), and antimicrobial therapy (i.e., topical agents: Silvadene, povidone iodine, mafenide, silver nitrate, pro-
teolytic enzymes) control bacterial proliferation and provide a wound capable of
producing granulation tissue and a capillary network.

14. **Split-thickness skin grafting:** Provides closure for full-thickness injuries. Biologic
dressings, such as cadaver skin or porcine or amniotic membranes, may be used for
temporary closure prior to autografting.

NURSING DIAGNOSES AND INTERVENTIONS

Impaired gas exchange related to hypoventilation and decreased diffusion of oxygen
secondary to circumferential burns to neck and thorax or swelling of the membranes of
the nasooropharyngeal passage due to smoke inhalation

Desired outcome: Patient exhibits adequate gas exchange as evidenced by Pao_2 ≥80
mm Hg; oxygen saturation ≥95%; RR 12-20 breaths/min with a normal pattern and
depth (eupnea); absence of stridor and other clinical indicators of respiratory dysfunction; and orientation to person, place, and time.

1. Assess and document respiratory status qh, noting rate and depth, breath sounds, and
LOC. Monitor for indicators of upper airway distress (e.g., severe hoarseness, stridor, dyspnea, and [less frequently] CNS depression) and lower airway distress (e.g.,
crackles, rhonchi, hacking cough, and labored and rapid breathing). Notify MD
promptly of all significant findings.

2. Monitor serial ABGs and pulse oximetry readings for decreasing Pao_2 and oxygen
saturation as evidence of worsening hypoxemia.

3. Place patient in high-Fowler's position to enhance respiratory excursion. Reposition
patient from side to side q1-2h to help mobilize secretions and prevent atelectasis.

4. Teach patient the necessity of coughing and deep-breathing exercises q2h, including incentive spirometry.
5. Administer oxygen therapy or bronchodilator treatment (i.e., theophylline, sympathomimetics) as prescribed.
6. As prescribed, administer percussion and postural drainage to facilitate airway clearance (this is contraindicated with fresh skin grafts).

Fluid volume deficit related to decreased circulating volume secondary to leakage of fluid, plasma proteins, and other cellular elements into the interstitial space and loss through the burn wound

Desired outcomes: Patient's circulating volume is restored without signs of fluid overload or excessive edema formation as evidenced by BP 110-120/70-80 mm Hg (or within patient's normal range), peripheral pulses >2+ (on a 0-4+ scale), urine output 30-50 ml/hr, urine specific gravity 1.010-1.030, and CVP 5-12 cm H_2O. Hematocrit is 40%-54% (male) or 37%-47% (female); hemoglobin is 14-18 g/dl (male) or 12-16 g/dl (female); serum sodium is 137-147 mEq/L; and serum potassium is 3.5-5.0 mEq/L.

1. Monitor patient for evidence of fluid volume deficit, including tachycardia, decreased BP, decreased amplitude of peripheral pulses, urine output <30 ml/hr, thirst, and dry mucous membranes.
2. Monitor I&O. Administer fluid therapy as prescribed. Notify MD of urine output <30-50 ml/hr. **Note:** In moderate burn injuries, the indwelling catheter usually is removed with onset of spontaneous diuresis, which usually occurs 3-7 days post-burn.
3. Monitor weight daily; report significant gains or losses. For example, 2 kg acute weight loss may signal a 2 L fluid loss. Following the acute phase, weight loss may be due to catabolism and an increased metabolic rate as the body attempts to heal itself.
4. Monitor urine specific gravity. As fluid resuscitation occurs, urine specific gravity will become normal, reflecting a normovolemic status; conversely, an elevated value occurs with a dehydrated state, and a decreased value reflects an overhydrated state.
5. Monitor serial hct, hgb, serum sodium, and serum potassium values. As the circulating volume is restored, the hct decreases to within normal limits. Hgb values may decrease secondary to hemolysis within the first 1-2 hours post-burn. Transfusions with packed red blood cells generally are required by the fifth day post-burn. Usually, potassium is elevated during the first 24-36 hours post-burn due to hemolysis and the lysis of cells.

Note: In the presence of elevated serum potassium do *not* add potassium to the IV fluids used for resuscitation.

After 72-96 hours, hypokalemia may be seen as cell membranes regain their integrity and the patient experiences diuresis. At this point, it may be necessary to add potassium to the IV solutions. Notify MD of significant findings.

6. Monitor patient for evidence of fluid volume excess secondary to rapid fluid resuscitation, especially in patients with preexisting respiratory or cardiac disease. Be alert to crackles (rales), SOB, tachypnea, and an increased CVP.
7. Confer with MD regarding use of mannitol in the presence of myoglobinuria to "flush" the kidney tubules. All other diuretics are avoided because they further deplete an already compromised intravascular volume, aggravating the shock state.
8. With the onset of spontaneous diuresis, discuss with MD the appropriate IV solutions, whether to add potassium, and infusion rate changes (usually a maintenance rate of 75 ml/hr).

Potential for injury related to risk of paralytic ileus

Desired outcome: Bowel sounds are auscultated and the patient demonstrates bowel elimination within his or her normal pattern.

1. Monitor bowel sounds q2h. Be alert to an absence of or decrease in bowel sounds indicative of paralytic ileus, which occurs in the presence of major trauma.

2. During period of absent or hypoactive bowel sounds, maintain NG tube to intermittent low suction as prescribed.
3. Maintain NPO status until return of bowel sounds. Provide mouth care at frequent intervals.

Potential for injury related to risk of development of gastric (Curling's) ulcer secondary to gastric pH <5

Desired outcome: Patient's gastric pH tests >5 and gastric aspirate is negative for blood.

Note: After return of bowel sounds, any major trauma victim is at high risk for development of gastric ulcers. In the burn patient acute ulceration of the stomach and duodenum is called Curling's ulcer.

---

1. Monitor gastric pH q2h. Administer antacids as prescribed to maintain pH >5.0.
2. Administer oral or IV H_2 receptor blocking agents q2-4h or as prescribed to prevent formation of gastric acids.
3. Test gastric aspirate for blood q8h. Promptly report presence of blood to MD.

Impaired tissue and skin integrity: Burn injury

Desired outcomes: Patient's wound exhibits evidence of granulation and healing by primary intention or split-thickness skin grafting within an acceptable time frame. Tissue perfusion in burned extremities is adequate as evidenced by peripheral pulses >2+ (on a scale of 0-4+), brisk capillary refill (<3 seconds), and skin temperature warm to the touch.

1. Assess and document time and circumstances of burn injury, as well as extent and depth of burn wound. See Tables 11-8 and 11-9, pp. 578-579.
2. In burned extremities, evaluate tissue perfusion by monitoring capillary refill, temperature, and peripheral pulses qh. Be alert to signs of decreased peripheral perfusion, including coolness of the extremity, weak or absent peripheral pulses (≤2+), and delayed capillary refill (>4 seconds). Report significant findings to MD.
3. Cleanse and debride wound as prescribed. Control ambient temperature carefully to prevent hypothermia.
4. Apply topical antimicrobial treatments as prescribed, using aseptic technique.
5. Elevate burned extremities above heart level to promote venous return and prevent excessive dependent edema formation.
6. Maintain immobility of grafted site for 3 days or as prescribed. This is achieved with a combination of positioning, splinting, or light pressure and sedation. In some instances, restraints, stents, bulky dressings, or occlusive dressings may be required to maintain immobilization and promote hemostasis of graft.
7. Elevate grafted extremity above heart level to promote venous return and decrease pooling of blood and plasma.
8. Utilize bed cradle to prevent bedding from coming into contact with open grafted area.
9. Monitor type and amount of drainage. Promptly report the presence of bright red bleeding, which would inhibit graft "take," and purulent exudate, which is indicative of infection.
10. Provide donor site care as prescribed and be alert to signs of donor site infection.
11. Apply elastic wraps to grafted legs to promote venous return when ambulation is permitted.

Potential for disuse syndrome related to immobilization secondary to pain or scar formation

Desired outcome: Patient displays complete range of motion without verbal or nonverbal indicators of discomfort.

1. Provide ROM exercises q4h. When possible, combine with hydrotherapy in a Hubbard tank.

2. Apply splints as recommended by physical therapy to maintain body parts in functional positions and prevent contracture formation.
3. For graft patient, institute ROM exercises and ambulation on tenth day post-graft, or as prescribed.

Potential for infection related to vulnerability secondary to bacterial proliferation in burn wounds, presence of invasive lines or urinary catheter, and immunocompromised status

Desired outcome: Patient is free of infection as evidenced by normothermia, WBC count <11,000 μl, negative cultures, well-defined burn wound margin, and absence of pockets containing purulent matter and other clinical indicators of burn wound infection.

1. For facial burns, shave all hair (except eyebrows) within 2 inches of wound margin to prevent wound contamination.
2. Monitor temperature q2h. Report temperatures >38.9° C (102° F).
3. Assess burn wound daily for status of eschar separation and granulation tissue formation, color, vascularity, sensation, and odor. Be alert to signs of infection, including fever, elevated WBC count, rapid eschar separation, increased amount of exudate, pockets containing purulent material, disappearance of a well-defined burn margin with edema formation, wound discoloration (e.g., black or dark brown), change in color of partial-thickness burn from pink or mottled red to full-thickness necrosis, superficial ulceration of burned skin at wound margins, pale and boggy granulation tissue, hemorrhagic discoloration of subeschar fat, and spongy and poorly demarcated eschar. Report significant findings promptly.
4. Assess appearance of grafted site, including adherence to recipient bed, appearance, and color. Be alert to erythema, hyperthermia, increasing tenderness, purulent drainage, and swelling around the grafted site.
5. Observe for clinical indicators of sepsis: tachypnea, hypothermia, hyperthermia, ileus, subtle disorientation, unexplained metabolic acidosis, and glucose intolerance, as evidenced by glycosuria and elevated blood sugar levels.
6. As prescribed, obtain wound, blood, sputum, and urine cultures in the presence of a temperature >38.9° C (102° F).
7. Administer systemic antibiotics and antipyretics as prescribed.
8. Ensure aseptic technique when administering care to burned areas and performing invasive techniques.
9. Place patients with burns >30% BSA in protective isolation.
10. For patients with skin grafts, monitor donor site for evidence of infection.

Alteration in nutrition: Less than body requirements of protein, vitamins, and calories related to hypermetabolic state secondary to burn wound healing

Desired outcome: Patient has adequate nutrition as evidenced by stable weight, balanced or positive nitrogen state per nitrogen studies, serum albumin ≥3.5 g/dl, and evidence of burn wound healing and graft "take" within an acceptable time frame.

1. Record all intake for daily calorie counts. Measure weight daily and evaluate based on patient's preburn weight.
2. Monitor serum albumin and urine nitrogen measurements. Burn patients undergo long periods of catabolism, with large amounts of nitrogen excreted in the urine. Serum values will be decreased from normal. Be alert to continuing deficiencies, weight loss, and poor graft "take," all of which are signals that nutritional needs are not being met.
3. Provide high-protein, high-calorie diet. When patient can take foods orally, promote supplemental feedings of milkshakes, ice cream, etc. between meals.
4. Confer with MD regarding need for enteral feedings in patients with burns >10% BSA, preinjury illness, or associated injuries, as they have calorie requirements that cannot be met orally. Patients with ileus that persists for more than 4 days or those unable to meet caloric needs enterally will require TPN as prescribed by MD.

Pain related to exposed sensory nerve endings secondary to burn injury

Desired outcome: Patient's subjective evaluation of pain improves, as documented by a pain scale.

1. Assess patient's level of discomfort at frequent intervals. Patients with partial-thickness burns may experience severe pain because of exposure of sensory nerve endings. Be aware that pain tolerance decreases with prolonged hospitalization and sleep deprivation. Establish a pain scale with patient, rating pain from 0 (no pain) to 10.
2. Monitor patient for clinical indicators of pain: increased BP, tachypnea, dilated pupils (unless patient has received narcotic analgesia), shivering, rigid muscle tone, or guarded position.
3. Administer narcotic analgesics or tranquilizers as prescribed and at least 20-30 minutes before painful procedures. Evaluate pain relief obtained, using the pain scale.
4. Provide a full explanation of procedures and honest feedback, using a calm, organized, and firm manner.
5. Employ nonpharmacologic interventions as indicated: relaxation breathing, guided imagery, soft music.
6. Ensure that patient receives periods of uninterrupted sleep (optimally 90 minutes at a time) by grouping care procedures when possible and limiting visitors.

Sensory/perceptual alterations related to tactile and visual deficits, medications, sleep-pattern disturbance, or pain secondary to severe burn injury

Desired outcomes: Patient verbalizes orientation to person, place, and time and describes rationale for necessary treatments.

1. Assess patient's orientation to person, place, and time.
2. Answer patient's questions simply and succinctly, providing information regarding immediate surroundings, procedures, and treatments. During the emergent phase of the burn injury, anticipate the necessity of having to repeat information at frequent intervals.
3. For patient with full-thickness injury, explain why tactile sensation is decreased or absent and that it will return with eschar separation and debridement.
4. If patient's eyelids are swollen shut due to facial edema, reassure patient that he or she is not blind and that swelling will resolve within 4-5 days.
5. Touch patient often on unburned skin to provide nonpainful tactile stimulation.
6. For more information, see the same nursing diagnosis in "Caring for Patients with Cancer and Other Life-Disrupting Illnesses," p. 690.

For other nursing diagnoses and interventions, see the following, as appropriate: "Providing Nutritional Support," p. 611, "Caring for Patients on Prolonged Bed Rest," p. 651, and "Caring for Patients with Cancer and Other Life-Disrupting Illnesses," p. 690.

PATIENT-FAMILY TEACHING AND DISCHARGE PLANNING

Burn patients usually are hospitalized for a prolonged period of time. Patient and family teaching efforts are directed toward the rehabilitative phases. Give patient and significant others verbal and written instructions for the following:

1. Splinting and exercise program for contracture prevention, as directed by physical therapist. Teach patient and significant others to monitor for pain or pressure due to improperly applied splint and to assess splinted extremity for coolness, pallor, cyanosis, decreased pulses, and impaired function.
2. Skin care
   □ Explain that a lubricating cream without alcohol (e.g., Nivea) should be applied several times a day and after bathing to promote soft and pliant skin and assist with control of pruritus.
   □ Explain that dressings or padding should be applied to areas that may be traumatized by pressure.
   □ Teach patient to avoid exposure to sun, as healed skin is highly sensitive to ultraviolet rays for up to a year.

☐ Explain to black patient that permanent pigmentation changes are likely due to destruction of melanocytes and that burned areas usually will stay pink.
☐ Wound care: Provide simplified dressing change procedure; explain indicators of infection and importance of notifying MD should they appear.
☐ Teach patient the importance of wearing pressure garment as prescribed to prevent excessive or hypertrophic scarring.
3. Nutrition: Explain the importance of maintaining an adequate intake of protein and calories for optimal wound healing.
4. Medications, including drug name, purpose, dosage, schedule, precautions, and potential side effects.
5. Home care and the importance of counseling to provide support for adjustment to life outside the hospital environment following disfiguring injury.
6. Importance of follow-up care; confirm date and time of first appointment if it has been established.

Section Four   ACQUIRED IMMUNE DEFICIENCY SYNDROME

Acquired immune deficiency syndrome (AIDS) is a life-threatening illness caused by the human immunodeficiency virus (HIV). AIDS is characterized by the disruption of cell-mediated immunity. This breakdown of the immune system is manifested by opportunistic infections, such as *Pneumocystis carinii* pneumonia (PCP), or tumors, such as Kaposi's sarcoma (KS).

The three confirmed routes of HIV transmission are the following:
1. Sexual contact that involves an exchange of body fluids.
2. Parenterally *via* receipt of contaminated blood or blood products, or IV drug abuse.
3. From an infected mother to a child during the perinatal period.

It is estimated that the average time span between infection with HIV and seroconversion (development of a positive HIV antibody test) is 6-8 weeks, although antibody response may be absent for a year or more. Therefore, a negative test does not guarantee the absence of infection. Individuals with a recent history of high-risk behavior and a negative HIV antibody test should be retested at 6-month intervals for one year and follow the guidelines for safer sex practices (see Table 11-10). Anyone with a positive HIV antibody test must be considered infectious and capable of transmitting the virus.

Individuals at highest risk for HIV infection are the following:
☐ homosexual or bisexual men.
☐ IV drug users.
☐ individuals with a history of multiple sexually transmitted diseases.
☐ recipients of blood or blood products prior to 1985.
☐ sexual contacts with individuals described above.
☐ children born to infected mothers.

See Figure 11-1, p. 588, for detail. To a minimal extent, health care workers who come into contact with the body substances of patients also are at some risk. Understanding and practice of universal precautions or variations, such as body substance isolation, are essential for all health care workers.

High-risk behaviors are primarily responsible for the transmission of HIV. Some of these behaviors include the following:
☐ having sexual relations with multiple partners.
☐ receptive anal intercourse, particularly, or any sexual practice that involves an exchange of body fluids.
☐ IV drug abuse.
☐ having sexual relations with persons practicing high-risk behaviors.

See Table 11-11 for more detail.

AIDS is the terminal phase of HIV infection. This is a chronic viral disease that covers a wide spectrum of illnesses and symptomatology over a variable course of time.

TABLE 11-10 Safer sex guidelines

Safe sexual practices include the following:
  Social (dry) kissing
  Hugging
  Massage
  Mutual masturbation
  Body-to-body contact, excepting mucous membrane areas
  Activities not involving direct body contact
Sexual practices of questionable safety include:
  French (wet) kissing
  Anal or vaginal intercourse using latex condoms*
  Fellatio (mouth to penis) without ejaculation
  Cunnilingus (mouth to vaginal area)
  Watersports (enemas, urination)
Unsafe sexual practices include:
  Anal or vaginal intercourse without latex condom
  Oral contact with bodily fluids (semen, urine, feces, vaginal secretions)
  Contact with blood
  Oral-anal contact (rimming)
  Manual anal penetration (fisting)
  Sharing sexual aids or needles

---

*Petroleum-based lubricants have been shown to increase the risk of condom rupture. Water-based products, such as K-Y jelly, are preferred. In addition, use of viricidal spermicides, such as nonoxynol 9, are strongly urged as added protection.

TABLE 11-11 Groups at higher risk for contracting AIDS

Group	Percent
Homosexual/bisexual males who are not IV drug abusers	62
IV drug users (males and females)	20
Homosexual males who also are IV drug abusers	7
Hemophiliacs/individuals with coagulation disorders	1
Heterosexuals	4
Individuals who have had transfusions/blood components	3
Undetermined	3

There is no classic disease progression. For example, some individuals procede from an asymptomatic, seropositive state to AIDS, while others may experience the symptoms of AIDS-related complex (ARC) for many years. Therefore, HIV disease should be considered as a continuum of infection. The stages of illness are described under "Assessment," below.

The mortality rate for those diagnosed with AIDS is grim but slowly improving. Early recognition and treatment of the complications of HIV infections, as well as promising experimental drug therapies, have given patients not only increased survival times, but also a better quality of life. Maintenance of a positive attitude by the patient and caregivers is an essential element in the therapeutic plan, but an honest approach to the realities of any life-threatening illness also must prevail.

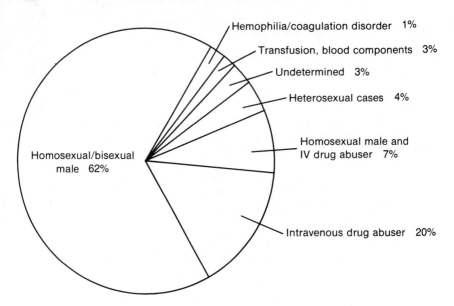

FIGURE 11-1. Approximate proportions of cases within each HIV classification.

ASSESSMENT

The four stages of HIV infection can be categorized as acute infection, asymptomatic stage, ARC, and AIDS.

Acute infection (a mononucleosis-like syndrome):

Signs and symptoms: Fever, malaise, muscle aches, night sweats, headache, nausea.
Laboratory results: HIV antibody test may not yet be positive.

Asymptomatic stage (may range anywhere from 5 to many more years):

Signs and symptoms: Generally none, but may have persistent, generalized lymphadenopathy.
Laboratory results: Positive HIV antibody test; T_4 or helper lymphocyte count usually >400/mm^3.

ARC (see Table 11-12):

Signs and symptoms: Persistent fever, involuntary weight loss, chronic diarrhea, fatigue, night sweats, thrush, hairy leukoplakia.
Laboratory results: Positive HIV antibody test, T_4 or helper lymphocyte count usually <400/mm^3, anemia, thrombocytopenia, leukopenia, or lymphopenia.

AIDS (as diagnosed by the presence of "indicator" diseases as defined by Centers for Disease Control [CDC]):

Signs and symptoms: Depend on the presenting opportunistic infection.
Laboratory results: Positive HIV antibody test, T_4 or helper lymphocyte count usually <200/mm^3, hematologic disorders (see data with ARC, above), multiple chemistry abnormalities.

History: If the patient is suspected of having HIV infection, the history would be incomplete without detailed social and sexual interviews, with special focus on determining high-risk behaviors. A complete review of body systems with careful attention to the common symptoms of HIV infection should be performed.

TABLE 11-12 CDC criteria for diagnosis of AIDS-related complex (ARC)

According to the CDC, definitive diagnosis of ARC can be made if the patient presents with any 2 clinical manifestations *plus* any 2 laboratory abnormalities from the following lists:

Clinical manifestations
  Lymphadenopathy in 2 or more extrainguinal sites existing for >3 months
  Fever >100 ° F for >3 months
  Weight loss >10% from preinfection state
  Persistent diarrhea
  Fatigue

Laboratory abnormalities
  Positive HIV antibody test
  CD4 (T_4 or helper cells) <400/mm^3
  CD4/CD8 ratio <1.0
  Anemia
  Leukopenia
  Thrombocytopenia
  Anergy to skin tests
  Elevated serum globulins
  Reduced blastogenesis

Physical assessment: Be aware of the following indicators that are seen frequently with HIV infection:

General: Fever, cachexia.

Cutaneous: Herpes zoster or simplex infection(s); seborrheic or other dermatitis; fungal infections of the skin (moniliasis, candidiasis) or nailbeds (onychomycosis); KS lesions.

Head/neck: "Cotton-wool" spots visualized on funduscopic examination; oral KS; *candida* infection (thrush); hairy leukoplakia; aphthous ulcers; enlarged, hard, and occasionally tender lymph nodes.

Respiratory: Tachypnea, dyspnea, diminished or adventitious breath sounds (crackles, rhonchi, wheezing).

Cardiac: Tachycardia, friction rub, gallops, murmurs.

Gastrointestinal: Enlargement of liver or spleen.

Genital/rectal: KS lesions, herpes, candidiasis.

Neuromuscular: Flattened affect, apathy, withdrawal, memory deficits, headache, muscle atrophy, speech deficits, gait disorders, generalized weakness, incontinence, neuropathy.

DIAGNOSTIC TESTS

AIDS patients may experience many signs and symptoms, as previously stated. The MD may prescribe other evaluations than those listed below, which are merely some of the more commonly performed diagnostic tests.

1. _HIV antibody:_ Tests for presence of antibody to the virus that causes AIDS. A positive result signals the individual's exposure to and ability to transmit HIV to others, not the presence of AIDS.

2. _CD cell subsets:_ CD cells are highly specialized lymphocytes that are invaded and destroyed by HIV. These include CD4 (T_4 or helper) cells and CD8 (T_8 or suppressor) cells. The CD4 count is greatly reduced and the normal CD4/CD8 ratio of 2:1 is inverted in HIV infection.

3. _CBC:_ May reveal leukopenia, anemia, thrombocytopenia, lymphopenia, granulocytopenia, or all of these manifestations (pancytopenia).

4. *Chemistry:* Multiple abnormalities are possible, depending on the opportunistic infection present, drug reactions, or overall condition. For example, the individual's chemistry results may reveal electrolyte imbalance or renal or hepatic dysfunction.

5. *Skin tests:* Anergy (lack of response) to common antigens (e.g., *candida*, mumps, PPD) applied intradermally is a signal of a damaged immune response.

6. *Serology:* May reveal a positive VDRL in the presence of syphilis; positive cryptococcal antigen in *Cryptococcus neoformans* infections of the CNS, lungs, and blood; and the presence of hepatitis antigens/antibodies.

7. *Viral titers:* A positive result confirms exposure to such viral organisms as herpes I or II, chlamydia, or cytomegalovirus (CMV).

8. *Microbiology:* Cultures of body fluids/tissues may reveal the presence of a wide variety of HIV-associated infections.

9. *Chest x-ray:* The most common AIDS opportunistic infection is *Pneumocystis carinii* pneumonia (PCP), which is seen on film as diffuse, interstitial infiltrates. Changes also will be seen in the presence of pulmonary TB or bacterial pneumonias. Signs of congestive heart failure or cardiomyopathy may appear, as well.

10. *Gallium scan:* Increased uptake of gallium in the lungs may aid in the diagnosis of PCP.

11. *Bronchoscopy:* To examine lungs and obtain lung tissue for culture to determine such conditions as PCP, KS, and TB.

12. *ABG values:* Done to assess pulmonary/metabolic status.

13. *Total protein, albumin, thyroxine-binding prealbumin:* Will be decreased if patient is in a malnourished state.

14. *Complete neurologic workup:* Indicated for individuals in whom central neurologic complications are evident (e.g., encephalitis, meningitis, herpes zoster radiculitis, dementia).

MEDICAL MANAGEMENT AND SURGICAL INTERVENTIONS

Medical management is limited primarily to chemotherapeutic intervention in an attempt to arrest the progression of the disease. Currently, there is no single drug or combination of drugs that has restored immunocompetency to afflicted patients. Medical treatment is palliative.

1. Zidovudine, AZT (Retrovir): The only FDA-approved retroviral drug available to date. This medication promises no cure for HIV infection, but has been shown to prolong life and reduce the number of opportunistic infections in individuals who can tolerate it. Retrovir has numerous side effects, most notably bone marrow suppression. Patients taking this drug need close monitoring of hematologic parameters.

2. Surgical interventions: May include resection of tumors; placement of venous access devices for TPN, chemotherapy, or frequent blood withdrawals; or, in selected instances, splenectomy for idiopathic thrombocytopenia (ITP). **Note:** IV gammaglobulin or prednisone therapy is also used for ITP.

NURSING DIAGNOSES AND INTERVENTIONS

Potential for infection related to vulnerability secondary to compromised immune system, malnutrition, or side effects of chemotherapy

Desired outcome: Patient is free of additional infections during hospitalization, as evidenced by negative cultures or biopsies.

1. Assess for indicators of opportunistic infections (e.g., persistent fevers, night sweats, fatigue, involuntary weight loss, persistent and dry cough, persistent diarrhea, headache). See Table 11-13, p. 550, for a description of the common opportunistic infections and organisms infecting AIDS patients.

2. Monitor laboratory data, especially CBC, differential, ESR, and cultures, to evaluate the course of infection. Be alert to abnormal results and notify MD of significant findings.

T A B L E   1 1 - 1 3   Opportunistic infections and organisms infecting AIDS patients

Viral	Fungal	Protozoal	Bacterial
Herpes (I&II)	*Candida*	*Pneumocystis carinii*	Syphilis
Cytomegalovirus	*Histoplasma*	*Toxoplasma gondii*	*Neisseria gonorrhoeae*
Varicella	*capsulatum*	*Entamoeba histolytica*	*Shigella*
Epstein-Barr	*Cryptococcus*	*Giardia lamblia*	*Salmonella*
Hepatitis A,B	Coccidioido-	*Cryptosporidium*	*Mycobacterium avium*
Hepatitis non-A/non-B	mycosis	*enteritisdis*	*intracellulare*
			Tuberculosis (TB)

3. Maintain strict asepsis for all invasive procedures to prevent introduction of new pathogens.
4. Assist patient in maintaining meticulous body hygiene to prevent spread of organisms from body secretions into skin breaks. This is especially critical if patient has diarrhea.
5. Monitor temperature and VS at frequent intervals for evidence of fever or sepsis. In addition to increased temperature, be alert to diaphoresis, confusion, decrease in LOC, increased HR, and decreased BP secondary to the vasodilatory effect of the increased body temperature. Perform a complete physical assessment at least q8h to identify changes from baseline assessment. Assess for changes in breath sounds, which may be indicative of an increasing level of infiltrates.
6. Promote pulmonary toilet by encouraging patient to engage in frequent breathing or incentive spirometry exercises. Use caution when performing postural drainage and chest physiotherapy, if prescribed, because patients may be too ill to tolerate these activities.
7. Monitor sites of invasive procedures for signs of infection, including erythema, swelling, tenderness, and purulent exudate.
8. Enforce good handwashing techniques before contact with patient to minimize the risk of transmitting infectious organisms from staff and other patients.

Potential for infection related to risk of transmitting patient's infectious organisms to others

Desired outcomes: Needlestick, "sharps," or other injuries do not occur. The risk of transmitting organisms causing infections or colonization in persons with AIDS to staff or other patients is minimized *via* meticulous handwashing and the use of gloves, masks, and gowns when they are indicated.

1. Put on a gown when it is anticipated that clothing will become soiled with patient's bodily secretions.
2. Wear gloves at *any time* it is likely that there will be direct contact with patient's bodily secretions, mucous membranes, or nonintact skin. Keep a box of gloves at patient's bedside.
3. Wash hands well before leaving patient's room, using soap, water, and friction.
4. Wear a mask if patient is positive for active pulmonary tuberculosis.
5. In situations during which there is risk of being splashed by bodily secretions, such as during bronchoscopy or wound irrigation, ensure that protective eyewear is worn.
6. Dispose of contaminated needles in a puncture-proof container. Do *not* attempt to recap needle prior to disposal.
7. To avoid the need for mouth-to-mouth resuscitation, keep disposable resuscitation equipment (manual resuscitator bag, mouth pieces) at patient's bedside.

Impaired gas exchange related to hyperventilation, increased oxygen requirements associated with sepsis, and decreased diffusion of oxygen secondary to pulmonary infiltrates

Desired outcome: Patient has adequate gas exchange as evidenced by Pao_2 ≥80 mm Hg, $Paco_2$ 35-45 mm Hg, pH 7.35-7.45, RR 12-20 breaths/min with normal depth and pattern (eupnea), and absence of adventitious sounds, nasal flaring, and other clinical indicators of respiratory dysfunction.

1. Assess patient's respiratory status frequently, noting rate, rhythm, depth, and regularity of respirations. Observe for use of accessory muscles, flaring of nares, presence of adventitious sounds, cough, or cyanosis, which occur with respiratory dysfunction.
2. Monitor ABG results closely for decreased $Paco_2$ (<35 mm Hg) and increased pH (>7.40), which can occur with hyperventilation.
3. Adjust oxygen therapy to attain optimal oxygenation, as determined by ABG values.
4. Instruct patient to report changes in cough, as well as dyspnea that increases with exertion.
5. To maintain adequate tidal volume, provide chest physiotherapy as prescribed; encourage use of incentive spirometry at frequent intervals.
6. Reposition immobile patient q2h to help prevent stasis of lung fluids.
7. Obtain sputum for culture and sensitivity as indicated.
8. Group nursing activities to provide patient with uninterrupted periods of rest, optimally 90-120 minutes at a time.
9. When administering sulfa for *Pneumocystis carinii,* monitor closely for side effects such as rash or bone marrow suppression (leukopenia, neutropenia). If administering pentamidine, be alert to side effects such as hypotension or hypoglycemia, which necessitate frequent BP checks and fingersticks for blood sugar levels.
10. To relieve mucous membrane irritation, which can predispose patient to coughing spells, deliver humidified oxygen to patient.
11. Administer sedatives and analgesics judiciously to help prevent or minimize respiratory depression.

Alteration in nutrition: Less than body requirements related to decreased intake and losses secondary to diarrhea and nausea associated with side effects of medications, malabsorption, anorexia, dysphagia, and fatigue

Desired outcome: Patient has adequate nutrition as evidenced by stable weights, serum albumin 3.5-5.5 g/dl, transferrin 180-260 mg/dl, thyroxine-binding prealbumin 200-300 μg/ml, retinol-binding protein 40-50 μg/ml, and a state of nitrogen balance or positive nitrogen state as revealed by nitrogen studies.

1. Assess nutritional status daily, noting weight, caloric intake, and protein and albumin values. Be alert to progressive weight loss, wasting of muscle tissue, loss of skin tone, and decreases in both total protein and albumin, which can adversely affect wound healing as well as impair the patient's ability to withstand infection.
2. Provide small, frequent, high-caloric, high-protein meals, allowing sufficient time for patient to eat. Offer supplements between feedings. As a rule, these patients are kept in a slightly positive nitrogen state (following resolution of the critical phases of this illness) by ensuring daily caloric intake equal to 50 kilocalories/kg of ideal body weight with an additional 1.5 g of protein/kg. For example, a man weighing 70 kg should receive 3,500 kilocalories, plus 105 g of protein per day.
3. Provide supplemental vitamins and minerals, as prescribed, to replace deficiencies.
4. To minimize anorexia and help treat stomatitis, which can occur as a side effect of chemotherapy, provide oral hygiene before and after meals.
5. If patient feels isolated socially, encourage significant others to visit at mealtimes and bring in patient's favorite high-caloric, high-protein foods from home.
6. If patient is nauseated, provide instructions for deep breathing and voluntary swallowing, which will help decrease stimulation of vomiting center.
7. If patient is dysphagic, encourage intake of fluids that are high in calories and protein; provide different flavors and textures for variation.
8. As prescribed, deliver isotonic tube feeding for patients unable to eat. Isotonic fluids will help prevent diarrhea associated with hypertonic or hypotonic fluids. Check

placement of NG tube before each feeding; assess absorption by evaluating amount of residual feeding q4h. Do not deliver feeding if residual is >100 ml. Keep HOB elevated 30 degrees while feeding and position patient in a right side-lying position to facilitate gastric emptying.

9. If patient's caloric intake is insufficient, discuss the potential need for TPN with MD.

Diarrhea related to gastrointestinal infection, chemotherapy, or tube feeding intolerance

Desired outcome: Patient has formed stools and a bowel elimination pattern that is normal for him or her.

1. Ensure minimal use of antidiarrheal medications, which promote intestinal concentration of infectious organism.
2. Teach patient to avoid large amounts (>300 mg/day) of caffeine, which increases peristalsis and can promote diarrhea.
3. Maintain accurate I&O records to monitor for changes in fluid volume status. Be alert to signs of hypovolemia, such as cool and clammy skin, increased HR (>100 bpm), increased RR (>20 breaths/min), and decreased urinary output (<30 ml/hr).
4. Assess stool for the presence of blood, fat, and undigested materials.
5. Monitor stool cultures for evidence of new infectious organisms.
6. Monitor patient for indicators of electrolyte imbalance, such as anxiety, confusion, muscle weakness, cramps, dysrhythmias, weak pulse, and decreased BP.
7. If patient is on tube feedings, dilute strength or decrease rate of infusion to prevent "solute drag," which may be the cause of the diarrhea.
8. Encourage foods high in potassium (see p. 555) and sodium (see p. 550) to replace any decrements of these ions.
9. Protect anorectal area by keeping it cleansed and using compounds such as zinc oxide to prevent or retard skin excoriation.

Potential for impaired skin and tissue integrity related to vulnerability secondary to cachexia and malnourishment, diarrhea, side effects of chemotherapy, Kaposi's skin lesions, negative nitrogen state, and decreased mobility due to arthralgia and fatigue

Desired outcome: Patient's skin and tissue remain intact.

1. Assess and document skin integrity, noting temperature, moisture, color, vascularity, texture, lesions, and areas of excoriation or poor wound healing. Evaluate Kaposi's lesions for location, dissemination, weeping, or significant changes. Note and record the presence of herpes lesions, especially those that are perirectal.
2. Avoid prolonged pressure to dependent body parts by turning and positioning patient q2h; encourage patient to change position at frequent intervals. Massage areas susceptible to breakdown (e.g., skin over bony prominences) with each position change.
3. Provide patient with an egg crate or flotation-type mattress, as indicated.
4. Teach patient to use mild, hypoallergenic, nondrying soaps or lanolin-based products for bathing, and to pat rather than rub the skin to dry it.
5. Use soft sheets on the bed, avoiding wrinkles. If patient is incontinent, use some type of rectal device (e.g., fecal incontinence bags, rectal tube) to protect the skin and prevent perirectal excoriation and skin breakdown.
6. To enhance skin and tissue healing, assist patient toward a state of nitrogen balance by promoting adequate amounts of protein and carbohydrates (see discussion with **Alteration in nutrition,** p. 592).
7. Ensure that patient receives minimum daily requirements of vitamins and minerals; supplement them as necessary.
8. Encourage ROM and weight-bearing mobility, when possible, to increase circulation to skin and tissue.

Pain related to prolonged immobility, side effects of chemotherapy, infections, and frequent venipunctures

Desired outcome: Patient's subjective evaluation of pain improves, as documented by a pain scale.

1. Assess and record the following: location, onset, duration, and factors that precipitate and alleviate patient's pain. With patient, establish a pain scale (e.g., with a rating of 0-10). Use the scale to evaluate degree of pain as well as to document the degree of relief achieved.
2. Provide heat or cold applications to affected areas, for example, apply heat to painful joints and cold packs to reduce swelling associated with infections or multiple venipunctures.
3. Encourage patient to engage in diversional activities as a means of increasing pain tolerance and decreasing its intensity. Examples include soothing music, quiet conversation, reading, and slow and rhythmic breathing.
4. To reduce pain intensity, teach patient techniques that decrease skeletal muscle tension, such as deep-breathing, biofeedback, and relaxation exercises (see **Health-seeking behavior:** Relaxation technique effective for stress reduction, p. 49).
5. If frequent venipunctures are the cause of the patient's discomfort, discuss with MD the desirability of a capped venous catheter for long-term blood withdrawal.
6. Promote relaxation and comfort with backrubs and massage.

Activity intolerance related to weakness and fatigue secondary to fluid and electrolyte imbalance, arthralgia, myalgia, dyspnea, fever, pain, hypoxia, and effects of chemotherapy

Desired outcomes: Patient tolerates activities as evidenced by HR ≤100 bpm, RR ≤20 breaths/min, and BP within patient's normal range. Patient verbalizes the absence of fatigue and extremity weakness following activity.

1. Assess patient's tolerance to activity by assessing HR, RR, and BP prior to and immediately after activity. Be alert to increased fatigue, such as extremity weakness following periods of activity.
2. Plan adequate (90-120 minute) rest periods between patient's scheduled activities. Adjust activities, as appropriate, to reduce energy expenditures.
3. As much as possible, encourage regular periods of exercise to help prevent cardiac intolerance to activities, which can occur quickly after periods of prolonged inactivity.
4. Monitor electrolyte levels to ensure that patient's muscle weakness is not caused by hypokalemia.
5. Monitor ABG values to ensure that patient is oxygenated adequately; adjust oxygen delivery accordingly.
6. For more information, see the same nursing diagnosis in the section "Caring for Patients on Prolonged Bed Rest," p. 651.

Anxiety related to diagnosis, fear of death or social isolation, and hospitalization

Desired outcome: Patient expresses feelings and is free of harmful anxiety as evidenced by HR ≤100 bpm, RR ≤20 breaths/min with a normal depth and pattern (eupnea), and BP within patient's normal range.

1. Monitor patient for verbal or nonverbal expressions of the following: inability to cope, apprehension, guilt for past actions, uncertainty, concerns about rejection and isolation, and suicide ideation.
2. Spend time with patient and encourage expressions of feelings and concerns.
3. Support effective coping patterns, for example, by allowing patient to cry or talk, rather than denying his or her legitimate fears and concerns.
4. Provide accurate information about AIDS and related diagnostic procedures.
5. If patient hyperventilates, teach him or her to mimic your normal respiratory pattern (eupnea).

Body image disturbance related to body changes secondary to Kaposi's lesions, side effects of chemotherapy, social stigmatization, isolation, and emaciation

Desired outcome: Patient expresses positive feelings about self to family, significant others, and primary nurse.

1. Encourage patient to express feelings, especially the way in which he or she views or feels about self.
2. Provide patient with positive feedback; help patient focus on facts, rather than myths or exaggerations about self.
3. Provide patient with access to clergy, psychiatric nurse, social worker, psychologist, or AIDS counselor as appropriate.
4. Encourage patient to join and share feelings with AIDS support group.

Knowledge deficit: Disease process, prognosis, lifestyle changes, and treatment plan

Desired outcome: Patient verbalizes accurate information regarding his or her disease process, prognosis, behaviors that increase the risk of transmission of the virus to others, and treatment plan.

1. Assess patient's knowledge about AIDS, including pathophysiologic changes that will occur, ways in which the disease is transmitted, necessary behavioral changes, and side effects of treatment. Correct misinformation and misconceptions, as necessary.
2. Inform patient of private and community agencies that are available to help with such tasks as handling legal affairs, cooking, housecleaning, and nursing care. Provide telephone numbers and addresses for AIDS support groups and self-help groups.
3. Provide literature that explores the myths and realities of the AIDS disease process.
4. Teach patient the importance of modifying high-risk behaviors known to transmit the virus (see Table 11-10); and informing sexual partners of AIDS condition.
5. Involve significant others in the teaching and learning process.
6. For more information, see "Patient-Family Teaching and Discharge Planning," p. 596.

Social isolation related to disease, societal rejection, loss of support system, fear, feelings of guilt and punishment, fatigue, and changed patterns of sexual expression

Desired outcome: Patient communicates and interacts with others.

1. Keep patient and significant others well informed of patient's status and treatment plan.
2. Provide private periods of time for patient to communicate and interact with significant others.
3. Encourage significant others to share in the care of the patient.
4. Encourage physical closeness between patient and significant others. Provide privacy, as much as possible.
5. Involve patient in unit or group activities, as appropriate.
6. Explain significance of isolation precautions to patient.

Alteration in thought processes related to mentation changes secondary to infection, space-occupying lesion in the CNS, or HIV dementia

Desired outcome: Patient verbalizes orientation to person, place, and time and correctly completes exercises in logical reasoning, memory, perception, concentration, attention, and sequencing of activities.

1. Assess patient for minor alterations in personality traits that cannot be attributed to other causes, such as stress or medication.
2. Assess patient for signs of dementia, which would include a slowing of all cognitive functioning: problems in attention, concentration, memory, perception, logical reasoning, and sequencing of activities.
3. Encourage patient to report persistent headaches, dizziness, or seizures, which may signal CNS involvement.
4. Note any cranial nerve involvement that differs from patient's past medical history. Most commonly, the 5th (trigeminal), 7th (facial), and 8th (acoustic) nerves are involved in infectious processes of the CNS.
5. Assess patient for signs of mental aberration, blindness, aphasia, hemiparesis, or ataxia, which may signal the presence of a demyelinating disease. Notify MD of all significant findings.

For other nursing diagnoses and interventions, see "Providing Nutritional Support," p. 611; "Caring for Patients on Prolonged Bed Rest," p. 651; "Caring for Patients with Cancer and Other Life-Disrupting Illnesses," p. 659.

PATIENT-FAMILY TEACHING AND DISCHARGE PLANNING

Give patient and significant others verbal and written instructions for the following:
1. Importance of avoiding use of recreational drugs, which are believed to potentiate the immunosuppressive process and lower resistance to infection.
2. Significance and importance of refraining from donating blood.
3. Necessity of modifying high-risk behaviors. See Table 11-10 p. 587, for specific information.
4. Principles and importance of maintaining a balanced diet; ways to supplement diet with multivitamins and other food sources, such as high-caloric substances (e.g., Isocal and Ensure).
5. Because of decreased resistance to infection, the importance of limiting contact with individuals known to have active infections.
6. Necessity of meticulous hygiene for preventing spread of any extant, or new infectious organisms.
7. Techniques for self-assessment of early signs of infection (e.g., erythema, tenderness, swelling, purulent exudate) in all cuts, abrasions, lesions, or open wounds.
8. Care of venous access device, including technique for self-administration of TPN or medications (see "Caring for Patients with Cancer and Life-Disrupting Illnesses," p. 659); care of NG tube and administration of enteral tube feedings, if appropriate.
9. Importance of avoiding fatigue by limiting participation in social activities, getting maximum amounts of rest, and minimizing physical exertion.
10. Prescribed medications, including name, dosage, purpose, and potential side effects.
11. Importance of maintaining medical follow-up appointments.
12. Advisability of keeping anecdotal notes (perhaps in journal format) on exacerbation and remission of signs and symptoms.
13. Importance of reporting changes in neurologic status (e.g., increasing severity of headaches, blurred vision, gait disturbances, or "black-outs").
14. Advisability of sharing feelings with significant others or within a support group.
15. In addition, provide the following information regarding AIDS resources:

Public Health Service
AIDS Hotline
(800) 342-AIDS
(800) 342-2437

National Gay Task Force
AIDS Information Hotline
(800) 221-7044

Local Red Cross or
American Red Cross
AIDS Education Office
1730 D Street, N.W.
Washington, DC 20006
(202) 737-8300

National Sexually Transmitted
Diseases Hotline/American
Social Health Association
(800) 227-8922

Centers for Disease Control (CDC)
AIDS Activity
Building 6, Room 292
1600 Clifton Road
Atlanta, GA 30333
(401) 329-3479

National AIDS Network
729 Eighth St., SE
Suite 300
Washington, DC 20003
(202) 546-2424

AZT Information Hotline
(800)-843-9388

Section Five   CHEMICAL DEPENDENCY

Alcoholism (CNS depressant)

Addiction to alcohol can be defined as follows: compulsive use, loss of control of the amount used, and continued use despite adverse consequences. The abuse of alcohol has physiologic, psychologic, and socioeconomic effects. Knowledge of what to expect and how to care for affected patients to prevent or minimize complications is important.

Alcoholism is a progressive, multifactorial disease with biogenetic and psychosocial components. The duration of time for its development and rate of its progression vary greatly. There are three main patterns of drinking: (1) regular daily intake of large amounts; (2) regular heavy weekend drinking; or (3) periods of sobriety interspaced with binges of daily heavy drinking.

ASSESSMENT

Nursing history should include the following: Time of last drink, amount and type of beverage consumed, length of time individual has consumed alcohol, other drug use, seizure history, and presence of other disease states. The length of time drinking has occurred and the amount of alcohol consumed on a consistent basis are important factors in determining the type of withdrawal to expect. There is a positive correlation between past withdrawal symptoms and their recurrence. Alcohol withdrawal is usually complete within 5-7 days.

Indicators of uncomplicated withdrawal: Onset within 6-12 hours after cessation of drinking, with duration of 24 hours or less. Signs and symptoms may include anxiety, agitation, depressed mood, irritability, autonomic hyperactivity (tachycardia, hypertension, increased RR, tremors, diaphoresis), anorexia, nausea, vomiting, malaise, weakness, headache, insomnia, and transient hallucinations or delusions. **Note:** Seizures may occur during this period but are considered evidence of complicated withdrawal. They are related to a decreased seizure threshold, are a part of the withdrawal progression, and may precede delirium tremens.

Indicators of complicated withdrawal: Develop 2-4 days after the last drink and continue for more than 24 hours. Signs and symptoms may include progressive tremors, diaphoresis, anxiety, and tachycardia. Disorientation, clouding of sensorium, hallucinations (most commonly visual and tactile), and delusions also can occur.

□ *Delirium tremens* (DTs): The most severe progression of withdrawal, which can result in death. Signs and symptoms can develop 72-96 hours after cessation of drinking and can include disorientation with loss of touch with reality, delirium, agitation, severe diaphoresis, tachycardia, cardiovascular collapse, and fever. Generally, DTs resolve within 3-5 days.

Criteria for diagnosis of alcoholism

1. Possible physiologic dependence (withdrawal symptoms seen with cessation of drinking).
2. Tolerance to the effects of alcohol.
3. Evidence of alcohol-associated illnesses.
4. Continued drinking in spite of consequences.
5. Impaired functioning (social and occupational).
6. Depression.
7. Inability to control the amount used.

DIAGNOSTIC TESTS

1. *Serum tests:* A concentration of blood alcohol 0.10% or more signals legal intoxication. If the concentration is greater and the patient does not appear intoxicated, this is evidence of tolerance. Liver enzymes (SGOT, SGPT, GGPT) will be elevated with

liver disease. Increased amylase can signal the presence of pancreatitis. CBC is done to rule out anemia, and glucose levels are obtained to rule out hypoglycemia. Electrolytes are measured to rule out abnormalities (hypokalemia and hypomagnesemia may be seen), and PT is obtained to rule out clotting disorders.
2. *Stool Hemoccult:* To rule out GI bleeding.
3. *Chest x-ray:* To rule out pneumonia.
4. *EKG:* To determine presence of cardiac abnormalities.

MEDICAL MANAGEMENT

1. **Complete physical examination:** Special emphasis on liver and nervous system.
2. **Pharmacotherapy**
   □ *Sedation:* Substitution of long-acting CNS depressant (benzodiazepine) for short-acting CNS depressant (alcohol) to produce a state of calm wakefulness. **Note:** Withholding sedation until severe symptoms develop is not effective with alcohol withdrawal. Increase in VS, especially pulse rate, is the most sensitive indicator of the need for medication. Dosage is tapered daily until it reaches zero, with each daily dosage at least half as much as that of the previous day.
   □ *IM thiamine on admission; supplemental PO thiamine and multivitamins and multiminerals high in C, B-complex, zinc, and magnesium:* Thiamine is given to prevent Wernicke-Korsakoff syndrome; multivitamins and multiminerals are given because of the potential for malnutrition related to inadequate food intake and malabsorption caused by alcohol's irritating effect on the GI tract. **Note:** IM thiamine should be given *stat* on admission. Patients should not be permitted to eat for 1 hour following injection to ensure absorption.
   □ *Disulfiram (Antabuse):* Often given as a deterrent for alcohol consumption in long-term treatment. It blocks the metabolism of alcohol, causing acetaldehyde to accumulate and produce unpleasant reactions, such as flushing, sweating, palpitations, dyspnea, tachycardia, hypotension, hyperventilation, nausea, and vomiting, with the alcohol consumption.
   □ *Beta blockers:* Helpful in reducing hyperadrenergic state (tachycardia, hypertension, tremors). Patients appreciate the effects of beta blockers, which may shorten the duration of treatment for acute withdrawal.
3. **Dietary management:** Foods high in protein and vitamins. Parenteral therapy with electrolytes may be indicated if the patient has had severe diarrhea, vomiting, and malnutrition.
4. **Promote rest and relaxation:** Provision of a calm, dimly lit environment.
5. **Treatment of complications**
   □ *Seizures:* Because alcohol-withdrawal seizures occur during the first 2 days, benzodiazepines are given to raise the seizure threshold during the withdrawal period. Alcohol withdrawal seizures mandate the use of a heparin lock and IV diazepam (drug of choice) to achieve control over the seizure(s). Additional seizure management should reflect institution protocol. If the patient has a history of a primary seizure disorder, an anticonvulsant agent is indicated.
   □ *Alcoholic hallucinosis (auditory hallucinations that usually are persecutory in nature in a person who is otherwise well oriented):* Reassurance, sleep, and continued treatment with benzodiazepines usually are therapeutic. Haloperidol (Haldol) may be added to the treatment if hallucinosis persists beyond cessation of the DTs.
   □ *DTs:* Continued sedation with benzodiazepines; rest and sleep; and frequent orientation to reality, using familiar terms.
   □ *Wernicke-Korsakoff syndrome:* Caused by thiamine deficiency and manifested by diplopia (the first real diagnostic clue), confusion, excitation, and peripheral neuropathy, severe recent memory loss, impaired thought processes, and confabulation. The prophylactic administration of thiamine is recommended. **Caution:** Ingestion of carbohydrates, either oral or parenteral, increases the body's demand for thiamine. In patients with minimal thiamine levels, use of IV glucose can precipitate the syndrome. If the syndrome progresses, lifetime custodial care might be the only treatment.

6. **Detoxification:** Although not a treatment in itself, it provides the opportunity to begin treatment for recovery from alcoholism. It entails withdrawing the patient from alcohol in a controlled environment, using a protocol specified by the institution. Generally, sedation is used (see pharmacotherapy above).

NURSING DIAGNOSES AND INTERVENTIONS

Sensory/perceptual alterations related to mentation and motor disturbances secondary to intoxication and withdrawal

Desired outcome: Patient verbalizes orientation to person, place, and time and interacts appropriately with the environment.

1. Assess and document patient's orientation to reality to determine safety needs.
2. Admit patient into a room near the nurses' station.
3. Monitor VS at frequent intervals. Be alert to indicators of increasingly severe withdrawal, including increasing pulse rate, respirations, and BP, and tremors, diaphoresis, and anxiety. Describe potential withdrawal symptoms to patient and significant others, and request that they alert you if they occur.
4. Administer benzodiazepines as prescribed, usually as VS increase.
5. Keep frequently used objects within patient's reach to minimize need for getting out of bed.
6. As necessary, assist patient with activities such as ambulation.
7. Obtain a prescription for restraints if indicated.

Sleep pattern disturbance related to agitation secondary to withdrawal from short-acting CNS depressant

Desired outcome: Patient relates the attainment of increasing amounts of sleep and rest.

1. Decrease environmental stimuli and minimize care activities, as appropriate, when patient is trying to sleep.
2. Consider use of low-volume, relaxing music during patient's awake time.
3. Administer sedation promptly, as prescribed; avoid undersedation. During detoxification, the amount of benzodiazepine is usually increased at the hour of sleep.

Alteration in nutrition: Less than body requirements related to history of poor intake and malabsorption secondary to alcoholism

Desired outcome: Patient attains optimal nutritional status as evidenced by stable or increasing weight and positive nitrogen state.

1. Determine patient's food preferences that are congruent with dietary management; provide small, frequent feedings, including nighttime snacks.
2. Encourage significant others to bring in desirable, acceptable foods.
3. Provide encouragement during mealtimes.
4. Record food intake daily; record weight daily, or as indicated.
5. As needed, administer prescribed medications that decrease gastrointestinal distress: antacids, antiemetics, antidiarrheals, cathartics.
6. If indicated, obtain prescription for vitamin and mineral supplements.
7. If appropriate, arrange for dietitian to meet with patient and significant others.

Ineffective individual coping related to anger, denial, and poor self-esteem secondary to inability to manage stressors without alcohol

Desired outcome: Patient relates an increase in self-esteem, participates in choices related to care, and begins to set appropriate short-term goals.

1. Encourage patient to verbalize anxieties and ask questions about the disease.
2. Dispel common stereotypes about the disease such as moral weakness and skid row personality. Avoid moralizing about the disease.
3. Provide reading material such as Alcoholics Anonymous (AA) publications and other relevant articles about the disease.

4. Emphasize patient's self-worth by providing choices related to his or her care where appropriate.
5. Assist patient with setting short-term goals.
6. Discourage patient from focusing on questions, such as "Why me?" Encourage focusing on methods for staying sober instead.
7. Explore alternative methods for dealing with stress, including communications with others (e.g., AA members) and relaxation techniques.
8. Emphasize that prognosis is directly related to abstinence.
9. Provide positive reinforcement when changes are made.
10. Assess for suicidal ideation and institute suicide precautions (as prescribed by institution) when indicated.
11. Assess for coexisting psychopathology, which may emerge as the alcohol becomes cleared from the patient's system.

See "Caring for Patients with Cancer and Other Life-Disrupting Illnesses," for **Alteration in family processes, p. 699.**

PATIENT-FAMILY TEACHING AND DISCHARGE PLANNING

Provide patient and significant others with verbal and written information for the following:
1. Medications, including drug name, dosage, purpose, schedule, precautions, and potential side effects. For patient taking Antabuse, explain the necessity of avoiding "hidden" alcohol found in some foods and cosmetics such as sauces, vinegars, cough mixtures, after-shave lotions, perfumes, mouthwashes, and astringents.
2. Appropriate referrals, such as AA, Al-Anon, Ala-Teen, halfway houses, inpatient and outpatient treatment centers, community alcohol centers, and counseling services.
3. Importance of adequate nutrition, stress management, structure, and exercise to promote optimal health.
4. Treatment, which consists of detoxification, relief of distress, and full participation in a 12-step program.
5. Cross-tolerance to other drugs (CNS depressants) and the likelihood of becoming dependent on other mood-altering drugs.
6. Dry drunk syndrome: During sobriety, an alcoholic may think, act, and feel as though intoxicated, e.g., by exhibiting grandiose, childish, or unrealistic behavior; a rigidly judgmental outlook; or tense impatience. Explain that this syndrome is common, and the patient should contact a support system such as AA if it occurs.

Sedative-hypnotic abuse (CNS depressant)

Sedative-hypnotic agents are used clinically in lower doses to decrease anxiety and in higher doses to produce sleep. Barbiturates, which are used as sedatives, hypnotics, anesthetics, and anticonvulsants, can cause respiratory depression and are contraindicated in patients with pulmonary disease. Benzodiazepines are used to decrease anxiety, relax muscles, and produce anticonvulsant effects. There is a great potential for abuse with these drugs that can result in physiologic and psychologic dependence. Tolerance has occurred when greater doses are required to produce the initial effect. When any CNS depressant is taken in combination with others (e.g., alcohol with diazepam), synergistic effects often are found and death can occur. This means that the combined effect of the drugs is greater than the summation of the single effects. Cross-tolerance to other CNS depressants such as sedative-hypnotics, alcohol, and anesthetics can be found in chronic users of benzodiazepines. Therefore, a patient who is tolerant to one will have a "built-in" tolerance to all.

Drug half-life: Withdrawal symptoms can be correlated with the half-life of the drug that was used (see Tables 11-14 and 11-15). Withdrawal from drugs with shorter half-lives produces intense symptoms that last for shorter periods of time, while withdrawal

TABLE 11-14   Common barbiturates

Generic name	Common brand names	Half-life (in hours)
amobarbital	Amytal	8-42
secobarbital	Seconal	19-34
pentobarbital	Nembutal	15-48
phenobarbital	Luminal & others	24-140
butabarbital	Butisol	34-42
secobarbital/amobarbital	Tuinal	8-42

TABLE 11-15   Common benzodiazepines

Generic name	Common brand names	Half-life (in hours)
chlordiazepoxide	Librium & others	7-28
diazepam	Valium & others	20-90
lorazepam	Ativan	10-20
oxazepam	Serax	3-21
prazepam	Centrax	24-200*
flurazepam	Dalmane	24-100*
chlorazepate	Tranxene, Azene	30-100
tenazepam	Restoril	9.5-12.4
clonazepam	Clonopin	18.5-50
alprazolam	Xanax	12-15
halazepam	Paxipam	14

*Includes half-life of major metabolites.

from drugs with longer half-lives produces less intense symptoms that can be prolonged. Moreover, the severity of the withdrawal is directly related to the drug's dosage.

ASSESSMENT

Nursing history: should include the following: Time of last drug; amount and type taken; length of time individual has used the drug; other drug/alcohol use; seizure history; and presence of other disease states.

Indicators of withdrawal: Anxiety, panic, tremors, nausea, vomiting, impaired concentration, irritability, incoordination, insomnia, restlessness, blurred vision, diaphoresis, anorexia, weakness, depersonalization, increased sensitivity to light and sound, perceptual distortions, depression, seizures, and delirium. Typically, there will be a reemergence of the symptoms that initially were treated by the drug.

DIAGNOSTIC TESTS

1. *Serum drug screen:* A quantitative and qualitative study that detects the presence of various drugs in the blood.
2. *Urine drug screen:* Can test a broad spectrum of drugs. Some urine drug screens are more sensitive than others. **Note:** Drugs can be excreted rapidly (within 24 hours as with alcohol), moderately (48-72 hours as with some barbiturates), or slowly (weeks or months as with PCP and marijuana).

MEDICAL MANAGEMENT

1. **Complete physical exam:** To detect coexisting health problems.
2. **Sedation:** Either phenobarbital or the drug from which the patient is withdrawing is administered in doses that are tapered daily to zero. Dosage may be increased if tapering appears to be too rapid and withdrawal symptoms are too uncomfortable. Tapering of hypnotics should be slower than that with alcohol. A "comedown" schedule should be set up in which the drug used is reduced by no more than 15%/day, even if symptoms disappear or are not obvious. Abrupt benzodiazepine discontinuation leads to more severe withdrawal.
3. **Management of complications**
   - □ *Delirium:* Increase in the dosage and frequency of sedation.
   - □ *Seizures:* If the patient has a history of a primary seizure disorder, an anticonvulsant agent is indicated. Withdrawal seizures mandate the use of a heparin lock and IV diazepam (drug of choice) to achieve control over the seizure(s). Additional seizure management should reflect institution protocol.

NURSING DIAGNOSES AND INTERVENTIONS

Sensory/perceptual alterations related to motor and mentation disturbances secondary to withdrawal from CNS depressant

Desired outcome: Patient verbalizes orientation to person, place, and time and interacts appropriately with the environment.

1. Monitor VS at frequent intervals to assess patient's degree of withdrawal. Be alert to the following indicators of increasing withdrawal: increased pulse rate, diaphoresis, tremors, anxiety, and nausea. Instruct patient about the potential for these symptoms.
2. Administer the prescribed sedative medication as indicated.
3. Institute seizure precautions.
4. Minimize environmental stimuli to help patient attain calmness.
5. Reorient patient to reality as necessary; do not support hallucinations.
6. Remove potentially harmful objects from patient.
7. Minimize the need for getting out of bed by keeping frequently used objects within patient's reach.

Anxiety related to withdrawal symptoms

Desired outcome: Patient's subjective evaluation of discomfort improves, as documented by a 0-10 scale.

1. Determine patient's degree of discomfort. Devise a scale with patient, rating discomfort from 0 (no discomfort) to 10. Administer prescribed sedatives promptly and document their effectiveness using the pain scale.
2. Speak with patient in a calm, unhurried manner.
3. Decrease environmental stimuli to promote a calm environment; be supportive of patient during withdrawal. Minimizing anxiety will enhance comfort.
4. Provide soft, relaxing music.
5. Provide leisure or work activity to distract patient from focusing on physical symptoms.

See "Seizure Disorders" for **Potential for trauma** related to oral, musculoskeletal, and airway vulnerability secondary to seizure activity, p. 244. See "Alcoholism" for **Sleep pattern disturbance,** p. 599, **Alteration in nutrition:** Less than body requirements, p. 599, and **Ineffective individual coping,** p. 599. See "Caring for Patients with Cancer and Other Life-Disrupting Illnesses" for **Altered family processes,** p. 699.

PATIENT-FAMILY TEACHING AND DISCHARGE PLANNING

Provide patient and significant others with verbal and written information for the following:

1. Referrals to outside agencies, including AA, Narcotics Anonymous, Al-Anon, Ala-Teen, halfway houses, inpatient and outpatient treatment centers, community drug abuse centers, and individual or family counseling.
2. Importance of a direct transfer to a treatment program upon discharge. If the patient returns to his or her old environment, the potential for resuming drug use is great.
3. Importance of adequate nutrition, stress management, structured routine, and exercise to promote optimal health.
4. Cross-tolerance to other CNS depressants (e.g., alcohol).
5. Treatment, which consists of detoxification, relief of distress, and full participation in a 12-step program.

Cocaine abuse (CNS stimulant)

Cocaine is an increasingly popular drug that once was believed to be the drug of the wealthy, but it is clear now that its use is popular among all socioeconomic classes. Cocaine addiction is associated with other drug use and often is accompanied by alcohol and marijuana use or abuse. The physical and mental effects of cocaine are dose-dependent and progress from (1) physical and mental overconfidence, elation, and euphoria to (2) agitation, anxiety, and irritability to (3) aggression, violence, paranoia, and toxic psychosis to (4) hyperthermia, cardiac dysrhythmias, seizures, coma, and death. Cocaine-induced deaths are totally unpredictable regardless of dose, blood levels, or route of administration.

Cocaine can be introduced orally, intranasally, IV, or inhaled through smoking. A process known as free-basing removes all the water-soluble impurities, leaving pure cocaine, which is then smoked. "Crack" is not pharmacologically different from free-base cocaine. "Crack" is made available in small amounts of high-quality cocaine that is cheaper and therefore more affordable to people of lower economic classes and adolescents. It is now widely believed that cocaine produces both psychologic and physical dependence.

ASSESSMENT

Nursing history should include the following: Last use, frequency and duration of use, route of use, and other drug or alcohol use (it is not unusual for patients to use alcohol to "come down" from a cocaine high). Implement other detoxification protocols as necessary.

Indicators of cocaine intoxication: Mydriasis, vasoconstriction, anxiety, diaphoresis, tachycardia, hypertension, hyperthermia, tremors, and hyperkinesis.

Indicators of cocaine withdrawal ("crashing"): Poor concentration, anergia, anhedonia, bradykinesis, sleep disturbance, decreased libido, intense cocaine craving, depression, and suicidality.

Indicators of cocaine psychosis: Tactile and visual hallucinations and paranoia. Typically, treatment is that of psychosocial support; however, pharmacologic therapy with antipsychotic agents, such as haloperidol or chlorpromazine, may be instituted to diminish psychosis.

Note: The degree of CNS stimulation is directly related to the amount used and the route of use. Smoking or free-basing is most intense and addictive.

DIAGNOSTIC TESTS

Specific
1. *Urine drug screen:* Confirms the presence of cocaine metabolites and ascertains the presence of unknown substances in the street preparation of the drug.

Nonspecific

1. *Hepatitis B surface antigen:* Assessed for in IV drug users because of the potential for needle-sharing.
2. *HIV:* Obtained after written permission of patient to assess for possible exposure to the AIDS virus.

MEDICAL MANAGEMENT

1. **Restriction of cocaine:** Unlike CNS depressants, which require tapering, cocaine can be stopped abruptly.
2. **Pharmacotherapy:** Treatment is aimed at affecting neurotransmitter changes at presynaptic, synaptic, and postsynaptic levels. L-Tryptophan, tyrosine, and alanine have been used to replenish depleted neurotransmitters. L-Tryptophan, an amino acid, also may be given to promote sleep. Pharmacologic treatment is still evolving and has not been proven conclusively in its effects for cocaine withdrawal.

Note: Pharmacologic treatment cannot substitute for drug rehabilitation and extensive lifestyle changes.

3. **Management of complications:** For example, toxic psychoses; seizures; cardiovascular crises; hepatitis, septicemia, or endocarditis (caused by unsterile IV administration); positive HIV result; perforated nasal septum (from "snorting" cocaine); pulmonary dysfunction (from smoking cocaine); and acute anxiety reactions.

NURSING DIAGNOSES AND INTERVENTIONS

Potential for violence related to hallucinations/paranoia secondary to cocaine use/withdrawal

Desired outcomes: Patient does not exhibit violent behavior. Patient verbalizes orientation to time, place, and person.

1. Because patient may be anxious and uncertain about unfamiliar actions, explain all procedures in a calm manner. Use simple language and speak softly and clearly.
2. Assess for hallucinations and psychosis. Orient patient to time, place, and person as needed; do not support hallucinations.
3. Assure patient that all information obtained is used for medical purposes only.
4. Remove potentially harmful objects from patient area.
5. Avoid moralizing or chastising patient about drug use.
6. To promote a calm, relaxed environment, minimize environmental stimuli.
7. Do not touch patient without first announcing your intention.
8. Visit patient at frequent intervals to provide reassurance and enhance patient's feelings of safety.

Ineffective individual coping related to depression, dysphoria, poor self-esteem, and denial secondary to inability to manage stressors without cocaine

Desired outcome: Patient relates an increase in self-esteem and begins to plan appropriate short-term goals.

1. Discourage patient from focusing on "Why me?" Encourage patient to focus on ways to remain drug free instead.
2. Avoid moralizing about drug use. Speak calmly and matter-of-factly.
3. Assist patient with formulating short-term goals.
4. Encourage patient to verbalize concerns; provide an atmosphere of acceptance.
5. Give positive enforcement when changes are made.
6. Educate patient that cocaine "crash" (dysphoria, irritability, and restlessness) will pass. Assess for suicidal ideation.
7. Be aware that craving cocaine is to be expected. Assist patient with talking through "drug hunger." If appropriate, arrange for individuals who also have experienced cocaine craving to speak with patient.
8. Encourage patient to participate in routine exercise.

See "Caring for Patients with Cancer and Other Life-Disrupting Illnesses," for **Altered family processes,** p. 699.

PATIENT-FAMILY TEACHING AND DISCHARGE PLANNING

Provide patient and significant others with verbal and written information for the following:

1. Referrals to outside agencies, such as Narcotics Anonymous, Cocaine Anonymous, Al-Anon, Ala-Teen, halfway houses, inpatient or outpatient treatment centers, community drug abuse centers, individual and family counseling, and AIDS support groups.
2. AIDS education: Focus on transmission of the disease (i.e., *via* needle-sharing and sexual contact) and emphasize that AIDS is not restricted to the male homosexual population. Significant others should be informed of the risk of AIDS and should be given referrals for HIV testing, along with the patient.
3. Importance of adequate nutrition, stress management, structure, and exercise to promote optimal health.
4. Treatment, which consists of detoxification, relief of distress, and full participation in the 12-step program.

Opioid abuse (CNS depressant)

Opioids, also known as narcotics, are the most effective drugs for pain relief. They cloud consciousness, tranquilize, and cause euphoria. Opioids are either synthetic or nonsynthetic and all are compared to morphine, which is found in the opium poppy. Other opioids include codeine, heroin, oxymorphone (Numorphan), oxycodone (found in Percodan), hydromorphone (Dilaudid), diphenoxylate (found in Lomotil), meperidine (Demerol), alphaprodine (Nisentil), propoxyphene (Darvon), pentazocine (Talwin), butorphanol (Stadol), nalbuphine (Nubain), and fentanyl citrate (Sublimaze). Opioids differ slightly from one another in regard to potency, duration of effects, severity of side effects, withdrawal symptoms, and absorption.

Opioids are either inhaled, smoked, swallowed, taken by suppository, or injected. They produce physical dependence, and tolerance can occur along with cross-tolerance to other opioids. Tolerance seems to diminish after withdrawal has occurred. Additive effects can occur when taken with other drugs, and respiratory depression can result when they are mixed with alcohol or other CNS depressants.

ASSESSMENT

Indicators of adverse effects: Constipation, nausea, vomiting, orthostatic hypotension, rashes, delirium, endocarditis, hepatitis, muscle and joint problems, and respiratory infections from suppression of the cough reflex (especially with codeine).

Indicators of withdrawal (can be compared to symptoms of influenza): Lacrimation, rhinorrhea, mydriasis, piloerection, diaphoresis, diarrhea, yawning, mild hypertension, tachycardia, fever, insomnia, cold/hot flashes, twitching, tremors, muscle spasms, blurred vision, irritability, restlessness, increased anxiety, and aching of joints and muscles. Symptoms of opioid withdrawal occur approximately 8-12 hours after the last dose, intensify in 36-48 hours, and are generally complete in 10-14 days, although some symptoms can last up to 10 weeks. Withdrawal from opioids is not considered to be life threatening except in the elderly, severely debilitated patients, or newborns.

DIAGNOSTIC TESTS

Specific

1. <u>Urine drug screen:</u> Confirms the presence of opioid metabolites and ascertains the presence of unknown substances.

Nonspecific

1. *Hepatitis B surface antigen:* Assessed for in IV drug users because of the potential for needle sharing.
2. *Serology test:* To rule out sexually transmitted diseases, which are often seen with drug addicts.
3. *HIV:* Obtained after written permission from the patient to assess for exposure to the AIDS virus.

MEDICAL MANAGEMENT

1. Methadone substitution: Implemented by physicians who are part of a licensed maintenance program. After patient stabilization, methadone is withdrawn from the patient gradually.
2. Adrenergic agonists such as clonidine: May be used to minimize withdrawal symptoms by decreasing sympathetic outflow from the brain. It is tapered off gradually. Clonidine lowers BP and pulse and can cause sedation (assess for orthostatic hypertension).
3. Pharmacologic treatment for symptomatic relief of discomfort: For example, sedative-hypnotics for relief of anxiety and sleeplessness; mild anticholinergics for rhinorrhea.
4. Follow-up care: For example, counseling, long-term treatment, and rehabilitation.

NURSING DIAGNOSES AND INTERVENTIONS

Anxiety related to withdrawal from opioid substance

Desired outcome: Patient's subjective evaluation of anxiety improves, as documented by a 0-10 scale.

1. Monitor for indicators of withdrawal, including increases in pulse rate, BP, and temperature as well as increasing anxiety, diaphoresis, and insomnia. Report significant findings to MD.
2. Determine patient's subjective evaluation of the discomfort. Devise a scale with patient, rating discomfort from 0 (no discomfort) to 10. To help minimize patient's discomfort, promptly administer prescribed medications. Rate the degree of relief obtained, using the scale.
3. Reinforce that detoxification is only the beginning of treatment. Educate patient that follow-up treatment is essential for remaining drug free.
4. Offer comfort measures such as warm blankets and soothing music if they are effective for the patient.
5. Ensure strict avoidance of narcotic antagonists, such as pentazocine (Talwin), which can precipitate abrupt withdrawal.

Potential for infection related to susceptibility secondary to repeated IV drug injections or antitussive effects of opioids

Desired outcome: Patient is free of infection as evidenced by normothermia, HR ≤100 bpm, RR ≤20 breaths/min with normal pattern and depth (eupnea), BP within normal range, and absence of erythema, swelling, and purulent drainage at the injection sites.

1. Inspect injection sites for evidence of infection such as erythema, warmth, and purulent drainage. Notify MD of significant findings.
2. Institute measures that promote healing, such as cleansing the area and applying prescribed antibacterial ointment.
3. Instruct patient in the care of skin infections.
4. Teach patient about complications that can result from unsterile IV techniques.
5. Teach effective coughing techniques for patients who were users of opioids that have antitussive effects.
6. Monitor VS for general indicators of infection, such as an increase in temperature and rising pulse rate. Report significant findings to MD.

Ineffective individual coping related to denial, poor self-esteem, and depression secondary to inability to handle stressors without opioids

Desired outcomes: Patient complies with treatment regimen, relates an increase in self-esteem, participates in self-care, and demonstrates efforts aimed at remaining drug free.

1. Encourage patient to verbalize anxieties and ask questions about the disease.
2. Discourage patient from focusing on questions such as "Why me?" Encourage patient to focus on methods of remaining drug free instead.
3. Provide positive reinforcement when changes are made.
4. Encourage patient to participate in self-care.
5. Avoid moralizing about drug use.
6. Do not hesitate to search visitors.
7. Do not reward patient's manipulations.
8. Set firm limits on patient's behavior in advance and on a continuous basis.
9. Establish one "caretaker" and confront patient's attempts to split the staff.
10. Communicate care plan with other staff members to help ensure consistency.
11. Involve patient in decision making.

See "Alcohol Abuse" for **Alteration in nutrition:** Less than body requirements, p. 599, and **Sleep pattern disturbance,** p. 599. See "Caring for Patients with Cancer and Other Life-Disrupting Illnesses," for **Altered family processes,** p. 699.

PATIENT-FAMILY TEACHING AND DISCHARGE PLANNING

Provide patient and significant others with verbal and written information for the following:
1. Referrals to outside agencies such as Narcotics Anonymous, Al-Anon, Ala-Teen, halfway houses, inpatient and outpatient treatment centers, community drug abuse centers, individual and family counseling, and AIDS support groups.
2. Importance of a direct transfer to a treatment program. Should the patient return to his or her old environment, the potential for resumption of the drug abuse is great.
3. AIDS education: Focus on transmission of the disease (i.e., needle-sharing and sexual contact) and emphasize that AIDS is not restricted to the male homosexual population. Significant others should be informed of the risk of AIDS and should be given referrals for HIV testing, along with the patient.
4. Importance of adequate nutrition, stress management, structure, and exercise to promote optimal health.
5. Treatment, which consists of detoxification, relief of distress, and full participation in the 12-step program.

SELECTED REFERENCES

Adams EH et al: Elevated risk of cocaine use in adults, Psychiatr Ann 18(9):523-527, 1988.
Ake JM and Perlstein LM: AIDS: impact on neuroscience nursing practice, J Neurosci Nurs 19(6):300-304, 1987.
American Psychiatric Association: Diagnostic and statistical manual of mental disorders, ed 3, Washington, DC, 1987, American Psychiatric Association.
Arieff Al and De Fronzo RA: Fluid, electrolyte, and acid-base disorders, New York, 1985, Churchill Livingstone, Inc.
Barta MA: Correcting electrolyte imbalances, RN, pp. 30-34, Feb 1987.
Beaufoy A et al: AIDS: what nurses need to know. Part II. Nursing care, Can Nurse 84(7):23-27, 1988.
Brater DC: Serum electrolyte abnormalities caused by drugs, Prog Drug Res 30:9-69, 1986.
Calloway C: When the problem involves magnesium, calcium, or phosphate, RN pp. 30-35, May 1987.
Centers for Disease Control: Revision of CDC surveillance case definition for acquired immunedeficiency syndrome, MMWR 36:3s-5s, 1987.

Centers for Disease Control: AIDS update, MMWR 38(14):233, 1989.

Cohen FL: Acquired immunodeficiency syndrome research in critical care: a review and future directions, Focus Crit Care 15(4):30-35, 1988.

Dackis CA et al: Psychopharmacology of cocaine, Psychiatr Ann 18(9):528-530, 1988.

Easterday U: Acid-base imbalances. In Swearingen PL et al: Manual of critical care: applying nursing diagnoses to adult critical illness, St. Louis, 1988, The CV Mosby Co.

Extein IL et al: The treatment of cocaine addicts, Psychiatr Ann 18(9):535-537, 1988.

Geheb MA: Clinical approach to the hyperosmolar patient, Crit Care Clin 5(4):797-815, 1987.

Goldberger E: A primer of water, electrolyte, and acid-base syndromes, ed 7, Philadelphia, 1986, Lea & Febiger.

Gong V and Rudnick N: AIDS: facts and issues, 1987, Rutgers University Press.

Govoni LA: Psychosocial issues of AIDS in the nursing care of homosexual men and their significant others, Nurs Clin North Am 23(4):749-765, 1988.

Hilton G: AIDS dementia, J Neurosci Nurs 21(1):24-29, 1989.

Holmes KK and Mutulsky AG: AIDS: a guide for the primary care physician, Seattle, 1988, University of Washington Press.

Horne M: Fluid and electrolyte disturbances. In Swearingen PL et al: Manual of critical care: applying nursing diagnoses to adult critical illness, St. Louis, 1988, The CV Mosby Co.

Horne M and Swearingen PL: Pocket guide to fluids and electrolytes, St. Louis, 1989, The CV Mosby Co.

Klahr S: The kidney and body fluids in health and disease, New York, 1983, Plenum Publishing Co.

Kokko JP et al: Fluids and electrolytes, Philadelphia, 1986, WB Saunders Co.

Koushanpour WK: Renal physiology: principles, structure, and function, ed 2, New York, 1986, Springer-Verlag New York, Inc.

Landesmen S et al: Management of HIV disease: treatment team workshop handbook, New York, 1988, World Health Communications.

Levy RM, Bredesen DE, and Rosenblum ML: Neurological manifestations of acquired immune deficiency syndrome (AIDS): experience at UCSF and review of the literature, J Neurosurg 475-495, 1985.

Maxwell MH et al: Clinical disorders of fluid and electrolyte metabolism, ed 4, New York, 1987, McGraw-Hill Book Co.

Metheny NM: Fluid and electrolyte balance—nursing considerations, Philadelphia, 1987, JB Lippincott Co.

Miller K: Acquired immune deficiency syndrome. In Swearingen PL et al: Manual of critical care: applying nursing diagnoses to adult critical illness, St. Louis, 1988, The CV Mosby Co.

Needleman P and Greenwald JE: Atriopeptin: a cardiac hormone intimately involved in fluid, electrolyte, and blood pressure homeostasis, N Engl J Med 314:828-834, 1986.

Noyes R et al: Benzodiazepine withdrawal: a review of the evidence, J Clin Psychiatry 49(10):382-388, 1988.

Nyamathi A and Van Servellen G: Maladaptive coping in the critically ill population with acquired immunodeficiency syndrome: nursing assessment and treatment, Heart Lung 18(2):113-120, 1989.

Rice V: Magnesium, calcium, and phosphate imbalances: their clinical significance, Crit Care Nurs 3:90-112, 1983.

Rose BD: Clinical physiology of acid-base and electrolyte disorders, ed 3, New York, 1989, McGraw-Hill Book Co.

Sande MA and Volberding PA: The medical management of AIDS, Philadelphia, 1988, WB Saunders Co.

Scherer YK et al: AIDS: what are nurses' concerns? Clin Nurse Spec 3(1):48-54, 1989.

Schwartz MW: Potassium imbalances, AJN 87:1292-1299, 1987.

Seldin DW and Giebisch G: The kidney—physiology and pathophysiology, vol 2, New York, 1985, Raven Press.

Stoops CM: Fluid and electrolyte disturbances in the perioperative period, Indiana Med 1:13-19, 1987.

Thompson JM et al: Clinical nursing, St. Louis, 1986, The CV Mosby Co.

Toto KH: When the patient was hyperkalemic, RN 34-38, April 1987.

Urrows ST: Physiology of body fluids, Nurs Clin North Am 15(3):537-547, 1980.

Verebey K et al: The effects of dose and routes of administration in abuse liability, Psychiatr Ann 18(9):513-520, 1988.

Vokes TJ and Robertson GL: Disorders of antidiuretic hormone, Endocrinol Metab Clin North Am 17(2):281-299, 1988.

Wooldridge-King M: Burns. In Swearingen PL et al: Manual of critical care: applying nursing diagnoses to adult critical illness, St. Louis, 1988, The CV Mosby Co.

12

CHAPTER

Providing care for patients with special needs

Section One   PROVIDING NUTRITIONAL SUPPORT

Many hospitalized patients are at nutritional risk or have malnutrition. Malnutrition not only increases the time of hospital stay, morbidity, and mortality, it compromises wound healing and immune function as well. Nutrition interventions minimize patient complications and the cost of health care. Nursing observations are vital to early identification of malnutrition and prevention of iatrogenic weight loss during the hospital stay. When oral intake is not possible, specialized nutritional support modalities, tube feeding, or parenteral support may be required.

Screening for patients at nutritional risk

IDENTIFYING THE HIGH-RISK PATIENT

Standard criteria are used to evaluate for nutritional risk. These include:
☐ Age: Infancy, childhood, advanced.
☐ Drug or alcohol abuse.
☐ History of inadequate nutrient intake.

☐ IV support with dextrose or saline alone for >5 days.
☐ Organ or system failure (e.g., ARDS, COPD, renal failure, diabetes mellitus, pancreatitis, neuromuscular dysfunction).
☐ Overweight status (>20% above ideal body weight).
☐ Pregnancy (especially in an adolescent).
☐ Recent, unplanned weight loss (>10 pounds).
☐ Serum albumin <3.5 gm/dl.
☐ Trauma, surgery, or disease of the oral cavity or GI tract (e.g., fractured mandible, radical head and neck resection, malabsorption syndrome).
☐ Underweight condition (≤80% of ideal body weight).

FORMS OF MALNUTRITION

Several varieties of malnutrition exist.
1. **Kwashiorkor:** Condition that develops when adequate calories are consumed but protein intake is inadequate. Typical signs are a low serum albumin level and edema. The patient may actually appear well-nourished, with edema masking weight loss. This type of malnutrition can occur in the patient who is maintained for a prolonged period on IV dextrose or maintenance electrolyte solutions alone.
2. **Marasmus:** Caused by chronic, inadequate intake of both calories and protein. The patient appears wasted and may have a skeleton-like appearance. Severe depletion of lean body mass and subcutaneous fat stores is evident on physical examination. Serum albumin level may be normal, however.
3. **Protein-calorie malnutrition (PCM):** A combination of kwashiorkor and marasmus, it is the type most commonly seen in hospitalized patients in the United States. Severe wasting may be present, in conjunction with edema. Serum albumin levels may be normal or low, depending on the severity of protein inadequacy.
4. **Obesity:** State of poor nutrition associated with increased risk for a number of diseases, including diabetes mellitus, hypertension, cardiovascular disease, and some forms of cancer. Although caloric intake may exceed needs, selected nutrient deficiencies can occur because food intake may lack nutrient density. This patient, though 20% or more over ideal body weight, may have marginal stores of protein, vitamins A and C, folic acid, iron, or calcium, among other potential deficiencies.
5. **Vitamin deficiencies:** Seen most often in severe or chronic malnutrition. Some deficiencies are also associated with certain conditions or dietary patterns (e.g., thiamine and folate deficiencies in the alcoholic, B_{12} deficiency in the strict vegetarian or patient with ileal resection, and vitamin C deficiency in the individual who avoids all fruits, juices, and vegetables).
6. **Mineral deficiencies:** Usually seen only after prolonged periods of inadequate intake or in certain disease states. Iron deficiency is seen more commonly in women, infants, and children. Calcium deficiency leading to rickets or osteoporosis may be seen if the diet excludes milk and milk products. Zinc deficiency, though rare, may be seen in patients with chronic diarrhea or malabsorption.

Nutritional assessment

DIETARY HISTORY

Dietary history is taken to reveal adequacy of usual and recent food intake. Excesses or deficiencies of nutrients should be noted. Unusual eating patterns may be revealed, as well (e.g., fad diets, vegetarian diet, extraordinary use of nutritional supplements). Of keen interest from a nutritional perspective is anything that impairs adequate selection, preparation, ingestion, digestion, absorption, and excretion of nutrients. Dietary history should include the following:
☐ Comprehensive review of usual dietary intake, including food allergies, food aversions, and use of nutritional supplements.

☐ Unplanned weight gain or loss.
☐ Chewing or swallowing difficulties.
☐ Nausea, vomiting, or pain with eating.
☐ Diarrhea, constipation, or any alteration in elimination pattern.
☐ Chronic disease affecting utilization of nutrients (e.g., malabsorption, pancreatitis, diabetes mellitus).
☐ Surgical resection or disease of the gut or accessory organs of digestion (pancreas, liver, gallbladder).
☐ Alcohol or drug addiction.
☐ Chronic use of drugs affecting appetite, digestion, utilization or excretion of nutrients (see Table 12-1 for detail).

Medical, surgical, and social history also should be obtained to complete this assessment of the patient's current nutritional status.

TABLE 12-1   Drugs affecting appetite, digestion, and nutrient use

Drug	Nutritional concern	Management suggestions
Aspirin	Gastric ulceration; nausea, vomiting	Give with water or food; use buffered or enteric-coated product when possible
Estrogen	Nausea, vomiting; sodium, water retention	Give with meals; restrict sodium intake
Furosemide	Increased excretion of potassium; fluid and electrolyte imbalance	Ensure high dietary potassium intake (e.g., apricots, bananas, oranges, orange juice, most meats, peas, beans, and nuts)
Mineral oil	Malabsorption of vitamins A, D, E, K	Avoid frequent use; avoid use at mealtime.
Methotrexate	Nausea, vomiting	Honor food preferences; provide small meals, cold beverages
Levodopa	Dietary protein may impair absorption	Avoid high-protein diet
Phenobarbital	Inactivates vitamin D; impairs folate utilization; may indirectly cause rickets or osteomalacia	Ensure adequate dietary intake of vitamin D and folate; administer vitamin supplements as prescribed
Phenytoin	See "Phenobarbital," above; may contribute to development of megaloblastic anemia, rickets, or osteomalacia	See "Phenobarbital," above
Tetracycline	Milk products may impair absorption	Restrict milk and milk products
Theophylline	Response increased with caffeine; decreased half-life with charcoal-broiled meats	Restrict caffeine-containing beverages (coffee, tea, colas) and charcoal-broiled meats
Warfarin	Vitamin K impairs hypoprothrombic effect	Avoid use of vitamin-K rich foods (e.g., green leafy vegetables, such as cabbage, cauliflower, and turnip greens)

PHYSICAL ASSESSMENT

Assessment may reveal important indicators of nutritional deficiencies or disorders. Examples are outlined in Table 12-2.

ANTHROPOMETRICS

Measurement of the body or its parts is termed anthropometrics. Certain measurements are very useful, such as height and weight; others, such as triceps skinfold and mid-upper arm muscle circumference, are used only in special circumstances.

1. **Measuring height and weight:** Should be done on admission. If the patient's condition is too critical, reported height and weight from family or significant others should be noted on the medical record. If necessary, estimates of height and weight are made by observing body size and comparing recumbent length to known length of the mattress.
   □ Estimates of desirable male weight can be made as follows: Allot 106 pounds for the first 5 feet of height, plus 6 pounds for each additional inch.
   □ Estimates of desirable female weight can be made as follows: Allot 100 pounds for the first 5 feet of height, plus 5 pounds for each additional inch.
   These estimates correspond fairly well with weights for heights reported by the Metropolitan Life Insurance Company, as seen in Table 12-3, p. 616.
2. **Monitoring weight changes:** The patient's maintenance of body weight is one of the most readily available and practical indicators of adequacy of nutritional status and provisions. In the hospitalized patient weight changes may reflect the following:
   □ Fluid shifts (edema, diuresis, third-spacing).
   □ Surgical resections or traumatic or surgical amputations.
   □ Weight of dressings or equipment.
   Interpretation of weight changes must be made with these factors in mind. One liter of fluid equals approximately 2 pounds, so being "ahead" or "behind" on a patient's fluids can be reflected readily in weight changes.
3. **Measurement of triceps skinfold thickness and mid-upper arm muscle circumference:** Previously was widely suggested for assessment of fat stores and lean body mass in hospitalized patients. However, for proper interpretation of these results, the measurements must be made by a trained clinician, the patient positioned in a standard manner, and the results compared to national norms specific to age and sex. As it often is impossible to position hospitalized patients appropriately to make these measurements and there is wide variability, even when specific standards are used, these measurements are not widely used at present. They do have value in the long-term patient who cannot be weighed. In this situation, serial measurements, using the patient as a control or standard, can be made and used as a crude indicator of adequate, inadequate, or excessive provision of nutritional support.

LABORATORY AND DIAGNOSTIC TESTING

Laboratory values pertinent to nutritional status are numerous.
1. **Visceral protein status:**

Laboratory test	Normal range
Serum albumin	3.5-5.5 g/dl
Transferrin	180-260 mg/dl
Thyroxine-binding prealbumin	200-300 μg/ml
Retinol-binding protein	40-50 μg/ml

Normal values may vary somewhat with different laboratory procedures and standards. Albumin and transferrin have relatively long half-lives of 19 and 9 days, respectively, whereas thyroxine-binding prealbumin and retinol-binding protein have very short half-lives of 24-48 hours and 10 hours, respectively. If hydration status is normal and anemia is absent, albumin and transferrin can be used as baseline indica-

TABLE 12-2 Physical assessment with nutritional implications

Body area	Abnormal appearance	Possible nutrient deficiency or disorder
Hair	Dull, dry, sparse, easily plucked	Protein, energy, zinc
Nails	Spoon-shaped, brittle ridged	Iron
Face	Rotundness, "moon face" appearance	Obesity, protein
	Presence of edema or decubiti	Protein
	Nasolabial seborrhea	Riboflavin, zinc
	Xerosis (dryness of mucous membranes)	Vitamin A
	Pallor, listlessness	Iron
Eyes	Redness or fissures at corners of eyelids	Riboflavin
	Dry cornea, Bitot's spots	Vitamin A
	Cloudy, pale conjunctiva	Iron
	Periorbital numbness	Phosphorus
Lips	Angular lesions at corners of the mouth	Riboflavin
Gums	Bleeding, spongy gums	Vitamin C
Tongue	Magenta in color	Riboflavin
	Scarlet, raw, swollen, fissures	Niacin
	Thick, difficulty with speaking	Phosphorus
Neck	Goiter	Iodine
Skin	Scrotal and vulvar dermatosis not accompanied by inflammation	Riboflavin
	Swollen pigmentation of areas exposed to sun	Niacin
	Pinhead size, purplish hemorrhagic spots (petechiae)	Vitamin C
	Excessive bruising	Vitamin C or K
	Poor wound healing, decubiti	Protein, energy
	Follicular hyperkeratosis (epidermal hypertrophy causing horny skin formation)	Vitamin A
Muscular system	Thinness, tissue wasting	Protein, energy
	Presence of edema	Obesity, protein, sodium
Skeletal system	Osteoporosis	Calcium, protein
	Circumscribed swelling or growth of frontal and parietal areas of skull; bowed legs	Vitamin D
Central nervous system	Mental irritability	Protein
	Hyporeflexia, foot and wrist drop	Thiamine
	Psychotic behavior	Niacin
	Peripheral neuropathy, forgetfulness	Pyridoxine
	Tremor, convulsions, tetany	Magnesium, calcium

Adapted from Horne M and Swearingen PL: Pocket guide to fluids and electrolytes, St Louis, 1989, The CV Mosby Co.

TABLE 12-3   Height and weight tables for men and women

Height	Men Small frame	Men Medium frame	Men Large frame	Women Small frame	Women Medium frame	Women Large frame
4 ft 10 in	—	—	—	102-111	109-121	118-131
4 ft 11 in	—	—	—	103-113	111-123	120-134
5 ft	—	—	—	104-115	113-126	122-137
5 ft 1 in	—	—	—	106-118	115-129	125-140
5 ft 2 in	128-134	131-141	138-150	108-121	118-132	128-143
5 ft 3 in	130-136	133-143	140-153	111-124	121-135	131-147
5 ft 4 in	132-138	135-145	142-156	114-127	124-138	134-151
5 ft 5 in	134-140	137-148	144-160	117-130	127-141	137-155
5 ft 6 in	136-142	139-151	146-164	120-133	130-144	140-159
5 ft 7 in	138-146	142-154	148-168	123-136	133-147	143-163
5 ft 8 in	140-148	145-157	152-172	126-139	136-150	146-167
5 ft 9 in	142-151	148-160	156-176	129-142	139-153	149-170
5 ft 10 in	144-154	151-163	158-180	132-145	142-156	152-173
5 ft 11 in	146-157	154-166	161-184	135-148	145-159	155-176
6 ft	149-160	157-170	164-188	138-151	148-162	158-179
6 ft 1 in	152-164	160-174	168-192	—	—	—
6 ft 2 in	155-168	164-178	172-197	—	—	—
6 ft 3 in	158-172	167-182	176-202	—	—	—
6 ft 4 in	162-176	171-187	181-207	—	—	—

Ages 25 through 59 for 5 pounds of indoor clothing for men and 3 pounds of indoor clothing for women and 1-inch heels for both. Data for 1983. Courtesy of the Metropolitan Life Insurance Company.

tors of adequacy of protein intake and synthesis. For evidence of response to nutritional therapy, the short turnover proteins, thyroxine-binding prealbumin and retinol-binding protein, are the most useful.

2. Anemia: Tested for *via* hgb, hct, and RBC indices. Data from these hematologic tests are useful in nutritional assessment when hydration state is normal. The usefulness of these tests in assessing nutritional status is invalidated by massive hemorrhage. Below normal hgb and hct, combined with appearance of microcytic and hypochromic RBCs, may denote iron deficiency anemia. Appearance of macrocytic RBCs may signal folate deficiency; megaloblasts are associated with vitamin B_{12} deficiency.

3. Serum levels of vitamins and minerals: Yield little information regarding overall body stores of these nutrients; test values require cautious interpretation.

4. Total lymphocyte count: While previously widely used as an indicator of protein status and immune competence, it is affected by so many variables common to critical illness, such as the leukocytosis seen in sepsis, trauma, burns, or surgery, that its use is diminishing.

5. Delayed cutaneous hypersensitivity: Involves the application of antigens to the skin and observation of cutaneous response or lack thereof (anergy). Many iatrogenic, disease-specific, and technical factors are now known to alter this response and the use of this form of testing is no longer widely recommended or implemented.

6. Nitrogen balance: State of equilibrium that exists when the intake and excretion of nitrogen are equal. If more is taken in than excreted, nitrogen is said to be positive and an anabolic state exists. If more nitrogen is excreted than taken in, nitrogen balance is said to be negative and a catabolic state exists. Most nitrogen loss occurs

through urinary urea nitrogen (UUN) loss, with a small, constant amount lost *via* skin and feces. Nitrogen balance is calculated as follows:

$$N_{bal} = N \text{ intake} - N \text{ excretion}$$

$$N_{bal} = \frac{\text{Protein intake (g)}}{6.25} (24 \text{ hr UUN} + 4)$$

Nitrogen balance studies are conducted more frequently for critically ill patients. Accurate results rely heavily on complete 24-hour urine collections.

In a true state of balance, needs for energy and nitrogen are being met and are adequate to provide for the following: (1) wound healing; (2) extraneous losses; (3) catabolism of stress; (4) usual synthesis of enzymes and hormones; (5) repair and replacement of worn-out cells; and (6) normal needs and physiologic functions. A positive nitrogen state is desired when anabolism is the goal, for example, following resolution of the critical phase of an illness. This is a state of "rebuilding," regaining weight and lean body mass.

Nutritional therapy

Following completion of a comprehensive nutritional assessment, a care plan can be developed to provide optimal nutritional support for the patient. The goal for the hospitalized patient is maintenance of existing lean body mass and adequate provision of energy and nutrients to sustain physiologic systems. Patients in this setting should not incur either weight loss or weight gain. Weight loss during this period is likely to cause loss of protein rather than fat stores. Attempts to facilitate weight gain during hospitalization may cause some of the complications of overfeeding during stress (e.g., increased CO_2 production, provision of excessive glucose and fluid load, elevation of liver enzymes, and weight gain of fluid or fat rather than repletion of lean body mass). Nutritional therapy should be provided in the most physiologic, safe, and efficacious manner possible, with cost-effectiveness considered as well.

ENERGY REQUIREMENTS

Energy expenditure is dependent on age, sex, body size, physical activity, and level of stress or catabolism. Basal energy expenditure (BEE) is defined as the energy required to support vital life functions (circulation, respirations, and other physiologic processes) in a healthy, normal, fasting individual, at rest in a neutral, thermal environment. Calculation of BEE can be made using the following equations developed by Harris and Benedict:

$$\text{BEE (male)} = 66.5 + (13.8 \times W) + (5 \times H) - (6.8 \times A)$$
$$\text{BEE (female)} = 655.1 + (9.6 \times W) + (1.9 \times H) - (4.7 \times A)$$
$$W = \text{weight in kg; } H = \text{height in cm; } A = \text{age in years.}$$

If the patient is being nourished, energy expenditure is increased approximately 5%-10% above BEE for the specific dynamic action of nutrient utilization. This combined figure is called the resting energy expenditure (REE). As the difference in BEE and REE is often only 5%, the BEE and REE are considered relatively equal in actual clinical practice.

1. **Adjustment of BEE and REE during physical activity, illness, or injury:** The following factors are applied to the BEE and REE as suggested by Calvin Long:

$$\text{BEE or REE} \times \text{Activity factor} \times \text{Injury factor} = \text{TEE (total energy expenditure)}$$

Activity factors	**Injury factors**
1.2 = bedridden patient	1.2 = surgery
1.3 = ambulatory patient	1.35 = trauma (blunt or skeletal)
	1.6 = sepsis
	2.1 = burns

Additional increases in TEE may be caused by temperature elevations, with an increase of 7% per degree of temperature elevation from normal in Fahrenheit or 13% per degree of temperature elevation from normal in Centrigrade, as reported by Kinney.

2. **Measuring energy needs directly:** Can be accomplished at the bedside by using a metabolic cart. This cart is an instrument that performs indirect calorimetry, the calculation of energy expenditure by measurement of respiratory gas exchange. This technique is based on the theory that oxygen consumption and carbon dioxide production profile intracellular metabolism. The gas collection device can be adapted to the exhalation unit of most mechanical ventilation systems; patients not requiring mechanical ventilation can have gas exchange measured using a plastic hood or canopy. A microcomputer utilizes the data on gas exchange, urinary urea nitrogen values, as well as some basic nutritional assessment data, and generates estimates of REE, protein requirements, utilization of energy substrates (carbohydrates, protein, and fat), as well as respiratory quotient (RQ). The RQ, which is a ratio of carbon dioxide production to oxygen consumption, provides information on the adequacy of nutritional provision, that is, whether the patient is well nourished (from an energy perspective) or whether a starved or overfed state exists.

$RQ \dfrac{VCO2}{VO2}$	Interpretation
0.7	Lipolysis or starvation; primary source of energy = fat.
0.8	Primary source of energy = protein.
0.85	Energy source = mixed substrates (carbohydrates, protein, fat).
1.0	Primary source of energy = carbohydrates.
>1.0	Overfeeding; lipogenesis (conversion of glucose to fat); increased CO_2 production.

Correct interpretation of this information on measured REE, protein needs, and substrate utilization is crucial so that proper nutritional therapy can be provided and errors in assessment avoided. For example, if measured REE represents a starved state for an individual unable to eat for several days posttrauma, the goal is not to provide support at a starvation level, but rather to adjust support to an adequate maintenance level. This may require an increase of 500 kilocalories/day or more over measured REE. To avoid the complications of rapid refeeding of a starved patient (e.g., cardiac failure, pulmonary compromise, or electrolyte imbalance), progression of feedings to maintenance level may have to proceed in small daily increments. The nonstarved patient, however, may require energy at levels 10%-30% greater than the measured REE if they are bathed, active in bed, or undergoing pulmonary treatments or painful stimuli from other treatments (e.g., dressing changes, debridement, multiple injections). These factors must be considered in the estimate of total energy needs for each patient. In addition, reassessment is necessary at frequent intervals. For example, in closed head injury, needs are very elevated initially, and then reduced when barbiturate therapy is begun. Unfortunately, metabolic cart measurements are performed over a brief period, often for only 20 minutes, and therefore cannot be expected to reveal total energy needs over a 24-hour period.

PROTEIN REQUIREMENTS AND DISTRIBUTION OF CALORIES

Once TEE has been determined, an estimate of quantities of protein, carbohydrates, and fat can be derived. Providing a relatively normal distribution of calories from these is desirable and usually adequate.

1. **Energy macronutrients and calorie: nitrogen ratio:** Percentages of total calories from carbohydrates, protein, and fat should equal approximately 50%, 15%, and 35% respectively. A nonprotein calorie per gram of nitrogen ratio of 150:1 to 100:1 usually will be achieved by providing 14%-20% of total calories as protein. This will provide a range of 0.8-2.0 g of protein/kg/day.
2. **Protein requirements:** The usual recommendation for protein intake for the hospitalized patient experiencing stress or surgery is 1.2-1.5 g of protein/kg/day.
3. **Providing glucose:** In TPN, glucose administration of 5 mg/kg/min is a suitable amount. Glucose provided in excess of this is not well utilized and may lead to hyperglycemia, excessive CO_2 production, hypophosphatemia, and fluid overload.
4. **Delivering fat:** If protein and glucose are supplied as outlined, providing the remainder of needed calories as fat will meet overall needs. Fat, particularly linoleic and linolenic acids, may be administered in minimal quantities to satisfy needs for essential fatty acids, or may be provided in larger quantities, as tolerated, to meet energy needs, especially in the patient who is glucose intolerant or being weaned from ventilator support with CO_2 retention as a complicator.

VITAMIN AND MINERAL REQUIREMENTS

It is an uncontested fact that a variety of vitamins and minerals is essential for optimal health. Even in health, quantities required vary widely, with some individuals' needs considerably higher than others. With deficiency, several responses occur, including mobilization of stores, increased absorption, reduced excretion, and improved utilization. Some deficiencies develop more rapidly than others, but in general, vitamin and mineral deficiencies take weeks, months, or years to develop. For hospitalized patients, the goals are the following:

□ Provide at least minimum quantities of vitamins and minerals as outlined in standard recommendations published by American Medical Association (parenteral) and the Food and Nutrition Board of the National Research Council in the Recommended Dietary Allowances (enteral).
□ Detect and treat existing deficiencies.
□ Supplement specific vitamins or minerals known to be needed in increased amounts in existing disease states (e.g., zinc and vitamins A and C in burns; thiamine and folate in alcoholism).
□ Observe patient for development of signs of deficiency (see Table 12-2).

FLUID REQUIREMENTS

Many factors affect fluid balance. A primary goal is to achieve equilibrium between I&O. Under usual circumstances, an estimate of fluid needs can be made by providing 1 ml of free water for each calorie provided. If 1 L of 1 cal/ml tube feeding provides 75%-80% free water (i.e., 750-800 ml), the patient then has a water deficit of 1,000 ml minus 750-800 ml, or a deficit of 250-200 ml. Therefore, 200-250 ml of additional free water should be provided per day. Water can be administered *via* flushing of the feeding tube to maintain patency or before or after medication administration to prevent precipitation and obstruction.

An awareness is required of all sources of intake (oral, enteral, IV fluids, and medications) as well as losses (urine, stool, drains, fistulas, emesis, and expiratory and evaporative losses). Renal failure, congestive heart failure, and progression of ascites are a few conditions that necessitate careful monitoring of fluid status and may require restriction of intake. In critically ill patients, third-spacing of fluid is common and makes estimates of fluid balance and weight difficult. Fluid management must be responsive to hemodynamic variables, electrolyte balance, and optimal functioning of all bodily organs and systems.

Usual fluid requirements are 1.5 L/m². The daily loss of water includes approximately 1,400 ml in urine (60 ml/hr), 350 ml *via* respiration, 350 ml as evaporative losses through skin, 100 ml in sweat, and about 200 ml in feces. If loss by any of these routes is increased, fluid needs will increase; if loss by any of these routes is impaired, fluid restriction may be necessary. **Note:** Urine output may be as high as 2-3 L under normal conditions. This represents a range of 80-125 ml/hr.

Nutritional support modalities

Specialized nutritional support refers to enteral and parenteral support, that is, tube feedings and intravenous delivery of nutrients. Hospitalized individuals frequently cannot eat enough to meet their needs. Often, several types of nutritional support are administered simultaneously when the patient is being weaned from one type of support to another. During these transition times, recording intake from all sources and obtaining calorie counts can help ensure that intake is adequate. The following are the various types of nutritional therapy.

ORAL DIET

An oral diet is based on guidelines for normal human nutrition and may be modified for consistency or for special disease states. Clear liquid and full liquid diets are nutritionally incomplete and usually are used for the purpose of testing tolerance of anything by mouth and should not be used without other nutritional supplementation for more than 5 days. For the patient with lactose intolerance, gastroenteritis (often accompanied by a lactose intolerance that can last 6-8 weeks), fat malabsorption, or pancreatitis (often accompanied by fat malabsorption), the full liquid diet is usually avoided because it contains many dairy products high in both lactose and fat. The regular hospital diet can be altered in texture to accommodate the patient with poor dentition, ill-fitting dentures, mucositis, stomatitis, oral surgery, or neuromuscular disorders. Other alterations can be made by the dietitian to provide diets for patients who are diabetics, in renal failure, with hepatic disease, or with numerous other disease states and conditions requiring alterations of specific nutrients or distribution of calories.

LIQUID NUTRITIONAL SUPPLEMENTS

These are plentiful and range from complete nutritional products capable of meeting total nutritional needs if provided in adequate quantity, to others that are incomplete and intended for use as supplementation to an oral diet or as an occasional meal replacement. Caution should be exercised in selecting these aids to ensure that the patient's dietary needs are met. Most of these products are more palatable when served cold or over crushed ice.

MODULAR ENTERAL COMPONENTS

These are available as individual nutrients (e.g., carbohydrates, protein, or fat; forms may vary, i.e., as long-chain triglycerides, medium-chain triglycerides, or a mixture of both) or as a carefully compounded combination of nutrients (e.g., vitamins or minerals or electrolytes). They can be used in a mix-and-match manner to produce individually tailored enteral products or to supplement other existing products. When added to foods they can enhance caloric density and protein intake, provide fat in an easy-to-absorb form, or supplement vitamins or minerals. Because deficiencies or toxicities of nutrients can occur unless requirements are carefully met and not exceeded, these products usually are used at the discretion of the clinical dietitian.

ENTERAL PRODUCTS

These products are usually prepared for administration *via* a feeding tube, although some also can be taken orally. These products may be nutritionally complete or incomplete, fiber enriched or low residue, isosmolar (300 mOsm/kg H_2O) or hyperosmolar (>300 mOsm/kg/H_2O), standard (1 cal/ml) or high calorie (1.5-2 cal/ml), restricted in protein or high in nitrogen, and containing intact or predigested nutrients. Choice of product is dependent on nutrient needs, fluid tolerance, digestive and absorptive ability, as well as route of administration (gastric, duodenal, jejunal) and lumen size of the feeding tube used. Length of the gut and function of all accessory organs of digestion are other key factors.

1. **Use of predigested products:** Currently reserved for deep jejunal feedings (in which most of the absorptive length of the gut is bypassed) and for short gut syndrome or severe malabsorption.

2. **Osmolarity and rate of administration:** Tube feeding products usually are introduced at isosmolarity (full strength for an isosmolar product, dilution with tap water to achieve an isosmolar state for hyperosmolar products). Rates are often initiated at 50 ml/hr and advanced at 25 ml/hr/day until desired nutrient goals are reached. A usual maximum infusion rate is 125 ml/hr.

   □ *Gastric infusions:* Increased first in concentration and then in volume as hyperosmolar solutions are better tolerated intragastrically. For example, 50 ml/hr half strength, 50 ml/hr full strength, 75 ml/hr full strength, then 100 ml/hr full strength.

   □ *Small bowel infusions:* Advanced in volume first and concentration second. For example, 50 ml/hr half strength, 75 ml/hr half strength, 100 ml/hr half strength, 100 ml/hr three-fourths strength, and 100 ml/hr full strength.

3. **Types of tubes used:** Temporary (oro- or nasogastric, duodenal, or jejunal) or more permanent (surgical or percutaneous endoscopically placed gastrostomy, standard jejunostomy, or needle catheter jejunostomy). The small diameter of the needle catheter jejunostomy often requires a predigested formula for lowered viscosity. It is predisposed to occlusion unless vigilant care is given to regular flushing for maintaining patency, especially if it is the only route for medication administration.

4. **Method of administration:** Gravity, syringe, or continual infusion device (pump) may be used, *via* bolus, intermittent, or continuous drip method. Of these, bolus is the most likely to cause discomfort (nausea, distention) or complications (vomiting, cramping, dumping syndrome, or diarrhea).

5. **Prevention of infection:** Hanging time should not exceed 8 hours because of the risk of bacterial proliferation at room temperature. Clean technique should be used when handling enteral products, containers, and feeding tube. Containers and tubing for enteral administration usually are changed q24h. All opened products should be dated (day, date, and time) and any unused product discarded after 24 hours.

PARENTERAL NUTRITION

Parenteral nutrition is the intravenous provision of nutrients. It may be accomplished either by peripheral or central veins.

1. **Peripheral therapy:** Used only when peripheral venous access is good and nutritional needs are low. It is used for short-term (7-10 days) delivery of nutrients or to supplement other nutritional support modalities.

2. **Central therapy:** For patients who are unable to tolerate oral or enteral feedings for a period exceeding 5-10 days.

3. **Types of parenteral solutions:** These solutions may contain dextrose, amino acids, electrolytes, vitamins, and minerals. Fat emulsions of soybean or safflower oils are available, also. The pharmacist may start with a solution of 50%-70% dextrose, to which he or she adds a quantity of 8.5%-10% amino acids, electrolytes, vitamins, and minerals. The final dilution of dextrose may range from 15%-47%, and the quantity of amino acids may range from 2%-5%, with the lower quantities provided in renal failure without dialysis, at which time only essential amino acids are provided. Amino acid solutions also may be enriched with the branched-chain amino acids or contain reduced quantities of aromatic amino acids. The former solution may be used in stress, while the latter is used in hepatic failure. IV fat emulsions are available in 10% and 20% solutions. These are used to provide essential fatty acids or for energy. In cases of glucose intolerance (e.g., diabetes, pancreatitis, sepsis, stress) or when carbon dioxide retention is a problem (e.g., COPD, weaning patient from the ventilator) carbohydrate kilocalories are replaced in part by fat.

NURSING DIAGNOSES AND INTERVENTIONS

Alteration in nutrition: Less than body requirements related to inadequate provision of nutrients

Desired outcome: Patient has adequate nutrition as evidenced by stable weight, serum albumin 3.5-5.5 g/dl, thyroxine-binding prealbumin 200-300 μg/ml, retinol-binding protein 40-50 μg/ml, and a positive nitrogen state as determined by nitrogen studies.

For parenteral nutrition:

1. Ensure nutritional screening and assessment of patient within 72 hours of admission. For guidelines, see p. 612.
2. Assist in central venous catheter placement and maintenance of sterility and patency of the line. Obtain x-ray confirmation of proper placement before commencing infusion of parenteral solutions.
3. Administer parenteral solutions as prescribed. Alert MD to
   □ Indicators of sepsis.
   □ Occlusion or malfunction of central line.
   □ Sudden cessation of infusion in central line.
   □ Factors causing impaired delivery of prescribed quantity of nutrients, for example, change in patient's status; discontinued infusion due to surgery, treatments, or therapy (OT/PT); delayed delivery due to broken bottle.
4. Test urine sugar q6h; notify MD of values ≥3.
5. Weigh patient daily at the same time of day, using the same scale. Notify MD if weight change is ≥1 kg.
6. Record I&O, noting 24-hour trends.
7. Monitor laboratory values for the following:
   □ At the beginning of parenteral therapy obtain baseline serum values for:
   *Na, K, Cl, CO_2
   Platelets, PT, PTT
   CBC with differential
   Total iron-binding capacity (TIBC)
   *Glucose
   *BUN, creatinine
   Ca, Mg, PO_4
   SGPT, alkaline phosphatase, total bilirubin
   Albumin, transferrin
   Thyroxine-binding prealbumin and retinol-binding protein
   □ Tests marked with an asterisk above often are ordered daily during initiation progression of TPN, then as needed based on individual tolerance.
   □ Laboratory tests cited above are repeated on a weekly basis.

For enteral nutrition:

1. Ensure nutritional screening and assessment of patient within 72 hours of admission. For guidelines, see p. 612.
2. Insert or assist in placement of enteral tube. If patient has a small-bore feeding tube with a guide wire, obtain x-ray confirmation of proper placement before initiating infusion of tube feeding. Check placement of large-bore feeding tube by aspirating gastric contents and auscultating over epigastric area for "whoosh" of air that is noted immediately after injection of 10-20 ml of air.
3. Administer enteral product as prescribed. Alert MD to
   □ Technical or mechanical complications (i.e., clogged or displaced feeding tube).
   □ Signs of aspiration.
   □ Metabolic complications (e.g., glycosuria, proteinuria, change in urine output or hydration status).
   □ Factors causing impaired delivery of prescribed quantity of nutrients (e.g., occlusion of tube, GI distress).
4. Test urine sugar q6h; notify MD of values ≥3+.

5. Weigh patient daily at the same time of day, using the same scale. Notify MD if weight change is ≥1 kg.
6. Record I&O, noting 24-hour trends.

For oral nutrition:

1. Ensure nutritional screening and assessment of patient within 72 hours of admission. See guidelines, p. 612.
2. Position patient properly for eating; assist with eating as needed. Involve significant others in meal rituals for companionship and caring.
3. Provide small, frequent feedings of diet compatible with disease state and patient's ability to ingest foods.
4. Respect food aversions and try to maximize on food preferences.
5. Provide liquid nutritional supplements as prescribed. Serve them cold or over ice to enhance palatability.
6. Provide psychologic support.

Potential for impaired skin and tissue integrity related to vulnerability secondary to malnourished state or presence of central venous catheters or enteral tube

Desired outcome: Patient's skin and tissue remain intact, with no evidence of decubitus ulcers, skin rashes, excoriation, mucous membrane breakdown, or necrosis.

1. Ensure adequate nutrition after assessing energy, protein, fat, vitamin, mineral, and fluid needs (see pp. 618-620).
2. Alter patient's position at least q2h; check for erythematous areas.
3. Examine central catheter insertion site daily or at each dressing change, noting erythema, swelling, irritation, rash. Consider tapes or antibacterial and antifungal ointments and solutions as possible irritants. Pursue alternatives as necessary.
4. Secure feeding tube so that there is no pressure on surrounding tissues. Use transparent tape when possible for enhanced patient body image and ease of viewing patient's insertion site. Provide regular oral and nasal hygiene. Be alert to pressure areas.

Potential for infection related to vulnerability secondary to malnourished state and presence of central venous catheter or enteral tube

Desired outcome: Patient is free of infection as evidenced by normothermia, HR ≤100 bpm, RR ≤20 breaths/min, WBC count ≤11,000 µl, and absence of erythema and swelling at catheter insertion site.

1. Ensure adequate nutritional support, based on patient's needs. For guidelines, see pp. 620-621.
2. Examine catheter insertion site daily or with each dressing change for presence of erythema or swelling.
3. Assess temperature and VS q6h; report temperature >38.3° C (101° F) or temperature spike and leukocytosis. Also be alert to increased HR and RR, which are other indicators of infection.
4. Test urine for sugar q6h; report values ≥3+.
5. Use meticulous sterile technique when changing central line dressing and hanging new bottle of feeding solution.
6. Avoid using central line that is being used for nutritional support for blood drawing, pressure monitoring, or administration of medications or other fluids.
7. Hang tube feeding solution a maximum of 8 hours at a time.
8. Use clean technique in handling feeding tube and enteral products and containers.
9. Change enteral administration set q24h.
10. Report signs of GI intolerance that may be related to enteral product contamination (i.e., nausea and vomiting, abdominal distention, cramping, diarrhea).

Potential for impaired swallowing related to pain or decreased ability to ingest secondary to disease or treatment of disease (e.g., surgery, chemotherapy, radiation)

Desired outcome: Patient demonstrates adequate cough and gag reflexes and the ability to ingest foods *via* the phases of swallowing as instructed.

1. Ensure nutritional screening and assessment as well as assessment of oral motor function within 72 hours of admission or progression to oral diet.
2. Provide small, frequent meals.
3. Provide foods at temperatures acceptable to patient.
4. Respect food aversions; honor food preferences whenever possible.
5. Provide oral supplements or tube feeding supplements as prescribed. Advise patient of transition status and praise his or her progress.
6. Order extra sauces, gravies, or liquids if dryness of the oral cavity impairs patient's swallowing ability. Suggest that patient moisten each bite of food with these substances.
7. In conjunction with physical or occupational therapist, assist in retraining or facilitating patient's swallowing. Assess cough and gag reflexes before the first feeding. Initially, liquids and solids may be difficult to manage. Offer foods with thickened consistency and progress to increased texture as tolerated. Assist patient through the phases of ingesting food: opening the mouth, achieving lip closure, chewing, transferring food from side to side in the mouth and then to the back of the oral cavity, elevating the tongue to the roof of the mouth (hard palate), and swallowing between breaths.

Potential for impaired gas exchange related to risk of aspiration secondary to administration of enteral feeding

Desired outcome: Patient's proper tube position is verified by x-ray, aspiration of gastric contents, and auscultation of "whoosh" of air over epigastric area.

1. Do not initiate enteral feeding until small-bore tube position has been documented by x-ray. For large-bore feeding tube, check position *via* aspiration and auscultation (see description p. 622, under enteral nutrition, **Alteration in nutrition**).
2. Elevate HOB at least 30 degrees. Maintain this position for 45-60 minutes after feeding. If this is not possible or comfortable for the patient, turn patient into a slightly elevated right side-lying position to enhance gravity flow from the greater stomach curve to the pylorus.
3. Utilize enteral pump to facilitate infusion.
4. Aspirate gastric contents at least q4h to measure residual feeding. If residual is <100 ml, return aspirate and continue feeding. If aspirate is >100 ml, return aspirate and notify MD or follow agency policy regarding whether to hold or continue feeding.
5. Assess rate of tube feeding hourly; reset to prescribed rate as indicated. If infusion lags behind prescribed quantity significantly, do not attempt to "catch up" by increasing infusion rate greatly.

Section Two   MANAGING WOUND CARE

A wound is a disruption of tissue integrity caused by trauma, surgery, or an underlying medical disorder. Wound management is directed at preventing infection and/or deterioration in wound status and promoting healing.

Wounds closed by primary intention

Clean, surgical, or traumatic wounds whose edges are closed with sutures, clips, or sterile tape strips are referred to as wounds closed by primary intention. Impairment of healing most frequently manifests as dehiscence, evisceration, or infection. Individuals at high risk for disruption of wound healing include those who are obese, diabetic, elderly, malnourished, receiving steroids, or undergoing chemotherapy or radiation therapy.

ASSESSMENT

Optimal healing: Immediately after injury, the incision line is warm, reddened, indurated, and tender. After 1 or 2 days, wound fluid on the incision line dries, forming a scab that subsequently falls off and leaves a pink scar. After 5-9 days a healing ridge, a palpable accumulation of scar tissue, forms. In patients who undergo cosmetic surgery, scab formation and a healing ridge are purposely avoided to minimize scar formation. See Table 12-4, below.

Impaired healing: Lack of an adequate inflammatory response manifested by absence of initial redness, warmth, and induration; continued drainage from the incision line 2 days after injury (when no drain is present); absence of a healing ridge by the ninth day after injury; presence of purulent exudate. See Table 12-4, below.

DIAGNOSTIC TESTS

1. *WBC with differential:* To assess for infection.
2. *Gram stain of drainage:* If infection is suspected, to identify the offending organism and aid in the selection of preliminary antibiotics.
3. *Culture and sensitivity of drainage:* To determine optimal antibiotic. Infection is said to be present when there are 10^5 organisms per gram of tissue or presence of fever and drainage.

MEDICAL MANAGEMENT AND SURGICAL INTERVENTIONS

1. Application of a sterile dressing in surgery: To protect wound from external contamination and trauma or provide pressure. Usually, surgeon changes the initial dressing.
2. High-calorie/high-protein diet: To promote positive nitrogen balance for optimal wound healing.
3. Multivitamins, especially C: To enhance tissue healing.
4. Minerals, especially zinc and iron: May be prescribed, depending on patient's serum levels.
5. Supplemental oxygen: Empirically, 2-4 L/min in high-risk patients. After injury, wound Po_2 is low and administration of oxygen may enhance healing.
6. Insulin: As needed to control glucose levels in diabetics.
7. Local or systemic antibiotics: Given when infection is present and sometimes used prophylactically as well.
8. Incision and drainage of the incision line: When infection is present and localized. This allows healing by secondary intention. Often, the wound is irrigated with antiinfective agents such as dilute Dakin's solution or povidone-iodine.

TABLE 12-4 Assessment of healing by primary intention

Expected findings	Abnormal findings
Edges well approximated	Edges not well approximated
Good inflammatory response (redness, warmth, induration, pain) initially post-injury	Decreased/absent inflammatory response
No drainage (without drain present) 48 hours after closure	Drainage continues 48 hours after closure
Healing ridge present by postoperative day 7-9	No healing ridge present by postoperative day 9

NURSING DIAGNOSES AND INTERVENTIONS

Potential impairment of tissue integrity: Wound healing by primary intention, related to risk of infection, metabolic alterations (e.g., diabetes mellitus), impaired oxygen transport, altered tissue perfusion, and alterations in fluid volume and nutrition

Desired outcome: Patient exhibits signs of wound healing within an acceptable time frame (7-9 postoperative days).

1. Assess wound for indications of impaired healing, including absence of a healing ridge after 5-9 days, presence of purulent exudate, and delayed inflammatory response. Monitor VS for signs of infection, including elevated temperature and pulse rate. Document findings.
2. Use aseptic technique when changing dressings. If a drain is present, keep it sterile, maintain patency, and handle it gently to prevent it from becoming dislodged. If wound care will be necessary after hospital discharge, teach the dressing change procedure to patient and significant others.
3. Maintain blood glucose within normal range for diabetics by performing serial monitoring of blood glucose and administering insulin on time, as indicated.
4. Explain to patient that deep breathing promotes oxygenation, which enhances wound healing. If indicated, provide incentive spirometry at least qid. Stress the importance of position changes and activity as tolerated to promote ventilation. Explain that if maximal inspiratory efforts are not sufficient to keep the lungs clear, coughing must be performed at frequent intervals to raise secretions.
5. Monitor perfusion status by checking BP, pulse, capillary refill time in the tissue adjacent to incision, moisture of mucous membranes, skin turgor, volume and specific gravity of urine, and I&O.
6. For nonrestricted patients, ensure a fluid intake of at least 2-3 L/day.
7. Encourage ambulation or ROM exercises as allowed to enhance peripheral circulation.
8. To promote positive nitrogen balance, which enhances wound healing, provide a diet high in protein and calories. Ensure sufficient dietary intake of vitamin C and encourage between-meal supplements that are high in protein. If patient complains of feeling full with three meals a day, give six small feedings instead.
9. Check protein status *via* serum protein and serum albumin levels. Optimal levels are 6-8 g/dl total protein and 3.5-5.5 g/dl serum albumin.
10. Obtain a dietary consult if intake is not adequate or will not be adequate during the first 7-10 days after the injury or if laboratory work indicates low protein status.
11. Provide prescribed vitamin supplements, as well as zinc and iron when indicated.
12. Weigh patient daily and evaluate trend of weight change.
13. Teach patient about nutrient needs for healing so that he or she can participate in the planning to meet requirements.
14. Teach patient to support wound as needed (e.g., using binder for obese individual; splinting incision with pillows or hands when coughing).

PATIENT-FAMILY TEACHING AND DISCHARGE PLANNING

Provide patient and significant others with verbal and written information for the following:
1. Local wound care, including type of equipment necessary, wound care procedure, and therapeutic and negative side effects of topical agents used. Have patient/significant other demonstrate dressing change procedure before hospital discharge.
2. Signs and symptoms that occur with improvement in wound status (see Table 12-4, p. 625).
3. Signs and symptoms that signal deterioration in wound status, including those that necessitate notification of MD or clinic (see Table 12-4, p. 625).
4. Diet that enhances wound healing. Provide information about high-calorie, high-protein diet. See "Providing Nutritional Support," p. 611. Involve dietitian as necessary.

5. Activities that maximize ventilatory status: a planned regimen for ambulatory patients and deep breathing and turning (at least q2h) for those on bed rest.
6. Importance of taking multivitamins, antibiotics, and supplements of iron and zinc as prescribed. For all medications to be taken at home, provide the following: name, purpose, dosage, schedule, precautions, and potential side effects.
7. Importance of follow-up care with MD; confirm time and date of next appointment if known.

In addition:

8. If needed, arrange for a visit by public health or visiting nurses before hospital discharge.

Surgical or traumatic wounds healing by secondary intention

Wounds healing by secondary intention are those with tissue loss or heavy contamination that form granulation tissue and contract in order to heal. Most often, impairment of healing is caused by increased contamination and impairment of perfusion, oxygenation, and nutrition, which results in a delay in the healing process. Individuals at risk for impaired healing include those who are obese, diabetic, malnourished, elderly, taking steroids, or undergoing radiation or chemotherapy.

ASSESSMENT

Optimal healing: Initially, the wound edges are inflamed, indurated, and tender. At first, granulation tissue on the floor and walls is pink, progressing to a deeper pink and then to a beefy red; it should be moist. Epithelial cells from the tissue surrounding the wound gradually migrate across the granulation tissue. As healing occurs, the wound edges become pink, the angle between surrounding tissue and the wound becomes less acute, and wound contraction occurs. Occasionally a wound has a tract or sinus that gradually decreases in size as healing occurs. See Table 12-5, below.

Impaired healing: Exudate appears on the floor and walls of the wound and does not abate as healing progresses. It is important to note the distribution, color, odor, volume, and adherence of the exudate. The skin surrounding the wound should be assessed for signs of tissue damage, including disruption, discoloration, and increasing pain. When a drain is in place, the volume, color, and odor of the drainage should be evaluated. See Table 12-5, below.

DIAGNOSTIC TESTS

1. *CBC with WBC differential:* To assess hematocrit level and for presence of infection. Increased WBC count signals infection, while a decrease occurs with immunosuppression. Watch the neutrophil count for a shift to the left, which indicates infection.

T A B L E   1 2 - 5   Assessment of healing by secondary intention

Expected findings	Abnormal findings
Initially post-injury, wound edges inflamed, indurated, and tender; with epithelialization, edges become pink	Initially post-injury, decreased inflammatory response; epithelialization slowed or mechanically disrupted so not continuous around wound
Granulation tissue moist and pink, becoming beefy red over time	Granulation tissue remains pale or is excessively dry or moist
No odor present	Odor present
No exudate or necrotic tissue present	Exudate or necrotic tissue present

Monitor the lymphocyte count; ≤1,800 μl is a sign of malnutrition. For optimal healing, the hematocrit should be >20%.

2. *Gram stain of drainage:* To determine the offending organism, if present, and aid in the selection of the preliminary antibiotic.

3. *Tissue biopsy or culture and sensitivity of drainage:* To determine presence of infection and the optimal antibiotic, if appropriate.

4. *Ultrasound, sonogram, or sinogram:* To determine wound size, especially when abscesses or tracts are suspected.

MEDICAL MANAGEMENT AND SURGICAL INTERVENTIONS

1. Debriding enzymes: To soften and remove necrotic tissue, for example, fibrinolysin plus desoxyribonuclease (Elase).

2. Dressings: To provide debridement, keep healthy wound tissue moist, or provide antiseptic agent to decrease wound surface bacterial counts. See Table 12-6, p. 629.

3. Hydrophilic agents: To remove contaminants and excess exudate, for example, dextran beads or paste (Envisan) or polymer flakes (Bard Absorption Dressing).

4. Hydrotherapy: To soften and remove debris mechanically.

5. Wound irrigation with or without antiinfective agents: To dislodge and remove bacteria and loosen necrotic tissue, foreign bodies, and exudate.

6. IV fluids: For patients unable to take adequate oral fluids.

7. Topical or systemic vitamin A: As needed to reverse adverse effects of steroids on healing.

8. Drain(s): To remove excess tissue fluid or purulent drainage.

9. Surgical debridement: To remove dead tissue and reduce debris and fibrotic tissue

10. Skin graft: To provide coverage of wound if necessary.

11. Tissue flaps: To fill tissue defect and provide wound closure with its own blood supply.

12. High-protein/high-calorie diet, supplemental oxygen, multivitamins and minerals, insulin, and incision and drainage: See discussion, "Wounds Closed by Primary Intention," p. 625.

NURSING DIAGNOSES AND INTERVENTIONS

Impaired tissue integrity: Wound, related to presence of contamination

Desired outcomes: Patient's wound exhibits signs of healing within an acceptable time frame. Patient or significant other successfully demonstrates wound care procedure, if appropriate.

1. Use dressings as prescribed. Insert dressing into all tracts to promote gradual closure of those areas. Dressings may be changed with sterile or clean technique, depending on agency policy, potential for external contamination, and patient's ability to mount an adequate immunologic response. Ensure good handwashing before and after dressing changes, and dispose of contaminated dressings appropriately, following Universal Precautions.

2. When a drain is used, maintain its patency, prevent kinking of the tubing, and secure the tubing to prevent the drain from becoming dislodged. Always use aseptic technique when caring for drains.

3. To help prevent contamination, cleanse the skin surrounding the wound with a mild disinfectant, e.g., soap and water. Do not use friction with cleansing if tissue is friable.

4. If irrigation is prescribed for reducing contaminants, use high-pressure irrigation with an ultrasonic water jet or a 35 ml syringe with an 18-gauge needle. If the tissue is friable or the wound is over a major organ or blood vessel, use extreme caution with the irrigation pressure. Both the patient and nurse should wear a surgical mask to prevent seeding of the nares with wound contaminants, thereby eliminating a potential reservoir for cross-contamination. To remove contaminants effectively, use a large volume of irrigant, for example, 100-150 ml.

TABLE 12-6 Dressings used for wound care

Dressing	Advantages	Limitations
Dry to Dry* Insert dry and remove dry	Highly absorbent; debridement	Excessively drying to tissue; disruption of new tissues; painful removal
Wet to Dry* Insert wet and remove dry	Good absorption but not as absorptive as dry to dry; good debridement	Drying of tissues but not as much as dry to dry; disruption of new tissue; painful removal
Moist to Moist* Insert and remove with moisture present	Provides topical antiinfective agent; no wound desiccation; good debridement. Not painful; inexpensive	Less effective removal of exudate; if excessively wet, can cause tissue maceration; if it dries out, dressing must be moistened before removal
Xeroform Gauze	Provides topical antiseptic; keeps tissue hydrated; minimal pain with removal	Can cause tissue maceration if it is excessively moist
Porcine Skin Dressing	Can provide topical antibiotic; keeps tissue hydrated; not painful when removed; often used before closure of wound with tissue grafts	Expensive; usually stored in refrigerator until use
Transparent Dressing: e.g., Op-Site, Tegaderm, Biooclusive	Prevents loss of wound fluid; protects wound from external contamination; minimal pain with removal; protects from friction and fluid loss	Must withdraw excessive drainage and reseal dressing; appearance of drainage erroneously suggests infection
Hydrocolloid Dressing: e.g., Duoderm, Restore, Intact	Maintains moist wound surface while minimizing pooling; easy to apply; minimal pain with removal	Cannot directly assess wound without removing dressing; "melts" when used under radiant heat; limited absorption
Hydrophilic Gel: e.g., Vigilon	Maintains moist wound surface; nonadherent; absorbs some exudate; compatible with topical medications; easy to apply; minimal pain with removal	Causes maceration when in direct contact with normal tissue; expensive; may require frequent changing

*All dressings are sterile, coarse mesh gauze without cotton fiber fill and are covered with dry sterile outer layer to prevent ingress of organisms. When moisture is prescribed, it is provided with an antiinfective agent or physiologic solution.

5. Topically applied antiinfective agents, such as neomycin and iodophors, are absorbed by the wound and can produce systemic side effects. When these agents are used, be alert to side effects such as toxicity to cells in the wound, nephrotoxicity, and acidosis.
6. When a hydrophilic agent such as Debrisan or Bard Absorption Dressing is prescribed, remove it with high-pressure irrigation. If the agent were to be removed with a 4×4 or surgical sponge, the friction would disrupt capillary budding and delay healing.
7. When topical enzymes are prescribed, use them on necrotic tissue only and follow package directions carefully. Be aware that some agents such as povidone-iodine deactivate the enzymes. Protect surrounding undamaged skin with zinc oxide or aluminum hydroxide paste.
8. Teach patient or significant other the prescribed wound care procedure, if indicated.

Impaired tissue integrity: Wound, related to alterations in perfusion, oxygenation, fluid volume, and nutrition

Desired outcome: Patient exhibits signs of wound healing within an acceptable time frame.

1. Compare energy expenditure and nutrient intake with daily weights until stable, and then twice a week thereafter. If weight loss is progressive or intake insufficient to offset demands during the first 7-10 days after injury, discuss supplemental enteral or parenteral nutrition with MD or dietitian. For more information, see "Providing Nutritional Support," p. 611.
2. Be alert to fluid and electrolyte losses that can occur with draining wounds (see "Fluid and Electrolyte Disturbances," p. 546).
3. If patient exhibits signs of dehydration or is unable to consume adequate amounts of oral fluids, discuss with MD the possibility of IV fluids.
4. For other interventions, see **Potential for impaired tissue integrity,** p. 626, in "Wounds Closed by Primary Intention."

PATIENT-FAMILY TEACHING AND DISCHARGE PLANNING

See teaching and discharge planning interventions in "Wounds Closed by Primary Intention," p. 626.

Pressure ulcers

Pressure ulcers result from a disruption in tissue integrity and are most often caused by excessive tissue pressure or shearing of blood vessels. High-risk patients include the elderly and those who have decreased mobility, decreased LOC, impaired sensation, debilitation, incontinence, sepsis/elevated temperature, or malnutrition.

ASSESSMENT

High-risk individuals should be identified upon admission assessment, with ongoing assessments during hospitalization. Assessment should include the patient's LOC, ability to perform ADL, degree of sensation and mobility, status of nutrition and continence, body temperature, and age. When pressure ulcers are present, their severity can be graded on a scale of I to IV:

Grade I: Irregular area of soft tissue swelling, pain, erythema, and heat. Erythema is not relieved by alleviation of pressure or stimulation of local circulation. In dark-skinned individuals, heat may be the only indication of a grade I pressure ulcer.

Grade II: Skin damage with heat, erythema, pain, and induration. The skin may be attached to or removed from the ulcer.

Grade III: Involves subcutaneous tissue down to fat; often infected or necrotic; muscle under the fat frequently inflamed; and skin surrounding the ulcer often affected. Induration and pain are present.

Grade IV: Involves extensive soft tissue damage, extending to the bone; often associated with osteomyelitis, profuse drainage, tissue necrosis, and pain.

See "Surgical or Traumatic Wounds Healing by Secondary Intention," p. 627, for other assessment data.

DIAGNOSTIC TESTS

See "Diagnostic Tests," p. 627, in "Surgical or Traumatic Wounds Healing by Secondary Intention."

MEDICAL MANAGEMENT AND SURGICAL INTERVENTIONS

1. Debriding enzymes: To soften and remove necrotic tissue.
2. Dressings: To provide debridement, keep healthy tissue moist, or apply an antiinfective agent. See Table 12-6, p. 629.
3. Hydrophilic agents: To remove contaminants and excess moisture.
4. Wound irrigation with antiinfective agents: To reduce contamination.
5. Hydrotherapy: To soften and remove debris mechanically.
6. Diet: Adequate protein and calories to promote positive nitrogen state for rapid wound healing.
7. Supplemental vitamins and minerals: As needed.
8. Supplemental oxygen: Usually 2-4 L/min to promote wound healing for high-risk patients or those with delayed wound healing.
9. Surgical debridement: Removal of devitalized tissue with a scalpel to reduce the amount of debris and fibrotic tissue.
10. Tissue flaps: Provide closure of wound as well as its own blood supply.

NURSING DIAGNOSES AND INTERVENTIONS

Potential for impaired skin/tissue integrity related to excessive tissue pressure

Desired outcomes: Patient's tissue remains intact. Patient participates in prevention measures and verbalizes understanding of the rationale for these interventions.

1. Assist patient with position changes. There is an inverse relationship between pressure and time in ulcer formation; therefore, heavier patients need to change position more frequently. Position changes include turning the bed-bound patient q1-2h as well as having the wheelchair-bound patient perform pushups in the chair q20min to ensure periodic relief from pressure on the buttocks. In addition, patients with history of previous tissue injury will require pressure relief measures more frequently. Use low-Fowler's position and alternate supine position with side-lying and prone positions.
2. Establish and post a position-changing schedule.
3. Minimize friction on tissue during activity. Friction causes shearing of vessels, which leads to tissue disruption. Lift rather than drag patient during position changes and transferring; use a draw sheet to facilitate patient movement.
4. Use a mattress that minimizes tissue pressure, such as the Clinitron bed, low air loss bed, water bed, or alternating pressure mattress.
5. When using foam mattress, make sure patient's weight and sheets do not compress the mattress. When the mattress is compressed, it cannot effectively reduce tissue pressure.
6. With every position change, massage susceptible areas, especially over bony prominences such as the sacrum and greater tuberosities. Be aware that massage of erythematous skin that does not blanch in response to digital pressure may exacerbate tissue damage. At this time, research does not indicate whether skin breakdown can be prevented with massage of blanchable erythematous skin or massage of skin surrounding the reddened areas.

7. To enhance circulation, encourage patient to perform ROM, ankle-circling, and iso-metric exercises unless contraindicated.

Impaired tissue integrity related to presence of pressure ulcer (with increased risk for further breakdown)

Desired outcomes: Patient exhibits signs of healing within an acceptable time frame. Patient verbalizes causes and preventive measures for pressure ulcers and successfully participates in the plan of care to promote healing and prevent further breakdown.

1. Maintain a moist environment to promote epithelialization on grade I and grade II pressure ulcers with dressings, such as Op-Site, Tegaderm, or Duoderm.
2. Be sure patient's skin is kept clean with regular bathing, and be especially conscientious about washing urine and feces from the skin. Soap should be used and then thoroughly rinsed from the skin.
3. If the patient has excessive perspiration, use absorptive pads to remove perspiration; change them often.
4. To absorb moisture and prevent shearing when the patient is moved, apply heel and elbow covers as needed.
5. Use lambswool to keep the areas between the toes dry. Change it periodically, depending on the amount of moisture present.
6. Do not use a heat lamp because it increases the metabolic rate of the tissues, resulting in increased demand for blood flow in an area with impaired perfusion. As a result, ulcer diameter and depth can be increased.
7. Teach patient and significant others the importance of and measures for preventing excess pressure as a means of preventing pressure ulcers.

See "Surgical or Traumatic Wounds Healing by Secondary Intention" for **Impaired tissue integrity: Wound,** related to presence of contamination, p. 628, and **Impaired tissue integrity: Wound,** related to alterations in perfusion, oxygenation, fluid volume, and nutrition, p. 630.

Note: Many products used on pressure ulcers have not been scientifically evaluated. Before initiating therapy, understand the mechanism by which all drugs and treatments produce their effects. Follow directions for new products carefully and monitor healing progress.

PATIENT-FAMILY TEACHING AND DISCHARGE PLANNING

Provide patient and significant others with verbal and written information for the following:
1. Location of local medical supply stores that have pressure-reducing mattresses and wound care supplies.
2. Planning a schedule for changing patient's position.

For other teaching and discharge planning interventions, see "Wounds Closed by Primary Intention," p. 626.

SELECTED REFERENCES

American Medical Association, Department of Foods and Nutrition: Guidelines for essential trace element preparations for parenteral use, JAMA 241:2051, 1979.

American Medical Association, Department of Foods and Nutrition: Multivitamin preparations for parenteral use: a statement by the Nutrition Advisory Group, J Parenter Enter Nutr 3:258, 1979.

Blackburn GL et al: Nutritional and metabolic assessment of the hospitalized patient, J Parenter Enter Nutr 3:17, 1977.

Committee on Dietary Allowances, Food and Nutrition Board, National Research Council: Recommended dietary allowances, Washington DC, 1980, National Academy of Sciences.

Fowler EM: Equipment and products used in management and treatment of pressure ulcers, Nurs Clin North Am 22(2):449-461, 1987.

Horne M and Swearingen PL: Pocket guide to fluids and electrolytes, St. Louis, 1989, The CV Mosby Co.

Hotter AN: Physiologic aspects and clinical implications of wound healing, Heart Lung 11(6):522-530, 1982.

Kamath SK et al: Hospital malnutrition: a 33-hospital screening study, J Am Diet Assoc: 203, 1986.

Kinney JM and Roe CF: Caloric equivalent of fever: patterns of postoperative response, Ann Surg 156:610, 1962.

Lang CE: Nutritional support in critical care, Rockville, Md, 1987, Aspen Systems Corp.

Lang CE: Providing nutritional support. In Swearingen PL et al: Manual of critical care, St Louis, 1988, The CV Mosby Co.

Long CL et al: Metabolic response to injury and illness: estimation of energy and protein needs from indirect calorimetry and nitrogen balance, J Parenter Enter Nutr 3:452, 1979.

Reed BR and Clark RA: Cutaneous tissue repaid: practical implications of current knowledge, II, J Am Acad Dermatol 13(6):919-941, 1985.

Stotts NA: Impaired wound healing. In Carrieri AM et al: Pathophysiologic phenomena in nursing, Philadelphia, 1986, WB Saunders Co.

Weissman C et al: Effects of routine intensive care interactions on metabolic rate, Chest 86:815, 1984.

Young ME: Malnutrition and wound healing, Heart Lung 17(1):60-67, 1988.

Appendices

1

APPENDIX

Patient care

Section One CARING FOR PREOPERATIVE AND POSTOPERATIVE PATIENTS

Knowledge deficit: Surgical procedure, preoperative routine, and postoperative care

Desired outcome: Patient verbalizes knowledge of the surgical procedure, including preoperative and postoperative care, and demonstrates relevant postoperative exercises and use of appropriate devices.

1. Assess patient's understanding of the diagnosis and surgical procedure. Evaluate patient's desire for knowledge regarding diagnosis and procedure (some individuals find detailed information helpful; others find very brief and simple explanations more helpful).
2. Based on your assessment, clarify and explain diagnosis and surgical procedure accordingly. Use anatomic models, diagrams, and other audiovisual aids when possible. Provide simply written information to reinforce learning. Provide written and verbal information in the patient's native language for non-English speaking patients. **Note:** Evaluate patient's reading comprehension before providing written materials.
3. Explain the perioperative course of events. Review the following with the patient and significant others:
   □ Physical site before, during, and immediately after surgery (i.e., postanesthesia recovery room, ICU, other speciality unit). If possible, take the patient to the new unit and introduce him or her to the nursing staff.
   □ Preoperative medications and timing of surgery (scheduled time, expected duration).
   □ Pain management, including sensations to expect and methods of relief. If patient-controlled anesthesia (PCA) will be prescribed, have patient return demonstration of the use of the delivery device.
   □ Placement of tubes, catheters, drains, and oxygen delivery devices. Enable patient to see these devices when possible.
   □ Use of antiembolic stockings or pneumatic compression stockings.
   □ Dietary alterations, including NPO status followed by clear liquids until return of full GI function.
   □ Restrictions of activity and positions.
   □ Visiting hours and location of waiting room.
4. Explain the postoperative activities, exercises, and precautions. Have patient return demonstration of the following devices and exercises, as appropriate:

□ Deep breathing and coughing exercises. **Note:** Individuals for whom increased intracranial, intrathoracic, or intraabdominal pressure is contraindicated should not cough. (See **Ineffective airway clearance,** below.)

□ Use of incentive spirometry and other respiratory devices.

□ Calf-pumping, ankle-circling, and footboard-pressing exercises to enhance circulation and prevent thrombophlebitis in the lower extremities (see "Thrombosis/Thrombophlebitis," p. 93, for more information).

□ Use of PCA infusion device.

□ Movement into and out of bed.

5. Provide time for patient to ask questions and express feelings of anxiety; be reassuring and supportive. Be certain to address the individual's main concern(s).

6. When possible, emphasize sensations (i.e., dry mouth, thirst, muscle weakness). This information is often more helpful in reducing stress and anxiety than simple information giving.

Pain related to disease process, injury, or surgical procedure

Desired outcomes: Patient's subjective evaluation of discomfort improves, as documented by a pain scale. Patient does not exhibit nonverbal indicators of pain (see Table A-1). Autonomic indicators (see Table A-2) are diminished or absent. Verbal responses, such as crying or moaning, are absent.

1. Monitor patient at frequent intervals for the presence of discomfort. Devise a pain scale with patient, rating discomfort on a scale of 0 (no discomfort) to 10.

2. Evaluate patients with acute and chronic pain for nonverbal indicators of discomfort (see Table A-1).

3. Evaluate patients with acute pain for autonomic indicators of discomfort (see Table A-2). Be aware that patients with chronic pain (>6 months duration) will not exhibit an autonomic response.

T A B L E   A - 1   Nonverbal indicators of pain

Facial expression: mask-like, grimace, tension
Guarding or protective behaviors
Restlessness or increase in motor activity
Withdrawal or decrease in motor activity
Skeletal muscle tension
Short attention span
Irritability
Anxiety
Sleep disturbances

T A B L E   A - 2   Autonomic indicators of pain

Diaphoresis
Vasoconstriction
Increased systolic and diastolic BP
Increased pulse rate (>100 bpm)
Pupillary dilatation
Change in respiratory rate (usually increased, >20 breaths/min)
Muscle tension or spasm
Decreased intestinal motility, evidenced by nausea, vomiting, abdominal distention, and possibly ileus
Endocrine imbalance, evidenced by sodium and water retention and mild hyperglycemia

4. Evaluate health history for evidence of alcohol and drug (prescribed and nonprescribed) use. A positive history of addiction to alcohol or drugs affects effective dosages of analgesics (i.e., may require more or less) and may be an indication of the need for psychiatric consultation.
5. Administer opioid and related mixed agonist-antagonist analgesics as prescribed (see Table A-3). Monitor for side effects, such as respiratory depression, excessive sedation, nausea, vomiting, and constipation. Be aware that meperidine (Demerol) may produce excitation, muscle twitching, and seizures, especially in conjunction with phenothiazines. For individuals receiving parenteral opioid, have naloxone (Narcan) readily available to reverse severe respiratory depression. **Note:** Due to respiratory depression and other side effects, opioid analgesics should be used cautiously in individuals with asthma, chronic obstructive pulmonary disease (COPD), and other respiratory disorders.
6. Check the patient's analgesia record for the last dose and amount of medication given during surgery and in the postanesthesia recovery room. Be careful to coordinate timing and dose of postoperative analgesics with previously administered medication. **Note:** Droperidol and fentanyl anesthesia potentiate the effects of opioids for up to 10 hours after administration and initial postoperative doses should be reduced by ¼ to ⅓ of the usual dose.
7. Administer prn analgesics before pain becomes severe. Prolonged stimulation of pain receptors results in increased sensitivity to painful stimuli and will increase the amount of drug required to relieve pain. Be aware that addiction to narcotics occurs infrequently in hospitalized patients.
8. Plan to administer intermittently scheduled analgesics prior to painful procedures, ambulation, and at bedtime, scheduling them so that their peak effect is achieved at the inception of the activity or procedure.
9. Augment analgesic therapy with sedatives and tranquilizers in order to prolong and enhance analgesia. Avoid substituting sedatives and tranquilizers for analgesics.

T A B L E   A - 3   Use of opioid and agonist-antagonist analgesia

Route	Commonly prescribed medications	Advantages	Disadvantages
Continuous infusion	morphine, fentanyl (Sublimaze)	*Useful for severe, predictable pain *Relieves pain with lower doses than IV bolus *Avoids peaks and valleys of pain present with IV bolus and IM injections	*Requires frequent observation to monitor flow rate *VS must be monitored often *Weaning necessary *Often reserved for critical care use
IV bolus	morphine, meperidine (Demerol)	*Useful for severe, intermittent pain (i.e., for procedures, treatments) *Rapid onset of action	*Relatively short duration of pain relief *Fluctuating levels *Possibility of excessive sedation as drug levels peak

Continued.

TABLE A-3   Use of opioid and agonist-antagonist analgesia—cont'd

Route	Commonly prescribed medications	Advantages	Disadvantages
Patient-controlled analgesic (PCA). May be delivered IV or sub-Q	morphine, meperidine (Demerol), buprenorphine (Buprenex)	*Useful for moderate to severe pain *Enables titration by patient for effective analgesia without excessive sedation *Relief of pain with lower dosages of medication *Immediate delivery of medication *Patient's sense of self-control lowers anxiety *Less nursing time spent preparing medications	*Pumps necessary to deliver drug are expensive *Patient must have clear mental status *Health provider resistance to self-administration by patient
IM injection	meperidine (Demerol) morphine, pentazocine (Talwin), nalbuphine (Nubain), butorphanol (Stadol), buprenorphine (Buprenex)	*Useful for moderate to severe pain *Longer duration of action than with IV route *Faster pain relief than with oral medication *Very commonly used for postoperative pain	*Variable absorption and fluctuating levels, especially in hypotensive and critically ill patients *Possibility of excessive sedation as drug levels peak *Potential delay in administration
Oral	codeine, oxycodone (Percodan), meperidine (Demerol), pentazocine (Talwin), propoxyphene (Darvon), hydromorphine (Dilaudid)	*Useful for mild to moderate acute pain or chronic severe pain (large doses necessary)	*Variable absorption *Cannot be used until GI function returns. Lengthy interval before onset of action

10. Wean patient from opioid analgesics by decreasing dosage or frequency of the drug. When changing route of administration or medication, be certain to employ equianalgesic doses of the new drug (see Table A-4, p. 642).
11. Administer nonnarcotic and nonsteroidal antiinflammatory drugs (NSAIDs) as prescribed for relief of mild to moderate pain during postoperative recovery (see Table A-5). NSAIDs are especially effective when pain is associated with inflammation and soft tissue injury. Be certain that GI function has returned before administering these oral agents. Monitor for side effects, such as epigastric pain, nausea, dyspepsia, and gastric bleeding. **Note:** Because NSAIDs have a specific peripheral action, they are combined or used in conjunction with centrally acting opioid analgesics.
12. Augment action of medication by employing nonpharmacologic methods of pain control (see Table A-6).
13. Maintain a quiet environment to promote rest. Plan nursing activities to enable long periods of uninterrupted rest at night.
14. Evaluate for and correct nonoperative sources of discomfort (i.e., position, full bladder, infiltrated IV site).
15. Position patient comfortably and reposition at frequent intervals to relieve discomfort due to pressure and improve circulation.
16. Document efficacy of analgesics and other pain control interventions, using the pain scale.

Potential ineffective airway clearance related to increased tracheobronchial secretions secondary to effects of anesthesia; ineffective coughing secondary to CNS depression or pain and muscle splinting; and possible laryngospasm secondary to endotracheal tube or allergic reaction to anesthetics

Desired outcome: Patient's airway remains clear as evidenced by clear breath sounds to auscultation, relaxed breathing, RR 12-20 breaths/min with normal depth and pattern (eupnea), normothermia, and normal skin color.

1. Assess respiratory status, including breath sounds q1-2h during the immediate postoperative period and q8h during recovery. Note and report the presence of rhonchi that do not clear with coughing, labored breathing, tachypnea (RR >20 breaths/min), restlessness, and the presence of fever ($\geq 38.33°$ C [$101°$ F]) and cyanosis.
2. Encourage deep breathing and coughing q2h or more often. Splint thoracic and abdominal incisions during coughing. **Note:** Vigorous coughing may be contraindicated for some individuals (e.g., those undergoing intracranial surgery, spinal fusion, eye and ear surgery, and similar procedures). Coughing after a herniorraphy and some thoracic surgeries should be done in a controlled manner, with the incision supported carefully.
3. Administer humidified oxygen as prescribed to prevent further drying of respiratory passageways and secretions.
4. Be certain that emergency airway equipment (i.e., intubation tray, endotracheal tubes, suctioning equipment, and tracheostomy tray) are on the floor and readily available in the event of sudden airway obstruction.

Potential for aspiration related to obstruction by secretions secondary to CNS depression, decreased GI motility, abdominal distention, recumbent position, presence of gastric tube, and possible impaired swallowing in individuals with oral, facial, or neck surgery

Desired outcome: Patient's upper airway remains unobstructed as evidenced by clear breath sounds, RR 12-20 breaths/min with normal depth and pattern (eupnea), and normal skin color.

1. See interventions 1-4 under **Potential ineffective airway clearance.**
2. If the sedated patient experiences nausea or vomiting, turn him or her immediately into a side-lying position. Fully alert patients may remain in an upright position. As necessary, suction the oropharynx with a Vankauer or similar suction device to remove vomitus.
3. Check placement and patency of gastric tubes q8h and prior to instillation of feedings

T A B L E A - 4   Equianalgesic doses of narcotic analgesics

Class/name	Route	Equianalgesic dose (mg)[*]	Average duration (hr)
Morphine-like agonists			
Codeine	IM, SC	130[†]	3
	PO	180[†]	3
Hydromor-phone	IM, SC	1.5-2.0	4
(Dilaudid)	PO	6.0-7.5	4
Levorphanol	IM, SC	2.0	6
(Levo-Dromoran)	PO	4.0	6
Morphine	IM, SC	10	4
Oxycodone	PO	30[†]	4
(Percodan)			
Oxymor-phone	IM, SC	1.0-1.5	4
(Numor-phan)	rectal	10	4
Meperidine-like agonists			
Fentanyl	IV, IM, SC	0.1-0.2	1[‡]
(Sublimaze)			
Meperidine	IM, SC	100	3
(Demerol)			
	PO	300[†]	3
Methadone-like agonists			
Methadone	IM, SC	10	6
(Dolophine)	PO	10-20	6
Propoxyphene	PO	130-250[†]	4
(Darvon)			
Mixed agonist-antagonist[§]			
Buprenor-phine (Bu-prenex)	IM	0.3-0.6	4
Butorphanol	IM, SC	2.0-3.0	3
(Stadol)			
Nalbuphine	IM, SC	10-20	4
(Nubain)			
Pentazocine	IM	30-60	3
(Talwin)			
	PO	10-200[†]	3

* = recommended starting dose; actual dose must be titrated to patient response.
† = starting doses lower (codeine 30 mg, oxycodone 5 mg, meperidine 50 mg, propoxyphene 65-130 mg, pentazocine 50 mg).
‡ = respiratory depressant effects persist longer than analgesic effects.
§ = mixed agonist/antagonist analgesics may precipitate withdrawal in narcotic-dependent patients.
Adapted from Baumann T and Lehman M: Pain management. In DiPiro J et al: Pharmacotherapy: a pathophysiologic approach, New York, 1988, Elsevier Science Publishing Co; and Young L and Koda-Kimble M, editors: Applied therapeutics: the clinical use of drugs, ed 4, Vancouver Wa, 1988, Applied Therapeutics, Inc.

TABLE A-5 Common nonnarcotic and nonsteroidal antiinflammatory analgesics

acetominophen (Tylenol, Tempra)
acetysalicylic acid (aspirin)
ibuprofen (Motrin, Advil, Nuprin)
indomethacin (Indocin)
naproxen (Naprosyn, Anaprox)

TABLE A-6 Common nonpharmacologic methods of pain control

Sensory interventions
☐ Massage: To relax muscular tension and increase local circulation. Back and foot massage are especially relaxing
☐ ROM exercises (passive, assisted, or active): To relax muscles, improve circulation, and prevent pain related to stiffness and immobility
☐ Transcutaneous nerve stimulation: A battery operated device used to send weak electric impulses *via* electrodes placed on the body. The sensation of pain is reduced during and sometimes after treatment

Emotional interventions
☐ Prevention and control of anxiety: Limiting anxiety reduces muscle tension and increases the patient's pain tolerance. Anxiety and fear contribute to autonomic stimulation and pain responses. Progressive relaxation exercises and encouraging slow, controlled breathing may be helpful
☐ Promoting self-control: Feelings of helplessness and lack of control contribute to anxiety and pain. Techniques, such as PCA and promoting self-helping behaviors, contribute to feelings of self-control

Cognitive interventions
☐ Cognitive preparations: Preparing the patient by explaining what can be expected, thereby reducing stress and anxiety. Preoperative teaching is an example of this technique
☐ Patient education: Teaching methods for preventing or reducing pain. Examples include suggesting comfortable postoperative positions, methods of ambulation, and splinting of incisions when coughing
☐ Distraction: Encouraging patient to focus on something unrelated to the pain. Examples include conversing, reading, watching TV or videos, listening to music, relaxation techniques (see **Health-seeking behavior:** Relaxation technique effective for stress reduction, p. 49)
☐ Humor: Can be an excellent distraction and may help the patient cope with stress
☐ Guided imagery: The patient employs a mental process that uses images to alter a physical or emotional state. This technique promotes relaxation and decreases pain sensations

Many of these techniques may be taught to and implemented by the patient and significant others.

and medications. **Note:** Use caution when irrigating and otherwise manipulating the gastric tubes of patients with recent esophageal, gastric, or duodenal surgery as the tube may become displaced or the surgical incision disrupted by such activity. Consult surgeon prior to irrigation for these individuals.
4. Encourage early and frequent ambulation to improve GI motility and reduce abdominal distention owing to accumulated gases.

5. Introduce oral fluids cautiously, especially in patients with oral, facial, and neck surgery.
6. Administer antiemetics and metochlorpramide (Reglan) as prescribed.

Potential ineffective breathing pattern related to decreased lung expansion secondary to CNS depression, pain, muscle splinting, recumbent position, and effects of anesthesia

Desired outcome: Patient exhibits effective ventilation as evidenced by relaxed breathing, RR 12-20 breaths/min with normal depth and pattern (eupnea), clear breath sounds, normal color, Pao_2 ≥80 mm Hg, pH 7.35-7.45, $Paco_2$ 35-45 mm Hg, and HCO_3^- 22-26 mEq/L.

1. See interventions, Nos. 1, 2, and 3, under **Potential ineffective airway clearance.**
2. Perform a preoperative baseline assessment of patient's respiratory system, noting rate, rhythm, degree of chest expansion, quality of breath sounds, and cough and sputum production. Note preoperative ABG values if available.
3. If appropriate, encourage patient to refrain from smoking for at least 1 week after surgery. Explain the effects of smoking on the body.
4. Evaluate ABG values and notify MD of low or decreasing Pao_2 and high or increasing $Paco_2$.
5. Assist patient with turning and deep-breathing exercises q2h for the first 72 hours postoperatively to promote lung expansion. In the presence of fine crackles (rales), and if not contraindicated, have patient cough to expectorate secretions. Facilitate deep breathing and coughing by demonstrating how to splint the incision with the hands or a pillow. If indicated, medicate patient a half-hour before deep breathing, coughing, or ambulation to enhance compliance. Be aware that opioid analgesics depress the respiratory system.
6. If patient has an incentive spirometer, provide instructions and ensure compliance with its use q2h or as prescribed.
7. Unless contraindicated, assist patient with ambulation by the second postoperative day to enhance ventilation.
8. For other interventions, see **Potential for ineffective breathing pattern** related to hypoventilation secondary to inactivity or omission of deep breathing (for all patients on bed rest or at risk for atelectasis), p. 3, in "Atelectasis."

Potential fluid volume deficit related to *loss of fluids* secondary to presence of indwelling drainage tubes, wound drainage, or vomiting; *inadequate intake of fluids* secondary to nausea, NPO status, CNS depression, or lack of access to fluids; or *intravascular fluid volume loss* secondary to altered regulatory mechanisms and third spacing of bodily fluids due to the effects of anesthesia and major surgery

Desired outcomes: Circulating fluid volume is maintained or restored as evidenced by BP ≥90/60 mm Hg (or within patient's preoperative baseline), HR 60-100 bpm, distal pulses >2+ on a 0-4+ scale, urinary output ≥30 ml/hr, stable or increasing weight, good skin turgor, warm skin, moist mucous membranes, and normothermia. Patient verbalizes orientation to person, place, and time.

1. Monitor VS q4-8h during the recovery phase. Be alert to indicators of dehydration, including decreasing BP, increasing HR, and slightly increased body temperature.
2. Assess patient's physical status q4-8h. Be alert to indicators of dehydration, including dry skin, dry mucous membranes, excessive thirst, diminished intensity of peripheral pulses, and alteration in mental status. Assess skin turgor by lifting a section of skin along the forearm, abdomen, or calf. Release the skin and watch its return to the original position. With good hydration, it will return quickly; with dehydration, the skin will remain in the lifted position (tenting) or return slowly. **Note:** This test may be less reliable in the older adult due to loss of skin elasticity and subcutaneous fat.
3. Monitor urinary output q4-8h. Be alert to a concentrated urine and low or decreasing output (the average normal output is 60 ml/hr or 1,400-1,500 ml/day).
4. Measure, describe, and document any emesis. Be alert to and document excessive

perspiration. Include your assessment of both with the documentation of urinary, fecal, and other drainage for a total picture of the patient's hydration status.

5. Measure and record output from drains, ostomies, wounds, and other sources. Ensure patency of gastric and other drainage tubes. Record quality and quantity of output. Report and replace excessive losses.

6. Monitor patient's weight daily, using the results as an indicator of the patient's hydration and nutritional status. Always weigh the patient at the same time every day, using the same scale and same type and amount of bed clothing. Be aware that this method is not useful in detecting intravascular fluid loss due to third spacing.

7. If nausea and vomiting are present, assess the potential causes, including administration of opioid analgesics, loss of patency of the NG tube, and environmental factors (e.g., unpleasant odors or sights). Administer antiemetics or metochlorpramide (Reglan) as prescribed.

8. Monitor serum electrolytes. Be alert to low potassium levels and the following signs and symptoms of hypokalemia: lethargy, irritability, anorexia, vomiting, muscle weakness and cramping, parasthesias, weak and irregular pulse, and respiratory dysfunction. Also assess for low calcium levels and the following signs and symptoms of hypocalcemia: Trousseau's or Chvostek's sign (for description, see p. 271), tetany, muscle cramps, fatigue, irritability, and personality changes.

9. Administer and regulate IV fluids and electrolytes as prescribed until patient is able to resume oral intake. When IV fluids are discontinued, encourage intake of oral fluids, at least 2-3 L/day in the nonrestricted patient. Honor patient's preference in oral fluids and keep them readily available in patient's room.

10. See "Hypovolemia," p. 546, for additional information and management.

Potential fluid volume deficit related to abnormal loss secondary to postoperative bleeding

Desired outcomes: Patient's circulating blood volume is maintained or restored as evidenced by BP ≥90/60 mm Hg (or within patient's preoperative baseline), HR 60-100 bpm, RR 12-20 breaths/min with normal depth and pattern (eupnea), brisk capillary refill (<3 seconds), warm extremities, distal pulses >2+ on a 0-4+ scale, and urinary output ≥30 ml/hr. Patient verbalizes orientation to person, place, and time.

1. Monitor VS at frequent intervals during the first 24 hours of the postoperative period. Be alert to indicators of internal hemorrhage and impending shock, including decreasing BP, decreasing pulse pressure (difference between systolic and diastolic BP), increasing HR, and increasing RR.

2. Assess patient at frequent intervals during the first 24 hours of the postoperative period for indicators of internal hemorrhage and impending shock, including pallor, diaphoresis, cool extremities, delayed capillary refill, diminished intensity of distal pulses, restlessness, agitation, and disorientation. Also note subjective complaints of thirst or a sense of impending doom.

3. Monitor and measure urinary output q4-8h during the initial postoperative period. Report average hourly output <30 ml/hr. Be alert to progressive urine concentration.

4. Inspect surgical dressing for evidence of frank bleeding (e.g., rapid saturation of dressing with bright red blood). Record saturated dressings and report significant findings to surgeon. If the initial postoperative dressing becomes saturated, reinforce and notify surgeon, as he or she may wish to perform the initial dressing change.

5. Note the amount of character of drainage from gastric and other tubes at least q8h. (See Table 6-10, p. 377, for normal characteristics of GI drainage). If drainage appears to contain blood (e.g., bright red, burgundy, dark coffee ground appearance), perform an occult blood test. If the test is newly or unexpectedly positive, report results to surgeon.

Note: After gastric and some other GI surgeries, the patient will have small amounts of bloody or blood-tinged drainage for the first 12-24 hours. Be alert to large or increasing amounts of bloody drainage.

---

6. Review CBC values for evidence of bleeding: decreases in hgb from normal (male

14-18 g/dl; female 12-16 g/dl); and decreases in hct from normal (male 40%-54%; female 37%-47%).
7. Maintain a patent IV catheter for use should hemorrhagic shock develop. See "Cardiac and Noncardiac Shock," p. 71, for management.

Potential fluid volume excess related to retention secondary to compensatory mechanisms following major surgery

Desired outcome: Patient's fluid balance is maintained as evidenced by BP within normal range of patient's preoperative baseline, distal pulses <4+ on a 0-4+ scale, presence of eupnea, clear breath sounds, absence of or barely detectable edema (≤1+ on a 0-4+ scale), and body weight near or at preoperative baseline.

1. Assess for and report any indicators of fluid overload, including elevated BP, bounding pulses, dyspnea, crackles (rales), and pretibial or sacral edema.
2. Maintain record of 8-hour and 24-hour I&O. Note and report significant imbalance. Remember that normal 24-hour output is 1,400-1,500 ml and normal hourly output is 60 ml/hr.
3. Weigh patient daily, using the same scale and same type and amount of bed clothing. Note significant weight gain. Remember that 1 liter of fluid equals approximately 2.2 pounds.
4. Anticipate postoperative diuresis at approximately 48-72 hours after surgery due to mobilization of third-space (interstitial) fluid.
5. Administer furosemide (Lasix) as prescribed to mobilize interstitial fluid. **Note:** Diuretic therapy may cause dangerous potassium depletion (see "Hypokalemia," p. 555).
6. Be aware that the older adult and individuals with cardiovascular disease are at high risk for developing postoperative fluid volume excess.
7. See "Hypervolemia," p. 549, or additional information and management.

Potential for infection related to vulnerability secondary to IV therapy, indwelling urethral catheter, surgical incision, or nature of disease process

Desired outcome: Patient is free of infection, as evidenced by normothermia; HR ≤100 bpm; RR ≤20 breaths/min with normal depth and pattern (eupnea); negative cultures; clear urine; clear and thin sputum; orientation to person, place, and time; and absence of unusual erythema, warmth, or drainage at the surgical incision.

1. Monitor VS for evidence of infection, such as elevated HR and RR and increased body temperature. Notify surgeon if these are new findings.
2. Evaluate orientation and LOC q8h. Consider infection if altered LOC is unexplained by other factors, such as medication or disease process.
3. Evaluate IV sites for evidence of infection (erythema, warmth, swelling, unusual drainage). Change IV line and site if evidence of infection is present and according to agency protocol (q48-72h).
4. Evaluate patency of all surgically placed tubes or drains. Irrigate or attach to low pressure suction as prescribed. Promptly report unrelieved loss of patency.
5. Note color, character, and odor of all drainage. Report the presence of foul-smelling or abnormal drainage.
6. Evaluate incisions and wound sites for evidence of infection: unusual erythema, warmth, delayed healing, and purulent drainage.
7. Change dressings as prescribed, using sterile technique. Prevent cross contamination of wounds in the same patient by changing one dressing at a time and washing hands between dressing changes.
8. If patient develops evisceration, do not reinsert tissue or organs. Place a sterile saline-soaked gauze over the evisceration and cover with a sterile towel until the wound can be evaluated by the surgeon.
9. Prevent reflux of urine into the bladder by keeping drainage collection container below the level of patient's bladder. Help prevent urinary stasis by avoiding kinks or obstructions in the drainage tubing.

10. Do not open closed urinary drainage system unless absolutely necessary; irrigate catheter only with MD prescription and when obstruction is the known cause.
11. Assess for indicators of UTI, including chills, high-grade fever (>37.78° C [100°F]), flank or labial pain, and cloudy or foul-smelling urine.
12. Encourage intake of 2-3 L/day in nonrestricted patients to minimize the potential for UTI by diluting the urine and maximizing urinary flow.
13. Ensure that the patient's perineum and meatus are cleansed during the daily bath and that the perianal area is cleansed after bowel movements. Do not hesitate to remind patient of these hygiene measures. Be alert to indicators of meatal infection, including swelling, purulent drainage, and persistent meatal redness. Intervene for the patient if he or she is unable to perform self-care.
14. Change the catheter according to established protocol, or sooner if sandy particles can be felt in the distal end of the catheter or patient develops UTI. Change the drainage collection container according to established protocol, or sooner, if it becomes foul-smelling or leaks.
15. Obtain cultures of suspicious drainage or secretions (e.g., sputum, urine, wound) as prescribed. For urine specimens, be certain to use the sampling port, which is at the proximal end of the drainage tube. Cleanse the area with an antimicrobial wipe and use a sterile syringe with a 25-gauge needle to aspirate the urine.
16. Prevent transmission of infectious agents by washing hands well before and after caring for patient and by wearing gloves when contact with blood, drainage, or other body substance is likely.

Constipation related to immobility, opioid analgesics and other medications, effects of anesthesia, lack of privacy, disruption of abdominal musculature, or manipulation of abdominal viscera during surgery

Desired outcome: Patient returns to presurgical bowel elimination pattern as evidenced by return of active bowel sounds, absence of abdominal distention or sensation of fullness, and the elimination of soft, formed stools.

1. Monitor for and document the elimination of flatus or stool, which signals returning intestinal motility. Bowel sounds and bowel function normally return within 48-72 hours following surgery.
2. Assess for evidence of decreased GI motility, including abdominal distention, tenderness, absent or hypoactive bowel sounds, and sensation of fullness. Report gross distention, extreme tenderness, and prolonged absence of bowel sounds.
3. To stimulate peristalsis, encourage in-bed position changes, exercises, and ambulation to patient's tolerance unless contraindicated.
4. If NG tube is in place, perform the following:
   □ Check placement of the tube after insertion, before any instillation, and q8h. Either insert air into the proximal end of the tube to elicit a "whoosh" sound, which can be heard while auscultating over the epigastric area, or aspirate gastric contents. If the tube is in the trachea, the patient will exhibit signs of respiratory distress and the tube should the repositioned immediately.
   □ Prevent migration of the tube by keeping it securely taped to the patient's nose and reinforcing placement by attaching the tube to the patient's gown with a safety pin or tape.
   □ Measure and record the quantity and quality of output. Typically, the color will be green. For patients who have undergone gastric surgery, it may be brownish initially due to small amounts of bloody drainage, but should change to green after about 12 hours. Test reddish or brown output for the presence of blood, which can signal the development of a stress ulcer or indicate that a tube opening is compressed against the stomach lining. Reposition the tube as necessary. **Caution:** For patient with gastric, esophageal, or duodenal surgery, notify MD before manipulating the tube.
   □ Maintain patency of the NG tube with gentle instillation of normal saline as prescribed. Ensure low, intermittent suction of gastric sump tubes by maintaining patency of sump port (usually blue). If sump port becomes occluded by gastric con-

tents, flush sump port with air until a "whoosh" sound is heard over the epigastric area. **Caution:** Never clamp or otherwise occlude sump port, as excessive pressure may accumulate and damage gastric mucosa. **Caution:** For patient with gastric, esophageal, or duodenal surgery, notify MD before irrigating tube.

☐ When the tube is removed, monitor patient for the presence of abdominal distention, nausea, and vomiting.

5. Monitor and document patient's response to diet advancement from clear liquids to a regular or other prescribed diet.
6. Encourage oral fluid intake, especially of prune juice.
7. Administer stool softeners, mild laxatives, and enemas as prescribed. Monitor and record results.
8. Arrange periods of privacy during patient's attempts at bowel elimination.

Sleep pattern disturbance related to preoperative anxiety, postoperative pain, altered environment, disruption of normal sleep pattern, immobility, and stress

Desired outcome: Patient relates minimal or no difficulty with falling asleep and describes a feeling of being well rested.

1. Administer sedative/hypnotic (see Table A-7) as prescribed. Be aware that these agents may cause CNS depression and contribute to the respiratory depressent effects of opioid analgesics. Also be aware that active metabolites of many of the benzodiazepines may accumulate and result in greater physiologic effects or toxicity. **Note:** Use caution when administering sedative/hypnotic to patients with COPD due to respiratory depressant effects. Monitor respiratory function at frequent intervals in these individuals.
2. After administering sedative/hypnotic, be certain to raise side rails and caution patient not to smoke in bed.
3. Administer analgesics at bedtime to reduce pain and augment effects of hypnotic.
4. Be certain that consent for surgery is signed before administering sedative/hypnotic.
5. Employ nonpharmacologic measures to promote sleep (see Table A-8, p. 649).

Impaired physical mobility related to postoperative pain, decreased strength and endurance secondary to CNS effects of anesthesia or blood loss, musculoskeletal or neuromuscular impairment secondary to disease process or surgical procedure, perceptual impairment secondary to disease process or surgical procedure (e.g., ocular surgery, neurosurgery), or cognitive deficit secondary to disease process or effects of opioid analgesics and anesthetics

Desired outcome: Patient returns to preoperative baseline physical mobility as evidenced by the ability to move in bed, transfer, and ambulate independently or with minimal assistance.

1. Assess patient's preoperative physical mobility by evaluating coordination and muscle strength, control, and mass. Be aware of medically-imposed restrictions against

---

T A B L E A - 7   Sedatives and hypnotics commonly used perioperatively

Antihistamine sedatives
diphenhydramine (Benadryl)
hydroxyzine (Vistaril)

Benzodiazepines
alprazolam (Xanax)
chlordiazepoxide (Librium)
diazepam (Valium)
flurazepam (Dalmane)
oxazepam (Serax)
triazolam (Halcion)

Other hypnotics
chloral hydrate

TABLE A-8 Nonpharmacologic measures to promote sleep

Activity	Example(s)
Mask or eliminate environmental stimuli	Use eyeshields, ear plugs Play soothing music Dim lights at bedtime Mask odors from dressings/drainage; change dressing or drainage container as indicated
Promote muscle relaxation	Encourage ambulation as tolerated throughout the day Teach and encourage in-bed exercises and position changes Perform back massage at bedtime If not contraindicated, use a heating pad
Reduce anxiety	Ensure adequate pain control Keep patient informed of his/her progress and treatment measures Avoid overstimulation by visitors or other activities immediately before bedtime Avoid stimulant drugs (e.g., caffeine)
Promote comfort	Encourage patient to use own pillows, bed clothes if not contraindicated Adjust bed; rearrange linens Regulate room temperature
Promote usual pre-sleep routine	Offer oral hygiene at bedtime Provide warm beverage at bedtime Encourage reading or other quiet activity
Minimize sleep disruption	Maintain quiet environment throughout the night Plan nursing activities to enable long periods (at least 90 minutes) of undisturbed sleep Use dim lights when checking on patient during the night

movement, especially with certain conditions or surgeries that are orthopaedic, neurosurgical, or ocular in nature.

2. Evaluate and correct factors limiting physical mobility, including oversedation with opioid analgesics, failure to achieve adequate pain control, and poorly arranged physical environment.

3. Initiate movement from bed to chair and ambulation as soon as possible after surgery, depending on postoperative prescriptions, type of surgery, and patient's recovery from anesthetics (usually 12-24 hours after surgery). Assist patient with moving slowly to a sitting position in bed and then standing position at bedside before attempting ambulation. For more information, see **Potential for altered tissue perfusion:** Cerebral, p. 656. **Note:** Many anesthetic agents depress normal vasoconstrictor mechanisms and can result in sudden hypotension with quick changes in position.

4. Encourage frequent movement and ambulation by postoperative patients. Provide assistance as indicated.

5. Explain the importance of movement in bed and ambulation in reducing postopera-

tive complications, including atelectasis, pneumonia, thrombophlebitis, and depressed GI motility.

6. For additional information, see "Caring for Patients on Prolonged Bed Rest" for **Potential activity intolerance,** p. 651, and **Potential for disuse syndrome,** p. 653.

Potential for trauma related to CNS depression secondary to anesthetics and postoperative opioid analgesics

Desired outcome: Patient remains free of trauma as evidenced by absence of bruises, wounds, or fractures.

1. Orient and reorient patient to person, place, and time during the initial postoperative period. Inform patient that surgery is over. Repeat information until patient is fully awake and oriented (usually several hours, but may be days in heavily sedated or otherwise obtunded individuals).
2. Maintain siderails on stretchers and beds in upright and locked positions. Be aware that some individuals experience agitation and thrash about as they emerge from anesthesia.
3. Secure all IV lines, drains, and tubing to prevent dislodgement.
4. Maintain bed in its lowest position when leaving patient's room.
5. Be certain that the call-for-aid mechanism is within patient's reach; instruct patient regarding its use.
6. Caution patient and visitors to avoid smoking in rooms when oxygen is in use.
7. Identify patients at high risk for falling by assessing individual factors contributing to the likelihood of falling (see Table A-9). Correct or compensate for risk factors.
8. Use restraints and protective devices if necessary and prescribed.

Potential for altered skin integrity related to irritation of skin by secretions/excretions around percutaneous drains and tubes

Desired outcome: Patient's skin around percutaneous drains and tubes remains clear and intact.

1. Change dressings as soon as they become wet. The surgeon may prefer to perform the first dressing changes at the surgical incision. Use sterile technique for all dressing changes.
2. Keep the area around drain or T-tube as clean as possible. The presence of bile, for example, can quickly lead to skin excoriation. Sterile normal saline or a solution of saline and hydrogen peroxide or other prescribed solution may be used to clean around the drain site.
3. If drainage is a problem, position a pectin-wafer skin barrier around the drain or tube. Ointments, such as zinc oxide, petrolatum, and aluminum paste, also may be used. Consult with enterostomal therapy (ET) nurse if drainage is excessive or skin excoriation develops. For additional information, see "Managing Wound Care," p. 624.

Potential for impaired tissue integrity: Oral and gastric mucosa secondary to NPO status and presence of gastric tube

Desired outcome: Patient's oral and gastric mucosa remain intact, without pain or evidence of bleeding.

TABLE A-9 Factors that may contribute to the likelihood of falling

Time of day	Night shift; peak activity periods, such as meals; bedtime
Medications	Opioid analgesics, sedatives, hypnotics, and anesthetics
Impaired mobility	Individuals requiring assistance with transfer and ambulation
Sensory deficits	Diminished visual acuity due to disease process or environmental factors; changes in kinesthetic sense due to disease or trauma

1. Provide oral care and oral hygiene q4h and prn. Arrange for patient to gargle, brush teeth, and cleanse the mouth with swabs as necessary to prevent excoration and excessive dryness. Use a cotton-tipped applicator to remove encrustations and lubricate the lips and nares with a water-soluble lubricant. If the patient's throat is irritated from the presence of an NG tube, obtain a prescription for a lidocaine gargling solution.
2. Ensure that the suction apparatus is decompressing at the prescribed pressure (usually low-continuous or intermittent). Ensure patency of ventilation ports in sump tubes to prevent excessive pressure. Be aware that high-vacuum pressure can result in mucosal damage.
3. Evaluate gastric drainage for the presence of blood. Test drainage for blood if it appears red or brown. Report positive findings to the MD.

For additional information regarding the prevention of surgical complications, see "Pneumonia," p. 3, "Atelectasis," p. 1, "Urinary Retention," p. 145, "Venous Thrombosis/Thrombophlebitis," p. 93, "Providing Nutritional Support," p. 611, "Managing Wound Care," p. 624, and "Caring for Patients on Prolonged Bed Rest," below. For psychosocial nursing diagnoses and interventions, see "Caring for Patients with Cancer and Other Life-Disrupting Illnesses," p. 690.

SELECTED REFERENCES

Cardona V et al: Trauma nursing: resuscitation through rehabilitation, Philadelphia, 1988, WB Saunders Co.

Devine E and Cook T: Clinical and cost-saving effects of psychoeducational interventions with surgical patients: a meta-analysis, Res Nurs Health 9:89-103, 1986.

DiPiro J et al: Pharmacotherapy: a pathophysiologic approach, New York, 1988, Elsevier Science Publishing Co.

Lange M et al: Patient-controlled analgesia versus intermittent analgesia dosing, Heart Lung 17(5):495-498, 1988.

Tack K et al: Patient falls: profile for intervention, J Neurosc Nurs 19(2):83-89, 1987.

Webster R and Thompson D: Sleep in hospital, J Adv Nurs 11:447-457, 1989.

Young L and Koda-Kimble M, editors: Applied therapeutics: the clinical use of drugs, ed 4, Vancouver, Wash, 1988, Applied Therapeutics, Inc.

Section Two CARING FOR PATIENTS ON PROLONGED BED REST

Potential for activity intolerance related to deconditioning secondary to prolonged bed rest

---

TABLE A-10 Physiologic effects of prolonged bed rest (Deconditioning)

Increased HR and BP for submaximal workload
Decrease in functional capacity
Decrease in circulating volume
Orthostatic hypotension
Reflex tachycardia
Modest decrease in pulmonary function
Increase in thromboemboli
Loss of muscle mass
Loss of muscle contractile strength
Negative protein state
Negative nitrogen state

Desired outcomes: Patient exhibits cardiac tolerance to exercise as evidenced by HR ≤20 bpm over resting HR, systolic BP ≤20 mm Hg over or under resting systolic BP, RR ≤20 breaths/min with normal depth and pattern (eupnea), normal sinus rhythm, warm and dry skin, and absence of crackles, murmurs, and chest pain. Patient rates his or her perceived exertion at ≤3 on a scale of 0 (low) to 10 (high).

1. Perform ROM exercises bid to qid on each extremity. Individualize the exercise plan based on the following guidelines:
   □ *Mode or type of exercise:* Begin with passive exercises, moving the joints through the motions of abduction, adduction, flexion, and extension. Progress to active-assisted exercises in which you support the joints while the patient initiates muscle contraction. When the patient is able, supervise him or her in active isotonic exercises, during which the patient contracts a selected muscle group, moves the extremity at a slow pace, and then relaxes the muscle group. Have the patient repeat each exercise three to ten times. **Caution:** Stop any exercise that results in muscular or skeletal pain. Consult with a physical therapist regarding necessary modifications. Avoid isometric exercises in cardiac patients.
   □ *Intensity:* Begin with three to five repetitions as tolerated by the patient. Assess exercise tolerance by measuring HR and BP at rest, peak exercise, and 5 minutes after exercise. If HR or systolic BP increases >20 bpm or mm Hg over the resting level, decrease the number of repetitions. If HR or systolic BP decreases >10 bpm or mm Hg at peak exercise, this could be a sign of left ventricular failure, denoting that the heart cannot meet this workload. For other adverse signs and symptoms, see "Assessment," below.
   □ *Duration:* Begin with 5 minutes or less of exercise. Gradually increase the exercise to 15 minutes as tolerated.
   □ *Frequency:* Begin exercises bid-qid. As the duration increases, the frequency can be reduced.
   □ *Assessment of exercise tolerance:* Be alert to signs and symptoms that the cardiovascular and respiratory systems are unable to meet the demands of the low-level ROM exercises. Excessive SOB may occur if (1) transient pulmonary congestion occurs secondary to ischemia or left ventricular dysfunction; (2) lung volumes are decreased; (3) oxygen-carrying capacity of the blood is reduced; or (4) there is shunting of blood from the right to the left side of the heart without adequate oxygenation. If cardiac output does not increase to meet the body's needs during modest levels of exercise, systolic BP may fall; the skin may become cool, cyanotic, and diaphoretic; dysrhythmias may be noted; crackles (rales) may be auscultated; or a systolic murmur of mitral regurgitation may occur. If the patient tolerates the exercise, increase the intensity or number of repetitions each day.
2. Ask the patient to rate perceived exertion (RPE) experienced during exercise, basing it on the following scale developed by Borg:
   0 nothing at all
   1 very weak effort
   2 weak (light) effort
   3 moderate
   4 somewhat stronger effort
   5 strong effort
   7 very strong effort
   9 very, very strong effort
   10 maximal effort
   The patient should not experience a RPE >3 while performing ROM exercises. Reduce the intensity of the exercise and increase the frequency until a RPE of ≤3 is attained.
3. As the patient's condition improves, increase activity as soon as possible to include sitting in a chair. Assess for orthostatic hypotension, which can occur as a result of decreased plasma volume and difficulty in adjusting immediately to postural change. Prepare the patient for this by increasing the amount of time spent in high-Fowler's position and moving the patient slowly and in stages. For more information about activity progression, see Table A-11.

APPENDIX **653**

TABLE A-11 Activity level progression in hospitalized patients

Level I: Bedrest	Flexion and extension of extremities qid, 15 times each extremity; deep breathing qid, 15 breaths; position change from side to side q2h
Level II: OOB to Chair	As tolerated, tid for 20-30 minutes; may perform ROM exercises bid while sitting in chair
Level III: Ambulate in room	As tolerated, tid for 3-5 minutes
Level IV: Ambulate in hall	Initially, 50-200 feet bid; progressing to 600 feet qid, may incorporate slow stair climbing in preparation for hospital discharge
Signs of activity intolerance:	Decrease in BP >20 mm Hg; increase in HR to >120 bpm (or >20 bpm above resting HR in patients on beta-blocker therapy)

4. Increase activity level by having patient perform self-care activities, such as eating, mouth care, and bathing as tolerated.
5. Teach significant others the purpose and interventions for preventing deconditioning. Involve them in the patient's plan of care.
6. To help allay fears of failure, pain, or medical setbacks, provide emotional support to patient and significant others as patient's activity level is increased.

Potential for disuse syndrome related to inactivity secondary to prolonged bed rest

Desired outcome: Patient exhibits complete ROM of all joints without pain, and limb girth measurements congruent with baseline measurements.

Note: ROM exercises should be performed every day for all immobilized patients with *normal* joints. Modification may be required for patients with flaccidity (i.e., immediately following CVA or spinal cord injury) to prevent subluxation; or for patient with spasticity (i.e., during the recovery period for patients with CVA or spinal cord injury) to prevent an increase in spasticity. Consult with physical therapist or occupational therapist for assistance with modifying the exercise plan for these patients. In addition, be aware that ROM exercises are contraindicated for patients with rheumatologic disease during the inflammatory phase and for joints that are dislocated or fractured.

1. Be alert to the following areas that are especially prone to joint contracture: *shoulder,* which can become "frozen" to limit abduction and extension; *wrist,* which can "drop," prohibiting extension; *fingers,* which can develop flexion contractures that limit extension; *hips,* which can develop flexion contractures that affect the gait by shortening the limb or develop external rotation or adduction deformities that affect the gait; *knees,* in which flexion contractures can develop to limit extension and alter the gait; and *feet,* which can "drop" as a result of plantarflexion, which limits dorsiflexion and alters the gait.
2. Ensure that patient changes position at least q2h. Post a turning schedule at patient's bedside accordingly. Position changes not only will maintain correct body alignment, thereby reducing strain on the joints, they will prevent contractures, minimize pressure on bony prominences, and promote maximal chest expansion as well.
   □ Try to place patient in a position that achieves proper standing alignment: head neutral or slightly flexed on the neck, hips extended, knees extended or minimally flexed, and feet at right angles to the legs. Maintain this position with pillows, towels, or other positioning aids.
   □ To prevent hip flexion contractures, ensure that the patient is sidelying with the hips extended for the same amount of time patient spends in the supine position.
   □ When the HOB must be elevated 30 degrees, extend the patient's shoulders and

arms, using pillows to support the position, and allow the fingertips to extend over the edge of the pillows to maintain normal arching of the hands. **Caution:** Because elevating the HOB promotes hip flexion, ensure that patient spends equal time with the hips in extension (see intervention, above).

☐ When patient is in the side-lying position, use the opportunity to extend the lower leg from the hip to help prevent hip flexion contracture.

☐ When able to place patient in the prone position, move patient to the end of the bed and allow the feet to rest between the mattress and footboard. This will not only prevent plantarflexion and hip rotation, it will prevent injury to the heels and toes as well. Place thin pads under the angles of the axillae and lateral aspects of the clavicles to prevent internal rotation of the shoulders and maintain anatomic position of the shoulder girdle.

3. To maintain the joints in neutral position, use the following as indicated: pillows, rolled towels, blankets, sandbags, antirotation boots, splints, and orthotics. When using adjunctive devices, monitor the involved skin at frequent intervals for alterations in integrity, and implement measures to prevent skin breakdown.

4. Assess for footdrop by inspecting the feet for plantarflexion and evaluating patient's ability to pull the toes upward toward his or her nose. Although feet posture naturally in plantarflexion, be particularly alert to the patient's inability to pull the toes up. Document this assessment daily.

5. Teach patient the rationale and procedure for ROM exercises, and have patient return the demonstrations. Review **Potential for activity intolerance**, p. 651, to ensure that patient does not exceed his or her tolerance. Provide passive exercises for patients unable to perform active or active-assistive exercises. In addition, incorporate movement patterns into care activities, such as position changes, bed baths, getting the patient on and off the bed pan, or changing the patient's gown. Ensure that joints especially prone to contracture are exercised more stringently. Provide patient with a handout that reviews the exercises and lists the repetitions for each.

6. Perform and document limb girth measurements, dynamography, ROM, and exercise baseline limits to assess patient's existing muscle mass and strength and joint motion.

7. Explain to patient that muscle atrophy occurs because of disuse or failure to use the joint, often due to immediate or anticipated pain. Eventually, this may result in a decrease in muscle mass and blood supply and a loss of periarticular tissue elasticity, which in turn can lead to increased muscle fatigue and joint pain with use.

8. Emphasize the importance of maintaining or increasing muscle strength and periarticular tissue elasticity through exercise. If unsure about patient's complicating pathology, consult with MD about the appropriate form of exercise for patient.

9. Explain the necessity of participating maximally in self-care as tolerated to help maintain muscle strength and enhance a sense of participation and control.

10. For noncardiac patients needing greater help with muscle strength, assist with resistive exercises (e.g., moderate weight lifting to increase the size, endurance, and strength of the muscles). For patients in beds with Balkan frames, provide the means for resistive exercise by implementing a system of weights and pulleys. First, determine patient's baseline level of performance on a given set of exercises, and then set realistic goals with the patient for repetitions. For example, if the patient can do 5 repetitions of lifting a 5-pound weight with the biceps muscle, the goal may be to increase the repetitions to 10 within a week, to an ultimate goal of 20 within three weeks, and then advance to 7.5-pound weights.

11. If the joints require rest, isometric exercises can be used. With these exercises, teach patient to contract a muscle group and hold the contraction for a count of five or ten. The sequence is repeated for increasing numbers or repetitions until an adequate level of endurance has been achieved. Thereafter, maintenance levels are performed.

12. Provide a chart to show patient's progress, and combine this with large amounts of positive reinforcement. Post the exercise regimen at the bedside to ensure consistency by all health care personnel.

13. As appropriate, teach transfer or crutchwalking techniques and use of a walker,

wheelchair, or cane so that patient can maintain the highest level of mobility possible. Include significant others in the demonstrations, and stress the importance of good body mechanics.

14. Seek a referral to a physical or occupational therapist as appropriate.

Potential for altered oral mucous membrane related to self-care deficit

Desired outcome: Patient's oral mucosa, lips, and tongue remain intact.

1. Assess patient's oral mucous membrane, lips, and tongue q2h, noting presence of dryness, exudate, swelling, blisters, and ulcers.

2. If patient is alert and able to take oral fluids, offer frequent sips of water or ice chips to alleviate dryness.

3. Perform mouth care q2-4h, using a soft-bristled toothbrush to cleanse the teeth and a moistened cloth or Toothette (small sponge on a stick) to moisten crusty areas or exudate on tongue and oral mucosa. If patient is intubated, suction mouth to remove fluid and debris.

4. Apply lip balm q2h and prn to prevent cracking of lips.

5. If indicated, use an artificial saliva preparation to assist in keeping mucous membrane moist. Avoid use of lemon and glycerine swabs, which can contribute to dryness.

6. As appropriate, have patient wear dentures as soon as he or she is able, to improve communication and enhance comfort.

7. Note: If it is necessary to put fingers in patient's mouth, wear gloves on both hands. This practice will reduce the risk of acquiring herpetic Whitlow.

Potential for altered tissue perfusion: Peripheral, related to compromised circulation secondary to prolonged immobility

Desired outcomes: Patient has adequate peripheral perfusion as evidenced by normal skin color and temperature, and adequate distal pulses ($>2+$ on a 0-4+ scale) in peripheral extremities. Patient performs exercises independently, adheres to the prophylactic regimen, and maintains an intake of 2-3 L/day of fluid unless contraindicated.

1. Teach patient that pain, swelling, warmth in the involved area, coolness distal to the involved area, superficial venous dilatation, and persistent redness are all indicators of deep-vein thrombosis (DVT) and should be reported to staff promptly if they occur.

2. Monitor for the same indicators listed above along with routine VS checks. If patient is asymptomatic of DVT, assess for a positive Homan's sign: Flex the knee 30 degrees and dorsiflex the foot. Pain elicited with the dorsiflexion may be a sign of DVT, and patient should be referred to MD for further evaluation. Additional signs of DVT may include fever, tachycardia, and elevated erythrocyte sedimentation rate (ESR). Normal ESR (Westergren method) in males under 50 years is 0-15 mm/hr, over 50 years 0-20 mm/hr; and in females under 50 years is 0-20 mm/hr, over 50 years 0-30 mm/hr.

3. Teach patient calf-pumping (ankle dorsiflexion-plantarflexion) and ankle-circling exercises. Instruct patient to repeat each movement ten times, performing each exercise qh during extended periods of immobility, provided that patient is asymptomatic of DVT. Help promote circulation by performing passive ROM or encouraging active ROM exercises.

4. Encourage deep breathing, which increases negative pressure in the lungs and thorax to promote emptying of large veins.

5. When not contraindicated by peripheral vascular disease, ensure that patient wears antiembolic hose or pneumatic stockings. Remove them for 10-20 minutes q8h and inspect underlying skin for evidence of irritation or breakdown. Reapply hose after elevating patient's legs 10-15 degrees for 10 minutes.

6. Instruct patient not to cross the feet at the ankles or knees while in bed because doing so may cause venous stasis. If patient is at risk for DVT, elevate the foot of the bed 10 degrees to increase venous return.

7. In nonrestricted patient, increase fluid intake to at least 2-3L/day to reduce hemoconcentration, which can contribute to the development of DVT. Educate patient about the need to drink large amounts of fluid.

8. Patients at risk for DVT, including those with chronic infection and a history of peripheral vascular disease, as well as the aged, obese, and anemic, may require pharmacologic interventions, such as aspirin, sodium warfarin, phenindione derivatives, or heparin. Administer medication as prescribed, and monitor appropriate laboratory values (e.g., PT, PTT).

9. In patients prone to DVT, acquire bilateral baseline measurements of the midcalf, knee, and midthigh and record them on patient's cardex. Monitor these measurements daily and compare them to the baseline measurements to rule out extremity enlargement caused by DVT.

Altered tissue perfusion: Cerebral, related to orthostatic hypotension secondary to prolonged bed rest

Desired outcome: Patient has adequate cerebral perfusion as evidenced by HR <120 bpm and BP ≥90/60 mm Hg immediately following position change (or within 20 mm Hg of patient's normal range), dry skin, normal skin color, and denial of vertigo and syncope, with return of HR and BP to resting levels within 3 minutes of position change.

1. Assess patient for factors that increase the risk of orthostatic hypotension secondary to fluid volume changes (recent diuresis, diaphoresis, or change in vasodilator therapy) or altered autonomic control (diabetic cardiac neuropathy, denervation post heart transplant, or advanced age).

2. Explain the cause of orthostatic hypotension and measures for preventing it.

3. Application of antiembolic hose, which are used to prevent DVT, may be useful in preventing orthostatic hypotension once the patient is mobilized. For patients who continue to have difficulty with orthostatic hypotension, it may be necessary to supplement the hose with elastic wraps to the groin during the period of time the patient is out of bed. Ensure that these wraps encompass the entire surface of the legs.

4. When patient is in bed, provide instructions for leg exercises as described under **Potential for activity intolerance,** p. 651.

5. Prepare patient for getting out of bed by encouraging position changes within necessary confines. It is sometimes possible and advisable to use a tilt table to reacclimate patient to upright positions.

6. Follow these guidelines for mobilization
   □ Check the BP in any high-risk patient for whom this will be the first time out of bed.
   □ Have the patient dangle legs at the bedside. Be alert to indicators of orthostatic hypotension, including diaphoresis, pallor, tachycardia, hypotension, and syncope. Question patient about the presence of lightheadedness or dizziness.
   □ If indicators of orthostatic hypotension occur, check the VS. A drop in systolic BP of 20 mm Hg and an increased pulse rate, combined with symptoms of vertigo and impending syncope, signal the need for return to a supine position.
   □ If leg dangling is tolerated, have patient stand at the bedside with two staff members in attendance. If no adverse signs or symptoms occur, have patient progress to ambulation as tolerated.

Constipation related to immobility, changes in normal bowel habits during hospitalization, positional restrictions, dietary alterations, and use of narcotic analgesics

Desired outcomes: Patient verbalizes knowledge of measures that promote bowel elimination. Patient relates the return of his or her normal pattern and character of bowel elimination.

1. Assess patient's bowel history to determine normal bowel habits and interventions that are used successfully at home.

2. Monitor and document patient's bowel movements, diet, and I&O. Be alert to the following indications of constipation: fewer than patient's usual number of bowel

movements, abdominal discomfort or distention, straining at stool, and patient complaints of rectal pressure or fullness.

3. Auscultate each abdominal quadrant for at least 1 minute to determine the presence of bowel sounds. Normal sounds are clicks or gurgles occurring at a rate of 5-34 per minute. **Note:** Bowel sounds are decreased or absent with paralytic ileus. High-pitched rushing sounds may be heard during abdominal cramping, indicating an intestinal obstruction.

4. If a rectal impaction is suspected, use a gloved, lubricated finger to remove stool from the rectum. This stimulation may be adequate to stimulate bowel movement.

5. Teach patient the importance of a high-roughage diet and a fluid intake of at least 2-3 L/day (unless this is contraindicated by a renal or cardiac disorder). High-roughage foods include bran, whole grains, nuts, raw and coarse vegetables, and fruits with skins.

6. Maintain patient's normal bowel habits whenever possible by offering the bedpan; ensuring privacy; providing warm oral fluids; and timing medications, enemas, or suppositories so that they take effect at the time of day patient normally has a bowel movement.

7. To promote peristalsis, maximize patient's activity level within the limitations of endurance, therapy, and pain.

8. Request pharmacologic interventions from MD when necessary. To help prevent rebound constipation, prioritize pharmacologic interventions to ensure minimal disruption of patient's normal bowel habits. A suggested hierarchy of interventions is the following:
   □ Bulk-building additives (psyllium), bran.
   □ Mild laxatives (apple or prune juice, milk of magnesia).
   □ Stool softeners (docusate sodium or docusate calcium).
   □ Potent laxatives and cathartics (bisacodyl, cascara sagrada).
   □ Medicated suppositories.
   □ Enemas.

Diversional activity deficit related to monotony of confinement secondary to prolonged illness and hospitalization

Desired outcome: Patient engages in diversional activities and relates the absence of boredom.

1. Be alert to patient indicators of boredom, including wishing for something to read or do, daytime napping, and expressed inability to perform usual hobbies because of hospitalization.

2. Assess patient's activity tolerance as described on p. 651.

3. Collect a data base by assessing patient's normal support systems and relationship patterns with significant others. Question patient about his or her interests, and explore diversional activities that may be suitable for the hospital setting and patient's level of activity tolerance.

4. Provide low-level activities commensurate with patient's tolerance. Examples include books or magazines pertaining to patient's recreational or other interests, television, or writing for short intervals.

5. Initiate activities that require little concentration and proceed to more complicated tasks as patient's condition allows. For example, if reading requires more energy or concentration than patient is capable of, suggest that significant others read to patient or bring in audio tapes of books, such as those marketed for the visually impaired.

6. As patient's endurance improves, obtain appropriate diversional activities, such as puzzles, model kits, handicrafts, and computerized games and activities; encourage patient to use them.

7. Encourage significant others to visit within limits of patient's endurance and to involve patient in activities that are of interest to him or her, such as playing cards or backgammon. Encourage significant others to stagger their visits throughout the day.

8. Spend extra time with patient.
9. Suggest that significant others bring in a radio, or, if appropriate, rent a TV or radio from the hospital if not part of the standard room charge.
10. If appropriate for patient, arrange for hospital volunteers to visit, play cards, read books, or play board games.
11. As appropriate for patient who desires social interaction, consider relocation to a room in an area of high traffic.
12. As patient's condition improves assist him or her with sitting in a chair near a window so that outside activities can be viewed. When patients are able, provide opportunities to sit in a solarium so that they can visit with other patients. If their conditions and weather permit, take patients outside for brief periods of time.
13. Request consultation from social services, occupational therapists, pastoral services, and psychiatric nurse for interventions as appropriate.
14. Increase patient's involvement in self-care to provide a sense of purpose and accomplishment. Performing in-bed exercises (e.g., deep breathing, ankle circling, calf pumping), keeping track of I&O, and similar activities, can and should be accomplished routinely by these patients.

Altered sexuality pattern related to actual or perceived physiologic limitations on sexual performance secondary to disease, therapy, or prolonged hospitalization

Desired outcome: Patient relates satisfaction with his or her own sexual activity.

1. Assess patient's normal sexual function, including the importance placed on sex in the relationship, frequency of interaction, normal positions used, and the couple's ability to adapt or change to meet requirements of patient's limitations.
2. Identify patient's problem diplomatically, and clarify it with patient. Indicators of sexual dysfunction can include regression, acting-out with inappropriate behavior, such as grabbing or pinching, sexual overtures toward the hospital staff, self-enforced isolation, and other similar behaviors.
3. Encourage patient and significant other to verbalize their feelings and anxieties about sexual abstinence, having sexual relations in the hospital, hurting the patient, or having to use new or alternative methods for sexual gratification. Develop strategies collaboratively among the patient, significant other, and yourself.
4. Encourage acceptable expressions of sexuality by the patient. For example, in a woman this can involve wearing makeup, jewelry, and her own clothing.
5. Inform patient and significant other that it is possible to have time alone together for intimacy. Provide that time accordingly by putting a "Do Not Disturb" sign on the door, enforcing privacy by restricting staff and visitors from the room, or arranging for temporary private quarters.
6. Encourage patient and significant other to seek alternate methods of sexual expression when necessary. This may include mutual masturbation, altered positions, vibrators, and identification of other erotic areas for the partner.
7. Refer patient and significant other to professional sexual counselling as necessary.

Altered role performance: Dependence versus independence

Desired outcome: Patient collaborates with caregivers in planning realistic goals for independence, participates in own care, and takes responsibility for self-care.

1. Encourage patient to be as independent as possible within limitations of endurance, therapy, and pain.
2. Ensure that all health care providers are consistent in conveying their expectations of independence.
3. Alert patient to areas of overdependence, and involve him or her in collaborative goal-setting to achieve independence.
4. Do not minimize patient's expressions of feelings of depression. Allow patient to express emotions, while providing support, understanding, and realistic hope for a positive role change.
5. If indicated, provide self-help devices to increase patient's independence with self-care.
6. Provide positive reinforcement when patient meets or advances toward goals.

For interventions related to prevention of atelectasis and pneumonia, see appropriate nursing diagnoses in "Respiratory Disorders," pp. 1-36. See "Pressure Ulcers" for **Potential impaired skin/tissue integrity** related to excessive tissue pressure secondary to prolonged immobility (for patients without pressure ulcers who are at risk because of immobility), p. 631. For psychosocial nursing diagnoses and interventions, see section "Caring for Patients with Cancer and Other Life-Disrupting Disorders," p. 690.

SELECTED REFERENCES

Borg GV: Psychòphysical basis of perceived exertion, Med Sci Sports Exercise 14:377-381, 1982.

Marshall JR and Hawrysio A: Inpatient recovery following myocardial infarction and coronary artery bypass graft surgery, J Cardiovasc Nurs 2(3):1-12, 1988.

Swearingen PL: Addison-Wesley photo-atlas of nursing procedures, ed 2, Redwood City, Calif, 1990, Addison-Wesley Publishing Co.

Wenger N and Hellerstein M: Cardiac rehabilitation, ed 2, Philadelphia, 1985, JB Lippincott Co.

Winslow, EH: Cardiovascular consequences of bed rest, Heart Lung 14(3):236-246, 1985.

Section Three CARING FOR PATIENTS WITH CANCER AND OTHER LIFE-DISRUPTING ILLNESSES

CHEMOTHERAPY AND IMMUNOTHERAPY

Potential for injury (to staff and environment) related to preparation, handling, administration, and disposal of chemotherapy agents

Desired outcome: Chemotherapy exposure to staff and environment is minimized by proper preparation, handling, administration, and disposal by individuals familiar with these agents.

1. Ensure that preparation and administration of chemotherapy is done by pharmacists or nurses familiar with the agents. Keep institutional guidelines readily available for safe preparation, handling, and potential complications, such as spills or individual contact with these drugs. **Note:** A chemotherapy approval course is highly recommended for nurses who will be administering these drugs.
2. Ensure that pregnant nurses exercise extreme caution when handling these agents. Check with individual agencies for policies regarding administration of these drugs by women who are pregnant or who are considering getting pregnant.
3. Implement measures to minimize aerosolization and direct contact with these drugs during preparation. These measures include using a biologic safety cabinet, absorbant pad placed on the work area, latex gloves, full length gown with cuffed sleeves, and goggles.
4. Prime IV tubing with a 50 ml bag of dilutent or prime the tubing into a sterile bag, using gauze to absorb excess liquid.
5. When removing the IV administration set, wrap sterile gauze around the needle to prevent direct contact with the drug. Place all needles, drugs, drug containers, and related material in a puncture-proof container that is clearly marked "biohazardous waste." **Note:** Follow this same procedure for disposal of immunotherapy waste.
6. Wear latex gloves when handling all body excretions for 48 hours following chemotherapy, since the drug is excreted through urine and feces.
7. To clean up a chemotherapy spill, double glove and wear a full length gown. Use absorbant pads to absorb liquid. Then, cleanse three times with a detergent solution. Dispose of all waste in a biohazardous waste container.
8. In the event of skin contact with the drug, wash the affected area with soap and water. Notify MD for follow-up care.

9. Should eye contact occur, irrigate the eye with water for 15 minutes and notify MD for follow-up care.

Potential/actual impaired tissue integrity related to irritation secondary to extravasation of vesicant or irritating chemotherapy agents

Desired outcome: Patient's tissue remains intact without evidence of inflammation or pain along the injection site.

Note: The following vesicant agents have the potential to produce tissue damage: dactinomycin, daunomycin, doxorubicin, mitomycin C, estramustine, mechlorethamine, vinblastine, and vincristine. The following irritants have the potential to produce pain along the injection site with or without inflammation: carmustine, dacarbazine, etoposide, streptozocin.

---

1. Ensure that vesicant chemotherapy is administered by a nurse who is experienced in venipuncture and knowledgeable about chemotherapy.
2. Select the IV site carefully, using a new site if possible. Avoid sites, such as the antecubital fossa, wrist, or dorsal side of the hand, with which there is an increased risk of damage to underlying tendons or nerves.
3. Check patency of the IV prior to and during administration of the drug. Instruct patient to report burning or pain immediately.
4. Give infusions of vesicant drugs through a central venous catheter to minimize risk of extravasation. Assess the entry site at frequent intervals. Pain, burning, and stinging are common with extravasation, as well as erythema and swelling around the needle site. Do not use blood return as an indicator that extravasation has not occurred, because it may be possible to get blood return in the presence of extravasation. Instruct patient to report discomfort at the site promptly.
5. Keep an extravasation kit readily available, along with institutional guidelines for extravasation management.
6. In the event of extravasation, follow these general guidelines:
   □ Stop the infusion immediately and aspirate any remaining drug from the needle. To do this, first apply latex gloves, then attach the syringe to the tubing, and aspirate the drug.
   □ Notify MD.
   □ Leave the needle in place if an antidote is to be used with the extravasated drug. See Table A-12 for suggested antidotes for specific agents.
   □ Attach a syringe containing the recommended antidote and instill the antidote. Remove the IV needle from the site.
   □ If recommended, inject the extravasated site with the antidote, using a TB syringe and a 25-27 gauge needle.
   □ Do not apply pressure to the site. Apply a sterile occlusive dressing, elevate the site, and apply heat or cold as recommended (see Table A-12, p. 662).
   □ Document the incident, noting the date, time, insertion site of the needle, drug, approximate amount of drug that extravasated, management of the extravasation, and appearance of the site. Check with institutional guidelines regarding necessity of photodocumentation. Monitor the site at frequent intervals.
   □ Provide patient with information regarding site care and follow-up appointments for evaluating severity of the extravasation.

Knowledge deficit: Chemotherapy, its purpose, expected side effects and potential toxicities associated with these drugs, appropriate self-care measures for minimizing side effects, and available community and educational resources

Desired outcome: Patient and significant others verbalize knowledge of the specific chemotherapy drugs, the potential side effects and toxicities, appropriate self-care measures for minimizing the side effects, and available community and educational resources.

1. Establish patient's current level of knowledge regarding his or her health status and prescribed therapies.
2. Assess patient's cognitive and emotional readiness to learn.

3. Recognize barriers to learning, such as ineffective communication, neurologic deficit, sensory alterations, fear, anxiety, or lack of motivation. In particular, clarify misunderstandings regarding the side effects and toxicities of chemotherapy. Define all terminology, as needed. Correct any misconceptions.
4. Assess patient's learning needs and establish short- and long-term goals with the patient and significant others. Identify the patient's preferred method of learning and the amount of information patient would like to receive. Develop a teaching plan based on this information.
5. Use individualized verbal and audiovisual strategies to promote learning and enhance understanding. Give simple, direct instructions; reinforce this information frequently.
6. Provide an environment that is free from distractions and conducive for teaching/ learning.
7. Discuss the drugs the patient will receive, including route of administration, duration of treatment, schedule, and the most common side effects and toxicities and the appropriate self-care should they occur. Provide written as well as verbal information. See Table A-12 for details.
8. Provide emergency phone numbers in the event the patient develops a fever or other side effects.
9. Provide materials from educational resources, such as the American Cancer Society, National Cancer Institute, and drug companies.
10. Identify appropriate community resources that assist with transportation, costs of care, and skilled care as appropriate.

Knowledge deficit: Immunotherapy and its purpose, potential side effects and toxicities, appropriate self-care measures to minimize side effects, and available community and education resources

Desired outcome: Patient and significant others verbalize understanding of immunotherapy, its purpose, potential side effects and toxicities, appropriate self-care measures to minimize side effects, and available community and education resources.

1. See interventions 1-6 with **Knowledge deficit,** above.
2. Provide information about the route of administration, the expected action, and potential side effects. Because these individuals often give their own injections of interferon, instruct them in the proper technique and site rotation schedule. Teach patient to record the site and time of administration, side effects, self-management of side effects, and any medications that were taken. Teach patient proper disposal of needles.
3. Arrange for pharmacy delivery of medication since it must be refrigerated. As appropriate, arrange for community nursing follow-up for additional supervision and instruction.
4. Teach patient to be alert to the following side effects of interferon: fever, chills, and flulike symptoms. Suggest that patient take acetaminophen, with MD approval, to manage these symptoms but to avoid aspirin and nonsteroidal antiinflammatory agents because they may interrupt the action of interferon.
5. Teach patient to monitor and record temperature twice a day and drink extra fluids. Anorexia and weight loss, which are dose-related, are other common side effects of interferon. Provide information about nutritional supplementation.
6. Provide patient educational materials that are available through drug companies.

VENOUS ACCESS DEVICES (VAD)

Nurses play a vital role in the identification of individuals who are appropriate candidates for a VAD. Use of a VAD can promote quality of life by minimizing the trauma associated with multiple venipunctures as well as maintaining tissue integrity, which otherwise may be compromised by long-term administration or continuous infusions of vesicant or irritating chemotherapy agents. Individuals who should be considered potential candidates for VAD include those with poor venous access, venous access limited to

TABLE A-12   Common chemotherapy and immunotherapy agents

Classification Generic/trade name	Route of administration	Dosage
Alkylating agents		
1. carmustine/BCNU	IV	40 mg/m^2 for 5 days; 200 mg/m^2 single dose
2. cisplatinum/Platinol	IV; intra-arterial intraperitoneal	20 mg/m^2 for 5 days; 120 mg/m^2 single dose
3. dacarbazine/DTIC[†]	IV	100-200 mg/m^2 for 5 days; 375 mg/m^2 single dose

Acute toxicity	Delayed toxicity	Special precautions
☐ nausea & vomiting ☐ flushing of skin if infused too rapidly ☐ pain at injection site	☐ hepatic toxicity ☐ delayed bone marrow depression ☐ skin hyperpigmentation ☐ pulmonary fibrosis ☐ renal damage ☐ rare: dizziness, stomatitis, alopecia	☐ drug unstable at room temperature; infuse within 2 hrs ☐ premedicate with antiemetics ☐ report symptoms of pulmonary fibrosis (see p. 33) promptly ☐ Monitor liver function tests, BUN, creatinine, CBC and platelets before each treatment
☐ severe nausea & vomiting ☐ anaphylaxis (uncommon)	☐ nephrotoxicity, neurotoxicity, ototoxicity ☐ bone marrow depression ☐ electrolyte imbalances	☐ monitor creatinine clearance, BUN, serum creatinine, Mg^{++}, Ca^{++}, and K^+ before each treatment ☐ maintain adequate hydration before, during, and after treatments ☐ maintain urine output at 100 ml/hr before administration and for at least 4 hrs after; keep fluid intake greater than output ☐ premedicate with antiemetics before treatment ☐ keep the following emergency drugs readily available: epinephrine, hydrocortisone, antihistamines ☐ this drug precipitates; do not use aluminum needles
☐ severe nausea & vomiting ☐ pain at injection site ☐ possible tissue damage with extravasation	☐ bone marrow depression ☐ flulike symptoms ☐ elevated liver enzymes ☐ rare: alopecia, anaphylaxis	☐ stable for 8 hrs at room temperature ☐ premedicate with antiemetics ☐ check CBC, platelets, and liver function enzymes before treatment ☐ keep emergency drugs readily available ☐ in the event of extravasation: apply ice for 24 hrs

Continued.

TABLE A-12 Common chemotherapy and immunotherapy agents—cont'd

Classification Generic/trade name	Route of administration	Dosage
Alkylating agents—cont'd		
4. cyclophosphamide/ Cytoxan	PO; IV	50-100 mg/m² PO daily; 500-1500 mg/m² IV q3-4 weeks
5. ifosfamide/IFEX	IV	1.2 G/m² daily for 5 consecutive days
6. mesna/MESNEX‡	IV	20% of ifosfamide dose on a mg/kg basis
7. lomustine/CCNU	PO	100-130 mg/m² q6 weeks

Acute toxicity	Delayed toxicity	Special precautions
□ nausea & vomiting □ nasal congestion, headache with high doses that are infused rapidly	□ bone marrow depression □ alopecia □ hemorrhagic cystitis □ amenorrhea and sterility □ stomatitis □ potentiation of doxorubicin □ cardiotoxicity □ interstitial pulmonary fibrosis □ liver dysfunction □ SIADH with high doses □ development of secondary cancer	□ fluid intake should be at least 2-3 L/day after treatment □ voiding should be frequent to avoid bladder irritation □ administer early in day to minimize risk of bladder irritation from not voiding at night □ high doses (>1.5 G) may require IV hydration □ maintain I&O for 48 hrs after treatment □ test urine for blood □ initiate oral care/saline rinses qid □ monitor CBC, liver function tests, BUN, and creatinine before and after treatment
□ nausea & vomiting	□ bone marrow depression □ alopecia □ hematuria/hemorrhagic cystitis □ confusion, lethargy □ rare: renal impairment, liver dysfunction	□ hydrate with at least 2 L/day □ administer MESNA before treatment and 4 & 8 hrs after to minimize hemorrhagic cystitis □ test urine for blood
□ bad taste in the mouth	□ diarrhea	□ give 15 min before ifosfamide, then again after 4 hrs and 8 hrs
□ nausea & vomiting	□ anorexia □ bone marrow depression □ rare: hepatic toxicity, stomatitis, alopecia	□ give before bed and on an empty stomach to minimize nausea & vomiting □ monitor CBC, platelets, and liver function tests

Continued.

TABLE A-12 Common chemotherapy and immunotherapy agents—cont'd

Classification Generic/trade name	Route of administration	Dosage
Alkylating agents—cont'd		
8. mechlorethamine/ nitrogen mustard*	IV intracavitary topical	1.6 mg/m^2 q3-4 weeks 0.8 mg/m^2 10 mg dissolved in 50 ml sterile water
Antibiotics		
9. bleomycin/Blenoxane	IV; IM; SQ	10-20 mg/m^2 weekly or biweekly
10. doxorubicin/ Adriamycin*	IV	15 mg/m^2 weekly; 20-30 mg/m^2 for 3 days; 50-75 mg/m^2 q3 weeks
11. mitomycin C*	IV	10-20 mg/m^2 repeated once q6-8 weeks

Acute toxicity	Delayed toxicity	Special precautions
□ severe nausea & vomiting □ burning sensation around injection site; tissue damage with extravasation □ chills, fever, and diarrhea may occur immediately after drug administration	□ bone marrow depression □ amenorrhea □ skin rash □ secondary cancers	□ premedicate with antiemetics before administration □ never give IM or SQ since severe tissue necrosis would occur □ extravasation management (antidote for vesicant): —mix 4 ml 10% sodium thiosulfate with 6 ml sterile water for injection —inject 5-6 ml IV through existing IV line and then SQ with multiple injections —repeat dosing over next several hours —apply cold compresses
□ mild nausea & vomiting □ anaphylaxis	□ fever and chills □ skin reactions, including rash, dermatitis, hyperpigmentation □ stomatitis □ alopecia □ pulmonary fibrosis	□ administer test dose of 1-2 U before treatment □ premedicate with acetaminophen and diphenhydramine □ pulmonary toxicity is dose-related; suggested total cumulative dose is 500 U □ monitor pulmonary function tests before treatment and after every 100 U □ initiate oral care/saline rinses qid
□ moderate nausea & vomiting □ tissue damage if extravasation occurs □ local erythematosus streaking with rapid infusion ("adria flare") □ moderate nausea & vomiting □ extravasation causes tissue damage	□ red urine □ alopecia □ bone marrow depression □ stomatitis □ cardiomyopathy □ potentiates radiation-induced skin damage □ bone marrow depression □ mouth ulcers □ hemolytic-uremic syndrome □ pulmonary fibrosis	□ cardiac toxicity is dose-related; suggested total cumulative dose is 550 mg/m^2 □ modify dose during radiation to minimize skin reaction □ initiate oral care/saline rinses qid □ extravasation management: apply ice □ extravasation management: apply ice □ initiate oral care/saline rinses qid □ report symptoms of pulmonary fibrosis

Continued.

T A B L E A - 1 2   Common chemotherapy and immunotherapy agents—cont'd

Classification Generic/trade name	Route of administration	Dosage
Antimetabolites		
12. 5 fluorouricil/5 FU	IV	300-450 mg/m^2 for 5 days 300-750 mg/m^2 q week
	intra-arterial	20-30 mg/kg/day for 4 days, followed by 15/mg/kg for 17 days
13. methotrexate/ Amethoptrin	PO IV, IM	50 mg/m^2 q week 20-40 mg/m^2 q week or every other week
	intrathecal	6-15 mg as a single dose or repeated weekly or twice a week
14. leucovorin/Wellcovorin (given with high-dose methotrexate)[‡]	PO, IM, IV	Dose calculated based on methotrexate dose

Acute toxicity	Delayed toxicity	Special precautions
☐ mild nausea & vomiting	☐ bone marrow depression ☐ stomatitis ☐ diarrhea ☐ photosensitivity ☐ hyperpigmentation ☐ excessive lacrimation	☐ initiate oral care/saline rinses qid ☐ instruct patient in use of sunscreen to protect the skin
☐ nausea & vomiting	☐ bone marrow depression ☐ stomatitis ☐ diarrhea ☐ photosensitivity ☐ infertility ☐ CNS reaction with intrathecal administration ☐ rare: hepatic, renal toxicity	☐ do not administer to patients with BUN >25 ☐ use with cautions in patients with "third-spacing" of fluids because elimination will be decreased, thereby enhancing toxicity ☐ administer high-dosage (>100 mg/m^2) with leucovorin to minimize toxicity ☐ ensure adequate hydration before, during, and after high-dose administration ☐ ensure alkaline urine (pH > 7) to promote excretion ☐ teach use of sunscreen during sun exposure ☐ check serum BUN, creatinine, CBC, platelets, and liver function tests before and after administration ☐ dose usually begins 24 hrs after infusion of methotrexate ☐ stress importance of taking all doses as prescribed; give written instructions about dose and schedule ☐ provide emergency number in case patient unable to take doses

Continued.

TABLE A-12 Common chemotherapy and immunotherapy agents—cont'd

Classification Generic/trade name	Route of administration	Dosage
Antimetabolites—cont'd		
15. cytosine arabinoside/ Ara-C	IV	100-200 mg/m^2; high dose = 1.5-4.5 G/m^2 q12h for 2-6 days
	SQ, IM	1 mg/kg q12h for 5-7 days
	intrathecal	10-30 mg/m^2 up to 3× week
Plant alkaloids		
16. vinblastine/Velban*	IV	5-10 mg/m^2 weekly or every other week
17. vincristine/Oncovin*	IV	0.5-2.0 mg/m^2 weekly or every other week
18. etoposide (VP-16)[†]	IV	50-100 mg/m^2 for 5 days, repeated q3-4 weeks
	PO	Twice the IV dose rounded to the nearest 50 mg

Acute toxicity	Delayed toxicity	Special precautions
☐ mild to moderate nausea & vomiting	☐ bone marrow depression ☐ stomatitis ☐ diarrhea ☐ hepatotoxicity ☐ rash ☐ ocular toxicity ☐ neurotoxicity with high doses	☐ initiate oral care/saline rinses qid ☐ SQ injection may cause pain at injection site; apply warm compresses ☐ administer high doses over 1 hr to minimize neurologic toxicity ☐ perform neurologic exam before high-dose administration and report signs of cerebellar dysfunction ☐ steroid eye drops usually given with high doses to minimize ocular toxicity ☐ pyrodoxine (B6) usually given to minimize neurotoxicity with high doses
☐ nausea & vomiting ☐ tissue damage with extravasation	☐ bone marrow depression ☐ alopecia ☐ neurotoxicity (peripheral neuropathy and constipation) ☐ infertility ☐ stomatitis	☐ assess for neurotoxicity prior to administration ☐ initiate prophylactic bowel regimen to minimize constipation ☐ extravasation management: —mix 1 ml NaCl with 150 U/ml of hyaluronidase —inject 1-6 ml (150-900 U) SQ into the extravasated site with multiple injections —repeat dose SQ over next several hours —apply warm compresses
☐ tissue damage with extravasation	☐ neurotoxicity (peripheral neuropathy and constipation) ☐ jaw pain ☐ alopecia ☐ bone marrow depression	☐ do not exceed 2.5 mg/dose ☐ assess for neurotoxicity prior to administration ☐ initiate prophylactic bowel regimen to minimize constipation ☐ extravasation management: see "vinblastine," above
☐ hypotension with rapid infusion ☐ mild nausea & vomiting	☐ stomatitis ☐ alopecia ☐ bone marrow depression ☐ rare: anaphylaxis	☐ administer over 1-hr period to minimize hypotension ☐ monitor BP q15 min during infusion ☐ extravasation management: see "vinblastine," above

Continued.

TABLE A-12 Common chemotherapy and immunotherapy agents—cont'd

Classification Generic/trade name	Route of administration	Dosage
Miscellaneous agents		
19. hydroxyurea/Hydrea	PO	60-75 mg/m^2 daily
20. L-asparaginase/Elspar	IV, IM, SQ	200-1,000 IU/kg daily or twice weekly
21. procarbazine/Matulane	PO	100-200 mg/m^2 daily
Immunotherapy *Biologic response modifiers*		
22. interferon/Intron	IM IV SQ, intra- lesional	3 × 10^6 U/day 30 × 10^6 U/day
23. monoclonal antibodies (I)	IV	

Note: This table is not meant to be comprehensive, but rather it provides a quick reference for the most common drugs in clinical practice, including the route of administration, dose, side effects, and precautions. Because the drug dose and schedule of administration varies with each protocol, check individual protocols for additional information and guidelines.

*Vesicant drug: An agent capable of producing tissue damage.

†Irritant drug: An agent that produces pain along the injection site with or without an inflammatory reaction.

‡Given along with certain chemotherapy agents to minimize toxicity.

(I) Investigational drug; not currently FDA-approved for routine use.

Acute toxicity	Delayed toxicity	Special precautions
□ nausea & vomiting □ anaphylaxis	□ bone marrow depression □ renal insufficiency □ hepatotoxicity	□ ensure adequate hydration (at least 2 L/day) □ have emergency drugs readily
□ nausea & vomiting	□ fever, malaise □ CNS toxicity □ renal dysfunction	available before administration □ MD should be available in the event of anaphylaxis; drug should be administered during the day in the hospital setting □ record baseline VS; record VS 15 min into the infusion and following infusion
□ nausea & vomiting	□ bone marrow depression □ CNS depression □ peripheral neuropathy □ amenorrhea □ dermatologic reactions	□ avoid foods with high tyramine content (bananas, fava beans, aged cheeses, yogurt, beer, chianti wine, chocolate, coffee, cola, yeast)
	□ flulike symptoms (fever, chills, fatigue, malaise) □ anorexia □ bone marrow depression □ CNS toxicity □ rare: nausea & vomiting, hypotension	□ avoid ASA and nonsteroidal antiinflammatory drugs □ premedicate with acetaminophen; administer q4h □ anorexia may be dose-related; arrange for nutritional consult □ refrigerate after first use
□ anaphylaxis	□ fever, chills, rigors, malaise □ serum sickness	□ keep emergency equipment readily available □ premedicate with acetaminophine and diphenhydramine □ check VS q15min for 1 hr, then q30min □ use infusion pump if giving over 4-6 hr □ IV meperidine used for rigors

one extremity, long-term treatment, previous damage to the nervous system or tissue integrity, and those who require frequent venous access or continuous infusions of vesicant chemotherapy.

Knowledge deficit: Purpose and management of VAD

Desired outcome: Patient verbalizes understanding of the VAD, including its purpose, appropriate management measures, and potential complications.

1. Determine patient's and significant others' level of understanding of the purpose of a VAD. As appropriate, explain that the device can be used for administration of drugs, fluids, and blood products; drawing of blood samples; and that it eliminates the necessity of frequent venipunctures.
2. Show patient a model of the device and explain the insertion procedure. The silastic atrial catheters and implanted venous ports are inserted in the operating room using local anesthetic. There may be mild discomfort, similar to a toothache, for 48 hours postprocedure. Reassure patient that the discomfort responds readily to mild pain medication.
3. If possible, introduce patient and significant others to another individual who has the device so that they can see first hand what the VAD looks like and discuss their concerns.
4. Teach patient about maintenance care. Provide both verbal and written instructions.
   □ Give patient a card or instruction sheet that describes the VAD and maintenance care.
   □ Give patient educational materials provided by the VAD manufacturer.
   □ Have patient or significant other demonstrate dressing care, flushing technique, and cap-changing routine before hospital discharge.
5. Discuss potential complications associated with VADs, along with appropriate self-management measures.
   □ *Infection:* Teach patient to assess exit site for erythema, swelling, discomfort, purulent drainage, and fever >38° C (100.5° F).
   □ *Bleeding:* Teach patient to apply pressure to the site. Instruct patient to notify health team member if bleeding does not stop in 5 minutes.
   □ *Clot in the catheter:* Teach patient to flush the catheter without using excessive pressure, which could damage or dislodge the catheter (particularly an implanted port). If flushing does not dislodge the clot, instruct patient to notify health team member. **Note:** It is not unusual for small blood clots or fibrin sheaths to develop on the end of the catheter. The most common manifestation of a fibrin sheath is the ability to infuse fluids with the inability to aspirate blood. Both fibrin sheaths and small blood clots respond readily to urokinase therapy.
   □ *Disconnected cap:* Instruct patients to tape all connections and to carry hemostats with them at all times.

RADIATION THERAPY

Potential for injury to staff, other patients, and visitors related to risk of exposure to sealed sources of radiation, such as $^{137}CS, ^{198}AU, ^{192}IR, ^{125}I$, or unsealed sources of radiation, such as ^{131}I or^{32}P

Desired outcome: Staff and visitors verbalize understanding about the potential dangers of radiation therapy and the measures that must be taken to ensure safety.

Note: Most institutions have a radiation safety committee that assists in providing and enforcing guidelines that minimize radiation risks to employees and the environment (committee guidelines should be kept readily available). The committee approves certain rooms that can be used for patients undergoing radioactive treatment in order to minimize exposure to employees and other patients.

1. Provide patient with a private room and place an appropriate radiation precaution sign on patient's chart, door, and ID bracelet.

2. Follow radiologist or agency protocol for visitor restrictions. Visitors usually are restricted to 1 hour per day and should stand 6 feet from the bed.
3. Ensure that pregnant women and children under age 18 do not enter the room.
4. To ensure optimal care planning, recognize the type and amount of the radiation source. The two major principles are time and distance.
   □ *Time:* Plan care to minimize the amount of time spent in the patient's room. Staff members should not spend more than 30 min/shift with patient and should not care for more than two patients with implants at the same time. Staff should perform nondirect care activities in the hall, for example, opening food containers, preparing food tray, opening medications. Linen should be changed only when it is soiled, rather than routinely, and complete bed baths should be avoided.
   □ *Distance:* Maximize distance from the implant. For example, if the implant is in the patient's prostate, stand at the HOB.
5. Wear gloves when in contact with secretions/excretions of all patients treated with unsealed radiation sources, which are radioactive. Flush toilet several times after depositing urine or feces in commode.

Note: Urine from individuals with sealed radiation is *not* radioactive and can be discarded in the usual manner. However, patients with implanted ^{125}I seeds should save all urine so that it can be assessed for the presence of seeds.

---

6. Save all linen, dressings, and trash from patients with sealed sources of radiation. They will be analyzed by the safety committee representative prior to discarding to ensure that seeds have not been misplaced.
7. Keep long, disposable forceps and a sealed box in the room at all times in the event displaced seeds are found. Caution all staff members to use forceps but never the hands to pick up the seeds.
8. Use disposable products for all patients with unsealed radiation. These patients will be radioactive for several days. Cover all articles in the room with paper to prevent their contamination.
9. Attach a radiation badge (dosimeter) to your clothing before entering the room to monitor the amount of radiation exposure. According to federal regulations, radiation should not exceed 400 mrem/mo. Nurses who care for patients with radiation implants rarely receive this much exposure.

Knowledge deficit: Type and purpose of radiation implant (internal radiation) and the measures for preventing and managing complications

Desired outcome: Patient verbalizes understanding of his or her type of radiation implant and identifies measures for preventing and managing complications.

1. Determine patient's level of understanding of the radiation implant. Explain the following, as indicated:
   □ *Afterloading:* The implant carrier is inserted in the operating room and the radioactive source is inserted later.
   □ *Preloading:* Radioactive source is implanted with the carrier.
2. Explain that the implant is used to provide high doses of radiation therapy to one area, thereby sparing normal tissue.
3. Explain that radiation precautions (see **Potential for injury,** above) are required to protect health care team, other patients, and visitors).
4. Explain the following assessment parameters and management interventions for specific types of implants:
   □ *Gynecologic implants*
      —Teach patient that the following can occur: vaginal drainage, bleeding, or tenderness; impaired bowel or urinary elimination; and phlebitis. Instruct patient to report any of these signs and symptoms.
      —Teach patient to perform isometric exercises while on bed rest to minimize the risk of contractures or muscle atrophy.
      —Ensure that patient wears antiembolic hose while on bed rest.
      —Assist patient with gradual ambulation when bed rest is no longer required (see

section "Caring for Patients on Prolonged Bed Rest," p. 651, for guidelines following prolonged immobility).

—Explain to patient that after the radiation source has been removed, she should dilate the vagina either *via* sexual intercourse or vaginal dilator to prevent fibrosis or stenosis.

☐ *Head and neck implants*

—Following a complete nutritional assessment and assessment of the oropharyngeal area, discuss measures for nutritional support during the implantation, for example, soft or liquid diet, a high-protein diet, and optimal hydration.

—Teach patient the signs and symptoms of infection: fever, pain, and erythema and purulent drainage at the site of implantation.

—Encourage patient to take analgesics routinely for pain, rather than when pain becomes too severe.

—Identify alternative means for communication systems if patient's speech deteriorates (e.g., cards, use of magic slate).

☐ *Breast implants*

—Teach patient the signs of infection that may appear over the breast: erythema, warmth, and drainage at the insertion site.

—Teach patient the importance of avoiding trauma at the implant site and keeping the skin clean and dry to help maintain skin integrity.

☐ *Prostate implants*

—Explain to patient that urinary output will be measured every shift and that staff will inspect urine for the presence of radiation seeds.

—Caution patient that linen, dressings, and trash will be saved and examined for the presence of seeds.

5. Explain that caregivers will limit the amount of time spent at the implant site.

Knowledge deficit: Purpose and procedure for external beam radiation therapy, appropriate self-care measures following treatment, and available educational and community resources

Desired outcome: Patient and significant others identify the purpose and procedure for external radiation beam therapy, the appropriate self-care measures, and the available educational and community resources.

1. See interventions Nos. 1-6 with **Knowledge deficit:** Chemotherapy, p. 660.
2. Provide information about treatment schedule, duration of each treatment, and the number of treatments planned.
   ☐ Radiation therapy usually is given 5 days a week, Monday through Friday.
   ☐ The treatment itself lasts only a few minutes; the majority of the time is spent preparing patient for treatment. Immobilization devices and shields are positioned before treatment to ensure proper delivery of radiation and minimize radiation to surrounding normal tissue.
3. Explain that the skin will be marked to facilitate delivery of radiation to the desired area. Usually, small skin tatoos (small pinpoint marks) are used. These are permanent and are used to ensure precise delivery of the radiation. However, if gentian violet is used, explain the importance of not washing the marks (see **Impaired skin integrity,** p. 686, for more information).
4. Discuss side effects that may occur with radiation treatment and the appropriate self-care measures. Systemic side effects include fatigue and anorexia. The most commonly occuring side effects appear locally, however. For example, side effects associated with head and neck radiation include mucositis, xerostomia, altered taste sensation, dental caries, sore throat, hoarseness, dysphagia, headache, and nausea and vomiting. See subsequent nursing diagnoses and interventions for more detail about local side effects.
5. Provide patient with a written copy of the side effects for his or her site of radiation therapy. Explain that the National Cancer Institute has a book entitled *Radiation and You,* which lists side effects and side effect management.
6. Provide information about community resources for transportation to and from the radiation center and for skilled nursing care, as needed.

PHYSICAL CARE OF PATIENTS WITH CANCER

Constipation related to VINCA alkaloid chemotherapy, narcotic analgesics, tranquilizers, antidepressants, anorexia, hypercalcemia, spinal cord compression, mental status changes, decreased mobility, or colonic disorders

For desired outcomes and interventions, see the same nursing diagnosis in "General Care of Patients with Neurologic Disorders," p. 252, "Caring for Patients on Prolonged Bed Rest," p. 656, and "Caring for Preoperative and Postoperative Patients," p. 647. **Note:** Patients should not go more than 2 days without having a bowel movement. Patients receiving VINCA alkaloid are at risk for ileus, in addition to constipation. Preventive measures, such as use of senna products (e.g., Pericolace or Sennokot), especially for patients taking narcotics, are highly recommended. In addition, all individuals taking narcotics should receive a prophylactic home regimen.

Diarrhea related to chemotherapy drugs, especially antimetabolite agents; antacids containing magnesium; radiation therapy to the abdomen or pelvis; tube feedings; food intolerances; and GI dysfunction, such as tumors, Crohn's disease, ulcerative colitis, and fecal impaction

For desired outcomes and interventions, see "Malabsorption/Maldigestion" for the same nursing diagnosis, p. 331; Table 6-1, p. 331, for lists of low-residue foods; and **Potential fluid volume deficit** related to loss secondary to diarrhea, p. 331. See "Ulcerative Colitis" for **Potential impairment of skin integrity:** Perineal/perianal area related to irritation secondary to prolonged diarrhea, p. 358. In addition, patient may experience hypokalemia due to loss of potassium with excessive diarrhea. See "Hypokalemia," p. 555. Instruct patient to notify health care member if experiencing more than 3 loose stools per day.

Ineffective breathing pattern related to decreased lung expansion secondary to fluid accumulation in the lungs (pleural effusion)

For desired outcome and interventions, see the same nursing diagnosis in "Pleural Effusion," p. 12. Patients at increased risk for pleural effusion are those with corresponding cancers, including lymphoma, leukemia, mesothelioma, lung and breast cancers, and metastasis to the lung from other primary cancers.

Ineffective breathing pattern related to dyspnea secondary to decreased lung expansion (pulmonary fibrosis)

For desired outcome and interventions, see the same nursing diagnosis in "Pulmonary Fibrosis," p. 34. Some chemotherapeutic agents can cause pulmonary toxicity, an inflammatory type of reaction that occurs, resulting in fibrotic lung changes, cellular damage, and decreased lung capacity. Examples of chemotherapeutic agents causing pulmonary toxicity include the following: busulfon, cyclophosphamide, chlorambucil, melphalan, carmustine, semustine, bleomycin sulfate, mitomycin, methotrexate, mercaptopurine, cytarabine, L-asparaginase, procarbazine hydrochloride, zinostatin, and chlorozotocin.

Pain: Acute or chronic related to the presence of cancer or its treatments

For desired outcome and interventions, see the same nursing diagnosis in "Caring for Preoperative and Postoperative Patients," p. 638. Explain that acute pain is of short duration and that relief will occur when the underlying cause is treated (see Table A-13). Describe the physiologic causes of pain for patients with chronic pain (see Table A-14) and stress noninvasive methods of pain relief for these patients (see Table A-6, p. 643).

Fatigue related to decreased oxygen-carrying capacity of the blood secondary to anemia due to chemotherapy with such drugs as chloramphenicol, radiation therapy, protein deficiency, or chronic disease

TABLE A-13 Physiologic causes of acute pain in the cancer patient

☐ Tumor compression or infiltration of nerves
☐ Tumor obstruction of hollow viscera or ductal system
☐ Infiltration/obstruction of blood vessels
☐ Exacerbations of alterated body functions unrelated to the cancer (e.g., pre-existing conditions such as chronic headaches, arthritis)
☐ Pain associated with the treatments
☐ Postsurgical pain, stomatitis, or peripheral neuropathies

TABLE A-14 Physiologic causes of chronic pain in the cancer patient

☐ Tumor that is no longer responding to therapy
☐ Postsurgical pain
☐ Postchemotherapy pain
☐ Postradiation pain
☐ Postherpetic neuralgia
☐ Altered body functions (e.g., chronic arthritis, back pain, or any musculoskeletal disorder)

For desired outcome and interventions, see the same nursing diagnosis in "Hypoplasic (Aplastic) Anemia," p. 406. Review the anemia disorders, pp. 396-407, which are discussed in "Hematologic Disorders." Advise patient that fatigue is a temporary side effect of chemotherapy or radiation therapy and that it will abate when therapy has been completed. Stress the importance of good nutrition, vitamin and iron supplements, and intake of foods high in iron, such as liver and other organ meats, seafood, green vegetables, cereals, nuts, and legumes.

Potential for infection related to risk of neutropenia secondary to malignancy, chemotherapy, radiation therapy, or immunotherapy

Desired outcomes: Patient is free of infection as evidenced by normothermia, BP ≥90/60 mm Hg, and HR ≤100 bpm. Patient identifies risk factors for infection, verbalizes early signs and symptoms of infection and reports them promptly to health care professional should they occur, and demonstrates appropriate self-care measures that minimize the risk of infection.

1. Identify patients at risk for infection by obtaining the absolute neutrophil count (ANC). Calculate ANC by using the following formula:
   ANC = (% of segmented neutrophils + % bands) × total WBC count.
   ☐ 1,500-2,000/mm^3 ANC = no significant risk.
   ☐ 1,000-1,500/mm^3 ANC = minimal risk.
   ☐ 500-1,000/mm^3 ANC = moderate risk. Initiate neutropenic precautions.
   ☐ <500/mm^3 ANC = severe risk. Initiate neutropenic precautions.
2. Assess each body system thoroughly to determine potential/actual sources of infection.
3. Monitor VS and temperature q4h. Be alert to temperature ≥38° C (100.4° F) × 2, temperature <35.56° C (96° F) × 1, temperature >38.33° C (101° F) × 1, increased HR, decreased BP, and the following clinical signs of infection: tenderness, erythema, warmth, swelling, and drainage at invasive sites; chills; and malaise.
   Note: Signs of infection may be absent in the presence of neutropenia.
4. Place sign on patient's door indicating that neutropenic precautions are in effect for patients with ANC ≤1,000/mm^3.
   ☐ Move patient to a private room, if possible.

☐ Instruct all persons entering patient's room to wash hands thoroughly.

☐ Restrict individuals from entering who have contagious diseases, such as colds or flu.

☐ Instruct patient to wear a mask when out of the hospital room.

5. Notify MD immediately if temperature is >100.4° F × 2, temperature >101° F × 1, or temperature <96° F. Initiate antibiotic therapy as prescribed within 1 hour when ANC is ≤500/mm³.

6. Implement oral care routine to minimize the risk of infection due to nonintact mucosa or tongue. Teach patient to use a soft-bristled toothbrush after meals and before bed (bristles may be softened even more by running them under hot water). Inspect oral cavity daily, noting presence of white patches on the tongue or mucous membrane. Mycostatin swish and swallow may be prescribed to prevent the development of oral or esophageal candida. Individuals with prolonged neutropenia are at high risk for candida as well as other bacterial and viral infections. Monitor for vesicles, which are crusted lesions that may signal herpes simplex. Acyclovir may be initiated, as prescribed, to prevent or minimize herpetic infections in patients with prolonged neutropenia, who are at risk for herpes.

7. Avoid the use of rectal suppositories, rectal temperature, or enemas to minimize the risk of traumatizing the rectal mucosa, thereby increasing the risk of infection. Be aware that patients with prolonged neutropenia are at increased risk for perirectal infection; monitor for it accordingly.

8. Implement measures that maintain skin integrity and instruct patient accordingly: use electric shaver rather than razor blade; avoid vaginal douche and tampons; use emery board rather than clipper for nail care; caution patient to check with MD prior to dental care; avoid all invasive procedures; use antimicrobial skin preparations prior to injections; change IV sites q48h; use steel-tipped rather than plastic catheters (minimizes the risk of infection); and advise use of water-soluble lubricant prior to sexual intercourse and avoidance of oral and anal manipulation during sexual activities.

9. Teach patient to avoid potential sources of infection during periods of neutropenia. For example, patient should avoid foods with high bacterial count (raw eggs, raw fruits and vegetables, foods prepared in a blender that cannot adequately be cleaned); bird, cat, and dog excreta; and plants, flowers, and sources of stagnant water.

10. Be alert to signs of impending sepsis, including subtle changes in mental status: restlessness or irritability; warm and flushed skin; chills, fever, or hypothermia; increased urine output; bounding pulse; tachypnea; and glycosuria. These symptoms often precede the classic signs of septic shock: cold, clammy skin; thready pulse; decreased BP; and oliguria.

Potential for injury related to increased risk of bleeding/hemorrhage secondary to thrombocytopenia (for all patients receiving chemotherapy and radiation therapy, as well as those with cancer, particularly that involving the bone marrow)

Desired outcome: Patient is asymptomatic of bleeding as evidenced by negative occult blood tests; HR ≤00 bpm; and systolic BP ≥90 mm Hg.

1. Identify individuals at increased risk for bleeding:

☐ Platelets 150,000-300,000 μl = normal risk for bleeding.

☐ Platelets <50,000 μl = moderate risk for bleeding; initiate thrombocytopenic precautions.

☐ Platelets <20,000 μl = severe risk of bleeding; may develop spontaneous bleeding; initiate thrombocytopenic precautions.

2. Perform a baseline physical assessment, monitoring for evidence of bleeding, including petechiae, ecchymosis, hematuria, coffee ground emesis, tarry stools, hemoptysis, heavy menses, headaches, and blurred vision. Also monitor VS q shift, being alert to hypotension and tachycardia. Avoid use of rectal thermometer, which can cause rectal bleeding.

3. Test all secretions for the presence of occult blood.

4. Perform a psychosocial assessment, including patient's past experience with throm-

bocytopenia; the effect of thrombocytopenia on patient's lifestyle; and changes in patient's work pattern, family relationships, and social activities. Identify learning needs and necessity of skilled care after hospital discharge.

5. Hang a sign on patient's door, indicating that thrombocytopenia precautions are in effect for patients with platelet count <50,000 μl.

6. In the presence of bleeding, begin pad count for heavy menses; measure quantity of vomiting and stool; apply direct pressure to site of bleeding (VAD, venipuncture); and deliver platelet transfusion as prescribed.

7. Initiate oral care at frequent intervals to promote integrity of gingiva and mucosa. Advise patient to brush with soft-bristled toothbrush after meals and before bed (hot water run over bristles may soften them further). In the presence of gum bleeding, teach patient to use Toothettes, avoid use of dental floss, and avoid mouthwash with greater than 6% alcohol content. Suggest use of normal saline solution mouthwashes qid and water-based ointment for lubricating the lips.

8. Implement bowel program and check with patient daily for bowel movement. Assess need for stool softeners to prevent constipation; encourage adequate hydration (at least 2 L/day) and high-fiber foods to promote bowel function; and avoid use of rectal suppositories, enemas, or harsh laxatives to minimize the risk of bleeding.

9. Implement measures that prevent bleeding. Teach patient to use electric shaver; apply direct pressure for 3-5 minutes after injections and venipuncture; avoid vaginal douche and tampons, constrictive clothing, aspirin or aspirin-containing products because of aspirin's antiplatelet action, alcohol ingestion, anticoagulants, and indomethacin (Indocin), which is a GI irritant. Caution patient to perform gentle nose-blowing, use emery board rather than clippers for nail care, check with MD prior to dental care, and avoid bladder catheterization if possible.

10. Caution patient to avoid activities that predispose to trauma or injury; remove hazardous objects or furniture from patient's environment. Assist patient with ambulating if patient's physical mobility is impaired. When the patient's platelet count is <20,000 μl, teach patient to avoid activities involving the Valsalva maneuver, which increases intracranial pressure. These activities include moving up in bed, straining at stool, bending at the waist, and lifting heavy objects. Suggest bed rest if patient's platelet count is <10,000 μl.

11. See "Thrombocytopenia," p. 409, for more information.

Alteration in nutrition: Less than body requirements related to decreased intake secondary to nausea and vomiting or anorexia occurring with chemotherapy or radiation therapy

Desired outcome: Patient has adequate nutrition as evidenced by stable weights and a positive or balanced nitrogen state.

For anorexia

1. Monitor for clinical signs of malnutrition. See Table 12-2, "Physical Assessment with Nutritional Implications," p. 615. Weigh patient daily.

2. Assess patient's food likes and dislikes, as well as the cultural and religious preferences related to food choices.

3. Explain to patient that anorexia can be caused by pathophysiology of cancer, surgery, and side effects of chemotherapy and radiation therapy.

4. Teach patient the importance of increasing caloric intake to increase energy and minimize weight loss.

5. Teach patient the importance of increasing protein intake to facilitate repair and regeneration of cells.

6. Suggest that patient eat several small meals at frequent intervals throughout the day.

7. Encourage use of nutritional supplements.

For nausea and vomiting

1. Assess patient's pattern of nausea and vomiting: onset, frequency, duration, intensity, and amount and character of emesis.

2. Explain to patient that nausea and vomiting are side effects of chemotherapy and radiation therapy (see Table A-15)

TABLE A-15 Antineoplastic agents with known emetic action

Mild emetic action	Moderate emetic action	Severe emetic action
L-asparaginase	hexamethylmelamine	nitrosureas
bleomycin	azacytidine	dactinomycin
chlorambucil	daunorubicin	cisplatin
hydroxyurea	doxorubicin	cyclophosphamide
melphan	etoposide (VP 16)	decarbazine
mercaptopurine	5-fluorouracil (5 FU)	mitomycin-C
tamoxifen	procarbazine	methotrexate
thioguanine	streptozotocin	mithramycin
thiotepa		mechlorethamine
vinblastine		
vincristine		
steroids		
cytarabine		
L-phenylalanine		

3. Teach patient to eat cold foods or food served at room temperature, since the odor of hot food may aggravate nausea.
4. Suggest intake of clear liquids and bland foods.
5. Teach patient to avoid sweet, fatty, highly salted, and spicy foods, as well as foods with strong odors, any of which may increase nausea.
6. Minimize such stimuli as smells, sounds, or sights, all of which may promote nausea.
7. Encourage patient to eat sour or mint candy during chemotherapy to decrease the unpleasant, metallic taste.
8. Encourage patient to experiment with various dietary patterns:
   □ Avoid eating or drinking for 1-2h prior to and after chemotherapy.
   □ Follow a clear liquid diet for 1-2h prior to chemotherapy and for 1-24h afterward.
   □ Avoid contact with food while it is being cooked; avoid being around people who are eating.
   □ Eat light meals at frequent intervals (5-6 times per day).
9. Suggest that patient sit near an open window to breathe fresh air when feeling nauseated.
10. Help patient find the appropriate distraction technique (e.g., music, TV, reading).
11. Teach patient to use relaxation techniques. See **Health-seeking behavior:** Relaxation technique effect for stress reduction, p. 49.
12. Administer antiemetics as prescribed (see Table A-16). Teach patient to take prescribed antiemetic 1-12h prior to chemotherapy and continue to take the drug q4-6h for at least 12-24h following chemotherapy, continuing for as long as nausea persists.
13. Teach patient to stay NPO for 4-8h if frequent episodes of vomiting occur.
14. Instruct patient to sip liquids, such as broth, ginger ale, cola, tea, or jello, slowly; suck on ice chips; and avoid large volumes of water.

Altered oral mucous membrane: Stomatitis secondary to chemotherapy agents (especially antibiotics), antimetabolites, and VINCA alkaloids; radiation therapy to head and neck; poor oral hygiene; and myelosuppression

For desired outcome and interventions, see the same nursing diagnosis in "Stomatitis," p. 315. Caution patient not to floss teeth in the presence of myelosuppression. For moderate-severe stomatitis, patient may require parenteral analgesics, such as morphine.

TABLE A-16   Common antiemetic agents

Agent	Generic name	Trade name
phenothiazine	prochlorperazine	Compazine
steroids	dexamethasone	Decadron
antihistamine	diphenhydramine	Benadryl
butyrophenon derivatives	haloperidol	Haldol
benzodiazepines	lorazepam	Ativan
miscellaneous	metoclopramide*	Reglan

*Metoclopramide blocks the neurotransmitter sites to decrease stimulation of an area in the medulla called the chemoreceptor trigger zone.

Impaired physical mobility related to altered motor ability secondary to bone metastasis or spinal cord compression

For desired outcome and interventions, see the same nursing diagnosis in "Osteoarthritis," p. 426. Also see related discussions in "Spinal Cord Injury," p. 196, "General Care for Patients with Neurologic Disorders," p. 248, "Fractures," p. 449, and "Malignant Neoplasms," p. 457. See discussions of care of patients at risk for pressure ulcers, p. 630, and care of patients on prolonged bed rest, p. 651.

Potential body image disturbance related to alopecia secondary to radiation therapy to the head and neck or administration of chemotherapy agents

Desired outcome: Patient discusses the effects that alopecia may have on his or her self-concept, body image, and social interaction and identifies measures that prevent, minimize, or enable adaptation to alopecia.

Note: Common chemotherapy agents that cause alopecia include the following: cyclophosphamide, doxorubicin, daunamycin, actinomycin D, bleomycin, vinblastine, vincristine, and VP 16.

1. Discuss the potential for hair loss with the patient prior to treatment.
   □ Radiation therapy of 1,500-3,000 rads to the head and neck will produce either partial or complete hair loss. Explain that this hair loss is temporary and that onset usually occurs within 5-7 days, with regrowth beginning 2-3 months after the final treatment.
   □ Radiation therapy greater than 4,500 rads usually results in permanent hair loss.
   □ Hair loss associated with chemotherapy is temporary and related to the specific agent, the dose, and the duration of administration. Regrowth usually begins 1-2 months after the last treatment. However, the hair often grows back a different color or texture.
2. Explore the impact hair loss will have/has on the patient's self concept, body image, and social interaction. Recognize that alopecia is an extremely stressful side effect for most patients.
3. Encourage the following measures that will minimize the impact or severity of alopecia: using a mild shampoo, hair conditioner, soft-bristled hair brush or a wide-toothed comb; sleeping on a silk pillowcase to minimize hair tangles; decreasing frequency of hairwashing; and avoiding irritants, such as dyes, permanent wave solutions, hair dryers, curling irons, clips, and hair sprays.
4. Explain that scalp hypothermia and tourniquet applications during IV infusion have been identified as measures that decrease the severity of hair loss. In particular, a significant decrease in alopecia has been found in individuals who use a hypothermia cap. These techniques are contraindicated in hematologic malignancy and in solid tu-

mors with scalp metastasis because these techniques may prevent adequate absorption of the drug where it is needed.

5. Suggest measures that may help minimize the psychologic impact of hair loss: cut the hair short prior to treatment; select a wig before hair loss occurs, which will enable patients to match color and style of their own hair; wear a hairnet or turban during hair loss to collect hair that falls out; use scarves, hats, caps, and turbans to cover the head; use makeup and accessories to enhance self concept. **Note:** Wigs are tax deductible and often are reimbursed by insurance with the appropriate prescription.

6. Inform patient that hair loss may occur on body parts as well as the head, including the axilla, groin, legs, facial hair, eyelashes, and eyebrows.

7. Instruct patient to keep head covered during the summer to minimize sunburn.

8. Provide information about alopecia that is available through community resources, such as the American Cancer Society.

Potential sensory/perceptual alterations related to auditory and kinesthetic impairment secondary to use of cisplatinum or VINCA alkaloids

Desired outcome: Patient reports early signs and symptoms of ototoxicity and peripheral neuropathy; measures are implemented promptly to minimize adverse side effects.

1. Explain that tinnitus or decreased hearing can occur with use of cisplatinum. Usually it is dose-related and a result of cumulative side effects. Most commonly, high frequency hearing loss occurs, although with cumulative doses, speech frequency hearing range also may be affected. Affected individuals may have difficulty hearing speech in the presence of background noise. Suggest that the patient face the speaker during conversation. A hearing aid also may be helpful. In instances of hearing loss from cisplatinum, which is usually irreversible, refer the patient to community resources for the hearing impaired.

2. Monitor patient for the development of peripheral neuropathy, which can occur with cisplatinum and vincristine use. The first symptom usually is numbness and tingling of the fingers and toes, which can progress to difficulty with fine motor skills, such as buttoning shirts or picking up objects. The most severely affected individuals may lose sensation at hip level and have difficulty with balance and ambulation. Instruct patient to report early signs and symptoms. Suggest consultation with physical and occupational therapist to assist with maintaining function.

3. Put individuals at risk for paralytic ileus associated with the neuropathy (i.e., those taking vincristine, vinblastine) on daily bowel checks. Administer stool softeners and laxatives daily if patient has not had a bowel movement within a 48-hour period, or as prescribed.

Potential sensory/perceptual alterations related to motor and sensorium changes secondary to hypercalcemia

For desired outcome and interventions, see the same nursing diagnosis in "Hypercalcemia," p. 56. Cancer patients at risk for hypercalcemia include those with bone metastasis, breast cancer, lung cancer, multiple myeloma, head and neck cancer, and hypernephroma. In addition, see "Hypercalcemia" for the following: **Alteration in pattern of urinary elimination,** p. 562.

Potential sexual dysfunction: Impaired sexual self concept and infertility secondary to radiation therapy to the lower abdomen, pelvis, and gonads; or chemotherapy agents, especially alkylating agents, vinblastine, bleomycin, actinomycin D, daunorubicin, mitomycin, procarbazine, and cytarabine

Desired outcome: Patient identifies potential side effects of treatment on sexual and reproductive function and identifies acceptable methods of contraception during treatment.

1. Initiate discussion about the effects of treatment on sexuality and reproduction. The PLISSIT model provides an excellent framework for discussion. This 4-step model includes the following: 1) **Permission**—give the patient permission to discuss issues

of concern; 2) **LImited** information—provide patient with information about expected treatment effects upon sexual and reproductive function, without going into complete detail; 3) **Specific Suggestions**—provide suggestions for managing common problems that occur during treatment; and 4) **Intensive Therapy**—although most individuals can be managed by nurses using the first 3 steps in this model, some patients may require referral to an expert counselor.

2. Assess the impact the diagnosis and treatment has on the patient's sexual functioning and self-concept.
3. Identify the possibility of pregnancy before treatment is initiated. Pregnancy will cause a delay in treatment. If treatment cannot be delayed, a therapeutic abortion may be recommended.
4. Discuss the possibilities of decreased sexual response or desire, which may result from side effects of chemotherapy. Encourage patients to maintain open communication with their partners regarding needs and concerns. Explore alternate methods of sexual fulfillment, such as hugging, kissing, talking quietly together, or massage. In the presence of symptoms related to therapy, such interventions as taking a nap before sexual activity or use of pain or antiemetic medication may help decrease symptoms. Other suggestions include use of a water-based lubricant if dyspareunia is a problem, or if fatigue is a problem, changing the usual time of day for intimacy or using supine or side-lying positions, which require the least expenditure of energy.
5. Discuss the possibility of temporary or permanent sterility resulting from treatment. Explore the possibility of sperm banking for men prior to treatment or utilization of oophoropexy (surgical displacement of the ovaries outside the radiation field) for women.
6. Teach male patients the importance of contraception during treatment and for 2 years after completion of therapy to ensure adequate time for renewal of sperm and to determine the individual's response to treatment.
7. Inform patients that healthy offspring have been born from parents who have received radiation therapy or chemotherapy. However, long-term effects have not been clearly identified. Suggest that patients have genetic counseling prior to parenting, as indicated.

Potential for impaired skin integrity related to cutaneous reactions secondary to chemotherapy

Desired outcome: Patient identifies the potential side effects of chemotherapy on the skin and measures that will promote comfort and skin integrity.

Note: Alterations of the skin or nails that occur in conjunction with chemotherapy are a result of the destruction of the basal cells of the epidermis (general) or due to cellular alterations at the site of chemotherapy administration (local). The reactions are specific to the agent used and vary in onset, severity, and duration. The skin reactions include the following: transient erythema/urticaria, hyperpigmentation, telangiectasis, photosensitivity, hyperkeratosis, acnelike reaction, ulceration, and radiation recall.

Transient erythema/urticaria: May be generalized or localized at the site of chemotherapy administration. Usually it occurs within several hours after chemotherapy and disappears in several hours. It is caused by the following agents: doxorubicin hydrochloride (Adriamycin), bleomycin, L-asparaginase, mithramycin, and mechlorethamine.

1. Perform and document a pretreatment assessment of the patient's skin for posttreatment comparison.
2. Assess the onset, pattern, severity, and duration of the reaction following treatment.
3. Compare posttreatment findings to those from the pretreatment assessment to determine if the cause of the erythema/urticaria is related to the chemotherapy or to herpes zoster, bacterial or fungal embolic lesions, skin metastasis, allergic reaction, or parasitic infestation.

Hyperpigmentation: This reaction is believed to be caused by increased levels of melanin-stimulating hormone. It can occur on the nail beds, oral mucosa, along the veins used for chemotherapy administration, or it can be generalized. It is caused by the following chemotherapeutic agents: doxorubicin hydrochloride (Adriamycin), carmustine, bleomycin, cyclophosphamide, daunorubicin, fluorouracil, and melphalan. In addition, it can occur with tumors of the pituitary gland.

1. Inform the patient pretreatment that this reaction is to be expected and that it will disappear gradually when the course of treatment is finished.

Telangiectasis (spider veins): This reaction is believed to be caused by destruction of the capillary bed and occurs as a result of applications of topical carmustine and mechlorethamine.

1. Inform patient that this reaction is permanent but that the configuration of the veins will become less severe after a period of time.

Photosensitivity: This reaction is enhanced when the skin is exposed to ultraviolet light. Acute sunburn and residual tanning can occur with short exposure to the sun. Photosensitivity can occur during the time the agent is administered or it can reactivate a skin reaction caused by sun exposure when the agent is administered in close proximity to the sun exposure. It is caused by dactinomycin, doxorubicin hydrochloride, bleomycin, dacarbazine, fluorouracil, methotrexate, and vinblastine.

1. Assess onset, pattern, severity, and duration of the reaction.
2. Teach patient to avoid exposing skin to the sun. Advise patient to wear protective clothing and use an effective sun-screening agent (SPF of 15 or greater).
3. In the event that burning takes place, advise patient to treat it like a sunburn (e.g., tepid bath, moisturizing cream, consultation with MD).

Hyperkeratosis: This reaction presents as a thickening of the skin, especially over the hands, feet, face, and areas of trauma. It is disfiguring and causes loss of fine motor function of the hands. It occurs with bleomycin administration and should be considered an indicator of the more severe fibrotic changes in the lungs. It is reversible when treatment with bleomycin is discontinued.

1. For patients taking bleomycin, assess for the presence of skin thickening and loss of fine motor function of the hands.
2. In the presence of skin thickening, be aware that fibrotic changes may be present in the lungs. Assess for this condition accordingly (see "Pulmonary Fibrosis," p. 32).
3. Reassure patient that this condition is reversible when bleomycin has been discontinued.

Acnelike reaction: This reaction presents as erythema, especially of the face, and progresses to papules and pustules, which are characteristic of acne. It occurs with administration of dactinomycin and will disappear when the drug has been discontinued.

1. Reassure patient that this reaction will disappear when treatment with dactinomycin has been discontinued.
2. Suggest that patient use a commercial preparation to conceal these blemishes.

Ulceration: This reaction presents as a generalized, shallow lesion of the epidermal layer. It is caused by bleomycin, methotrexate, and mitomycin-C.

1. Assess for the presence of ulceration.
2. If present, cleanse the ulcers with a solution of ¼ strength hydrogen peroxide and ¾ strength normal saline q4-6h.
3. Expose the ulcer to the air, if possible.
4. Be alert to the presence of infection at the ulcerated site, as evidenced by local warmth, erythema, and purulent drainage.
5. Teach patient the treatment and assessment interventions.

Radiation recall reaction: This occurs when chemotherapy is given at the same time or following treatment with radiation therapy. It presents as erythema, followed by dry desquamation. More severe reactions can progress to vesicle formation and wet desquamation. After the skin heals, it is permanently hyperpigmented. This reaction is caused by doxorubicin hydrochloride, bleomycin, cyclophosphamide, dactinomycin, fluorouracil, hydroxyuria, and methotrexate.

1. Teach patient the following skin care routine:
   □ Cleanse the skin gently at the site of recall reaction, using mild soap, tepid water, and a soft cloth; pat dry.
   □ Use A&D ointment or topical steroids on areas with dry desquamation.
   □ If edema and wet desquamation are present, cleanse the area with half strength hydrogen peroxide and normal saline.
2. Teach patient to protect the skin at the site of recall reaction in the following ways:
   □ Avoid wearing tight-fitting clothes.
   □ Avoid harsh fabrics, such as wool or corduroy.
   □ Use mild detergents, such as Ivory Snow.
   □ Avoid sun exposure.
   □ Avoid exposing the site of recall reaction to heat and cold.
   □ Avoid swimming in salt water or chlorinated pools.
   □ Avoid use of all medications (with the exceptions of A&D ointment and topical steroids), deodorants, perfumes, powders, or cosmetics on the skin at the recall site.
   □ Avoid shaving the site of recall reaction; if shaving is absolutely necessary, use an electric razor.

Impaired skin integrity related to cutaneous reactions secondary to radiation therapy

Desired outcome: Patient identifies potential skin reactions and the management interventions that will promote comfort and skin integrity.

1. Assess the degree and extensiveness of the skin reaction.
2. Teach patient the following skin care over the treatment field:
   □ Cleanse skin gently and in a patting motion, using a mild soap, tepid water, and a soft cloth. Rinse the area and pat it dry.
   □ Apply A&D ointment to skin with stage II reaction (see Table A-17).
3. For patients with stage III skin reaction, teach the following regimen:
   □ Cleanse the area with ½ strength hydrogen peroxide and normal saline, using an irrigation syringe. Rinse with saline or water and pat dry gently.
   □ Use nonadhesive absorbent dressings, such as Telfa or Adaptic and ABD for draining areas. Be alert to indicators of infection.
4. Teach the following interventions for protecting the patient's skin:
   □ Avoid tight-fitting clothing.
   □ Avoid wearing harsh fabrics, such as wool and corduroy.
   □ Avoid sun exposure.
   □ Use mild detergents (e.g., Ivory Snow).
   □ Avoid exposure to heat and cold.
   □ Avoid swimming in chlorinated pools or salt water.
   □ Avoid using medications, deodorants, perfumes, powders, or cosmetics on the skin in the treatment field.
   □ Avoid shaving the hair on the skin in the treatment field; if shaving is absolutely necessary, use an electric razor.

TABLE A-17 Stages of the effects of radiation on the skin

Stage I:	Inflammation, mild erythema, slight edema
Stage II:	Inflammation; dry desquamation; dry, scaly, itchy skin
Stage III:	Inflammation, edema, wet desquamation, blisters, peeling
Stage IV:	Permanent loss of hair in the treatment field, suppression of sebaceous glands. *Late effects:* Fibrosis and atrophy of the skin, fibrosis of the lymph glands

5. For stage IV reaction, see interventions for alopecia under **Body image disturbance,** p. 682.

Altered skin integrity: Malignant skin lesions

Desired outcome: Patient verbalizes measures that promote comfort and skin integrity.

1. Identify populations at risk for malignant lesions: individuals with primary tumors of the breast, lung, colon/rectum, ovary, or oral cavity; and those with malignant melanoma, lymphoma, or leukemia.
2. Identify common sites of cutaneous metastases: anterior chest, abdomen, head (scalp), and neck.
3. Inspect skin lesions and note and document the following: general characteristics, location and distribution, configuration, size, morphologic structure (e.g., nodule, erosion, fissure), drainage (color, amount, and character), and odor.
4. Monitor for indicators of infection: local warmth, erythema, tenderness, purulent drainage.
5. Perform the following skin care for nonulcerating lesions, and teach these interventions to the patient and significant others, as indicated.
   ☐ Wash affected area with tepid water and pat dry.
   ☐ Avoid pressure on the area.
   ☐ Apply dry dressing to protect the area against exposure to irritants and mechanical trauma (e.g., scratching).
   ☐ To enhance penetration of topical medications, apply occlusive dressings, such as Telfa, using paper tape.
   ☐ Teach patient not to wear irritating fabrics, such as wool and corduroy.
6. Perform the following skin care for ulcerating lesions, and teach these interventions to the patient and significant others, as indicated:
   ☐ *For cleansing and debriding*
      —May use half strength hydrogen peroxide and normal saline for irrigation.
      —May use cotton swabs or sponges to apply gentle pressure, thereby debriding the ulcerated area.
      —If the ulcerated area is prone to bleeding, irrigate only, using a syringe.
      —May use soaks (wet dressings) of saline, water, Burrow's solution (aluminum acetate), hydrogen peroxide, and Dakin's solution for debridement.
      —May use wet-to-dry dressings for gentle debridement.
   ☐ *For prevention and management of local infection*
      —Irrigate and scrub with antibacterial agents, such as acetic acid solution or Betadine.
      —Perform wound cultures as prescribed.
      —Apply topical antibacterial agents as prescribed.
      —Administer systemic antibiotics as prescribed.
   ☐ *To maintain hemostasis*
      —For capillary oozing, use silver nitrate sticks.
      —For larger surface area bleeding, use oxidized cellulose or pack the wound with Gelfoam or other such product.
   ☐ *To control odor*
      —Cleanse wound and change dressings as frequently as necessary.
      —Perform cultures and sensitivities of the wound, as prescribed.
      —Use antiodor agents (e.g., open a bottle of oil of peppermint or place a tray of activated charcoal) in patient's room.
7. For more information, see "Providing Nutritional Support," p. 611, and "Managing Wound Care," p. 644.

Impaired swallowing: Esophagitis secondary to radiation therapy to the neck, chest, and upper back; chemotherapy agents, especially the antimetabolites; infection due to immunosuppression; or tumors of the esophagus

Desired outcomes: Patient exhibits the gag reflex and is asymptomatic of aspiration, as evidenced by RR 12-20 breaths/min with normal depth and pattern (eupnea), normal skin color, and the ability to speak. Patient verbalizes the early signs and symptoms of esophagitis, alerts health care team as soon as they occur, and identifies measures for maintaining nutrition and comfort.

1. Monitor patient for evidence of impaired swallowing with concomitant respiratory difficulties.
2. Teach patient the early signs and symptoms of esophagitis and the importance of reporting them promptly to the staff should they occur: sensation of lump in the throat with swallowing, difficulty with swallowing solid foods, discomfort or pain with swallowing.
3. Monitor patient's dietary intake and provide the following guidelines: maintain a high-protein diet; eat foods that are soft and bland; add milk or milk products to the diet to coat the esophageal lining (for individuals without excessive mucus production); and add sauces and creams to foods, which may facilitate swallowing.
4. Ensure an adequate fluid intake of at least 2 L/day.
5. Implement the following measures that promote comfort and discuss them with the patient accordingly:
   □ Use a local anesthetic, as prescribed, to minimize pain with meals. Lidocaine 2% or diclone and diphenhydramine may be taken *via* swish and swallow before eating. **Caution:** These anesthetics may decrease the patient's gag reflex.
   □ Suggest that patient sit in an upright position during meals and for 15-30 minutes after eating.
   □ Mild analgesics, such as liquid ASA or acetaminophen, can be very helpful. Administer them as prescribed.
   □ For severe discomfort, narcotic analgesics may be required. Administer as prescribed. **Note:** If pain is severe or persistent, a barrium swallow may be performed to evaluate for the presence of an infection. Common causative agents are candida and herpes. Appropriate medical treatment, such as low-dose amphotericin or IV acyclovir, may be initiated.
6. Keep suction equipment readily available in the event that patient experiences aspiration.

Altered tissue perfusion: Cardiopulmonary, related to impaired circulation secondary to pericardial tamponade

Pericardial tamponade, caused by an accumulation of fluid in the pericardial space, tumor, invasion of the mediastinum, pericardial fibrosis, and effusion from radiotherapy, can occur. Patients at increased risk for pericardial tamponade include those with corresponding cancers, such as mesothelioma, sarcoma, leukemia, lymphoma, melanoma, primary gastrointestinal cancer, and metastatic lung and breast tumors.

For desired outcome and interventions, see the same nursing diagnosis in "Pericarditis," p. 59.

Altered tissue perfusion: Peripheral, related to impaired circulation secondary to lymphedema

Desired outcome: Patient exhibits adequate peripheral perfusion as evidenced by edema <2+ on a 0-4+ scale, peripheral pulses >2+ on a 0-4+ scale, normal skin color, decreasing or stable circumference of edematous site, bilaterally equal sensation, and ability to perform complete ROM in the involved extremity.

Note: Patient populations at risk include those who have had a radical mastectomy, lymph node dissection (upper and lower extremities), blockage of the lymphatic system from tumor burden, radiation therapy to the lymphatic system, or any combination of the above.

1. Assess the involved extremity for the degree of edema, quality of the peripheral pulses, color, circumference, sensation, and ROM.
2. Assess for signs of infection: tenderness, erythema, and warmth at the edematous site.

3. Elevate and position the involved extremity on a pillow in slight abduction.
4. Encourage wearing of loose-fitting clothing.
5. Consult with physical therapist and MD regarding development of exercise plan for ensuring mobility.

Potential for altered pattern of urinary elimination: Hemorrhagic cystitis secondary to cyclophosphamide/phosphamide treatment; oliguria or renal toxicity secondary to cisplatinum or high-dose methotrexate administration; renal calculi secondary to hyperurecemia; or dysuria secondary to cystitis

Desired outcomes: Patients receiving cyclophosphamide/ifosfamide test negatively for blood in their urine and patients receiving cisplatinum exhibit urine output of ≥ 100 ml/hr 1 hour prior to treatment and 4-12 hours following treatment. Patients with leukemia and lymphomas and those taking methotrexate exhibit urine pH of 7.5.

1. Ensure adequate hydration during treatment and for at least 24 hours following treatment for patients taking cyclophosphamide (Cytoxan), ifosfamide, methotrexate, and cisplatinum. Teach patient the importance of drinking at least 2-3 L/day. IV hydration also may be required, especially with high-dose chemotherapy.
2. Administer cyclophosphamide early in the day to minimize the retention of antimetabolites in the bladder during the night. Encourage patients to void q2h during the day and before going to bed. Test urine for the presence of blood and report positive results to MD. Monitor I&O q8h during high-dose treatment for 48 hours posttreatment. Be alert to decreasing urinary output.
3. MESNA is administered before ifosfamide and then 4 hours and 8 hours after the infusion to minimize the risk of hemorrhagic cystitis. Test all urine for the presence of blood. Promote fluid intake to maintain urine output at 100 ml/hr. Monitor I&O during infusion and for a 24-hour period after therapy to ensure that this urinary output is attained.
4. For patients receiving cisplatinum, prehydrate with ≥ 150-200 ml/hr of IV fluid. Cisplatinum can be administered as soon as the patient's urine output is ≥ 100-150 ml/hr. Monitor I&O qh for 4-12 hours following therapy to ensure urine output is maintained at ≥ 100-150 ml/hr. Patients may require diuretics to maintain this output. Promote fluid intake to ensure a positive fluid state for at least 24 hours following treatment, especially for patients taking diuretics. Notify MD promptly if urine output drops to <100 ml/hr. Urine output should be kept at a relatively high level because nephrotoxicity can occur as a side effect of this treatment.
5. An alkaline urine will enhance excretion of methotrexate as well as uric acid that results from tumor lysis, which is associated with leukemia and lymphoma. Monitor I&O q8h, being alert to a decreasing output, and test urine pH with each voiding to ensure it is 7.5. Sodium bicarbonate or acetazolamide (Diamox) will be used to alkalinize the urine. Allopurinol prevents uric acid formation and is often used prior to chemotherapy for patients with leukemia or lymphoma.
6. Renal calculi can occur due to hyperuricemia as a result of chemotherapy treatment for leukemia and lymphoma, which causes rapid cell lysis and increased excretion of uric acid. For more information, see "Renal Calculi," p. 110, and "Urinary Calculi," p. 131.
7. Teach patient the signs of cystitis, which can occur as a result of cytoxan and ifosfamide treatment: fever, pain with urination, malodorous or cloudy urine, and urinary frequency and urgency. Instruct patient to notify health care professional if these signs and symptoms occur.

In addition, see nursing diagnoses and interventions in "Pneumonia," p. 8, and "Atelectasis," p. 12 (for patients with myelosuppression); "Pulmonary Fibrosis," p. 34, (for patients on bleomycin therapy); "Heart Failure," p. 55, (for patients experiencing cardiotoxicity and who are on chemotherapeutic agents, such as doxorubicin or daunorubicin); "Hepatic and Biliary Disorders," p. 380, (for patients on hepatotoxic medications, such as cyclophosphamide and methotrexate); "Hypovolemia," p. 546, (for patients experiencing nausea, vomiting, and dehydration); and "Hypokalemia," p. 555, (for patients on steroid therapy).

PROVIDING PSYCHOSOCIAL CARE

Anxiety related to actual or perceived threat to biologic integrity, self concept, or role; unfamiliar people and environment; or the unknown

Desired outcome: Patient's anxiety is absent or reduced as evidenced by HR ≤100 bpm, RR ≤20 breaths per minute with normal depth and pattern (eupnea), and an absence of or decrease in irritability and restlessness.

1. Engage in honest communication with the patient; provide empathetic understanding. Establish an atmosphere that allows free expression.
2. Assess the patient's level of anxiety. Be alert to verbal and nonverbal cues.
   - □ *Mild:* Restlessness, irritability, increase in questions, focusing on the environment.
   - □ *Moderate:* Inattentiveness, expressions of concern, narrowed perceptions, insomnia, increased HR.
   - □ *Severe:* Expressions of feelings of doom, rapid speech, tremors, poor eye contact. Patient may be preoccupied with the past; unable to understand the present; and may present with tachycardia, nausea, and hyperventilation.
   - □ *Panic:* Inability to concentrate or communicate, distortion of reality, increased motor activity, vomiting, tachypnea.
3. For patients with severe anxiety or panic state, refer to psychiatric clinical nurse specialist or other as appropriate.
4. If patient is hyperventilating, encourage slow, deep breaths by having patient mimic your own breathing pattern.
5. Validate the nursing assessment of anxiety with the patient. ("You seem distressed; are you feeling uncomfortable now?")
6. Following an episode of anxiety, review and discuss with patient the thoughts and feelings that led to the episode.
7. Identify coping behaviors currently being used by patient (e.g., denial, anger, repression, withdrawal, daydreaming, or dependence on narcotics). Review coping behaviors patient has used in the past. Assist patient with using adaptive coping to manage anxiety. ("I understand that your wife reads to you to help you relax. Would you like to spend a part of each day alone with her?")
8. Encourage patient to express fears, concerns, and questions. ("I know this room looks like a maze of wires and tubes; please let me know when you have any questions.")
9. Reduce sensory overload by providing an organized, quiet environment. See nursing diagnosis **Sensory/perceptual alterations,** p. 691.
10. Introduce self and other health care members, explaining each individual's role as it relates to the patient's care.
11. Teach patient relaxation and imagery techniques. See the following: **Health-seeking behavior:** Relaxation technique effective for stress reduction, p. 49.
12. Enable support persons to be in attendance whenever possible.

Impaired verbal communication related to dysarthria secondary to neurologic deficit or physical barrier (e.g., tracheostomy)

Desired outcome: Patient communicates needs and feelings and relates decreased or absence of frustration over communication barriers.

1. Assess etiology of the impaired communication (e.g., tracheostomy, cerebrovascular accident, cerebral tumor, Guillain-Barré syndrome).
2. Along with patient and significant others, assess patient's ability to read, write, and comprehend English. If patient speaks a language other than English, collaborate with English-speaking family member or interpreter to establish effective communication.
3. When communicating with patient, use eye contact; speak in a clear, normal tone of voice; and face the patient.
4. If patient is unable to speak because of a physical barrier (e.g., tracheostomy, wired mandibles) provide reassurance and acknowledge his or her frustration. ("I know this is frustrating for you, but let's not give up. I want to understand you.")

5. Provide slate, word cards, pencil and paper, alphabet board, pictures, or other device to assist patient with communication.
6. Explain the source of the patient's communication impairment to significant others; teach them effective communication alternatives (listed above).
7. Be alert to nonverbal messages, such as facial expressions, hand movements, and nodding of the head. Validate their meaning with patient.
8. Recognize that the inability to speak may foster maladaptive behaviors. Encourage patient to communicate needs; reinforce independent behaviors.
9. Be honest with patient; do not relate understanding if you are unable to interpret patient's communication.

Sensory/perceptual alterations related to environmental overload or monotony, socially-restricted environment, psychologic stress, or pathophysiologic alterations

Desired outcomes: Patient verbalizes orientation to person, place, and time; relates the ability to concentrate; and expresses satisfaction with the degree and type of sensory stimulation being received.

1. Assess factors contributing to patient's sensory-perceptual alteration.
   □ *Environmental:* Excessive noise in the environment; constant, monotonous noise; restricted environment (immobility, traction, isolation); social isolation (restricted visitors, impaired communication); therapies.
   □ *Physiologic:* Decreased organ function, sleep or rest pattern disturbance, medication, previous history of altered sensory perception.
2. Determine the appropriate sensory stimulation needed for the patient, and plan care accordingly.
3. Control factors that contribute to environmental overload. For example, avoid constant lighting (use blindfolds, if necessary); decrease noise whenever possible (e.g., decrease alarm volumes, avoid loud talking, close room door occasionally, provide ear plugs for patient).
4. Provide meaningful sensory stimulation.
   □ Display clocks and large calendars and photographs and objects from home.
   □ Provide a radio, music, reading materials, tape recordings of family and significant others.
   □ Position patient toward window when possible.
   □ Discuss current events, time of day, holidays, and topics of interest during patient care activities. ("Good morning, Mr. Smith. I'm Ms. Stone, your nurse for the afternoon and evening, 3 PM to 11 PM. It's sunny outside. Today is the first day of summer.")
   □ As needed, orient patient to surroundings. Direct patient to reality as necessary.
   □ Touch patient frequently.
   □ Encourage significant others to communicate with patient frequently, using a normal tone of voice.
   □ Convey concern and respect for the patient. Introduce self and call patient by name.
   □ Stimulate patient's vision with mirrors, colored decorations, and pictures.
   □ Stimulate patient's sense of taste with sweet, salty, and sour substances as allowed.
   □ Encourage use of eyeglasses and hearing aids.
5. Explain routines, therapies, and equipment simply and directly. Individuals in crisis often cannot comprehend complex information.
6. Encourage patient to participate in health-care planning and decision making whenever possible.
7. Assess patient's sleep-rest pattern to evaluate its contribution to patient's sensory-perceptual disorder. Ensure that patient attains at least 90 minutes of uninterrupted sleep as frequently as possible. For more information, see next nursing diagnosis.

Sleep pattern disturbance related to environmental overload, therapeutic regimen, pain, immobility, or psychologic stress

Desired outcomes: Patient identifies factors that promote sleep, attains 90-minute periods of uninterrupted sleep, and verbalizes satisfaction with his or her ability to rest.

1. Assess patient's usual sleeping patterns (e.g., bedtime routine, hours of sleep per night, sleeping position, use of pillows and blankets, napping during the day, nocturia).
2. Explore relaxation techniques that promote patient's sleep-rest pattern (e.g., imagining relaxing scenes, listening to soothing music or taped stories, using muscle relaxation exercises).
3. Identify causative factors and activities that contribute to patient's insomnia, awaken patient, or adversely affect sleep pattern. Examples include pain, anxiety, therapies, depression, hallucinations, medications, underlying illness, sleep apnea, respiratory disorder, caffeine use, and fear.
4. Organize procedures and activities to allow for 90-minute periods of uninterrupted sleep-rest. Limit visiting during these periods.
5. Whenever possible, maintain a quiet environment by providing ear plugs or decreasing alarm levels. The use of "white noise" (e.g., low-pitched, monotonous sounds; electric fan; soft music) may facilitate sleep. Dim the lights for a period of time each day by drawing the drapes or providing blindfolds.
6. If appropriate, put limitations on patient's daytime sleeping. Attempt to establish regularly scheduled daytime activity (e.g., ambulation, sitting in chair, active ROM), which may promote nighttime sleep.
7. Investigate and provide comfort measures that are known to promote patient's sleep (e.g., soft music, massage, reading to patient, personal hygiene, such as a bath at bedtime, snack).
8. For more information, see Table A-8, p. 649, "Nonpharmacologic Measures to Promote Sleep."

Fear related to threat to biologic integrity, potential for loss, altered body image, loss of control, or therapeutic regimen

Desired outcomes: Patient communicates fears and concerns, relates the attainment of increased psychologic and physical comfort, and does not exhibit ineffective coping techniques.

1. Assess patient's perceptions of the environment and his or her health status and determine contributing factors to patient's feelings of fear. Evaluate patient's verbal and nonverbal responses.
2. Acknowledge patient's fears. ("I understand that all this equipment frightens you. Let me explain its function to you.")
3. Assess patient's history of coping behavior to determine sources of strength. ("What helps you get through stressful situations?") Identify negative coping behaviors, including severe depression, withdrawal, prolonged denial, hostility, and violence.
4. Provide opportunities for the patient to express fears and concerns. ("You seem very concerned about receiving more blood today.") Listen actively to the patient. Recognize that anger, denial, occasional withdrawal, and demanding behaviors may be coping responses. Be supportive of significant others who may misinterpret patient's coping mechanisms.
5. In addition to verbal communications of fear, be alert to somatic complaints, such as frequent urination; abdominal discomfort; and such behaviors as repetitive questioning, irritability, inability to concentrate, appetite changes, and sleeplessness.
6. Encourage patient to ask questions and gather information about the unknown. Provide ongoing information about equipment, therapies, and unit routines according to patient's ability to understand. Because fear tends to inhibit learning, provide recurring instructions and obtain validation of learning to ensure that appropriate information has been retained.
7. To promote an increased sense of control over self, encourage patient to participate in and plan his or her care whenever possible. Provide continuity of care by establishing a routine and arranging for consistent caregivers whenever possible.
8. Discuss with health-care team the appropriateness of medication therapy for patient's disabling fear or anxiety.

9. Explore patient's desire for spiritual or other counseling.
10. If there is a possibility of survival of the illness or surgery, collaborate with MD regarding a visit by another individual with the same disorder who has survived the surgery or disorder.
11. Assess your own feelings about cancer (or other grave prognoses). If you feel that the diagnosis is a death sentence, your attitude may be reflected to the patient. Recognize that your own positive attitude can be very therapeutic.

Ineffective individual coping related to threat to biologic integrity, knowledge deficit, unsatisfactory support systems, or hospitalization

Desired outcomes: Patient verbalizes feelings, identifies strengths and coping behaviors, and does not demonstrate ineffective coping behaviors.

1. Assess patient's perceptions and ability to understand his or her current health status.
2. Establish honest communication with the patient. ("Please tell me what I can do to help you.") Assist patient with identifying strengths, stressors, inappropriate behaviors, and personal needs.
3. Support positive coping behaviors. ("I see that reading that book seems to help you relax.")
4. Provide opportunities for the patient to express concerns, fears, and anxieties; gather information from nurses and other support systems. Provide patient with explanations regarding the unit routine, therapies, and equipment. Acknowledge patient's feelings and assessment of his or her current health status and environment.
5. Identify factors that inhibit patient's ability to cope (e.g., unsatisfactory support system, knowledge deficit, grief, fear).
6. Recognize maladaptive coping behaviors (e.g., severe depression, dependence on narcotics, hostility, violence, suicidal ideations). Confront patient about these behaviors. ("You seem to be requiring more pain medication. Are you experiencing more physical pain, or does it help you to remove yourself from reality?") Refer patient to psychiatric liaison, clinical nurse specialist, or clergy, as appropriate.
7. As patient's condition allows, assist with reducing anxiety. See **Anxiety,** p. 690.
8. Help reduce patient's sensory overload by maintaining an organized, quiet environment. See **Sensory/perceptual alterations,** p. 691.
9. Encourage regular visits by significant others. Encourage them to engage in conversation with patient to help minimize patient's emotional and social isolation.
10. Assess significant others' interactions with patient. Attempt to mobilize support systems by involving them in patient care whenever possible.
11. As appropriate, explain to patient and significant others that increased dependency, anger, and denial may be adaptive coping behaviors used by patient in early stages of crisis until effective coping behaviors are learned.
12. Seek referrals to social services, chaplains, psychiatric nurse, or hospice as appropriate.
13. When necessary, ensure that the patient is assisted with bringing closure to his or her affairs and relationships. For example, provide privacy for patient and significant others, call patient's attorney as needed, and request that patient's chaplain visit.

Anticipatory grieving related to expected loss of body function or body part, changes in self-concept or body image, or terminal illness

Desired outcomes: Patient and significant other(s) express grief, participate in decisions regarding the future, and communicate concerns to health-care team and to one another.

1. Assess factors contributing to anticipated loss.
2. Assess and accept patient's stage in the grieving process and behavioral response. Expect reactions, such as disbelief, denial, guilt, ambivalence, and depression.
3. Assess religious and sociocultural expectations related to loss. ("Is religion an important part of your life? How do you and your family deal with serious health problems?") Refer to the clergy or community support groups as appropriate.

4. Encourage patient and significant others to explore and communicate feelings regarding anticipated or actual loss of significant relationships. ("Is there anything you'd like to talk about today?") Also, respect their desire not to speak.
5. Demonstrate empathy. ("This must be a very difficult time for you and your family.") Provide an open and supportive environment. Be as comfortable as possible with crying, anger, and regressive behavior.
6. In selected circumstances, provide individuals with an explanation of the grieving process. This may assist them to better understand and acknowledge their feelings.
7. Assess grief reactions of patient and significant others and identify those individuals who may have a potential for dysfunctional grieving reactions (e.g., absence of emotion, hostility, avoidance). If the potential for dysfunctional grieving is present, refer the individual to psychiatric clinical nurse specialist, clergy, or other as appropriate.
8. When appropriate, assist patient and significant other(s) through the grieving process by providing a referral to a therapist trained in this process (e.g., a psychologist or psychiatric nurse).
9. As appropriate, arrange for a visit by patient's clergy.

Dysfunctional grieving related to actual or perceived loss or change in body function, body image, lifestyle, relationships, or lack of support systems

Desired outcomes: Patient and significant other(s) express grief, explain the meaning of the loss, and communicate concerns with each other. The patient completes necessary self-care activities.

1. Assess grief stage and previous coping abilities. Discuss with patient and significant others their feelings, the meaning of the loss, and their goals. ("How do you feel about your condition/illness? What do you hope to accomplish in these next few days/weeks?")
2. Because of the loss of body part (or function) and perceived mutilation of the body, expect and accept patient's behavioral responses, including initial shock and disbelief, sad and angry feelings, and statements expressing resistance and dislike. Reassure patient that these responses are normal.
3. Acknowledge and permit anger; set limits on the expression of anger to discourage destructive behavior. ("I understand that you must feel very angry, but for the safety of others, you may not throw equipment.")
4. Identify suicidal behavior (e.g., severe depression, statements of intent, suicide plan, previous history of suicide attempt). Ensure patient safety and refer patient to psychiatric clinical nurse specialist, psychiatrist, clergy, or other support system.
5. Encourage patient and significant others to participate in daily and diversional activities. Identify physiologic problems related to loss (e.g., eating or sleeping disorders) and intervene accordingly.
6. If there is a possibility of the patient's survival of the illness, collaborate with MD regarding a visit by another individual with the same disorder who has survived the surgery or illness.

Powerlessness related to lack of control over self-care, health care status, or outcome secondary to nature of health care environment, therapeutic regimen, or life-threatening illness

Desired outcomes: Patient makes decisions regarding care and therapies and relates an attitude of realistic hope and a sense of control over self.

1. Assess with patient his or her personal preferences, needs, values, and attitudes.
2. Before providing information, assess patient's knowledge and understanding of his or her condition and care.
3. Recognize patient's expressions of fear, lack of response to events, and lack of interest in information, any of which may signal patient's sense of powerlessness.
4. Evaluate caregiver practices and adjust them to support patient's sense of control. For example, if the patient always bathes in the evening to promote relaxation before bedtime, modify the care plan to include an evening bath rather than follow the hospital routine of giving a morning bath.

5. Assist patient to identify and demonstrate activities he or she can perform independently.
6. Whenever possible, offer alternatives related to routine hygiene, diet, diversional activities, visiting hours, or treatment times.
7. Ensure patient's privacy and preserve his or her territorial rights whenever possible. For example, when distant relatives and casual acquaintances request information about the patient's status, check with patient and family members before sharing that information.
8. Discourage patient's dependency on staff. Avoid overprotection and parenting behaviors toward patient.
9. Assess support systems; enable significant others to be involved in patient care whenever possible.
10. Offer realistic hope for the future. On occasion, encourage patient to direct thoughts beyond the present.
11. Provide referrals to clergy and other support systems as appropriate.

Spiritual distress related to altered health state, separation from religious ties, life-threatening illness, or conflict between religious beliefs and therapeutic regimens

Desired outcomes: Patient verbalizes his or her religious beliefs and expresses hope for the future, the attainment of spiritual well-being, and that conflicts have been resolved or diminished.

1. Assess patient's spiritual or religious beliefs, values, and practices. ("Do you have a religious preference? How important is it to you? Are there any religious or spiritual practices you wish to participate in while in the hospital?") If the patient expresses a desire, volunteer to read scripture or other religious literature.
2. Inform patient and significant others of the availability of spiritual aids, such as a chapel or volunteer chaplain.
3. Display a nonjudgmental attitude toward patient's religious or spiritual beliefs and values. Attempt to create an environment that is conducive to free expression.
4. Identify available support systems that may assist in meeting the patient's religious or spiritual needs (e.g., clergy, fellow church members, support groups).
5. Be alert to comments related to spiritual concerns or conflicts. ("I don't know why God is doing this to me." "I'm being punished for my sins.")
6. Use active listening and open-ended questioning to assist patient in resolving conflicts related to spiritual issues. ("I understand that you want to be baptized. We can arrange to do that here.")
7. Provide privacy and opportunities for religious practices, such as prayer and meditation.
8. If spiritual beliefs and therapeutic regimens are in conflict, provide patient with honest, concrete information to encourage informed decision making. ("I understand that your religion discourages the transfusion of blood. Do you understand that by refusing blood your risk of disability increases greatly?")

Social isolation related to prolonged hospitalization, altered health status, inadequate support systems, terminal illness

Desired outcome: Patient demonstrates interaction and communication with others.

1. Assess factors contributing to patient's social isolation.
   □ Restricted visiting hours.
   □ Absence of or inadequate support system.
   □ Inability to communicate (e.g., neurologic deficit or physical barrier).
   □ Physical changes that affect self-concept.
   □ Patient denial or withdrawal.
2. Recognize patients at high risk for social isolation: the elderly, disabled, chronically ill, economically disadvantaged.
3. Assist patient with identifying feelings associated with loneliness and isolation. ("You seem very sad when your family leaves the room. Can you tell me more about your feelings?")

4. Determine patient's need for socialization, and identify available and potential support systems. Explore methods for increasing social contact (e.g., TV, radio, tapes of loved ones, intercom system, more frequent visitations, scheduled interaction with nurse or support staff).
5. Provide positive reinforcement for socialization that lessens the patient's feelings of isolation and loneliness. ("Please continue to call me when you need to talk to someone. Talking will help both of us to better understand your feelings.")
6. Facilitate patient's ability to communicate with others (see **Impaired verbal communication,** p. 690).

Body image disturbance related to loss or change in body parts or function, physical trauma, or hospitalization

Desired outcomes: Patient acknowledges body changes and demonstrates movement toward incorporating changes into self-concept. Patient does not demonstrate maladaptive response, such as severe depression.

1. Establish open, honest communication with the patient. Promote an environment that is conducive to free expression. ("Please feel free to talk to me whenever you have any questions.")
2. Provide time for patient to verbalize feelings regarding actual or perceived changes in body function, as well as perceived changes in lifestyle, fear of rejection from others, and feelings of helplessness, hopelessness, guilt, and shame. Encourage patient to share these feelings with significant others.
3. When planning patient's care, be aware of therapies that may influence patient's self-concept (e.g., medications, chemotherapeutic agents; radiation therapy; invasive procedures; and monitoring).
4. Assess patient's knowledge of the pathophysiologic process that has occurred and his or her present health status. Clarify any misconceptions.
5. Discuss the loss or change with the patient and significant others. Recognize that what may seem to be a small change may be of great significance to the patient (e.g., arm immobilizer, catheter, hair loss, facial abrasions).
6. Explore with patient his or her concerns, fears, and feelings of guilt. ("I understand that you are frightened. Your face looks very different now, but you will see changes and it will improve. Gradually you will begin to look more like yourself.")
7. Encourage patient and significant others to interact with one another. Help family to avoid reinforcement of their loved one's changed body part or function. ("I know your son looks very different to you now, but it would help if you speak to him and touch him as you would normally.")
8. Encourage patient to participate gradually in self-care activities, as he or she becomes physically and emotionally able. Allow for some initial withdrawal and denial behaviors.
9. Discuss opportunities for reconstruction of the loss or change (i.e., surgery, prosthesis, physical therapy, cosmetic therapies, organ transplant). Discuss options for coping with change (e.g., use of wigs, prosthesis).
10. Recognize manifestations of severe depression (i.e., sleep disturbances, change in affect, change in communication pattern). As appropriate, refer to psychiatric clinical nurse specialist, clergy, or support group.
11. Help patient attain a sense of autonomy by offering choices and alternatives whenever possible. Emphasize patient's strengths and encourage activities that interest patient.
12. Offer realistic hope for the future.
13. If appropriate, consult with MD regarding visitation by an individual who has successfully undergone a similar surgery (e.g., amputation, mastectomy, ileostomy).
14. Provide information about support groups.

Potential for violence related to sensory overload, rage reactions, perceived threats, or physiologic imbalance

Desired outcome: There is no evidence that the patient has harmed self or others.

1. Assess factors that may contribute to or precipitate violent behavior (e.g., medication reactions, inability to cope, suicidal behavior, confusion, hypoxia, postictal states).
2. Attempt to eliminate or treat causative factors. For example, provide patient teaching, reorient patient, ensure delivery of prescribed oxygen therapy, and reduce or prevent sensory overload (see **Sensory/perceptual alterations,** p. 691).
3. Recognize that maladaptive behavior may be a response to patient's fears, grief, and feelings of powerlessness.
4. Monitor for early signs of increasing anxiety and agitation (i.e., restlessness, verbal aggressiveness, inability to concentrate). Assess for body language that is indicative of violent behavior: clenched fists, rigid posture, increased motor activity.
5. Approach patient in a positive manner and encourage verbalization of feelings and concerns. ("I understand that you are frightened. I will be here from 3 PM to 11 PM to care for you. Please call me if you need to talk.")
6. Offer patient as much personal and environmental control as the situation allows. ("Let's discuss the care you will need today. What fluids would you like to drink? Would you prefer a bath in the morning or evening?")
7. Help patient distinguish reality from altered perceptions. Orient patient to person, place, and time. Alter the environment to promote reality-based thought processes (e.g., provide clocks, calendars, pictures of loved ones, familiar objects).
8. Initiate measures that prevent or reduce excessive agitation.
   □ Reduce environmental stimuli (e.g., alarms, loud or unnecessary talking).
   □ Before touching patient, explain procedures and care, using short, concise statements.
   □ Speak quietly (but firmly, as necessary) and project a caring attitude toward the patient. ("We are very concerned for your comfort and safety. Can we do anything to help you feel more relaxed?")
   □ Avoid crowding (i.e., of equipment, visitors, health-care personnel) in patient's personal environment.
9. Explain and discuss patient's behavior with significant others. Acknowledge frustration, concerns, fears, and questions. Review safety precautions with significant others (see next intervention).
10. In the event of violent behavior, institute safety precautions.
    □ Remove harmful objects from the environment, such as heavy objects, scissors.
    □ Apply padding to side rails.
    □ Use restraints as necessary and prescribed.
    □ Never turn back toward violent patient.
    □ Do not approach violent patient without adequate assistance from others.
    □ Set limits on patient's behavior. ("I understand you must feel very frustrated, but you cannot continue to throw supplies or strike the siderails with your fists.")
    □ Explain safety precautions to patient. ("We are placing these restraints on your wrists to prevent you from harming yourself.")

Hopelessness related to prolonged hospitalization or life-threatening or terminal illness

Desired outcomes: Patient verbalizes hopeful aspects of health status and relates that feelings of despair are absent or lessened.

1. Develop open, honest communication with the patient, providing empathetic understanding of fears and doubts and promoting an environment that is conducive to free expression.
2. Assess patient's and significant others' understanding of patient's health status and prognosis; clarify any misperceptions.
3. Assess for indicators of hopelessness: unwillingness to accept help, pessimism, withdrawal, lack of interest, silence, loss of gratification in roles, previous history of hopeless behavior, hypoactivity, inability to accomplish tasks, expressions of incompetence, entrapment, irritability.
4. Provide opportunities for the patient to feel cared for, needed, and valued by others. For example, emphasize importance of relationships. ("Tell me about your grandchildren." "It seems that your family loves you very much.")

5. Support significant others who seem powerful in sparking or maintaining patient's feelings of hope. ("Your husband's mood seemed to improve after your visit today.")
6. Recognize discussions and factors that promote patient's sense of hope (i.e., discussions about family members, reminiscing about better times).
7. Explore patient's coping mechanisms; assist patient with expanding positive coping behavior (see **Ineffective individual coping**, p. 693).
8. Assess patient's spiritual state and needs (see **Spiritual distress**, p. 695).
9. Promote anticipation of positive events (i.e., mealtime, grandchildren's visits, bath time, discontinuation of chemotherapy or radiation therapy).
10. When appropriate, help patient recognize that although there may be no hope for returning to original lifestyle, there *is* hope for a new, but different, life.
11. Avoid insisting that the patient assume a positive attitude. Encourage hope for the future, even if it is the hope for a peaceful death.

CARING FOR THE PATIENT'S FAMILY AND SIGNIFICANT OTHERS

Ineffective family coping: Disabling, related to ambivalent family relationships, unexpressed feelings, lack of communication with family, lack of support systems, or patient dependence on family

Desired outcomes: Family members verbalize feelings, identify sources of support as well as ineffective coping behaviors that create ambivalence and disharmony, and do not demonstrate destructive behaviors.

1. Establish open, honest communication and rapport with family members. ("I am here to care for your mother and to help your family as well.")
2. Assess previous coping behaviors and identify those that were ineffective (e.g., violence, depression, substance abuse, withdrawal). ("You seem to be angry. Would you like to talk to me about your feelings?") Refer to psychiatric clinical nurse specialist, clergy, or support group as appropriate.
3. Identify perceived or actual conflicts. ("Are you able to talk freely with your family members?" "Are your brothers and sisters able to help and support you during this time?")
4. Assist family to search for healthy functioning within the family unit. For example, facilitate open communication among family members and encourage behaviors that support family cohesiveness. ("Your mother enjoyed your last visit.")
5. Assess the family's knowledge of patient's current health status. Provide opportunities for questions; reassess family's understanding at frequent intervals.
6. Provide the patient and family with accurate information and guidance related to the patient's health status. Assist family with developing realistic goals, plans, and actions. Refer them to clergy, psychiatric nurse, social services, financial counseling, and family therapy as appropriate.
7. Encourage family members to spend time outside of the hospital environment and to interact with support individuals. Respect the family's need for occasional withdrawal.
8. Include the family in the patient's plan of care. Offer them opportunities to become involved in patient care, for example, ROM exercises, patient hygiene, and comfort measures (e.g., backrub).

Ineffective family coping: Potential for growth, related to use of support systems and referrals, and renewed strength of family unit

Desired outcomes: Family members express their intent to use support systems and resources and identify alternative behaviors that enhance family communication and strengths. Family members express realistic expectations and do not demonstrate ineffective coping behaviors.

1. Assess family relationships, interactions, support systems, and individual coping behaviors. Permit a period of denial; then encourage further positive coping.

2. Acknowledge family expressions of hope, future plans, and growth among family members.

3. Develop open, honest communication with the family. Provide opportunities in a private setting for family interactions, discussions, and questions. ("I know the waiting room is very crowded. Would your family like some private time together?")

4. Refer the family to community or support groups (e.g., ostomy support group, head injury rehabilitation group).

5. Encourage the family to explore outlets that foster positive feelings (e.g., periods of time outside the patient care area, meaningful communication with the patient or support individuals, and relaxing activities, such as showering, eating, and exercising).

Altered family processes related to inability of patient and family to cope with crisis, lack of open and honest communication among family members, lack of support systems, or impending death of family member

Desired outcomes: Patient and family express feelings of conflict, demonstrate effective coping mechanisms, seek external support when necessary, and share concerns among the family unit.

1. Assess the family's character: social, environmental, ethnic, and cultural factors; relationships; and role patterns. Identify family developmental stage. For example, the family may be dealing with other situational or maturational crises, such as an elderly parent or teenager with a learning disability.

2. Assess previous coping behaviors. ("How does your family react in stressful situations?") Discuss observed conflicts and communication breakdown. ("I noticed that your brother would not visit your mother today. Has there been a problem we should be aware of? Knowing about it may help us better care for your mother.")

3. Acknowledge the family's involvement in patient care and promote strengths. ("You were able to encourage your wife to turn and cough. That is very important to her recovery.") Encourage family to participate in patient care conferences. Promote frequent, regular patient visits by family members. Provide opportunities for patient and significant others to spend time alone.

4. Provide the patient and family with accurate information and guidance related to patient's status. Discuss the stresses of hospitalization and encourage the family to discuss feelings of anger, guilt, hostility, depression, or sorrow. ("You seem to be upset since having been told that your husband is not showing significant improvement.") Refer to clergy, clinical nurse specialist, or social services as appropriate.

5. Evaluate patient and family responses to one another. Encourage family to reorganize roles and establish priorities as appropriate. ("I know your husband is concerned about his insurance policy and seems to expect you to investigate it. I'll call the financial counselor to come and talk with you.")

6. Encourage the family to schedule periods of rest and activity outside the hospital environment and to seek support when necessary. ("Your neighbor volunteered to stay with your wife this afternoon. Would you like to rest at home? I'll call you if anything changes.")

7. Encourage patient and significant others to verbalize fears and concerns regarding patient's illness, impaired level of functioning, or impending death. Assist significant others with recognizing and understanding patient's behavior as it relates to the disease process or disability.

Fear: Family, related to situational crisis of patient's life-threatening condition

Desired outcomes: Family members communicate and discuss fears and concerns, do not demonstrate ineffective coping behaviors, and relate feelings of increased well-being and lessened fear.

1. Assess the family's fear and their understanding of the patient's clinical situation. Evaluate verbal and nonverbal responses.

2. Acknowledge the family's fear. ("I understand these machines must frighten you, but they are necessary to treat your son's illness.")

3. Assess the family's history of coping behavior. ("How does your family react to difficult situations?") Determine resources and significant others available for support. ("Who usually helps your family during stressful times?")

4. Provide opportunities for family members to express fears and concerns. Recognize that anger, denial, withdrawal, and demanding behavior may be adaptive coping responses during initial period of crisis.

5. Provide information at frequent intervals regarding patient's status and the therapies and equipment used.

6. Encourage the family to use positive coping behaviors by identifying the fear(s), developing goals, identifying supportive resources, facilitating realistic perceptions, and promoting problem-solving.

7. Recognize anxiety and encourage family members to describe their feelings. ("You seem very uncomfortable tonight. Can you describe your feelings?")

8. Be alert to maladaptive responses to fear: potential for violence, withdrawal, severe depression, hostility, and unrealistic expectations of staff or of patient's recovery. Provide referrals to psychiatric clinical nurse specialist or other as appropriate.

9. Offer realistic hope, even if it is the hope for the patient's peaceful death.

10. Explore the family's desire for spiritual or other counseling.

11. Assess your own feelings about the patient's life-threatening illness. Acknowledge that your attitude and fear may be reflected to the family.

12. For other interventions, see nursing diagnoses **Altered family processes** and **Ineffective family coping.**

Knowledge deficit: Family: Patient's current health status or therapies

Desired outcome: Family members verbalize knowledge and understanding of the patient's current health status or therapies.

1. At frequent intervals, inform the family about the patient's current health status, therapies, and prognosis. Use individualized verbal and audiovisual strategies to enhance family's understanding.

2. Evaluate the family at frequent intervals for understanding of information that has been provided. Assess factors for misunderstanding and adjust teaching as appropriate. Some individuals in crisis need multiple explanations before comprehension can be assured. ("I have explained many things to you today. Would you mind summarizing what I've told you so that I can be sure you understand your husband's status and what we are doing to care for him?")

3. Encourage family to relay correct information to the patient. This will reinforce comprehension for family and patient, as well.

4. Ask family members if their needs for information are being met. ("Do you have any questions about the care your mother is receiving or about her condition?")

5. Help family members to use the information they receive to make health-care decisions regarding family member (e.g., surgery, resuscitation, organ donation.)

6. Promote family's active participation in patient care when appropriate. Encourage family to seek information and express feelings, concerns, and questions.

SELECTED REFERENCES

Ahano DN and Kuniski MM: Cancer care protocols for hospital and home care use, New York, Springer-Verlag, 1986.

Baird S: Decision making in oncology nursing, Toronto, 1988, BC Decker, Inc.

Batist G and Andrews J: Pulmonary toxicity of antineoplastic drugs, JAMA 246(13):1449-1453, 1981.

Brager B and Yasko J: Care of the client receiving chemotherapy, Reston, Va, 1984, Reston Publishing Co, Inc.

Cancer chemotherapy guidelines: module V, recommendations for the management of extravasation and anyphylaxis, Pittsburgh, 1988, Oncology Nursing Society.

Carlson A: Infection prophylaxis in patients with cancer, Oncol Nurs Forum 12(3):56-64, 1985.

Carrieri V et al: Pathophysiological phenomena in nursing: human responses to illness, Philadelphia, 1986, WB Saunders Co.

Cooley M et al: Sexual and reproductive issues for women with Hodgkin's disease: application of PLISSIT model, Cancer Nurs 9(5):248-255, 1986.

Coyle N and Foley K: Pain in patients with cancer: profile of patients and common pain syndromes, Semin Oncol Nurs 1(2):93-99, 1985.

Dean J et al: Scalp hypothermia: ice versus Kold Kap in the prevention of adriamycin induced alopecia. Abstract published in Proceedings of the sixth annual congress of the oncology nursing society (Baltimore), Pittsburgh, 1981, Oncology Nursing Society.

Dillman J: Toxicity of monoclonal antibodies in the treatment of cancer, Semin Oncol Nurs 4(2):107-111, 1988.

Engelking C and Steele N: A model for pretreatment nursing assessment of patient's receiving chemotherapy, Cancer Nurs 7(3):203, 1984.

Frytak S and Moertel C: Management of nausea and vomiting in the cancer patient, J Am Med Assoc 245(4):393-396, 1981.

Goodman M: Cisplatin: outpatient and office hydration regimens, Semin Oncol Nurs 3(1):36, 1987.

Goodman M and Wickham R: Venous access devices: an overview, Oncol Nurs Forum 11(5):16-23, 1984.

Groenwald S: Cancer nursing: principles and practice, Boston, 1987, Jones & Bartlett Publishers.

Hagle M: Implantable devices for chemotherapy: access and delivery, Semin Oncol Nurs 3(2):96-105, 1987.

Hahn M and Jassak P: Nursing management of patients receiving interferon, Semin Oncol Nurs 4(2):95-102, 1988.

Hassey K: Principles of radiation safety and protection, Semin Oncol Nurs 3(1):23-29, 1987.

Higgs D et al: Ifosfamide: a clinical review, Semin Oncol Nurs 5(2), Suppl 1:70-77, 1989.

Miller S: Issues of cytotoxic drug handling safety, Semin Oncol Nurs 3(2):133-141, 1987.

Montrose P: Extravasation management, Semin Oncol Nurs 3(2):128-132, 1987.

Preston F and Wilfinger C: Memory bank for chemotherapy, Baltimore, 1988, Williams & Wilkins.

Schulmeister L: Developing guidelines for bleomycin test dosing, Oncol Nurs Forum 16(2):205-212, 1989.

Stone S: Caring for the critically ill with life-threatening disorders. In Swearingen PL et al: Manual of critical care: applying nursing diagnoses to adult critical illness, St Louis, 1988, The CV Mosby Co.

Welch-McCafferty P: Evolving patient education needs in cancer, Oncol Nurs Forum 12(5):62-65, 1985.

Yasko JM: Care of the client receiving external radiation therapy, Reston Va, 1982, Reston Publishing Co.

Yasko JM: Guidelines for cancer care: symptom management, Reston Va, 1983, Reston Publishing Co.

Ziegfield C: Core curriculum for oncology nursing, Philadelphia, 1987, WB Saunders Co.

2

APPENDIX

Abbreviations used in this manual

AA: Alcoholics Anonymous
ABA: American Burn Association
ABG: arterial blood gas
ac: before meals
ACBaE: air contrast barium enema
ACL: anterior cruciate ligament
ACS: American Cancer Society
ACTH: adrenocorticotropic hormone
AD: autonomic dysreflexia
ADH: antidiuretic hormone
ADL: activity(ies) of daily living
AFP: alpha-fetoprotein
AIDS: acquired immune deficiency syndrome
ALL: acute lymphoblastic leukemia
ALS: amyotrophic lateral sclerosis
ALT: alanine aminotransferase
ANC: absolute neutrophil count
AP: anterior posterior
APR: abdominoperineal resection
ARC: AIDS-related complex
ARDS: adult respiratory distress syndrome
ARF: acute respiratory failure
ASA: acetylsalicylic acid
ATN: acute tubular necrosis
A-V: atrioventricular
AVM: arteriovenous malformation

BCNU: carmustine
BEE: basal energy expenditure
B&O: belladonna and opium
BP: blood pressure
bpm: beats per minute
BSE: breast self-examination
BUN: blood urea nitrogen
bid: twice a day

C: cervical
CABG: coronary artery bypass grafting
CAD: coronary artery disease
CAPD: continuous ambulatory peritoneal dialysis
CBC: complete blood count
CBI: continuous bladder irrigation
CCNU: lomustine
CCPD: continuous cycling peritoneal dialysis
CCU: coronary care unit
CDCA: chemodeoxycholic acid
CEA: carcinoembryonic antigen
CHF: congestive heart failure
CIN: cervical intraepithelial neoplasia
Cl: chloride
cm: centimeter
CMC: carpometacarpal
CNS: central nervous system
CO$_2$: carbon dioxide
COPD: chronic obstructive pulmonary disease
CPK: creatinine phosphokinase
CPM: continuous passive movement
CPR: cardiopulmonary resuscitation
CRF: chronic renal failure
CSF: cerebrospinal fluid
CT: computerized axial tomography
CVA: cerebrovascular accident
CVP: central venous pressure

D&C: dilatation and curettage
DES: diethylstilbestrol
DIC: disseminated intravascular coagulation
DIP: distal interphalangeal
DJD: degenerative joint disease
DKA: diabetes ketoacidosis
dl: deciliter
DPL: diagnostic peritoneal lavage
DSA: digital subtractive angiography
DTs: delirium tremens
DTR: deep tendon reflex
DVT: deep vein thrombosis
D$_5$W: 5% dextrose in water

EBV: Epstein-Barr virus
ECF: extracellular fluid
EEG: electroencephalogram
e.g.: for example
EKG: electrocardiogram
ELISA: enzyme-linked immunosorbent assay
EMG: electromyography
ERCP: endoscopic retrocholangiopancreatography
ERT: estrogen replacement therapy
ESR: erythrocyte sedimentation rate
ESRD: end-stage renal disease
ESWL: extracorporeal shock wave lithotripsy
ET: enterostomal therapy

FBS: fasting blood sugar
FEV: forced expiratory volume

FSH: follicle-stimulating hormone
FSP: fibrin split products
FTI: free thyroxine index

g: gram
GGTP: gammaglutamyl transpeptidase
GH: growth hormone
GI: gastrointestinal
GN: glomerulonephritis
GOT: glutamic oxalacetic transaminase

h: hour
HCG: human chorionic gonadotropin
HCO₃: bicarbonate
hct: hematocrit
hgb: hemoglobin
HHNC: hyperosmolar hyperglycemic nonketotic coma
HIV: human immunodeficiency virus
HOB: head of bed
HR: heart rate
hs: hour of sleep

ICF: intracellular fluid
ICP: intracranial pressure
ICSH: interstitial cell-stimulating hormone
ICU: intensive care unit
IDDM: insulin-dependent diabetes mellitus
IgG: immunoglobulin G
IICP: increased intracranial pressure
IM: intramuscular
I&O: intake and output
IPD: intermittent peritoneal dialysis
IPPD: intermittent positive pressure breathing
ITP: idiopathic thrombocytopenic purpura
IUD: intrauterine device
IV: intravenous
IVP: intravenous pyelogram

K: potassium
kg: kilogram
KUB: kidney, ureter, bladder

L: liter; lumbar
LATS: long-acting thyroid stimulator
lb: pound
LDH: lactate dehydrogenase
LES: lower esophageal sphincter
LH: luteinizing hormone
LLQ: left lower quadrant
LMN: lower motor neuron
LOC: level of consciousness
LPA: latex particle agglutination
LTH: luteotropic hormone

MCP: metacarpophalangeal
MCT: medium chain triglycerides
MD: physician
mEq: milliequivalent

mg: milligram
MI: myocardial infarction
min: minute
ml: milliliter
mm Hg: millimeters of mercury
mOsm: milliosmol
MRC: medical research council
MRI: magnetic resonance imaging
MS: multiple sclerosis
MSG: monosodium glutamate
MSH: melanocyte-stimulating hormone
MSU: monosodium urate
MTBE: methyltert-butyl ether
MTP: metatarsophalangeal
μg: microgram

N: nitrogen
Na: sodium
ng: nanogram
NG: nasogastric
NIDDM: non-insulin-dependent diabetes mellitus
NPO: nothing by mouth
NSAID: nonsteroidal antiinflammatory drug
NSCLC: non-small cell lung cancer

O_2: oxygen
OGTT: oral glucose tolerance test
ORIF: open reduction with internal fixation
OT: occupational therapist
OTC: over-the-counter

$Paco_2$: partial pressure of dissolved carbon dioxide in arterial blood
Pao_2: partial pressure of dissolved oxygen in arterial blood
pc: after meals
PCA: patient-controlled analgesia
PCM: protein-calorie malnutrition
PCP: pneumocystis carinii pneumonia
PEEP: positive end-expiratory pressure
PET: positron emission tomography
pg: picogram
PID: pelvic inflammatory disease
PIP: proximal interphalangeal
PMI: point of maximal impulse
PO: by mouth
PPG: postprandial blood glucose
prn: as needed
PSA: prostatic-specific antigen
PT: physical therapist; prothrombin time
PTH: parathyroid hormone
PTHC: percutaneous transhepatic cholangiogram
PTT: partial thromboplastin time
PTV: propylthiouracil
PUL: percutaneous ultrasonic lithotripsy

q: every
qid: four times a day

RA: rheumatoid arthritis
RBC: red blood cell
RDA: recommended daily allowance
REE: resting energy expenditure
RIA: radioimmunoassay
RLQ: right lower quadrant
ROM: range of motion
RPE: rate perceived exertion
RQ: respiratory quotient
RR: respiratory rate
RUQ: right upper quadrant

SC: subcutaneous
SCI: spinal cord injury
SCLC: small cell lung cancer
SGOT: serum glutamic oxaloacetic-acid-transaminase
SGPT: serum glutamic pyruvic transaminase
SIADH: secretion of inappropriate antidiuretic hormone
SOB: shortness of breath
stat: immediately
STH: somatotropic hormone

T: thoracic
TB: tuberculosis
TBSA: total body surface area
TEE: total energy expenditure
TENS: transcutaneous electrical nerve stimulation
THA: total hip arthroplasty
TIA: transient ischemic attack
TKA: total knee arthroplasty
TKO: to keep open
TOPS: Take Off Pounds Sensibly
TPN: total parenteral nutrition
TPR: temperature, pulse, respirations
TRH: thyrotropin-releasing hormone
TSH: thyroid-stimulating hormone
TTP: thrombotic thrombocytopenic purpura
TUR: transurethral resection
TURP: transurethral resection of the prostate
TURBT: transurethral resection of the bladder and tumor

U: unit
UA: urinalysis
UDCA: ursodeoxycholic acid
UMN: upper motor neuron
UOA: United Ostomy Association
URI: upper respiratory infection
UTI: urinary tract infection
UUN: urine urea nitrogen

VAD: venous access device
VMA: vanillamandelic acid
VS: vital signs

WBC: white blood cell
WOB: work of breathing

3

<u>APPENDIX</u>

Heart and breath sounds

Assessing heart sounds

Sound	Auscultation site	Timing	Pitch	Clinical occurrence	End-piece/patient position
S_1 (M_1 T_1)	Apex	Beginning of systole	High	Closing of mitral and tricuspid valves; normal sound	Diaphragm/patient supine
S_1 split	Apex	Beginning of systole	High	Ventricles contracting at different times due to electrical or mechanical problems. For example, a longer time span between M_1 T_1 caused by right bundle-branch heart block, or reversal (T_1 M_1) caused by mitral stenosis	Same as S_1
S_2 (A_2 P_2)	A_2 at 2nd ICS, RSB; P_2 at 2nd ICS, LSB	End of systole	High	Closing of aortic and pulmonic valves; Normal sound	Diaphragm/patient supine
S_2 Physiologic split	2nd ICS, LSB	End of systole	High	Accentuated by inspiration; disappears on expiration. Sound that corresponds with the respiratory cycle due to normal delay in closure of pulmonic valve during inspiration. It is accentuated during exercise or in individuals with thin chest walls; heard most often in children and young adults	Same as S_2
S_2 Persistent (wide) split	2nd ICS, LSB	End of systole	High	Heard throughout the respiratory cycle; caused by late closure of pulmonic valve or early closure of aortic valve. Occurs in atrial septal defect, right ventricular failure, pulmonic stenosis, hypertension, or right bundle-branch heart block	Same as S_2

S$_2$ Paradoxic (reversed) split (P$_2$ A$_2$)	2nd ICS, LSB	End of systole	High	Because of delayed left ventricular systole, the aortic valve closes after the pulmonic valve rather than before it. (Normally during expiration the two sounds merge.) Causes may include left bundle-branch heart block, aortic stenosis, severe left ventricular failure, MI, and severe hypertension	Same as S$_2$
S$_2$ Fixed split	2nd ICS, LSB	End of systole	High	Heard with equal intensity during inspiration and expiration due to split of pulmonic and aortic components, which are unaffected by blood volume or respiratory changes. May be heard in pulmonary stenosis or atrial septal defect	Same as S$_2$
S$_3$ (ventricular gallop)	Apex	Early diastole just after S$_2$	Dull, low	Early and rapid filling of ventricle, as in early ventricular failure, CHF; common in children, during last trimester of pregnancy, and possibly in healthy adults over age 50	Bell/patient in left lateral or supine position
S$_4$ (atrial gallop)	Apex	Late in diastole just before S$_1$	Low	Atrium filling against increased resistance of stiff ventricle, as in CHF, coronary artery disease, cardiomyopathy, pulmonary artery hypertension, ventricular failure. May be normal in infants, children, and athletes	Same as S$_3$

ICS = intercostal space; RSB = right sternal border; LSB = left sternal border.

Commonly occurring heart murmurs

Type	Timing	Pitch	Quality	Auscultation site	Radiation
Pulmonic stenosis	Systolic ejection	Medium-high	Harsh	2nd ICS, LSB	Toward left shoulder, back
Aortic stenosis	Midsystolic	Medium-high	Harsh	2nd ICS, RSB	Toward carotid arteries
Ventricular septal defect	Late systolic	High	Blowing	4th ICS, LSB	Toward right sternal border
Mitral insufficiency	Holosystolic	High	Blowing	5-6th ICS, left MCL	Toward left axilla
Tricuspid insufficiency	Holosystolic	High	Blowing	4th ICS, LSB	Toward apex
Aortic insufficiency	Early diastolic	High	Blowing	2nd ICS, RSB	Toward sternum
Pulmonary insufficiency	Early diastolic	High	Blowing	2nd ICS, LSB	Toward sternum
Mitral stenosis	Mid-late diastolic	Low	Rumbling	5th ICS, left MCL	Toward axilla
Tricuspid stenosis	Mid-late diastolic	Low	Rumbling	4th ICS, LSB	Usually none

ICS = intercostal space; RSB = right sternal border; LSB = left sternal border; MCL = mid-clavicular line.

Assessing normal breath sounds

Type	Normal site	Duration	Characteristics
Vesicular	Peripheral lung	I > E	Soft and swishing sounds. Abnormal when heard over the large airways
Bronchial	Trachea and bronchi	E > I	Louder, coarser, and of longer duration than vesicular. Abnormal if heard over peripheral lung
Bronchovesicular	Sternal border of the major bronchi	E = I	Moderate in pitch and intensity. Abnormal if heard over peripheral lung

I = inspiration; E = expiration.

Assessing adventitious breath sounds

Type	Waveform	Characteristics	Possible clinical condition
Coarse crackle		Discontinuous, explosive, interrupted. Loud; low in pitch	Pulmonary edema; pneumonia in resolution stage
Fine crackle		Discontinuous, explosive, interrupted. Less loud than coarse crackles, lower in pitch, and of shorter duration	Interstitial lung disease; heart failure; atelectasis
Wheeze		Continuous, of long duration, high-pitched, musical, hissing	Narrowing of airway; bronchial asthma; COPD
Rhonchus		Continuous, of long duration, low-pitched, snoring	Production of sputum (usually cleared or lessened by coughing)
Pleural friction rub		Grating, rasping noise	Rubbing together of inflamed parietal linings; loss of normal pleural lubrication

Assessing respiratory patterns

Type	Waveform	Characteristics	Possible clinical condition
Eupnea		Normal rate and rhythm for adults and teenagers (12-20 breaths/min)	Normal pattern while awake
Bradypnea		Decreased rate (<12 breaths/min); regular rhythm	Normal sleep pattern; opiate or alcohol use; tumor; metabolic disorder
Tachypnea		Rapid rate (>20 breaths/min); hypo- or hyperventilation	Fever; restrictive respiratory disorders; pulmonary emboli
Hyperpnea		Depth of respirations greater than normal	Meeting increased metabolic demand (e.g., exercise)
Apnea		Cessation of breathing; may be intermittent	Intermittent with CNS disturbances or drug intoxication; obstructed airway; respiratory arrest if it persists

Assessing respiratory patterns

Type	Waveform	Characteristics	Possible clinical condition
Cheyne-Stokes		Alternating patterns of apnea (10-20 seconds) with periods of deep and rapid breathing	CHF, narcotic or hypnotic overdose, thyrotoxicosis dissecting aneurysm, subarachnoid hemorrhage, increased ICP, aortic valve disorders, may be normal in elderly during sleep
Biot's		Irregular (can be slow and deep or rapid and shallow) followed by periods of apnea	CNS abnormalities (e.g., meningitis, increased ICP)
Kussmaul's		Deep, rapid (>20 breaths/min), sighing, labored	Renal failure, DKA, sepsis, shock
Apneustic		Prolonged inspiration followed by short expirations	Anoxia, meningitis

4

APPENDIX

Nursing diagnosis used in this manual

Activity intolerance related to decreased energy levels secondary to ineffecient work of breathing, *"Emphysema,"* p. 32; related to fatigue and weakness secondary to right and left ventricular failure, *"Pulmonary Hypertension,"* p. 41; related to weakness and fatigue secondary to decrease in cardiac contractility, *"Cardiomyopathy,"* p. 44; related to weakness and fatigue secondary to tissue ischemia (myocardial infarction), *"Coronary Artery Disease,"* p. 47; related to fatigue and weakness secondary to decreased strength of cardiac contraction and decreased cardiac output, *"Myocardial Infarction,"* p. 52; related to weakness and fatigue secondary to decreased strength of cardiac contraction, *"Heart Failure,"* p. 55; related to weakness and dyspnea secondary to inflammation of the cardiac muscle and restriction of contraction, *"Pericarditis,"* p. 59; related to weakness and fatigue secondary to dysfunction of the myocardial muscle, *"Myocarditis,"* p. 61; related to fatigue and weakness secondary to decreased left ventricular filling, *"Mitral Stenosis,"* p. 66; related to fatigue and weakness secondary to decreased cardiac output with valvular regurgitation, *"Mitral Regurgitation,"* p. 68; related to weakness secondary to cardiac surgery, *"Cardiac Surgery,"* p. 84; related to weakness secondary to prolonged bed rest and disease process, *"Glomerulonephritis,"* p. 103; related to fatigue and weakness secondary to uremia and anemia, *"Acute Renal Failure,"* p. 119; related to weakness and fatigue secondary to anemia and uremia, *"Chronic Renal Failure,"* p. 122; related to weakness and fatigue secondary to slowed metabolism and decreased cardiac output caused by pericardial effusions, atherosclerosis, and decreased adrenergic stimulation, *"Hypothyroidism,"* p. 265; related to neuromuscular weakness and joint pain secondary to increased serum calcium and altered phosphorus levels, *"Hyperparathyroidism,"* p. 269; related to weakness and fatigue secondary to decreased cardiac contractility, *"Hypoparathyroidism,"* p. 273; related to weakness and fatigue secondary to decreased cardiac output, *"Addison's Disease,"* p. 276; related to weakness and fatigue secondary to fluid and electrolyte imbalance, arthralgia, myalgia, dyspnea, fever, pain, hypoxia, and effects of chemotherapy, *"Acquired Immune Deficiency Syndrome,"* p. 594; related to deconditioning secondary to prolonged bed rest, *"Caring for Patients on Prolonged Bed Rest,"* p. 652.

Airway clearance, ineffective, related to presence of viscous pulmonary secretions or pain and fatigue secondary to lung consolidation, *"Pneumonia,"* p. 8; related to impaired coughing ability secondary to fatigue or decreased LOC, *"Acute Respiratory Failure,"* p. 23; related to excessive mucus production and ineffective coughing, *"Chronic Bronchitis,"* p. 29; related to neuromuscular paralysis/weakness or restriction of chest expansion secondary to halo vest traction, *"Spinal Cord Injury,"* p. 201; related to imposed inactivity secondary to the risk of aneurysm rupture and rebleeding, *"Cere-*

bral Aneurysm," p. 225; related to coughing and swallowing deficits secondary to facial and throat muscle weakness or decreasing LOC, *"General Care of Patients with Neurologic Disorders,"* p. 251; related to increased tracheobronchial secretions secondary to effects of anesthesia; ineffective coughing secondary to CNS depression or pain and muscle splinting; and possible laryngospasm secondary to endotracheal tube or allergic reaction to anesthetics, *"Caring for Preoperative and Postoperative Patients,"* p. 641.

Anxiety related to anticipated loss of body part/function and threat to self-concept secondary to urinary diversion surgery,*"Urinary Diversions,"* p. 152; related to actual or perceived threats or changes secondary to degeneration of intellectual functioning, *"Alzheimer's Disease,"* p. 187; related to untoward response to sympathetic nervous system stimulation, *"Hyperthyroidism,"* p. 261; related to diagnosis, fear of death or social isolation, and hospitalization, *"Acquired Immune Deficiency Syndrome,"* p. 594; related to withdrawal symptoms, *"Sedative-Hypnotic Abuse,"* p. 602; related to withdrawal from opioid substances, *"Opioid Abuse,"* p. 606; related to actual or perceived threat to biologic integrity, self-concept, or role; unfamiliar people and environment; or the unknown, *"Caring for Patients with Cancer and Other Life-Disrupting Illnesses,"* p. 690.

Aspiration, potential for, related to obstruction by secretions secondary to CNS depression, decreased GI motility, abdominal distention, recumbent position, presence of gastric tube, and possible impaired swallowing in individuals with oral, facial, or neck surgery, *"Caring for Preoperative and Postoperative Patients,"* p. 641.

Body image disturbance related to odor, discomfort, and embarrassment secondary to incontinence, *"Urinary Incontinence,"* p. 144; related to exophthalmos or surgical scar, *"Hyperthyroidism,"* p. 261; related to physical changes secondary to increased ACTH production, *"Cushing's Disease,"* p. 279; related to presence of fecal diversion, *"Fecal Diversions,"* p. 368; related to presence of jaundice, *"Hepatitis,"* p. 384; related to loss of limb, *"Amputation,"* p. 468; related to small breast size, *"Breast Augmentation,"* p. 482; related to body changes before and following breast reconstruction surgery, *"Breast Reconstruction,"* p. 485; related to loss of a breast, *"Malignant Disorders of the Breast,"* p. 492; related to actual and perceived changes in sexual functioning secondary to impending orchiectomy, *"Testicular Neoplasm,"* p. 522; related to presence of the penile implant, *"Penile Implants,"* p. 524; related to body changes secondary to Kaposi's lesions, side effects of chemotherapy, social stigmatization, isolation, and emaciation, *"Acquired Immune Deficiency Syndrome,"* p. 594; related to alopecia secondary to radiation therapy to the head and neck or administration of chemotherapy agents, *"Caring for Patients with Cancer and Other Life-Disrupting Illnesses,"* p. 682; related to loss or change in body parts or function, physical trauma, or hospitalization, *"Caring for Patients with Cancer and Other Life-Disrupting Illnesses,"* p. 696.

Bowel incontinence or defecating in inappropriate places related to inability to find bathroom or decreased awareness of or loss of sphincter control secondary to cognitive deficit, *"Alzheimer's Disease,"* p. 185; Disruption of normal function secondary to fecal diversion, *"Fecal Diversions,"* p. 367.

Breastfeeding, ineffective, related to breast augmentation procedure, *"Breast Augmentation,"* p. 482.

Breathing pattern, ineffective, related to hypoventilation secondary to inactivity or omission of deep breathing, *"Atelectasis,"* p. 3; related to decreased lung expansion secondary to fluid accumulation in the pleural space, *"Pleural Effusion,"* p. 12; related to malfunction of chest drainage system, *"Pneumothorax/Hemothorax,"* p. 20; related to dyspnea secondary to chronic airflow limitations, *"Emphysema"* p. 31; related to dyspnea secondary to decreased lung expansion, *"Pulmonary Fibrosis,"* p. 34; related to guarding secondary to pericardial pain, *"Pericarditis,"* p. 60; related to neuromuscular weakness or paralysis of the facial, throat, and respiratory muscles, *"Guillain-Barré*

Syndrome," p. 166; related to hypoventilation secondary to decreased ventilatory drive or upper airway obstruction occurring with myxedematous infiltration, *"Hypothyroidism,"* p. 264; related to hypoventilation secondary to respiratory depression with use of narcotics or guarding secondary to painful abdominal incision, *"Pancreatic Tumors,"* p. 294; related to guarding secondary to pain of thoracic incision or chest tube insertion, *"Hiatal Hernia and Reflux Esophagitis,"* p. 319; related to guarding or decreased depth of respirations secondary to abdominal pain and distention, *"Peritonitis,"* p. 339; related to limited ventilatory excursion secondary to pain from injury or surgical incision; chemical irritation of blood or bile on pleural tissue; and diaphragmatic elevation due to abdominal distention, *"Abdominal Trauma,"* p. 377; related to weakness or paralysis of respiratory muscles secondary to *severe* hypokalemia (potassium <2-2.5 mEq/L), *"Fluid and Electrolyte Disturbances,"* p. 557; related to decreased lung expansion secondary to CNS depression, pain, muscle splinting, recumbent position, and effects of anesthesia, *"Caring for Preoperative and Postoperative Patients,"* p. 644.

Cardiac output, decreased, related to impaired contractility secondary to cardiac muscle changes, *"Cardiomyopathy,"* p. 44; related to decreased strength of contractions secondary to ventricular dysfunction, *"Mitral Stenosis,"* p. 65; related to ineffective ventricular contractions secondary to cardiac arrest, *"Cardiac Arrest,"* p. 76; related to relative hypovolemia secondary to decreased vasomotor tone due to SCI, *"Spinal Cord Injury,"* p. 204; related to risk of ventricular dysrhythmias secondary to hypokalemia or too rapid correction of hypokalemia with resulting hyperkalemia, *"Fluid and Electrolyte Disturbances,"* p. 556; related to risk of ventricular dysrhythmias secondary to severe hyperkalemia or too rapid correction of hyperkalemia with resulting hypokalemia, *"Fluid and Electrolyte Disturbances,"* p. 558.

Communication, impaired verbal related to aphasia and altered sensory reception, transmission, and integration secondary to cognitive deficits, *"Alzheimer's Disease,"* p. 186; related to aphasia or dysarthria secondary to cerebrovascular insult, *"Cerebrovascular Accident,"* p. 237; related to dysarthria secondary to facial/throat muscle weakness, intubation, or tracheostomy, *"General Care of Patients with Neurologic Disorders,"* p. 252; related to dysarthria secondary to neurologic deficit or physical barrier (e.g., tracheostomy), *"Caring for Patients with Cancer and Other Life-Disrupting Illnesses,"* p. 690.

Constipation related to restrictions of fresh fruits and fluids, prolonged bed rest, and negative side effects of drugs (e.g., phosphate binders), *"Acute Renal Failure,"* p. 120; or fecal impaction related to immobility and decreased peristalsis, atonic bowel, and loss of sensation and voluntary sphincter control secondary to sensorimotor deficit, *"Spinal Cord Injury,"* p. 201; related to inability to chew and swallow a high-roughage diet, side effects of medications, and immobility, *"General Care of Patients with Neurologic Disorders,"* p. 252; related to decreased peristalsis secondary to slowed metabolism, *"Hypothyroidism,"* p. 265; related to decreased peristalsis secondary to increased serum calcium level, *"Hyperparathyroidism,"* p. 270; related to gastrointestinal mucosal atrophy secondary to reduced hct, *"Pernicious Anemia,"* p. 398; related to immobility, opioid analgesics and other medications, effects of anesthesia, lack of privacy, disruption of abdominal musculature, or manipulation of abdominal viscera during surgery, *"Caring for Preoperative and Postoperative Patients,"* p. 647; related to immobility, changes in normal bowel habits during hospitalization, positional restrictions, dietary alterations, and use of narcotic analgesics, *"Caring for Patients on Prolonged Bed Rest,"* p. 656.

Constipation, colonic related to fear of pain with postoperative defecation, *"Hemorrhoids,"* p. 345; Diminished frequency of bowel elimination with resultant hard, dry, or painful stools, *"Hemorrhoids,"* p. 344; related to restriction against straining, low-residue diet, or pain with defecation secondary to surgical procedure, *"Rectocele,"* p. 503; related to postsurgical discomfort or fear or exerting pressure on the prostatic capsule, *"Benign Prostatic Hypertrophy,"* p. 513.

Coping, ineffective family: Disabling, related to ambivalent family relationships, unexpressed feelings, lack of communication with family, lack of support systems, or patient dependence on family, *"Caring for Patients with Cancer and Other Life-Disrupting Illnesses,"* p. 698; Potential for growth, related to use of support systems and referrals, and renewed strength of family unit, *"Caring for Patients with Cancer and Other Life-Disrupting Illnesses,"* p. 698.

Coping, ineffective individual, related to grief or stress secondary to diagnosis of breast cancer, *"Malignant Disorders of the Breast,"* p. 490; related to anger, denial, and poor self-esteem secondary to inability to manage stressors without alcohol, *"Alcoholism,"* p. 599; related to depression, dysphoria, poor self-esteem, and denial secondary to inability to manage stressors without cocaine, *"Cocaine Abuse,"* p. 604; related to denial, poor self-esteem, and depression secondary to inability to handle stressors without opioids, *"Opioid Abuse,"* p. 607; related to threat to biologic integrity, knowledge deficit, unsatisfactory support systems, or hospitalization, *"Caring for Patients with Cancer and Other Life-Disrupting Illnesses,"* p. 693.

Diarrhea, bloating, excessive flatus, and abdominal cramping related to malabsorption disorder, *"Malabsorption/Maldigestion,"* p. 331; related to inflammatory process of the intestines, *"Ulcerative Colitis,"* p. 358; related to intestinal inflammatory process, *"Crohn's Disease,"* p. 363; related to gastrointestinal mucusal atrophy secondary to reduced hct, *"Pernicious Anemia,"* p. 398; related to gastrointestinal infection, chemotherapy, or tube feeding intolerance, *"Acquired Immune Deficiency Syndrome,"* p. 593.

Disuse syndrome, potential for, related to inactivity or spasticity secondary to SCI, *"Spinal Cord Injury,"* p. 202; related to prolonged inactivity secondary to sensorimotor deficits and decreased LOC, *"Head Injury,"* p. 212; related to imposed activity restrictions secondary to risk of aneurysm rupture or rebleeding, *"Cerebral Aneurysm,"* p. 226; related to pain and immobility secondary to amputation, *"Amputation,"* p. 466; related to physical alterations in the upper extremities secondary to mastectomy, *"Malignant Disorders of the Breast,"* p. 491; related to immobilization secondary to pain or scar formation, *"Burns,"* p. 583; related to inactivity secondary to prolonged bed rest, *"Caring for Patients on Prolonged Bed Rest,"* p. 653.

Diversional activity deficit related to monotony of confinement secondary to prolonged illness and hospitalization, *"Caring for Patients on Prolonged Bed Rest,"* p. 657.

Dysreflexia, potential for related to untoward response to noxious stimuli for individuals with SCI at or above T-6, *"Spinal Cord Injury,"* p. 200.

Family processes, altered related to illness of family member, *"Alzheimer's Disease,"* p. 188; related to inability of patient and family to cope with crisis, lack of open and honest communication among family members, lack of support systems, or impending death of family member, *"Caring for Patients with Cancer and Other Life-Disrupting Illnesses,"* p. 699.

Fatigue related to intestinal inflammatory process, *"Crohn's Disease,"* p. 364; related to diminished energy levels secondary to decreased oxygen-carrying capacity of the blood, *"Pernicious Anemia,"* p. 397; related to diminished energy level secondary to decreased oxygen-carrying capacity of the blood, *"Hypoplastic Anemia,"* p. 406; related to diminished energy level secondary to decreased oxygen-carrying capacity of the blood, *"Acute Leukemia,"* p. 420; related to pathophysiology of RA and immobility, *"Rheumatoid Arthritis,"* p. 433.

Fear related to life-threatening situation, *"Pulmonary Edema,"* p. 77; related to threat to bioligic integrity, *"Guillain-Barré Syndrome,"* p. 167; related to possibility of cancer, change in body image, surgical or diagnostic procedure, and pain, *"Benign breast disease,"* p. 487; related to the possibility of cancer and its treatment, *"Malignant Disorders of the Breast,"* p. 490; related to threat to biologic integrity, potential for loss, altered body image, loss of control, or therapeutic regimen, *"Caring for Patients with*

Cancer and Other Life-Disrupting Illnesses," p. 692; (Family), related to situational crisis of patient's life-threatening condition, *"Caring for Patients with Cancer and Other Life-Disrupting Illnesses,"* p. 699.

Fluid volume deficit related to increased need secondary to infection or loss secondary to tachypnea, fever, or diaphoresis, *"Pneumonia,"* p. 9; related to risk of hemorrhage or hematoma formation secondary to arterial puncture, *"Cardiac Catheterization,"* p. 82; related to loss secondary to postsurgical bleeding/hemorrhage, *"Aneurysms,"* p. 91; related to decreased vascular volume secondary to pharmacotherapy, *"Nephrotic Syndrome,"* p. 106; related to decreased intake secondary to anorexia or abnormal loss secondary to vomiting and diaphoresis, *"Acute Pyelonephritis,"* p. 109; related to abnormal loss secondary to postoperative bleeding, *"Renal Calculi,"* p. 111; related to abnormal loss secondary to postobstructive diuresis, *"Hydronephrosis,"* p. 113; related to abnormal loss secondary to excessive urinary output: diuretic phase, *"Acute Renal Failure,"* p. 118; related to a abnormal loss secondary to hypertonicity of the dialysate, *"Renal Dialysis,"* p. 128; related to excessive fluid removal or increased risk of bleeding secondary to dialysis, *"Renal Dialysis,"* p. 129; related to excessive urinary loss or hematuria secondary to postobstructive diuresis or rapid bladder decompression after catheterization procedure, *"Urinary Tract Obstruction,"* p. 136; related to loss secondary to postsurgical hemorrhage after TURBT or segmental resection, *"Cancer of the Bladder,"* p. 139; related to abnormal blood loss secondary to surgical procedure, *"Urinary Diversions,"* p. 156; related to abnormal loss secondary to osmotic diuresis, vomiting, or diarrhea caused by oral phosphate supplements, *"Hyperparathyroidism,"* p. 269; related to abnormal loss secondary to diuresis, *"Addison's Disease,"* p. 276; related to abnormal loss secondary to polyuria, *"Diabetes Insipidus,"* p. 281; related to abnormal loss secondary to NG suctioning, vomiting, diaphoresis, or pooling of fluids in the abdomen and retroperitoneum, *"Pancreatitis,"* p. 289; related to loss secondary to postsurgical hemorrhage and risk of fluid shift to third-space compartments, *"Pancreatic Tumors,"* p. 292; related to decreased circulating volume secondary to hyperglycemia and osmotic diuresis, *"Diabetic Ketoacidosis,"* p. 301; related to decreased intake secondary to nausea, anorexia, or bloating and loss secondary to vomiting, *"Gastric Neoplasm,"* p. 327; related to increased need secondary to impaired absorption or abnormal loss secondary to diarrhea, *"Malabsorption/Maldigestion,"* p. 331; related to abnormal losses secondary to obstructive process and subsequent vomiting or gastric decompression of large volumes of GI fluids and decreased intake secondary to fluid restrictions, *"Obstructive Processes,"* p. 335; related to abnormal blood loss secondary to slipped ligatures, *"Hemorrhoids,"* p. 346; related to abnormal loss secondary to diarrhea and active GI bleeding/hemorrhage, *"Ulcerative Colitis,"* p. 357; related to abnormal loss secondary to diarrhea or GI fistula, *"Crohn's Disease,"* p. 362; related to decreased circulating volume secondary to active bleeding; GI drainage through gastric, intestinal, or drainage tubes; diarrhea; or fistulas, *"Abdominal Trauma,"* p. 375; related to increased risk of esophageal bleeding secondary to altered clotting factors and portal hypertension, *"Cirrhosis,"* p. 388; related to abnormal loss secondary to postsplenectomy bleeding/hemorrhage, *"Thrombocytopenia,"* p. 411; related to risk of bleeding secondary to hemorrhagic component of DIC, *"Disseminated Intravascular Coagulation,"* p. 416; related to abnormal loss secondary to postsurgical hemorrhage or hematoma formation, *"Meniscal Injuries,"* p. 442; related to abnormal loss secondary to postsurgical hemorrhage, *"Amputation,"* p. 468; related to abnormal blood loss secondary to postsurgical hemorrhage or hematoma formation, *"Breast Reconstruction,"* p. 485; related to abnormal blood loss secondary to operative, postoperative, or postimplant bleeding, *"Cancer of the Cervix,"* p. 495; related to abnormal blood loss secondary to abortion or surgical intervention, *"Spontaneous Abortion,"* p. 506; related to abnormal loss secondary to bleeding or hemorrhage with ectopic rupture, *"Ectopic Pregnancy,"* p. 508; related to abnormal blood loss secondary to surgical procedure or pressure on the prostatic capsule, *"Benign Prostatic Hypertrophy,"* p. 511; related to risk of abnormal blood loss secondary to the surgical procedure, *"Testicular Neoplasm,"* p. 522; related to decreased circulating volume secondary to abnormal loss of ECF or reduced intake, *"Fluid and Electrolyte Disturbances,"* p. 548; related to abnormal fluid loss, *"Fluid and Electrolyte Disturbances,"* p. 553; related to decreased circulating volume secondary to leakage of fluid, plasma proteins, and other cellular elements into the interstitial space and loss through the burn wound, *"Burns,"* p. 582; related to *loss of fluids* secondary to presence of indwelling drainage tubes, wound drainage, or vomiting; *indadequate intake of fluids* secondary to nausea, NPO status, CNS depression, or lack of access to fluids; or *intravascular fluid volume loss* secondary to altered regulatory mechanisms and third spacing of bodily fluids due to the effects of anesthesia and major surgery, *"Caring for Preoperative and Postoperative Patients,"* p. 644; related to abnormal loss secondary to postoperative bleeding, *"Caring for Preoperative and Postoperative Patients,"* p. 645.

Fluid volume excess: Edema (pulmonary or peripheral) related to retention of fluids secondary to decreased cardiac output, *"Myocardial Infarction,"* p. 552; Edema related to retention secondary to decreased cardiac output, *"Heart Failure,"* p. 56; Edema related to retention of fluid secondary to right-sided heart failure, *"Mitral Stenosis,"* p. 66; Edema related to retention secondary to decreased cardiac output, *"Pulmonary Edema,"* p. 78; Edema and hypertension related to retention secondary to decreased renal function, *"Glomerulonephritis,"* p. 103; related to fluid retention secondary to decreased serum albumin and renal retention of sodium and water, *"Nephrotic Syndrome,"* p. 106; Edema related to fluid retention secondary to renal dysfunction: oliguric phase, *"Acute Renal Failure,"* p. 118; related to fluid retention or inadequate exchange secondary to catheter problems or peritonitis, *"Renal Dialysis,"* p. 128; related to fluid retention secondary to renal failure, *"Renal Dialysis,"* p. 129; related to fluid retention secondary to irrigation, *"Cancer of the Bladder,"* p. 139; related to retention secondary to decreased metabolic rate and adrenal insufficiency, *"Hypothyroidism,"* p. 264; Extravascular, related to edema and ascites secondary to sequestration of fluids with portal hypertension and hepatocellular failure; and intravascular, related to retention secondary to sodium and electrolyte disturbances, *"Cirrhosis,"* p. 389; related to risk of water intoxication secondary to administration of high volumes of irrigating fluid, *"Benign Prostatic Hypertrophy,"* p. 511; Edema (peripheral and pulmonary) related to surplus of circulating fluid secondary to expanded ECF volume, *"Fluid and Electrolyte Disturbances,"* p. 550; related to intake of hypertonic solutions or abnormal retention of water, *"Fluid and Electrolyte Disturbances,"* p. 553; related to retention secondary to compensatory mechanisms following major surgery, *"Caring for Preoperative and Postoperative Patients,"* p. 646.

Gas exchange, impaired, related to decreased diffusion of oxygen or increased retention of CO_2 secondary to ventilation-perfusion mismatch occurring as a result of alveolar collapse, *"Atelectasis,"* p. 2; related to decreased diffusion of oxygen secondary to inflammatory process in the lungs, *"Pneumonia,"* p. 8; related to decreased diffusion of oxygen secondary to ventilation-perfusion mismatch occurring with pulmonary embolus, *"Pulmonary Embolus,"* p. 15; related to decreased diffusion of oxygen secondary to ventilation-perfusion mismatch, *"Pneumothorax/Hemothorax,"* p. 20; related to decreased alveolar ventilation secondary to narrowed airways, *"Asthma,"* p. 25; related to reduced oxygen transport secondary to pulmonary capillary constriction and restricted blood flow, *"Pulmonary Hypertension,"* p. 41; related to decreased diffusion of oxygen secondary to fluid accumulation in the lungs, *"Myocardial Infarction,"* p. 53; related to decreased diffusion of oxygen secondary to decreased respiratory muscle function occurring with altered metabolism, *"Cardiac and Noncardiac Shock,"* p. 74; related to decreased diffusion of oxygen secondary to fluid accumulation in the alveoli, *"Pulmonary Edema,"* p. 78; related to decreased diffusion of oxygen secondary to shallow breathing occurring with pressure on the diaphragm caused by ascites; retention of sodium and water associated with pleural effusion; and erythrocytopenia, *"Cirrhosis,"* p. 387; related to decreased diffusion of oxygen secondary to pulmonary vascular congestion occurring with ECF expansion, *"Fluid and Electrolyte Disturbances,"* p. 551; related to decreased availability of oxygen secondary to laryngeal spasm occurring with severe hypocalcemia, *"Fluid and Electrolyte Disturbances,"* p. 561; related to trapping of CO_2 secondary to pulmonary tissue destruction, *"Acid-Base Imbalances,"* p. 571; related to hypoventilation and decreased diffusion of oxygen secondary to circumferential burns to neck and thorax or swelling of the membranes of the oronasopharyngeal passage due to smoke inhalation, *"Burns,"* p. 581; related to hyperventilation, increased oxygen requirements associated with sepsis, and decreased diffusion of oxygen secondary to pulmonary infiltrates, *"Acquired Immune Deficiency Syndrome,"* p. 591; related to risk of aspiration secondary to administration of enteral feeding, *"Providing Nutritional Support,"* p. 624.

Grieving, related to actual of perceived loss or changes in body image, body function, or role performance secondary to diagnosis of cancer, *"Cancer of the Cervix,"* p. 495; related to anticipated or actual fetal loss, *"Spontaneous Abortion,"* p. 507; (anticipatory) related to expected loss of body function or body part, changes in self-concept or body image, or terminal illness, *"Caring for Patients with Cancer and Other Life-Disrupting Illnesses,"* p. 693; (dysfunctional) related to actual or perceived loss or change in body function, body image, lifestyle, relationships, or lack of support systems, *"Caring for Patients with Cancer and Other Life-Disrupting Illnesses,"* p. 694.

Health-seeking behavior: Relaxation technique effective for stress reduction, *"Coronary Artery Disease,"* p. 49; Dietary regimen and its relationship to stone formation, *"Ureteral Calculi,"* p. 134; Proper body mechanics and other measures that prevent back injury, *"Intervertebral Disk Disease,"* p. 193; Prevention of osteoporosis, its treatment, and the importance of choosing and using calcium supplements effectively, *"Osteoporosis,"* p. 460.

Hopelessness related to prolonged hospitalization or life-threatening or terminal illness, *"Caring for Patients with Cancer and Other Life-Disrupting Illnesses,"* p. 697.

Incontinence, functional, related to impaired mobility secondary to bed rest or impaired motor, sensory, or cognitive capacity, *"Urinary Incontinence,"* p. 143.

Incontinence, reflex: Involuntary passage of urine occurring with neurologic impairment following injury or disease that affects the transmission of signals from the reflex arc to the cerbral cortex, *"Neurogenic Bladder,"* p. 149; related to spasticity or flaccidity secondary to SCI, *"Spinal Cord Injury,"* p. 203.

Incontinence, stress: Loss of urine <50 ml secondary to decreased pelvic muscle tone due to menopause, childbirth, obesity, or surgical procedure interfering with the posterior urethrovesical angle, *"Urinary Incontinence,"* p. 142; Loss of small ($\leq$50 ml) amounts of urine secondary to temporary loss of muscle tone in the urethral sphincter following prostatectomy, *"Prostatic Neoplasm,"* p. 519.

Incontinence, total: Continuous and unpredictable loss of urine occurring with lower motor neuron disturbance secondary to SCI below S-3–S-4 or neurologic dysfunction caused by disease, *"Neurogenic Bladder,"* p. 150.

Incontinence, urge: Involuntary passage of urine secondary to bladder irritation or reduced bladder capacity following radiation treatment for bladder cancer, UTI, increased urine concentration, use of caffeine or alcohol, or enlarged prostate, *"Urinary Incontinence,"* p. 143; related to frequency and dribbling of urine secondary to urethral irritation following removal of urethral catheter, *"Benign Prostatic Hypertrophy,"* p. 513.

Infection, potential for, (nosocomial pneumonia) related to high risk secondary to recent thoracoabdominal surgery, aspiration, exposure to contaminated respiratory equipment, respiratory instrumentation, colonization of oropharynx with aerobic gram-negative bacilli, or immunosuppression, *"Pneumonia,"* p. 9; (secondary) related to decreased immune response secondary to prolonged antibiotic therapy and vulnerability secondary to invasive procedures, *"Infective Endocarditis,"* p. 63; (with concomitant endocarditis) related to increased susceptibility secondary to valvular disorder, *"Mitral Stenosis,"* p. 66; related to increased susceptibility secondary to corticosteroid therapy, immobility, invasive techniques, and impaired skin integrity, *"Glomerulonephritis,"* p. 104; related to vulnerability secondary to treatment with immunosuppressive agents, prolonged immobility, invasive procedures, and disease process, *"Nephrotic Syndrome,"* p. 107; (or its recurrence) related to increased susceptibility secondary to disease process, *"Acute Pyelonephritis,"* p. 109; related to vulnerability secondary to insertion/presence of nephrostomy tube, *"Hydronephrosis,"* p. 113; related to increased susceptibility secondary to uremia, *"Acute Renal Failure,"* p. 120; related to vulnerability secondary to invasive procedures, exposure to infected individuals, and immunosuppression, *"Care of the Renal Transplant Patient,"* p. 125; related to vulnerability secondary to direct access of the catheter to the peritoneum, *"Renal Dialysis,"* p. 127; related to susceptibility secondary to creation of the vascular access for hemodialysis, *"Renal Dialysis,"* p. 130; related to vulnerability secondary to presence of suprapubic catheter and opening of a closed drainage system, *"Cancer of the Bladder,"* p. 139; related to vulnerability secondary to invasive procedure and contact of pouch with suture line, *"Urinary Diversions,"* p. 155; related to increased susceptibility secondary to basilar skull fractures, penetrating or open head injuries, or surgical wounds, *"Head Injury,"* p. 211; related to increased susceptibility secondary to alterations in adrenal function, *"Hypothyroidism,"* p. 265; related to lowered resistance secondary to decreased adrenal function, *"Addison's Disease,"* p. 275; related to increased susceptibility secondary to disease process, *"Diabetes Mellitus,"* p. 298; related to susceptibility secondary to protein depletion and hyperglycemia, *"Diabetic Ketoacidosis,"* p. 302; related to risk of rupture, peritonitis, and abscess formation secondary to inflammatory process, *"Appendicitis,"* p. 342; related to vulnerability secondary to deeply inflamed colonic mucosa and risk of perforation, *"Ulcerative Colitis,"* p. 357; related to risk of complications (intraabdominal injury) secondary to intestinal inflammatory disorder, *"Crohn's Disease,"* p. 363; related to vulnerability secondary to disruption of the GI tract, particularly of the terminal ileum and colon; traumatically inflicted open wound; multiple indwelling catheters and tubes; and compromised immune state due to stress of trauma and blood loss, *"Abdominal Trauma,"* p. 376; related to increased susceptibility secondary to decreased leukocyte production, *"Pernicious Anemia,"* p. 397; related to increased susceptibility secondary to decreased leukocyte production, *"Hypoplastic Anemia,"* p. 402; related to increased susceptibility secondary to myelosuppression from disease process or therapy, *"Acute Leukemia,"* p. 419; related to risk secondary to large skin deficit following fasciotomy and the presence of devitalized muscle tissue, *"Ischemic Myositis,"* p. 444; (for others) related to cross-contamination; (for patient) related to disease chronicity, *"Osteomyelitis,"* p. 446; related to increased susceptibility secondary to retention of some or all of the products of conception, *"Spontaneous Abortion,"* p. 506; (septic shock) related to susceptibility secondary to introduction of gram-negative bacteria occurring with cystoscopy or TURP, *"Benign Prostatic Hypertrophy,"* p. 510; related to increased susceptibility secondary to surgical procedure, *"Corneal Ulceration/Trauma,"* p. 529; related to susceptibility secondary to invasive procedure and nonsterile field, *"Otosclerosis,"* p. 542; related to vulnerability secondary to bacterial proliferation in burn wounds, presence of invasive lines or urinary catheter, and immunocompromised state, *"Burns,"* p. 584; related to vulnerability secondary to compromised immune system, malnutrition, or side effects of chemotherapy, *"Acquired Immune Deficiency Syndrome,"* p. 590; related to risk of transmitting patient's infectious organisms to others, *"Acquired Immune Deficiency Syndrome,"* p. 591; related to susceptibility secondary to repeated IV drug injections or antitussive effects of opioids, *"Opioid Abuse,"* p. 606; related to vulnerability secondary to malnourished state and presence of central venous catheter or enteral tube, *"Providing Nutritional Support,"* p. 623; related to vulnerability secondary to IV therapy, indwelling urethral catheter, surgical incision, or nature of disease process, *"Caring for Preoperative and Postoperative Patients,"* p. 646; related to risk of neutropenia secondary to malignancy, chemotherapy, radiation therapy, or immunotherapy, *"Caring for Patients with Cancer and Other Life-Disrupting Illnesses,"* p. 678.

Injury, potential for related to increased risk of bleeding or hemorrhage secondary to anticoagulation therapy, *"Pulmonary Embolus,"* p. 16; related to lack of access for external cardiac compression, incorrect neck position, irritation of cranial nerves, and impaired lateral vision secondary to presence of halo vest traction, *"Spinal Cord Injury,"* p. 202; related to risk of increased intracranial pressure and herniation secondary to positional factors, increased intrathoracic or intraabdominal pressure, fluid volume excess, hyperthermia, or discomfort, *"General Care of Patients with Neurologic Disorders,"* p. 253; related to risk of thyrotoxic crisis secondary to emotional stress, trauma, infection, or surgical manipulation of the gland, *"Hyperthyroidism,"* p. 260; related to risk of myxedema coma secondary to inadequate response to treatment of hypothyroidism or stressors, such as infection, *"Hypothyroidism,"* p. 266; related to risk of hypercalcemia, hypocalcemia, tetany, and thyroid storm secondary to surgical procedure or manipulation of the gland, *"Hyperparathyroidism,"* p. 270; related to risk of tetany, respiratory distress, and seizures secondary to hypocalcemia, *"Hypoparathyroidism,"* p. 273; related to risk of Addisonian crisis or side effects from the drug therapy used to treat it, *"Addison's Disease,"* p. 276; related to negative side effects of vasopressin, *"Diabetes Insipidus,"* p. 284; related to increased intracranial pressure, cerebrospinal fluid leak, hemorrhage, infection, and diabetes insipidus secondary to transsphenoidal hypophysectomy, *"Pituitary Tumor,"* p. 285; related to confusion, obtundation, coma, or seizures secondary to cerebral edema or dehydration, *"Diabetic Ketoacidosis,"* p. 303; related to risk of brain damage secondary to hypoglycemia, *"Hypoglycemia,"* p. 309; related to risk of gastrointestinal complications (obstruction, recurring reflux, esophageal tear, or perforation) secondary to surgery, *"Hiatal Hernia and Reflux Esophagitis,"* p. 319; Gastrointestinal complications (bleeding, obstruction, and perforation) secondary to ulcerative process, *"Peptic Ulcer,"* p. 325; related to risk of worsening peritonitis or development of septic shock secondary to inflammatory process, *"Peritonitis,"* p. 339; related to risk of complications (intraabdominal injury) secondary to intestinal inflammatory disorder, *"Crohn's Disease,"* p. 363; related to increased risk of bleeding secondary to decreased vitamin K absorption, *"Hepatitis,"* p. 384; related to use of T-tube or recurrence of biliary obstruction, *"Cholelithiasis and Cholecystitis,"* p. 392; related to risk of sensorimotor deficit secondary to inability to absorb and use vitamin B$_{12}$, *"Pernicious Anemia,"* p. 397; related to sensorimotor deficit secondary to peripheral nerve hypoxia, *"Hemolytic Anemia,"* p. 400; related to sensorimotor alterations secondary to tissue hypoxia occurring with decreased production of erythrocytes, *"Hypoplastic Anemia,"* p. 406; related to increased risk of bleeding secondary to decreased platelet count, *"Thrombocytopenia,"* p. 410; related to increased risk of bleeding secondary to clotting factor deficiency, *"Hemophilia,"* p. 412; related to risk of bleeding secondary to decreased platelet count, *"Acute Leukemia,"* p. 419; related to increased risk of bleeding secondary to hypervascularity of ocular tissue, *"Retinal Detachment,"* p. 538; related to risk of paralytic ileus, *"Burns,"* p. 582; related to risk of development of gastric (Curling's) ulcer secondary to gastric pH <5, *"Burns,"* p. 583; (to staff and environment) related to preparation, handling, and disposal of chemotherapy agents, *"Caring for Patients with Cancer and Other Life-Disrupting Illnesses,"* p. 659; to staff, other patients, and visitors related to risk of exposure to sealed or unsealed sources of radiation, *"Caring for Patients with Cancer and Other Life-Disrupting Illnesses,"* p. 674; related to increased risk of bleeding/hemorrhage secondary to thrombocytopenia (for all patients receiving chemotherapy and radiation therapy, as well as those with cancer, particularly that involving the bone marrow, *"Caring for Patients with Cancer and Other Life-Disrupting Illnesses,"* p. 679.

Knowledge deficit: Oral anticoagulant therapy, potential side effects, and foods and medications to avoid during therapy, *"Pulmonary Embolus,"* p. 16; Disease process and treatment, *"Pulmonary Hypertension,"* p. 42; Precautions and negative side effects of nitrates, *"Coronary Artery Disease,"* p. 49; Precautions and negative side effects of beta blockers, *"Coronary Artery Disease,"* p. 50; Precautions and negative side effects of diuretic therapy, *"Heart Failure,"* p. 56; Precautions and negative side effects of digitalis therapy, *"Heart Failure,"* p. 56; Precautions and negative side effects of vasodilators, *"Heart Failure,"* p. 57; Disease process, therapeutic regimen, and assessment for infection, *"Infective Endocarditis,"* p. 63; Potential for development of endocarditis, *"Mitral Stenosis,"* p. 66; Pacemaker insertion procedure and pacemaker function, *"Pacemakers,"* p. 80; Catheterization procedure and postcatheterization regimen, *"Cardiac Catheterization,"* p. 82; Diagnosis, surgical procedure, preoperative routine, and postoperative care, *"Cardiac Surgery,"* p. 84; Potential for infection and impaired skin and tissue integrity due to decreased arterial circulation, *"Ath-*

erosclerotic Arterial Occlusive Disease," p. 88; Potential for aneurysm rupture (if surgery is not immediately planned), "Aneurysms," p. 90; Signs and symptoms of fluid and electrolyte imbalance (caused by decreased renal function or diuretic therapy), "Glomerulonephritis," p. 104; Negative side effects of corticosteroids and cytotoxic agents, "Glomerulonephritis," p. 104; Rationale for frequent assessments after angioplasty, endarterectomy, or resection and the importance of measuring BP, "Renal Artery Stenosis," p. 115; Need for frequent BP checks and adherence to antihypertensive therapy and the potential for change in insulin requirements, "Chronic Renal Failure," p. 123; Signs and symptoms of rejection, negative side effects of immunosuppressive agents, and importance of protecting the fistula, "Care of the Renal Transplant Patient," p. 126; Function and care of long-term indwelling catheters after continent vesicostomy, "Neurogenic Bladder," p. 151; Pubococcygeal (Kegel) exercise program to strengthen perineal muscles, "Urinary Incontinence," p. 144; Use of external (condom) catheter, "Urinary Incontinence," p. 144; Self-care regarding urinary diversion, "Urinary Diversions," p. 156; Factors that aggravate and exacerbate MS symptoms, "Multiple Sclerosis," p. 162; Precautions and potential side effects of prescribed medications, "Multiple Sclerosis," p. 162; Side effects and precautions for the prescribed antibiotics, "Bacterial Meningitis," p. 169; Methods for overcoming difficulty with initiating movement, "Parkinsonism," p. 178; Side effects of and precautionary measures for taking anti-Parkinson medications, "Parkinsonism," p. 179; Facial and tongue exercises that enhance verbal communication and help prevent choking, "Parkinsonism," p. 180; Pain control measures, "Intervertebral Disk Disease," p. 193; Surgical procedure, preoperative routine, and postoperative regimen, "Intervertebral Disk Disease," p. 193; Caretaker's responsibility for observing the patient who is sent home with a concussion, "Head Injury," p. 211; Aneurysms and the potential for rebleeding, rupture, or vasospasm, "Cerebral Aneurysm," p. 225; Effects of aminocaproic acid drug therapy, "Cerebral Aneurysm," p. 225; Life-threatening environmental factors and preventive measures for seizures, "Seizure Disorders," p. 245; Purpose, precautions, and side effects of antiepilepsy medications, "Seizure Disorders," p. 245; Potential for negative side effects from steroids, phosphate supplements, and mithramycin, "Hyperparathyroidism," p. 271; Proper insulin administration, "Diabetes Mellitus," p. 299; Disease process, diagnostic testing, indicators of hypoglycemia, and therapeutic regimen, "Hypoglycemia," p. 310; Disease process, treatment, and factors that potentiate bleeding, "Stomatitis," p. 316; Disease process and treatment for hiatal hernia and reflux esophagitis, "Hiatal Hernia and Reflux Esophagitis," p. 318; Disease process and therapeutic regimen for achalasia, "Achalasia," p. 322; Potential for gastrointestinal complications associated with presence of a hernia and measures that can prevent their occurrence, "Hernia," p. 337; Potential for recurrence of hemorrhoids and measures that help prevent it, "Hemorrhoids," p. 346; Colostomy irrigation procedure, "Fecal Diversions," p. 369; Causes of hepatitis and modes of transmission, "Hepatitis," p. 382; Factors that precipitate hemolytic crisis and measures that can help prevent it, "Hemolytic Anemia," p. 401; Potential for bleeding (caused by low platelet count) and measures that can help prevent it, "Hypoplastic Anemia," p. 406; Use of a heating device, "Osteoarthritis," p. 425; Disease process and medication regimen, "Gouty Arthritis," p. 428; Proper care of inflamed joints, "Gouty Arthritis," p. 429; Assessments and preventive measures for uric acid renal calculi, "Gouty Arthritis," p. 429; Need for elevation of the involved extremity, use of thermotherapy, and exercise, "Ligamentous Injuries," p. 435; Care and assessment of the casted extremity, "Ligamentous Injuries," p. 435; Potential for joint weakness, and the techniques for applying external supports and assessing neurovascular status, "Ligamentous Injuries," p. 436; Adverse side effects from prolonged use of potent antibiotics, "Osteomyelitis," p. 447; Potential for infection and air embolus related to use of Hickman catheter or similar device for long-term intermittent antibiotic therapy, "Osteomyelitis," p. 448; Potential for disuse osteoporosis (appropriate for patient with cast or traction), "Fractures," p. 453; Potential for infection related to orthopaedic procedure or presence of internal or external device (appropriate for patients with ORIF or external fixators), "Fractures," p. 454; Potential for refracture owing to vulnerability secondary to presence of internal fixator (applies to patients with

ORIF), *"Fractures,"* p. 454; Function of external fixator, pin care, transport, and signs of symptoms of pin site infection, *"Fractures,"* p. 454; Disease process and potential for recurrence, *"Benign Neoplasms,"* p. 456; Potential complications of Paget's disease, *"Paget's Disease,"* p. 462; Disease process and therapeutic regimen, *"Bunionectomy,"* p. 464; Postsurgical exercise regimen, *"Amputation,"* p. 467; Care of the stump and prosthesis; signs and symptoms of skin irritation or pressure necrosis, *"Amputation,"* p. 467; Potential for and mechanism of THA dislocation, preventive measures, positional restrictions, prescribed ambulation regimen, and use of assistive devices, *"Total Hip Arthroplasty,"* p. 474; Potential for infection caused by foreign body reaction to endoprosthesis, *"Total Hip Arthroplasty,"* p. 475; Incisional site care and the potential for postoperative capsular contracture, *"Breast Augmentation,"* p. 483; Surgical procedure, preoperative care, and postoperative regimen, *"Breast Reconstruction,"* p. 484; Potential for postoperative fibrotic capsular contracture and the technique for breast massage, *"Breast Reconstruction,"* p. 484; Side effects of estrogen therapy or bilateral orchiectomy, *"Prostatic Neoplasm,"* p. 519; Diagnosis and treatment plan, *"Corneal Ulceration/Trauma,"* p. 529; Importance of avoiding increased intraocular pressure and activities that can cause it, *"Corneal Ulceration/Trauma,"* p. 530; Diagnosis, surgery, precautionary measures, and treatment plan, *"Keratoplasty,"* p. 532; Diagnosis, surgery, and treatment plan, *"Vitreous Disorders/Vitrectomy,"* p. 533; Diagnosis, surgery, and treatment plan, *"Glaucoma,"* p. 536; Diagnosis, surgical procedure, and treatment plan, *"Retinal Detachment,"* p. 538; Surgical procedure, postsurgical precautions, and function of the ocular prosthesis, *"Enucleation,"* p. 540; Surgical procedure, postsurgical regimen, and expected outcomes, *"Otosclerosis,"* p. 542; Disease process, prognosis, lifestyle changes, and treatment plan, *"Acquired Immune Deficiency Syndrome,"* p. 595; Surgical procedure, preoperative routine, and postoperative care, *"Caring for Preoperative and Postoperative Patients,"* p. 637; Chemotherapy, its purpose, expected side effects, and potential toxicities associated with these drugs, appropriate self-care measures for minimizing side effects, and available community and educational resources, *"Caring for Patients with Cancer and Other Life-Disrupting Illnesses,"* p. 660; Immunotherapy and its purpose, potential side effects and toxicities, appropriate self-care measures to minimize side effects, and available community and education resources, *"Caring for Patients with Cancer and Other Life-Disrupting Illnesses,"* p. 661; Purpose and management of venous access devices (VAD), *"Caring for Patients with Cancer and Other Life-Disrupting Illnesses,"* p. 674; Type and purpose of radiation implant and the measures for preventing and managing complications, *"Caring for Patients with Cancer and Other Life-Disrupting Illnesses,"* p. 675; Purpose and procedure for external beam radiation therapy, appropriate self care measures following treatment, and available educational and community resources, *"Caring for Patients with Cancer and Other Life-Disrupting Illnesses,"* p. 676; (Family): Patient's current health status or therapies, *"Caring for Patients with Cancer and Other Life-Disrupting Illnesses,"* p. 700.

Mobility, impaired physical, related to alterations in the upper or lower limbs secondary to weakness, hemiparesis, or hemiplegia occurring with CVA, *"Cerebrovascular Accident,"* p. 236; related to adjustment to a new walking gait secondary to the use of an assistive device, *"Osteoarthritis,"* p. 426; related to immobilization device or nonweightbearing secondary to bunionectomy, *"Bunionectomy,"* p. 464; related to altered stance secondary to amputation of the lower limb, *"Amputation,"* p. 467; related to postoperative pain, decreased strength and endurance secondary to CNS effects of anesthesia or blood loss; musculoskeletal or neuromuscular impairment secondary to disease process or surgical procedure, perceptual impairment secondary to disease process or surgical procedure (e.g., ocular surgery, neurosurgery), or cognitive deficit secondary to disease process or effects of opioid analgesics and anesthetics, *"Caring for Preoperative and Postoperative Patients,"* p. 648.

Noncompliance with the therapy related to denial of the illness or perceived negative consequences of the treatment regimen secondary to social stigma, negative side effects of antiepilepsy medications, or difficulty with making necessary lifestyle changes, *"Sei-*

zure Disorders," p. 247; related to frustration secondary to frequency of antibiotic administration and lack of knowledge of its importance, *"Corneal Ulceration/Trauma,"* p. 531; related to frustration secondary to extensiveness of pharmacologic regimen and lack of knowledge of its importance, *"Glaucoma,"* p. 536.

Nutrition, altered: *Less than body requirements* related to decreased intake secondary to anorexia, *"Pneumonia,"* p. 9; related to decreased intake secondary to fatigue and anorexia, *"Chronic bronchitis,"* p. 29; related to decreased intake secondary to anorexia and increased need secondary to urinary losses of protein, *"Nephrotic Syndrome,"* p. 106; related to decreased intake secondary to nausea and anorexia, *"Acute Pyelonephritis,"* p. 109; related to nausea, vomiting, anorexia, and dietary restrictions, *"Acute Renal Failure,"* p. 118; related to increased need secondary to protein loss in the dialysate, *"Renal Dialysis,"* p. 128; related to decreased intake secondary to NPO status with adynamic ileus, *"Guillain-Barré Syndrome,"* p. 166; related to decreased intake secondary to cognitive and motor deficit; and increased need secondary to constant pacing and restlessness, *"Alzheimer's Disease,"* p. 185; related to decreased intake secondary to chewing and swallowing deficits, fatigue, weakness, paresis, paralysis, visual neglect, or decreased LOC, *"General Care of Patients with Neurologic Disorders,"* p. 249; related to increased need secondary to hypermetabolic state, *"Hyperthyroidism,"* p. 259; related to decreased intake secondary to anorexia and dietary restrictions, and increased need secondary to digestive dysfunction, *"Pancreatitis,"* p. 290; related to decreased intake secondary to discomfort with chewing and swallowing, *"Stomatitis,"* p. 316; related to decreased intake secondary to dysphagia or surgery, *"Achalasia,"* p. 321; related to decreased intake secondary to nausea, vomiting, bloating, and anorexia, *"Gastric Neoplasm,"* p. 327; related to loss secondary to vomiting and intestinal suctioning and increased need secondary to NPO status, *"Peritonitis,"* p. 340; related to decreased intake secondary to disruption of GI tract integrity (traumatic or surgical) and increased need secondary to hypermetabolic posttrauma state, *"Abdominal Trauma,"* p. 378; related to decreased intake secondary to anorexia, nausea, and gastric distress, *"Hepatitis,"* p. 383; related to decreased intake secondary to anorexia and nausea; and increased need secondary to malabsorption, *"Cirrhosis,"* p. 387; related to decreased intake secondary to fatigue, impairment of oral mucosa, or anorexia, *"Pernicious Anemia,"* p. 397; related to decreased intake secondary to anorexia associated with feelings of "fullness" (owing to congestion of organ systems, *"Polycythemia,"* p. 408; related to increased need for calcium and vitamin D, *"Osteoporosis,"* p. 460; related to hypermetabolic state secondary to burn wound healing, *"Burns,"* p. 584; related to decreased intake and losses secondary to diarrhea and nausea associated with side effects of medications, malabsorption, anorexia, dysphagia, and fatigue, *"Acquired Immune Deficiency Syndrome,"* p. 592; related to history of poor intake and malabsorption secondary to alcoholism, *"Alcoholism,"* p. 599; related to inadequate provision of nutrients, *"Providing Nutritional Support,"* p. 622; related to decreased intake secondary to nausea and vomiting or anorexia occurring with chemotherapy or radiation therapy, *"Caring for Patients with Cancer and Other Life-Disrupting Illnesses,"* p. 680.

Nutrition, altered: *More than body requirements* related to excessive intake of calories, sodium, or fats, *"Coronary Artery Disease,"* p. 49; of calories related to decreased need secondary to slowed metabolism, *"Hypothyroidism,"* p. 265; of purine or alcohol, *"Gouty Arthritis,"* p. 429.

Oral mucous membrane, altered, related to stomatitis, *"Stomatitis,"* p. 315; related to self-care deficit, *"Caring for Patients on Prolonged Bed Rest,"* p. 655.

Pain related to impaired pleural integrity, inflammation, or presence of chest tube, *"Pneumothorax/Hemothorax,"* p. 21; related to compression of nerves by the tumor, *"Bronchogenic Carcinoma,"* p. 36; related to angina secondary to decreased oxygen supply to the myocardium, *"Coronary Artery Disease,"* p. 47; related to ischemia and infarction of myocardial tissue, *"Myocardial Infarction,"* p. 52; related to friction rub secondary to inflammatory process, *"Pericarditis,"* p. 59; related to pacemaker insertion, *"Pacemakers,"* p. 81; related to inflammatory process secondary to thrombus formation, *"Venous Thrombosis/Thrombophlebitis,"* p. 94; related to preoperative venous engorgement or surgical procedure, *"Varicose Veins,"* p. 97; related to dysuria secondary to infection, *"Acute Pyelonephritis,"* p. 108; related to presence of a calculus or the surgical procedure to remove it, *"Ureteral Calculi,"* p. 133; related to bladder spasms, *"Urinary Tract Obstruction,"* p. 137; related to headaches secondary to head injury, *"Head Injury,"* p. 212; related to tissue compression secondary to tumor growth, *"Spinal Cord Tumor,"* p. 220; related to spasms, headache, and photophobia secondary to neurologic dysfunction, *"General Care of Patients with Neurologic Disorders,"* p. 254; related to surgical procedure, *"Hyperthyroidism,"* p. 262; related to surgical procedure or arthralgia secondary to bone demineralization, *"Hyperparathyroidism,"* p. 271; related to inflammatory process of the pancreas, *"Pancreatitis,"* p. 289; related to major abdominal surgery, *"Pancreatic Tumors,"* p. 293; nausea and feeling of fullness related to gastroesophageal reflux and increase in intraabdominal pressure, *"Hiatal Hernia and Reflux Esophagitis,"* p. 319; related to epigastric discomfort secondary to ulcerative process, *"Peptic Ulcer,"* p. 325; abdominal fullness, weakness, and diaphoresis after meals related to postgastrectomy dumping syndrome, *"Peptic Ulcer,"* p. 325; nausea and distention related to obstructive process and presence of NG or intestinal tube, *"Obstructive Processes,"* p. 334; related to hernia condition or surgical intervention, *"Hernia,"* p. 336; abdominal distention and nausea related to the inflammatory process, fever, and tissue damage, *"Peritonitis,"* p. 339; and nausea related to the inflammatory process, *"Appendicitis,"* p. 343; and itching related to hemorrhoidectomy, *"Hemorrhoids,"* p. 345; abdominal cramping and nausea related to intestinal inflammatory process, *"Ulcerative Colitis,"* p. 358; abdominal cramping and nausea related to intestinal inflammatory process, *"Crohn's Disease,"* p. 363; related to irritation secondary to intraperitoneal blood or secretions, actual trauma or surgical incision, and manipulation of organs, *"Abdominal Trauma,"* p. 376; spasms, nausea, and itching related to obstructive or inflammatory process, *"Cholelithiasis and Cholecystitis,"* p. 392; related to hemolysis in the joints secondary to hemolytic crisis, *"Hemolytic Anemia,"* p. 401; related to headache, angina, and abdominal and joint discomfort secondary to altered circulation occurring with hyperviscosity of the blood, *"Polycythemia,"* p. 408; related to joint discomfort secondary to hemorrhagic episodes or blood extravasation into the tissues, *"Thrombocytopenia,"* p. 411; related to swollen joints (hemarthrosis), *"Hemophilia,"* p. 413; related to joint changes and corrective therapy, *"Osteoarthritis,"* p. 425; related to joint changes and corrective therapy, *"Bunionectomy,"* p. 464; related to phantom limb sensation, *"Amputation,"* p. 468; related to surgical procedure, *"Breast Augmentation,"* p. 482; related to surgical biopsy, *"Benign Breast Disease,"* p. 487; related to surgical procedure, *"Malignant Disorders of the Breast,"* p. 491; related to surgery or radiation implant, *"Cancer of the Cervix,"* p. 495; related to uterine contractions, *"Spontaneous Abortion,"* p. 506; related to bladder spasms, *"Benign Prostatic Hypertrophy,"* p. 512; related to dysuria secondary to the infectious process, *"Prostatitis,"* p. 515; related to scrotal swelling secondary to orchiectomy or lymphadenectomy, *"Testicular Neoplasm,"* p. 522; related to surgical procedure, *"Penile Implants,"* p. 523; related to corneal ulceration, *"Corneal Ulceration/Trauma,"* p. 530; related to surgical procedure, *"Keratoplasty,"* p. 532; related to surgical procedure, *"Enucleation,"* p. 540; related to exposed sensory nerve endings secondary to burn injury, *"Burns,"* p. 584; related to prolonged immobility, side effects of chemotherapy, infections, and frequent venipunctures, *"Acquired Immune Deficiency Syndrome,"* p. 593; related to disease process, injury, or surgical procedure, *"Caring for Preoperative and Postoperative Patients,"* p. 638.

Pain, chronic, and spasms related to tissue ischemia secondary to atherosclerotic obstructions, *"Atherosclerotic Arterial Occlusive Disease,"* p. 88; related to motor and sensory nerve tract damage, *"Multiple Sclerosis,"* p. 163.

Parenting, altered, related to treatment with radiation therapy and chemotherapy secondary to breast malignancy, *"Malignant Disorders of the Breast,"* p. 492.

Post-trauma response related to stress reaction secondary to life-threatening accident or event resulting in trauma, *"Abdominal Trauma,"* p. 379.

Powerlessness related to lack of control over self-care, health care status, or outcome secondary to nature of health care environment, therapeutic regimen, or life-threatening illness, *"Caring for Patients with Cancer and Other Life-Disrupting Illnesses,"* p. 694.

Role performance, altered, related to loss of limb, *"Amputation,"* p. 468; related to fetal loss, *"Spontaneous Abortion,"* p. 506; Dependence vs. independence, *"Caring for Patients on Prolonged Bed Rest,"* p. 658.

Self-care deficit: Inability to perform ADL related to memory loss and coordination problems secondary to cognitive and motor deficits, *"Alzheimer's Disease,"* p. 185; related to imposed activity restrictions secondary to risk of aneurysm rupture and rebleeding, *"Cerebral Aneurysm,"* p. 226; related to spasticity, tremors, weakness, paresis, paralysis, or decreasing LOC secondary to sensorimotor deficits, *"General Care of Patients with Neurologic Disorders,"* p. 251; Oral hygiene related to sensorimotor deficit or decreased LOC, *"Stomatitis,"* p. 315; related to physical limitations secondary to cast or surgical procedure (applies to patients with casts, ORIF, and external fixators), *"Fractures,"* p. 452; Inability to perform ADL related to imposed restrictions and visual deficit, *"Corneal Ulceration/Trauma,"* p. 530.

Sensory/perceptual alterations related to mentation and motor disturbances secondary to uremia, electrolyte imbalance, and metabolic acidosis, *"Acute Renal Failure,"* p. 119; related to mentation and motor disturbances secondary to electrolyte and acid-base imbalance, *"Chronic Renal Failure,"* p. 123; related to mentation and motor changes secondary to uremia and serum electrolyte imbalance, *"Renal Dialysis,"* p. 128; related to impaired mentation or motor function secondary to loss of sodium and potassium (ileal conduit), *"Urinary Diversions,"* p. 153; related to impaired pain, touch, and temperature sensations secondary to sensory deficit or decreased LOC, *"General Care of Patients with Neurologic Disorders,"* p. 249; related to visual disturbances secondary to diplopia, *"General Care of Patients with Neurologic Disorders,"* p. 254; related to sensorium changes secondary to cerebral retention of water, *"Hypothyroidism,"* p. 266; related to mentation and motor disturbances secondary to hepatic coma occurring with cerebral accumulation of ammonia or GI bleeding, *"Cirrhosis,"* p. 388; related to mentation changes secondary to decreased oxygenation in the brain occurring with the infectious process, *"Prostatitis,"* p. 516; related to visual deficit secondary to disease process or presence of eye shield, eye patch, or other measure that distorts or diminishes vision, *"Corneal Ulceration/Trauma,"* p. 529; related to auditory deficit secondary to disease process, postoperative earplug, or tissue edema, *"Otosclerosis,"* p. 543; related to mentation changes secondary to sodium level <120-125 mEq/L, *"Fluid and Electrolyte Disturbances,"* p. 553; related to mentation changes and risk of seizures secondary to cerebral edema occurring with too rapid correction of hypernatremia, *"Fluid and Electrolyte Disturbances,"* p. 554; related to motor and sensorium changes secondary to hypercalcemia, *"Fluid and Electrolyte Disturbances,"* p. 562; related to tactile and visual deficits, medications, sleep-pattern disturbance, or pain secondary to severe burn injury, *"Burns,"* p. 585; related to mentation and motor disturbances secondary to intoxication and withdrawal, *"Alcoholism,"* p. 599; related to motor and mentation disturbances secondary to withdrawal from CNS depressant, *"Sedative-Hypnotic Abuse,"* p. 602; Auditory and kinesthetic impairment, secondary to cisplatinum or VINCA alkaloids, *"Caring for Patients with Cancer and Other Life-Disrupting Illnesses,"* p. 683; related to environmental overload or monotony, socially-restricted environment, psychologic stress, or pathophysiologic alterations, *"Caring for Patients with Cancer and Other Life-Disrupting Illnesses,"* p. 691.

Sexual dysfunction related to physiologic limitations secondary to abnormal hormone levels, *"Pituitary Tumor,"* p. 286; related to impotence (risk if 85%-90%) secondary to radical prostatectomy, *"Prostatic Neoplasm,"* p. 578; Impaired sexual self-concept and infertility secondary to radiation therapy to the lower abdomen, pelvis, and gonads; or chemotherapy agents, especially alkylating agents, vinblastine, bleomycin, actinomycin D, daunorubicin, mitomycin, procarbazine, and cytarabine, *"Caring for Patients with Cancer and Other Life-Disrupting Illnesses,"* p. 683.

Sexuality pattern, altered, related to loss of aspects of sexual functioning secondary to SCI, *"Spinal Cord Injury,"* p. 205; related to fear of impotence secondary to lack of knowledge of postsurgical sexual function, *"Benign Prostatic Hypertrophy,"* p. 512; related to actual or perceived physiologic limitations on sexual performance secondary to disease, therapy, or prolonged hospitalization, *"Caring for Patients on Prolonged Bed Rest,"* p. 658.

Skin integrity, impaired, related to tissue ischemia secondary to decreased arterial circulation, *"Atherosclerotic Arterial Occlusive Disease,"* p. 87; related to impaired tissue nutrition secondary to venous engorgement, *"Varicose Veins,"* p. 97; related to irritation secondary to wound drainage, *"Renal Calculi,"* p. 111; related to pruritus and dry skin secondary to uremia and edema, *"Chronic Renal Failure,"* p. 123; related to irritation secondary to wound drainage, *"Ureteral Calculi,"* p. 134; related to chemical irritation from urine on the skin, improperly fitting appliance, or sensitivity to the appliance material, *"Urinary Diversions,"* p. 153; related to irritation or pressure secondary to cervical or pelvic traction, *"Intervertebral Disk Disease,"* p. 195; related to irritation and pressure secondary to presence of halo vest traction, *"Spinal Cord Injury,"* p. 203; related to vulnerability secondary to thinning of skin and fragility of capillaries, *"Cushing's Disease,"* p. 279; related to irritation secondary to wound drainage or pressure on incision, *"Pancreatic Tumors,"* p. 293; related to increased susceptibility secondary to peripheral neuropathy and vascular pathology, *"Diabetes Mellitus,"* p. 299; Perineal/perianal area related to irritation secondary to persistent diarrhea, *"Ulcerative Colitis,"* p. 358; Stoma and peristomal area, related to erythema, improper appliance, or sensitivity to appliance material, *"Fecal Diversions,"* p. 366; related to direct trauma and surgery; hypermetabolic, catabolic posttraumatic state; impaired tissue perfusion; or exposure to irritating GI drainage, *"Abdominal Trauma,"* p. 378; related to pruritus secondary to hepatic dysfunction, *"Hepatitis,"* p. 384; related to vulnerability secondary to occlusion of the vessels and impaired oxygen transport to the tissues and skin, *"Hemolytic Anemia,"* p. 400; related to decreased blood circulation to the tissues secondary to bleeding, *"Hemophilia,"* p. 413; related to decreased circulation secondary to hemorrhage and thrombosis, *"Disseminated Intravascular Coagulation,"* p. 416; related to irritation secondary to the presence of a cast (applies to patients with casts and ORIF), *"Fractures,"* p. 453; related to risk of maceration of the axillary skin secondary to shoulder immobilization, *"Repair of Recurrent Shoulder Dislocation,"* p. 472; related to irritation secondary to presence of CPM device, *"Total Knee Arthroplasty,"* p. 477; related to risk of irritation secondary to wound drainage from suprapubic or retropubic prostatectomy, *"Benign Prostatic Hypertrophy,"* p. 512; related to imposed position restrictions and frequent removal of eye patch, *"Retinal Detachment,"* p. 539; Burn injury, *"Burns,"* p. 583; related to vulnerability secondary to cachexia and malnourishment, diarrhea, side effects of chemotherapy, Kaposi's skin lesions, negative nitrogen state, and decreased mobility due to arthralgia and fatigue, *"Acquired Immune Deficiency Syndrome,"* p. 593; related to vulnerability secondary to malnourished state or presence of central venous catheters or enteral tube, *"Providing Nutritional Support,"* p. 623; related to excessive tissue pressure, *"Managing Wound Care,"* p. 631; related to irritation of skin by secretions/excretions around percutaneous drains and tubes, *"Caring for Preoperative and Postoperative Patients,"* p. 650; related to cutaneous reactions secondary to chemotherapy, *"Caring for Patients with Cancer and Other Life-Disrupting Illnesses,"* p. 684; related to cutaneous reactions secondary to radiation therapy, *"Caring for Patients with Cancer and Other Life-Disrupting Illnesses,"* p. 686; Malignant skin lesions, *"Caring for Patients with Cancer and Other Life-Disrupting Illnesses,"* p. 687.

Sleep pattern disturbance related to awakening for VS assessment or medication administration, *"Myocardial Infarction,"* p. 53; related to restlessness and disorientation secondary to cognitive deficits, *"Alzheimer's Disease,"* p. 187; related to agitation secondary to accelerated metabolism, *"Hyperthyroidism,"* p. 260; related to agitation secondary to hepatic dysfunction (faulty absorption, metabolism, and storage of nutrients), *"Hepatitis,"* p. 382; related to frequent antibiotic and steroid administrations, *"Corneal*

Ulceration/Trauma," p. 531; related to agitation secondary to withdrawal from short-acting CNS depressant, *"Alcoholism,"* p. 599; related to preoperative anxiety, postoperative pain, altered environment, disruption of normal sleep pattern, immobility, and stress, *"Caring for Preoperative and Postoperative Patients,"* p. 648; related to environmental overload, therapeutic regimen, pain, immobility, or psychologic stress, *"Caring for Patients with Cancer and Other Life-Disrupting Illnesses,"* p. 691.

Social isolation related to disease, societal rejection, loss of support system, fear, feelings of guilt and punishment, fatigue, and changed patterns of social expression, *"Acquired Immune Deficiency Syndrome,"* p. 595; related to prolonged hospitalization, altered health status, inadequate support systems, or terminal illness, *"Caring for Patients with Cancer and Other Life-Disrupting Illnesses,"* p. 695.

Spiritual distress related to altered health state, separation from religious ties, life-threatening illness, or conflict between religious beliefs and therapeutic regimens, *"Caring for Patients with Cancer and Other Life-Disrupting Illnesses,"* p. 695.

Swallowing, impaired, potential for related to postoperative edema or hematoma formation secondary to anterior cervical fusion, *"Intervertebral Disk Disease,"* p. 195; related to edema or laryngeal nerve damage secondary to surgical procedure, *"Hyperthyroidism,"* p. 262; related to pain or decreased ability to ingest secondary to disease or treatment (e.g., surgery, chemotherapy, radiation), *"Providing Nutritional Support,"* p. 623; Esophagitis secondary to radiation therapy to the neck, chest, and upper back; chemotherapy agents, especially the antimetabolites; infection due to immunosuppression; or tumors of the esophagus, *"Caring for Patients with Cancer and Other Life-Disrupting Illnesses,"* p. 687.

Thought processes, altered, related to impaired sensory reception, transmission, integration, and evaluation secondary to degeneration of intellectual functioning, *"Alzheimer's Disease,"* p. 186; related to mentation changes secondary to infection or space-occupying lesion in the central nervous system (CNS), *"Acquired Immune Deficiency Syndrome,"* p. 595.

Tissue integrity, impaired, related to tissue ischemia secondary to decreased arterial circulation, *"Atherosclerotic Arterial Occlusive Disease,"* p. 87; related to impaired tissue nutrition secondary to venous engorgement, *"Varicose Veins,"* p. 97; related to insertion/presence of nephrostomy tube, *"Hydronephrosis,"* p. 113; related to chemical irritation from urine on the skin, improperly fitting appliance, or sensitivity to appliance material, *"Urinary Diversions,"* p. 154; related to irritation or pressure secondary to cervical or pelvic traction, *"Intervertebral Disk Disease,"* p. 195; related to irritation and pressure secondary to presence of halo vest traction, *"Spinal Cord Injury,"* p. 203; related to risk of corneal irritation/abrasion secondary to diminished blink reflex or inability to close the eyes, *"General Care of Patients with Neurologic Disorders,"* p. 249; Corneal damage secondary to exophthalmos, *"Hyperthyroidism,"* p. 261; related to irritation secondary to wound drainage or pressure on incision, *"Pancreatic Tumors,"* p. 293; related to increased susceptibility secondary to peripheral neuropathy and vascular pathology, *"Diabetes Mellitus,"* p. 299; Stoma and peristomal area, related to erythema, improper appliance, or sensitivity to appliance material, *"Fecal Diversions,"* p. 366; related to direct trauma and surgery; hypermetabolic, catabolic posttraumatic state; impaired tissue perfusion; or exposure to irritating GI drainage, *"Abdominal Trauma,"* p. 378; related to vulnerability secondary to occlusion of the vessels and impaired oxygen transport to the tissues and skin, *"Hemolytic Anemia,"* p. 400; related to vulnerability secondary to decreased blood circulation to the tissues due to bleeding, *"Hemophilia,"* p. 413; related to decreased circulation secondary to hemorrhage and thrombosis, *"Disseminated Intravascular Coagulation,"* p. 416; related to imposed position restrictions and frequent removal of eye patch, *"Retinal Detachment,"* p. 539; Burn injury, *"Burns,"* p. 583; related to vulnerability secondary to cachexia and malnourishment, diarrhea, side effects of chemotherapy, Kaposi's skin lesions, negative nitrogen state, and decreased mobility due to arthralgia and fatigue, *"Acquired Immune Deficiency Syndrome,"* p. 593; related to vulnerability secondary to malnourished state or presence of central venous catheters or enteral tube, *"Providing Nutritional Sup-*

port," p. 623; Wound healing by primary intention, related to risk of infection, metabolic alterations (e.g., diabetes mellitus), impaired oxygen transport, altered tissue perfusion, and alterations in fluid volume and nutrition, *"Managing Wound Care,"* p. 626; Wound, related to presence of contamination, *"Managing Wound Care,"* p. 628; Wound, related to alterations in perfusion, oxygenation, fluid volume, and nutrition, *"Managing Wound Care,"* p. 630; related to excessive tissue pressure, *"Managing Wound Care,"* p. 631; related to presence of pressure ulcer (with increased risk for further breakdown), *"Managing Wound Care,"* p. 632; Oral and gastric mucosa, secondary to NPO status and presence of gastric tube, *"Caring for Preoperative and Postoperative Patients,"* p. 650; related to irritation secondary to extravasation of vesicant or irritating chemotherapy agents, *"Caring for Patients with Cancer and Other Life-Disrupting Illnesses,"* p. 660.

Tissue perfusion, altered: Cardiopulmonary and peripheral, related to impaired circulation secondary to embolus formation, *"Cardiomyopathy,"* p. 45; Peripheral, cardiopulmonary, cerebral, and renal, related to impaired circulation secondary to dysfunctional cardiac muscle, *"Pericarditis,"* p. 59; Peripheral, cardiopulmonary, cerebral, and renal related to impaired circulation secondary to decreased circulating blood volume, *"Cardiac and Noncardiac Shock,"* p. 73; Cardiopulmonary, peripheral, and cerebral, related to impaired circulation secondary to decreased cardiac output, *"Pulmonary Edema,"* p. 77; Peripheral and cardiopulmonary, related to impaired circulation secondary to pacemaker malfunction, *"Pacemakers,"* p. 80; Peripheral, cardiopulmonary, and cerebral, related to impaired circulation secondary to catheterization procedure, *"Cardiac Catheterization,"* p. 82; Peripheral, related to impaired circulation secondary to embolization, *"Cardiac Catheterization,"* p. 82; Renal, related to impaired circulation secondary to decreased cardiac output or reaction to contrast dye, *"Cardiac Catheterization,"* p. 83; related to tissue ischemia secondary to decreased arterial circulation, *"Atherosclerotic Arterial Occlusive Disease,"* p. 88; Peripheral, related to impaired circulation secondary to graft occlusion, *"Atherosclerotic Arterial Occlusive Disease,"* p. 89; Renal, related to impaired circulation secondary to decreased blood supply during surgery and potential embolization, *"Atherosclerotic Arterial Occlusive Disease,"* p. 89; Peripheral, related to impaired circulation secondary to postoperative embolization, *"Aneurysms,"* p. 91; Peripheral, related to impaired circulation secondary to embolization (preoperative period), *"Arterial Embolism,"* p. 92; Pulmonary, related to impaired circulation secondary to embolization from thrombus formation, *"Venous Thrombosis/Thrombophlebitis,"* p. 94; Peripheral, related to impaired circulation secondary to venous engorgement or edema, *"Venous Thrombosis/Thrombophlebitis,"* p. 95; related to susceptibility secondary to the creation of the vascular access for hemodialysis, *"Renal Dialysis,"* p. 130; Peripheral and cardiopulmonary, related to risk of thrombophlebitis and pulmonary emboli formation secondary to venous stasis occurring with immobility and decreased vasomotor tone, *"Spinal Cord Injury,"* p. 204; Peripheral, cardiopulmonary, renal, cerebral, and gastrointestinal related to impaired circulation secondary to development and progression of macroangiopathy and microangiopathy, *"Diabetes Mellitus,"* p. 297; Peripheral, related to risk of thromboembolism secondary to increased viscosity of the blood, increased platelet aggregation and adhesiveness, and patient immobility, *"Diabetic Ketoacidosis,"* p. 303; GI tract, related to risk of interruption of blood flow to abdominal viscera from vascular disruption or occlusion or moderate to severe hypovolemia caused by hemorrhage, *"Abdominal Trauma,"* p. 377; Peripheral and cardiopulmonary, related to decreased circulation secondary to inflammatory process and occlusion of blood vessels with RBCs, *"Hemolytic Anemia,"* p. 400; Cardiopulmonary and cerebral, related to decreased circulation secondary to phlebotomy, *"Polycythemia,"* p. 408; Renal, peripheral, and cerebral, related to decreased circulation secondary to hyperviscosity of the blood, *"Polycythemia,"* p. 408; Cerebral, peripheral, and renal, related to decreased circulation secondary to occlusion of small vessels owing to thombotic component (TTP), *"Thrombocytopenia,"* p. 411; Cardiopulmonary, peripheral, renal, and cerebral, related to altered circulation secondary to coagulation/fibrinolysis processes, *"Disseminated Intravascular Coagulation,"* p. 415; Peripheral, cerebral, or cardiopulmonary, related to impaired circulation secondary to fat embolization (applies to patients with multiple trauma, multiple fractures, or surgical repair of fractures), *"Fractures,"* p. 453; Peripheral, related to impaired circulation secondary to compression from circumferential cast or dressing, *"Bunionectomy,"* p. 464; Peripheral, related to impaired circulation to and compression of the musculocutaneous nerve secondary to pressure from the immobilization device, *"Repair of Recurrent Shoulder Dislocation,"* p. 472; Peripheral, related to impaired circulation secondary to compression from traction or abduction device, *"Total Hip Arthroplasty,"* p. 475; Cerebral and peripheral, related to decreased circulation secondary to hypovolemia, *"Fluid and Electrolyte Disturbances,"* p. 548; Peripheral, related to compromised circulation secondary to prolonged immobility, *"Caring for Patients on Prolonged Bed Rest,"* p. 655; Cerebral, related to orthostatic hypotension secondary to prolonged bed rest, *"Caring for Patients on Prolonged Bed Rest,"* p. 656; Peripheral, related to impaired circulation secondary to lymphedema, *"Caring for Patients with Cancer and Other Life-Disrupting Illnesses,"* p. 688.

Trauma, potential for, related to unsteady gait secondary to bradykinesis, tremors, and rigidity, *"Parkinsonism,"* p. 178; related to lack of awareness of environmental hazards secondary to cognitive deficit, *"Alzheimer's Disease,"* p. 184; related to oral, musculoskeletal, and airway vulnerability secondary to seizure activity, *"Seizure Disorders,"* p. 244; related to unsteady gait secondary to sensorimotor deficit, *"General Care of Patients with Neurologic Disorders,"* p. 248; related to risk of pathologic fractures secondary to bone demineralization, *"Hyperparathyroidism,"* p. 270; related to alterations in LOC and risk of seizures secondary to hypoglycemia, *"Hypoglycemia,"* p. 309; related to risk of falling secondary to equilibrium disturbance, *"Otosclerosis,"* p. 542; related to risk of tetany and seizures secondary to severe hypocalcemia, *"Fluid and Electrolyte Disturbances,"* p. 560; related to CNS depression secondary to anesthetics and postoperative opioid analgesics, *"Caring for Preoperative and Postoperative Patients,"* p. 650.

Unilateral neglect related to disturbed perceptual ability secondary to neurologic insult, *"Cerebrovascular Accident,"* p. 235.

Urinary elimination, altered patterns: Dysuria, urgency, or frequency in the presence of a ureteral calculus, *"Ureteral Calculi,"* p. 133; Obstruction or positional problems of the ureteral catheter, *"Ureteral Calculi,"* p. 133; Obstruction of the suprapubic catheter or anuria/dysuria secondary to removal of the catheter, *"Cancer of the Bladder,"* p. 140; Disruption in normal function secondary to postoperative use of ureteral stents, catheters, or drains, and actual urinary diversion surgery, *"Urinary Diversions,"* p. 154; related to urinating in inappropriate places or incontinence secondary to cognitive deficit, *"Alzheimer's Disease,"* p. 185; Anuria or dysuria related to local swelling or presence of rectal packing secondary to hemorrhoidectomy, *"Hemorrhoids,"* p. 345; Oliguria or anuria occurring with inadequate intake, obstruction of indwelling catheter, or ureteral ligation, *"Cancer of the Cervix,"* p. 495; Anuria, dysuria, or frequency occurring with obstruction associated with prostatitis, *"Prostatitis,"* p. 515; Dysuria, urgency, frequency, and polyuria secondary to administration of diuretics, calcium stone formation, or changes in renal function occurring with hypercalcemia, *"Fluid and Electrolyte Disturbances,"* p. 562; Hemorrhagic cystitis, secondary to cyclophosphamide/phosphamide treatment; oliguria or renal toxicity secondary to cisplatinum or high-dose methotrexate administration; renal calculi secondary to hyperurecemia; or dysuria secondary to cystitis, *"Caring for Patients with Cancer and Other Life-Disrupting Illnesses,"* p. 689.

Urinary retention: Incomplete emptying of or inability to empty the bladder secondary to weak detrusor muscle, blockage, inhibition of reflex arc, or anxiety, *"Urinary retention,"* p. 146; related to spasticity or flaccidity secondary to SCI, *"Spinal Cord Injury,"* p. 203; related to pain, trauma, and use of anesthetic secondary to lower abdominal surgery, *"Hernia,"* p. 337.

Violence, potential for, related to irritability, frustration, and disorientation secondary to degeneration of cognitive thinking, *"Alzheimer's Disease,"* p. 187; related to hallucinations/paranoia secondary to cocaine use/withdrawal, *"Cocaine Abuse,"* p. 604; related to sensory overload, rage reactions, perceived threats, or physiologic imbalance, *"Caring for Patients with Cancer and Other Life-Disrupting Illnesses,"* p. 696.

Index

735